MANIPAL
Manual of
SURGERY
SECOND EDITION

Dr Rajgopal Shenoy K MBBS, MS

Consultant Surgeon

Kasturba Medical College Hospital, Manipal

Professor of Surgery, Kasturba Medical College

Manipal Academy of Higher Education

Manipal – 576104 (India)

E-mail : shenoyrajgopal@yahoo.com

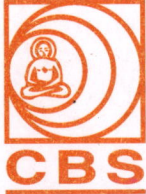

CBS PUBLISHERS & DISTRIBUTORS
NEW DELHI ● BANGALORE (INDIA)

Medical knowledge is constantly changing. As new information becomes available, changes in treatment, procedures, equipment and the use of drugs become necessary. The authors and the publisher have, as far as it is possible, taken care to ensure that the information given in this text is accurate and up to date. However, readers are strongly advised to confirm that the information, especially with regard to drug usage, complies with the latest legislation and standards of practice.

ISBN : 81-239-1237-4

First Edition : 2000
Reprint : 2001
Reprint : 2002
Reprint : 2003
Reprint : 2004
Second Edition : 2005
Reprint : 2006
Reprint : 2007

Publishing Director : Vinod K. Jain

Published by :
Satish Kumar Jain for CBS Publishers & Distributors,
4596/1-A, 11 Darya Ganj, New Delhi - 110 002 (India)
E-mail : cbspubs@del3.vsnl.net.in
Website : http://www.cbspd.com

Branch Office :
2975, 17th Cross, K.R. Road,
Bansankari 2nd Stage, Bangalore - 560 070
Fax : 080-26771680 • E-mail : cbsbng@vsnl.net

Printed at :
SDR Printers, Delhi - 110 094 (India)

Dedicated

To

My Wife, Dr. Anitha Shenoy,
And
My children, Ranjan and Rachana

Foreword

Surgery is an ever-progressive, continuously changing facet of medicine which in the face of its ever-widening horizon poses a real challenge for an author of a text book. Dr. K. Rajgopal Shenoy, author of Manipal Manual of Surgery has stood up to the challenge and come out with a comprehensive, yet simplified text book. Any darn fool can make something complex but it takes a genius to make something simple. Dr. Shenoy has proved to be a genius.

Dr. K. Rajgopal Shenoy, known to me for the last two decades is an excellent teacher and a proven leader. His collection of clinical photographs may shortly outnumber the stars in the sky. The previous edition of his book was highly appreciated, and has been amply rewarded and accepted by the entire medical student community.

The popularity of the book can be attributed to the effort to keep it simple in language and content but at the same time complete, explicit but not exhaustive, explanatory but not redundant, enlivened by real-life examples but bereft of exaggeration – all helping to sustain and retain the essence of the subject.

I have no doubt that this book will make a lucid reading and will elicit a lot of appreciation and acceptance by both undergraduate and postgraduate students in surgery.

Dr. B. H. Anand Rao,
Professor and Head of Surgery,
Kasturba Medical College, Manipal

Contributors

Dr. Anitha Shenoy
Additional Professor, Dept. of Anaesthesiology
Principles of Anaesthesiology

Dr. Deepak Shetty and Dr. Chandrakanth Shetty
Associate Professors, Dept. of Radiodiagnosis
Principles of Radiology

Dr. Donald Fernandes
Additional Professor, Dept. of Radiation Oncology
Principles of Radiation Oncology

Dr. Ganesh Kamath
Professor and Head, Dept. of Cardiothoracic Surgery
Cardiothoracic Surgery

Dr. Raja A
Professor and Head, Dept. of Neurosurgery
Neurosurgery

Dr. Rajesh Kumar and Dr. Nandini Pandit
Associate Professors, Dept. of Nuclear Medicine
Nuclear Medicine in Surgery

Preface

It gives me great pleasure to write the preface of the second edition of my book 'Manipal Manual of Surgery'. The first edition has enjoyed immense popularity among both undergraduate and postgraduate students of surgery. The book is being read by students not only in Manipal or Karnataka but all along the length and breadth of India and a few SAARC countries. I am very grateful to the positive responses and suggestions that have come from students from all over India through e-mail. The simplicity and point-wise summarisation has made the manual popular with students for a 'quick' reading before exams. The manual is also being used by other health professionals such as students of Ayurveda and Homeopathy because of its simplicity. It has become a ready-reckoner even for private practitioners.

The second edition is born simply out of compulsion from students who want the book to be more comprehensive, complete and up-to-date. The second edition has each of its chapters re-edited carefully and revised as necessary. Visual impressions last longer in the mind and to aid memory, a large number of clinical photographs have been added. The second edition also includes details of many investigations such as CT scan, ERCP and endoscopy. Emphasis has been placed on management strategies of various clinical problems and is **evidence-based.** The success of the earlier book was also its layout. Features such as key boxes, figures, simple sketches and clinical notes that aided easy grasp and retention of the subject have been maintained. A new chapter on radionuclear scan in general surgery has been added. The specialty topics have also been revised for the benefit of those who aim for the top marks. Some **pearls of wisdom (Blue shade)** have been added for interest and the book is in colour to make it visually more pleasing.

The information available to the student of surgery as of any subject has seen a boom. This has aided to make information search easy but also has been successful in confusing the students and create a degree of panic among them. The limited time frame available to the students makes it necessary for them to be able read one good comprehensive book reliably. The second edition of Manipal Manual of Surgery achieves just that requirement. The multitude of clinical photographs along with the content would be most helpful to even the postgraduate students of surgery and the practising surgeons.

The credit of shaping this book into its present form is shared by many individuals. Foremost among them is my wife, Dr Anitha Shenoy, who has been a constant source of inspiration to me. Apart from contributing the chapter on Anaesthesiology, she has helped me immensely in editing this manual. I am extremely grateful to Dr Mahesh Gopa Setty, Assistant Professor of Surgery and my colleague who helped me a great deal in editing the book. I am also thankful to Dr Joseph Thomas, Professor of Urology for editing chapters on urology and Dr Natarajan, Associate Professor of Urology for contributing photographs. Dr Stanley Mathew, Associate Professor and Dr Vikas Jain, Assistant Professor from dept of Surgery have also helped me a lot in editing the book. Dr Chandrakanth Shetty, Associate Professor, dept. of Radiology also contributed significant photographs to the book. I appreciate the important role of proof-reading and corrections done by (Dr) Priyank Tyagi, (Dr) Anjali Singh, (Dr) Anu, and many other undergraduate students, Dr Devanjali, Dr Hethal, Interns and Dr Madhu, Dr Basant, Dr Kirun, Dr Rohit Jain and Dr Sanjeev and other postgraduate students. Dr Ullas Kamath, Professor of Biochemistry, Deputy Registrar of Examinations, MAHE and my brother-in-law kindly found the time, in spite of his busy schedule, and meticulously weeded out spelling and printing errors and I am thankful to him.

I also thank Mr Umesh Acharya, artist from Dental College, MAHE, for drawing simple and beautiful diagrams. I extend my thanks to Mr Sandeep and Miss Netravathi who helped in the preliminary stages of computer-work. I am very grateful to Mr Wilfred Lobo who did the major part of page-making, very patiently working for long hours, trying to meet deadlines and schedules even through Christmas! Without him, this enormous task would not have been possible.

I greatly appreciate the constant support and encouragement given to me by Mr S.K. Jain, managing Director and Mr B.R. Sharma of CBS Publishers and Distributors, New Delhi. Mr. V.K. Jain, Production Director, deserves special thanks for the excellent production of the book.

I sincerely hope that the expectations of the students are met and the book will help them to achieve greater laurels in their future career. **Any criticisms, suggestions and contributions to this book are welcome. I wish all my dear students the very best. Do enjoy reading this book.**

Dr. K. Rajgopal Shenoy

Professor of Surgery, Kasturba Medical College
Manipal Academy of Higher Education,
(University MAHE)
Manipal, India 576104
E-mail: shenoyrajgopal@yahoo.com

Contents

UROLOGY

SPECIALITIES

VIVA VOCE EXAMINATION IN SURGERY

Wound, Sinus and Fistula

1

- Wound
- Asepsis and Antisepsis
- Nosocomial infections
- Sinus and Fistula
- Hypertrophic scar and Keloid
- Clinical notes
- Classification of surgical wounds

WOUND

Wound is discontinuity or break in the surface epithelium. A wound is simple when only skin is involved. It is complex when it involves underlying nerves, vessels, tendons etc.

TYPES OF WOUNDS

I. Closed Wounds

Contusion

Abrasion

Haematoma

Contusion: Can be minor soft tissue injury without break in the skin or sometimes it can be major due to run over by a vehicle. Generally it produces discolouration of skin due to collection of blood underneath.

Abrasion: In this wound, epidermis of the skin is scraped away thus exposing dermis. They are painful as dermal nerve endings are exposed. These wounds need cleaning, antibiotics and proper dressings.

Haematoma: This refers to collection of blood. It follows injury or spontaneously as in patients who have bleeding tendencies such as **haemophilia**. Depending upon the site, it can be subcutaneous, intramuscular or even subperiosteal. Haematoma in the knee joint may have to be aspirated followed by compression bandage. Small haematomas get absorbed, if not may get infected.

II. Open Wounds

Incised

Lacerated

Penetrating

Crushed

Incised wounds: They are caused by sharp objects like knife, blade, glass, etc. This type of wound has a sharp edge and is less contaminated. Primary suturing is ideal for such wounds, as it gives a neat and clean scar.

Lacerated wounds: They are caused by blunt objects like fall on a stone or due to road traffic accidents. Edges are jagged. The injury may involve only skin and subcutaneous tissue or sometimes deeper structures also. Due to the blunt nature of the object, there is crushing of the tissue which may result in haematoma, bruising or even necrosis of the tissue. These wounds are treated by wound excision and primary suturing provided they are treated within six hours of the injury.

Penetrating wounds: They are not uncommon nowadays. Stab injuries of abdomen are very notorious. It may look like an innocent injury with a small, one or two cm. long, cut. But internal organs like intestines, liver, spleen or mesenteric blood vessels might have been damaged. All penetrating wounds of the abdomen should be admitted and observed for at least 24 hours. Layer by layer exploration and repair, though recommended, may not be possible at times due to oblique track of the wound.

Crushed or contused wounds: They are caused by blunt trauma due to run over by vehicle, wall collapse, earthquakes or industrial accidents. These wounds are dangerous as they may cause severe haemorrhage, death of the tissues and crushing of blood vessels. These patients are more prone for gas gangrene, tetanus etc. Adequate treatment involves a good debridement and removal of all dead and necrotic tissues.

GENERAL PRINCIPLES OF MANAGEMENT OF WOUND (Fig.1.1)

Admission or observation in the hospital.

Monitoring of temperature, pulse and respiration.

Systemic antibiotics depending upon the contamination of wound.

Injection tetanus toxoid for prophylaxis against tetanus.

Treatment of the wound in the form of cleaning, dressing or suturing.

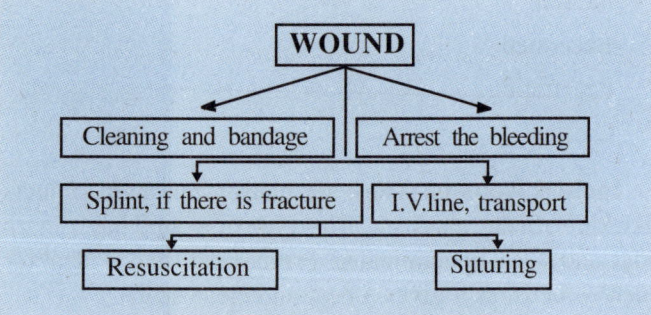

Fig. 1.1 Wound management

HEALING OF THE WOUND

Healing by primary intention occurs in a clean incised wound such as a surgical incision where in there is only a potential space between the edges. It produces a clean, neat, thin scar.

Healing by secondary intention refers to a wound which is infected, discharging pus or wound with skin loss. Such wounds heal with an ugly scar.

Components of wound healing

1. **Epithelialisation** occurs mainly from the edges of the wound by a process of cell migration and cell mul-

tiplication. This is mainly brought about by marginal basal cells. Thus, within 48 hours entire wound is re-epithelialised. When there is a wound with skin loss, skin appendages also help in epithelialisation. Slowly, surface cells get keratinised.

2. **Wound contraction:** It starts after 4 days and is usually completed by 14 days. It is brought about by specialised fibroblasts. Because of their contractile elements, they are called myofibroblasts. It is the nature's way of reducing the size of defect thereby helping the wound healing. Wound contraction readily occurs when there is loose skin as in back, gluteal region etc. Skin contraction is greatly reduced when it occurs over tibia (skin) or malleolar surface. Corticosteroids, irradiation, chemotherapy delay wound contraction.

3. **Connective tissue formation:** Formation of granulation tissue is the most important and fundamental step in wound healing. (It can be compared to concrete slab laying).

Injury results in the release of mediators of inflammation, mainly histamine from platelets, mast cells and granulocytes. This results in increased capillary permeability.

Later kinins and prostaglandins act and they play a chemotactic role for white cells and fibroblasts.

In the first **48 hours**, polymorphonuclear leukocytes dominate. They play the role of scavengers by removing the dead and necrotic tissue.

Between 3rd and 5th day, polymorphonuclear leukocytes diminish in number but monocytes increase. They are the specialised scavengers.

By 5th or 6th day, **fibroblasts** appear, proliferate and eventually give rise to a protocollagen which is converted into collagen in the presence of an enzyme protocollagen hydroxylase. O_2, ferrous ions and ascorbic acid are necessary for this step.

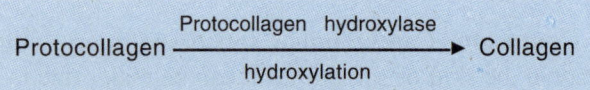

Fibroplasia along with capillary budding give rise to granulation tissue.

Secretion of ground substance - mucopolysaccharides by fibroblasts. These are called proteoglycans. They help in binding of collagen fibres. Thus, wound is FIBRE – GEL – FLUID SYSTEM (iron rods + Cement + Water used for concrete slab).

4. Scar formation: Following changes take place during scar formation.

Fibroplasia and laying of collagen is increased.

Vascularity becomes less (devascularisation).

Epithelialisation continues

Ingrowth of lymphatics and nerve fibres takes place.

Remodelling of collagen takes place with cicatrisation, resulting in a scar.

COMPLICATIONS OF WOUND HEALING

1. **Infection**: It is the most important complication which is responsible for delay in wound healing. Majority of bacteria are endogenous. Depending upon pus/culture sensitivity report, appropriate antibiotics are given.

2. **Ugly scar**: It is the result of infections

3. **Keloid** and hypertrophic scar

4. **Incisional hernia** and wound dehiscence

5. **Pigmentation** of the skin

6. **Marjolin's ulcer**

WOUND CLOSURE OR WOUND SUTURING

1. **Primary suturing**: Suturing the wound within a few hours following an injury (six hours is ideal) is called primary suturing.

Primary suturing can be done provided:

It is an incised or cut wound with a sharp object like knife or razor blade.

Minimal injury to structures on either side.

There should not be any infection. If a wound is sutured in the presence of infection the suture material is eaten away (digested) by organisms which results in gaping of the wound.

Precautions to be taken while doing a primary suturing:

Foreign body, if present in the deeper aspect of the wound, should be removed.

Associated injury to blood vessel, nerve or tendons to be recognised and repaired.

Wound on the abdomen may have associated visceral injuries.

Prevention of tetanus by using tetanus toxoid 0.5 ml intramuscularly.

2. **Wound excision and primary suturing of skin**: This is indicated when –
Wound edges are jagged

Contamination of wound with organisms or foreign body.

Tissues are crushed and devitalised.

In such situations, wound is explored, devitalised tissues and foreign body, if present, are removed. The wound is irrigated with antiseptic agents. Thus, lacerated wound is converted into an incised wound and then sutured.

Precautions to be taken are:

Should be done within 6 hours.

Tetanus and gas gangrene prophylaxis.

Repair of tendons and nerves can be done at a later date, if contamination is excessive.

3. **Wound excision and delayed primary suture:** This is indicated in lacerated wounds with major crush injuries. Primary suturing within 6 hours is not done in these wounds because of –

Gross oedema of the part

Increased tissue tension

Haematoma

Contamination with bacteria

In such situations, excision of all dead tissue is done. The wound is irrigated with antiseptic agents like betadine, hydrogen peroxide solution, etc., and is left open without suturing and dressing is applied.

Wound is re-examined 4-6 days later. If there is no infection, or no nonviable tissues, wound is sutured. This two stage procedure is called **delayed primary suturing**.

4. **Wound with skin loss** (Fig. 1.2): It can follow surgical procedures or accidents etc.

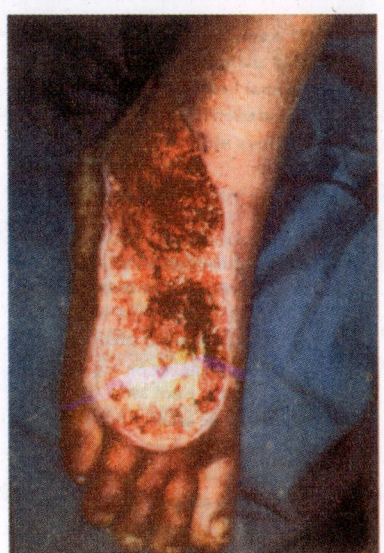

Fig. 1.2 Wound with skin loss

Complications of skin loss

Secondary infection of the wound.

The underlying structures like tendons and nerves are in danger.

Diabetic patients can develop septicaemia.

Deformity and disability can occur at a later date.

Hence, as soon as possible, skin grafting should be done.

5. **Secondary suturing:** After operations, sutures may give way because of severe infection with persistent discharge of pus. In such cases 7-14 days later, after controlling infection, skin is freed from the edge of the wound from the granulation tissue and the skin is approximated. This type of suturing is called as secondary suturing.

FACTORS AFFECTING WOUND HEALING

A. General factors

1. **Age:** In children, wounds heal faster. Healing is delayed in old age.

2. **Debilitation** results in malnutrition. Wound healing is delayed probably because of vitamin C deficiency. Following injury, vitamin C deficiency can occur after 3-4 weeks. Vitamin C is necessary for the synthesis and maintenance of collagen. Zinc deficiency is known to delay the healing of pilonidal sinus.

3. In **diabetic** patients, wound healing is delayed because of several factors such as microangiopathy, atherosclerosis, decreased phagocytic activity, proliferation of bacteria due to high blood sugar etc.

4. **Jaundiced** and **uraemic** patients have poor wound healing because fibroblastic repair is delayed.

5. **Cytotoxic** drugs and **malignancy**.

6. **Generalised infection:** Pus in some part of body delays wound healing.

7. **Corticosteroids** given early may delay wound healing because of anti-inflammatory activity. Once healing is established they do not interfere.

B. Local factors

1. **Poor blood supply:** Wound over the knee and shin of tibia heal very slowly but wound on the face heals fast.

2. **Local infection:** Organisms eat away the suture material, destroy granulation tissue and cause slough and purulent discharge. Collagen synthesis is reduced and collagenolysis is increased.

3. **Haematoma** precipitates infection.

4. **Faulty technique** of wound closure.

5. **Tension** while suturing.

6. **Oxygen:** Killing property of macrophages and increased production of fibroblasts can occur due to oxygen. If contamination occurs, antibiotics should be given immediately or within 2 hours to prevent infection.

ASEPSIS AND ANTISEPSIS

Strictly speaking, they are equivalent, there is not much of a difference between these.

ASEPSIS means precautions taken before any surgical procedure, against development of infection.

Examples

Wearing gloves before any procedure.

Cleaning the patient's abdomen with iodine and spirit.

Sterilisation of instruments.

Autoclaving.

ANTISEPSIS: All the surgical procedures done today are after taking precautions.

Dressing of an already contaminated wound using carbolic acid, iodine.

Broad-spectrum antibiotics used in presence of infection.

Wearing mask and cap in the operation theatre.

NOSOCOMIAL INFECTIONS

Acquired infection from the hospital is called as nosocomial infection.

Infection can be from the patient's own organisms (self infection) or organisms from other place.

Examples: In surgical wards, discharging wounds, infected urine, faeces, sputum are all sources of nosocomial infection.

Common organisms: Staphylococci and gram-negative organisms. Thus, wound infection, bronchopneumonia, urinary tract infection and even septicaemia can occur. Gas gangrene can occur due to patient's own intestinal clostridium.

Prevention of hospital infection

Avoid unnecessary antibiotics to prevent development of resistant organisms

Autoclaving, sterilisation, etc.

Proper ventilation of the wards

Proper scrubbing before any procedure

Proper disposal of urine, faeces, sputum

Use of disinfectants

SINUS AND FISTULA

SINUS

It is a blind track leading from the surface down into the tissues. It is lined with granulation tissue. Following are a few examples (Fig. 1.3).

1. *Congenital sinus*: Preauricular sinus
2. *Acquired sinus*:

Median mental sinus: Occurs as a result of tooth abscess.

Pilonidal sinus: Occurs in the midline in the anal region.

Osteomyelitis: Gives rise to sinus discharging pus with or without bony spicules.

Commonest sinus in the neck is due to tubercular lymphadenitis. It discharges cheesy material. Skin surrounding the sinus shows bluish discolouration.

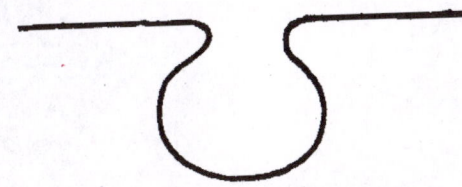

Fig. 1.3 Sinus

FISTULA

It is an abnormal communication between the lumen of one viscus and the lumen of another (internal) or communication of one hollow viscus with the exterior i.e. body surface (external fistula).

Examples of internal fistula

Tracheo-oesophageal fistula
Colovesical fistula

Examples of external fistula

Orocutaneous fistula due to carcinoma of the oral cavity infiltrating the skin

Branchial fistula

Thyroglossal fistula

Causes of persistence of a sinus or fistula

1. Presence of foreign body
2. Persistent infection
3. Distal obstruction
4. Absence of rest
5. Epithelialisation of the track
6. Malignancy
7. Non-dependent drainage, inadequate drainage
8. Dense fibrosis
9. Irradiation
10. Specific causes - Tuberculosis, Actinomycosis

CLINICAL EXAMINATION OF SINUS AND FISTULA

INSPECTION

1. **Location** gives the diagnosis in the majority of the cases of sinus or fistula.

FISTULAS

Branchial fistula: Anterior border of lower third of sternomastoid

Parotid fistula: In the parotid region

Thyroglossal fistula: Midline of neck below hyoid bone

Appendicular fistula: Right iliac fossa

SINUSES

Preauricular sinus: Front of root of helix of ear due to failure of fusion of ear tubercles. Direction of the sinus is upwards and backwards.

Median mental sinus – Symphysis menti

Tubercular sinus – Neck

Lymphogranuloma – Groin

2. **NUMBER** – can be single or multiple

3. **OPENING**
Sprouting granulation tissue – Foreign body

Flush with skin – Tuberculosis

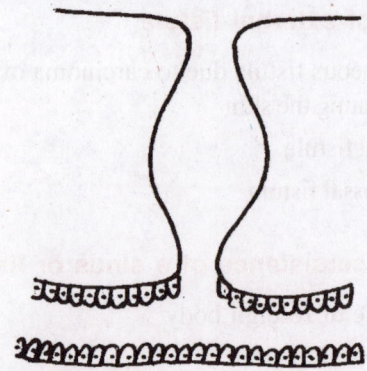

Fig. 1.4 Enterocutaneous fistula

4. **DISCHARGE**

   White thin caseous – Tuberculosis

   Yellow purulent – Staphylococci

   Faecal – Faecal fistula (Fig. 1.4)

   Yellow granules – Actinomycosis

   Thin mucus discharge – Branchial fistula

   Urine – Urinary fistula

5. **SURROUNDING SKIN**

   Red, angry looking - Inflammatory.

   Bluish discolouration - Tuberculosis.

   Pigmentation - Chronic sinus.

   Skin excoriation - Faecal fistula.

PALPATION

1. Temperature and tenderness is increased if there is inflammation of the sinus, e.g., pilonidal sinus

2. Discharge after application of pressure. It suggests nature of fluid

3. Induration is present in chronic fistula, actinomycosis, osteomyelitis, etc.

   In tubercular sinus, induration is absent

4. **Fixity**

   Osteomyelitis sinus is fixed to the bone and median mental sinus may be fixed to the jaw bone.

5. **Palpation at a deeper plane**

   Enlarged nodes in tuberculosis or lymphogranuloma venereum

   Thickening of mandible or bone

   Submandibular stone may be palpable as in submandibular fistula

Relevant clinical examination

Submandibular gland enlargement can be made out by bidigital examination.

Alveolar abscess can be found as in median mental sinus.

Per rectal examination and proctoscopy may reveal internal opening of the fistula.

Investigations

1. Complete blood picture (**CBP** - Haemoglobin %, total and differential count, erythrocyte sedimentation rate - **ESR**): **ESR** may be increased as in tuberculosis. Increased total count suggests infection.

2. Urine sugar, fasting blood sugar (**FBS**) and post-prandial blood sugar (**PPBS**) to rule out diabetes.

3. **X-ray** of the part: Osteomyelitis of mandible; toe, also to look for foreign body (Fig. 1.5).

4. X-ray kidney, ureter, bladder region (**KUB**) - Staghorn calculi as in lumbar urinary fistula.

5. Fistulography or sinusography is done to know the exact extent or origin of the sinus or fistula. Dye such as **lipoidal (poppy seed oil contains 40% iodine)** is used.

6. Biopsy from the edge of sinus is done if specific etiology is suspected e.g. tuberculosis, malignancy etc.

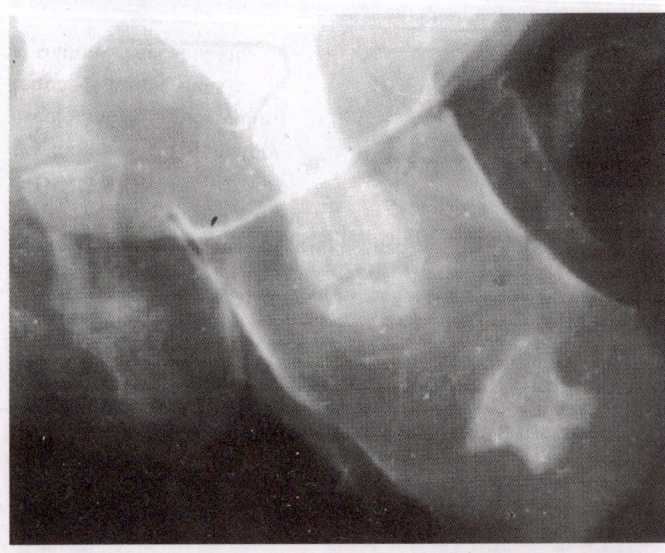

Fig. 1.5 Persisting sinus due to osteomyelitis of distal phalanx of great toe

Management (Key Box 1.1)

Following are a few examples:

    Sequestrectomy for osteomyelitis

    Control of tuberculosis for tubercular sinus in neck

    Removal of the foreign body

Key Box 1.1
BASIC PRINCIPLES
• Antibiotics • Adequate rest • Adequate excision • Adequate drainage

CLINICAL NOTES

1. A patient who underwent surgery for varicose veins, had persistent seropurulent discharge from the inguinal incision. Initially, it was thought to be due to infection. The discharge persisted for a period of two months. The wound was explored. A gauze piece was found and removed. The wound healed well. Retrospective analysis of the surgery revealed slipping of the ligature applied to the long saphenous vein and several gauze pieces were used to control the bleeding point.

2. We had a sixty year old man who had a small sinus in the loin discharging watery fluid. He had seen many doctors for many years. He was treated with antibiotics and even antituberculous treatment without any relief. X-ray KUB revealed a staghorn calculus.

Few clinical cases are shown below (Fig. 1.6, 1.7, 1.8, 1.9).

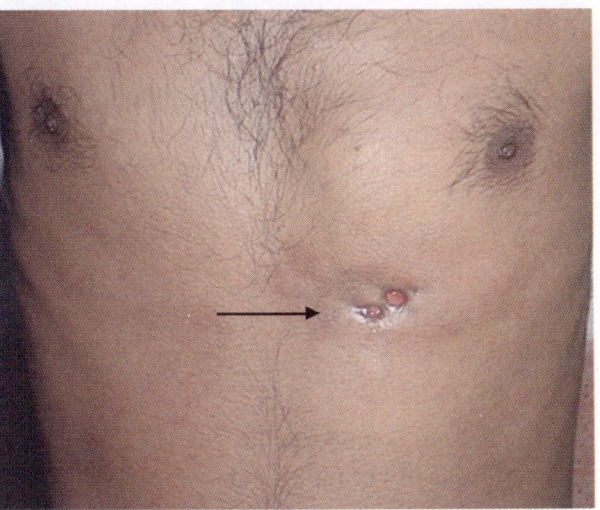

Fig. 1.7 Tuberculous sinuses in the chest wall, observe edge of the sinuses are in flush with the skin.

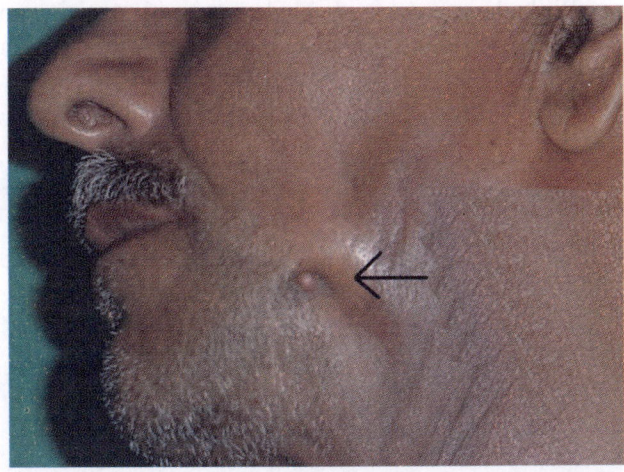

Fig. 1.8 Mandibular sinus due to badly infected caries teeth

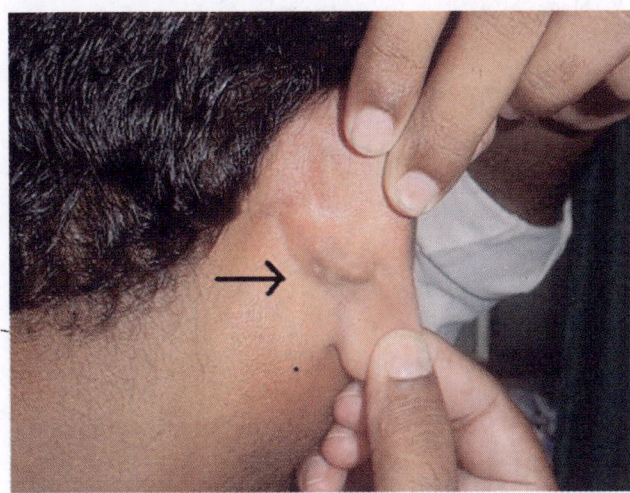

Fig. 1.6 Post auricular sinus

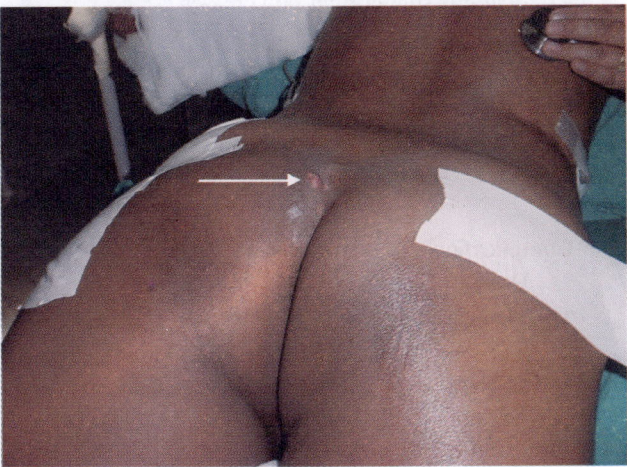

Fig. 1.9 A case of pilonidal sinus positioned in jack-knife position for excision

HYPERTROPHIC SCAR AND KELOID

As the name suggests there is hypertrophy of mature fibroblasts in hypertrophic scar. Blood vessels are minimal in this condition. However in keloid, proliferation of immature fibroblasts with immature blood vessels are found. These two conditions represent variations in the normal process of wound healing (refer Table 1.1).

Keloid is very common in **Negroes** and least common in Caucasians.

Keloid is **not a true tumour** but has a marked tendency to **local recurrence** after excision.

Keloid takes the shape of a butterfly over the sternum. It is the commonest site for a keloid. It is extremely difficult to treat the keloid over the sternum. We had one patient who underwent wide excision and grafting 6 times for a sternal keloid (Fig. 1.10 and Fig.1.11).

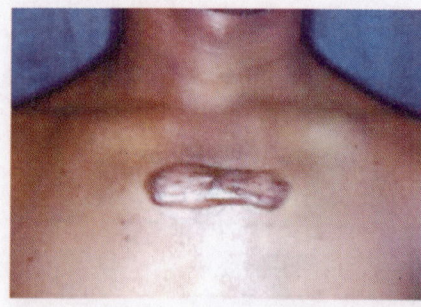

Fig. 1.10 Keloid over the sternurm

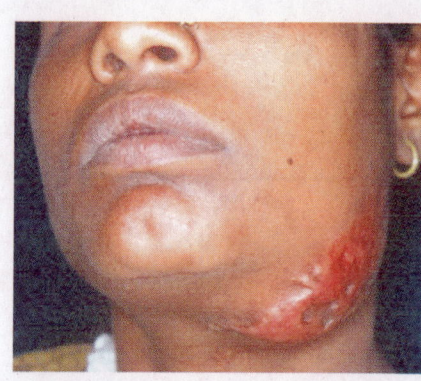

Fig. 1.11 Keloid over the jaw

Table 1.1. Comparison of hypertrophic scar and keloid

HYPERTROPHIC SCAR	KELOID
• It never gets worse after 6 months	• It continues to get worse even after 1 year and up to few years.
• Itching is not usually present. If present, it is not severe.	• Severe itching is present
• Non-tender	• Margin is tender
• Not vascular	• Vascular, red, erythematous (immature blood vessels)
• Does not spread to normal tissues	• Spreads to normal tissues, has claw-like process. Hence the name
Precipitating factors:	
1. Scar crossing normal skin creases	1. Negro race
2. Over sternum, over joints	2. Tuberculosis patients
3. Young persons	3. Over the sternum
	4. Women
	5. Hereditary and familial
	6. Vaccination sites
Complications	
• Do not occur	• Ulceration, infection
Treatment	
• It is often not necessary. Stocking, armlets, gloves, elastic bandage may help. Excision can be done.	• It is difficult. Injection of steroid preparation like triamcinolone acetate (Kanacort) has been found extremely useful. It flattens the keloid. **Intrakeloidal excision** and skin grafting is to be tried last. Recurrence is common. Care should be taken not to extend the incision on to the normal surrounding tissues.

Table 1.2 Classification of surgical Wounds

WOUNDS CLASS	DEFINITION	EXAMPLES OF TYPICAL PROCEDURES	WOUND INFECTION. RATE (%)	USUAL ORGANISM
CLEAN (Fig. 1.12)	• Non-traumatic • Elective surgery • Gastro intestinal, Respiratory or genito urinary tract not entered	• Mastectomy • Vascular procedures	2%	Staphylococcus aureus
CLEAN CONTAMINATED (Fig. 1.13)	• Respiratory • Genito-urinary or Gastro-intestinal tracts entered but minimal contamination	• Gastrectomy • Hysterectomy • Cholecystectomy	<10%	Related to viscous entered
CONTAMINATED (Fig. 1.14)	• Open, fresh, traumatic wounds • Uncontrolled spillage from an unprepared viscous • Minor break in sterile technique	• Ruptured appendix • Resection of unprepared bowel	20%	Depends on underlying cause
DIRTY (Fig. 1.15)	• Open, traumatic dirty wounds • Traumatic perforated viscous • Pus in operative field	• Resection of gangrene	30-70%	Depends on underlying cause

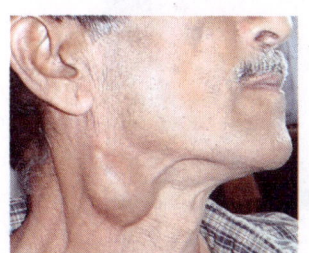

Fig. 1.12 Excision of neck swelling - Clean

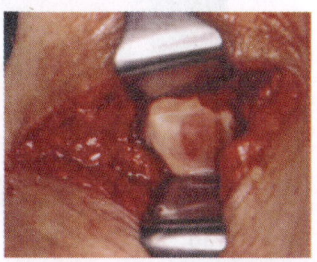

Fig. 1.14 Appendicular abcess - Contaminated

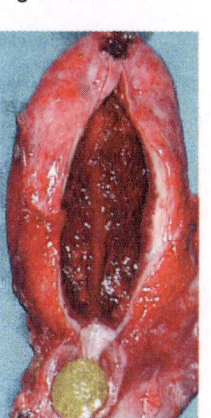

Fig. 1.13 Cholecystectomy - Clean contaminated

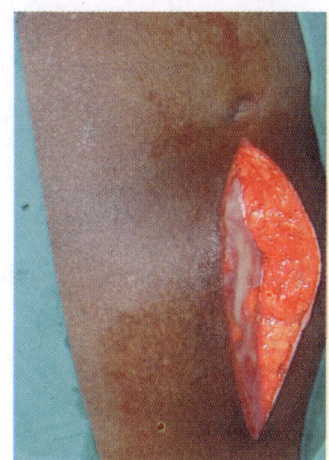

Fig. 1.15 Peritonitis - Dirty

HEALING OF SPECIALISED TISSUES (Key Box 1.2)

Key Box 1.2

HEALING OF SPECIALISED TISSUES ONCE DESTROYED

• Nerve cells of brain and spinal cord	• Cannot be replaced by proliferation of other nerve cells
• Peripheral nerves	• Regenerative capacity is present
• Stomach and intestines	• Healing is good after anastomosis - rarely leaks
• Colon and oesophagus	• Healing is precarious, chances of leakage are high.
• Wounds on the face	• Healing is excellent due to good vascularity
• Muscles	• Can heal completely or may be replaced by fibrosis
• Bone	• Rapid proliferation of osteoblasts (refer orthopaedic books)

2

Acute Infections

- Cellulitis
- Ludwig's angina
- Abscess
- Tuberculous lymphadenitis
- Boil
- Carbuncle
- Erysipelas
- Chronic abscess
- Clinical notes
- Necrotising fascitis
- Acute pyomyositis

Since the time surgery has evolved as a speciality, infection and haemorrhage have been recognised as two well known enemies of surgeons. Over a period of time, many newer antibiotics have come into existence. However, infection still dominates and it is one of the major causes of mortality and morbidity in a patient who has a 'benign disease'. This is the sad part of disease. Hence, it is important to diagnose and treat infections effectively as early as possible.

CELLULITIS (Fig. 2.1)

Cellulitis is a spreading subcutaneous inflammation caused by haemolytic streptococcus. Streptococci produce hyaluronidase and streptokinase. Net result is that the inflammatory exudate spreads in the subcutaneous and fascial planes resulting in a gross swelling of the affected part. Wherever there is loose subcutaneous tissue as in scrotum or loose connective and interstitial tissue as in face, forearm, it spreads fast.

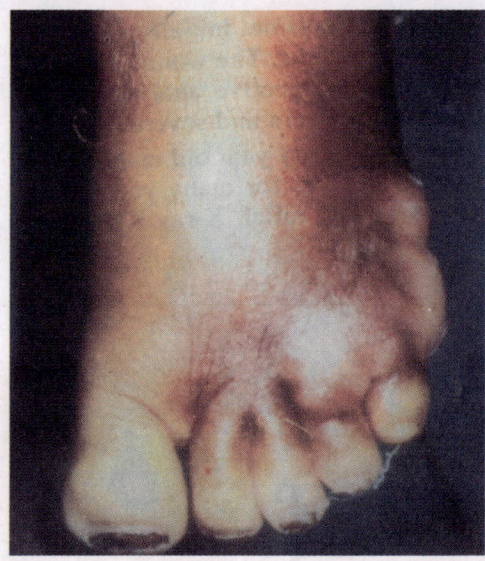

Fig. 2.1 Cellulitis of the foot with abscess

Sources of Infection

- Injuries - minor or major
- Graze or scratch
- Snake bite, scorpion bite, etc.

Precipitating factors

- Diabetes
- Low resistance of an individual

Common sites

- Lower limbs
- Face
- Scrotum

Clinical features

The affected part shows evidence of inflammation such as redness and itching followed by diffuse swelling. Skin is stretched and shiny. Pain, fever, toxaemia follow later. It is differentiated from an abscess by features mentioned below (Key Boxes 2.1 and 2.2).

Key Box 2.1
CELLULITIS
• No edge (diffuse swelling)
• No limit
• No pus
• No fluctuation

Key Box 2.2
ABSCESS
• Well-circumscribed, has an edge
• Limit is present
• Pus is present
• Fluctuation is positive

- In untreated cases, suppuration, sloughing and gangrene can occur.

Treatment

- Bed rest with legs elevated. This reduces oedema of legs.
- Glycerine MgSo₄ dressing which reduces oedema of part by osmotic effect.
- Diabetes mellitus, if present, is treated with injection **plain Insulin** given **subcutaneously**.
- Appropriate antibiotics such as Injection Crystalline Penicillin 10 lakh units, intramuscular (I.M.) or intravenous (I.V.), 6th hourly for 5-7 days or Ciprofloxacin 500 mg twice a day can be given.
- Anti-snake venom is given in snake bite cases.

Complications

1. Cellulitis can turn into an abscess which needs to be drained.
2. **Necrotising fascitis:** Certain highly invasive strains of *Streptococcus pyogenes* can cause extensive necrosis of skin, subcutaneous tissues and may result in necrotising fascitis. It is treated by debride-ment and skin grafting later (Page 19).
3. **Toxaemia and septicaemia**: *Streptococcal toxic shock syndrome* can result if exotoxins are produced by the organisms.
4. Cellulitis can precipitate ketoacidosis in a patient who has diabetes.

LUDWIG'S ANGINA

It refers to cellulitis of submental and submandibular regions combined with inflammatory oedema of the mouth. Virulent streptococcal organisms are responsible for infection surrounding submandibular region. Anaerobes also play a major role.

Precipitating factors

- Caries tooth
- Cancer of the oral cavity
- Calculi in the submandibular gland
- Chemotherapy
- Cachexia
- Chronic disease - diabetes

Clinical features

- Elderly patient who presents with diffuse swelling in the submandibular and submental region (Brawny oedema).
- **Oedema of the floor of the mouth**, as a result of which tongue is pushed upwards resulting in difficulty in swallowing.
- High grade fever with toxicity
- **Putrid halitosis** is characteristic of this condition.

Treatment

- Rest and hospitalisation
- Appropriate antibiotics
- Intravenous fluids to correct the dehydration and Ryle's tube feeding
- If it doesn't respond to conservative treatment, surgical intervention is recommended.

Surgery

- Under general anaesthesia, 5-6 cm curved incision is made below the mandible in the submandibular region over the most prominent part of the swelling. Submandibular gland is mobilised, mylohyoid muscle is divided and the pus is drained. ***Even if pus is not found, the oedematous fluid comes out greatly improving the condition of the patient.*** Wound is closed with loose sutures, after irrigating the cavity with antiseptic agents and a drainage tube is kept in place.

Complications

1. Mediastinitis and septicaemia
2. Oedema of the glottis due to spread of the cellulitis via a tunnel occupied by stylohyoid to submucosa of the glottis

ABSCESS

An abscess is a localised collection of pus (dead and dying neutrophils plus proteinaceous exudate).

Classification

1. **Pyogenic abscess**. It is the commonest form of an abscess, subcutaneous, deep, or it can occur within the viscera such as liver or kidney, etc. In this chapter pyogenic abscess refers to soft tissue abscess.
2. **Pyaemic abscess** occurs due to circulation of pyaemic emboli in the blood (pyaemia).
3. **Cold abscess**. Usually refers to tubercular abscess either due to involvement of lymph nodes or involvement of spine.

PYOGENIC ABSCESS

It is usually produced by *staphylococcal infections*. The organisms enter soft tissues by an external wound, minor or major. It can also be due to haematogenous spread from a distant focus such as tonsillitis or caries tooth etc. Pyogenic abscess can also be due to cellulitis.

Pathophysiology

- Following an injury, there is inflammation of the part brought about by the organism such as Staphylococcus. Pathological events are summarised in Fig. 2.2.
- The end result is production of pus which is composed of dead leukocytes, bacteria and necrotic tissue. The area around the abscess is encircled by fibrin products and it is infiltrated with leukocytes and bacteria. It is called **pyogenic membrane**.

Symptoms

- The patient feels ill and complains of **throbbing pain** at the site. Throbbing pain is indicative of pus and is due to pressure on the nerve endings by the pus. Fever, with or without chills, rigors can be present.

Signs

1. **Calor** – heat. The affected part is warmer due to

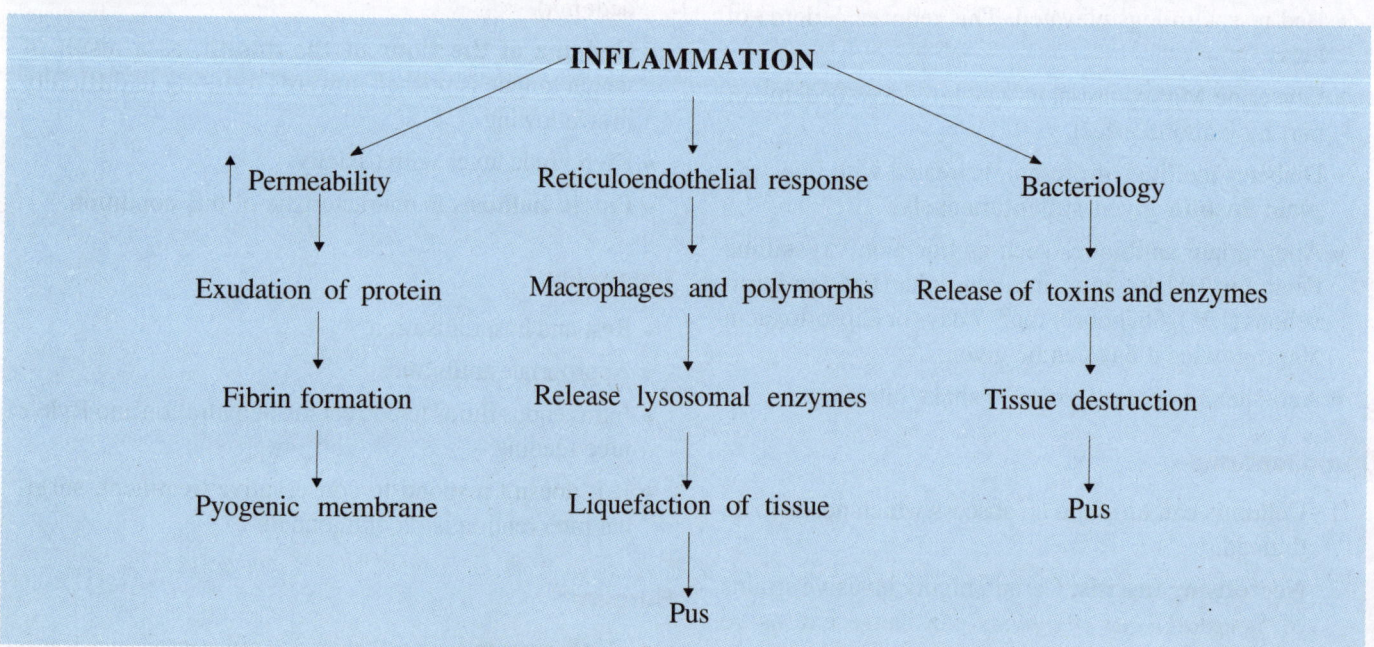

Fig. 2.2 Pathological events during inflammation

local rise in temperature.

2. **Rubor** – redness. It is due to inflammation resulting in hyperaemia.

3. **Dolor** – pain. An abscess is extremely tender.

4. **Tumor** – swelling. It consists of pus. It is tensely cystic with surrounding brawny oedema.

5. **Loss of function** – The function of the part is impaired, due to pain.

6. **Fluctuation** can be elicited. However, in a deep seated abscess it may be negative, as in breast abscess.

Treatment

- Untreated abscess tend to point spontaneously the area of least resistance – nearest an epithelial surface. e.g. Skin, gut, oral cavity, etc. However deep seated abscess - such as beast abscess, may cause much tissue destruction before pointing.

- **Incision and drainage (I and D)** under general anaesthesia. General anaesthesia is preferred because in the presence of infection, local anaesthesia may not act and it is difficult to break all the loculi of an abscess without causing pain.

Procedure

- A **stab** incision is made over the most prominent (pointing) part of an abscess. The pus which comes out is collected and sent for culture and sensitivity. A sinus forceps or a finger is introduced within the abscess cavity and all the loculi are broken down. Fresh bleeding which is seen is an indication of completeness of the procedure. The abscess cavity is irrigated with mild antiseptic agents like iodine solution or hydrogen peroxide. Hydrogen peroxide acts by liberating nascent oxygen.

$$H_2O_2 \rightarrow H_2O + [O]$$

- Nascent oxygen bubbles out and thus helps in separating the slough. The cavity, if large may need to be packed with roller gauze dipped in iodine solution which is removed 1–2 days later. Roller gauze packing prevents the premature closure of the skin, thus facilitates the healing to take place from the depth of the cavity by granulation tissue. With appropriate antibiotics and proper dressings the wound heals within 5–7 days.

- Antibiotic of choice is cloxacillin for staphylococcus abscess. Dosage - 500 mg 6th hourly for 5-7 days.

- **Modified Hilton's method** for I & D. This method is followed where an abscess is situated in the vicinity of important anatomical structures like vessels or nerves (Table 2.1).

- In this method skin and superficial fascia are incised, instead of a stab incision, followed by opening the abscess by sinus forceps, so as to avoid damage to vital structures like vessels and nerves.

Differential diagnosis (Table 2.2)

1. **Ruptured aneurysm** can present as subcutaneous abscess with pain, redness and local rise in temperature. There may be leukocytosis also. Ruptured vertebral artery aneurysm in the posterior triangle and

Table 2.1 Relationship of nerves or vessels with an abscess	
SITE	**ANATOMICAL STRUCTURE**
Axilla	→ Axillary vessels
Neck	→ Subclavian vessels and brachial plexus
Parotid region	→ Facial nerve
Mid Palmar space	→ Median nerve

Table 2.2 Differences between acute abscess and ruptured aneurysm	
ACUTE ABSCESS	**RUPTURED ANEURYSM**
No previous history of the swelling	Previous history of the swelling will be present
Throbbing pain is characteristic	Throbbing pain is usually absent
High grade fever with chills and rigors is present	Low grade fever is present
Extremely tender	Tender

popliteal artery aneurysm in the popliteal fossa have been incised, mistaking them for an abscess (Table 2.2).

Caution: When in doubt, before incising an abscess, aspirate with a wide bore needle.

2. **Soft tissue sarcoma** in the thigh can be confused for a deep-seated abscess. However, throbbing pain, high grade fever with chills and rigors and short duration of the swelling clinches the diagnosis of an abscess.

ANTIBIOMA

It is antibiotic induced swelling (oma). However once an abscess is formed, antibiotics seldom effect a cure if given because pus gets partially sterilised. Antibiotics also produce fibrosis, resulting in thickening of the abscess wall. Clinically, this may result in a **hard lump**.

Sites of antibioma are **breast, thigh, ischiorectal fossa,** etc. Antibioma in the breast may mimic carcinoma of the breast.

PYAEMIC ABSCESS

This is due to pus-producing organisms in the circulation (Pyaemia). It is the systemic effect of sepsis. It commonly occurs in diabetics and patients receiving chemotherapy and radiotherapy. Pyaemic abscess is characterised by following features.

- They are multiple
- They are deep-seated
- Tenderness is minimal
- Local rise in temperature is not present

Hence, it is called **nonreactive abscess** to differentiate it from pyogenic abscess. This is treated by multiple incisions over the abscess site and drainage (like a pyogenic abscess) with antibiotic cover.

COLD ABSCESS

- Even though it is a chronic abscess due to a chronic disease (tuberculosis), for the completeness of the chapter on abscess and for the convenience of reading, it is discussed here.

Key Box 2.3
COLD ABSCESS - CAUSES
• Tuberculosis
• Actinomycosis
• Leprosy
• Madura foot

- Cold abscess means an abscess which has no signs of inflammation. Usually, it is due to tuberculosis e.g. following tubercular lymphadenitis or due to tuberculosis of spine. However, other chronic diseases like leprosy, actinomycosis, Madura foot etc., also produce abscess which are 'cold' in nature. In this chapter, cold abscess due to tubercular lymphadenitis in the neck is discussed (Key Box 2.3).

TUBERCULOUS LYMPHADENITIS

- Etiopathogenesis: In 80% of the cases, mycobacteria pass through tonsillar crypts and affect tonsillar node or jugulodigastric group of nodes, in the anterior triangle of the neck.

- In 20% of the cases, lymph nodes in the posterior triangle are affected due to involvement of adenoids.

- Rarely, infection can spread from tuberculosis of apex of lung. Organisms directly penetrate Sibson's fascia (suprapleural membrane) and can cause enlargement of supraclavicular node.

STAGES OF TUBERCULOUS (TB) LYMPHADENITIS

1. Stage of lymphadenitis (Fig. 2.3)

- Common in young adults between 20 to 30 years
- Upper anterior deep cervical nodes are enlarged
- Non-tender, discrete, mobile, firm lymph nodes are palpable.

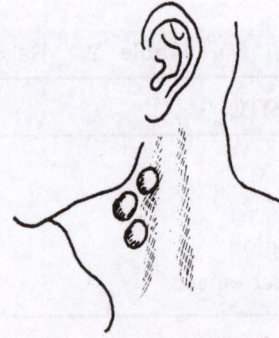

Fig. 2.3 TB lymphadenitis - discrete nodes

2. Stage of periadenitis/Stage of matting (Fig. 2.4)

- Results due to involvement of capsule
- Nodes move together

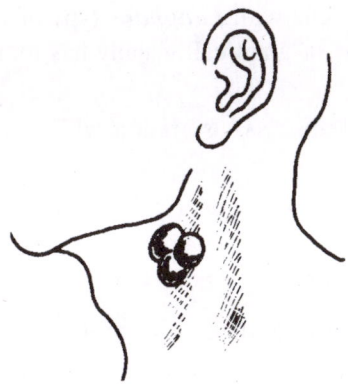

Fig. 2.4 TB lymphadenitis - matted nodes

- Firm, non-tender
- Matting is pathognomonic of tuberculosis.
- Other rare causes of matting are chronic lymphadenitis, anaplastic variety of lymphoma.

3. Stage of cold abscess (Fig. 2.5)

It occurs due to caseation necrosis of lymph nodes resulting in fluctuant swelling in the neck. Clinical features of cold abscess in the neck are:

- No local rise in temperature
- No tenderness
- No redness
- Soft, cystic and fluctuant swelling
- Transillumination is negative
- On sternocleidomastoid contraction test, it becomes less prominent indicating that it is deep to deep fascia.

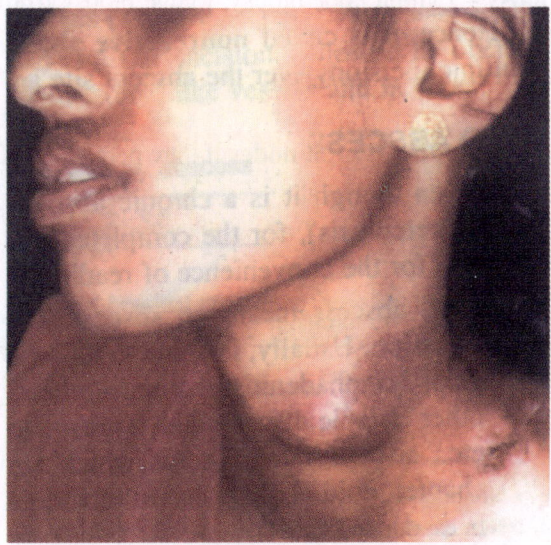

Fig. 2.5 TB lymphadenitis - Cold abscess

Differential diagnosis

- **Branchial cyst** can be confused for cold abscess in the anterior triangle. Branchial cyst is of longer duration and patients with cold abscess may have other lymph nodes in the neck.

Treatment of cold abscess (Fig. 2.6)

- **NON-DEPENDENT ASPIRATION** by using a wide bore needle to avoid a persistent sinus.
- Wide bore needle is preferred because caseous material is thick.
- Incision and drainage should not be done as it causes persistent tuberculous sinus.
- Antituberculous treatment is given.

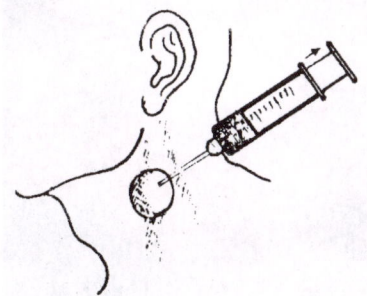

Fig. 2.6 Non-dependent aspiration

4. Stage of collar stud abscess (Fig. 2.7)

It results when a cold abscess which is deep to deep fascia ruptures through the deep fascia and forms another swelling in the subcutaneous plane which is fluctuant. Cross fluctuation test may be positive. It is treated like a cold abscess.

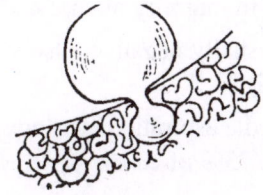

Fig. 2.7 Collar stud abscess.

5. Stage of sinus (Fig. 2.8)

- Sinus is a blind tract leading from the surface down into the tissues.
- It occurs when collar stud abscess ruptures through the skin
- Tubercular sinus is the commonest sinus in the neck in India.

- Common in young females
- It can be multiple
- Tubercular sinus will have wide opening
- Resembles an ulcer with undermined edge
- No induration
- Skin surrounding the sinus shows pigmentation and sometimes it is bluish in colour.
- A group of lymph nodes is usually palpable underneath the sinus.

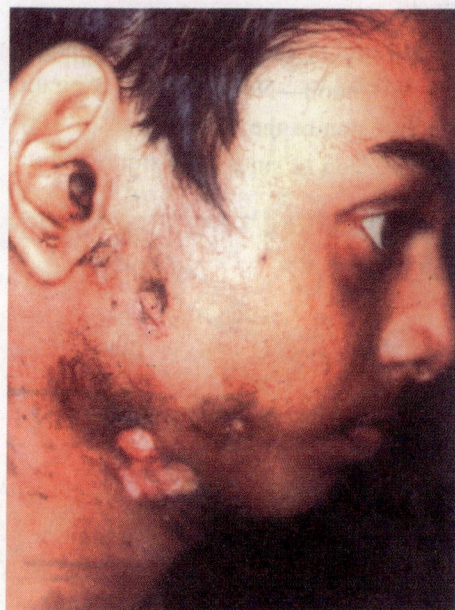

Fig. 2.8 Multiple tubercular sinuses in the neck and in front of the ear

INVESTIGATIONS IN TUBERCULAR LYMPHADENITIS

- Complete blood picture may reveal low Hb%.
- ESR is elevated in majority of cases.
- Chest X-ray is usually negative, also sputum for AFB (Acid-fast bacilli).
- FNAC (Fine needle aspiration cytology) can give a diagnosis in about 75% of cases.
- Lymph node biopsy reveals central caseation surrounded by epitheloid cells with **Langhans** type of giant cells. Langhans type of giant cell usually has more than 20 nuclei.
- If it is a cold abscess, aspiration will reveal **cheesy material**.
- Edge biopsy from the sinus

TREATMENT (Summary Table 2.3)

- After confirming the diagnosis anti-tuberculous treatment is given.

Antituberculous treatment (ATT) for lymphatic tuberculosis

The World Health Organisation recommendation for extra-pulmonary tuberculosis is as follows:

- The three-drug regime – INH, rifampicin, pyrazinamide (H.R.Z.) – for two months followed by INH and Rifampicin for another four months.
- The dosage is as given below:

  INH: 6 mg/kg body weight – usual adult dose is 300 mg/day.

  Rifampicin: 10 mg/kg body weight – usual adult dose is 450-600 mg/day.

  Pyrazinamide: 30 mg/kg body weight – usual adult dose is 1,500 mg/day.

- Detailed dosage of ATT, side effects of these drugs are discussed in medicine textbooks.

Role of surgery in tuberculous lymphadenitis

- **Biopsy** – Lymph node biopsy, wedge biopsy from the edge of the sinus.
- **Aspiration** – Non-dependent aspiration of cold abscess.
- **Excision of the lymph nodes** if they persist inspite of antituberculous treatment.
- **Excision of sinus wall** along with the tract.

STAGE	INVESTIGATIONS	TREATMENT
Lymphadenitis	Lymph node biopsy/FNAC	Antituberculous treatment (ATT)
Periadenitis	Lymph node biopsy/FNAC	Antituberculous treatment
Cold abscess	Aspirated cheesy material for AFB	Nondependent aspiration with ATT
Collar stud abscess	Aspirate for AFB	Non-dependent aspiration followed by ATT
Sinus	Edge biopsy of the sinus	ATT

Table 2.3 Summary of the management of various stages of tuberculous lymphadenitis

Other special types of pyogenic infections

BOIL (Key Boxes 2.4 & 2.5)

- This is also called furuncle. It is a hair follicle infection caused by *Staphylococcus aureus* or secondary infection of a sebaceous cyst.
- It starts with painful indurated swelling with surrounding oedema. After about 1-2 days, softening occurs in the centre and pustule develops which bursts spontaneously discharging pus. Necrosis of subcutaneous tissues produces a greenish slough. Skin overlying the boil also undergoes necrosis. ***Hence, boil is included under acute infective gangrene.***
- Furuncle of the external auditory meatus is a very painful condition because of the rich nerve supply of the skin. Pain is also due to dense adherence of skin to the perichondrium (subcutaneous tissue is not there).

Key Box 2.4	
PRECIPITATING FACTORS	**COMMON LOCATIONS**
Scratching	Face and back of the neck
Diabetes	Axilla
Poor immunity	Gluteal region

Key Box 2.5	
FACTS ABOUT A BOIL	
• Dangerous boil	: On the skin of face
• Tender boil	: External auditory
• Sweet boil	: Diabetic patients
• Boil likes	: Oily skin
• Blind boil or dull boil	: Subsides without suppuration

Treatment of boil

Incision and drainage with excision of slough. Antibiotic cloxacillin is given. Diabetes, if present, is treated.

Complications of boil

- Necrosis of the skin
- Pyaemic abscess and septicaemia
- Cavernous sinus thrombosis due to boil on the face or stye on the eyelid

CARBUNCLE (Fig. 2.9)

- This is an **infective gangrene** of the subcutaneous tissue caused by *Staphylococcus aureus*. It commonly occurs in diabetic patients. Poor immunity, radiotherapy patients can also develop carbuncle.

Key Box 2.6
STAPHYLOCOCCAL INFECTIONS OF SURGICAL IMPORTANCE
• Boil
• Carbuncle
• Breast abscess
• Parotitis
• Osteomyelitis

- **Sites: Nape of the neck** is the commonest site followed by back and shoulder region. Skin of these sites is coarse and has poor vascularity.

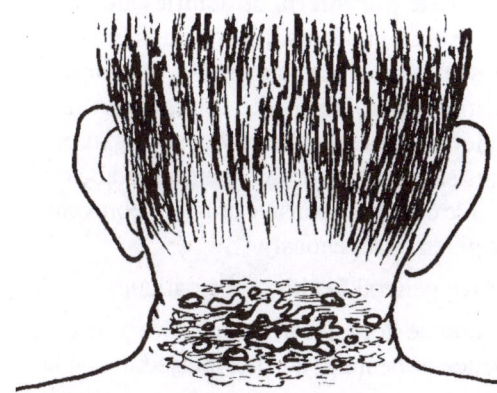

Fig. 2.9 Carbuncle of the back of neck - common site

Pathology

The initial lesion is similar to a boil in the form of hair follicle infection with perifolliculitis. Since majority of patients are diabetics, infection takes a virulent course and results in necrosis of subcutaneous fat which gives rise to multiple abscesses. These abscesses are **intercommunicating** and they open to the exterior by multiple openings which are called sieve-like openings. This appearance is described as **cribriform** appearance which is pathognomonic of carbuncle.

Clinical features

- Typically, the patient is a diabetic.
- Severe pain and the swelling in the nape of the neck
- Constitutional symptoms like fever with chills and rigors are severe.
- Surface is red, angry looking like a **red hot coal**.
- Surrounding area is indurated.
- Later, skin on the centre of carbuncle softens and peripheral satellite vesicles appear, which rupture discharging pus and give rise to **cribriform** appearance.
- The end result is development of large crateriform ulcer with central slough.

Complications

1. Worsening of the diabetic status resulting in diabetic ketoacidosis.
2. Extensive necrosis of skin overlying carbuncle. Hence, it is included under acute infective gangrene.
3. Septicaemia, toxaemia

Treatment (Key Box 2.7)

- Diabetes control preferably with injectable **insulin**
- Appropriate **parenteral antibiotics** are given till complete resolution occurs. Most strains of staphylococcal aureus are sensitive to cloxacillin, flucloxacillin, erythromycin and some of the cephalosporins. However Methicillin Resistant Staphylococcal Aureus (MRSA) are resistant to the drugs mentioned above. They are sensitive only to expensive drug Vancomycin which has to be given intravenously.
- Improve general health of the patient
- If carbuncle does not show any softening or if it shows evidence of healing, it is not incised. It can be left open

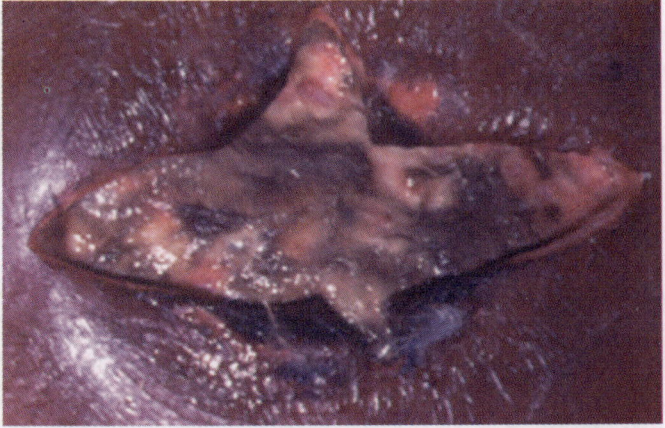

Fig. 2.10 observe central slough and cruciate incision

to the exterior or saline dressings are applied to reduce oedema. Complete resolution may take place within 10-15 days.

- Surgery is required when there is pus. *Cruciate incision* is preferred because of multiple abscesses and extensive subcutaneous necrosis. Edges of the skin flap are excised, pus is drained, loculi are broken down, slough is excised, and cavity is treated with antiseptic agents. Like pyogenic abscess, wound heals with granulation tissue from the depth (Fig. 2.10).

ERYSIPELAS

- It is an acute inflammation of the skin and subcutaneous tissues associated with severe lymphangitis. Causative organism is streptococcus pyogenes. Precipitating factors are malnourishment, chronic diseases etc. Thus, children and old people are commonly affected.
- Infection sets in after a small scratch or abrasion and spreads very rapidly resulting in toxaemia. Sites: Face, eyelids, scrotum and in infants, the umbilicus.

Clinical features

- **Rose-pink** rash with raised edge, appreciated on palpation and has a consistency of button hole.
- **Vesicles** appear later, rarely become pustular.
- Oedema of eyelids or scrotum depending upon the site.
- Features of **toxaemia**
- When it occurs in the face, it involves pinna because erysipelas is basically a **cuticular lymphangitis**. This is described as *Milian's ear sign positive*. This sign is used to differentiate cellulitis of face from facial erysipelas. In cellulitis of face, pinna does not get involved because of close adherence of skin to the cartilage.

Complications

1. Toxaemia and septicaemia
2. Gangrene of skin and subcutaneous tissue
3. Lymphoedema of face and eyelids due to lymphatic obstruction causing fibrosis of lymphatics.

Treatment

- Injection crystalline penicillin 10 lakh units 6th hourly I.M./I.V. for 5-10 days.

CHRONIC ABSCESS

- It results when initial infective process or the cause is not fully identified and treated.

Sites

- Foot, hand, etc.

Causes

1. **Foreign bodies:** These are the most common causes for chronic abscess. Typical history of a recurrent swelling discharging pus is present. Wooden pieces injected in the thigh or in the foot are common. Synthetic mesh used in repair of hernias can get infected is an another example.
2. **Dead tissue:** As it occurs in diabetes patients.
3. **Pilonidal sinus:** This condition gives rise to recurrent abscesses. Typical history of pain and swelling which ruptures followed by spontaneous recovery is present. However, the sinus persists.
4. **Chronic disease:** All features of cold abscess are present but in an unusual situation. (Not a Cold Abscess arising from the lymph nodes.)

CLINICAL NOTES

40-year-old female presented with swelling of the left thigh of 8 months duration, no signs of inflammation. FNAC was inconclusive. At surgery, thick walled, localised abscess with fleshy tissue was removed. The final report was tubercular abscess.

There was no evidence of tubeculosis anywhere in the body. In many cases tuberculosis can present in different forms as in this case. Detailed investigations could not reveal any evidence of pulmonary tuberculosis.

NECROTISING FASCITIS

It is a spreading destructive invasive infection of skin and soft tissues including deep fascia with **relative sparing of muscle.**

Common sites

- Genitalia, groin, lower abdomen. In these places it is comparable or similar to and called as Meleney's gangrene. Other sites are limbs.

Causative organism

Two types have been identified:

- **Monomicrobial:** It is due to Group A beta-haemolytic streptococci. It is also called as **Type II Necrotising fascitis**.

Key Box 2.8
SPECIFIC FEATURES OF TYPE II NECROTISING FASCITIS
• Caused by *Streptococcus pyogenes* • Occur in young healthy people • Minor abrasions, laceration may be a precipitating factor • Severe systemic illness with multiorgan failure – Streptococcal toxic shock syndrome

- **Polymicrobial:** It is due to synergistic combination of anerobes and coliforms or nongroup A streptococci – **Type I Necrotising fascitis**.
- Very often there is **no history of injury** when it occurs in the lower limbs.

Risk factors for Type I Necrotising fascitis

Key Box 2.9
NECROTISING FASCITIS - RISK FACTORS
• Diabetes mellitus, malnutrition • Obesity, corticosteroids • Immune deficiency

Clinical features

- Sudden pain in the affected area with gross swelling of the part

- The part is swollen, red erythematous, oedematous with skip lesions of skin necrosis and ulceration.
- High degree fever, jaundice, renal failure can occur soon in untreated cases. Often crepitus is palpable (Refer Key Box 2.8).

Diagnosis

- Full thickness biopsy taken at bedside can give full diagnosis. Watery pus (**dishwater liquid**) is also characteristic.

Treatment

- Early, aggressive treatment includes supportive and surgical treatment.

Supportive treatment

- This includes hospitalisation, adequate hydration, broad spectrum antibiotics.
- Surgery involves wide excision, generous debridement followed few days or weeks later by skin grafting
- **In Type II Cases (Streptococcal)**: High dose penicillins along with clindamycin is the treatment of choice. **Clindamycin** has special affect as it is a **potent suppressor of bacterial toxin synthesis.**

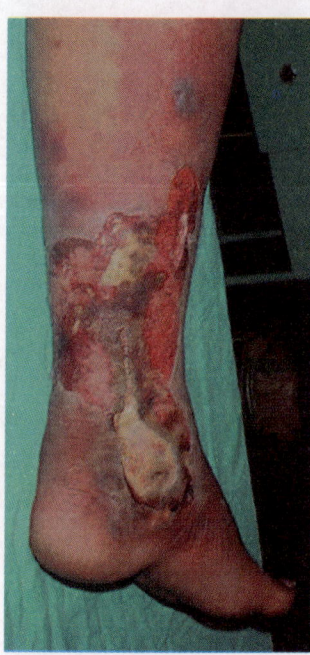

Fig. 2.11 type II Necrotising fascitis in a healthy man. Inspite of debridement and intensive care, he died of multiorgan failure

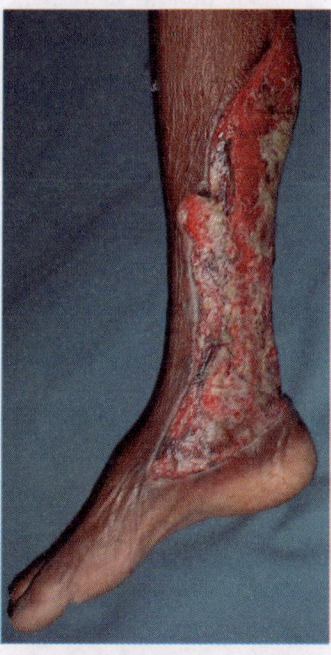

Fig. 2.12 This patient presented with features of cellulitis with renal failure. There were no precipitating factors. After debridement, recovery was complete

ACUTE PYOMYOSITIS

Definition: Localised area of suppuration **within striated muscle** is pyomyositis.

Aetiology

- Trauma
- Transient bactraemia
- Common in tropical countries
- IV drug abusers are affected often
- Immunocompromised conditions
- Abnormality of the immune system

Pathogenesis

Trauma
↓
Release of iron
↓
Profuse growth of bacteria
↓
Intramuscular abscess

Bacteriology

- Staphylococcus aureus - 90%, Streptococcus pyogenes
- E.coli

Clinical features

- Classically, quadriceps, gluteus, shoulder and upper arm muscle are affected. Pain over the part, oedema, fever, jaundice are common. Tenderness, induration and spasm of muscles are characteristic.
- **Renal failure results in soon.**

Investigations

- Sonographic aspiration of pus followed by culture
- CT, MRI are ideal investigations to know the spread of the infection.
- Creatine kinase can go up to 50,000 to 2,00,000 units/L during acute phase due to **rhabdomyolysis**

Treatment

- Early diagnosis and early aggressive treatment
- Antibiotics
- Exploration - as a treatment and for diagnosis
- Wide excision of muscles, compartmental excision till viable tissues are visible

Tetanus and Gas Gangrene

3

- Tetanus
- Gas gangrene
- Types of gas infections

TETANUS

A nonimmunised, eighteen year old girl was admitted with moderate tetanus following a nail prick in her foot. In the hospital she developed convulsions, laryngeal oedema and cardiac arrest from which she was resuscitated and shifted to intensive care unit under **anaesthesiologist's** care. Tracheostomy, ventilation and paralysing agents were used. Unlike others, she was lucky. She walked home after two months of stay in intensive care unit after a lot of suffering and spending a large amount of money. The case history has been written here to impress upon the students.

1. How important is immunisation to prevent tetanus

2. How serious is this disorder

3. Is it possible to save these patients who are critically ill?

AETIOPATHOGENESIS

- Tetanus is a serious disorder with very high mortality even with treatment. The disease is caused by **Clostridium tetani**, an anaerobic spore-forming bacillus with terminal spore which has a drumstick like appearance.

Possible routes of infection are

- **Umbilical cord - in neonates**, seen in communities which practice cowdung application on the umbilical stump.

- Wound - as a complication of road traffic accidents where other aerobic organisms reduce oxygen tension in the wound, thereby facilitating growth of anaerobic clostridium tetani.

- **Minor injuries** with **rusted nails**, piercing of the ear lobes, tattooing, injections etc.

- Endogenous infection after **septic abortion or surgical operations** on gastrointestinal tract.

- Tetanus due to infection acquired in the operation theatre.

- Thus, tetanus is a wound infection. **"NO WOUND, NO TETANUS"** is true. Having entered the wound, the organisms multiply and produce powerful exotoxins which produce the disease. Thus, the organisms by themselves, do not produce the disease. The toxins produced by the organisms are tetanospasmin (Neurotoxin) and tetanolysin (Haemolysin).

- **Tetanospasmin has affinity towards nervous tissues**. It reaches the central nervous system along the axons of motor nerve trunks. The toxin gets fixed to motor cells of the anterior horn cells. The toxin, which is fixed to the motor end plate, acts in the following ways:

1. It **inhibits the release of cholinesterase** which causes accumulation of acetylcholine at the motor end plate which is responsible for tonic rigidity of the limb, trunk, abdominal and neck muscles.

2. It acts at *the spinal level* and causes reflex contraction of muscles due to minor stimuli.

- **The toxin which is fixed to the nervous tissue cannot be neutralised**. However, the circulating toxin can be neutralised. Incubation period may vary from few days to months or years. Hence, it is not important. The interval between first symptom (dysphagia and stiffness of jaw) to a reflex spasm is called the **period of onset**. If this is less than 48 hours, the prognosis is poor and if more than 48 hours, prognosis is better.

Favourable conditions for development of tetanus

- No immunisation
- Foreign body
- Injury
- Improper sterilisation
- Devitalised tissues
- Anaerobic conditions

SPECIAL TYPES OF TETANUS

1. **Tetanus neonatorum**: It occurs due to contamination of umbilical cord in children born to non-immunised mothers. It manifests usually around 6-8 days of birth and is called as **Eighth day disease**. It carries almost 100% mortality.

2. **Local tetanus**: In this, contraction of muscles occurs in the neighbourhood of the wound.

3. **Cephalic tetanus** : Usually occurs after wound of head and face. Cranial nerves like facial nerve and oculomotor nerve can get **paralysed**. It carries poor prognosis.

4. **Bulbar tetanus** : It is a condition wherein muscles of deglutition and respiration are involved. It is fatal.

5. **Latent tetanus**: It develops after few months to years following a wound which might have been forgotten.

6. **Puerperal tetanus**: It occurs as a complication of abortion or puerperal sepsis.

7. **Postoperative tetanus**: Occurs due to improper sterilisation of instruments and carries 100% mortality. In an ideal operation theatre, this type of tetanus should not occur.

8. **Otitis tetanus**: It is due to chronic suppurative otitis media. In these cases, the wound is a tear in the tympanic membrane. It can occur in any age group, but commonly in children and young adults.

CLINICAL FEATURES : (Refer Table 3.1)

- **Autonomic dysfunction** : Increased basal sympathetic tone manifesting as tachycardia and bladder, bowel dysfunction, labile hypertension, pyrexia, pallor, sweating and cyanosis of the digits can occur.

- Episodes of bradycardia, low central venous pressure CVP and even cardiac arrests have been reported due to parasympathetic dysfunction.

- They can develop complications such as pneumonia, urinary tract infection etc.

Table 3.1 Clinical features with differential diagnosis	
SYMPTOMS AND SIGNS	**DIFFERENTIAL DIAGNOSIS**
• **Trismus or lock jaw,** occurs due to severe contraction of the masseter muscle, resulting in inability to open the mouth. It is the most common symptom of tetanus.	• Alveolar abscess or temporomandibular joint involvement
• **Dysphagia** occurs due to spasm of pharyngeal muscles.	• Tonsillitis
• **Neck rigidity**	• Meningitis
• **Rigidity of back muscles**	• Orthopaedic disorder
• **Risus sardonicus** due to spasm of facial muscles and jaw muscles.	• Anxiety neurosis
• **Generalised convulsions** wherein every muscle is thrown into contraction, with severe clenching of teeth, arched back and extended limbs is described as opisthotonos (bow-like body; hence the name **Dhanurvatha**).	• Epilepsy
• Mild temperature and tachycardia	• Sympathetic hyperactivity

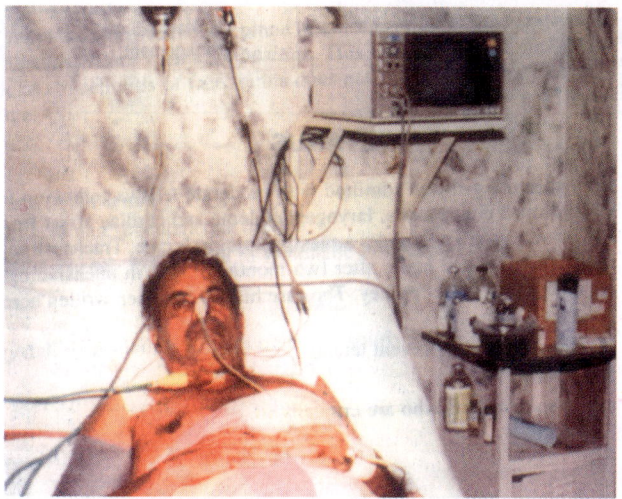

Fig. 3.1 Tetanus patient recovering in an intensive care unit

TREATMENT OF ESTABLISHED TETANUS

I. General management

II. Specific management.

I. General management (Fig 3.1)

- **Admission and isolation**[1] in a quiet room, to avoid minor stimuli which precipitate spasm.
- **Wound care** which includes drainage of pus, excision of necrotic tissue, removal of foreign body and proper dressing.
- **Inj. tetanus toxoid** 0.5 ml to be given I.M.
- **Antitetanus serum** (A.T.S.) 50,000 units intramuscular (I.M.) and 50,000 units intra-venous (I.V.). This should be given only after giving a test dose which consists of diluting a small dose of serum with ten times saline and inject a small amount in the subcutaneous tissue. It has become less popular due to availability of human antitetanus globulin.
- **Instead of A.T.S.**, human **antitetanus globulin** is better and safe. It does not cause anaphylaxis. It is given in the dose of 3000 to 4000 units **I.V.** No test dose is required.
- **Inj. crystalline penicillin** 10 lakh **units every** 6 hours is the drug of choice against clostridium tetani. It may have to be given for a period of 7-10 days.

- **Metronidazole** 500mg IV 8th hrly. for 10 days. It has been shown to be more effective than penicillin.
- After recovery, full immunisation with tetanus toxoid is a must.

II. Specific management

A. MILD CASES

- There is only tonic rigidity without spasm or dysphagia. These patients are managed by heavy sedation by using a combination of the drugs so as to avoid spasm or convulsions. An example of the method of treatment followed in our hospital is given in the next page (Table 3.2).
- Benzodiazepines and morphine act centrally to minimise the effects of tetanospasmin.
- Chlorpromazine being α - receptor blocker, can decrease sympathetic activity, other α blockers such as phenoxybenzamine, phentolamine also have been used.
- These drugs are repeated in such a way that every two hours the patient receives some sedative. The dosage of the drugs is adjusted once in 2 or 3 days so as to get the maximum effect of sedation or relaxation.
- Injection diazepam 10mg, tracheostomy set, resuscitation set which includes laryngoscope and endotracheal tube should be kept ready by the side of the patient.

B. SERIOUSLY ILL CASES

- They have dysphagia and reflex spasms
- A nasogastric tube is introduced for feeding purposes and to administer the drugs.
- Tracheostomy, if breathing difficulty arises.

C. DANGEROUSLY ILL CASES

- This group includes patients with major cyanotic convulsions. In addition to continuing sedatives, these patients are paralysed with muscle relaxants (neuromuscular blocking agents) and positive pressure ventilation is given till they recover. One cannot predict exactly how many days a patient requires ventilatory support. During this period adequate nutrition, care of the urinary bladder, care of the bowel, frequent change of position to avoid bed sore, have to be taken care of.

---

1. *Isolation for tetanus has been misunderstood by surgeons. It is a fact that in majority of the hospitals, tetanus patients are isolated in a remote corner of the hospital, well away from the reach of a skilled person. Many cases die due to convulsions and laryngeal spasm before they are intubated and resuscitated. The critically ill patients are admitted in an intensive care unit under the supervision of anaesthesiologist's care in our institution. (Fig. 3.1). Tetanus is NOT COMMUNICABLE from person to person.*

Key Box 3.1		
DRUG	**DOSAGE**	**TIME**
Chlorpromazine	50-100 mg	8 AM - 2 PM – 8 PM - 2 AM
Phenobarbitone	30-60 mg	10 AM - 4 PM – 10 PM - 4 AM
Diazepam	10-20 mg	12 Noon - 6 PM – 12 MN - 6 AM

PROPHYLAXIS

1. Tetanus neonatorum can be prevented by immunisation of the mother with two tetanus toxoid injections, **half ml** I.M. given in the third trimester of pregnancy.

2. Infants and children are immunised with tetanus toxoid, diphtheria and pertussis vaccine (DPT) three doses at 6, 10, 14 weeks of age. This is called triple antigen. A booster dose is given at 18 months and school going time (5 years), and once in five years 1 ml of tetanus toxoid is given to achieve active immunity.

3. Immunised individual who receives a provocative injury is administered a booster dose if he has not been given in the previous 5 years.

4. Tetanus can be prevented by giving tetanus antitoxin in the following situations :

   - Wounds of head and face, penetrating wounds
   - Wounds with contused and devitalised tissues
   - War wound and road traffic accidents

   In such patients, a dose of 250 units of human antitetanus globulin will give adequate protection.

CAUSES OF DEATH

1. Aspiration of pharyngeal contents into the lungs resulting in aspiration pneumonia

2. Laryngeal spasm and respiratory arrest resulting in cardiac arrest

3. Autonomic disturbances resulting in cardiac arrythmias

GAS GANGRENE

- It is a highly fatal spreading infection caused by clostridial organisms which results in myonecrosis.

Other names for gas gangrene are

- Clostridial myositis, clostridial myonecrosis, infective gangrene of the muscles.

AETIOLOGY

- The disease is caused by *Clostridium perfringens* (Clostridium welchii) - the commonest organism (60%). Other organisms are *Clostridium septicum, Clostridium oedematiens, Clostridium histolyticum.*

Source of infection

1. Manured soil or cultivated soil, normal intestines.

   Risk Group: Lower limb amputations performed for ischaemic gangrene of limb infection from patient's own bowel organisms. High velocity gun shot wounds with perforation of hollow viscus are also associated with risk of developing gas gangrene.

PATHOGENESIS (Table 3.2)

- Gas gangrene develops in wounds where there is heavy contamination with soil or foreign body or which is associated with laceration and devitalised muscle mass. This type of situation is common today following road

Table 3.2 Predisposing factors

FACTORS	HOW IT HELPS
Foreign body such as soil, clothing, bullets, glass pieces.	Soil supplies calcium and silicic acid which causes tissue necrosis.
Anoxia due to crushing of the arteries.	Necrosis of the tissues results in proliferation of the organism.
Dead and devitalised tissues.	Anaerobic organisms multiply.
Blood clots.	Supplies calcium
Extravasated haemoglobin and myoglobin	Cease to carry oxygen.

traffic accidents. Endogenous infection from patient's faecal matter may be responsible for gas gangrene, in certain cases of contamination of a surgical wound such as below knee amputation done for some other cause. Having entered the wound, clostridia multiply and produce powerful toxins.

- All these factors contribute to create a low oxygen tension. Under these favourable conditions clostridial organisms multiply and produce toxins which cause further tissue damage. The toxins produced by the organisms and their effects are given in Table 3.3.

- Once powerful toxins start acting, various pathological events occur like inflammation, oedema, muscle necrosis and gangrene of the muscles. These events are summarised below.

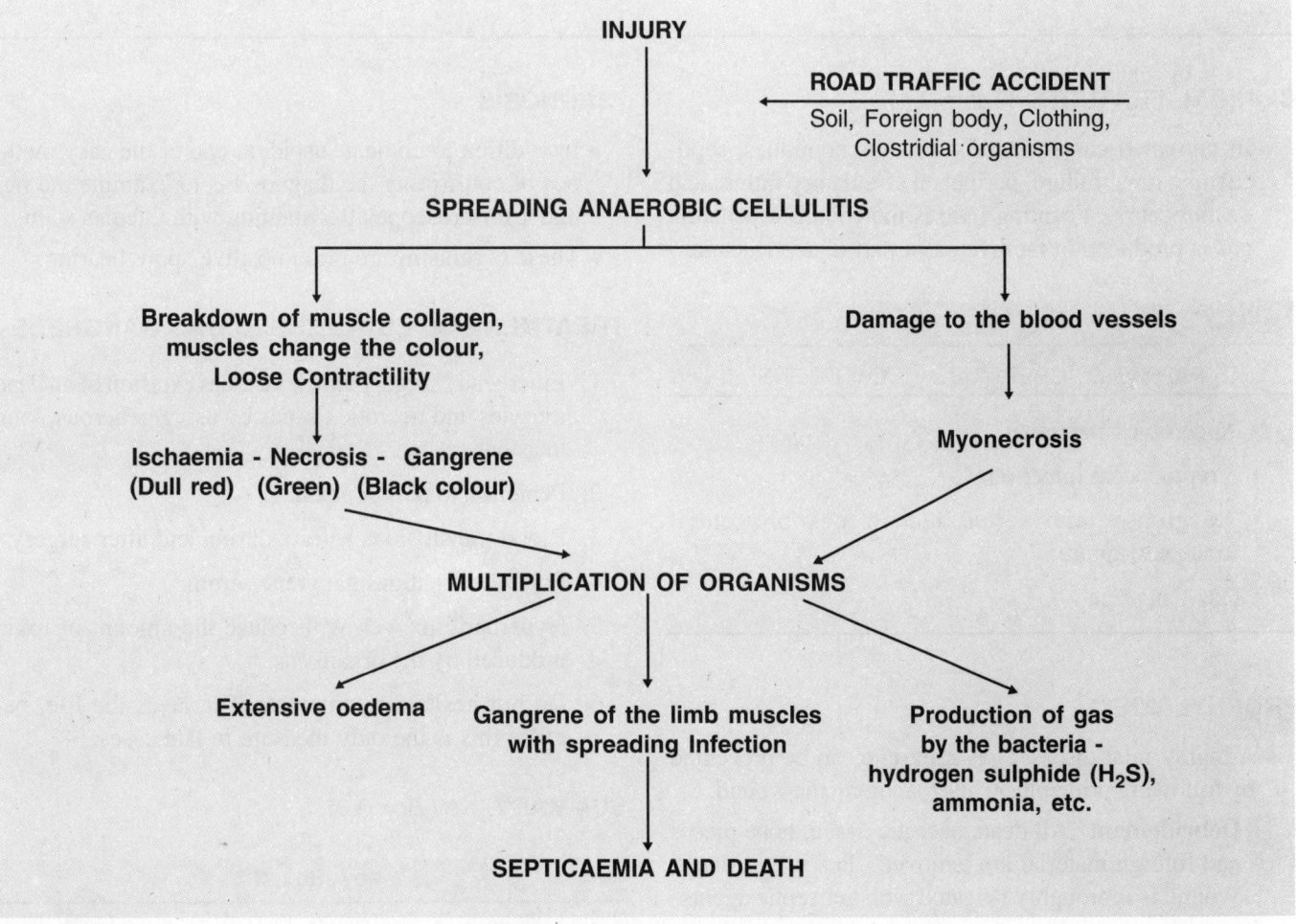

Fig. 3.2 Pathological Changes

Table 3.3 Toxins and their effect

TOXINS	EFFECT
1. Lecithinase (Alphatoxin)	• Dermonecrosis
	Haemolysis
	Profound toxaemia
2. Beta toxin	• Necrosis of the tissues
3. Proteinase	• Breakdown of collagen fibers
4. Hyaluronidase	• Break the cement substance of the muscle cells - hyaluronic acid

Table 3.4 Clinical features

LOCAL FEATURES	GENERAL FEATURES
Severe pain and gross oedema of the wound	Anxious and alert
Sutured wound is under tension	Toxic and ill
Thin brownish fluid escapes which has sickly sweet odour	Rapid increase in the pulse rate
Palpable crepitus	Hypotension due to suppression of adrenals
Colour changes in the muscles	Vomiting
Skin becomes khaki coloured due to haemolysis	Low grade fever

CLINICAL FEATURES (Table 3.4)

- In untreated cases, necrotic process continues, septicaemia, renal failure, peripheral circulatory failure and death occurs. Foaming liver is the condition wherein gas is produced in the liver, as a part of septicaemia.

Key Box 3.2

PALPABLE CREPITUS - CONDITIONS

- Anaerobic infections
- Streptococcal infections
- Surgical emphysema due to oesophageal, tracheal rupture
- Gas gangrene

PROPHYLAXIS

- A highly fatal disease, gas gangrene can be prevented by following principles while managing the wound.

1. **Debridement** : All dead, necrotic tissue, bone pieces and foreign material are removed. Pus is evacuated. Wound is thoroughly irrigated with antiseptic agents.

When in doubt do not suture the wound.

2. **Prophylactic antibiotics** : Penicillin is the drug of choice. Injection Crystalline Penicillin 10-20 lakh units, 4-6 hourly is given for a period of seven days.

3. **Judicious and minimal** use of **tourniquet**.

   If possible, avoid tourniquet while managing such a wound in the leg.

4. **Gentle** but **effective application of** *plaster cast* with or without treatment of associated fractures to avoid compression on the blood vessel.

DIAGNOSIS

- In addition to clinical suspicion one of the easy methods of confirming the diagnosis is to examine the pus under miscroscope after staining with Giemsa stain.
- These organisms are gram positive spore bearing.

TREATMENT OF ESTABLISHED GAS GANGRENE

1. Emergency surgery which includes excision of all dead muscles and necrotic tissues by using generous, long incisions.
2. Penicillin to be continued.
3. Blood transfusions before, during and after surgery.
4. Polyvalent antigas gangrene serum.
5. Hyperbaric oxygen will reduce the amount of toxin produced by the organisms.
6. Do not hesitate to amputate if it saves the life, because this is the only measure in late cases.

SUMMARY (Key Box 3.3)

Key Box 3.3

SUMMARY

Correct hypotension

Control infection

Treat dehydration

Conduct operation

Administer hyperbaric oxygen

Give blood transfusion

Passive immunisation

To save life do amputation

TYPE OF GAS INFECTIONS

1. **Clostridial cellulitis**: In this condition healthy muscle is not involved. It involves necrotic tissue and produces features of cellulitis such as tense, swollen parts with palpable crepitus. However, it is a mild infection, which can be managed by antibiotics without surgery (Key Box 3.4).

2. **Local type**: It refers to infection confined to a single muscle.

3. **Group type**: It refers to infection confined to one group of muscles in the compartment. Such cases get benefit after a compartmental excision.

4. **Massive Type** : Gas gangrene involving the entire limb, needs to be treated by amputation.

CLINICAL NOTES

This forty year old gentleman (Fig. 3.3) presented to the hospital with massive gas gangrene involving upper limb, chest wall, abdominal wall and back. It started after an injury to the elbow. Patient received initial treatment in the local hospital. However it was too late when we saw the patient. He was having severe hypotension and renal failure. Within six hours of admission to the hospital, he expired.

Key Box 3.4

INFECTIONS BY CLOSTRIDIUM WELCHII

- Gas gangrene of the limb
- Gas gangrene of the abdominal wall
- Gangrenous appendicitis, Cholangitis
- Necrotising enteritis, Food poisoning
- Infection of the uterus following septic abortion

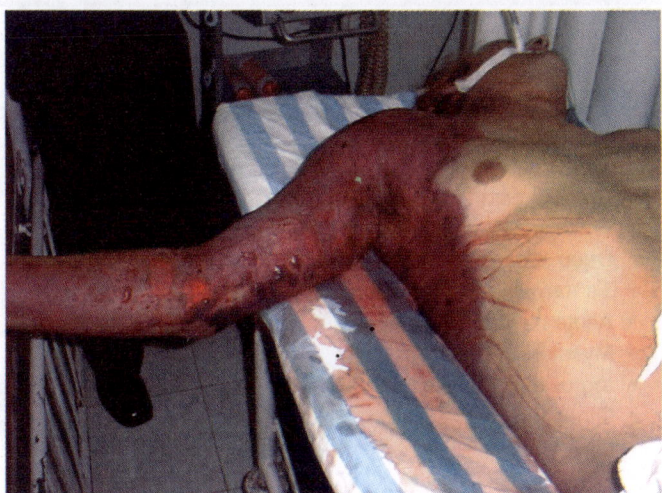

Fig. 3.3. Gas Gangrene

Hand and Foot Infections

4

- Paronychia
- Terminal pulp space infections
- Apical subungual infection
- Web space infections
- Deep palmar abscess
- Tenosynovitis
- Acute lymphangitis
- Mycetoma pedis
- Ingrowing toe nail
- Other hand infections

Hand infections are commonly encountered in manual labourers and is precipitated by injury such as a thorn prick, cut injuries, etc. In 80-90% of cases the causative organisms are *staphylococcus aureus* which is sensitive to *cloxacillin*. In remaining cases, streptococci, gram negative bacilli, anaerobic organisms also may play a role. Irrespective of the site of infection, oedema is commonly encountered on dorsal aspect because of the following reasons:

- Lymphatics from the palmar aspect of the hand travel through the dorsal aspect to the corresponding lymph node.
- Presence of the loose areolar tissue in the dorsum of the hand.

Oedema is the chief cause of stiffness of the fingers. Hence early physiotherapy should be encouraged.

SUPERFICIAL INFECTIONS

PARONYCHIA

It means near the nail. It is the commonest type of hand infection. There are two types of paronychia, acute and chronic.

ACUTE PARONYCHIA (Fig. 4.1)

- It occurs due to trimming of the nail or ingrowing nail.

Key Box 4.1	
SUPERFICIAL INFECTIONS	**DEEP INFECTIONS**
1. Paronychia	1. Terminal pulp space infection
2. Subcutaneous infections	2. Apical subungual infection
3. Infection of dorsal space	3. Volar space infection
4. Acute lymphangitis	4. Web space infection
	5. Mid palmar space infection
	6. Tenosynovitis

- Infection which is subcuticular starts in the lateral sulcus and spreads all around (Paronychia means 'run around'). This is because eponychium (skin overlying the nail base) is adherent to the nail base. Hence the infection spreads beneath the nail base. The affected finger is painful. Throbbing pain suggests presence of pus. Even collections of 0.5 ml pus produces severe pain. Low grade fever may be present.

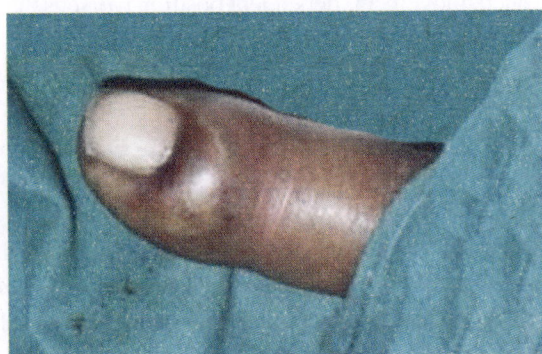

Fig. 4.1 Acute paronychia

Treatment

- Using a digital block (with 2% *plain lignocaine* 5ml injection into the root of the digit) incision and drainage is done by incising the eponychium. (In the finger, penis and ear lobule **adrenaline should not be used**, as it is a vasoconstrictor and can cause gangrene.) Pus is sent for culture and sensitivity. Antibiotics are given.

CHRONIC PARONYCHIA

- It is *not due to bacterial infection*. It is due to **fungal infection** - moniliasis or due to candida infections.
- It is common in women who wash the clothes, utensils resulting in constant wetting of fingers. As a result of this, fungal infection takes place. The infection is slow, onset is insidious and chronic. It is difficult to eradicate the infection. It produces a dull nagging pain in the fingers. The eponychium is faintly pink and nail is ridged.
- Antifungal agents such as nystatin or tolnaftate solution helps the patient. Rubber gloves should be worn while using hand for washing.

SUBCUTANEOUS INFECTIONS (Fig. 4.2-4.4)

a. **Intraepidermal abscess:** It is also called as purulent blister. Cuts, pricks and burns are also the cause of this condition.

b. **Intradermal:** This variety does not produce dome shaped elevation.

c. **Subcutaneous abscess:** This type of lesion is like that of cellulitis.

d. **Collar stud abscess:** It results when the epidermal component is connected to dermal component.

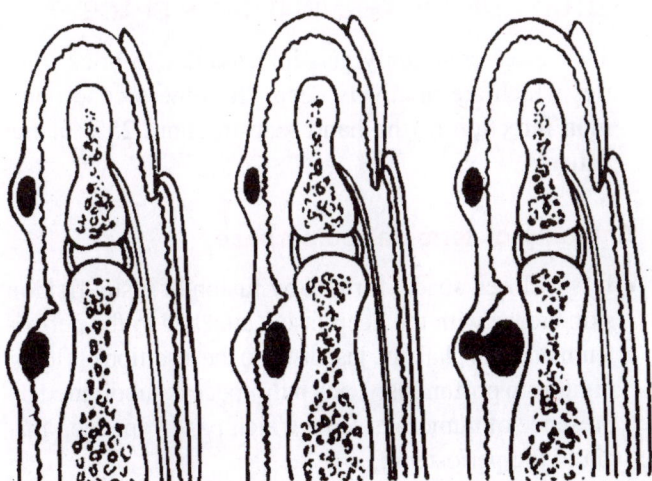

Fig. 4.2, 4.3, 4.4 Intraepidermal abscess, intradermal abscess and subcutaneous abscess respectively. **Fig. 4.4** also shows collar-stud abscess.

Treatment

- Incision and drainage under antibiotic cover. Care should be taken to drain the deeper cavity.

ACUTE LYMPHANGITIS OF HAND

- It is caused by an injury, which may be a minor abrasion.
- The causative organism is *streptococcus*.

Clinical features

1. Severe pain in the hand with fever, chills and rigors
2. Gross oedema of dorsum of hand
3. Red, hot streaks over the limb which indicates route of lymphatics.
4. Regional lymph nodes are swollen, tender.
   - Infection of little finger - epitrochlear lymph nodes are enlarged.
   - Ring and middle finger - nodes above the clavicle are affected.
   - Index and thumb - axillary nodes are enlarged.

Treatment

- Injection crystalline penicillin 10 lakh units **IV** or **IM** for 5-7 days.

DEEP INFECTIONS

INFECTION OF THE TERMINAL PULP SPACE

- This space commonly gets infected due to prick injuries which are relatively deep. It is the second common infection of the hand seen in about 25% of the patients.

Anatomy of terminal pulp space

- It is a closed space, formed by fusion of distal flexion skin crease with the deep fascia attached to the periosteum of distal phalanx, just distal to the insertion of flexor digitorum profundus. Each pulp space is subdivided by presence of numerous septa which pass from deep fascia to the periosteum.

- In this closed space, the digital artery runs which is an **end artery.**

Clinical features (Key Box 4.2)

1. Injury to the affected finger is usually present, thumb and index are commonly involved.
2. Throbbing pain is worse in the dependent position, with nocturnal exacerbations.
3. Indurated pulp, which is red and tense is characteristic of this condition.

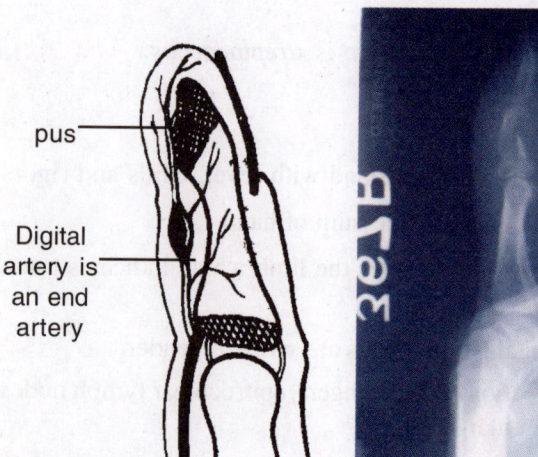

Fig. 4.5 Pulp space infection

pus

Digital artery is an end artery

Fig. 4.6 Osteomyelitis of terminal phalanx

Key Box 4.2
TERMINAL PULP SPACE INFECTIONS

- Extremely painful
- Loss of normal resilience of the pulp
- Early drainage should be done
- Osteomyelitis of terminal phalanx—late cases

4. Touch, movement, dependent position worsens the pain.

Treatment

- Incision and drainage under digital block.

Complications

1. If the pus is not released early, *thrombosis of digital artery* takes place *resulting in osteomyelitis and necrosis* of the *terminal* phalanx and may result in shortening of the finger (Fig. 4.5 & 4.6).
2. Pyogenic arthritis of distal interphalangeal joints
3. Tenosynovitis secondary to pus

APICAL SUBUNGUAL INFECTION

- Infection is confined to the space between the distal quarter of the subungual epithelium and the periosteum of the distal phalanx. Sharp object penetration is the cause for this condition. It manifests very often as a tender yellow spot beneath the distal portion of the nail. Pain, redness and minimal swelling are the features.

- Tenderness is maximum at the free edge of the nail. Pulp and distal parts of fingers are relatively painless. Treated by "V" excision of a portion of nail and opening of the abscess cavity with antibiotic cover (Fig. 4.7).

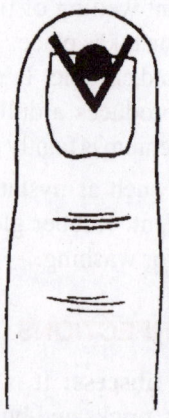

Fig. 4.7 V-excision of the nail, for apical infection

Middle and proximal volar space infections (Fig. 4.8)

- These spaces are loose when compared to terminal pulp space. They are filled with fibrofatty tissue.
- Middle volar space is closed, but proximally communicates with web space.
- Swelling is tender and indurated. Finger is held in the position of flexion.
- Treated by transverse incision and drainage of the pus.

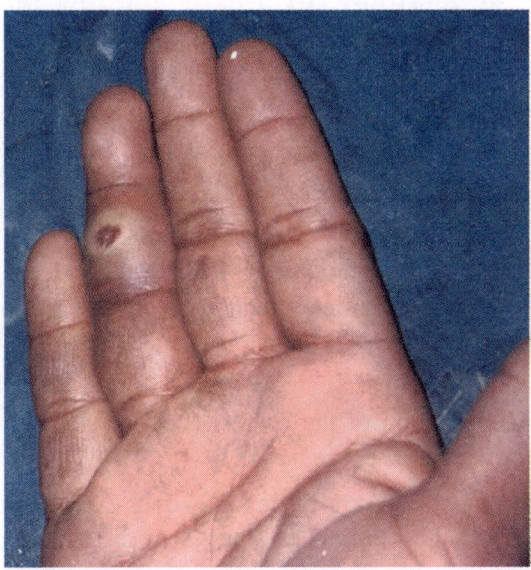

Fig. 4.8 Middle and proximal volar space infections

WEB SPACE INFECTIONS

- Web spaces are the triangular spaces in between the four divisions of the palmar aponeurosis. *They are 3 in number* (Fig. 4.9). Thumb has no palmar aponeurosis. They are filled with subcutaneous fat and posteriorly by metacarpal bones.

Causes of web space infection

- Penetrating injuries.
- Spread of proximal volar space (palmar space) infection.
- Lumbrical canal infection - suppurating tenosynovitis.

Clinical features

- Pain and swelling of palm in the region of web space.
- Extremely tender and hot swelling
- **Finger separation sign** - Adjacent fingers are separated due to oedema.

Key Box 4.3
WEB SPACE INFECTIONS
• 3 web spaces • Finger separation sign • Gross oedema of dorsum • Spread to other web space

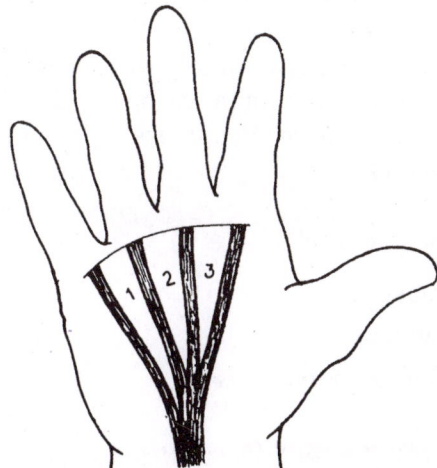

Fig. 4.9 Three web spaces

- Gross oedema of the dorsum of hand
- If untreated, pus from one web space can spread to the other web space and to the other proximal volar space.

Treatment

- Under anaesthesia, a transverse skin incision is made and the pus is drained. The cavity is treated like any other abscess cavity. The skin edge is trimmed in such

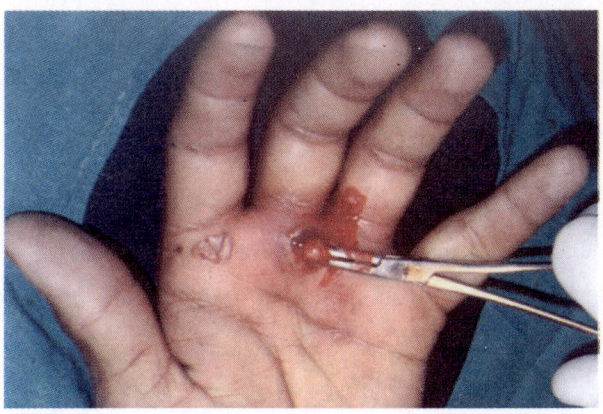

Fig. 4.10 Web space pus being drained

a way as to leave a *diamond* shaped opening to get better drainage.

DEEP PALMAR ABSCESS

- Infection of midpalmar space results in deep palmar abscess.
- Midpalmar space is the space behind the palmar aponeurosis and in front of the metacarpal bones.
- Since palmar fascia is thick, strong and unyielding, pus collects deep to palmar fascia. If it is due to penetrating injuries it collects in the subcutaneous plane like collar-stud abscess. In the centre of palm, there is no subcutaneous tissue. Hence, pus collects beneath the thick dermis.

Source of Infection

- Penetrating injuries
- Haematoma
- Suppurative tenosynovitis

Clinical features (Key Box 4.4)

- Obliteration of *normal concavity of the palm*
- *Gross oedema* of the dorsum of the hand
- *Extreme tenderness* in midpalmar space
- Fingers are held in *flexion* at the *metacarpo- phalangeal (MP)* joint because the palmar aponeurosis gets relaxed in the position. *MP joint movements are painful.*
- IP (interphalangeal) joint movements are not painful.

Thus, swollen palm, oedema of the dorsum of the hand, flexed attitude of MP joint, separated fingers give the picture of frog hand.

Key Box 4.4
DEEP PALMAR ABSCESS
• Midpalmar space infection
• Concavity of palm is lost
• Oedema of the dorsum of hand
• MP joint movement painful
• IP Joint movement painless
• Frog-hand appearance

1. Henry Hamilton Bailey lost his left index finger because of acute tenosynovitis.

Treatment

- Under anaesthesia, transverse crease incision is made and once the palmar aponeurosis is seen, it is split *longitudinally* in the direction of the fibres *to avoid damage to nerves and vessels.*
- Abscess cavity is treated in the usual manner.

ACUTE SUPPURATING TENOSYNOVITIS[1]

Surgical anatomy of flexor tendon sheath arrangements

- The flexor tendon sheaths which enclose the tendons run along the whole length of the finger. In the palm, the medial tendons are enclosed by a common synovial pocket called "ulnar bursa" and on the lateral side by "radial bursa" (Fig. 4.11).
- These two are communicating in 80% of the cases. In 25% of cases, the flexor tendon sheath of the thumb is communicating with radial bursa and of the little finger with ulnar bursa.
- Thus, infection of the fingers (flexor tendon sheath) can involve the entire hand.
- The synovial sheaths of flexor tendons extend from the bases of the terminal phalanges to the heads of the metacarpal bones.

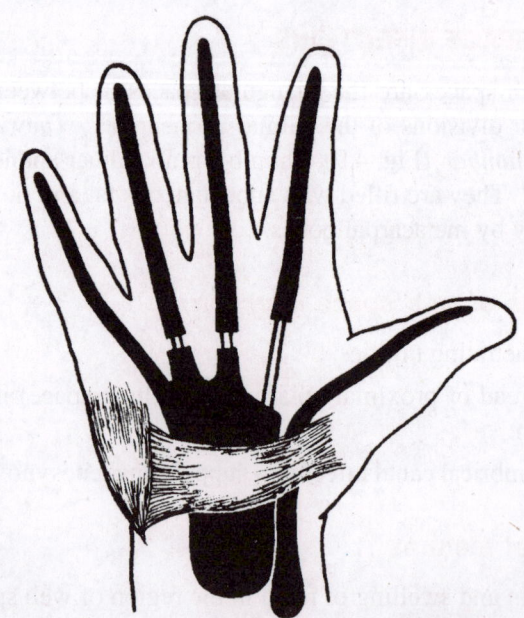

Fig. 4.11 Flexor tendon sheath arrangements

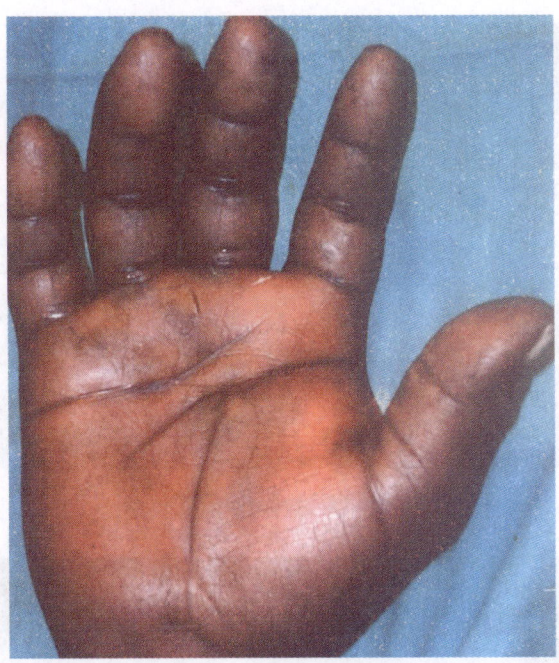

Fig. 4.12 Suppurating tenosynovitis

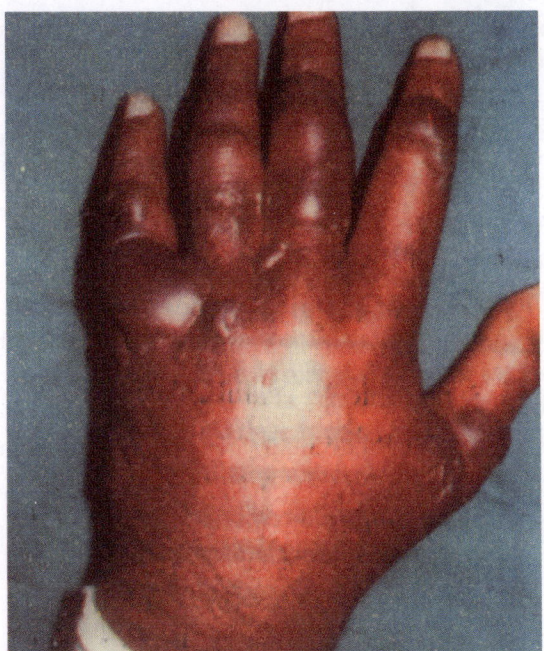

Fig. 4.13 Grossly swollen hand in a diabetic patient. It was looking dangerous, but responded to conservative line of treatment

Clinical features (Key Box 4.5)

1. The patient gives history of pricking type of injuries.

2. Symmetrical, painful enlargement of finger

3. Finger is bent - ***HOOK SIGN***

4. *IP joint movements are very painful.*

5. *MP joint movements are not painful* - Sign which differentiates suppurating tenosynovitis from deep palmar abscess.

6. When there is infection of ulnar bursa, the maximum tender spot is in between the two palmar creases. This sign is described as ***KANAVEL SIGN.***

7. Similarly, there is tenderness over lateral side, over the flexor pollicis longus sheath when radial bursa is involved (Fig 4.12, 4.13).

Key Box 4.5
SUPPURATING   TENOSYNOVITIS
• Sharp prick injuries • Hook sign - bent finger • IP joint movements painful • MP joint movements need not be painful • Kanavel sign - Ulnar bursa infection

Treatment

- Under anaesthesia, multiple incisions may have to be given to decompress the flexor tendon sheaths, so as to relieve tension to drain the pus, exudate etc.

- The cavity is irrigated with antiseptic solution.

- Postoperatively, appropriate antibiotics are given for about 2 weeks.

- Hand is positioned in elevated position to reduce oedema.

Complications

1. Stiffness of the fingers

2. Suppurating arthritis of the joints

3. Osteomyelitis

4. Loss of digit

5. Spread of infection to ***space of Parona***. It is the space deep to the flexor profundus and superficial to pronator quadratus in the lower end of forearm. Patients present with swelling of the forearm along with gross oedema of the hand.

   In addition to the treatment mentioned above, a separate incision may have to be given in the lower forearm for a better drainage of the pus.

General principles and management of hand infection

- Early diagnosis
- Early proper drainage
- Proper incision - preferably a crease incision
- **Elevation** of hand to reduce oedema
- Pus culture and sensitivity
- **Cloxacillin** 500 mg 6th hourly for 7-10 days, with metronidazole 400 mg 8th hourly for 7-10 days. Otherwise higher antibiotics such as **cephalosporins** may have to be given.
- Physiotherapy to decrease the stiffness of the fingers

OTHER HAND INFECTIONS

1. Compound palmar ganglion
2. Barber's pilonidal sinus
3. Madura mycosis
4. Orf : Highly contagious pustular dermatitis due to parapox virus infection.
5. Milker's nodes : It is a viral disease transmitted by handling Cow's udder.
6. Human bites, snake bites

FOOT INFECTIONS

MYCETOMA PEDIS

- It refers to chronic granulomatous lesions of the foot involving skin and subcutaneous tissues. The disease not only involves skin and subcutaneous tissue but also the deeper structures like bones resulting in osteomyelitis.
- **Gross thickening of subcutaneous tissue results in convexity of the instep of the foot** is characteristic of this condition. Chronic suppuration, **multiple sinuses**, sulphur granules in the discharge are characteristic of mycetoma pedis (Fig. 4.14).
- Bare foot walking which results in repeated minor trauma, implants the organisms within subcutaneous tissue. It starts as a **pale, painless single nodule.** Later multiple nodules develop, which rupture resulting in multiple sinuses.

Types

1. **Bacterial mycetoma** : It is due to **Nocardia madurae**

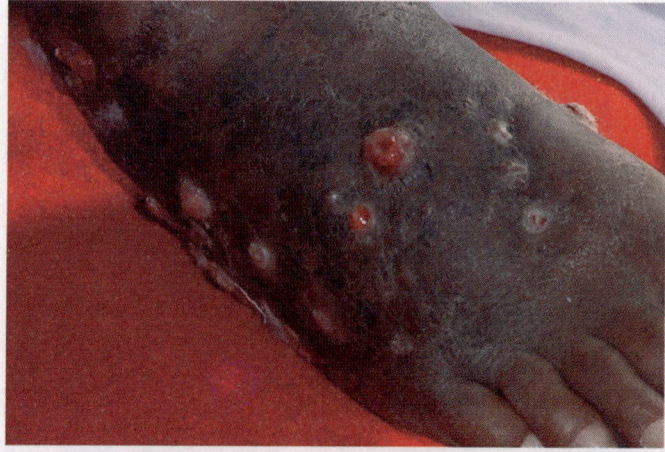

Fig. 4.14 Mycetoma pedis

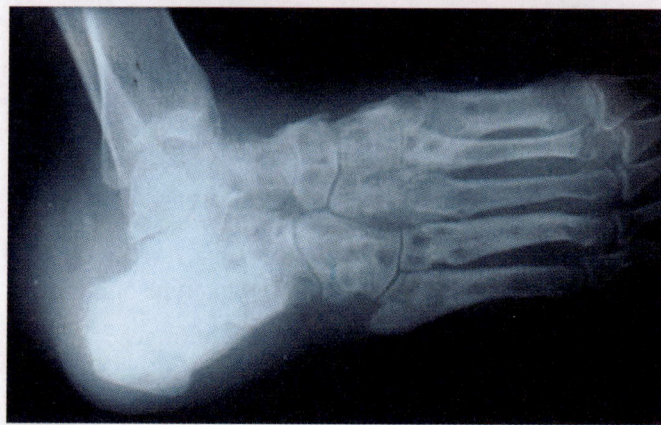

Fig. 4.15 X-ray of the foot showing extensive rarefaction of the bones

or due to actinomyces. These organisms are normally present in the soil.

2. **Fungal mycetoma** : It is caused by Madurella mycetoma, etc.

Diagnosis

- Sulphur granules in the discharge, X-ray of the foot (Fig. 4.15)

Treatment

1. Broad-spectrum antibiotics to treat secondary infection along with **Dapsone 100 mg twice daily is the choice**. Treatment may have to be continued for 1-2 years.

2. Fungal mycetoma may not respond to antibiotics.

3. Amputation may be necessary, in refractory cases, to get rid of a deformed, diseased limb.

INGROWING TOE NAIL (Onychocryptosis)

- It is also described as embedded toe nail. Exact aetiology is not clear. However, a few patients have family history of this condition. Trimming the nail too much, may result in ingrowing toe nail.

- As the nail grows inside, some degree of infection sets in, resulting in development of granulation tissue which starts pouting. The condition is painful, disturbing and unsightly.

Treatment

- **Conservative** : Dressing with the antiseptic agents like Iodine. Copper sulphate can be applied to treat extra granulation tissue. Appropriate antibiotics are given.

- **Surgical:** Under local anaesthesia, a portion of the involved nail upto the base is removed followed by application of phenol to the growing point of the nailbed at its base. It takes about 10-15 days for complete healing.

- **Zadik's or Fowler's operation:** The principle of this radical procedure is to expose the lateral spike and germinal matrix. This is achieved by incising the skin in lateral margin and root.

HAND INFECTIONS - FEW PHOTOGRAPHS

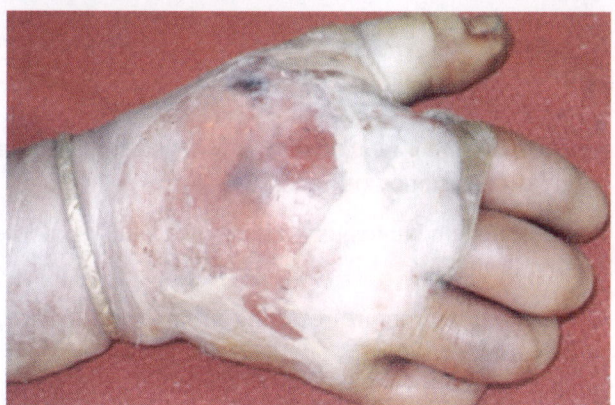 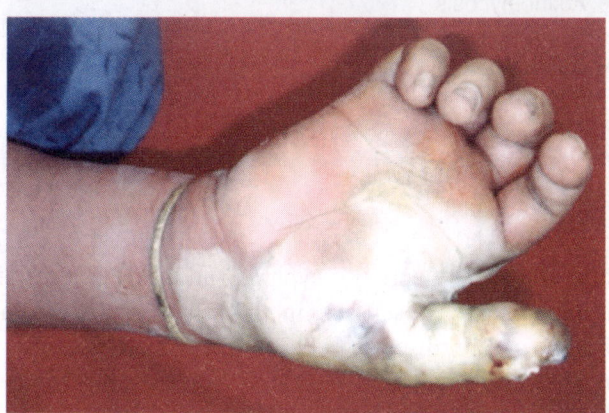

Fig. 4.16, 4.17 Very severe dorsal space infection in a diabetic patient. Observe the constriction effect caused by bangle. They need to be removed in all cases of hand infections

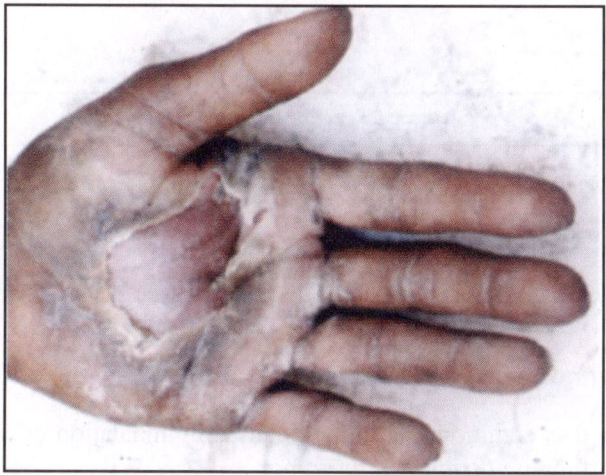 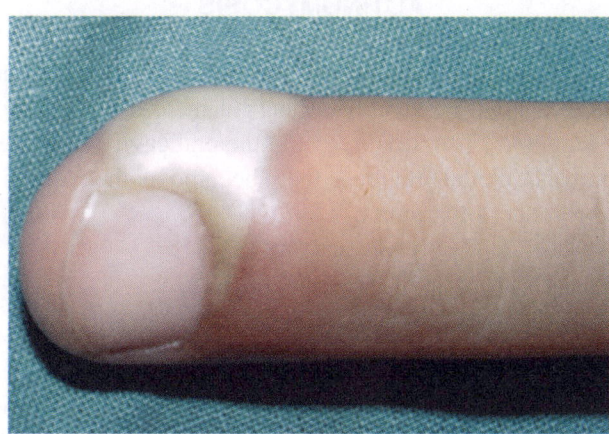

Fig. 4.18 Healing palmar space infection. Observe the cuticle being raised

Fig. 4.19 Acute paronychia - very painful condition, can be treated very easily

All the photographs in this chapter are contributed by Dr. P. Sreenivasa, Postgraduate student (2000-2003) and Prof. Mahimanjan Singh, Head of the Dept. of Surgery, Govt. Medical College, Mysore, Karnataka

Chronic Infectious Disease

5

- Actinomycosis
- Leprosy
- Deformities in leprosy
- Syphilis
- AIDS

Actinomycosis, leprosy, syphilis and AIDS are the chronic diseases discussed in this chapter. Actinomycosis is a rare disease, leprosy is of more interest to the skin specialists and AIDS is an interesting topic to all clinicians. Hence, the only relevant aspect of each of these diseases as far as general surgeons are concerned are being discussed here.

ACTINOMYCOSIS

Actinomycosis is caused by Actinomyces israelii, an anaerobic, gram-positive branching filamentous organism (ray fungus). Normally present in the oral cavity, tonsillar crypts and dental cavities, they become pathogenic in the presence of trauma.

TYPES OF ACTINOMYCOSIS

Facio-cervical actinomycosis

- It is common in patients with poor oral hygiene, bad caries tooth, etc.

- The organisms produce a subacute or chronic inflammation for many months to years and produce lumpy jaw (Key Box 5.1 for differential diagnosis).

- Eventually cheek, mandible, jaws, salivary glands are involved resulting in suppuration.

Clinical features

- Extensive induration of lower jaw (mandible) and gums gives consistency of bone.

- Multiple subcutaneous nodules over bluish coloured skin of the jaw.

- The nodules rupture resulting in *multiple discharging sinuses*.

- The discharge contains *sulphur granules* which are gram-positive mycelia surrounded by gram-negative clubs.

- **Lymph nodes are not involved.**

Key Box 5.1
DIFFERENTIAL DIAGNOSIS

- Jaw tumour
- Osteomyelitis of jaw
- Malignancy of oral cavity

Actinomycosis of thorax and lung

- It is common in children, caused by inhalation of ray fungus, *through diaphragm.*

- Over a period of years, it produces actinomycosis of lung with involvement of pleura. Later it involves the chest wall, resulting in multiple discharging sinuses.

- There may be associated empyema and can easily spread to liver.

Actinomycosis of the right iliac fossa and liver

- It commonly occurs after surgery when there is **mucosal injury**, discontinuity, etc.

  Example : After appendicectomy.

- The organisms which are normally present in the gut slowly migrate into pericaecal tissue, then into the soft tissue, subcutaneous tissue, and produces subacute or chronic low grade inflammation.

- No compromise with bowel lumen.

- Once the portal venous radical gets involved, spread to the liver occurs.

Clinical features

- History of appendicectomy is present in almost all cases.

- 3-6 months later swelling in right iliac fossa and fever occurs. Fever is probably due to pyaemia.

- On examination, there is a mass in the right iliac fossa, indurated, nodular and fixed.

- Late stages produce multiple discharging sinuses-sometimes fecal matter and sulphur granules. Unlike tuberculosis, the lymph nodes are not enlarged.

Differential diagnosis

- Carcinoma caecum, Crohn's ileocolitis, pericolic abscess

Treatment of actinomycosis in general

- It is low grade chronic disease, difficult to eradicate.

- Inj. crystalline penicillin - 10 lakh units once a day for 6-12 months. Tetracycline, lincomycin are the other alternatives.

- Sinuses in the jaw may have to be excised and osteomyelitis has to be curetted out.

- Actinomycosis of the right iliac fossa may need right hemicolectomy.

LEPROSY (HANSEN'S DISEASE)

- Leprosy is caused by **Mycobacterium leprae**, an acid-fast bacillus. Poverty, poor hygiene and population (overcrowding) facilitate the spread of the disease.

- The disease is contacted in childhood or adolescence, but it manifests after a latent period of 2-5 years.

- **Nasal secretions** are the main source of infection but *active ulcers, sweat* also contain lepra bacilli.

- Leprosy predominantly affects **skin, upper respiratory tract (nasal cavity) and nerves**. Thus, characteristic lesions of leprosy include an anaesthetic patch of skin, thickened nerves, a deformed leonine face and collapsed nose.

TYPES (Table 5.1)

1. Tuberculoid leprosy : It occurs in patients with good immunity with strong tissue response.

2. Lepromatous leprosy : It occurs in patients with poor immunity with poor tissue response.

3. Borderline leprosy : It can be borderline lepromatous or borderline tuberculoid leprosy depending upon the immune response.

TREATMENT

1. Lepromatous and borderline lepromatous leprosy (Multibacillary disease)

- 3-drug regimen is the most ideal treatment.

Dapsone 100 mg/day, Clofazimine 50 mg/day. Rifampicin 600 mg once monthly, supervised. Clofazimine 300 mg once monthly, supervised.	For a minimum of 2 years. Skin smear should be negative.

2. Tuberculoid and borderline tuberculoid leprosy (Paucibacillary disease)

• Dapsone 100mg daily. • Rifampicin 600mg once a month, supervised.	For a period of 6 months.

DEFORMITIES IN LEPROSY

I. Primary deformity (Fig. 5.1, 5.2, 5.3)

It occurs directly due to the disease.

- **Face** : It is involved in lepromatous leprosy and it is described as leonine facies with multiple nodules over

Table 5.1 Comparision of tuberculoid leprosy with lepromatous leprosy

	TUBERCULOID LEPROSY	LEPROMATOUS LEPROSY
1. Cell mediated immunity	Strong	Low
2. Histology	Giant cells, epitheloid cells, histiocytes, lymphocytes are present. Bacilli are few.	Bacilli distending the macrophages - 'GLOBI'. Plenty of bacilli invading nerves, adnexa, sweat glands, etc.
3. Clinical	Localised. Anaesthetic, hypopigmented, raised skin patch. Early nerve damage, nerve thickening is a characteristic feature. Involvement of face and nose is not seen.	Generalised. Erythematous multiple macular rashes. Nerve involvement is usually not seen. Leonine facies, collapse of the bridge of the nose are characteristic.
4. Prognosis	Good	Not good

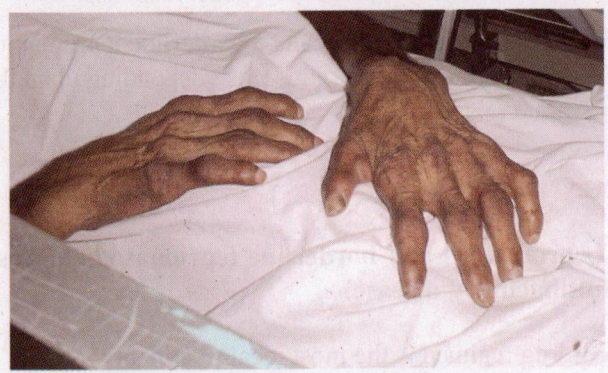

Fig. 5.1 Observe small muscle wasting in the both hands

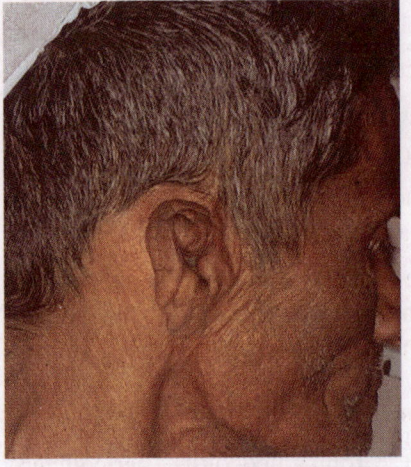

Leonine facies, collapse of the bridge of the nose are the few other features of lepromatous leprosy

Fig. 5.3 Observe deformed ear

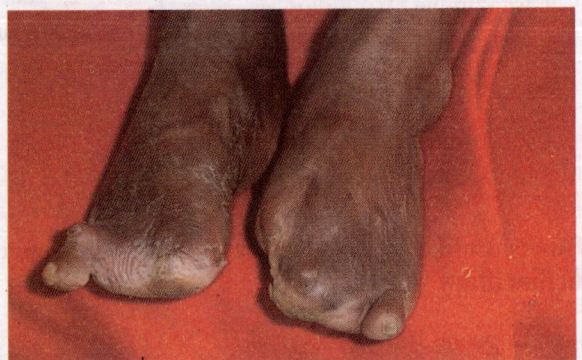

Fig. 5.2 Auto amputation of the toes in a case of leprosy

the face, pigmentation, *loss of lateral portion* of the eyebrows (Madarosis), collapse of bridge of the nose due to destruction of nasal cartilages (Warm and moist area) and paralysis of facial nerve.

- **Hands** : Involvement of ulnar nerve at the elbow and median nerve at wrist giving rise to *Claw Hand*.

- **Foot** : Posterior tibial nerve is involved at the ankle

leading to clawing of the toes. Foot drop occurs when lateral popliteal nerve below the knee joint is involved.

Correction of deformity of the face by

Plastic reconstruction
1. A prosthesis to correct the nose
2. Lateral tarsorrhaphy, to prevent exposure keratitis.
3. Temporalis muscle flap to the upper eye lid to prevent exposure keratitis.

Correction of deformity of the hand and foot

- Claw hand can be corrected by extensor carpi radialis brevis muscle (Paul Brand's procedure).

- Otherwise flexor digitorum profundus can be used (**Bunnell's procedure**).

- Foot drop can be corrected by using tibialis posterior muscle tendon transfer (**Ober's and Barr's procedure**).

II. Secondary deformity

- Because of involvement of the nerves, sensations are impaired or lost. As a result of this, ulcers on the fingers, a deep penetrating, *perforating* ulcer over sole of the foot, even auto amputation of toes can occur.

Treatment of secondary deformity

- Non-healing ulcer over the sole of foot is corrected by applying a POP (Plaster of Paris) posterior slab. It takes off the pressure and thus the ulcer heals. If calcaneous is involved due to osteomyelitis, the bone has to be curetted out followed by regular dressings.

SYPHILIS : FRENCH DISEASE, GREAT POX

- This is a sexually transmitted disease caused by *Treponema pallidum*. It is a delicate spiral organism (Spirochaete).
- Syphilis is infective only in its early stage. Early lesions are predominantly situated in moist areas like genitalia and oral cavity.

CLINICAL PRESENTATION

- Refer Key Box 5.2 for congenital syphilis

I. Early syphilis
II. Late syphilis

I. EARLY SYPHILIS

1. **Primary syphilis**: Classically, a genital chancre occurs in the penis or vulva after 3-4 weeks of sexual exposure.

   - This chancre is shallow, indurated, painless, ulcer - called as Hunterian chancre. Associated inguinal nodes which are shotty, multiple, nontender, clinches the diagnosis.

   - Extragenital chancres can occur in the lips, tongue, nipple etc. They produce large enlargement of the corresponding lymph nodes. Chancres in the rectum and perianal region are common in homosexuals. They are painful, resemble anal fissures.

Investigations

Serological tests for syphilis

I. **Non-specific**: VDRL, KAHN, MEINICKE, WASSERMAN.

Key Box 5.2

CONGENITAL SYPHILIS

Early :
- Snuffles (rhinitis), epiphysitis, periostitis, osteochondritis.

Late :
- HUTCHINSON'S TRIAD
- – Interstitial keratitis
- – 8th nerve deafness
- – Hutchinson's teeth

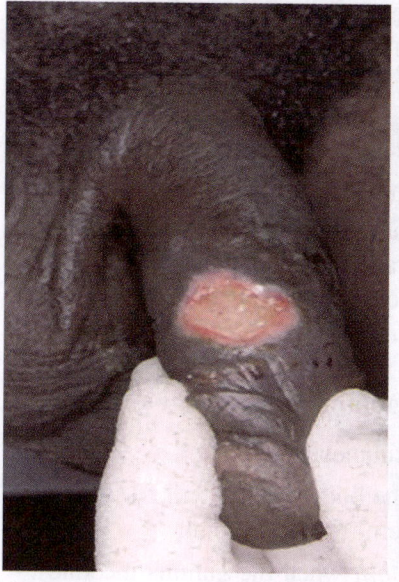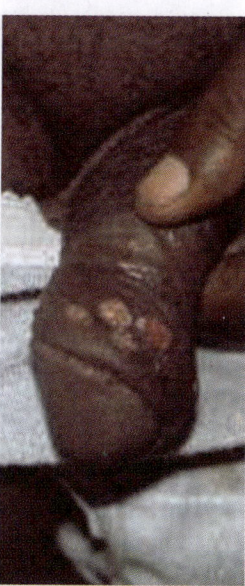

Fig. 5.4 Genital chancres

II. **Specific treponemal antigen tests:**

- CFT - Complement fixation test
- TPHA - T.P. haemagglutination test
- TPI - T.P. immobilization test
- FTA - Abs – Fluorescent treponema antibody absorption test
- Demonstration of *Treponema pallidum* in the clear exudate from the lesion by dark field microscopy confirms the diagnosis.

2. **Secondary Syphilis** : It appears after 6-12 weeks of spirochaetaemia.

   - It is characterised by **bilateral, symmetrical, coppery red rashes** which are generalised.

   The *rash* is macular or papular, *never vesicular*.

Papules on moist sites like vulva and perineum enlarge to form condylomata lata - flexy wartlike growths.

- Small superficial ulcers in the mouth join to form *snail track ulcers.*
- Generalised lymphadenopathy involving epitrochlear and occipital nodes can occur.
- Moth-eaten alopecia, iritis, bone and joint pains.

3. **Latent Syphilis**: If secondary syphilis is not treated, it will develop into latent syphilis. There are no signs but serum tests are positive.

II. LATE SYPHILIS

It is also called as tertiary syphilis. It basically affects vessels causing inflammatory reactions and the end result is as follows:

'Endarteritis obliterans' $\rightarrow$ tissue necrosis $\rightarrow$ ulcers or fibrosis

This stage develops after 5-15 years of primary syphilis. It causes neurosyphilis and cardiovascular syphilis. Lesser form, a benign lesion is called *GUMMA*. Gumma is a syphilitic hypersensitivity reaction consisting of granuloma with central necrosis and sloughing.

Clinical features of gumma

- Typically it is a subcutaneous swelling.
- Affects midline of the body, e.g. posterior 1/3 tongue, sternum, over the sternoclavicular joint.
- Edges are *punched out* when the gumma ulcerates.
- Floor contains *wash leather slough*
- On healing, it leaves a **silvery, tissue paper scar** (thin scar).

Gumma can also involve bone, testis and liver (Ovary is not involved).

Treatment

1. Primary and secondary syphilis are treated by injection procaine penicillin 10 lakh units I.M. x 14 days.
2. In late syphilis : Treatment is continued for a period of 21 days. With the current effective treatment of syphilis, it is highly unusual to find late cases now.

AIDS AND THE GENERAL SURGEON

- Acquired Immuno Deficiency Syndrome (AIDS) is the end stage of a progressive state of immunodeficiency. Causative organism: Human Immuno-deficiency Virus (HIV).
- The details regarding etiopathogenesis and immunology about AIDS is discussed in medicine books. Topics of surgeon's interest are discussed below.

Prophylactic measures to be adopted by surgeons (Healthcare workers) while treating AIDS Patients (UNIVERSAL PRECAUTIONS)

I. In the outpatient department (OPD)

- Any patient with open wound, gloves[1] are worn when examining a patient.
- During proctoscopy or sigmoidoscopy, gloves should be worn.
- Hand gloves and eye protection during flexible endoscopy.
- Use disposable instruments
- Re-usable instruments like endoscopes are cleaned in soap and water and immersed in glutaraldehyde.
- No surgical procedure involving sharp instruments is performed in the OPD.

II. In the operating room

- Operating table is covered with a single sheet of polythene.
- The number of theatre personnel is reduced to minimum.
- The **Staff** with abrasions or lacerations on their hands are not allowed inside the theatre.
- Staff who enter the theatre wear over- shoes, gloves and disposable, water resistant gowns and eye protection.
- **Double Gloves and Eye Protection** - by Staff directly involved with the operation (Surgeon, Assistant, Scrub nurse).
- Surgical technique:
  1. Avoid Sharp Injury
  2. Prefer scissors or diathermy, to the scalpel
  3. Use **skin clips**

---

1. Gloves were introduced by William Halstead to protect his nurse's hands from the harmful effects of carbolic acid. (The nurse became his wife).

4. Avoid 'needlestick' injuries

5. Proper autoclaving at the end of surgery

6. AZT–Zidovudine, Lamivudine and Indinavir should be given for health workers following exposure of susceptible areas to infected material from AIDS patients.

Range of surgery in HIV-positive patients

I. **Anorectal disease** is the most frequent reason for surgical treatment in HIV positive patients. This is common in homosexuals and AIDS is also common in homosexuals. They have been grouped together as "AIDS ANUS SYNDROME". Anorectal disease can be classified into :

- Anal warts, diarrhoea
- Perianal sepsis - abscesses
- Anal ulceration, fissures
- Reduced sphincter tone and anal incontinence in homosexuals.

II. Abdominal pain

This is due to gastrointestinal opportunistic infection usually caused by cytomegalovirus (CMV). It is a type of colitis and produces abdominal pain, cramps, loose stools, blood and mucus in the stools resulting in emaciation. Flexible sigmoidoscopy can reveal severe proctitis due to cytomegalovirus infection, severe colitis may lead to acute toxic dilatation of colon.

- Biliary tract infection by cryptosporidium can cause **acute cholecystitis**. AIDS related sclerosing cholangitis can occur resulting in right upper quadrant pain.
- **Abdominal lymphoma** with involvement of liver and spleen also causes abdominal pain.
- Severe abdominal pain, may be due to **perforation** of small or large bowel which should be treated as an emergency.

- **Appendicitis** is also common due to CMV infection.

III. Lymphomas and Kaposi's sarcoma, etc.

- They are due to reduced cellular immunity due to following reasons:

  1. Immunosuppression used in organ transplantation
  2. Severe malnourishment
  3. HIV infection
  4. Lymphoproliferative disease
  5. Kaposi's sarcoma can affect skin surface, gastrointestinal tract from mouth to anus, lungs etc. It presents as pigmented multifocal skin lesions.

IV. **Oesophageal ulcers** can present as dysphagia and odynophagia. Endoscopy should be done by using a glove and the scope should be washed thoroughly with soap and water and immersed in cetrimide solution for 15 minutes.

V. Very often surgeons are called for lymph node biopsy for evaluation of fever or generalised **lymphadenopathy**. All universal precautions have to be taken.

CLINICAL NOTES

23 year old lady, carrying a 6-month old child, presented to us with severe dysphagia and odynophagia. Endoscopy revealed extensive, unusual oesophageal ulcers which prompted us to conduct HIV test. It was positive. We called her husband and wanted to convey the message to him. Before we conveyed, he said - I am HIV positive, my wife is HIV positive and even my child is HIV positive!!!

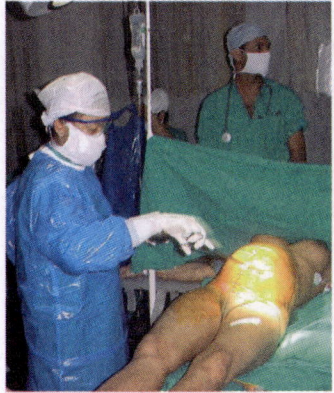
Fig. 5.5 Water resistant gowns

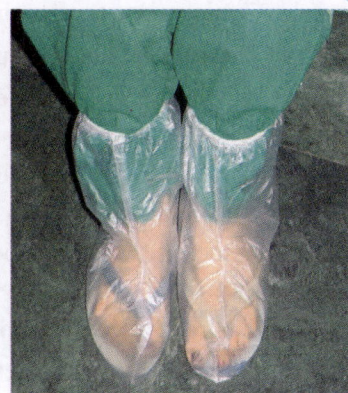
Fig. 5.6 Protection of feet

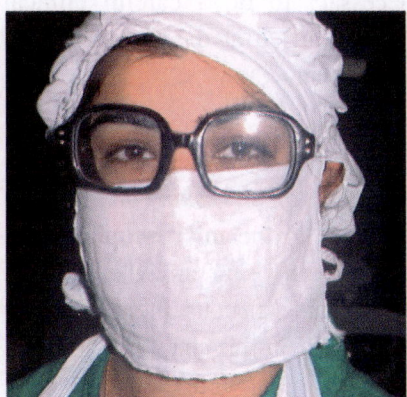
Fig. 5.7 Eye protection

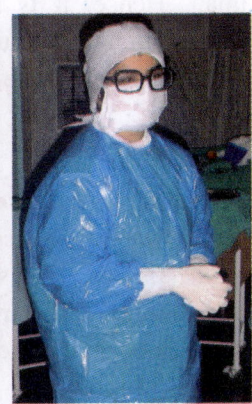
Fig. 5.8 Double glove

Differential Diagnosis of Leg Ulcer, Pressure Sore

6

- Classification
- Clinical examination
- Management
- Traumatic ulcer
- Venous ulcer
- Trophic ulcer
- Tropical ulcer
- Post thrombotic ulcer
- Rare ulcers
- Diabetic ulcer foot
- Pressure sore

Leg ulcers are one of the important topics in surgery. They can occur in children, adults and old people. No age is spared, no sex is spared. The varying aetiological factors, presence of complicated systemic diseases make the treatment of ulcers very difficult. Chronic ulcers in old people definitely cause considerable morbidity and diabetic ulcer of the leg can cause life-threatening complications such as diabetic ketoacidosis and septicae-mia. Hence, it is necessary to do a careful clinical examination of the ulcer to arrive at the diagnosis and plan for appropriate treatment.

Definition

An ulcer is a *discontinuity of the skin or mucous membrane* which occurs due to the **microscopic death** of the tissues. Thus, ulcer can occur anywhere in the body (skin), oral cavity, penis (mucous membrane) or in the duodenum, intestine, etc. In this chapter, leg ulcers will be discussed.

CLASSIFICATION

PATHOLOGICAL CLASSIFICATION (Key Box 6.1)

I. NONSPECIFIC

1. **Traumatic**: Trauma can be mechanical. This is the commonest cause of leg ulcer. It can be physical trauma due to burns or radiation. It can also be due to chemicals such as acids.

2. **Venous ulcers**: They include varicose ulcers and post thrombotic ulcers which can occur following deep vein thrombosis.

3. **Arterial ulcers**: Following are a few examples of arterial ulcers.

   Buerger's disease - common

   Atherosclerotic vascular disease - common

   Vasospastic disorders like Raynaud's disease - uncommon

   Martorell's ulcers or hypertensive ulcers - rare

   Rheumatoid arthritis patients can develop leg or foot ulcers due to vasculitis.

4. **Neurogenic** ulcer (Neuropathic ulcer, Trophic ulcers)

   Leprosy and diabetes are the common causes

   Paraplegia, meningomyelocoele, posterior tibial nerve injury, tabes dorsalis are the other causes.

5. **Tropical ulcer**: It is a rare ulcer due to malnutrition associated with infection caused by Vincent's organisms.

6. **Diabetic ulcer foot or diabetic ulcer leg**

7. **Blood Dyscrasias**: Sickle cell anaemia, thalassaemia,

I NONSPECIFIC ULCERS

1. Traumatic
2. Venous
3. Arterial
4. Neurogenic - Trophic
5. Tropic
6. Diabetic
7. Blood dyscrasias

II SPECIFIC ULCERS

III MALIGNANT ULCERS

leukaemia, etc. can produce recurrent ulcerations in the leg.

II. SPECIFIC ULCER : This is due to specific type of organisms, e.g., tubercular ulcers, syphilitic ulcers, actinomycotic ulcers, etc.

III. MALIGNANT ULCERS are squamous cell carcinoma, basal cell carcinoma, malignant melanoma. Malignant ulcers are discussed in Chapter 11.

CLINICAL CLASSIFICATION (Table 6.1)

CLINICAL EXAMINATION OF THE ULCER

INSPECTION

1. **Location of the ulcer**

    Arterial ulcer[1] - Tip of the toes, dorsum of the foot, etc.

    Long saphenous varicosity with ulcer - Medial side of the leg.

Short saphenous varicosity with ulcer - Lateral side of the leg just above the lateral malleolus.

Perforating ulcers - Over the sole at pressure points.

Nonhealing ulcer - Over the shin and lateral malleolus.

2. **Floor of the ulcer : This is the part of the ulcer which is exposed or seen.**

    Red granulation tissue - Healing ulcer (Fig. 6.1)

    Necrotic tissue, slough - Spreading ulcer

    Pale, scanty granulation tissue - Tuberculous[2] ulcer.

    Wash-leather slough - Gummatous ulcer

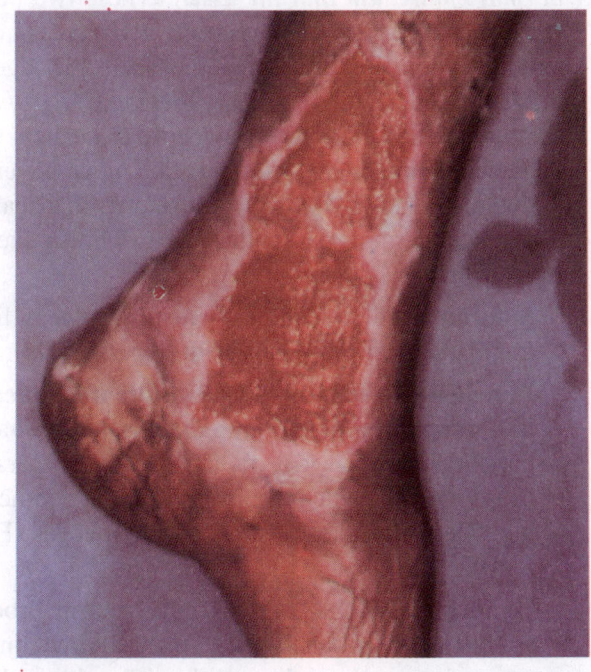

Fig. 6.1 Traumatic ulcer with red granulation tissue in the floor

Table 6.1		
A. SPREADING	**B. CALLOUS**	**C. HEALING**
No granulation tissue	Pale granulation tissue	Red granulation tissue
Plenty of discharge	Serous discharge	Minimal serous discharge
Excessive slough	Slough present	Slough absent
Surrounding area inflamed and oedematous	Induration at the base, edge and surrounding area.	Signs of inflammation are minimal.
Purulent smell present	Smell can be present	Smell is absent.

1. When there is a block in the pipelines supplying water, distal houses suffer the maximum. Is it not?
2. It is described as apple jelly granulation tissue.

Part of the bone - Neuropathic ulcer

Nodular - Epithelioma

Black tissue - Malignant melanoma

3. Discharge from the ulcer

Serous discharge - Healing ulcer

Purulent discharge - Spreading ulcer

Bloody discharge - Malignant ulcer

Discharge with bony spicules - Osteomyelitis

Greenish discharge - Pseudomonas infection

4. **Edge** : This is between the floor of the ulcer and the margin. ***The margin is the junction between the normal epithelium and the ulcer.*** These two parts represent the **areas of maximum activity**. If destruction dominates as in spreading ulcers, the edge is inflamed, oedematous and angry looking (*stage of extension*). When ulcer shows evidence of healing, the edge will be bluish due to granulation tissue covered with thin epithelium (*stage of transition*). In a healed ulcer, the outermost part of the edge is whitish due to fibrosis (*stage of repair*).

Sloping edge is seen in all **healing ulcers** like traumatic ulcers, venous ulcers (Fig. 6.2A).

Punched out edge is seen in **gummatous ulcers and trophic ulcers**. Gummatous ulcers have punched out edge due to endarteritis obliterans caused by syphilitic organisms. Chronic non-healing ulcers also may have punched out edges (Fig. 6.2B).

Undermined edge (Fig. 6.2C) is seen in **tuberculous** ulcers, probably due to more destruction of subcutaneous tissues than the skin. The edge is classically thin and bluish in colour.

Raised edge (beaded edge) is seen in rodent ulcers or **basal cell carcinoma** (Fig. 6.2D).

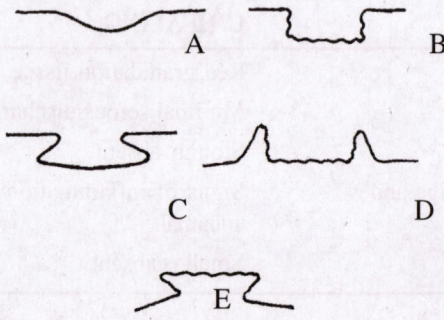

Fig. 6.2 Different types of edges

Everted edge (rolled out) is diagnostic of **squamous cell carcinoma**. The edge grows very rapidly and it occupies the normal skin and thus gets everted (Fig.6.2E).

5. Surrounding area

Thick and pigmented - Varicose ulcer.

Thin and dark - Arterial ulcer.

Red and oedematous - Spreading ulcers like diabetic ulcer.

Scar around the ulcer - Marjolin's ulcer.

PALPATION

1. **Edge** : Induration (hardness) of the edge is very characteristic of squamous cell carcinoma. Some degree of induration can also be seen in chronic ulcers and long standing varicose ulcers. Induration occurs due to extensive fibrosis. It is said to be a host defense mechanism. *By causing fibrosis, lymphatic spread is delayed.* Tenderness of the edge is characteristic of infected ulcers and arterial ulcers.

2. **Base** : *It is the area on which ulcer rests.* Pick up the ulcer between thumb and index finger and tissues beneath are appreciated. If the ulcer cannot be lifted up, the base cannot be made out. The base can be tendons, muscles or bone depending upon the site of ulcer. *Marked induration at the base is diagnostic of squamous cell carcinoma.* Hunterian chancre is a benign ulcer and produces significant induration. Hence, it is also called a hard chancre. (Key Box 6.2)

Key Box 6.2
INDURATION

- It means hardness.
- Maximum induration - Squamous cell carcinoma
- Minimal induration - Malignant melanoma.
- Brawny induration - Abscess.
- Cyanotic induration - Chronic venous congestion as in varicose ulcer.
- **The edge, base and the surrounding area should be examined for induration.**

3. **Mobility** : Gentle attempt is made to move the ulcer to know its fixity to the underlying tissues. Malignant ulcers are usually fixed, benign ulcers are not.

4. **Bleeding** : Malignant ulcer is friable like a cauliflower. On gentle palpation, it bleeds. Granulation[1] tissue as in a healing ulcer also causes bleeding.

5. **Surrounding area** : Thickening and induration is found in squamous cell carcinoma. Tenderness and pitting on pressure indicates spreading inflammation surrounding the ulcer.

RELEVANT CLINICAL EXAMINATION

1. **Regional lymph nodes**

   Tender and enlarged - Acute secondary infection.

   Non-tender and enlarged - Chronic infection.

   Non-tender and hard -Squamous cell carcinoma.

   Non-tender, large, firm, multiple - Malignant melanoma.

2. **Peripheral vessels**: Detailed examination of peripheral vessels is discussed under peripheral vascular disease. However, dorsalis pedis, posterior tibial, popliteal and femoral arteries should be palpated in cases of lower limb ulcers. Presence of weak pulses or absent pulses indicate peripheral vascular disease.

3. **Sensations**: Loss of vibration sense and loss of ankle jerk occurs early in cases of diabetic neuropathy. Later, touch and pain are lost. ***Totally anaesthetic feet are characteristic of leprosy***.

4. **Function of the joint**: The involved joint movements are restricted either due to the pain, involvement of the joint or due to infiltration into the joint by malignant ulcers.

5. **Varicose veins**: If present, it is most-probably a varicose ulcer. However, A-V fistula can present as distal ulcers, with arterialisation of veins and a continuous murmur.

SYSTEMIC EXAMINATION

1. **Central nervous system** (CNS) and spine in neuropathic ulcers. There may be gibbus as in cases of TB spine or operated scar due to myelo-meningocoele etc.

2. **Splenomegaly** in blood dyscrasias like early stages of sickle cell anaemia, etc.

3. **Cardiovascular system** (CVS) may reveal murmur as in cases of arteriovenous fistula or features suggestive of cardiac diseases.

CLINICAL NOTES

An 18 year old girl with a nonhealing trophic ulcer was examined by a post-graduate student. He gave a diagnosis of trophic ulcer (neuropathic ulcer) due to leprosy as first diagnosis followed by polyneuropathy. He failed. It was a case of myelomeningocoele and the candidate had not examined the spine! The patient had an operated myelomeningocoele.

Key Box 6.3
CLINICAL EXAMINATION OF AN ULCER

INSPECTION:
- Location, size, shape, floor, edge, discharge, surrounding area.

PALPATION:
- Tenderness, local rise of temperature, bleeding on touch, consistency of the ulcer, edge, surrounding area - oedema, mobility.
- Regional lymph nodes
- Sensations
- Pulsations
- Function of the joint
- Systemic examination

MANAGEMENT

Investigations

1. **Complete blood picture**: Hb%, TC, DC, ESR, peripheral smear

   Low Hb% is found in chronic ulcer. It is either nutritional or due to frequent blood loss during dressings as in diabetic ulcer.

   High total count indicates infection

   Peripheral smear to rule out anaemia and sickle cell disease

2. **Urine** and blood examination to rule out diabetes

3. **Chest X-ray** - P.A. view to rule out pulmonary tuberculosis.

4. **Pus** for culture/sensitivity

5. Lower limb angiography in cases of arterial diseases

---

1. Granulation tissue is made up of capillaries and fibroblasts. Hence, it gives rise to fresh blood loss.

6. **X-ray of the part** to see for

    Osteomyelitis - Common in diabetic ulcers

    Periostitis tibia - Varicose ulcers

7. **Biopsy**: Non-healing/malignant ulcers

TREATMENT OF THE ULCERS

It can be discussed under following headings:

1. Treatment of spreading ulcers
2. Treatment of healing ulcers
3. Treatment of chronic ulcers
4. Treatment of the underlying disease

1. **Treatment of spreading ulcer**: After obtaining pus culture/sensitivity report, appropriate antibiotics are given. Many solutions are available to treat the slough, like hydrogen peroxide and **EUSOL**.

    Hydrogen peroxide (diluted) when poured over the wound, liberates nascent oxygen which bubbles out and helps in separating the slough.

    Eusol[1] also separates the slough.

    Partially separated slough needs to be removed daily or on alternate days, in the wards.

    Excessive granulation tissue or pouting granulation tissue (proud flesh) needs to be decapitated by excision or by application of copper sulphate or silver nitrate solution.

    Thus, by repeated dressings, slough gets separated, discharge becomes minimal resulting in a healing ulcer with healthy red granulation tissue. Management thereafter is like a healing ulcer.

2. **Treatment of healing ulcer**

    Regular dressings are done for a few days with antiseptic creams like liquid iodine, zinc oxide or silver sulphadiazine preparation.

    A swab is taken to rule out the presence of Streptococcus haemolyticus which is a contraindication for skin grafting.

If the ulcer is small, it heals by itself with epithelialisation, from the cut edge of ulcer.

If the ulcer is large, free split skin graft is applied as early as possible. (Key Box 6.4)

Key Box 6.4
ADVANTAGES OF SPLIT SKIN GRAFT
• Wound healing occurs fast
• Secondary infection is avoided because of early skin cover
• It prevents contractures
• It prevents Marjolin's ulcer - squamous cell carcinoma arising from scar tissues

3. **Treatment of chronic ulcers** : These are the ulcers which do not respond to conventional methods of treatment. Some special forms of treatment are available; their usefulness is doubtful. They are as follows :

    Infrared radiation, short-wave therapy, ultraviolet rays decrease the size of the ulcer.

    Amnion helps in epithelialisation.

    Chorion helps in granulation tissue. These ulcers ultimately may require skin grafting.

4. **Treatment of the underlying disease** : (Vide infra)

DIFFERENTIAL DIAGNOSIS (Table 6.2)

TRAUMATIC ULCER (Fig. 6.3)

They can occur anywhere in the body. However, they are more common where skin is closely applied to bony prominences, e.g. shin, malleoli, over which there are no muscles. They are usually single, very painful ulcers

Table 6.2		
COMMON CAUSES	**UNCOMMON CAUSES**	**RARE CAUSES**
Traumatic ulcer	Neurogenic ulcer	Martorell's ulcer
Varicose ulcer	Tropical ulcer	Bazin's disease
Arterial ulcer	Post-thrombotic ulcer	
Diabetic ulcer	Malignant skin ulcer	

---

1. **EUSOL** - *Edinburgh University Solution (Hypochlorite solution).*

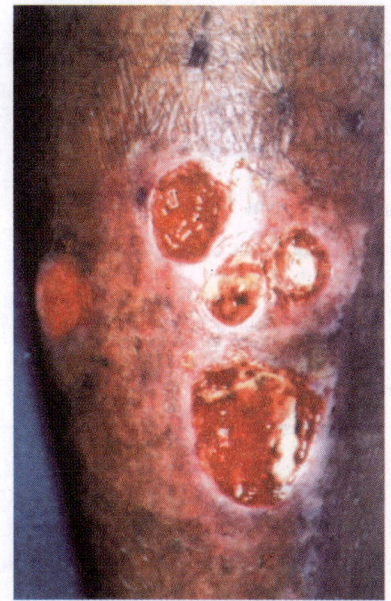

Fig. 6.3 Traumatic ulcers over the shin - observe multiple ulcers

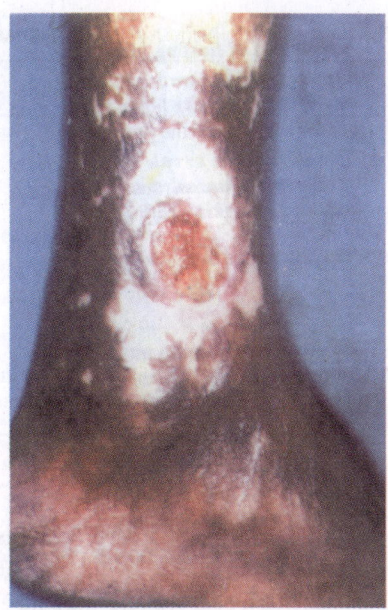

Fig. 6.4 Varicose ulcer - pigmentation due to chronicity

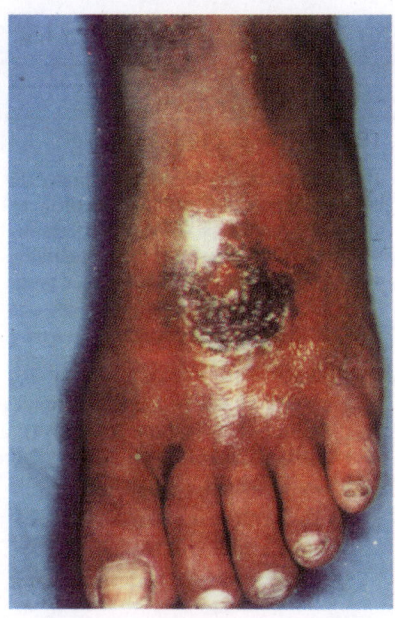

Fig. 6.5 Ischaemic ulcer on the dorsum of the foot

of healing type. With proper dressings and antibiotics, they usually heal within 5-7 days. **Footballer's ulcer** is the name given to those nonhealing ulcers which occur in the leg over the shin due to direct trauma caused by the football. If not treated properly, it gets adhered to the bone.

VARICOSE ULCER (Fig. 6.4)

It occurs due to increased venous hydrostatic pressure.

Located on the medial side of lower 1/3 leg in cases of long saphenous varicosity and on the lateral aspect of the leg in short saphenous varicosity.

It is shallow and superficial.

Never penetrates deep fascia

Usually painless unless it is infected or causes periostitis tibia

Shows evidence of healing

Usually associated with varicose veins

Typically lower leg around the ulcer is pigmented.

ARTERIAL ULCER (ISCHAEMIC ULCER) (Fig. 6.5)

They are very painful and occur in young patients who have Buerger's disease or occur in elderly patients due to atherosclerotic vascular disease. It commonly occurs

on the tips of toes and fingers. The ulcer is dry, deep and penetrates deep fascia. Evidence of chronic ischaemia in the rest of the foot clinches the diagnosis (see Table 6.3 for differences between arterial and venous ulcers).

NEUROGENIC ULCER, NEUROPATHIC ULCER, TROPHIC ULCER (Fig. 6.6)

This type of ulcer develops in an anaesthetic limb. The causes of neuropathy are:

Diabetic neuropathy

Meningomyelocoele

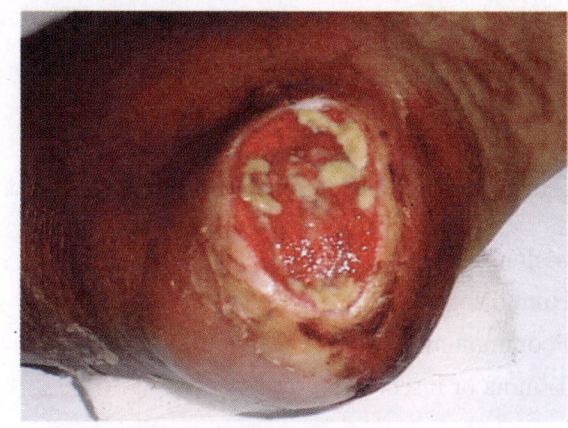

Fig. 6.6 Neuropathic ulcer - Classical site over the heel

	ARTERIAL ULCER	VENOUS ULCER
Location	Tip of toes	Medial or lateral side of leg
Pain	Very painful	Absent
Number and shape	Many and irregular	Single and oval
Depth	Deep, penetrates deep fascia	Superficial, does not penetrate deep fascia
Pigmentation	Not a feature	Usually present
Nature of the vessels	Peripheral pulses are weak or absent; veins are not dilated.	Peripheral pulses are normal; veins are dilated

Table 6.3 Differences between arterial and venous ulcers

Leprosy

Alcoholic neuropathy

Nerve injuries

Transverse myelitis

Ulcer develops on the pressure points like heel, beneath the first and fifth metatarsals and gluteal region (Decubitus ulcer). It develops as a callosity, gets infected, suppurates and leaves a central hole discharging pus. Slowly, it burrows deep inside, may involve bone and cause osteomyelitis. Hence, it is also called as **perforating ulcer.**

Trophic ulcers are caused by inadequate blood supply, malnutrition, and neurological deficit. They are also included in this group.

Treatment

Immobilisation of the foot in a plaster of paris posterior slab with a walking boot almost cures the ulcer within 2-3 weeks, provided the primary disease is also controlled, e.g. leprosy. If the ulcer is non-healing with slough, initial management should include desloughing agents, and surgical removal of the slough.

TROPICAL ULCER

It occurs in tropical countries. The precipitating factors are :

Malnutrition

Humid zones

Poor immunity

Trauma or insect bite

The infection is caused by Vincent's organisms like bacteroides, fusiformis and *Borrelia vincentii*. It starts as a pustule with extensive inflammation. The pustule bursts and the ulcer spreads rapidly and causes destruction of surrounding tissue. Hence, it is also called **Phagedenic ulcer[1].** The edges are undermined, floor contains slough, and there is copious seropurulent discharge. Healing is delayed for days to a month. Metronidazole may be quite useful in bringing down the inflammation. If healing takes place, it leaves behind a scar.

POST-THROMBOTIC ULCER

It occurs due to deep vein thrombosis. It may affect calf veins or it may be due to femoral vein thrombosis. It is an example of venous ulcer or gravitational ulcer.

Precipitating factors

Accidents involving lower leg

Following child birth

After abdominal operation

Clinical features

Bursting pain in the limb

Extensive induration of the leg or thigh depending upon site of thrombosis

Ulcer is non-healing with scanty granulation tissue.

Ulcer is deep and always infiltrates deep fascia.

Due to increased hydrostatic venous pressure, the part is significantly indurated (Cyanotic induration) pigmented, thickened with a rise in local temperature.

Ulcer is not associated with superficial varicosity.

---

1. Phagedenic (to eat). Rapidly spreading ulcerative destructive lesion. It can occur in the oral cavity and also over the penis.

Homan's sign is positive in calf vein thrombosis. It is elicited by forcible dorsiflexion of the foot with the knee extended causing pain in the region of calf.

Moses sign : Squeezing of the calf muscles from side to side also produces pain.

Treatment

Rest and elevation of the leg

Appropriate antibiotics

Elastic crepe bandage

With conservative treatment for a few days to a few weeks, veins may get canalised and the ulcer may heal. The treatment can be very very difficult (Refer varicose veins chapter for details on deep vein thrombosis).

RARE ULCERS[1]

MARTORELL'S ULCER

Affects elderly patients over the age of 50 years.

Commonly affects hypertensive patients, hence the name hypertensive ulcers.

Atherosclerosis is also a precipitating factor even though all peripheral pulses are usually present.

It occurs due to sudden obliteration of end-arterioles of the skin on the back or outerside of calf region.

Severe pain, ischaemic patch of skin which later develops into a deep punched out non healing ulcer are other clinical features.

Healing is delayed due to vascular insufficiency.

BAZIN'S ULCER

These ulcers exclusively occur in young females and occur in the lower third of leg and ankle region.

Usually seen in those patients who are obese with thick ankles and abnormal amount of subcutaneous fat.

It begins with erythematous purplish nodules (hence the name **erythrocyanosis frigida**) on the calves which later rupture producing non-healing ulcer.

Etiology of these ulcers is not clear. It is supposed to be due to ischaemia of lower leg due to spasm of branches of posterior tibial and peroneal arteries. These vessels are abnormally sensitive to hot and cold weather similar to Raynaud's disease. In some cases, tubercle

bacilli have been isolated, with ulcers responding to antituberculous treatment.

These ulcers are managed conservatively.

Sympathectomy may be beneficial in those patients who are hypersensitive to weather changes.

DIABETIC ULCER FOOT

Diabetic patients are more prone for development of ulcers in the foot because of the following reasons.

1. It usually produces a **NEUROPATHY** which can be distal and diffuse with a stocking type of distribution. It commonly manifests after about 10 years of diabetes. Loss of vibration sense and deep tendon reflexes occur early. Later, joint position, touch, pain and temperature sensations are lost. As a result of this, trophic ulcer develops which progresses and can penetrate deeper and deeper. Very often the patient is unaware of this. Diabetic neuropathy of the tibial nerve is dangerous. **Clawing of the toes and hammer toe result due to paralysis of the intrinsic muscles of the foot.** Sensation is absent over the entire sole of the foot due to involvement of medial and lateral plantar nerves. These two factors predispose to the pressure sore over the plantar surface of the head of the metatarsals.

2. **RESISTANCE TO INFECTION** is lowered due to diabetes. Uncontrolled diabetic patients are more susceptible for infection. Eventhough leukocytosis occurs in diabetic patients with infection, the **phagocytic activity of the leukocytes is greatly reduced. In ketoacidosis, granulocyte mobilization is impaired.**

3. Diabetes is usually associated with **ATHERO SCLEROSIS** involving major vessels resulting in ischaemia of the foot (**macroangiopathy**). In addition, it also produces small vessel disease in the form of non-specific thickening of the basement membrane. It is described as **microangiopathy**.

Thus, neuropathy or microangiopathy singly or in combination with secondary infection favours the development of diabetic ulcer. Ulcer starts due to minor trauma like thorn prick, trimming of the nail or due to shoe bite. It may also start as a callosity in the sole of the neuropathic foot.

---

1. *Students should not offer these ulcers as clinical diagnosis. They are rare ulcers, with rare clinical interest.*

SEQUENCE OF EVENTS IN DIABETIC ULCER FOOT (Fig. 6.7)

1. Following an injury or due to infection, an ulcer develops along with swollen, oedematous foot - **Stage of cellulitis.**

2. Cellulitis stage takes up a virulent course, spreads deeper and also upwards along fascial planes - **Stage of spreading cellulitis.**

3. Secondary infection caused by mixed organisms along with anaerobes and non-clostridial gas forming organisms produce multiple abscesses - **Stage of abscesses.**

4. Tense oedema along with vascular compromise which is already existing produce ischaemia and gangrenous patches of skin, toes, etc. - **Stage of gangrene.**

5. Infection involves deeper tissues like bone, producing osteomyelitis - **Stage of osteomyelitis.**

6. Untreated cases develop rapidly spreading cellulitis and **gangrene of the limb** producing septicaemia and diabetic ketoacidosis - **Stage of septicaemia.**

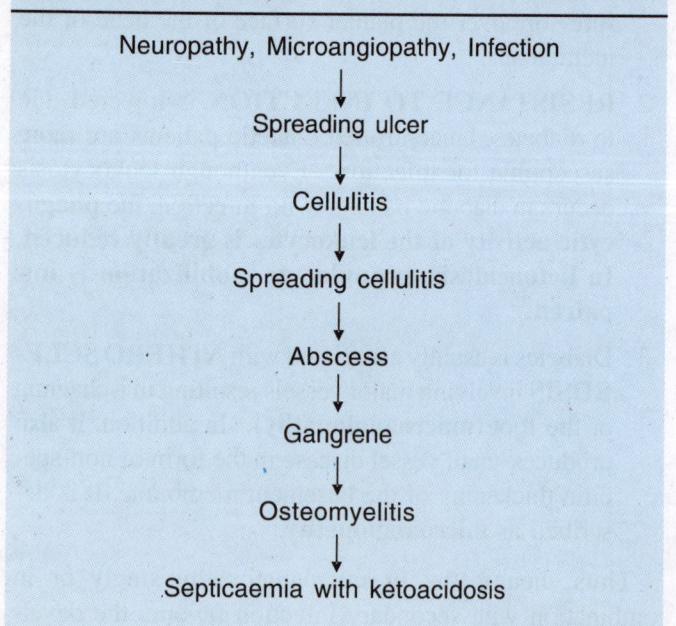

SUMMARY OF CLINICAL EVENTS IN DIABETIC FOOT

Neuropathy, Microangiopathy, Infection
↓
Spreading ulcer
↓
Cellulitis
↓
Spreading cellulitis
↓
Abscess
↓
Gangrene
↓
Osteomyelitis
↓
Septicaemia with ketoacidosis

Fig. 6.7 Various stages of infection of the leg, in diabetic patients

INVESTIGATIONS

1. Complete blood picture usually demonstrates high total count with low Hb% (Infection).

2. Blood and urine sugar estimations

3. Pus for culture/sensitivity

4. X-ray of the foot to rule out osteomyelitis which may be the cause for chronicity of the ulcer.

5. Liver function test (LFT), ECG, Chest X-ray, blood urea, creatinine as a routine in diabetic patients.

6. Lower limb angiography is an important investigation to check the patency of vessels.

TREATMENT[1] OF DIABETIC ULCER FOOT

It can be discussed under five headings:

1. Control of diabetes
2. Control of infection
3. Local treatment of the ulcer
4. Various types of surgery for diabetic ulcer foot
5. Care[2] of the patient as a whole

1. **Control of diabetes**: It is an important part of the treatment of diabetic ulcer foot. Diabetes precipitates infection and infection worsens the diabetic status. These ulcers are better managed, at least in the initial period by insulin rather than oral antidiabetic drugs. Injection plain insulin is given 3-4 times/day depending upon the requirement. At the time of admission after measuring blood levels of glucose, urine is checked 3-4 times/day by Benedict's test and a urine sugar chart is maintained. Depending upon the change in the colour of the reagent, insulin is given (Key Box 6.5).

   This method is described as a **SLIDING SCALE METHOD**. After starting the dosage, a careful watch is made regarding blood sugar values and urine colour changes in the Benedict's test. If the patient is not improving, insulin dosage is increased everyday, at each time, by 4-8 units till all the urine sugar samples show either blue or green colour.

2. **Control of infection** : Once culture/sensitivity report is available, appropriate antibiotics are started. Commonly gram-positive, gram-negative and anaerobic infection exists. Antibiotics may have to be continued for a long time depending upon the nature, type and

---

1. Even a small negligible diabetic ulcer should be treated properly, otherwise a patient may have to Pay through his foot" for it.
2. This is an important aspect forgotten many a time by the treating physicians and surgeons.

Key Box 6.5					
SLIDING SCALE METHOD - TREATMENT WITH INSULIN[1]					
Blue	**Green**	**Yellow**	**Orange**	**Red**	**Red precipitate**
No insulin	4 units	8 units	12 units	16 units	20 units

severity of infection. **Presence of high grade fever with chills and rigors suggest development of multiple abscess pockets which needs to be drained rather than indiscriminate change and usage of antibiotics.** If infection is not controlled properly, keto-acidosis results.

3. **Local treatment of diabetic ulcer foot** : Diabetic ulcer is a non-healing ulcer. Hence, initial treatment is with hydrogen peroxide or Eusol or iodine solution and when the ulcer is converted into a healing ulcer, with pink granulation tissue, a split skin graft is applied. Small ulcers heal by granulation tissue.

4. Various types of surgery[2] for diabetic foot (Table 6.4).

5. **Care of the patient as a whole** : Recovery from healing of diabetic ulcer foot may range from few weeks to few months. During this period there are various other aspects to be looked after apart from infection and insulin (Table 6.5).

Table 6.4 AIM - TO SAVE THE LEG	
1. Spreading ulcer with slough	• Debridement
2. Healing ulcer	• Skin grafting
3. Abscess	• Incision and drainage
4. Gangrene toe	• Disarticulate toe
5. Involvement of metatarsal bones	• Excision of metatarsal bones
6. Gangrene confined to toes	• Forefoot amputation
7. Spreading cellulitis	• Multiple fasciotomy
8. Spreading cellulitis with gangrene	• Amputation below knee or above knee.

Table 6.5 Various problems and their solutions	
PROBLEM	**SOLUTIONS**
Nutritional factors	Diabetic diet should be given
A bed ridden patient may have difficulty in passing urine, situation worsened by preexisting benign prostatic hypertrophy.	Catheterisation (Foley) under aseptic measures, frequent change of catheter and catheter care
Chest infection like pulmonary tuberculosis or static pneumonia	Control of tuberculosis, pneumonia, chest physiotherapy.
Development of bed sores	Frequent change of position and nursing care
More sensitive to carbohydrate metabolism, protein depletion and changes in water and electrolyte metabolism	Frequent checking of Hb%, total proteins, blood glucose and electrolyte levels, etc.

---

1. *Various types of insulin, dosage, resistance to insulin, complications like hypoglycaemic coma, etc. are given in Medicine text books.*
2. *Unfortunately in some patients, in an attempt to save the limb, all these surgeries will be done and at last, they may end up with amputation of the leg.*

Patient/Public education to protect the foot

Never walk barefoot, preferably use **Microcellular rubber shoes** which are not only soft, but also allow oxygenation.

Keep the foot dry after proper cleaning of the foot.

Paring of the nails, trimming should be done carefully, if infection sets in consult the physician at the earliest.

Avoid applying herbal/local medicines or lotions to a corn. Consult the surgeons for the corn.

Proper and regular control of diabetes by diet, frequent self examination of urine and regular blood sugar estimation.

Don't consult the neighbours[1].

Reassurance and good rapport with the treating doctors.

Since these patients have peripheral neuropathy, they will not be able to appreciate temperature of water. Pouring hot water over the foot can cause burns without the patient being aware of it. Hence, a bystander has to check the temperature of water before being used by the patient.

Thus, the best way to avoid complications related to diabetes is by controlling the sugar levels with diet alone or diet with insulin or oral hypoglycaemic agents.

Causes of death in diabetic ulcer foot

Septicaemia with ketoacidosis

Severe electrolyte abnormalities

Other causes like silent myocardial infarction

VARIOUS ASPECTS OF DIABETIC ULCER FOOT

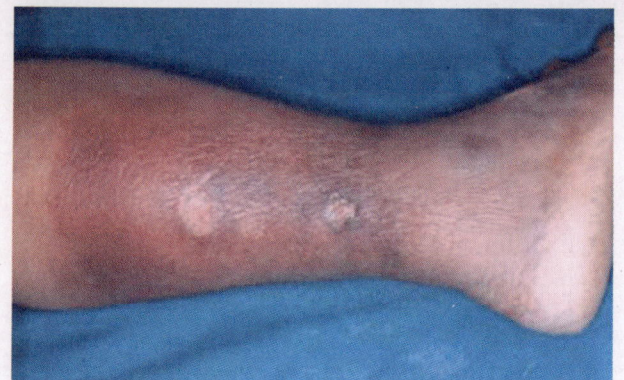

Fig. 6.8 Cellulitis leg

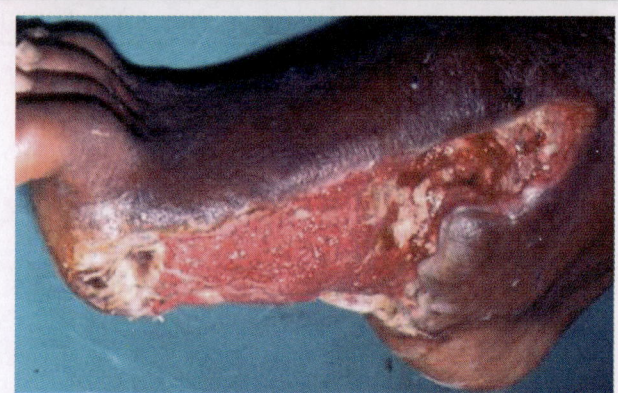

Fig. 6.10 Observe clawing of toes

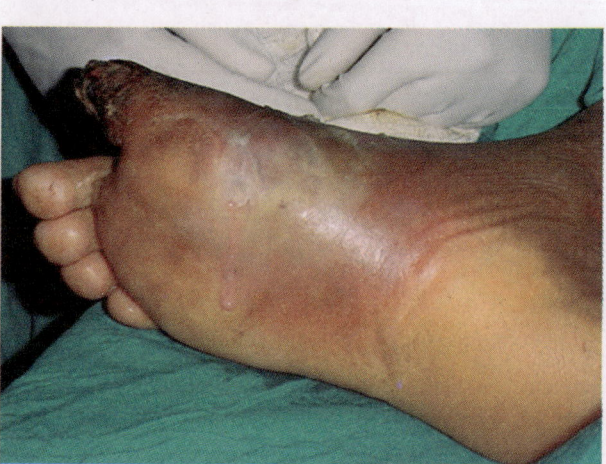

Fig. 6.9 Wet gangrene with abscess foot

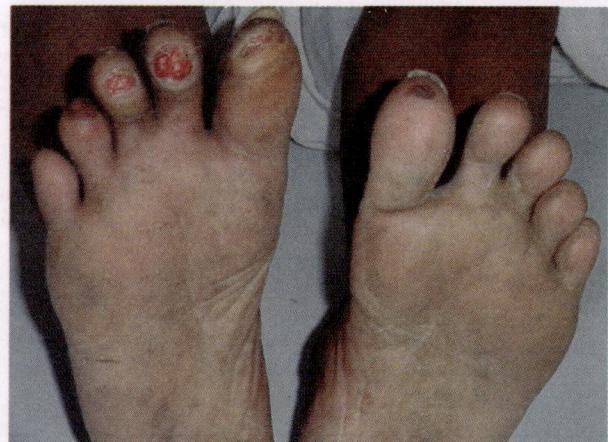

Fig. 6.11 This patient had hot burns following barefoot walking resulting in gangrene of all ten toes

---

1. *Remember it is the patient's leg that may have to be amputated and not the neighbours'.*

VARIOUS ASPECTS OF DIABETIC ULCER FOOT

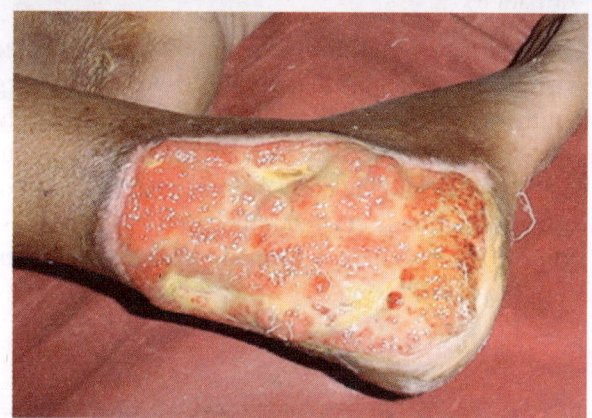

Fig. 6.12 Observe pale granulation tissue, purulent discharge

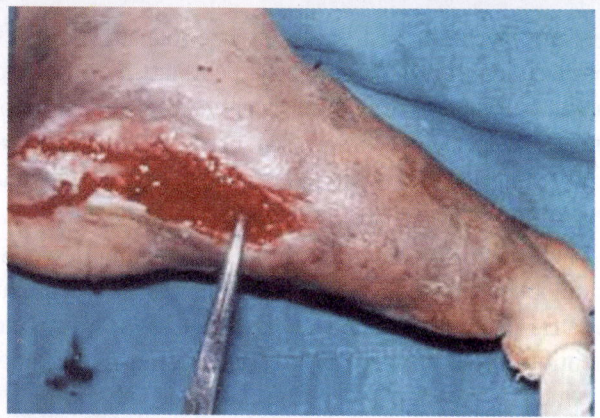

Fig. 6.13 Observe red granulation tissue - healing after control of diabetes and regular dressings

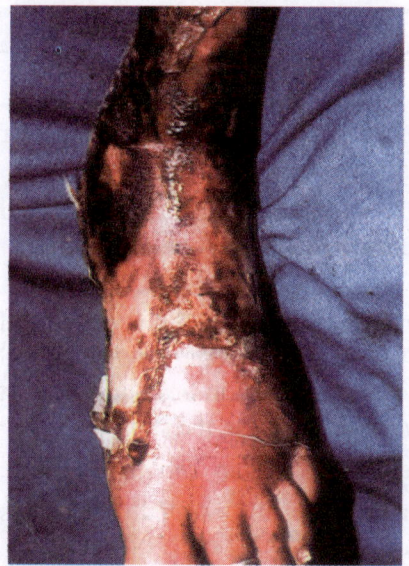

Fig. 6.14 Diabetic ulcer with moist gangrene. Patient had ketoacidosis with septicaemia. Inspite of amputation, patient died

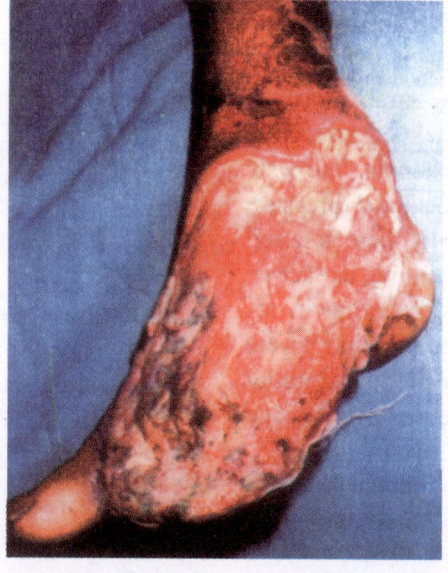

Fig. 6.15 Extensive diabetic ulcer foot - needed below knee amputation

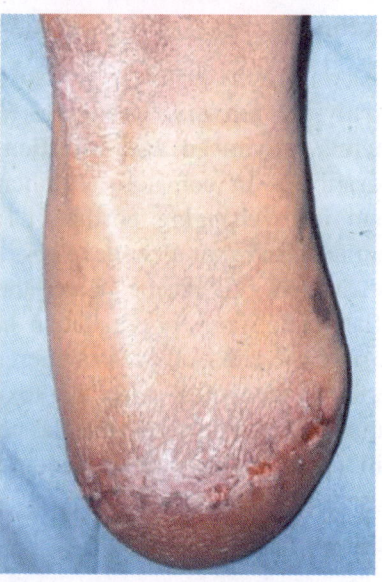

Fig. 6.16 Below knee amputation

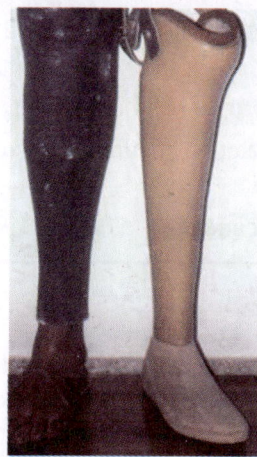

Fig. 6.17 Artificial limb - prosthesis

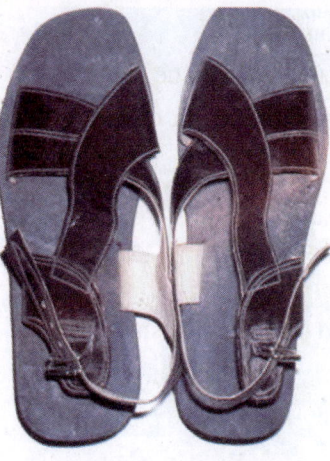

Fig. 6.18 Microcellular rubber (MCR) chapples specially designed for patients with neuropathic foot. They avoid pressure points

PRESSURE SORE – Prevention and Treatment

Pressure ulcers, or bed sores are a serious and frustrating complication for the paralyzed, debilitated or comatose patient confined to a bed or wheel chair. The ulcers form when soft tissue is compressed between a bony prominence such as the ischium, sacrum or trochanter and a supporting structure – the bed or wheel chair.

The growing incidence of spinal cord injuries due to automobile accidents and increased numbers of debilitated geriatric patients admitted to hospitals have drawn more attention to the problem of pressure ulcer prevention and treatment. Pressure ulcer is usually the most important factor that delays rehabilitation of the paraplegic or quadriplegic patient.

Factors predisposing to formation of pressure sore

Most important factor is **pressure**, other factors being **paralysis, paresis, shearing forces, malnutrition, anemia, advanced age, infection**. Lack of protective sensation – in comatose, debilitated patients, prevents them from changing posture. The localized pressure continues and skin ulcer develops. Initially there is tissue anoxia and cell death. Later there will be an active inflammation and vasodilatation occurs, resulting in re-active hyperemia. If pressure is removed allowing tissue perfusion and thus wash out toxic by-products, initial damage may be reversible, if not, permanent damage will occur. This can happen in one to six hours.

Clinical features

1. Early superficial ulceration

Erythema, oedema and punctate haemorrage. Moist irregular ulceration with surrounding erythematous halo.

2. Late superficial ulceration

Full thickness skin ulceration

Spreading necrosis of subcutaneous tissue

Deep inflammatory response spreads in cone shaped fashion to deeper tissues.

3. Early deep ulceration

Cicatrization of rolled ulcer edges

Eschar at base of ulcer

Spread of inflammation and bacterial invasion

4. Late deep ulceration

Breakdown of fascial plane

Chronic inflammation and fibrosis of deep tissue (Bursa formation)

There is no such thing as a small pressure ulcer. The visible skin wound is merely the "**tip of the iceberg**". 70% of the ulcer is below the skin. Pressure is transmitted in a cone-shaped or pyramidal manner from the skin through each layer of tissue to the bony prominence, so that a cone of tissue destruction is created – the point of the cone is at the skin surface, and base is formed by larger undermined defect overlying the bone.

Preventive measures

Pressure ulcers can be avoided by meticulous skin care and relief of pressure over bony prominence (Key Box 6.6)

Key Box 6.6
SKIN CARE
1. Regular, periodical skin inspection, especially over the bony prominences
2. Any sign of redness, irritation or abrasion – if noted – all pressure must be taken off the area immediately.
3. **Keeping the skin clean and dry** : Moist areas lead to maturation. Fine talcum powder may be applied to areas where moisture tends to develop. It must be dusted everyday after drying the skin.
4. **Gentle massage** of valuable skin with lanolin lotion.
5. Care of perineum and genitalia especially in patients with incontinence
6. Clothing and bedding must be wrinkle free, made of porous absorbent material to allow air circulation and avoid accumulation of perspiration.
7. Pressure relief – in bedridden patients
a. Frequent change of posture round the clock every 2 hours
b. Avoid localized pressure by proper body alignment.
c. Use of air or fluid filled floatation mattresses also lessen risk of ulcer formation.
d. Patient and patient party education

Treatment

1. Superficial ulceration: Debridement and allow it to heal by secondary intention. It will take many weeks to heal.

2. **Deep ulceration** or large superficial ulceration

Bed side debridement of obviously necrotic material

'Wet to dry' dressing

Use of **desloughing agents**

Systemic **antibiotics**

Nutritional consideration

Correction of spasm and contractures if present.

Once it is ready, the defect is closed.

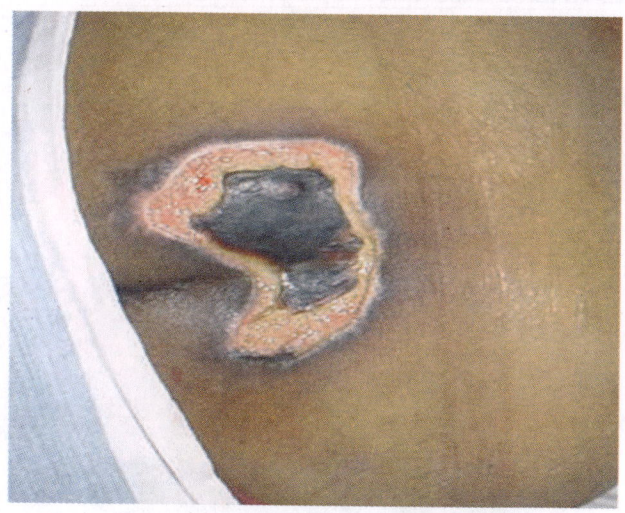

Fig. 6.19 Pressure sore

Methods of closure

a. Primary closure – undermine and approximate the cut edges

b. SSG – in selected cases only

c. Skin flaps

Transposition flap

Rotation flap

Advancement flap

Cultured muscle interposition for severe and ischial pressure sores.

3. Education of patient and patient attenders to prevent pressure sores

Lower Limb Ischaemia

7

- Causes of lower limb ischaemia
- Collateral circulation
- Clinical features
- Clinical examination
- Investigations
- Treatment
- Acute arterial occlusion
- Critical limb ischaemia
- Popliteal aneurysm
- Ainhum
- Frost bite
- Reperfusion injuries

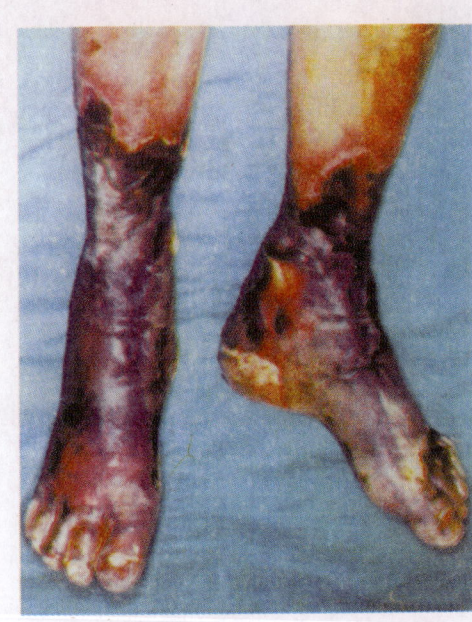

Fig. 7.1 Bilateral gangrene due to atherosclerosis

- Majority of the individuals are conscious about the chest pain caused by myocardial ischaemia. However, patients present relatively late to the hospital with ischaemia of the lower limb (Fig. 7.1). The disease, even though benign, is not curable totally, thus causing financial, social and psychological burden to the patient and his relatives.

- Other rare causes of lower limb ischaemia include popliteal entrapment syndrome and cystic medial degeneration. One should not forget that **diabetes** is also one of the common causes of peripheral vascular disease in elderly patients.

CAUSES OF LOWER LIMB ISCHEMIA

Table 7.1. Causes of lower limb ischaemia

CHRONIC LOWER LIMB ISCHAEMIA	ACUTE LOWER LIMB ISCHAEMIA
• Atherosclerosis	• Acute embolism
• **T**hrombo **A**ngitis **O**bliterans (TAO)	• Trauma to the vessels
• Collagen vascular disorders	• Aneurysm
• Diabetes	

COLLATERAL CIRCULATION

- Collateral circulation is present in most of the organs. Hence, even if a major vessel is occluded the organ can still survive provided collaterals are well developed.

- Chronic ischaemia caused by TAO or atherosclerosis, allows sufficient time for collaterals to develop. Hence necrosis or gangrene which occurs is minimised. Thus, limbs often survive.

- In acute ischaemia caused by thrombus or embolism there is no time for collaterals to develop. This results in gangrene of the limb, in untreated cases.

CLINICAL FEATURES

SYMPTOMS

1. **Pain** in the limb is the chief symptom of lower limb ischaemia. It is a severe cramp like pain, due to ischaemia of the muscles, brought on mainly by exertion. It is called intermittent claudication.

Key Box 7.1
GRADES OF INTERMITTENT CLAUDICATION

Grade-I Patient walks for a distance, gets the pain, continues to walk and the pain disappears. As a result of ischaemia, anaerobic metabolism takes place, which produces **substance P, Lactic acid**, etc. These produce vasodilatation and the pain disappears.

Grade-II Patient walks for a distance, gets the pain, continues to walk with the pain. He has a limp.

Grade-III Patient walks, gets the pain. He has to take rest. This grade indicates severe muscle ischaemia.

Grade-IV Pain at rest is due to ischaemia of nerves* in addition to ischaemia of the muscles.

Cry of the dying nerves, due to involvement of vasa nervorum

Rest pain

It is an intractable type of pain usually felt in the foot, toes etc. It is an indication of severe ischaemia of the foot with impending gangrene. Typically, a patient with rest pain sits on the bed, holds his foot with both hands or may hang the foot out of bed. This gives him some kind of relief. Rest pain is worse at night time[1]. It may lead to suicidal tendency.

- Claudication distance refers to the distance a patient is able to walk before the onset of pain. A patient with severe claudication may not be able to walk for a few yards.

- Site of claudication depends upon the level of arterial occlusion (Table 7.2).

Table 7.2	
LEVEL OF OCCLUSION	**CLAUDICATION SITE**
Aortoiliac obstruction	Claudication of both gluteal regions, thighs and calves
Iliofemoral obstruction	Claudication of thigh muscles
Femoropopliteal obstruction	Claudication of calf muscles
Popliteal obstruction	Claudication of the foot muscles

Intermittent claudication in a young patient can be due to some rare causes such as

- *Popliteal artery entrapment due to abnormal origin of gastroenemius muscle.*
- *Cyst in the media of the popliteal artery*

2. **Nonhealing ulcer** is the next common presenting symptom. It is usually precipitated by a minor trauma and it occurs in the most distal part of the body like tip of toes. Ischemic ulcers are very painful and deep ulcers.

3. Some patients present with **gangrenous patches** of skin or subcutaneous tissue. Gangrene affects distal parts like toes. However, gangrene is minimal because of collaterals (Figs. 7.2 and 7.3)

4. History of **bilateral gluteal claudication** with impotence can occur in a young patient due to a saddle thrombus at the bifurcation of aorta. It is called as **Leriche's syndrome.** Impotence is due to failure to achieve an erection due to paralysis of L_1 nerve.

   - **Gluteal claudication** is confused for sciatica and many patients are referred to orthopaedic department. This is **neurogenic claudication** which is present even at rest and aggravated on movements of the spine. Causes of neurogenic claudication are slipped disc, fracture vertebrae, tuberculosis of spine etc.

5. Coldness, numbness, paraesthesia and colour changes indicates chronic ischaemia.

---

1. *One of our TAO patients with sleepless nights due to rest pain comitted suicide by jumping from the 2nd floor of the hospital.*

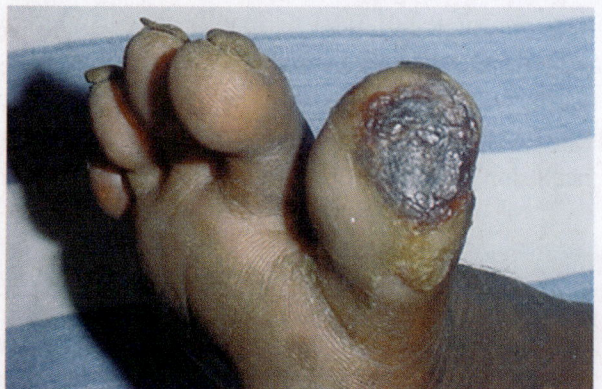

Fig. 7.2 TAO with dry gangrene

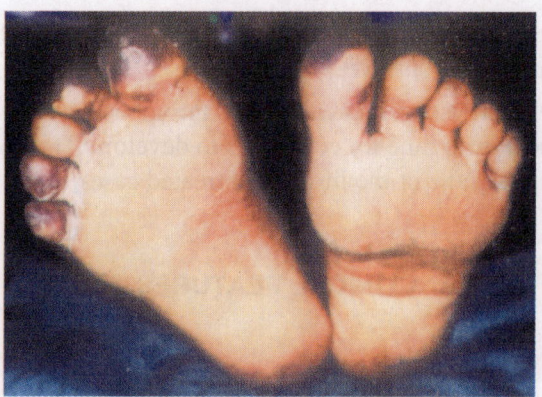

Fig. 7.3 Vasculitis with collagen vascular disorder. It had affected all the ten toes

6. Majority of patients with peripheral vascular disease are smokers. TAO occurs exclusively in male smokers[1].

SIGNS (CLINICAL EXAMINATION)

INSPECTION

The *findings are appreciated* better if a comparison is made with the opposite limb. Evidence of chronic ischaemia of the leg are:

- Flattening of the terminal pulp spaces of toes
- Fissures, cracks in between the toes
- Ulceration of toes, interdigital ulcers
- Brittle, flat and ridged nails, and shiny skin
- Loss of hair and loss of subcutaneous fat
- Limb may appear more dark in dark skinned patients or markedly pale in fair skinned patients with vasospastic disease like TAO
- Gangrene is usually dry with a clear line of demarcation. It indicates the junction of dead and living tissue. Since the blood supply to the muscle is better, usually the **line of demarcation involves skin and subcutaneous tissue**. Line of demarcation is very well appreciated in senile gangrene **where it can be skin, muscle or bone deep**.
- The limb may show atrophy of muscles.

PALPATION

1. **Ulcer** : Examination should be done as described in the Chapter 6. Ischaemic ulcers are very tender.

2. **Gangrene** is described according to its size, shape and extent. In dry gangrene, the part is dry and mummified or shrunken. Features of dry gangrene are summarised in the Key Box 7.2.

3. **Limb** above[2]

   - **Ischaemic limb is cold.** Careful palpation from above downwards will reveal the change in temperature from warm to the cold area. Temperature changes are appreciated better with the dorsum of the hand which is more sensitive as it has a lot of cutaneous nerve endings.

   - **Tenderness** : It is tender due to the presence of inflammation.

Key Box 7.2
GANGRENE
• Loss of temperature
• Loss of pulsation
• Loss of sensation
• Loss of colour
• Loss of function

---

1. *A 26-year old female, nonsmoker patient presented to the hospital with ischaemic features of the right upper limb. All causes of upper limb ischaemia were ruled out (Raynaud's, cervical rib, etc.). On careful questioning, she admitted to using SNUFF DIPPING for 10 years (snuff contains nicotine).*

2 *It is better to palpate the entire limb from the thigh downwards.*

- **Sensation** : Due to the irritation of nerve endings, ischaemic limb is hypersensitive[1].

- **Pitting oedema** can be due to thrombophlebitis or due to nonfunctioning of limb.

4. **Palpation of pulses**.[2] (Table 7.3).

- After examining the pulses, results are interpreted in **pulses chart** as shown in the next page.

- In a similar manner, upper limb pulses, head and neck pulses are also recorded in the pulses chart.

Other tests of minor importance

1. **Buerger's postural test** is relevant in fair skinned patients. The patient (supine) is asked to raise his legs vertically upwards keeping the knees straight.

Table 7.3 Examination of peripheral vessels

ARTERY	SITE WHERE IT IS FELT	REMARKS
EXAMINATION OF LOWER LIMB PULSES		
1. **Dorsalis pedis** is the continuation of anterior tibial artery.	At the level of ankle joint lateral to extensor hallucis longus. It should not be felt distally where it dips into the plantar space.	In 10% of cases it can be absent.
2. **Posterior tibial artery** is a branch of popliteal artery.	In between the medial malleolus and medial border of the tendoachilles.	For the foot circulation, anyone of these vessels are sufficient
3. **Popliteal artery** is a continuation of femoral artery extends from the hiatus in adductor magnus to the fibrous arch in soleus. It is about 20 cm long.	It is felt in the prone or supine position with knee flexed. It is felt against lower end of femur or against tibial condyles.	**Knee is flexed to relax popliteal fascia.** Dorsalis pedis, posterior tibial, popliteal artery are usually not palpable in TAO patients.
4. **Femoral artery** is the continuation of external iliac artery.	It is felt midway between anterior superior iliac spine and pubic tubercle, just below the inguinal ligament in the upper thigh.	Flexion, abduction and external rotation of hip joint may facilitate the palpation in obese patients.
EXAMINATION OF HEAD AND NECK VESSELS		
1. **Subclavian artery** arises from arch of aorta on the left side and brachiocephalic on the right side.	It is felt in the supraclavicular region in the posterior triangle against the first rib.	Difficult to feel in obese patients
2. **Common carotid artery** arises from arch of aorta on the left side and from brachiocephalic artery on the right side.	It is felt against the carotid tubercle of sixth cervical vertebra (C6) in the carotid triangle (at the upper border of the thyroid cartilage).	At the upper border of the lamina of thyroid cartilage (C3 vertebra) carotid artery bifurcates.
3. **Superficial temporal artery** is the terminal branch of the external carotid artery.	It is felt in front of tragus of the ear against the zygoma..	This is involved in temporal arteritis, a type of giant cell arteritis.

- See Key Box 7.3 for Pulses Chart (Next page)

---

1. *Ischaemic limb is like irritable personalities.*
2. *A thorough clinical examination of pulses include not only lower limb vessels, also head, neck and upper limb vessels.*

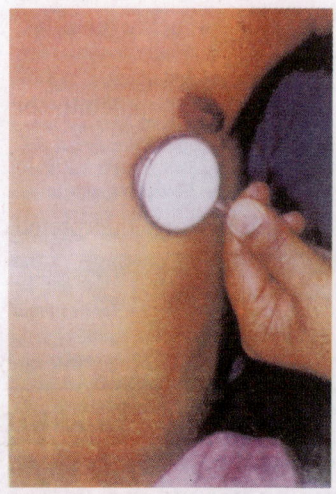
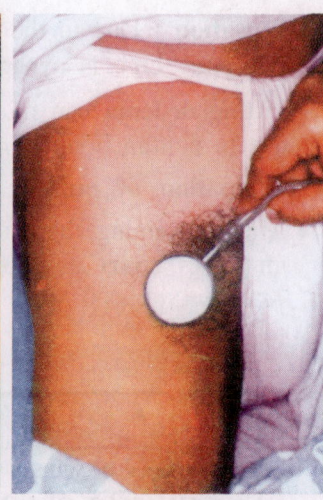

Fig. 7.4 Auscultation of the heart to rule out valvular heart diseases,

Fig. 7.5 Auscultation over the femoral artery

Key Box 7.3		
PULSES CHART		
(For example, classical case of TAO left lower limb)		
LOWER LIMB PULSES	**Right**	**Left**
Dorsalis pedis	++++	-
Posterior tibial	++++	-
Popliteal	++++	++
Femoral	++++	++++
++++ : Normal; **++** : Weak; **-** : Absent.		

In cases of chronic ischaemia, marked pallor develops within 2-3 minutes. The angle at which pallor develops is Buerger's angle of circulatory insufficiency. In ischaemic limb, pallor develops even on elevation of leg upto 15-30 degrees.

2. **Capillary refilling test** : Apply pressure over the tip of the terminal pulp space for a few seconds and release the pressure. Rapid return of circulation is observed in normal persons.

- The test can also be done in the ischaemic foot by asking the patient to sit up and hang his legs down and observe for colour changes. The time taken for the ischaemic foot to become pink is described capillary filling time. This is prolonged in an ischaemic foot.

Auscultation (Figs. 7.4 and 7.5)

1. Systolic bruit over the femoral artery can be heard in atherosclerotic occlusion of ilio-femoral segment, due to turbulence created by the blood flow.

2. Auscultation of the heart to rule out mitral stenosis (middiastolic murmur, loud 1st heart sound, etc.).

An eighteen-year girl was kept in the MBBS examination with ischaemia of lower limb of 6 days duration. The candidate offered collagen vascular disorder as the first diagnosis and failed. He had missed the cardiac history and findings totally, and had not auscultated the heart. It was a case of mitral stenosis with acute embolic gangrene of the lower limb.

CLINICAL NOTES

75 year old lady, known case of polycythaemia vera presented to the hospital with multiple gangrenous patches of skin in the upper limbs and in the lower limbs. Conservative surgery was attempted by debriding gangrenous portion of the skin. Polycythemia is also one of the causes of gangrene.

DIFFERENTIAL DIAGNOSIS

- Eventhough there are many causes of lower limb ischaemia, thromboangitis obliterans (TAO) and atherosclerotic vascular disease are the commonest causes. Hence they have to be considered first before giving other diagnosis

- TAO is also called as Buerger's disease - the details are given in Key Box 7.4 and Table 7.4.

- Atherosclerotic vascular disease is the commonest cause of lower limb ischaemia. It can manifest as simple ulcer to massive gangrene.

Key Box 7.4		
CLASSIFICATION OF BUERGER'S DISEASE		
Type I	:	Upper extermity
Type II	:	Crural (leg and foot)
Type III	:	Femoral type – femoropopliteal
Type IV	:	Aortoiliac
Type V	:	Generalised type

Table 7.4 DIFFERENTIAL   DIAGNOSIS[1]

	TAO (Buerger's disease)	ATHEROSCLEROSIS
1. Age	20-40 years	Around 50 years
2. Sex	Exclusively males	Females are also affected
3. Etiology	1. It is a smoker's disease. Excessive tobacco (nicotine) produces severe vasospasm of the vessels. 2. Excessive smoking produces increased levels of carboxy haemoglobin which damages these vessels. 3. Low socioeconomic group, recurrent trauma to the foot, poor hygiene are additional factors. 4. Hypercoagulable state 5. Autonomic hyperactivity 6. Autoimmune factors	1. Atherosclerosis is a rich man's disease, who is usually a smoker, diabetic and, hypertensive. 2. Strong family history is also present in a few cases. 3. Consumption of high fat diet leading onto obesity, lack of regular exercises and hypercholesterolaemia are other factors.
4. Pathology	Diffuse inflammatory reaction involving all three coats of vessel (panarteritis) causing a thrombus, resulting in occlusion of lumen (obliterans). Polymorphs, giant cells and micro-abscesses are found within the thrombus. In severe cases, vein and nerve are bound by fibrous tissue.	Deposition of lipid rich atheromatous plaque in the intima is the hallmark of atherosclerosis. Plaques tend to be more in **lower abdominal aorta**, coronary arteries, etc. Plaques may undergo **calcification**. ulceration and thrombosis or **dislodge** cholesterol emboli or may weaken the media and produce **aneurysm**.
5. Vessels involved	Small and medium-sized vessels like dorsalis pedis, posterior tibial, popliteal are commonly involved.	Medium-sized and large vessels like aorta, common iliac, femoral, common carotid etc are involved.
6. Upper limb involvement	Not uncommon	Rare
7. Nature of vessel wall	Not thickened	Thickened
8. Blood pressure	Normal in the normal limb and low in diseased limb.	Hypertension is commonly present
9. Superficial[2] migrating thrombophlebitis	Seen in about 30% of cases of TAO Veins of lower limb are involved and are tender and thickened.	Not seen
10. Auscultation-femoral artery	Bruit is not heard	Bruit can be present as in aortoiliac disease
11. Angiography	Cork-screw pattern of vessels	Shows site of block

INVESTIGATIONS

1. **Complete blood picture**

2. **Blood sugar estimation**
   - Normal levels - FBS 80-120 mg/dl and PPBS 120-180 mg/dl. Mainly help in diabetic patients.

3. **Serum cholesterol**
   - Normal levels - 150-250 mg/100 ml. Usually they are altered in atherosclerotic patients.

4. **Angiography (Arteriography)** (Fig. 7.6)
   - It is not usually indicated in TAO patients where direct arterial surgery is not done. However, a few

---

1. *From M.B.B.S. examination point of view TAO and atherosclerotic vascular disease are to be differentiated.*
2. *Migrating thrombophlebitis is also seen in pancreatic malignancy where it is called Trousseau's sign.*

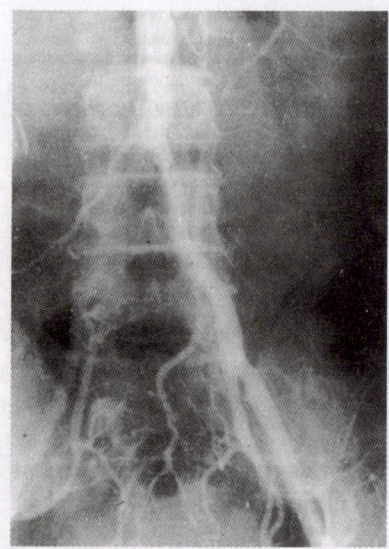

Fig. 7.6 Angiography showing block in the common iliac artery on the right side

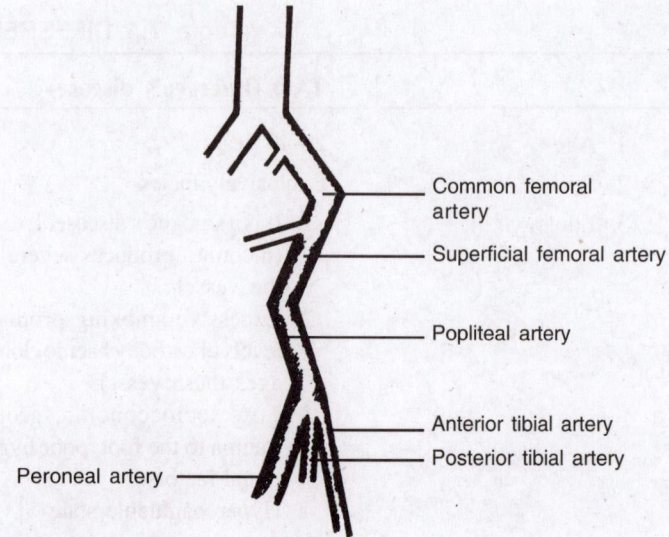

Common femoral artery
Superficial femoral artery
Popliteal artery
Anterior tibial artery
Posterior tibial artery
Peroneal artery

Fig. 7.7 Extensive narrowing of popliteal artery and branches

cases of presenile atherosclerosis who are mis-diagnosed as TAO will require angiography to locate the site of obstruction which is suitable for an arterial reconstruction. Angiography is indicated in patients with atherosclerotic vascular disease, to know the exact site of block, type of obstruction, to define the collaterals, so as to plan for arterial reconstruction.

Small vessel bypass is becoming popular today as in selected cases of diabetes and atherosclerosis.

Types of angiography

A. Percutaneous transfemoral retrograde angiography : This is done in unilateral obstruction. An incision is made in the upper thigh to expose the femoral artery on the normal[1] side. A Seldinger needle and guide wire are used to introduce arterial catheter and radio-opaque dye is introduced after placing the catheter into the aorta. It visualises the entire aortoiliac segment and below.

B. Direct translumbar angiography or aortography: It is indicated when obstruction is bilateral, both femoral pulses are not palpable, clinically manifesting as bilateral lower limb ischaemia. Aorta is directly punctured from behind (translumbar) by using ultrasound image intensifier.

Results : Arteriography establishes the site of block and nature of collaterals.

Complications of angiography

Thrombosis at the puncture site resulting in ischaemia.

Haemorrhage from the puncture site which needs to be stopped by pressure packing.

Arterial dissection if catheter is wrongly placed and advanced.

Anaphylaxis - can be avoided by a trial injection.

Paraplegia due to spasm of spinal arteries

Infection

5. **Digital subtraction angiography (D.S.A.)**: This can be done by arterial or venous route. The arterial route is preferred.

   DSA gives **excellent pictures in carotid and large central vessels**. However, the peripheral vessels may not reveal adequate information. Thus, conventional arteriography still has an important role in atherosclerotic vascular disease.

6. **Doppler ultrasound blood flow detector**: This test is based on Doppler principle. An ultrasound signal is beamed at an artery and the reflected beam is picked

---

1. *Normal limb is selected for two reasons:*
   - *Femoral pulse is palpable. hence easy to locate the artery and introduce the catheter.*
   - *If a thrombus occurs in the diseased limb due to angiography, it will worsen the ischaemia. may lead to gangrene.*

up by a receiver. Frequency changes of the beam due to the moving blood are converted into audio signals which can be heard by using a probe. Thus, Doppler probe can be used to detect the pulse even when the pulse is clinically not palpable.

- By using sphygmomanometer, systolic blood pressure (BP) of the limb can be measured by positioning the cuff at a suitable level and pressure index can be calculated.

$$\text{Pressure Index (PI)} = \frac{\text{Ankle blood pressure}}{\text{Brachial blood pressure}}$$

- Normal values are above 1. However in patients with peripheral vascular disease values are below 1. Values below 0.9 indicate vascular obstruction.
- When ankle pressure is less than 30 mmHg, gangrene may be imminent.

Uses of Doppler probe

- To feel the normal pulse as in operation theatres.
- To feel clinically non detectable pulse as in peripheral vascular disease.
- To measure B.P. in ischaemic limb.
- Remeasuring B.P. in lower limb after exercise to differentiate ischaemic claudication from neurogenic claudication.

7. **Duplex scan**
   - This is the investigation of choice today. Duplex scan is a combination of Doppler with B mode ultrasound. With the availability of colour Duplex, the direction of blood flow can be assessed. Red colour means direction of flow towards transducer and blue means away.

8. **Plethysmography** : In this method changes in the volume of the limb or digit can be assessed
   - It is performed by placing the limb in an air and water tight metal container which is connected to a floating needle. As the pressure pulse passes through one segment of the limb, a wave is generated and it is recorded.
   - Thus, it is an accurate method to assess the changes in blood volume in limb, indirectly estimating vasodilatation

- Oculoplethysmography is used to evaluate carotid artery disease.

TREATMENT OF PERIPHERAL VASCULAR DISEASE (TAO AND ATHEROSCLEROSIS)

- In all patients with peripheral vascular disease, following general measures to be taken which will help in better perfusion of the lower limb tissues.
- Anemia to be treated with hematinics and blood transfusion. If ejection fraction is low, drugs are given to improve cardiac output.

PRINCIPLES (Key Box 7.6)

Key Box 7.6
PRINCIPLES OF THE TREATMENT
• To relieve the pain • To arrest the progress of the disease • Role of vasodilators • Chemical sympathectomy • Surgical methods

I. To relieve the pain

As already discussed, the pain is very severe and distressing. Some amount of pain relief can be obtained as follows:

a. **Analgesics**: Simple analgesics may not help these patients.
   - **Aspirin** (300 mg) one tablet 3 times a day can be used. It has also anti adhesive effect on platelets.
   - **Ketorolac** 10-20 mg one tablet 3 times a day can be given in severe cases.
   - Narcotic analgesics can be used judiciously in cases with rest pain.

b. **Buerger's position** by elevating head end of the bed, causes venous congestion and reflex vasodilatation.

c. **Buerger's exercises** by elevation and dependency of the limb for a few minutes.

d. **Heel raise**: By raising the heels of shoes by 1-2 cm, claudication distance can be increased as it decreases work load on the calf muscles.

---

1. Because of these complications, angiography should be done carefully only when it is indicated.

II. To arrest the progression of the disease

- Stop smoking. This is more beneficial in TAO patients than atherosclerotic patients.
- Regular exercises
- Reduce obesity
- Diet : To avoid fatty food to avoid cholesterol. It is more useful in patients with hyperlipidaemia.
- Avoid injuries

III. Role of vasodilators

- Vasodilators have not been found to be useful in atherosclerotic vascular disease.
- Some degree of improvement in reducing pain and healing of cutaneous ulcers have been found in TAO patients.
- The drugs are pentoxyphylline, prostacyclin or Xanthinol nicotinate (Complamina).
- Few cases of Buerger's disease are benefited with injection xanthinol nicotinate (Complamina) given in a graded dose, e.g. 3000 mg on the 1st day, 4500 mg on 2nd day, 6000 mg on the 3rd day, 7500 mg on 4th day and 9000 mg on 5th day followed by an injection of low molecular weight dextran. **Injection xanthinol nicotinate helps in following ways** :
  - In a few cases, it helps in healing of cutaneous ulcers.
  - To improve claudication distance
  - To postpone lumbar sympathectomy
  - Repeat courses of vasodilator are necessary to control the disease.
  - However, it should be remembered that the treatment is only temporary.

IV. Chemical sympathectomy

- It acts by producing vasodilatation of the blood vessels of the lower limb.
- In this procedure, 5 ml of phenol in water is injected beside the bodies of 2nd, 3rd and 4th lumbar vertebrae.
- The effect of the drug can be judged immediately by feeling the warm feet.
- It helps in healing of ulcers and may improve rest pain probably by interfering with afferent sensory circuits.

Precautions

1. **Lateral injection** by using a lumbar puncture needle
2. Injection should be **in front of lumbar fascia** which contains the sympathetic trunk.
3. **Avoid injuries** to aorta and inferior vena cava
4. Procedure is to be done **under x-ray control** (Screening)

   Since phenol has replaced lignocaine because of its long lasting effect, it is also called **phenol sympathectomy**.

V. Surgical procedures in TAO

1. **Lumbar sympathectomy** is the indirect surgery done for TAO patients since direct arterial surgery is not possible.

Key Box 7.7

SALIENT FEATUES OF LUMBAR SYMPATHECTOMY

- Transverse loin incision
- Extraperitoneal approach, and it is a pre-ganglionic sympathectomy.
- Lumbar sympathetic trunk is identified in the paravertebral gutter lateral to the psoas muscle as a cord like structure.
- **2nd lumbar ganglion is large** and has white rami joining it.
- Sympathetic trunk is divided below the first lumbar vertebra and removed up to the 4th lumbar vertebra.
- This is a **preganglionic sympathectomy** because fibres supplying the vessels of the limb have their cell stations in the sacral ganglia which are not disturbed.

- **Indications : Cutaneous ulcer and rest pain.**
- **Structures which can be confused** for lumbar sympathetic trunk are –
  1. Genitofemoral nerve
  2. Tendon strip of psoas muscle
  3. Lymphatic chain and fatty tissue
- **One should be careful not to damage lumbar veins[1] which join inferior vena cava.**
- By depriving the sympathetic nerve supply to lower

---

1. *Lumbar veins, if cut accidentally, retract and troublesome bleeding can occur from inferior vena cava. Pressure packing and wait for 3-5 minutes and then see and ligate should be the policy.*

limb blood vessels, vasomotor tone is reduced so that some amount of vasospasm is reduced. Thus, rest pain improves, minor ulcerations heal due to cutaneous vasodilatation. However, the duration of effect of lumbar sympathectomy is not clear.

- Both sides can be done in one sitting. However, during bilateral operation, the 1st lumbar ganglion on one side should be left since removal of both ganglia may cause sterility due to paralysis of ejaculatory mechanism.

2. **Omentoplasty** has been tried in TAO patients. In most of these patients vasodilator therapy and lumbar sympathectomy has been done with almost no relief of symptoms. In such cases, before a merciful amputation is done, omentoplasty is done.

- By careful division of vascular arcade of omentum, it can be lengthened based on one of the epiploic arteries, brought out of the laparotomy incision, tunnelled in the subcutaneous plane and can be brought up to calf or even to the ankle joint level in some patients.

- Greater omentum is supposed to produce neovascularisation and thus helps in healing of the cutaneous ulcers. The effect seems to be temporary (Not done nowadays).

3. **Conservative amputations** should be done if the toes are gangrenous.

4. **Below knee amputation**[1] is the last resort. It is indicated in severe rest pain cases where in all other modalities of treatment have failed. **Risk of amputation after ten years of the disease is around 10%.**

VI. Surgery in atherosclerotic vascular disease

- The decision to revascularise the limb is taken after an angiography. The success of reconstruction depends upon a number of factors. They are given in Key Box 7.8.

- **Intermittent claudication alone is not an indication for surgery**. Rest pain and pregangrenous changes in the limb are definite indications for reconstruction with accepted mortality and morbidity.

- Surgery can be classified into surgery for aortoiliac disease and surgery for iliofemoral stenotic disease.

AORTOILIAC DISEASE

- It is treated by bypass grafts or endarterectomy.

---

1. *Students are requested not to tell this first as a treatment.*

Key Box 7.8

PROGNOSTIC FACTORS FOR LIMB REVASCULARISATION

- Severity of the disease
- Presence of collaterals
- Presence of diabetes
- Chronic smoking
- Site of occlusion
- Age of the patient
- Angina pectoris
- Fitness for anaesthesia

---

1. **Bypass grafts**
- Usually, it is bilateral and it is treated by using aortobifemoral graft to bypass the stenosis. The graft either made from teflon or dacron is used. It is also called y-graft or trouser graft. It has commonly 16 mm trunk and two 8 mm diameter limbs (Fig. 7.8).
- In unilateral cases unilateral graft is applied.

2. **Aortoiliac endarterectomy** is indicated when the disease affects
- Short segment
- Big artery like aorta
- One artery

Types

A. Open endarterectomy: An arteriotomy is done first and the diseased intima, atheromatous plaque and the thrombus are removed. An arteriotomy incision can be closed directly or a vein patch graft is used to close the defect, so as to avoid narrowing.

B. Closed endarterectomy is indicated in a longer diseased segment. In this procedure, after an arteriotomy, a wire loop is used to strip out a core of atheroma by introducing it through the lower arteriotomy and removing the atheromatous plaque from the upper end.

- However, results of bypass graft are better than endarterectomy and modern tendency is to do bypass graft.

ILIOFEMORAL STENOTIC DISEASE

- This can be repaired by a bypass graft which is sutured to the normal common iliac above and to the normal femoral artery below (Fig. 7.9).
- If patients are unfit for a major vascular bypass, angioplasty can be done.
- In this procedure, a balloon catheter is inserted into the artery and it is inflated and its correct position is confirmed by radio-opaque markers which are present in

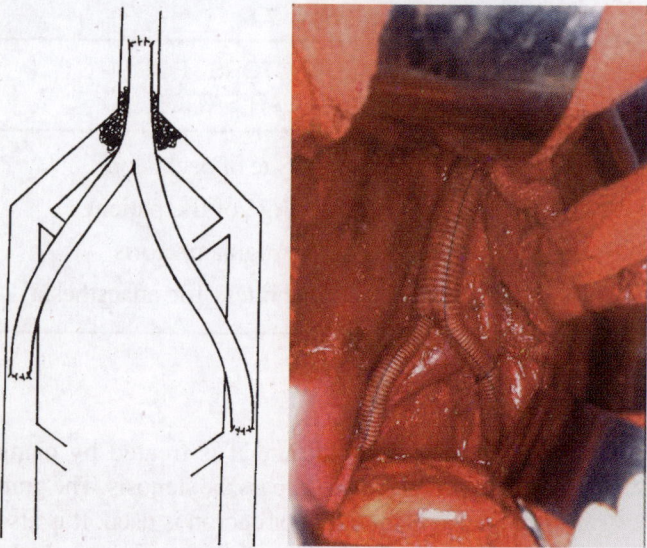

Fig. 7.8 & 7.9 Aortobifemoral graft- contributed by Dr. Ganesh Kamath - Professor, Cardiothoracic Surgery

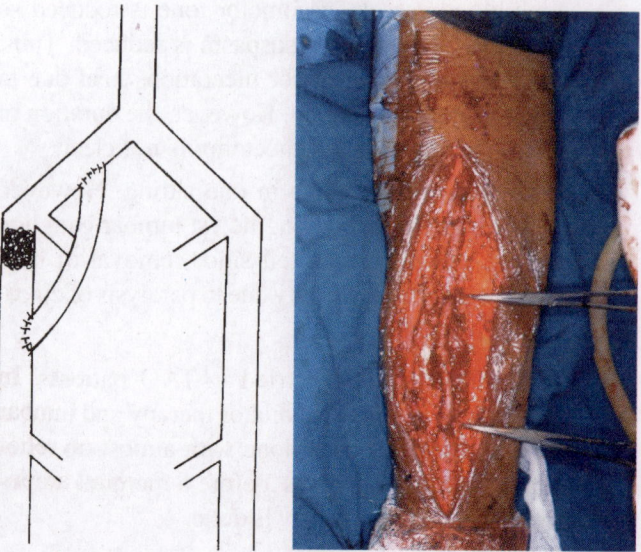

Fig. 7.10 & 7.11 Iliofemoral graft by using reversed saphenous vein

the balloon. By inflation and dilation technique 2-3 times, the stenosed segment can be dilated.

- Any arterial stenosis can be dilated in angioplasty.
- Technique can be repeated if stenosis recurs.
- The procedure is done under local anaesthesia and is indicated in poor risk patients.
- **Ideally suitable for iliofemoral segment**, not suitable for below knee stenosed vessels.
- Internal dissection, distal embolization, thrombosis and even rupture of vessel can occur.
- Recently, angioplasty combined with LASER to drill holes through short stenosis have been employed.

FEMOROPOPLITEAL OCCLUSION

- This is treated by using a graft extending from the femoral artery above, to the popliteal artery below
- Reversed long saphenous vein is better than other grafts.
- Dacron graft, polytetrafluoroethylene graft (PTFE), human umbilical vein graft are the other grafts.

PROFUNDA ARTERY STENOSIS

- Significant occlusion of profunda is demonstrated by oblique views in an arteriography. If there are no significant vessels available below the stenosis for reconstruction, profundoplasty is considered. It is done by using a patch of Dacron or vein to widen the origin of this vessel after doing endarterectomy.

Key Box 7.9	
SUMMARY OF THE REVASCULARIZATION SURGERY	
Aortoiliac disease	Aortobifemoral or aortofemoral graft and endarterectomy
Iliofemoral disease	Iliofemoral bypass graft Balloon angioplasty
Femoropopliteal disease	Bypass graft
Profunda artery stenosis	Profundoplasty

ACUTE ARTERIAL OCCLUSION

- Sudden occlusion of an artery is commonly due to emboli, increased incidence of road traffic accidents, fall or war injuries. Trauma to the artery also produces occlusion.

EMBOLIC OCCLUSION (Key Box 7.10)

- This commonly occurs in the peripheral arteries such as the common iliac, femoral and popliteal.
- An embolus is a foreign body to the bloodstream, it gets lodged in a vessel and produces obstruction and clinically manifests as severe ischaemia or gangrene, resulting in **Critical Limb Ischaemia (CLI)**.

- Mural thrombus following a myocardial infarction (MI)
- Mural thrombus due to mitral stenosis and atrial fibrillation
- Atheromatous plaque
- Aneurysm
- Emboli from myxoma of the heart
- Valve vegetations

What is Critical Limb Ischaemia (CLI) ?

It is defined as persistently recurring ischaemic rest pain requiring regular, adequate analgesia for more than 2 weeks or ulceration or gangrene of foot or toes with an ankle pressure of < 50 mmHg or a toe systolic pressure of < 30 mm Hg.

- Atherosclerotic vascular disease, thrombo-angitis obliterans, acute embolic ischaemia and even diabetes etc. at one stage or other can present as CLI.

Clinical features

- No previous history suggestive of intermittent claudication
- Sudden dramatic symptoms which are described in the form of 5P's
    - **Pain**
    - **Pallor**
    - **Paresis**
    - **Pulselessness**
    - **Paraesthesia**

1. **Pain** is severe, unbearable. burning or bursting type.
2. Limb is **pale**, cold and superficial veins are collapsed.
3. **Paresis** : Depending on the level of occlusion, the function of the limb is lost. Movement of the toes becomes difficult, followed by total paralysis.
4. **Pulselessness** : Characteristically, peripheral pulses below the level of embolism are not palpable.
5. **Altered sensation** in the limb.
    - If left untreated, necrosis of the muscles followed by gangrene of the limb can occur within a few hours (6-24 hours).
    - Cardiac examination may reveal the source of emboli.

Intravenous drug abuse remains a major risk factor for endocarditis and embolic complications.

Pathology (Fig. 7.12)

Investigations

- Peripheral circulation should be assessed by Doppler ultrasound, which is an excellent noninvasive investigation to judge the severity, level, position, length of superficial femoral artery stenosis.
- Digital subtraction angiography is indicated in aortoiliac lesions.

Treatment

I. Angioplasty : Percutaneous transluminal angioplasty (PTA) is **indicated in short stenotic lesions in large vessel.** eg. : Iliac and femoro-popliteal lesions.

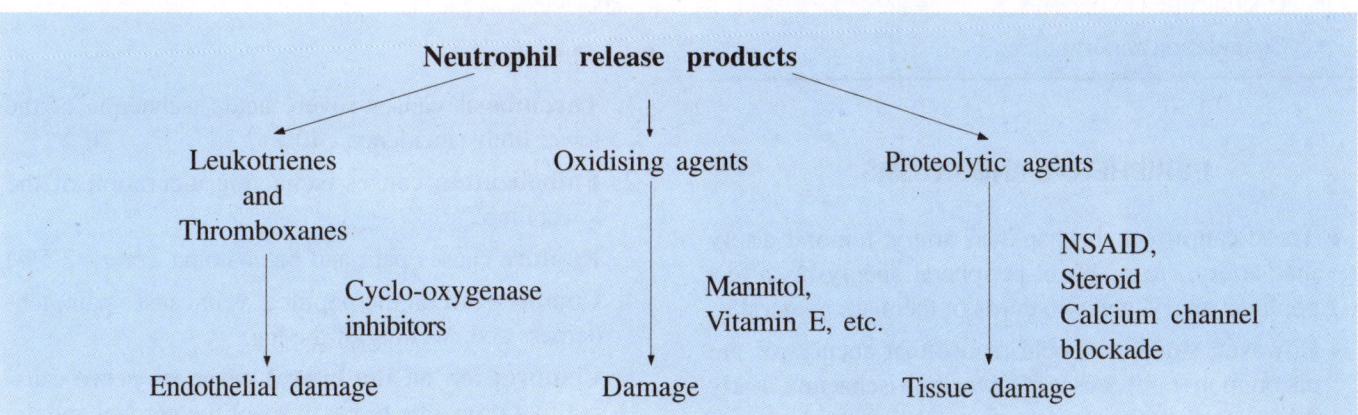

Fig. 7.12 Pathogenesis of tissue damage

- First, the balloon catheter is introduced percutaneously over a guidewire across the lesion. Under fluoroscopic control, the balloon is dilated, till satisfactory widening of lumen is achieved.

- Relatively safe and simple procedure.

- Immediate intravenous infusion of heparin (5000-10000 units) is necessary to reduce the extension of the thromboembolism.

II. Emergency embolectomy is done under G/A or local anaesthesia either by direct arteriotomy incision removing the clot or by using a Fogarty balloon catheter to remove an embolus from a vessel remote from arteriotomy.

III. Thrombolysis: It is indicated in acute or acute on chronic ischaemia. A fine lysis catheter is passed percutaneously into blocked vessel. Streptokinase is infused at a rate of 5000 I.U. in 10 ml per hour. It will reopen the occluded lumen within 24 hours. Repeat angiogram is necessary to check for patency.

- For contraindications see Key Box 7.11.

Key Box 7.11

CONTRAINDICATIONS TO THROMBOLYTIC THERAPY

Absolute
- Recent major bleeding
- Recent major surgery
- Recent ophthalmologic procedure
- Recent stroke

Relative
- Active peptic ulcer disease
- Pregnancy
- Uncontrolled hypertension
- Coagulation abnormalities

PERIPHERAL ANEURYSMS

- These can affect the popliteal artery, femoral artery iliac artery, etc., 70% of peripheral aneurysms affect popliteal artery, and two thirds of them are bilateral.

- However, students should realise that aneurysms are uncommon (rare) causes of lower limb ischaemia. Early diagnosis and effective treatment is essential to save the limb.

POPLITEAL ANEURYSMS

They are the **commonest peripheral aneurysms** because of following reasons:

1. Turbulence beyond stenosis at the adductor magnus hiatus
2. Repeated flexion at the knee

Clinical features

- They affect elderly patients and atherosclerosis is the cause. One third of the cases are associated with aortic aneurysm.

- Age at presentation is 65 years

- Striking preponderance in males - male female ratio is 20-30:1. Presents as a swelling behind the knee

- Dull aching pain is common

- Severe bursting pain indicates rapid expansion and impending rupture.

- Pulsatile, tense, cystic, fluctuant swelling behind the knee, in the popliteal fossa in the line of popliteal artery.

- Size diminishes on extending the knee as the aneurysm is deep to popliteal fascia.

- **Proximal compression test** : On occluding the femoral artery proximally the swelling may diminish in size.

In all cases of popliteal aneurysm please search for femoral and aortic aneurysm

Investigations

- Duplex ultrasonography is the investigation of choice which can measure diameter and determine extent of mural thrombus.

- Angiography can demonstrate the extent of involved segment to look for patency and quality of runoff vessels.

Complications

1. **Thrombosis** causes severe acute ischaemia of the lower limb. (incidence - 40%)
2. **Embolization** causes ischaemic ulceration of the lower limb.
3. **Rupture** causes pain and haematoma. (rare - 2-5%)
4. **Compression** on the popliteal vein causes pain, tenderness and swelling of the leg.
5. **Compression on the lateral peroneal nerve** causing foot drop, due to paralysis of the peronei and the extensors of the foot.

Treatment

- **Proximal and distal ligation of the artery** followed by reversed saphenous vein bypass graft is the treatment of choice. This method results in total obliteration of the sac with revascularisation of the limb.
- **Excision of the sac is better avoided** because of chances of injury to the popliteal vein and nerves. Lateral popliteal nerve injury causes foot drop and tibial (medial popliteal) nerve injury causes thinning of the calf region, inability to plantar flex the ankle and clawing of the toes due to paralysis of the intrinsic muscles of the foot.

Miscellaneous

AINHUM

It affects those who do not use footwear or walk barefoot. Starts as a fissure at the level of interphalyngeal joint of a toe, usually fifth. Repeated trauma of minor degree may be present. The tissue becomes a fibrous band resulting in tight constriction and necrosis. If it continues it may land with autoamputation.

- The division of band or early Z-plasty may be needed to avoid amputation.
- Thrombolysis with catheter in situ, in early cases

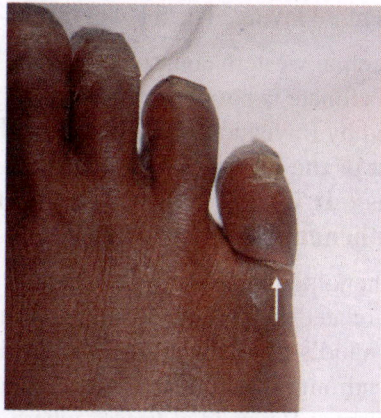

Fig. 7.13 Ainhum

FROSTBITE

- It occurs due to too much of exposure to cold weather.
- High altitudes with excessive cold precipitates vasospasm and damage to the blood vessel wall. It causes sludging of blood and thrombosis.
- Malnutrition, ageing process are the other precipitating

factors. Severe burning pain, discolouration of foot, development of blisters suggest gangrene is imminent.

Treatment

- Slow warming of the parts and protection with cotton wool
- Analgesics, antibiotics
- Paravertebral injection into the sympathetic chain helps in a few patients
- Elevation of the foot to reduce oedema
- Frank cases of frost bite with gangrene require conservative amputation.

REPERFUSION INJURIES OR SYNDROME

- This dangerous event follow revascularisation of limbs, resulting in **acute compartment syndrome** with pressure beyond capillary pressure (30 mm Hg)
- Sequence of events are as follows:

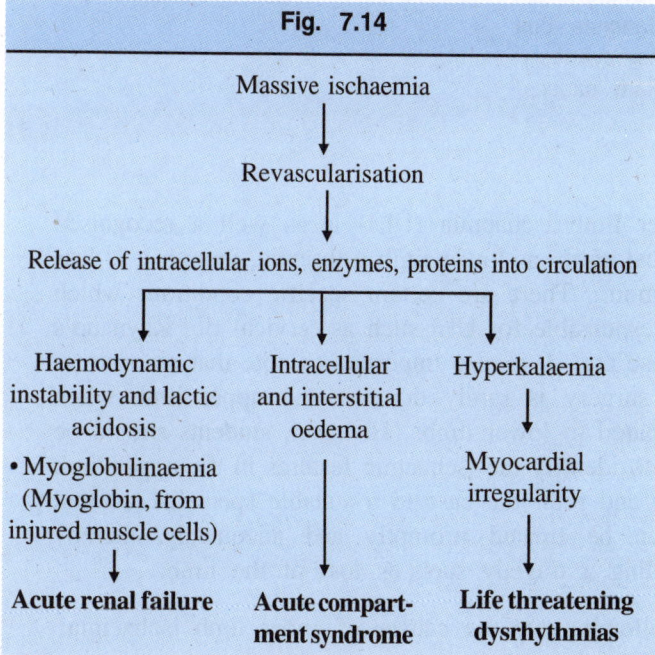

Fig. 7.14

Massive ischaemia
↓
Revascularisation
↓
Release of intracellular ions, enzymes, proteins into circulation

Haemodynamic instability and lactic acidosis
- Myoglobulinaemia (Myoglobin, from injured muscle cells)
↓
Acute renal failure

Intracellular and interstitial oedema
↓
Acute compartment syndrome

Hyperkalaemia
↓
Myocardial irregularity
↓
Life threatening dysrhythmias

- However most of the injury is believed to be due to oxygen derived free radicals - the most important ones include superoxide radical, hydrogen peroxide and hydroxyl radical. These radicals attach unsaturated bonds of fatty acids within the phospholipid membranes resulting in damage.

Management

- Diagnosis by severe pain in the limb, oedema of the leg, muscle tenderness, raised intra compartmental pressure measured by transducer cannula.
- Treated by multiple fasciotomy

Upper Limb Ischaemia and Gangrene

8

- Raynaud's disease
- Thoracic outlet syndrome
- Axillary vein thrombosis
- Vasculitis syndrome
- Gangrene
- Cancrum oris
- Acrocyanosis
- Rare causes

Upper limb ischaemia (ULI) is as well a recognised clinical entity as lower limb ischaemia, though it is less common. There are certain specific conditions which are responsible for ULI such as cervical rib, Raynaud's disease etc. It is also important to note that reconstructive surgery is rarely done in the upper limb when compared to lower limb. However, students should be able to identify the ischaemic features in the upper limb early and refer the case to a suitable specialist, so that it can be treated promptly and adequately, thereby avoiding a tragedy such as loss of the limb.

Following are the causes of upper limb ischaemia:

1. Raynaud's disease and Raynaud's syndrome
2. Embolic causes (Page 67)
3. Thoracic outlet syndrome
4. Trauma
5. Buerger's disease
6. Atherosclerotic vascular disease of upper limb
7. Axillary vein thrombosis

8. **Vasculitis syndromes**

   Takayasu's arteritis

   Giant cell arteritis

   Polyarteritis nodosa

   Systemic sclerosis - Scleroderma,- **CREST Syndrome**

RAYNAUD'S DISEASE (PRIMARY RAYNAUD'S PHENOMENON)

It occurs in young women, commonly

Upper limb is more involved than lower limb

Commonly seen in western countries in white-skinned people. Cold climate is possibly a precipitating factor. First described by Raynaud as **bilateral episodic digital ischaemia of the upper limb** on exposure to cold and emotions. **It is also referred to as primary Raynaud's phenomenon**.

Raynaud's phenomenon is the blanket term used to describe cold-related digital vasospasm (see pathophysiology). Raynaud's phenomenon is subdivided into Raynaud's syndrome where there is an associated disorder, and primary Raynaud's disease where there is NOT.

CREST syndrome: **C**alcinosis circumscripta, **R**aynaud's phenomenon, (O) **E**sophageal defects, **S**clerodactyly, **T**elangiectasia.

Causes of **Secondary Raynaud's** phenomenon are given in the Key Box 8.1.

Key Box 8.1

SECONDARY RAYNAUD'S PHENOMENON CAUSES

- Atherosclerosis
- Scleroderma
- Systemic lupus
- Cervical rib
- Carpal tunnel syndrome
- Vibrating tools - **Vibration white finger**

PATHOPHYSIOLOGY

On exposure to cold[1], some kind of discomfort and colour changes are observed. This is due to abnormal sensitivity of the arterioles to cold. Three stages have been described.

1. **Stage of syncope** : Arterioles undergo constriction as an abnormal response to cold. As a result of this, the part becomes blanched and severe pallor develops.

2. **Stage of asphyxia** : After a brief period of vasoconstriction, capillaries dilate, filling with deoxygenated blood resulting in bluish discolouration of the part (cyanosis).

3. **Stage of recovery or stage of rubor** : As the attack passes off, relaxation of the arterioles occur, circulation improves and redness occurs. Because of dilatation of capillaries, red engorgement of the part occurs, which causes tingling, burning or bursting pain in the fingers.

CLINICAL FEATURES

Affects young women

Typically causes bilateral episodic digital ischaemia on exposure to cold

Thumb is usually spared

Peripheral pulses are normal

Pallor, cyanosis and rubor are the colour changes during the attack along with the pain

In a few patients, because of recurrent attacks, gangrenous patches occur on the tip of the fingers (superficial necrosis).

DIFFERENTIAL DIAGNOSIS

Cervical rib

Vasculitis syndromes

TAO affecting the upper limb usually affects male smokers. Peripheral pulses are feeble or weak.

TREATMENT

I. **Conservative line of treatment**:

Reassurance

Avoid unnecessary exposure to cold

Avoid smoking

Calcium antagonists such as nifedipine 10-20 mgs, two times a day may be beneficial.

If these measures fail, surgery is undertaken.

II. **Cervical sympathectomy** : (Key Box 8.2 and 8.3)

In this operation sympathetic trunk from the lower half of the stellate ganglion to just below the 3rd thoracic ganglion is removed.

Upper 1/2 of the stellate ganglion is preserved to avoid Horner's syndrome.

All rami communicantes associated with the 2nd and 3rd ganglion are removed.

Nerve of Kuntz, a grey ramus which springs from the 2nd thoracic ganglion to the 1st thoracic nerve is also divided.

Commonly done through a supraclavicular route and axillary route. Lap sympathectomy is becoming popular.

Effect seems to be temporary

However, the severity of the disease is reduced.

Sympathectomy raises the threshold at which spasm occurs.

Key Box 8.2

INDICATIONS FOR CERVICAL SYMPATHECTOMY

1. Raynaud's disease
2. Cervical rib
3. TAO
4. Causalgia
5. Hyperhidrosis

---

1. Cold refers to temperature - cold climate (winter) cold enviornment (refrigerator), or cold substance like cold water or ice piece.

Key Box 8.3

COMPLICATIONS OF CERVICAL SYMPATHECTOMY

1. Perforation of pleura causing pneumothorax
2. Lymph fistula due to injury to thoracic duct
3. Horner's syndrome
4. Injury to the accessory nerve
5. Haemorrhage

THORACIC OUTLET SYNDROME

CAUSES

Cervical rib

Scalenus anticus syndrome

Costoclavicular syndrome

Hyperabduction syndrome

Abnormal rib and clavicle

Malaligned fracture clavicle

Long C_7 transverse process

Hypertrophy of subclavius muscle as in **butterfly swimmers.**

Surgical anatomy of thoracic outlet and pathophysiology of cervical rib with compression (Key Box 8.4 and 8.5)

Thoracic outlet is a tight space with bony structures all around such as manubrium sternum in the front, spine posteriorly and first rib laterally.

At the root of the neck, brachial plexus and subclavian artery pass through scalene triangle into the axilla.

Scalenus triangle is the posterior compartment of costoclavicular space, the division of anterior and posterior is by scalenus anticus. The anterior compartment contains subclavian vein.

Boundaries of scalene triangle (Fig.8.1).

- Base : First thoracic rib
- Anteromedially : Scalenus anticus
- Posterolaterally : Scalenus medius

If the base (the first thoracic rib) is raised by interposition of cervical rib, it results in compression of the subclavian artery (Key Box 8.4).

Due to slow compression, artery distal to the compression dilates due to jet like effect and turbulence of blood flow. This is described as post-stenotic dilatation (VENTURI effect) (Fig. 8.2 and Key Box 8.5).

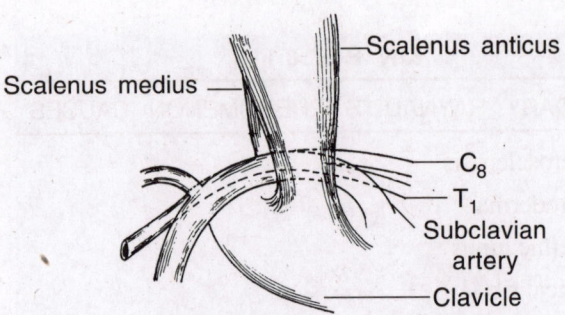

Fig. 8.1 Scalene triangle

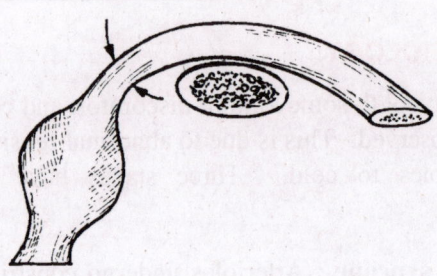

Fig. 8.2 Post-stenotic dilatation

In this dilated segment, small multiple thrombi develop, which, when dislodged, result in ischaemia. Vascular symptoms are strictly unilateral.

Key Box 8.4

CAUSES OF SUBCLAVIAN ARTERY COMPRESSION

- Cervical rib
- Clavicle
- Callus due to fracture
- Congenital abnormality - abnormal first rib
- Scalenus anticus muscle

Key Box 8.5

SUBCALVIAN ARTERY OCCLUSION - EFFECTS

Lumen narrowing
↓
Fibrosis or thickening of arterial wall
↓
Stenosis
↓
Post-stenotic dilatation
↓
Multiple thrombi→ Embolism→ Ischaemia

CERVICAL RIB

This is an extra rib present in the neck in about 1-2% of the population.

Commonly unilateral and in some cases it is bilateral.

It is more frequently encountered on the right side.

It is the anterior tubercle of the transverse process of the 7th cervical vertebra which attains excessive development and results in cervical rib.

Types of Cervical Rib (Fig. 8.3)

Type I   The free end of the cervical rib is expanded into a hard, bony mass which can be felt in the neck.

Type II   Complete cervical rib extends from C7 vertebra posteriorly to the manubrium anteriorly.

Type III Incomplete cervical rib, which is partly bony, partly fibrous.

Type IV A complete fibrous band which gives rise to symptoms but cannot be diagnosed by X-ray.

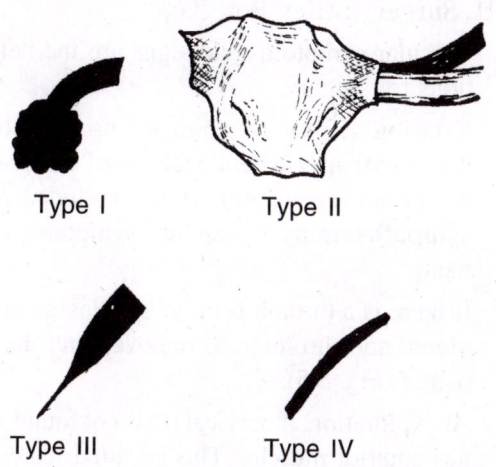

Type I   Type II

Type III   Type IV

Fig. 8.3 Four types of cervical rib

Clinical features

1. Common in **young females**. Even though congenital, symptoms appear only at or after puberty. This is because of the development of shoulder girdle muscles and sagging of the shoulder which narrows the root of the neck. Nerve roots C_8, T_1 are stretched by completion of growth around 25 years.

2. Dull aching pain in the neck is caused by expanded bony end of cervical rib.

3. **Features of upper limb ischaemia**

   Claudication pain is brought about by usage of arm

with muscle wasting. Low temperature, pallor, excessive sweating (vasomotor disturbances), **splinter haemorrhages**, ischaemic ulcers in fingers and gangrene of the skin of the fingers are the other features. Peripheral pulses may be absent/feeble. Oedema and venous distension are very rare. These are called vascular symptoms of cervical rib.

4. **Features of ulnar nerve paralysis** or weakness (lower nerve roots involvement, mainly first thoracic nerve) manifest as paralysis of interosseus muscles, wasting of hypothenar muscles, tingling and numbness, or paraesthesia in the distribution of C_8, T_1.

   The following are the tests which confirm ulnar nerve weakness. It includes sensory disturbances and motor disturbances (performing fine action - writing, buttoning, etc.)

a. **Card test**: Patient is asked to hold a thin paper or a card in between the fingers. In cases of ulnar nerve paralysis, due to weakness of interossei muscles, patient is unable to hold the card tightly.

b. **Froment's sign**: Patient is asked to hold a book between the hand and the thumb. In cases of ulnar nerve paralysis, since the adductor pollicis is paralysed, there is flexion at the distal interphalangeal joint of the thumb. This is because **flexor pollicis longus** which is **supplied by median nerve, contracts**.

5. **A hard mass** may be visible or may be palpable in the root of the neck. (Type I).

6. On palpation of supraclavicular region, a **thrill** and on auscultation, a **bruit** can be heard in cases of post-stenotic dilatation.

7. **Adson's test**: Feel radial pulse, ask the patient to take deep inspiration and turn the neck to the same side. The pulse may disappear or it may become feeble. This test indicates compression on subclavian artery.

8. **Hyperabduction test (Halsted test)**: This test is done to rule out hyperabduction syndrome caused by pectoralis minor. The radial pulse becomes weak on hyperabduction due to angulation of axillary vessels and brachial plexus, which gets compressed between pectoralis minor and its attachment to the coracoid process.

9. **Military attitude test**: When shoulders are set in backward and downward position the radial pulse becomes weak, this is due to the compression of subclavian artery between the clavicle and first rib. **This is seen in costoclavicular syndrome**.

10. **Allen's test**: Patient is asked to clench his fist tightly,

compress the radial artery and ulnar artery at the wrist with the thumbs. Wait for 10 seconds, ask the patient to open his hands. Pallor can be seen in the palm. Now release radial artery pressure and watch for the blood flow. If there is digital artery occlusion it will be evident when colour changes occur in the fingers slowly.

11. **Elevated Arm Stress Test-EAST (Roos)**: Patient is asked to abduct the shoulders to 90° and to flex the elbow. Then he is asked to pronate/supinate forearms continuously. Appearance of symptoms suggest thoracic outlet syndrome.

Differential diagnosis

A patient who presents with a few neurological symptoms and signs in the upper limb with a cervical rib may be having some other causes for those symptoms. Hence, it is important to exclude other causes.

1. **Cervical spondylosis**: This should be considered as a possibility in patients above the age of 40 years.

2. **Cervical disc protrusion and spinal cord tumours** may mimic cervical rib with predominant neurological feature.

3. **Carpal tunnel syndrome** can occur due to various causes like myxoedema, rheumatoid arthritis, malunited Colle's fracture, etc. Predominant features of median nerve involvement, more so in menopausal women gives a clue to the diagnosis.

4. **Raynaud's phenomenon**

5. **Costovertebral anomalies**

6. **Pancoast tumour**

Investigations

1. X-ray neck may show a cervical rib (Type I, II & III). Interestingly Type IV variety, a fibrous band which cannot be diagnosed by X-ray or by any other investigation, usually gives rise to symptoms.

2. Cervical disc protrusion and spinal cord tumours may mimic cervical rib with predominant neurological features.

Treatment: (Summary - Table 8.1)

I. Conservative:

Patients with mild neurological symptoms are managed by shoulder girdle exercises or correction of faulty posture.

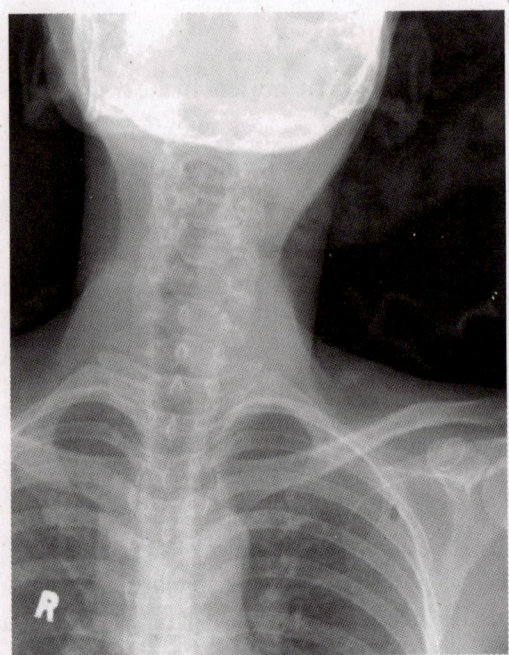

Fig. 8.4 X-ray of the neck showing cervical rib

II. Surgery : (Key Box. 8.6)

Vascular symptoms and signs are the definite indications for surgery.

Excision of cervical rib including periosteum: This is called **extraperiosteal excision** of cervical rib (so that it will not regenerate). This is included with **cervical sympathectomy** if vascular symptoms are predominant.

If there is a thrombus in the subclavian artery, it is explored and thrombus is removed and the artery is repaired (Fig. 8.5).

At exploration, if cervical rib is not found, divide scalenus anterior muscle. This is called scalenotomy (Key Box 8.7).

- If **hyperabduction syndrome** is diagnosed, **pectoralis minor is divided** from its insertion into the coracoid process.

Key Box 8.6
CERVICAL RIB SURGERY
• Remove cervical rib
• Repair subclavian artery
• Restore circulation
• Reduce vasospasm - Sympathectomy
• Recognise other causes

Table 8.1 Flowchart of summary of cervical rib

CERVICAL RIB

↓

SYMPTOMS

↓

LOCAL	**NEUROLOGICAL**	**VASCULAR**
• Pain	• Tingling and numbness	• Claudication pain
• Visible lump	• Muscle wasting	• Cold and pale hand
• Asymptomatic	• Muscle paralysis	• Ulcers of the fingers

SIGNS

• Visible lump	• Weakness	• Weak pulses
• Hard lump	• Wasting of hypothenar muscles	• Ulcer or gangrene
• Fixed lump	• Card test, Froment's sign	• Adson's test positive

TREATMENT

↓

Exercises ——— Failure ———→

Cervical sympathectomy
+
Extraperiosteal excision

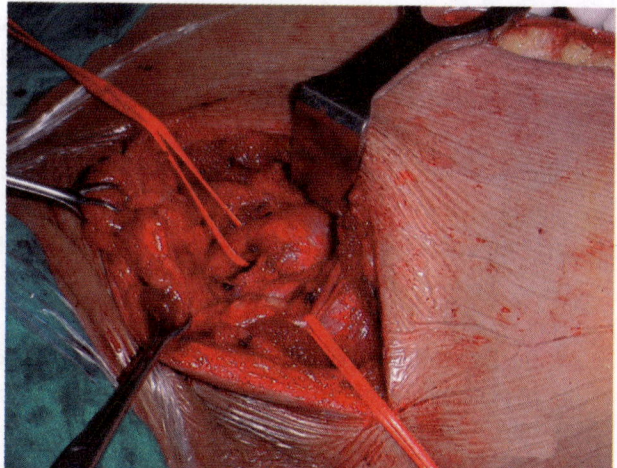

Fig. 8.5 Subclavian artery exposed to repair the dilatation and removal of the thrombus

Key Box 8.7
IF CERVICAL RIB IS NOT FOUND

• Scalenotomy
• Division of pectoralis minor
• Extraperiosteal resection of the first rib

AXILLARY VEIN THROMBOSIS

Patients present with swelling of arm after intense activity from the dominant hand.

Hypertrophy of subclavius muscle also can cause compression of subclavian-axillary vein (Sportsman).

Peripheral pulses will be normal.

Venography to diagnose thrombus

Thrombolysis or if necessary venotomy, removal of the thrombus and 1st rib (if it is the cause of obstruction) are the treatment modalities.

VASCULITIS SYNDROMES

TAKAYASU'S ARTERITIS (Pulseless disease)

It is of unknown etiology.

Commonly affects females (85%)

It is a panarteritis involving aortic arch and its branches - subclavian artery is involved in 85% of the cases.

Clinical features : It starts as a generalised inflammatory disease - fever, body ache, malaise, arthralgia, etc.

Key Box 8.8
VASCULITIS SYNDROMES

- Etiology is inflammatory or immunological
- Uncommon causes of upper and lower limb ischaemia
- Women are affected more than men.
- Multiple small vessel involvement
- Symptoms are confusing - depending upon organ involvement
- Ischaemic changes are minimal and superficial when it involves the limbs
- Steroids are useful in controlling the disease
- Immunosuppression should be tried carefully

Upper limb claudication (Key Box 8.8)

Absence of peripheral pulses

Hypertension is common in 50% of the cases due to renal artery involvement.

Bruit may be heard over the subclavian artery.

Visual disturbances can occur due to involvement of retinal arteries - late blindness can occur.

Pathology

It is a **panarteritis**, involving all layers of elastic arteries - Later thrombosis and stenosis can occur.

Investigations

C - reactive protein is elevated as a part of acute phase response (nonspecific).

Duplex-Doppler Ultrasound, MR angiography can diagnose the site of obstruction and blood flow pattern.

Treatment

Very early cases are benefitted with tablet **prednisolone 30 to 50 mg/day** (antiinflammatory effect). Cyclophosphamide can be tried when other measures fail (Immunosuppressive effect).

Vascular reconstruction - difficult

GIANT CELL ARTERITIS

It is also called as temporal arteritis

Elderly women presenting with severe headache is the common presentation.

Fever, malaise may also be present.

Key Box 8.9	
VESSEL INVOLVED	SYMPTOMS

- Temporal artery — headache
- Facial artery — jaw pain
- Retinal artery — sudden blindness
- Upper limb artery — claudication
- Coronary artery — myocardial infarction

Involvement of various arteries will result in various symptoms. (Key Box 8.9)

Palpable, pulsatile, tender temporal arteries will clinch the diagnosis.

Biopsy of the temporal arteries will reveal giant cell granuloma, comprising mainly CD_4+T lymphocytes.

Treated by prednisolone 60-80mg/day slowly tapered over 1-2 years.

Relapses and remissions are common.

POLYARTERITIS SYNDROME

This includes microscopic polyarteritis (commonly) and polyarteritis nodosa (less often).

This syndrome also has an inflammatory reaction.

Ischaemia of the lower limbs and upper limbs can occur due to involvement of small vessels.

Abdominal pain is due to involvement of visceral vessels.

Involvement of renal arteries cause loin pain, haematuria and hypertension.

Treatment is similar to other diseases mentioned above.

SYSTEMIC SCLEROSIS – SCLERODERMA

Earlier called as collagen vascular disorder because of obstruction of the small vessels by collagen deposition.

Now included under vasculitis syndromes because of their association with inflammatory reaction.

Ischaemic changes occur in the fingers and toes - necrosis and ulceration is common.

Oesophageal involvement results in dysphagia.

Small bowels sclerosis results in disordered motility and malabsorption.

Sympathectomy and vasodilators may be useful.

Raynaud's symptoms can be controlled by calcium channel blockers and nitrates.

GANGRENE

DEFINITION

Macroscopic death of tissue with superadded putrefaction. It affects the limbs (Figs. 8.5 and 8.6), intestines, appendix, etc. In this chapter differential diagnosis of causes of gangrene of the limbs is considered.

PREGANGRENE

Rest pain, colour changes at rest and at exercises, oedema, hyperaesthesia, skin ulcerations are due to inadequate blood supply to the limb. These changes are described as pregangrenous changes in the limb.

CLASSIFICATION OF GANGRENE

1. **Cardiovascular causes**
   TAO (Page 61)
   Atherosclerotic gangrene
   Acute embolic gangrene
   Syphilitic gangrene
   Raynaud's disease
   Cervical rib
   Vasculitis syndrome
   Polycythaemia

2. **Neurological causes**
   Hemiplegia, paraplegia, bed sore

3. **Traumatic gangrene**
   Direct - thrombosis; indirect - crushing injuries

4. **Physical causes**
   Sun rays, radiation, corrosive acids

5. **Drugs** - Ergotamine

6. **Diabetic** gangrene

7. **Acute infective gangrene**
   Boil, carbuncle, cancrum oris, gas gangrene

CLINICAL FEATURES OF GANGRENE

A part which is gangrenous is a dead portion of the body. It has **no arterial pulsations**, venous return or capillary filling.

It has no sensation.

The colour initially will be pale and later it changes to dusky grey and finally black. The **black colour** is due to disintegration of haemoglobin and formation of iron sulphide.

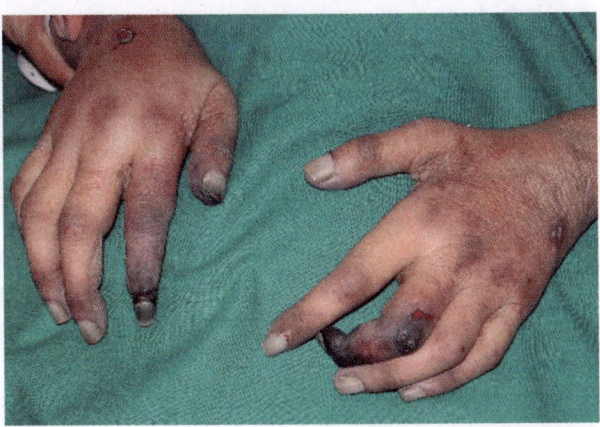

Fig. 8.6 Gangrene of the two fingers in a case of vasculitis syndrome (uncommon)

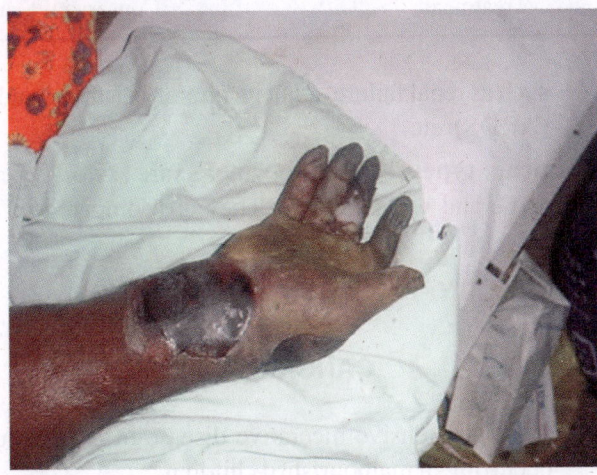

Fig. 8.7 Gangrene of the upper limb following acute embolism

The gangrenous part has to be treated by surgical excision or debridement, which may amount to either disarticulation of the toe or even an amputation.

The gram-positive, gram-negative and anaerobic organisms multiply in this segment and can produce septicaemia. Thus, this may precipitate multi-organ failure

Key Box 8.10
SIGNS OF GANGRENE
• Loss of pulsation
• Loss of colour
• Loss of temperature
• Loss of sensation
• Loss of function

Table 8.2 Comparison of dry gangrene and wet gangrene

	DRY GANGRENE	WET GANGRENE
Cause	Slow occlusion of the arteries	Sudden occlusion of the arteries
Involvement of part	Small area is gangrenous due to presence of collaterals	Large area is affected due to absence of collaterals
Local findings	Dry, shrivelled and mummified	Wet, turgid, swollen, oedematous
Line of demarcation	Usually present	Absent
Crepitus	Absent	May be present
Odour	Absent	Foul odour due to sulphurated hydrogen produced by putrefactive bacteria
Infection	Not present	Usually present
Diseases	TAO, atherosclerosis	Emboli, ligatures, crush injuries, etc.
Treatment	Conservative amputation	Major amputation is necessary

such as renal failure, adult respiratory distress syndrome (ARDS) etc.

Clinical types: Basically there are two types-dry gangrene and wet gangrene. They are compared in Table 8.2.

SPECIAL TYPES OF GANGRENE

CANCRUM ORIS

It is an extensive ulcerative disease of cheek mucosa occurring in malnourished children.

Precipitating factors are :

- Malnourishment

- Major disease like diphtheria, whooping cough, typhoid, measles, kala azar, etc.

As a result of these factors the opportunistic organisms like Vincent's organisms - *Borrelia vincentii* and fusiformis multiply and cause multiple ulcers, erosions, later fibrosis.

As the disease progresses sometimes the whole thickness of the cheek may be lost.

Treatment of cancrum oris

1. Ryle's tube feeding
2. Improve the nutrition
3. Appropriate antibiotics: Metronidazole 400 mg three times a day for 7-10 days
4. Reconstructive surgery may be necessary later.

Complications of cancrum oris

1. Fibrosis causing restriction of the movement of jaw.
2. Septicaemia, toxaemia and death.

ACROCYANOSIS

It is also called as hereditary cold extremities

Persistent cyanotic discolouration of hands when exposed to cold is a feature.

This is brought about by intermittent spasm of small peripheral vessels - commonly affects hands, rarely feet also.

Generally it is mild and nonprogressive.

DRUG ABUSE AND GANGRENE

Abuse of the drugs is an important cause of gangrene in the modern days.

Inadvertent injection of drugs into artery, results in thrombosis of the artery resulting in acute ischaemia-commonly in the femoral artery.

Emergency treatment in symptomatic cases include - heparinisation, infusion of dextran.

In severe cases, emergency angiography and intra-arterial thrombolysis is considered.

Iatrogenic drug induced gangrene

Inadvertent intra-arterial injection of thiopentone into one of the high divisions of brachial artery, (*congenital anomaly*) usually the ulnar, will result in severe burning and blanching of the hand.

VARIOUS TYPES OF GANGRENE

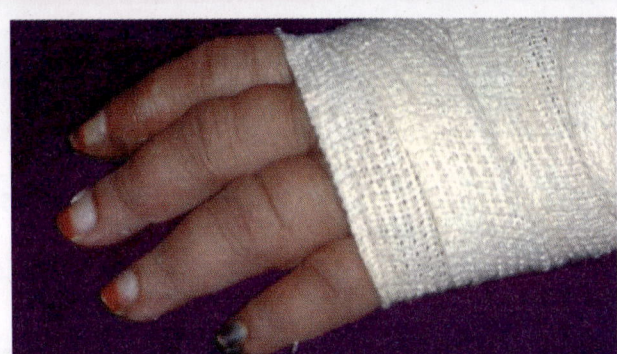

Fig. 8.10 Gangrene of the fingers in a case of polycythaemia vera

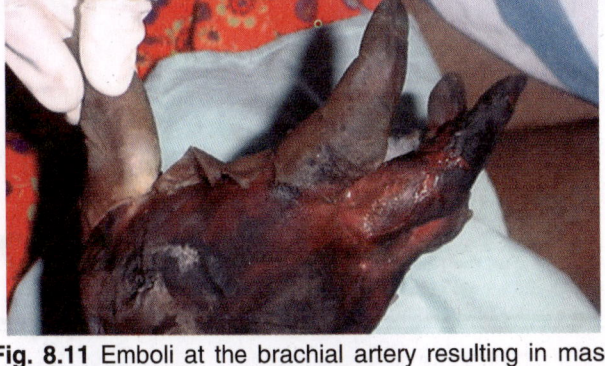

Fig. 8.11 Emboli at the brachial artery resulting in massive gangrene of the hand (wet gangrene)

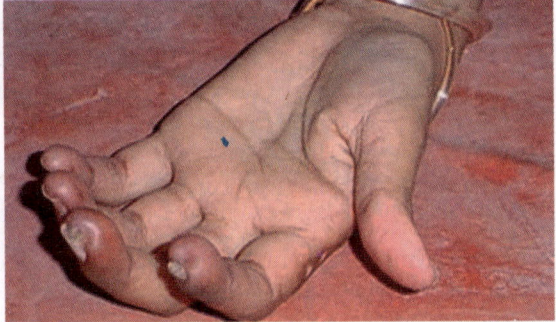

Fig. 8.9 Case of SLE - Observe pulp of the fingers

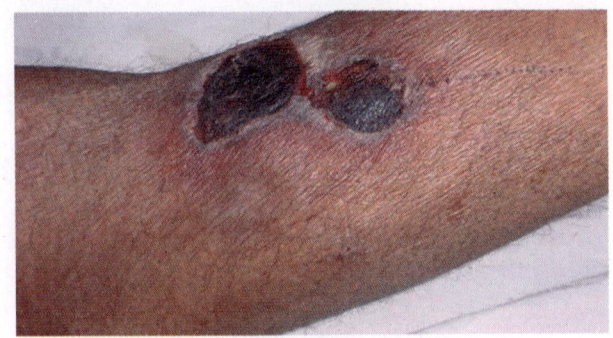

Fig. 8.12 Drug induced gangrene - caused by Ibuprofen

- If this complication is noticed following steps (measures) have to be taken immediately)

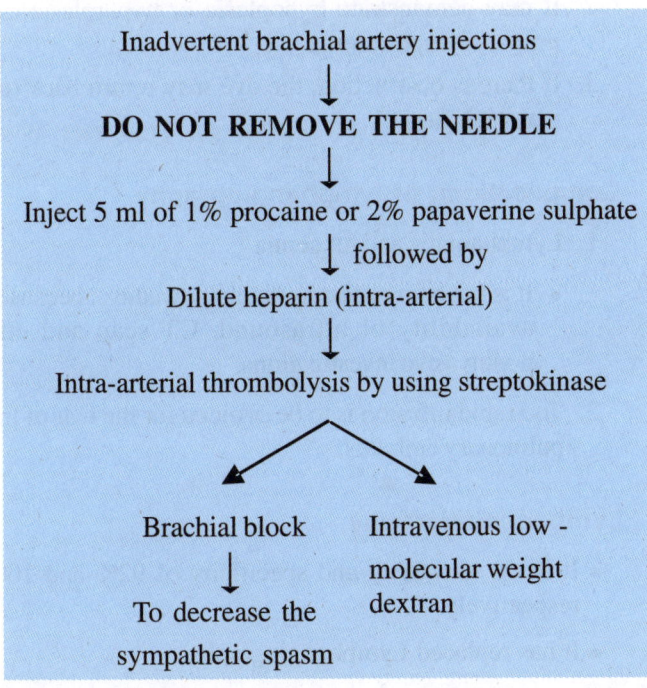

Inadvertent brachial artery injections

↓

DO NOT REMOVE THE NEEDLE

↓

Inject 5 ml of 1% procaine or 2% papaverine sulphate

↓ followed by

Dilute heparin (intra-arterial)

↓

Intra-arterial thrombolysis by using streptokinase

Brachial block

↓

To decrease the sympathetic spasm

Intravenous low - molecular weight dextran

Fig. 8.8 Management of Inadvertent brachial artery injections

Ergot and gangrene

Ergot preparations are used by patients with migraine over a long period.

Ergotamine gangrene occurs in those who eat bread infected with claviceps purpurea. Example : dwellers on the shores of the Mediterranean sea and the **Russian Steppes.**

Lymphatics, Lymph Vessels, Lymphoma

9

- Lymphangiography
- Lymphoedema leg
- Hodgkin's lymphoma
- Non-Hodgkin's lymphoma
- Lymphoscintigraphy
- Burkitt's lymphoma
- Sezary's syndrome
- Chyluria

Lymphatics and lymph vessels play the role of draining the waste fluid from the body. Hence they are vulnerable for various infections. The lymphatics drain into the veins and they are connected to a group of lymph nodes. Hence, infections of the lymphatics give rise to enlargement of lymph nodes. In this chapter, significant surgical diseases affecting the lymphatics and lymph nodes are discussed.

LYMPHANGIOGRAPHY

Lymphangiography is an investigation wherein a dye is injected into the lymphatics and the entire draining lymphatics and lymph nodes are visualised.

Indications for lymphangiography

1. Lymphoedema, if surgery is planned.
2. In cases of lymphoma, to detect pelvic nodes, paraaortic nodes etc.

Procedure

- Commonly, pedal lymphangiograms are done.
- 5-10 ml of methylene blue (patent blue) is injected into

the web spaces intradermally between the toes. This delineates the lymphatics of the dorsum of the foot which are identified. Then, oily dye such as "ultra fluid lipoidol" is injected (10-15 ml).

- It may take 12-24 hours to delineate inguinal nodes and paraaortic nodes.

- Isotope lymphangiography refers to injection of albumin labelled with technetium 99 colloid or I^{131}. (See next page)

Results

1. Metastasis appear as irregular filling defects in the lymph nodes.
2. It may demonstrate hypoplasia or hyperplasia as in primary lymphoedema.
3. If there is obstruction, the dye may return back (dermal back flow).

Complications of lymphangiography

1. Lymphangitis and toxaemia

   - It is not being done routinely nowadays, because of availability of ultrasound, CT scan and other noninvasive investigations.

2. Too rapid infusion is to be avoided for the fear of lipid pulmonary embolus.

Lymphoscintigraphy

- It has a sensitivity and specificity of 92% and 100% respectively.
- It has replaced Lymphangiography.

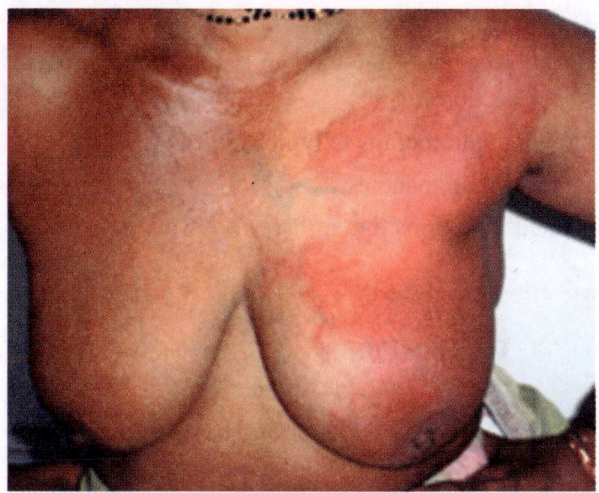

Fig. 9.1 Case of carcinoma of the breast presented with lymphangitis

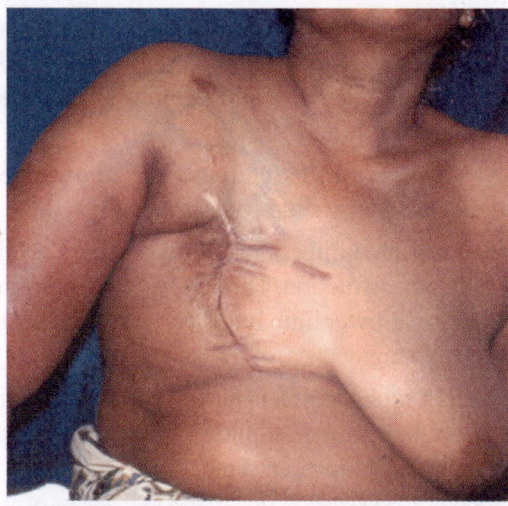

Fig. 9.2 Post mastectomy lymphoedema of the right upper limb

- Radiolabelled (technetium 99^m) colloid is injected into web space between 2nd and 3rd toes or fingers. Limb is exercised periodically and images are taken.

- If there is abnormal accumulation of tracer with collaterals, it is the sign of lymphoedema.

- MRI and CT scan are the latest investigations in addition to lymphangiography for the evaluation of gross swelling of the limb.

LYMPHOEDEMA OF LEG

Accumulation of the lymph in the subcutaneous tissues results in enlargement of the limb. Fluid collects in the **extracellular, extravascular compartment**.

COMMON SITES OF LYMPHOEDEMA

1. Lower limbs are the most common sites.

2. Upper limbs

3. Scrotum: Elephantiasis of the scrotum is caused by filarial organism *(Wuchereria bancrofti)*.

4. Elephantiasis of penis caused by filarial organisms produces *RAM'S HORN PENIS*.

CAUSES OF LOWER LIMB ELEPHANTIASIS

I. **Primary** :

- *Lymphatic aplasia* : Number of lymphatic channels and nodes are grossly reduced.

- *Lymphatic hypoplasia* : In this variety the lymphatic channels are of small calibre.
- **Milroy's disease** is a type of lymphoedema congenita which runs in families.
- Depending upon the time at which the lymphoedema appears, it can be classified as follows :

Birth	– Lymphoedema congenita.
Puberty	– Lymphoedema precox.
Later life	– Lymphoedema tarda.

II. **Acquired (Secondary lymphoedema)** :

1. **Filarial elephantiasis** (Fig. 9.3) is caused by *Wuchereria bancrofti*, transmitted by the mosquito *(Culex fatigans)*. The disease is caused by adult worms which have the affinity towards lymphatic vessels and lymph nodes. **Microfilariae do not produce any lesion**.

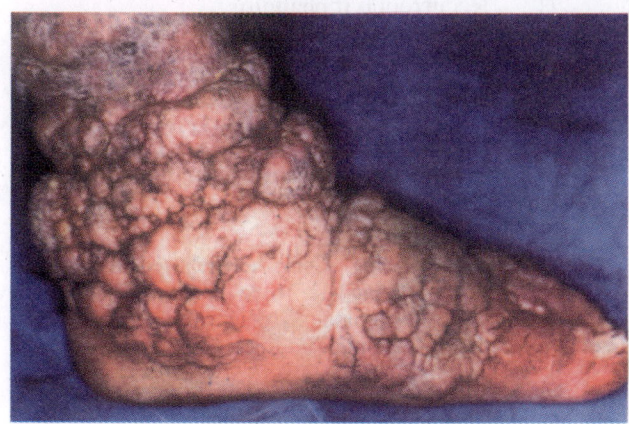

Fig. 9.3 Filarial lymphoedema

- Initially, it causes Iymphangitis which clinically presents with high grade fever with chills and rigors. red streaks in the limb, with tenderness and swelling of the spermatic cord and scrotum.

- The lymph nodes are swollen and tender. Retroperitoneal lymphangitis produces acute abdominal pain.

- Due to such repeated infections, fibrosis occurs resulting in lymphatic obstruction. This later gives rise to lymphatic dilatation. Lower limb lymphatics are dilated and tortuous (lymphangiectasis).

- To start with, lymphoedema is pitting in nature and after some time becomes non-pitting in nature. Lymph (protein) provides good nourishment for fibroblasts.

- After repeated infections, the skin over the limb becomes *dry, thickened,* thrown into folds and even *nodules* which *break open* and result in ulcers, hence called "Elephant leg". Lack of nutrition and infection precipitate lymphoedema. Oedema is also due to reflux of lymph from para-aortic vessels into the smaller lymphatics draining the lower limb. Subcutaneous tissue is grossly thickened. The presence of deep fascia prevents involvement of the deep muscles of the lower limb (Key Box 9.1).

Key Box 9.1

ELEPHANT LEG

Filarial lymphangitis
↓
Lymphatic obstruction
↓
Lymph stasis
↓
Recurrent lymphangitis
↓
Transudation of albumin
↓
Lymphoedema (Pitting)
↓
Coagulation of fluid
↓
Repeated infection
↓
Lymphoedema (Non-pitting)

---

2. After inguinal block dissection for secondaries in lymph nodes (Upper limb lymphoedema following axillary block dissection).

3. Following radiotherapy to lymph nodes.

4. Advanced malignancies.

5. Repeated infections due to bare-foot walking.

GRADES OF FILARIAL IYMHOEDEMA

Grade I - **Oedema-Pitting** – Completely relieved on rest and elevation. No skin changes.

Grade II - **Oedema-Pitting – Partially relieved** on rest and elevation. No skin changes.

Grade III - **Oedema-Non-pitting –** Skin involvement, subcutaneous thickening present.

Grade IV - **Oedema-Non-pitting** – Not relieved, warty projections, elephantiasis, lymphorrhoea present.

DIFFERENTIAL DIAGNOSIS OF UNILATERAL ELEPHANTIASIS OF THE LEG

1. **Filariasis** is the most common cause of elephantiasis of the leg in endemic areas like Coastal Karnataka, Coastal Andhra Pradesh, Tamilnadu, etc.

2. **Congenital A-V Fistula** can present with unilateral gigantism of the leg. Dilated veins, continuous murmur, gigantism, non-healing ulcer in the leg in a young boy gives the clue to the diagnosis.

3. **Elephantiasis neuromatosa** of the leg can cause diffuse enlargement of the leg. The leg is tender on palpation with soft to firm diffuse swelling.

4. **Extensive lipomatosis** of the leg.

TREATMENT OF FILARIAL LYMPHOEDEMA

I. Conservative line of management

- **Combination of physical therapies (CPT)**: This includes gentle massage of limbs, physical exercises, elastic compression bandage and rest and elevation of the limb.

- **Skin care and good hygiene** is an important part of the treatment. To avoid injury and not to apply any irritants to the skin.

- **Drugs** :

  1. **Diuretics** - 20mg of Furosemide every day/alternate days, this helps in early cases of lymphoedema.

2. Antifilarial treatment : Diethyl Carbamazine Citrate (DEC) 100g 3 times/day for 21 days with every attack of lymphangitis and once in 6 months.

Warfarin has been used in reducing lymphoedema due to filariasis. It acts by enhancing macrophage activity and extralymphatic absorption of interstitial fluid.

Antibiotics are used in cases of cellulitis and lymphangitis – Cephalosporins are being used against Staphylococci and Streptococci.

II. Surgery : (Fig.9.4)

Aim : To reduce the limb size.

1. **Swiss roll operation (Thompson's)** : In this a skin flap is raised containing dermis and it is buried into the deep tissues (close to vascular bundle). This is a dermal flap prepared by denuding epidermis (Fig. 9.5).

2. **Charle's excision operation**: It is indicated in primary lymphoedema. It is performed for extensive swelling and skin changes (Fig. 9.6).

   In this operation, thickened, diseased skin and subcutaneous tissue are excised till the healthy underlying structures are seen followed by split skin grafting.

   The skin has **dermal lymphatics which are never involved in filariasis.** Thus, the subcutaneous lymph may flow via dermal lymphatics.

3. **Nodovenous shunt**: Dilated, enlarged lymph node in the inguinal region is anastomosed to a vein nearby, e.g., long saphenous vein or femoral vein, etc (Fig. 9.7)

Thus, these are the 3 types of surgery commonly done for filarial leg. There are many other surgeries which are of historical interest. However, the results of the

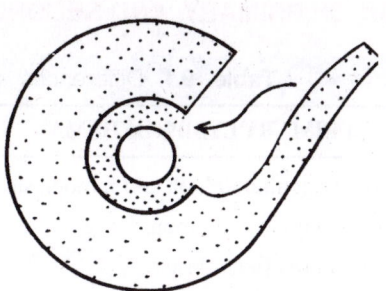

Fig.9.5 Swiss-roll operation

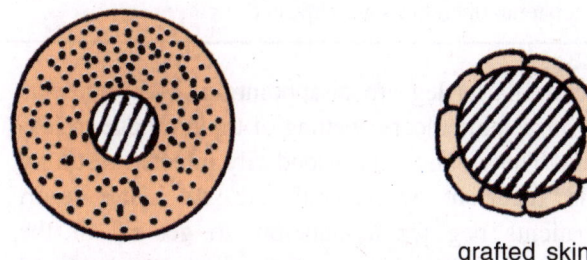

grafted skin

Fig.9.6 Excision and grafting

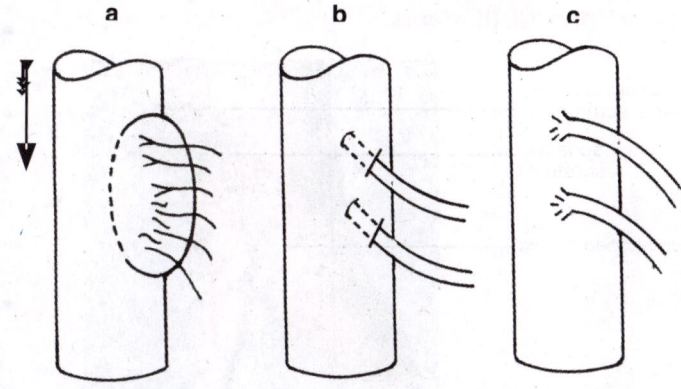

Fig.9.7 a Node to vein **b** Lymphatics threaded into a vein **c** Microvascular anastomosis

TYPES OF SURGERY		
Reduction procedures ↓	**Lymphatic bypass procedures**	**Excision combined with bypass** ↓
1. Charle's total subcutaneous excision and skin grafting	Lymphovenous anastomosis	Omental transposition	Lymphatic transposition (Swiss role operation)
2. Homan's excision and primary suturing of skin flaps	Nodovenous shunt (O'Brien's)	Spontaneous lympho-lympho anastomosis	Burial of dermal skin flap into the deep tissues

Fig. 9.4 Various surgeries for lymphoedema

COMPARISON OF PRIMARY AND SECONDARY LYMPHOEDEMA (Table 9.1)

Table 9.1 Differences between primary and secondary lymphoedema	
PRIMARY LYMPHOEDEMA	**SECONDARY LYMPHOEDEMA**
• It is due to congenital aplasia and hypoplasia.	Filariasis is the common cause
• It is seen in younger age group.	Middle age group.
• Females are more often affected.	Males are more commonly affected.
• Unilateral, begins distally, spreads proximally.	Sometimes it can start proximally.
• Capillary haemangioma may be present.	Absent.
• Regional lymph nodes are absent.	The lymph nodes are grossly enlarged.
• Excisional operations are indicated.	Excisional operations and other types of surgery.

surgery for filarial leg are disappointing. Many patients develop intractable ulcers, wetting of the limb due to loss of protein. The wound gets secondarily infected resulting in sepsis, recurrent lymphangitis etc. As a last resort many patients beg for amputation, to get rid of the "useless limb". After amputation the limb can be fitted with prosthesis. (For other manifestation refer Table 9.2)

Complications of filariasis

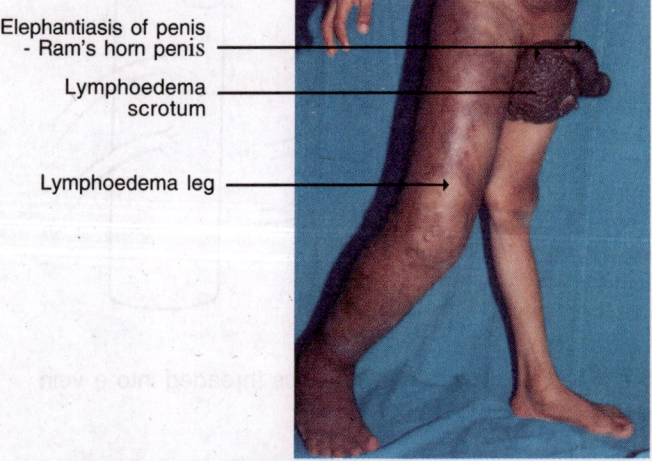

Elephantiasis of penis - Ram's horn penis

Lymphoedema scrotum

Lymphoedema leg

Fig.9.8 Complications of Filariasis

HODGKIN'S LYMPHOMA (DISEASE)

DEFINITION

This is a malignant neoplasm of lymphoreticular system. Thus, it can involve the lymph nodes, spleen, liver, etc.

PATHOLOGY

- Disease starts usually in one of the lymph nodes as a painless swelling.

- Commonly, it involves the left supraclavicular region. The nodes are **enlarged without matting**. It spreads to other nodes in a downstream lymphatic drainage. Cut surface of lymph nodes are smooth and homogenous.

- **The axial lymphatic system is almost always affected in Hodgkin's disease**.

- Microscopy : "Cellular pleomorphism" - lymphocytes, histiocytes, eosinophils and fibrous tissue with **REED STERNBERG CELLS** - a giant cell containing mirror image nucleus.

Table 9.2 Clinical manifestations of lymphatic filariasis		
SITE OF INVOLVEMENT	**ACUTE**	**CHRONIC**
Lower limbs	Lymphangitis, Lymphadenitis	Lymphoedema , Chronic lymphadenitis
Scrotum	Lymphangitis	Lymphoedema, Chylocoele
Spermatic cord	Acute funiculitis	Chronic thickened cord
Epididymis and testis	Acute epididymo-orchitis	Chronic epididymoorchitis
Abdomen	Acute retroperitoneal lymphangitis	Chyluria, Lymphadenovarix
Breast	Lymphangitis	Lymphoedema

CLASSIFICATION: (Ryle's classification is no longer used).

- **REAL (1994)** – **R**evised **E**uropean **A**merican **L**ymphoma

I. **Lymphocyte Predominance, nodular** (both Hodgkin's Lymphoma and low grade B Cell lymphomas)

II. **Classic Hodgkin's Lymphoma (HL)**

Nodular Sclerosis
Lymphocyte Rich
Lymphocyte Depletion
Mixed Cellularity

CLINICAL FEATURES

1. Age–Bimodal distribution. In children and middle age (30-50 years).

2. Sex–Increased incidence is found in males.

3. It presents as generalised lymphadenopathy. Generalised lymphadenopathy means when more than one group of lymph nodes are enlarged and are significant. Significant lymphadenopathy means:

   - Lymph node > 2 cm in size
   - Node is hard in consistency
   - Palpable left supraclavicular node

   Disease starts in the left posterior triangle as a group of lymph nodes with a 'bunch of grapes' appearance (Fig. 9.9 and 9.10). This is seen in about 80% of cases.

Key Box 9.2

PARA-AORTIC NODE ENLARGEMENT COMMON CAUSES

- Lymphoma
- Testicular tumours
- Malignant melanoma
- Gastrointestinal malignancy

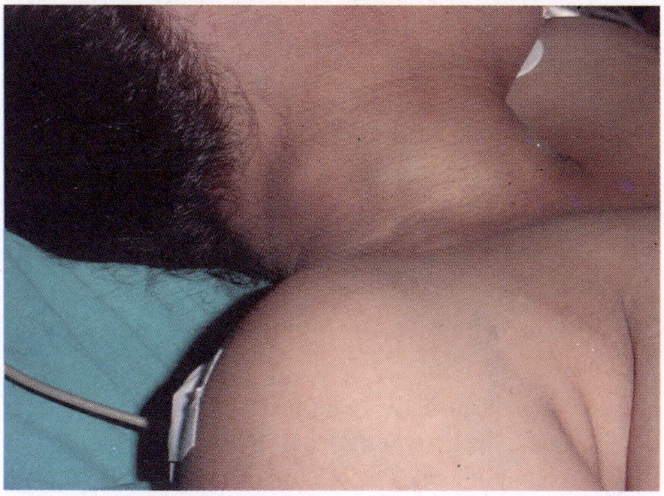

By means of contiguous and centripetal spread, other lymph nodes in the neck, axillary, mediastinal, para-aortic and inguinal lymph nodes get enlarged.

The **nodes are firm (India rubber consistency)** without matting. In advanced cases and in poorly differentiated variety, matting can occur.

4. Abdominal pain can occur due to hepato-splenomegaly, which are smooth and firm with round borders.

5. **Para-aortic nodes** are felt in the umbilical region, more so on the left side. Its clinical features are: (Key Box 9.2)

   - Nodular
   - Firm to hard mass
   - Fixed mass
   - Does not move with respiration
   - Being retroperitoneal, the mass does not fall forward on knee elbow position.

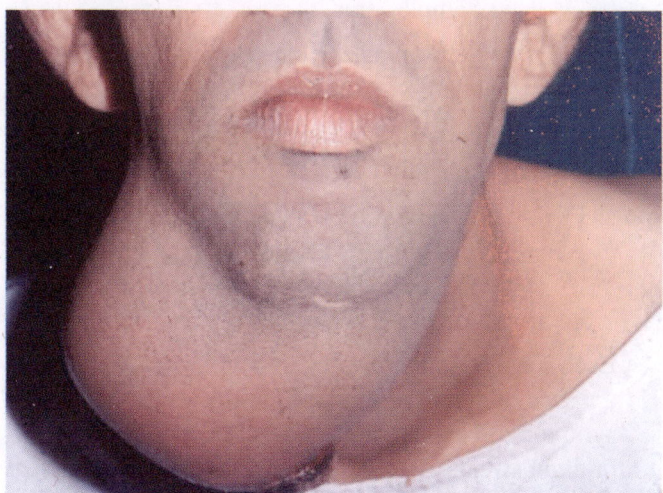

Fig. 9.9 Cervical lymphadenopathy due to Hodgkin's lymphoma - lymph nodes are firm or rubbery in consistency

Fig. 9.10 Advanced stage of Hodgkin's lymphoma

---

1. ***Mycosis fungoides:*** *It is not a fungal infection but is caused by non-Hodgkin's lymphoma with infiltration of the skin with malignant lymphocytes. Dermatitis, papular rashes are common which progresses to the tumour formation. It is a variety of cutaneous T-cell lymphoma.*

6. There may be ascites.

7. **Intermittent fever** (irregular) is sometimes seen. Skin rashes[1] are rare in Hodgkin's lymphoma.

8. **Multiple bony pains** can occur due to secondary deposits, especially in the lumbar vertebrae. The secondary deposits are usually osteoblastic giving rise to **ivory vertebrae**.

9. **Superior vena caval obstruction** indicates enlarged mediastinal nodes. This is tested by asking the patient to raise the hand above the head. Engorgement of the veins indicates obstruction and the test is said to be positive **(Pemberton's test)**.

CLINICAL STAGING OF LYMPHOMA

Stage I : Lymph node involvement in one anatomical region or involvement of single extralymphatic organ or site (I.E).
e.g.: Palpable left supraclavicular nodes.

Stage II : Involvement of two or more anatomical group of lymph nodes confined to same side of diaphragm. Examples are:
• Left supraclavicular and left axillary node.
• Left supraclavicular, left axillary and right supraclavicular.

Stage III : Involvement of the lymph nodes on both sides of the diaphragm, with or without spleen. Examples are:
• Left supraclavicular and left inguinal lymph nodes.
• Left supraclavicular lymph nodes with splenomegaly (III. S).

Stage IV : Diffuse involvement of one or more extra-lymphoid organs with or without lymph nodes involvement (Fig 9.9, 9.10) Liver (H), marrow (M), pleura (P), bones (O), etc.

• Each stage is further divided into group A which means absence of symptoms and group B means presence of symptoms. The symptoms are: (1) Fever, above 38°C or night sweats. (2) Pruritis, may be the presenting feature of nodular sclerosis. (3) Weight loss more than 10% of body weight in the last 6 months. (4) Bony pains. (5) Anaemia.

INVESTIGATIONS

1. **Complete blood picture (CBP)** : Peripheral smear

to rule out leukaemia. Anaemia indicates wide spread metastases.

2. **Elevated creatinine and blood urea nitrogen (BUN)** indicate ureteral obstruction or due to the direct involvement of kidneys. (Increased uric acid levels indicate aggressive non-Hodgkin's lymphoma.)

3. **Chest X-ray** is taken to rule out mediastinal lymph nodes, mediastinal widening, pleural effusion.

4. **Abdominal USG**
   • To look for para-aortic nodes
   • To look for splenomegaly
   • To rule out secondaries in the liver
   • However CT scan of the abdomen is better to define paraaortic nodes when there is minimal enlargement (0.5 cm).

5. **Intravenous pyelography (IVP)** is done to look for hydronephrosis as a result of back-pressure caused by para-aortic node mass pressing on the ureter (left side) and to assess the function of kidney.

6. **Lymph node biopsy** : Incision biopsy is done and a neck node is usually removed. Fine needle aspiration cytology (FNAC) may give the diagnosis but the definite histological pattern cannot be made out by FNAC. A trucut biopsy also can give the diagnosis.

7. **Mediastinoscopy (Chamberlain procedure)** is done if peripheral nodes are not available.

8. **Bipedal lymphangiography** can be done in doubtful cases. A foamy appearance is characteristic of lymphoma.

TREATMENT

• **Stage I, II are treated by RADIOTHERAPY** considering that the disease is still curable, not spread to blood stream and five-year survival rate is as high as 80%.

• **Dose of radiotherapy**: 3500-4500 Centigray (cGy) units.

   a. When the disease is confined to one group of lymph nodes, **local regional radiotherapy** is given.

   b. When both sides of neck nodes involved - **Mantle field of therapy** is given.

   c. Neck nodes with the mediastinal nodes are given - **Extended mantle field of therapy**.

   d. When paraaortic nodes and bilateral inguinal nodes are enlarged - **inverted Y field radiotherapy** is given.

- Stage IIIA, IIIB and IV are treated by chemotherapy because it is considered as a systemic disease. Following drugs are used in combination. Hence, it is called combination chemotherapy. There are various chemotherapy regimes available. These drugs have to be, used judiciously and carefully, depending upon the merits of the case. Age and weight of the patient, systemic illness and other factors also decide the chemotherapy. One example of a **chemotherapy regime** is given below.

MOPP regime

M. Mechlorethamine 6 mg/m^2 body area on 1st day and 8th day.

O. Oncovin (Vincristine) 1.4mg/m^2 I.V. on 1st day and 8th day.

P. Procarbazine 100 mg orally 1 to 10 days.

P. Prednisolone 15 mg 8th hourly orally 1 to 10 days.

- Minimum of 6 cycles or at least 2 extra cycles after attaining complete remission should be given. Inspite of stage III and stage IV disease, survival of 10 years with disease free interval is about 80%.

Side effects of MOPP therapy

- Infertility both in men and women
- Development of acute myeloid leukaemia
- Hematosuppression. (Bone marrow suppression)

Other alternative regimen which is as good as MOPP is **ABVD**: (Adriamycin, Bleomycin, Vinblastine and dacarbazine) less incidence of leukaemia and infertility.

STAGING LAPAROTOMY FOR LYMPHOMAS

- It is not done routinely nowadays because of sophisticated investigations like USG, CT scan, MRI scan (**M**agnetic **R**esonance **I**maging) which can detect lesions as small as 1-2 cm.
- Staging laparotomy is indicated in stage I and II early cases, specially supradiaphragmatic cases. Following procedures are done in a staging laparotomy (Fig.9.11):

1. Splenectomy and biopsy and removal of splenic hilar lymph nodes
2. Liver biopsy-wedge and needle biopsies of both lobes
3. Para-aortic node biopsy
4. Iliac node biopsy and coeliac node biopsy
5. Iliac crest bone biopsy
6. In females, strap the ovaries behind the uterus prevent radiation effect on the ovaries (Oophoropexy).

Advantages of staging laparotomy

- It avoids irradiation to the spleen. Thus, irradiation damage to lower lobe of the left lung and kidney are prevented.

Disadvantages

- It is an invasive procedure and may result in pneumonia, embolism, pancreatitis, etc.

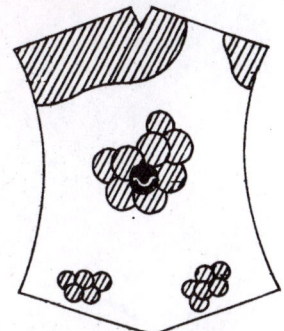

Fig. 9.11 Staging laparotomy (Refer text)

CAUSES OF DEATH IN LYMPHOMA

1. Recurrent respiratory tract infection both, bacterial and fungal because they are immunocompromised patients.
2. Disseminated disease - involvement of liver, hepatocellular failure, etc.
3. Multiple bony metastasis, pathological fracture, paraplegia, etc., with spine involvement.

NON-HODGKIN'S LYMPHOMA (NHL)

ETIOLOGY

1. **Age and sex**
   - Small lymphocytic lymphoma – Elderly patients
   - Lymphoblastic lymphoma – Male adolescents and young adults
   - Follicular lymphoma – Mid-adult age group
   - Burkitt's lymphoma – Children, young adults
2. **Viruses**
   - RNA viruses–Human immuno-deficiency virus (HIV) produces AIDS. These patients can develop high grade B cell lymphoma
   - DNA viruses–Epstein-Barr viruses (EBV) can produce Burkitt's lymphoma
3. **Bacteria**
   - H.Pylori – Gastric extra nodal marginal zone B-cell lymphomas of MALT type
4. **Immuno-deficiency states**
   - AIDS
   - Organ transplantation

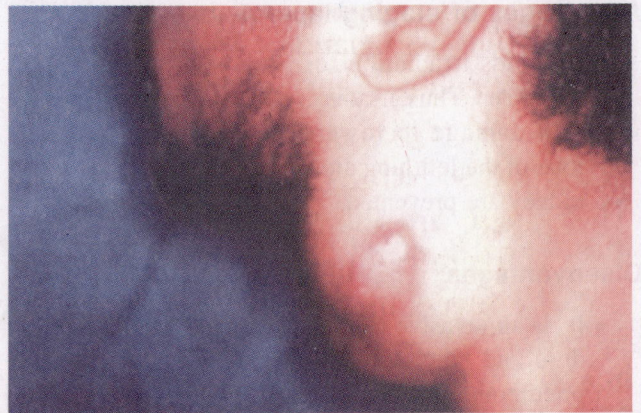

Fig. 9.12 Non Hodgkin's lymphoma with skin involvement

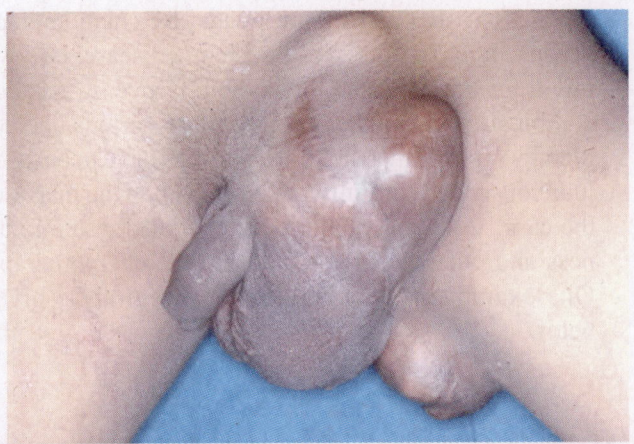

Fig. 9.13 Advanced case of non Hodgkin's lymphoma with involvement of groin nodes, testicle and skin deposits in the thigh

CLASSIFICATION OF NON-HODGKIN'S LYMPHOMA

Working formulation of NHL

I. Low grade
- Small lymphocytic
- Follicular, predominently small cleaved cell

II. Intermediate grade
- Follicular, predominantly large cell
- Diffuse, small cleaved cell
- Diffuse mixed small and large cell
- Diffuse large cell

III. High grade
- Large cell immunoblastic
- Lymphoblastic
- Burkitt's or Non-Burkitt's lymphoma

Pathological classification

I. B cell NHL – Small lymphocytic lymphoma, follicular lymphoma, Burkitt's lymphoma.

II. T cell NHL – Cutaneous T cell lymphoma-Mycosis fungoides and Sezary syndrome, lymphoblastic lymphoma, etc.

TREATMENT OF NON-HODGKIN'S LYMPHOMA

It depends on following factors:
- Grade of tumour.
- Stage of disease.

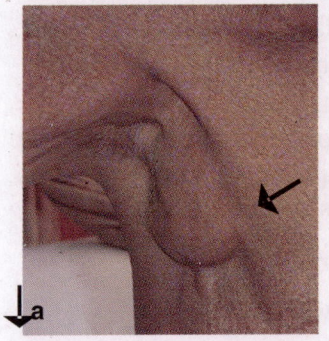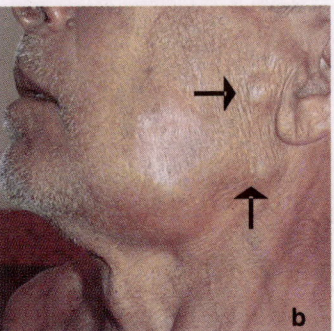

Fig. 9.14 a,b Observe massive axillary lymphadenopathy and enlargement of submandibular, upper deep cervical and preauricular lymph nodes

Stage I and II – Low grade: Radiotherapy

Stage I and II – Intermediate and high grade: Chemotherapy

Stage III and IV : Chemotherapy

Combination chemotherapy

- CHOP regime, cyclophosphamide, adriamycin, vincristine, prednisolone.
- Combination chemotherapy has its side effects hence has to be administered carefully.
- Cyclophosphamide can cause haemorrhagic cystitis, adriamycin can cause cardiac toxicity. Epirubicin has lesser cardiac toxicity.
- Vincristine can give rise to bone marrow depression.

Note: Lymphoma is a big chapter in pathology books. However, what is relevant to an undergraduate student has been given in this chapter in a simplified manner. Complex pathology, complex classification and complicated treatment modalities are of interest to the oncologists.

Table 9.2 Comparision of Hodgkin's and Non-Hodgkin's Lymphoma

	HODGKIN'S LYMPHOMA	NON-HODGKIN'S LYMPHOMA
Age	• Bimodal age	• More than 50 years
Involvement of lymph nodes	• Left supraclavicular, axillary, inguinal	• External Waldayer's ring, submental, sub mandibular, preauricular, postauricular, occipital nodes.
Tonsil enlargement	• Not enlarged	• Tonsils may be enlarged
Epitrochlear node	• Not enlarged	• Can be enlarged
Hepatomegaly	• Uncommon	• Common in low grade
Involvement of bone	• Uncommon (10%)	• In 40% of cases, iliac crest is involved by the time of diagnosis
Alcohol induced pain	• Characteristic	• Absent
Fluctuating fever	• Present	• Absent
Prognosis	• Better prognosis	• Poor prognosis
Common presentation	• **Lymphatic organ**	• **Extra lymphatic**

Comparison of Hodgkin's and Non-Hodgkin's Lymphoma (Table 9.2)

BURKITT'S LYMPHOMA
(Small Noncleaved Lymphoma)

- It is a type of high grade Non-Hodgkin's lymphoma first described by Burkitt affecting jaw bone (Maxilla, mandible).
- It is rare everywhere except in a few places where malarial infestation is heavy.
- It is caused by **Epstein - Barr Virus** (EBV) which multiplies in presence of heavy malarial infestation.

Types

- **Endemic** : Parts of Africa and other tropical locations. It is associated with EBV. Affects jaw and orbit. It has good prognosis.
- **Sporadic** : Throughout the world. It is not associated with EBV. It affects abdomen and GI tract than bones, has poor prognosis.

Diagnosis

- Biopsy will reveal typical 'starry sky' appearance with primitive lymphoid cells with large clear histiocytes.

Treatment

- Endemic cases respond well to cyclophosphamide.
- Sporadic cases need to be treated with combination chemotherapy.

SEZARY'S SYNDROME

It is also a type of cutaneous T-Cell lymphomas. Here skin involvement is manifested clinically as a generalised exfoliative erythroderma along with an associated leukaemia of SEZARY Cells. These cells are characterised by cerebriform nucleus. These are indolent tumours having good survival time.

Miscellaneous

CHYLURIA

- It is the most common manifestation of rupture of lymph vessels due to filriasis. (others being chylocoele, chylous ascits, chylothrax etc.
- It occurs when intestinal lymphatics are obstructed by filarial fibrosis and the lymphatics are diverted to renal lymphatics.
- The dilated and tortuous lymphatics due to high pressure, rupture into renal pelvis and ureter giving rise to chyluria. Passage of large amount of **chyle** results in loss of protein and fat resulting in malnutrition. Such patients are also debilitated with loss of immunity.
- Oral ingestion of fat labelled with sudan red III turns the urine pink in these cases.
- It is treated by DEC, bed rest, elevation of foot end of bed and administration of high protein diet.

Varicose Veins, Deep Vein Thrombosis

10

- Primary varicose veins
- Secondary varicose veins
- Anatomy of long saphenous vein
- Clinical examination
- Treatment
- Complications
- Short saphenous varicosity
- Deep vein thrombosis

"Varicosity is the penalty for verticality against gravity." This is the common statement made in lecture classes. The blood has to flow from the lower limbs into the heart against gravity because of the upright posture of human beings. In many cases, varicose veins are asymptomatic. The raised intra-abdominal pressure also precipitates varicose veins, more commonly in females due to repeated pregnancy. The complications of varicose veins are responsible for hospitalisation of the patient.

Definition

Dilated, tortuous and elongated superficial veins of the limb are called as varicose veins.

Following are the **examples of varicosity**

- Long saphenous varicosity
- Short saphenous varicosity
- Oesophageal varices and fundal varices
- Haemorrhoids
- Varicocoele
- Vulval varix and ovarian varix

In this chapter varicosity of the leg is discussed.

PRIMARY VARICOSE VEINS

They occur as a result of *congenital weakness* in the vessel wall.

It can also be due to muscular weakness or due to *congenital absence of valves*.

Very often, the valve at the saphenofemoral (SF) junction is incompetent/absent. The valves can also be absent where the superfical veins join the deep veins.

Klippel Trenuaney Syndrome is a congenital venous abnormality wherein superficial and deep veins do not have any valves. It is also called as **Valveless syndrome**.

Primary varicosity can also be familial. These factors, in addition to prolonged standing (agriculturists, hotel workers), help in development of the varicose veins.

SECONDARY VARICOSE VEINS

Women are more prone for varicose veins because of the following reasons.

- **Pregnancy and pelvic tumours** cause proximal obstruction to the blood flow.
- **Pills** (oral contraceptive pills) alter the viscosity of blood.
- **Progesterones dilate vessel wall**

Congenital arterio-venous (AV) fistula increases blood flow and increases venous pressure.

Deep vein thrombosis can occur as a result of road traffic accidents, post-operatively, etc., and can result in destruction of valves resulting in varicose veins.

SURGICAL ANATOMY OF THE VENOUS SYSTEM OF LEG

It can be discussed under following headings

1. Superficial system - long and short saphenous veins and their tributaries
2. Perforators
3. Deep system of veins

SUPERFICIAL VENOUS SYSTEM (Key Box 10.1)

Key Box 10.1

SALIENT FEATURES

- As the name suggests, they are in the superficial fascia, often are visible (saphenous means easily seen)
- They are low pressure and poorly supported system
- They are provided with numerous valves
- The middle coat of these veins consists mostly of smooth muscles.
- The middle coat is also thicker than that of other veins
- Normal blood flow is from superficial to deep system of veins.

Anatomy of the long saphenous vein (Fig. 10.1)

It starts in the foot from the tributaries of dorsal venous arch, permits reverse flow through its competent valves ascends in front of medial malleolus and runs along the medial side of the leg. It then ascends in the thigh and ends at the saphenofemoral junction (SF) by joining the femoral vein, which is 1½ inches (4 cm) below and lateral to the pubic tubercle. It has 15 to 20 valves. Absence of valves results in varicose veins.

TRIBUTARIES

Tributaries near the termination

1. Superficial circumflex iliac vein
2. Superficial epigastric vein
3. Superficial external pudendal vein

Tributaries in the leg

1. Anterior vein of the leg.
2. Posterior arch vein lies parallel to and behind the main trunk of long saphenous vein. It anastamoses with small venous arches connecting the medial perforating veins.

Tributaries in the lower thigh

1. Lateral superficial femoral
2. Medial superficial femoral
3. Transverse suprapatellar
4. Transverse infrapatellar

These tributaries connect the long saphenous with short saphenous veins. They are also called communicators.

PERFORATORS

These are the veins which connect long saphenous vein with deep system of veins. Since they perforate deep fascia; they are called perforators. There are 5 constant perforators in the lower limb on the medial side.

Leg perforators: They are 3 in number. The lowest perforator is situated below and behind the medial malleolus. The middle perforator is 10 cm above the tip of the medial malleolus. The upper perforator is 15 cm above the medial malleolus.

Knee perforator: It is situated just below the knee.

Thigh perforator: It is situated palm breadth above the knee.

The knowledge of perforators forms the basis behind **multiple tourniquet test**. Most of perforators are provided with valves. Weakness of these valves or damage to valves results in varicosity.

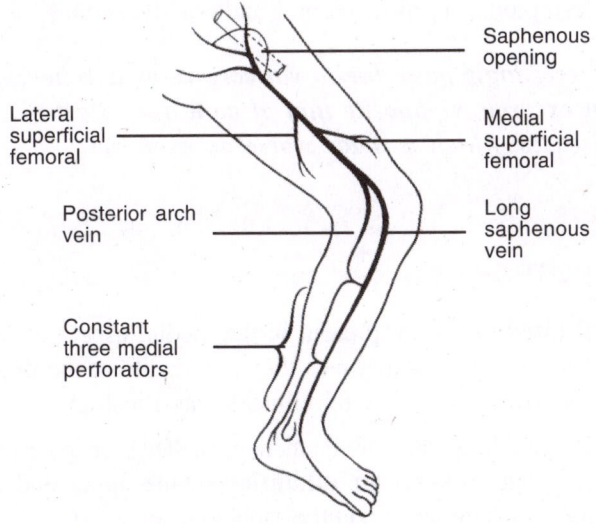

Lateral superficial femoral

Posterior arch vein

Constant three medial perforators

Saphenous opening

Medial superficial femoral

Long saphenous vein

Fig. 10.1 Long saphenous vein and its tributaries

DEEP VENOUS SYSTEM

This comprises the femoral and the popliteal veins, veins or venae comitantes accompanying anterior tibial, posterior tibial and peroneal arteries and valveless veins draining the calf muscles (Soleal venous sinus)

Salient features of deep venous system

They are high pressure and well supported system by powerful muscles.

They are connected to superficial veins by means of perforators.

It is the powerful calf muscle contraction that returns the blood to the heart.

The deep veins are also provided with valves.

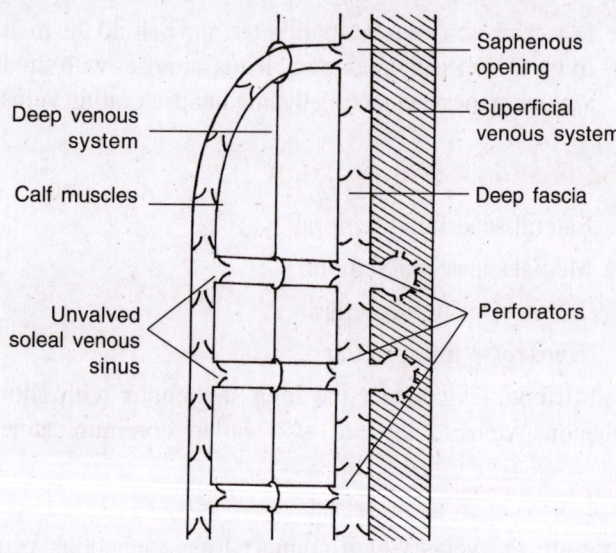

Fig. 10.2 Deep venous system

SURGICAL PHYSIOLOGY

Blood is returned to the heart from the lower limbs by the following mechanism:

Calf muscle pump: It is the alternate contraction and relaxation of the muscles of the leg (the major factor). The pressure within the calf compartment rises to 200-300 mm Hg during walking.

Competent valves (unidirectional) in the leg (Key Box 10.2) When these valves are absent or weak, perforator incompetence develops resulting in varicose veins.

Vis-a-tergo of the circulation, that is the pressure transmitted from the arterial tree passes the capillary bed to

Key Box 10.2		
DISTRIBUTION OF VALVES		
• Inferior Vena Cava	:	No valve
• Common Iliac Vein	:	No valve
• Long Saphenous Vein	:	10-14 valves
• Short Saphenous Vein	:	1 Valve

the venous side. This helps in return of blood to heart at resting position.

Negative intrathoracic pressure

Venae comitantes

CLINICAL EXAMINATION OF A CASE OF VARICOSITY OF THE LEG

SYMPTOMS

Majority of the patients come, with dilated veins in the leg. They are minimal to start with and at the end of the day they are sufficiently large because of the venous engorgement.

Dragging pain in the leg or dull ache is due to heaviness. Night cramps occur due to change in the diameter of veins. Aching pain is relieved at night on taking rest or elevation of limbs.

Sudden pain in the calf region with fever and oedema of the ankle region suggests deep vein thrombosis (DVT)

Patients can present with ulceration, eczema, dermatitis, bleeding, etc.

Symptoms of pruritis/itching and skin thickening

Interestingly pain due to varicose veins is relieved on excercises opposite that of pain due to arterial diseases, which is made worse on exercises.

SIGNS

INSPECTION (Should be done in standing position)

Dilated veins are present in the medial aspect of leg and the knee. Sometimes they are visible in the thigh also (refer next page for clinical classification)

Single dilated varix at SF junction is called saphena varix. It is due to **saccular dilatation** of the upper end of long saphenous vein at the saphenous opening.

(For classification see next page - Table 10.1, 10.2)

Table 10.1 Classification[1] of chronic lower-extremity venous disease

CLASSIFICATION	DEFINITION
C	Clinical signs (grade$_{0-6}$)[*] : A - for asymptomatic or S - for symtomatic
E	(O) Etiologic classification (congenital, primary, or secondary)
A	Anatomic distribution (superficial, deep, or perforator, alone or in combination)
P	Pathophysiologic dysfunction (reflux or obstruction; alone or in combination)

Table 10.2 Clinical Classification of chronic lower-extremity venous disease

GRADE	CHARACTERISTICS
0	No visible or palpable signs of venous disease
1	Telangiectases, reticular veins, or malleolar flare
2	Varicose veins
3	Edema without skin changes
4	Skin changes ascribed to venous disease (e.g., pigmentation, venous eczema, or lipodermatosclerosis)
5	Skin changes as defined above with healed ulceration
6	Skin changes as defined above with active ulceration

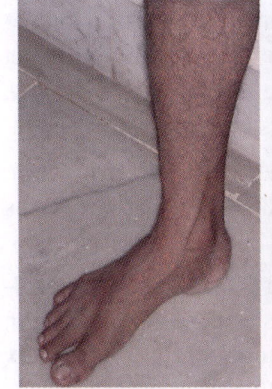

Fig. 10.3 Grade 0

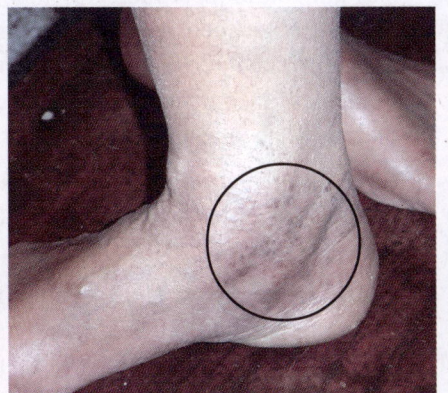

Fig. 10.4 Grade 1

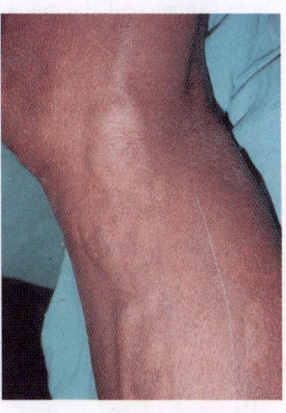

Fig. 10.5 Grade 2

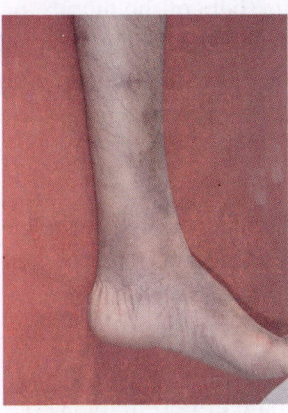

Fig. 10.6 Grade 3

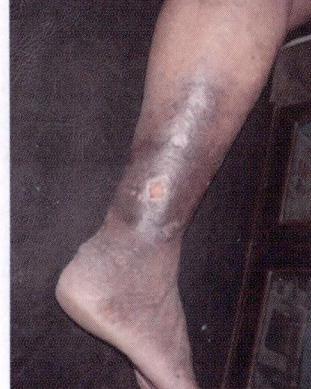

Fig. 10.7 Grade 4

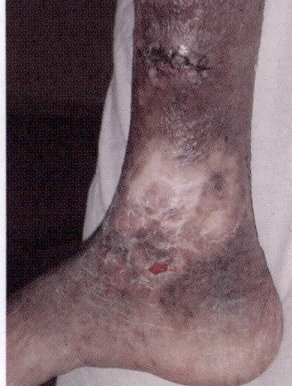

Fig. 10.8 Grade 5

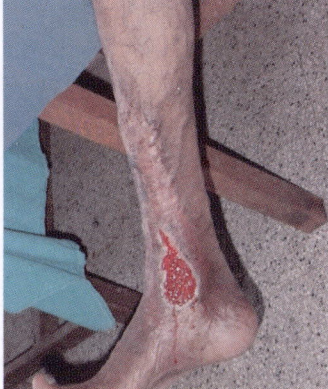

Fig. 10.9 Grade 6

Refer text above for description of the various grades of chronic lower extremity venous disease

---

1. *This classification is from International Consensus Committee on Chronic Venous Diseases*

Veins are tortuous and dilated.

A localised, dilated segment of the vein, if present, is an indication of a **BLOW OUT**. It signifies underlying perforator.

Ankle flare is a group of veins nearer the medial malleolus.

Complications like ulceration, bleeding, eczema, dermatitis may be present

Healed scar indicates previous ulceration.

PALPATION

1. **Cough impulse test (Morrissey's test)** : This test should be done in the standing position. The examiner keeps the finger at SF junction and the patient is asked to cough. Fluid thrill, an impulse felt by the fingers, is indicative of *"saphenofemoral incompetence"*.

2. **Trendelenburg test** : This test is done in 2 parts.

   Method: Patient is asked to lie on the couch in the supine position. The leg is elevated above the level of heart and the vein emptied. SF junction is occluded with the help of the thumb (or a tourniquet) and the patient is asked to stand. In Trendelenburg I, release the thumb or tourniquet immediately. *Rapid gush of blood from above downwards indicates sapheno femoral incompetence*.

   Trendelenburg II : The pressure at the SF junction is maintained without releasing the thumb or tourniquet. The patient is then asked to stand. *Slow filling of the long saphenous is seen. It is due to perforator incompetence*. (retrograde flow of blood)

3. **Multiple tourniquet test** is done to find out exact site of perforators (Fig. 10.10).

   Method : Patient is asked to lie supine on the couch. The vein is emptied by elevation. As the name suggests, 3-5 tourniquets (multiple) can be applied. However, if more tourniquets are applied the exact localisation of the perforators can be made out. It is not practical. There are mainly ankle, knee and thigh perforators. Hence, four tourniquets can be applied at various levels as mentioned below :

   1st Tourniquet: At the level of saphenofemoral junction. (SF junction)

   2nd Tourniquet : At the level of middle of the thigh, to occlude perforator in the Hunter's canal.

   3rd Tourniquet : Just below the knee.

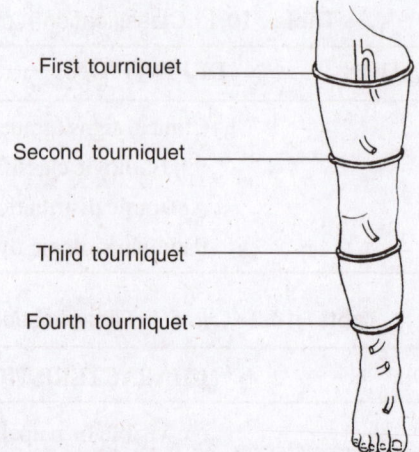

Fig.10.10 Multiple tourniquet test

4th Tourniquet : Palm breadth (lower third of the leg) above medial malleolus/ankle.

Patient is asked to stand and observe appearance of veins.

Inference : Appearance of veins between first and second tourniquets indicates incompetence of thigh perforators, between second and third indicates incompetence of knee perforators and below the fourth tourniquet indicates incompetence of ankle perforators. Usually, below knee and ankle perforators will be incompetent.

   On releasing the tourniquets one by one from below upwards, sudden retrograde filling of the veins occurs.

4. **Schwartz test** : It is done with the patient in the standing position. Place the fingers of the left hand over a dilated segment of the vein and with the right index finger tap the vein below. A palpable impulse suggests superficial column of blood in the vein and it also suggests incompetence of the valves in between the segment of the vein.

5. **Modified Perthes[1] test** is done to rule out deep vein thrombosis. Patient is asked to stand and the tourniquet is applied at SF junction and he is asked to have a brisk walk.

   Inference: If patient complains of severe pain in calf region or if superficial veins become more prominent, it is an indication of **deep vein thrombosis** and it is a contraindication for surgery.

Please note : Vein is not emptied in this test

---

[1] *In original Perthes Test the limb is wrapped and elastic bandage is applied.*

6. **Fegan's method (test)** : It is done to detect the site of perforators. The patient is asked to stand. Varicosity is marked with methylene blue and he is asked to lie down. The leg is elevated to empty the vein and the vein is palpated throughout its course. The defects in the deep fascia have a circular, button hole consistency (Summary - Key Box 10.3).

Key Box 10.3

TESTS FOR VARICOSE VEINS

- Cough impulse test – SF incompetence
- Trendelenburg 1 – SF incompetence
  Trendelenburg 2 – Perforator incompetence
- Multiple tourniquet test – Site of perforator incompetence
- Schwartz test – Superficial column of blood
- Modified Perthes test – Deep vein thrombosis
- Fegan's test – To locate the perforators in the deep fascia.

Examination of varicose ulcer: In the form of inspection and palpation should be done.

Evidence of deep vein thrombosis: Homan's test and Moses's test (vide infra) to be done.

Examination of the abdomen: To rule out pelvic tumours and inferior vena caval obstruction in the form of dilated veins in the lateral abdominal wall.

CLINICAL DISCUSSION

At the end of clinical examination you should be ready to answer following questions:
1. **Which system is involved?**
   - LSV - Medial veins
   - SSV - Lateral veins
2. **Is SF juntion incompetent?**
   Yes - Trendelenburg 1 is positive
   No - Trendelenburg 1 is negative
3. **Is there perforator incompetence?**
   Yes - Trendelenburg 2 is positive
   No - Trendelenburg 2 is negative
4. **Which group of perforators are incompetent?**
   - According to the results of multiple tourniquet test

5. **Is there deep vein thrombosis?**
   Yes - Perthes test is positive
   No - Perthes test is negative
6. **Is there any abdominal mass?**
   - Pelvic tumours
7. **Any complications are present?**
   - Eczema, dermatitis, ulcer etc
8. **Is it unilateral or bilateral?**

INVESTIGATIONS

1. **Doppler ultrasound** is the most important, mimimum level investigation to be done before treating a patient with venous disease (Key Box 10.4).

Key Box 10.4

DOPPLER ULTRASOUND

- This investigation is carried out with the patient standing.
- Incompetance of SFJ and saphenopopliteal junction (SPJ) can be assessed by this method.
- Gentle squeezing of calf muscles helps in detecting the incompetance.
- It also helps to rule out arterial diseases.
- It can detect patency of veins.

---

2. **Duplex ultrasound imaging:** In this investigation high resolution B - mode ultrasound imaging and Doppler ultrasound are used.

   It helps in getting images of veins

   It can also measure flow in these vessels
   All lower limb veins can be imaged
   Origin of venous ulcers and varicose veins can also be assessed.
   Importantly it can detect a thrombus.
3. **Venography** - Both ascending and descending venography can be done as in case of deep vein thrombosis. Dupex ultrasonography has largely replaced this investigation (rarely done nowadays).

TREATMENT

Varicose veins can be treated by three methods:
1. Conservative line of treatment
2. Injection line of treatment
3. Surgery

CONSERVATIVE TREATMENT

Elastic crepe bandage and elevation of leg forms the fundamental steps in treating varicose veins. This can be advised in asymptomatic cases of varicose veins and in secondary varicose veins.

Indications

Pregnancy

Pelvic tumour

Perthes test positive patient

AV fistula

INJECTION LINE OF MANAGEMENT (Compression Sclerotherapy)

Indications

1. Below knee varicosity

2. Recurrent varicosity after surgery

Varicose veins are marked in the standing position. The veins are punctured with a needle attached to a syringe containing sclerosant agent and the patient is asked to lie down. 3% Sodium tetradecyl sulphate or 1-2 ml of ethanolamine oleate or hypertonic saline is injected into the column of vein. Aseptic thrombosis occurs and when fibrosis occurs, the vein shrinks. Tight elastic compression bandage is applied. Success of sclerotherapy depends upon **effective sclerosant**, injection into an **empty vein** and **compression with exercise**.

SURGERY[1]

1. Trendelenburg's operation (Fig. 10.11)

An inguinal incision is made, long saphenous vein identified and the 3 tributaries are ligated. Long saphenous vein is ligated close to the femoral vein *JUXTA FEMORAL FLUSH LIGATION*.

An incision is given in front of the medial malleolus and long saphenous is isolated. The lower end is ligated and the vein incised. A long metallic stripper is introduced within the vein and brought out from the long saphenous vein in the inguinal incision. A metallic head is connected to the stripper and the vein is avulsed. Tight crepe bandage is applied, inguinal incision sutured and the limb is elevated.

During the procedure, the perforators get avulsed from the long saphenous vein and get thrombosed. Hence,

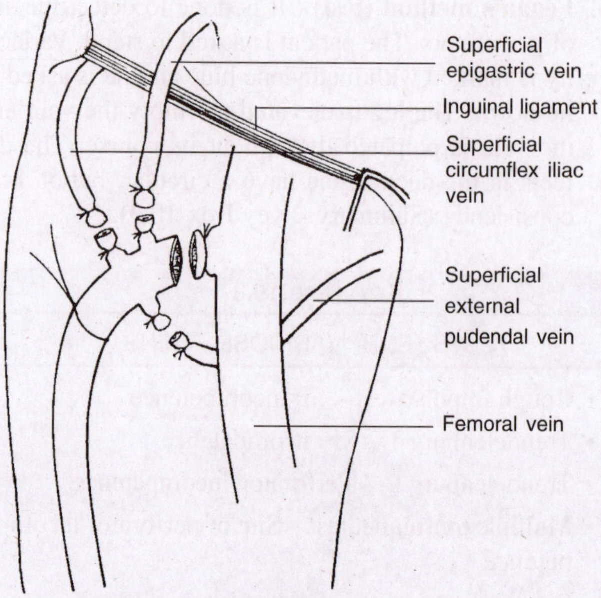

1. Only when there are complications, surgery is advisable.

Fig. 10.11 Trendelenburg operation

Superficial epigastric vein
Inguinal ligament
Superficial circumflex iliac vein
Superficial external pudendal vein
Femoral vein

this procedure is called ligation with stripping operation. It is indicated in cases of saphenofemoral incompetency.

2. Subfascial ligation of Cockett and Dodd

In this operation perforators are identified deep to deep fascia and they are ligated subfascially. This is indicated in cases of perforator incompetence with saphenofemoral competence. This is also done by an endoscope.

3. Subfascial Endoscopic Perforator Surgery (SEPS)

Small port incisions are made in the skin of calf region, deepened through the fascia.

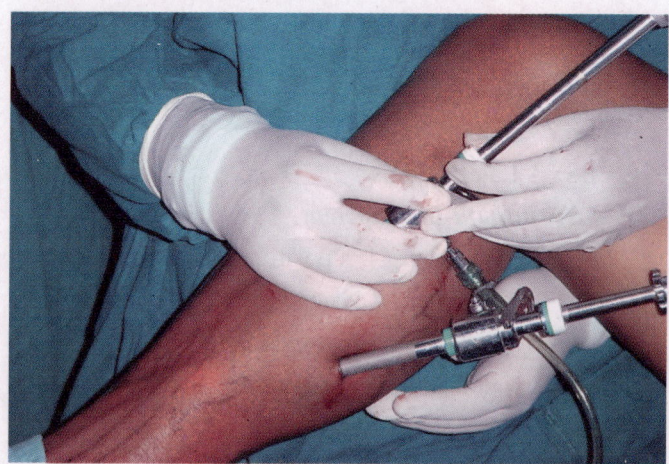

Fig. 10.12 SEPS

Carbon dioxide insufflation is done otherwise balloon expander is used to distend the subfascial plane.

2-6 perforators are identified and ligated

Procedure is simple, quick with least morbidity and is becoming popular.

Indicated for below knee perforators

Recent technique for the management of varicose veins

Vnus closure

By using an ultrasound control, an ablation catheter is inserted into saphenofemoral junction and slowly with drawn.

In this process, veins are destroyed.

This procedure has the advantage of lesser incidence of thigh haematoma and pain.

Complications include - deep vein thrombosis, recurrence and damage to overlying skin.

Trivex

In this method, veins are indentified by subcutaneous illumination, followed by injection of large quantities of fluid.

Then superficial veins are sucked.

Complications include induration, bruising and subcutaneous grooves.

COMPLICATIONS OF VARICOSE VEINS

1. **Eczema and dermatitis**: It occurs due to extravasation and break down of RBCs in the lower leg. It gives rise to itching which precipitates varicose ulcer. It is treated by application of zinc oxide cream or silver sulfadiazine cream (stasis dermatitis).

2. **Lipodermatosclerosis** refers to various skin changes in the lower leg associated with varicose veins such as **thickening of subcutaneous tissue, indurated feel like wood,** pigmentation etc. It is due to increased venous pressure resulting in capillary leakage with extravasation of blood and fibrin into surrounding tissues. Blood is broken down and haeme is released. This combines with iron giving rise to haemosiderin which is responsible for pigmentation. Classically this affects gaiter area of leg just above the malleoli.

3. **Haemorrhage**: It occurs due to trauma or eczema. It can be controlled by elevation of the leg and crepe bandage.

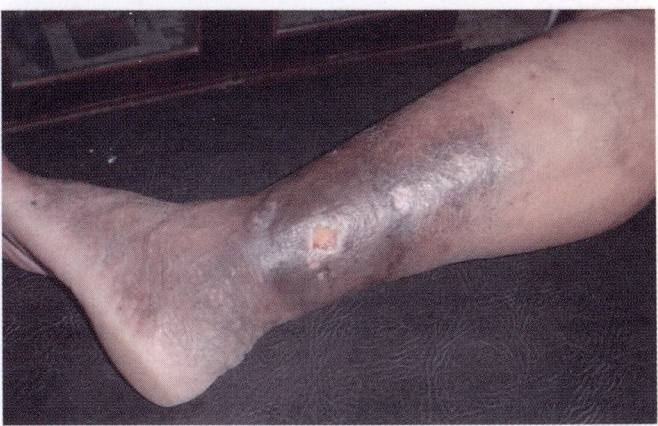

Fig. 10.13 Observe pigmentation, lipodermatosclerosis and ulcer formation

4. **Thrombophlebitis**: It refers to inflammation of superficial vein. The vein is tender, hard and cord-like. The skin is inflamed and pyrexia is usually present. It is treated by bed rest, elevation, crepe bandage, antibiotics and anti inflammatory drugs. (Key Box 10.5)

Key Box 10.5
THROMBOPHLEBITIS – CAUSES
• Spontaneous – TAO, malignancy • Trauma • Blood transfusion • IV Fluids, chemotherapeutic drugs • Varicose veins

5. **Venous ulcer** : It is also called **gravitational ulcer**. Precipitating factors are **venous stasis and tissue anoxia**. *Deep vein thrombosis* is also an important cause of venous ulcer where in valves are either destroyed or incompetent due to damage. **Sustained venous pressure** results in extravasation of cells, activation of capillary endothelium resulting in **release of free radicals**. These free radicals causes tissue destruction and ulceration – **Lipodermatosclerosis, tissue anoxia** are the other factors. Following hypothesis may explain genesis of varicose ulcers.

Fibrin cuff hypothesis

• The combination of capillary proliferation and inflammation in the form of presence of macrophages is a major factor in the development of venous ulcer. As a result of chronic

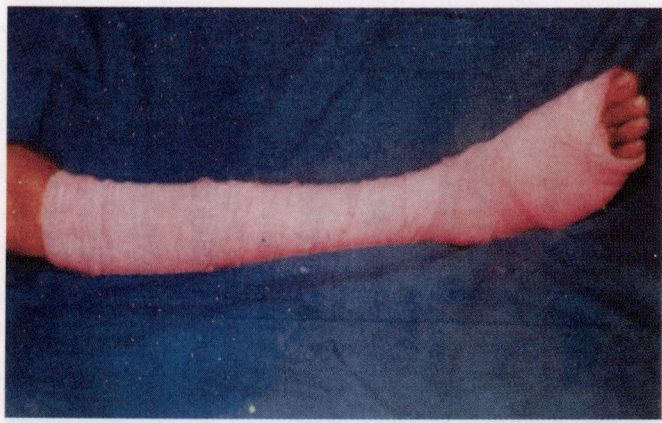

Fig. 10.14 Elastic crepe bandage for varicose ulcer - elevation of the leg is the most important factor for healing of the ulcer

inflammation, perivascular cuff develops around the capillaries. This perivascular cuff is made up of many connective tissue proteins including fibrin, collagen IV and fibronectin. Slowly venous ulcer results.

White cell trapping hypothesis

• Venous hypertension causes trapping of leucocytes. These leucocytes become activated and release proteolytic enzymes thus causing damage to capillary endothelium.

Features of venous ulcer

Typically, ulcers are situated just above the medial malleolus

The ulcers are oval, small, painless, superficial with pigmentation all around.

Dilated veins above the ulcer gives the clue to the diagnosis

Treatment of varicose ulcer: Bisgaard's method

Rest with **elevated limb** (Fig. 10.14).

Elastic crepe bandage helps in venous return

Active exercises should be taught to the patients (to contract calf muscles).

Passive exercises

Correct way of walking with the **heel down first**

If the ulcer is infected, antibiotics are given and dressing of the ulcer is done. Once the ulcer heals, Trendelenburg's operation is done.

6. **Calcification** can be seen in the walls of the vein

7. **Periostitis** of the tibia can occur due to the ulcer situated on the medial surface of the leg. Due to involvement of the periosteum, the ulcer gives rise to severe pain.

8. **Equinovarus deformity** results due to improper habit of walking on the toes which results in shortening of the tendo Achilles.

9. **Marjolin's ulcer** is a squamous cell carcinoma arising from healed varicose ulcer with scarring.

SHORT SAPHENOUS VARICOSITY

They are uncommon causes of varicosity in the leg. Short saphenous vein originates from the lateral part of the dorsal venous arch and ends in the popliteal vein in the popliteal fossa. Incompetence of sapheno popliteal valve results in short saphenous varicosity. It produces prominent veins on the lateral aspect of the leg with or without ulceration. They are treated by ligation of the short saphenous vein in the popliteal fossa (refer Table 10.3).

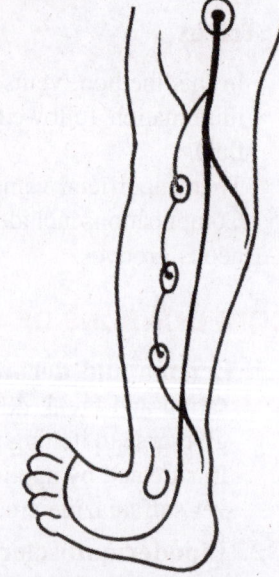

Fig. 10.15 Short saphenous vein and its perforators

	Table 10.3 Comparison between long saphenous and short saphenous veins		
FEATURES		**LONG SAPHENOUS VEIN**	**SHORT SAPHENOUS VEIN**
1.	Origin	Medial part of dorsal venous arch	Lateral part of dorsal venous arch
2.	Location	Front of medial malleolus	Behind lateral malleolus
3.	Relation with nerve	Saphenous nerve	Sural nerve
4.	Number of valves	15-20 valves	10-15 valves
5.	Termination	Saphenofemoral junction	Saphenopopliteal junction

Ligation of Saphenopopliteal junction

Preoperative ultrasonographic marking is very essential.

Vein should be ligated deep to deep fascia.

Branches – Giacomini vein and **gastrocnemius** veins may be seen – to be ligated.

It can be stripped upto mid-calf so as to avoid **injury to sural nerve**.

It is important to close the deep fascia to avoid unsighty cosmetic bulge behind the knee.

DEEP VEIN THROMBOSIS (DVT)

It is also called phlebothrombosis. It is an acute thrombosis of deep veins. Deep vein thrombosis is very common in the western countries, the exact cause of which is not known. Post operative immobilisation, pressure on the calf muscles, sluggish blood flow and prolonged bed rest are the various factors which precipitate deep vein thrombosis. Commonly, it affects venous sinuses in the soleal muscles. It is a common starting place. It can also involve pelvic veins. Various factors responsible for deep vein thrombosis can be remembered as T.H.R.O.M.B.O.S.I.S. (Key Box 10.6 and 10.7)

Key Box 10.6

THROMBOSIS – VIRCHOW'S TRIAD

- Endothelial injury
- Stasis
- Increased Coagulability

Key Box 10.7

CAUSES OF DEEP VEIN THROMBOSIS

Trauma–Injury to the vessel wall

Hormones–Increased coagulability

Road traffic accidents

Operations–Cholecystectomy

Malignancy–Sluggish blood flow

Blood disorders–Polycythaemia

Orthopaedic surgery, **obesity**, old age

Serious illness – Stroke, M.I.

Immobilisation

Splenectomy

Clinical features

The maximum incidence occurs on 2nd day and 5th-6th days in the post-operative period.

First complaint is usually oedema, erythema, dilated veins of the leg.

Dull aching or nagging pain in the calf muscles is present.

Superficial blebs in the skin

Low grade fever with increased pulse rate is characteristic.

Phlegmasia alba dolens refers to white leg. It occurs when the thrombus extends from calf region to ileo-femoral vein.

Phlegmasia coerulea dolens refers to blue leg with loss of superficial tissues of the toes.

Signs (Acute DVT)

1. **Homan's test**: Forcible dorsiflexion of foot results in severe pain in the calf region.
2. **Moses test** (Ideally should not be done for fear of embolism): Tenderness over calf muscle on squeezing the muscle from side to side.

Investigations

1. **Doppler study**: It is ideal for femoral vein thrombosis or when thrombus extends into popliteal vein. Normal femoral vein gives a wind storm sound which completely disappears at the end of inspiration. No sound is heard if there is femoral thrombosis.
2. **Contrast venography** is done by injecting radio-opaque dye into dorsal venous arch with an inflatable cuff both above the ankle and above the knee. Clot appears as a filling defect. However. venography is not routinely done because it is expensive and invasive.

Treatment

1. Bed rest and elevation of limbs
2. Injection HEPARIN 10,000 units IV bolus with continuous infusion of 30,000 to 45,000 units per day. During heparin therapy activated partial thromboplastin time should be double the normal value. International Normalized Ratio (INR) should be between 2.0 and 3.0. Heparin is given for a period of 7-10 days.

Warfarin, as oral anticoagulant is started 2-3 days before heparin is withdrawn because of the slow onset time of warfarin. Treatment with warfarin should continue for 6 to 12 months. Repeat duplex scan should be done to see for recanalisation of the veins. The dose of warfarin is 10mg twice a day.

3. **Inferior Vena Caval filters**: They can be inserted percutaneously via femoral vein in patients where in **lytic therapy** is contraindicated.

4. **Surgery** is not done regularly. However in chronic cases venous bypass has been attempted with moderate success.

   Palma operation is done in ileo-femoral thrombosis wherein common femoral vein below the block is anastomosed to the opposite femoral vein through opposite long saphenous vein.

   May-Husni operation wherein popliteal vein is connected to long saphenous vein above.

Complications

1. **Permanent oedema** of the limb. The limb has an **inverted beer bottle** appearance.
2. **Pulmonary embolism** because the thrombus is not attached to vessel wall.
3. Secondary varicosity and **non-healing ulcer**

PROPHYLAXIS OF DVT (Key Box 10.7)

Decrease obesity and exercises before surgery

Low dose heparin 5,000 units subcutaneous, 2 hours before surgery and 24 hours after surgery, and then every 12 hours for 5 days is given, during major surgeries like cholecystectomy, abdominoperineal resection, etc.

Intermittent pneumatic compression of the calf throughout the operation, maintains the blood flow in the lower limbs. Inflation pressure is around 30-50 mm Hg.

Dextran 70 inhibits sludging of red blood cells and platelet aggregation.

Aspirin along with dipyridamole has been used (antiplatelet agents).

Early mobilisation, walking, adequate hydration

Low molecular weight heparin decreases chances of bleeding.

Key Box 10.7		
PROPHYLAXIS : RISK GROUPS		
Low Risk	:	Young patients
		Minor illness
		Operation <30 minutes
Moderate Risk	:	> 40 years
		Debilitating illness
		Major Surgery
High Risk	:	> 50 years, medical conditions M.I., Strokes, Major Surgery, Malignancy, Obesity.

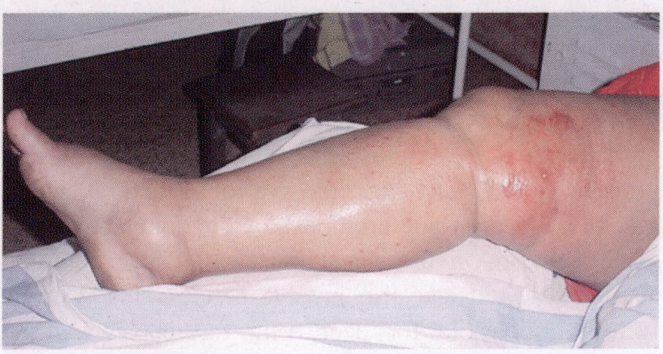

Fig. 10.16 Acute DVT : Grossly swollen, oedematous leg, skin is red and warm with superficial blisters

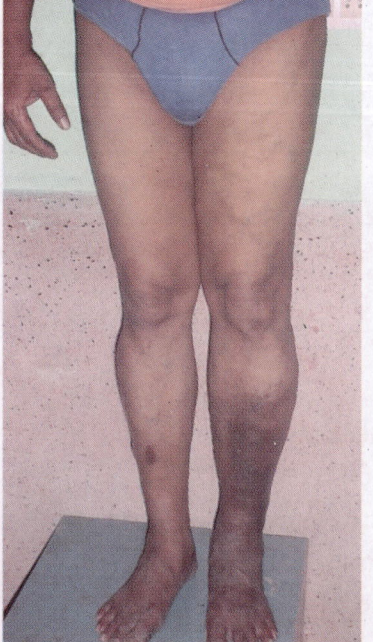

Observe the differences between acute DVT and chronic DVT. Such swollen legs have been mistaken for filariasias and treated also without any results.

Fig. 10.17 Grossly swollen leg, pigmentation, eczema and secondary varicosity in a case of chronic DVT

Skin Tumours

11

- Classification
- Premalignant lesions
- Basal cell carcinoma
- Squamous cell carcinoma
- Melanocytic tumours
- Malignant melanoma
- Keratoacanthoma
- Turban tumour
- Corn
- Wart
- Merkel cell carcinoma

The skin, the outermost coat of the human body, functions as a protective cover against various insulting agents such as ultraviolet radiation of sunlight, excessive heat and various chemical agents.

Hence, no wonder it is one of the commonest cancers in elderly patients. However, more than 90% of skin tumours are curable because of the following reasons:

- They are diagnosed early, easily (unlike intra abdominal malignancies) and they are low grade cancers.

Among skin cancers about 70% are basal cell carcinomas, 20% are squamous cell carcinomas and 5% are melanocarcinomas. Other rare skin cancers are sebaceous carcinomas, dermoid cystic carcinomas, dermato-fibrosarcomas etc. In this chapter only common malignant skin tumours are discussed.

Also some common skin leisons such as corn and wart are also discussed in this chapter.

CLASSIFICATION OF SKIN TUMOURS

I. Epidermal tumours
A. Benign
- Papilloma
- Seborrhoeic keratosis
- Verrucous naevus

B. Malignant
- Basal cell carcinoma
- Epithelioma, Marjolin's ulcer

II. Melanocytic tumours
A. Benign
- Junctional naevus
- Compound naevus
- Intradermal naevus
- Hutchinson's freckle
- Hairy naevus
- Blue naevus

B. Malignant
- Superficial spreading melanoma
- Nodular melanoma
- Lentigo maligna melanoma

III. Sweat gland tumours (malignant)
- Hidradenocarcinoma
- Adenoid cystic carcinoma

IV. Sebaceous gland tumours
- Sebaceous adenoma
- Sebaceous carcinoma

V. Other tumours

- Dermatofibrosarcoma protuberans
- Trichofolliculoma (hair follicle tumour)

PREMALIGNANT LESIONS OF THE SKIN

1. **Chronic irritation** to the skin can occur due to various chemicals like dyes, tar, inorganic arsenic, etc., which contain various carcinogens. Coal tar contains polycyclic aromatic hydrocarbons like benzopyrenes, which are carcinogenic.

2. **Solar keratosis (senile keratosis)**:   Prolonged exposure to sunrays can cause *hyperkeratosis* of the skin which is called solar keratosis. Skin changes occur due to accumulated effect of ultraviolet rays over a period of many years. Ultraviolet rays are also present in phototherapy given in the treatment of psoriasis (**PUVA** therapy –**P**soralen **U**ltra **V**iolet-**A**). **Common sites** : Back of hands, face, rim of ears.

- Age group: Middle age, more than 50 years.
- Clinically the lesion is irregular, firm and irritating patch which is flat or raised.
- Malignancy should be suspected when the lesion becomes indurated, when a non-healing ulcer develops, when the central crust is shed and when regional lymph nodes are palpable.

3. **Chronic scar** : Squamous cell carcinoma which develops in a scar tissue is called *Marjolin's ulcer* (Fig.11.1). **Burns scar** is the commonest cause of Marjolin's ulcer followed by scar due to varicose ulcer, snake bite scar, chronic osteomyelitis scar, lupus vulgaris (tuberculosis of face) scar.

- Marjolin's ulcer differs from squamous cell carcinoma by following characteristics (Table 11.1).

4. **Radiodermatitis** : Increased incidence of skin can-

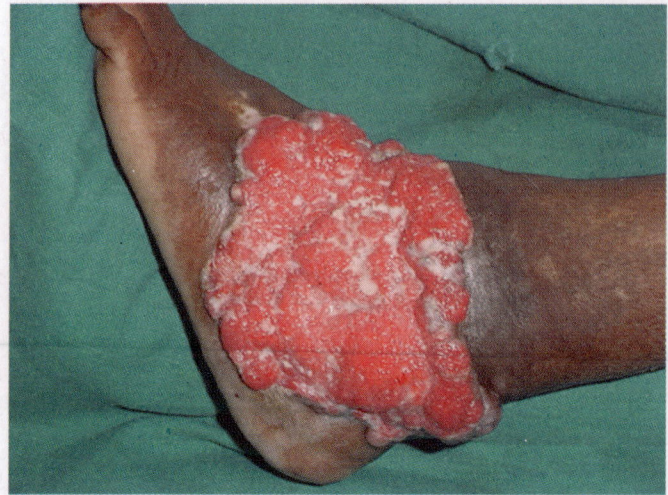

Fig. 11.1 Marjolin's ulcer arising in a burns scar

cer was found in persons who worked in the X-ray department initially. Now, the incidence is less due to the usage of protective gear. Radiation change in the skin may vary from a simple erythema initially to atrophy or hyperpigmentation. Later, this lesion changes into squamous cell carcinoma.

5. **Bowen's disease** is an intraepidermal carcinoma. It is rare and occurs in middle-aged patients. It occurs on the skin of the trunk as scaly, erythematous plaques which are often multiple. They are brownish patches with raised margin. Microscopically, large clear cells are found (these cells are also found in Paget's disease of the nipple).

6. **Leukoplakia** (Page 206)

7. **Autosomal recessive disorders**: In this group one or more of the DNA repair enzymes is defective or deficient. As a result of this, sites exposed to sun are vulnerable for the development of various skin cancers. **Xeroderma pigmentosum** and **albinism** have increased predisposition to skin cancer (Fig. 11.3).

Table 11.1 Comparison of Marjolin's ulcer and squamous cell carcinoma

MARJOLIN'S ULCER	SQUAMOUS CELL CARCINOMA
• Grows very slowly because of scar tissue	• Grows slowly
• It is painless as scar does not contain nerves	• It can be painful if it infiltrates the nerve fibres
• Lymphatic metastasis does not occur because lymphatics are destroyed or occluded	• Lymphatic metastasis is the chief method of spread
• It is less malignant	• Comparatively more malignant
• Surgery cures the disease, radiotherapy is *not very useful*	• Both surgery and radiotherapy are used

BASAL CELL CARCINOMA (RODENT ULCER)

It is the most common malignant skin tumour. Generally, it is a slow-growing neoplasm which can present as an ulcer of many years duration. In some cases, it can present as locally penetrating, ulcerative and destructive lesion. It arises from basal cell of the pilosebaceous adnexa and occurs only on the skin.

- Location: Majority of the lesions are found on the face above a line from lobule of the ear to the angle of mouth.

COMMON SITES

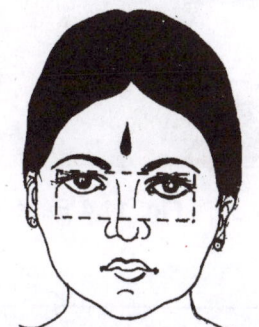

1. Inner canthus of the eye
2. Outer canthus of the eye
3. Eyelids
4. Bridge of the nose
5. Around nasolabial fold
- These sites are the areas where the tears roll down. Hence it is also called **tear cancer** (Fig. 11.3a, 11.3b).

Fig. 11.2 Sites of basal cell carcinoma

Basal cell carcinoma cannot occur in the mucosal surfaces which do not have pilosebaceous adnexa, e.g., cervix, lips, tongue.

PRECIPITATING FACTORS

- Ultraviolet rays : Basal cell carcinoma is common in Australia[1] and New Zealand because of ultra violet rays.
- Fair skin is vulnerable for the development of basal cell carcinoma.
- Arsenic once used in skin ointments, also increases the risk of basal cell carcinoma.

CLINICAL FEATURES

- The most common clinical presentation is an ulcer that never heals. Sometimes healing takes place with scabbing and later it breaks down and forms ulcer again. The ulcer has raised and beaded edge, induration may be present, and bleeds on touch. The base can be subcutaneous fat or deeper structures like muscle or bone depending upon invasion.

Scabbing occurs only in benign ulcers. Basal Cell carcinoma is the only malignant ulcer which shows scabbing.

- It can also present as a painless, firm, nodule, which is pigmented with fine blood vessels on its surface. (Key Box 11.1)

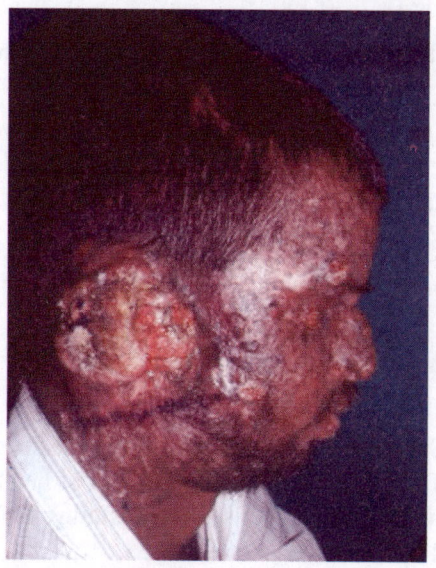

A brother and sister with **xeroderma pigmentosa** developed 33 and 26 skin malignancies respectively which included basal cell, squamous cell carcinoma and malignant melanoma, since the age of 5 till 22 years. Eventually boy died at 22 years of age (Fig. 11.3a). This is the sad part of this distressing and frustrating disease.

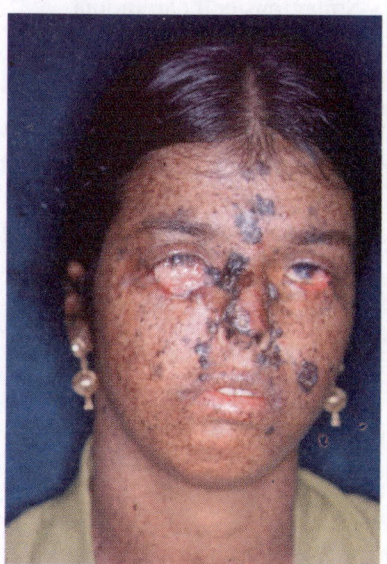

Fig. 11.3a Basal cell carcinoma involving the right ear

Fig. 11.3b Basal cell carcinoma involving nasolabial fold

---

1. This may be the reason why Australian and New Zealand cricket players apply some protective cream to the potential risky sites while playing the match.

Key Box 11.1

BASAL CELL CARCINOMA - TYPES

- Nodular
- Pigmented
- Superficial
- Cystic
- Infiltrative

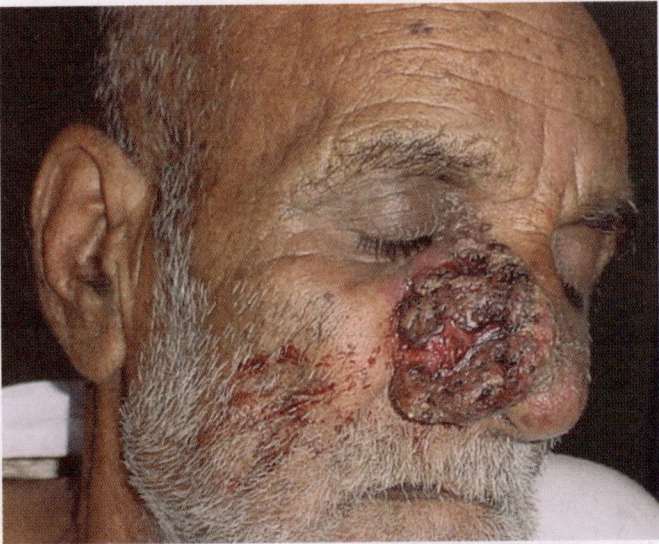

Fig. 11.4 Basal cell carcinoma - typical site

- It can present as nodular ulcerative form (Fig.11.4).

- Rarely, it can be cystic variety which does not show fluctuation.

- Field fire rodent ulcer is a rapidly growing rodent ulcer with destruction and disfigurement of the facial skin. It has an advancing edge with healed central scar.

DIFFERENTIAL DIAGNOSIS

- **Keratoacanthoma:** It ocurs only in the face. Edge can be raised with ulceration, thus resembling basal cell carcinoma (Page 116)

- **Sclerosing angioma**

- **Malignant melanoma** - Pigmented basal cell carcinoma may be mistaken for malignant melanoma.

- Squamous cell carcinoma

SPREAD

- It spreads by **local invasion**. Even though slow growing, it slowly penetrates deep inside, destroys the underlying tissues like bone, cartilage or even eyeball. Hence the name rodent ulcer. It **does not spread by lymphatics** because the size of tumour emboli are big. Blood spread is extremely rare.

INVESTIGATIONS

- Wedge biopsy from the edge of the ulcer (Key Box 11.2). The edge is selected because of following reasons:

1. Edge is the growing part, malignant cells are numerous

2. Centre has slough or scab which may not reveal malignancy

3. Comparison with the normal skin is possible.

Key Box 11.2

MICROSCOPIC PICTURE

- Central mass of polyhedral cells
- Cells are darkly stained
- With peripheral palisade layer of columnar cells. Cell nests, keratinisation and mitotic figures are absent.

TREATMENT (Refer also Fig. 11.5)

- Basal cell carcinoma responds well to radiation. Surgical excision also cures the disease.

1. **Radiation** is indicated in elderly patients who have an extensive lesion which requires a complicated plastic reconstruction. **Dosage** : 4000-6000 cGy units.

2. **Surgery** is indicated when the lesion is :

- Very close to the eye, adherent to the cartilage or bone

- In easily, accessible sites like neck, hand etc

- In radiation failure cases

Types of Surgery: Wide excision. This means excision of the growth with at least 1 cm of healthy margin and at the depth also. The resulting defect is closed by :

A. **Primary suturing** of the defect if the lesion is small

B. **Skin grafting** if defect is big as in neck or dorsum of hand

C. **Rotation flap**s as in face for better cosmetic effect.

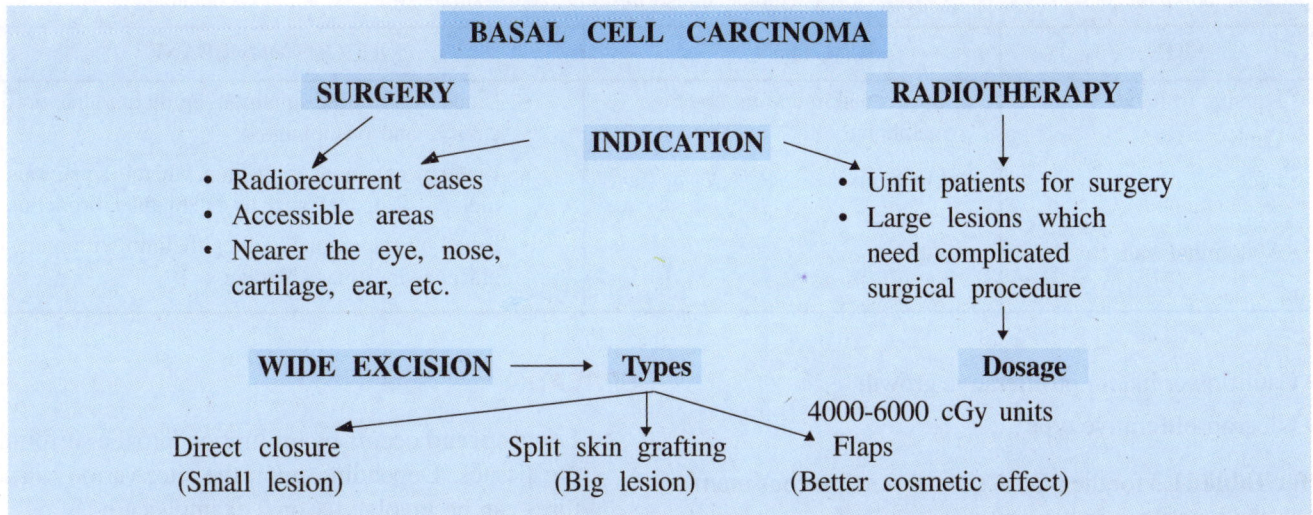

BASAL CELL CARCINOMA

SURGERY   **INDICATION**   **RADIOTHERAPY**

- Radiorecurrent cases
- Accessible areas
- Nearer the eye, nose, cartilage, ear, etc.

- Unfit patients for surgery
- Large lesions which need complicated surgical procedure

WIDE EXCISION ⟶ **Types**   **Dosage**

4000-6000 cGy units

Direct closure (Small lesion)   Split skin grafting (Big lesion)   Flaps (Better cosmetic effect)

Fig. 11.5 Summary of the treatment of basal cell carcinoma

SQUAMOUS CELL CARCINOMA (EPITHELIOMA)

It is the second common malignant skin tumour after basal cell carcinoma. It arises from prickle cell layer of the Malpighian layer of the skin. It usually affects elderly males. All the pre-malignant conditions listed earlier applies to this condition. It can also occur de novo in the skin. Basosquamous carcinoma is the term applied when squamous cell carcinoma arises in a pre-existing basal cell carcinona. It is interesting to note that a variety of names have been given to squamous cell carcinoma when it occurs in different places. They are given in Table 11.2.

PATHOLOGICAL TYPES

- Ulcerative variety-Commonest

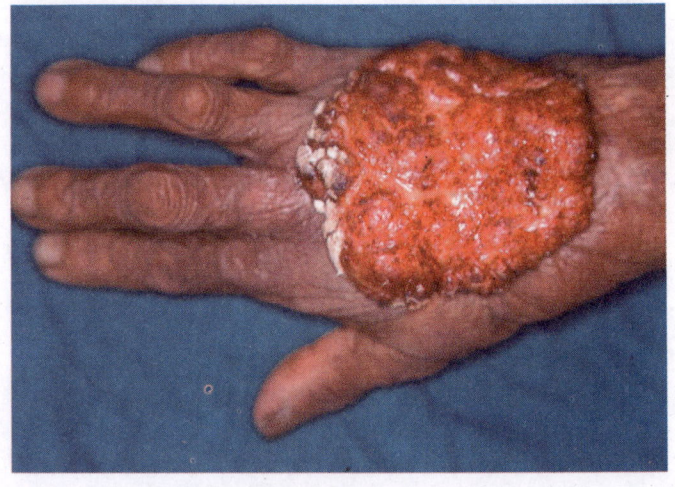

Fig. 11.6 Squamous cell carcinoma affecting dorsum of the hand - ulceroproliferative lesion

Table 11.2 Sites of Squamous cell carcinoma

SITE	NAME	REASON/EXPLANATION
1. Skin of the abdomen or back of thigh in Kashmiri patients	**Kangri** cancer	**Kangri** is the name given to the pot containing **hot charcoal** which is applied to the abdominal wall because of excessive cold in Kashmir (India).
2. Buttocks, heels, elbows	**Kang** cancer	Tibetans sleep on the **oven bed** due to the excess cold.
3. Scrotum	**Chimney sweep** cancer	Seen in chimney sweepers due to prolonged **irritation by chemicals** like tar or pitch in.
4. Abdominal wall	**Saree cancer** and **dhothi** cancer	Due to **chronic irritation** caused by wearing dhothi or saree too tight.
5. Lower lip	**Countryman's lip**	Carcinoma lower lip is common in **agriculturists** (outdoor occupation)

Table 11.3 Sites of Squamous cell carcinoma

SKIN	JUNCTION	MUCOUS MEMBRANE
• Dorsum of hand • Limbs • Face • Abdominal wall, etc.	• Between skin and mucous membrane • Lip, penis • Vulva	• Lined by stratified squamous epithelium like oral cavity and oesophagus • Lined by columnar epithelium, wherein squamous metaplasia occurs, such as gall bladder, bronchus • Lined by transitional cell epithelium with metaplasia as in urinary bladder

- Cauliflower like or proliferative growth
- Ulceroproliferative type

Refer Table 11.3 for the typical sites of skin, mucous membrane and junction involvement.

CLINICAL FEATURES

- Typically, it is an ulcerative or cauliflower like lesion (Fig. 11.6).
- Edge is everted and indurated (Fig. 11.7).
- Base is indurated and it may be subcutaneous tissue, muscle or bone.
- Floor contains **cancerous tissue which looks like granulation tissue.** It is pale, friable, bleeds easily on touch. (Fig.11.8)
- Surrounding area is also indurated.
- Mobility is usually restricted due to infiltration of underlying structures. In very early cases, ulcer can be moved along with skin over the underlying structures.
- Regional lymph nodes like inguinal lymph nodes (both vertical and horizontal group) can get enlarged when squamous cell carcinoma affects lower limb or abdominal wall. Hard lymph nodes are suggestive of secondaries.

SPREAD

1. **Local spread** occurs by infiltration into the surrounding tissues. Depending upon the site, various structures can be involved. Some examples are :

- Tendon involvement in the dorsum of the hand.
- Muscle involvement in the abdominal wall.
- Bone involvement like tibia in carcinoma developing in a varicose ulcer or mandible in carcinoma cheek.

2. **Lymphatic spread** is the chief method of spread even though it occurs relatively late. Regional nodes are involved first.

- Nodes which are soft to firm and tender are due to secondary infection.
- Nodes which are hard, non-tender, with or without fixity are due to secondary deposits.
- In untreated cases nodes start ulcerating through the skin resulting in bleeding and pain.
- As already stated, nodes do not get involved in Marjolin's ulcer.

3. **Blood spread** is rare and late.

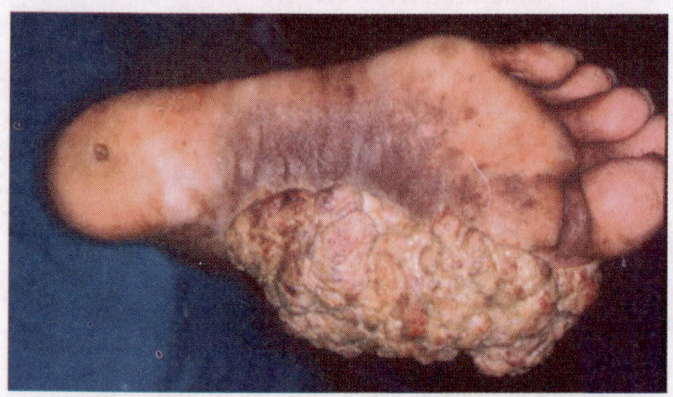

Fig. 11.7 Squamous cell carcinoma of the sole

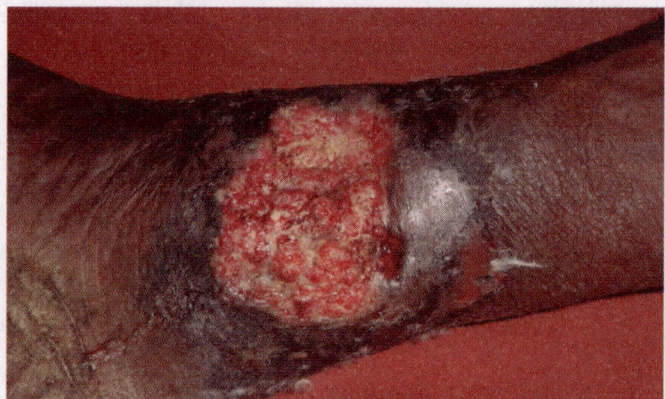

Fig. 11.8 Squamous cell carcinoma - bleeds on touch

Differential diagnosis (Key Box 11.3)

Key Box 11.3
DIFFERENTIAL DIAGNOSIS
• Basal cell carcinoma
• Keratoacanthoma
• Papilloma
• Pyogenic granuloma
• Tuberculous ulcer

INVESTIGATIONS

- A wedge biopsy from the edge of the ulcer or growth is taken.
- Microscopic picture: 80% of these cancers are well differentiated. (Key Box 11.4)
- It is characterised by central structureless mass of keratin surrounded by normal looking squamous cells which are arranged in concentric manner like onion skin. This whole appearance is called epithelial pearl or cell nest. In 20% of cases, cells are undifferentiated with numerous mitoses, without keratinization.

Key Box 11.4	
BRODER'S CLASSIFICATION	
I. Well differentiated	75% keratin pearls
II. Moderately differentiated	50% keratin pearls
III. Poorly differentiated	25% keratin pearls
IV. ---	< 25% keratin pearls

TREATMENT

- Treatment can be classified as treatment of the primary and treatment of the secondaries.

I. TREATMENT OF THE PRIMARY: Squamous cell carcinoma is treated by wide excision or radiotherapy.

A. SURGERY

- It involves removal of growth along with 2 cm of normal healthy tissue from the palpable indurated edge of the tumour.

Indications of surgery

- When the lesion is small and superficial
- When the lesion has involved deeper tissues like muscles, cartilage or bone, etc.
- Radio recurrent cases

  Reconstruction : After wide excision, the defect can be closed primarily or with split skin graft or a flap to reconstruct the part depending upon the extent of resection. If the growth is fixed to tibia, below knee amputation is the treatment.

B. RADIOTHERAPY

Indications for radiotherapy

- Well differentiated carcinoma
- Patients who are not fit for surgery

  Dosage: 6000 cGy units over 6 weeks, 200 units/day.

II. TREATMENT OF SECONDARIES

1. 30-40% of the enlarged regional nodes are due to secondary infection. Once the primary is treated or controlled along with antibiotics, lymph nodes regress. In such cases, 'wait and watch policy' is observed.

2. If lymph nodes do not regress or are hard and mobile, FNAC can be done to confirm the diagnosis followed by radical block dissection. Thus, squamous cell carcinoma of the leg requires inguinal block dissection.

3. If lymph nodes are hard and fixed to the femoral vessels, palliative radiotherapy is given. Even in advanced fungating lesions, the response rate to radiotherapy is reasonably good.

- Dose: 3000-4000 cGy units over 3-4 weeks, 200 units/day.

Structures removed in inguinal block dissection

- The superficial group of nodes which consist of horizontal chain which lies below inguinal ligament and vertical chain which lies along upper 5-6 cm of long saphenous vein. These two group of nodes form the letter T.
- The deep glands are located alongside the proximal end of the femoral vein, and one lying within femoral canal.
- Fat, fascia, lymphatics are cleared from 2 cm above the inguinal ligament up to 2 cm below saphenofemoral junction. The medial clearance is important upto femoral canal. 8-10 cm of long saphenous vein near its termination is removed to facilitate lymph node clearance.

Complications of inguinal block dissection and treatment

- Wound infection → Broad-spectrum antibiotics

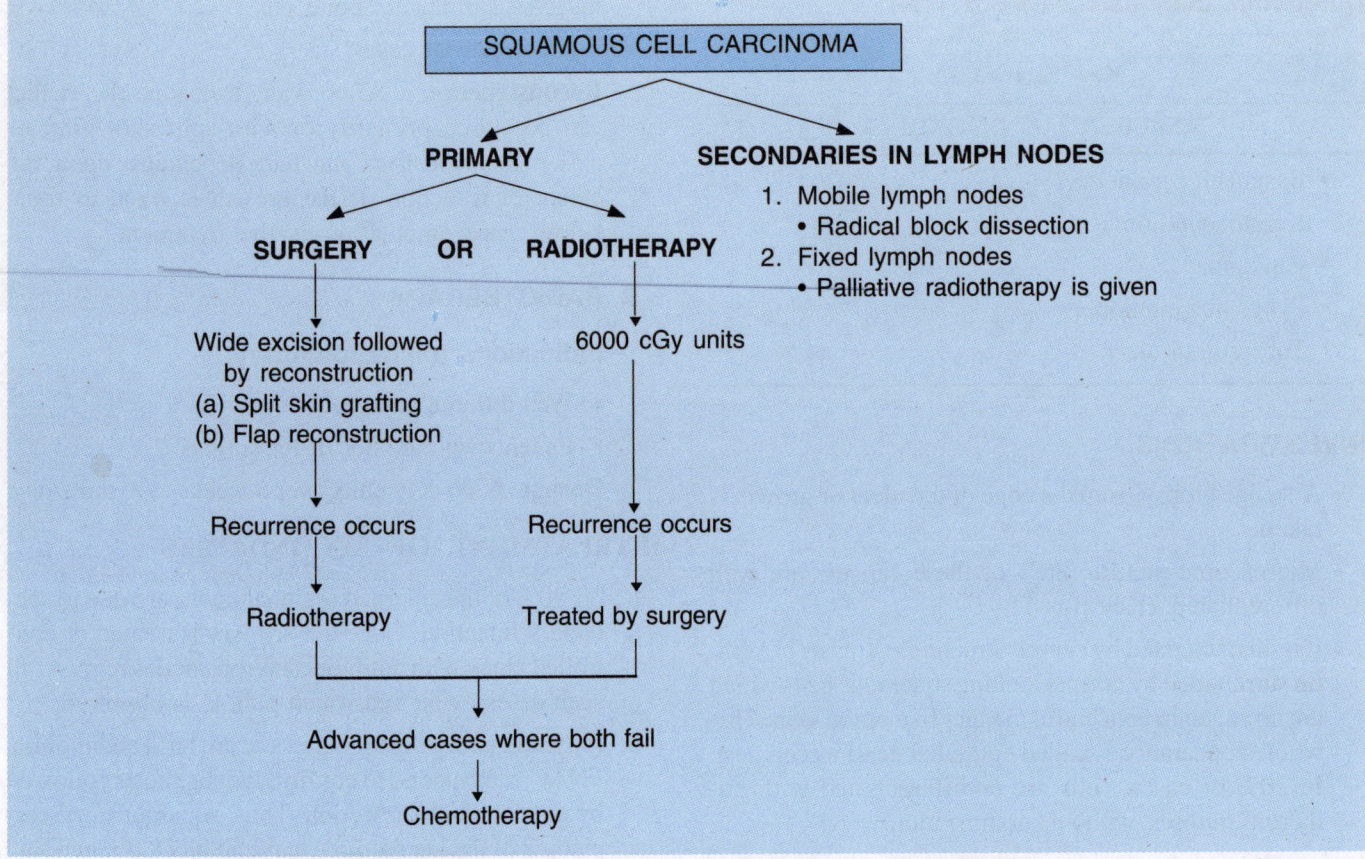

Fig. 11.9 Summary of the treatment of squamous cell carcinoma

- Lymphorrhoea → Adequate drainage
- Haemorrhage → Perfect haemostasis
- Femoral blow out → Sartorius muscle slide to cover femoral vessels at the end of surgery

Summary of the treatment of squamous cell carcinoma is given in Fig. 11.9.

MELANOCYTIC TUMOURS AND MALIGNANT MELANOMA

SIMPLE MELANOCYTIC TUMOURS

These are also called pigmented naevi which are composed of modified melanocytes derived from the neural crest. All naevi have excess melanin pigmentation because of which they are tan brown or black in colour. They are located in the basal layer of the epidermis. They are benign. They are of following types :

1. **Junctional naevus**: Located within the epidermis at the dermoepidermal junction. They are common in children. They appear as tanbrown to black macules. They are smooth, flat and hairless moles. As they enlarge, they become slightly raised and can evolve into an intradermal or a compound naevus or a malignant melanoma.

   Junctional naevus commonly occurs on the palm, sole, digits and genitalia and majority of malignant melanoma develop from junctional naevus.

2. **Compound naevus** : As the mole enlarges, naeval cells also appear in the dermis along the intraepidermal cells. Such moles are described as compound naevi. These are found usually in adolescents and are usually benign (Fig. 11.10).

3. **Intradermal naevus** : It is the most common mole in adults. Because of its deep seated nature, it appears blue, hence the name blue naevus. It is seen on the scalp and face. It contains hair and it does not become malignant.

4. **Congenital pigmented naevus** which is present at birth, has a **greater potential for malignant change.** It can involve extensive areas of the skin (**Giant**).

5. **Dysplastic naevi** are different from acquired naevi by the following way :
   - Malignant potential is more (Fig. 11.11)
   - Family members may have such lesions.
   - Such syndrome is described as **familial dysplastic naevus syndrome.**

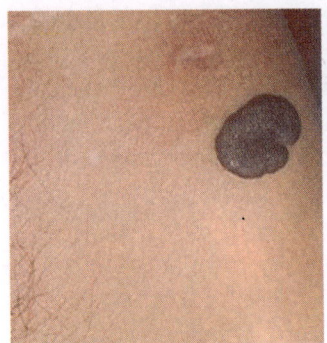
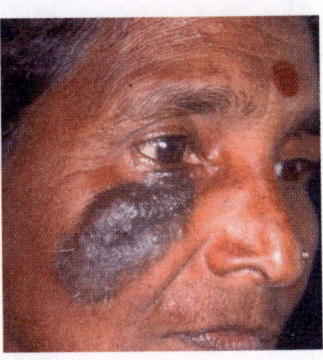

Fig. 11.10 Compound naevus

Fig. 11.11 Dysplastic naevi over the face

MALIGNANT MELANOMA (MELANOCARCINOMA)

It is a malignant tumour arising from pigment-forming cells (melanoblasts) which are derived from the neural crest. Melanoblasts and Melanocytes convert dihydroxyphenylalanine (DOPA) into melanin. This is called positive DOPA reaction (Key Box 11.5).

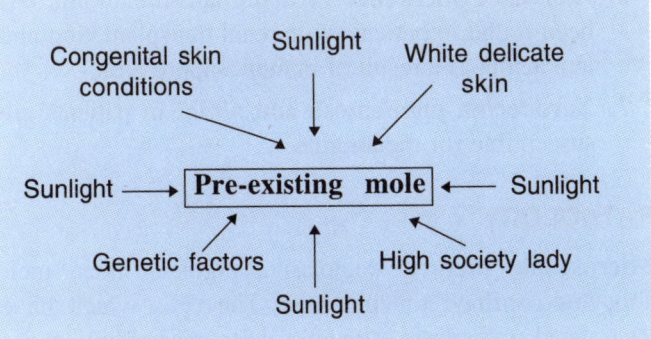

Fig. 11.12 Aetiopathogenesis

Key Box 11.5
POSITIVE DOPA REACTION
TYROSINE
↓ ← **TYROSINASE**
DOPA
↓ ← **OXIDASE**
MELANIN

- It is a potentially curable tumour in early stages. If left untreated or if not treated properly, it disseminates rapidly, showers the body with tumour emboli and offers a very painful death.

Common sites of malignant melanoma:
- Head and neck 20-30%
- Lower extremity 20-30%
- Trunk 20-30%
- Remaining cases occur in upper extremities, genitalia, choroid of the eye, etc.

AETIOPATHOGENESIS (Fig. 11.12)

1. **Ultraviolet rays** : It is more common in white skinned people. There is a linear correlation between intensity of exposure to sunlight and malignant melanoma

in white skinned people[1]. White skinned people who live close to the equator have increased tendency of developing malignant melanoma. Thus, the highest incidence is found in Queensland (Australia). For the same reasons, malignant melanoma is common in United Kingdom, North America, Australia, etc.

2. **Age and sex** : Malignant melanoma is more common in females. The higher incidence of the disease is found during reproductive age period. Eventhough oestrogen and progesterone receptors are found in malignant melanoma in some patients, their true role is not yet established.

3. **Genetic factors** : Increased incidence has been found in patients with familial dysplastic naevus syndrome. The disease is also common in individuals with Celtic race who give family history of malignant melanoma (3-5%).

4. **Trauma** : Malignant melanoma occurs in the sole of the foot in African Negroes. Whether trauma is the cause is not clear.

---

1. Malignant melanoma is the killer skin cancer of whites.

"Bronzed Body Beautiful" concept should be discouraged.

5. **Pre-existing mole**: Approximately 50% of melanomas arise in a preexisting mole, remaining 50% arise de novo in the normal skin. Malignant change occurs in the junctional or compound naevus. Malignancy should be suspected where following changes occur in a mole.

- Enlargement
- More pigmentation
- Ulceration
- Itching
- Bleeding
- Development of the halo surrounding the lesion.

6. **Increased incidence** of malignant melanoma has been found in patients with renal transplantation and leukaemia as a result of immunosuppression.

7. **Xeroderma pigmentosa and albinism** patients are susceptible for melanomas.

PATHOLOGY

Microscopic picture: Anaplastic, pigment laden melanocytes confined to epidermis. The cells which have vacuolated cytoplasm (Paget's cells resembling those seen in Paget's disease of the breast) are found. Cells also invade the dermis. Along with pigment-laden macrophages, dermal infiltration of lymphocytes[1] may be present. Rarely, anaplastic melanocytes do not form pigment (**amelanotic melanoma**).

- All melanomas (except nodular) show **radial growth initially** in the form of intraepidermal growth. However, **nodular melanoma** has **vertical growth phase** thus involving dermis leading to nodule formation. This has poor prognosis.

PATHOLOGICAL GRADING OF MALIGNANT MELANOMA

Clarke's level of invasion is represented in the diagram (Fig. 11.13).

Level 1 Tumour cells confined to basement membrane
Level 2 Tumour extension into papillary dermis
Level 3 Tumour reaches the interface between papillary dermis and reticular dermis
Level 4 Tumour reaches reticular dermis
Level 5 Tumour invades subcutaneous fat

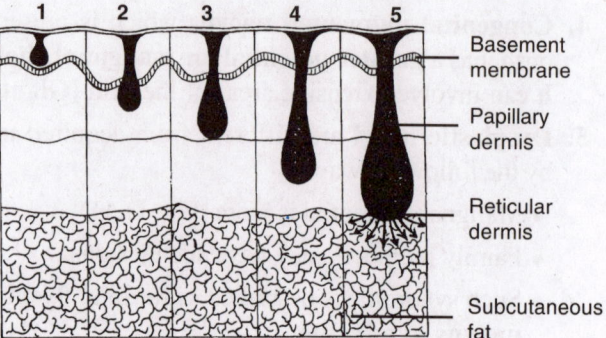

Fig. 11.13 Clarke's level of invasion

Breslow described the staging depending upon the maximum thickness at the centre of the lesion.

Stage I   Thickness less than 0.75 mm
Stage II   0.76 to 1.5 mm
Stage III   1.51 to 3 mm
Stage IV   More than 3 mm

CLINICAL FEATURES

1. Malignant melanoma can present as changes in the pre-existing mole which are already described.

2. The patient can present as a non-healing ulcer of the sole of the foot.

- It is a painless ulcer
- Edges are irregular
- Floor is irregular
- Bleeds on touch
- Typically, the ulcer is pigmented (Fig. 11.14). In 10% of patients, pigment is absent. They are called amelanotic melanoma.
- Lesion is firm in consistency and induration is absent.
- A halo may be present surrounding the ulcer.
- The lesion moves with the skin and is usually not fixed to underlying structures.
- Satellite nodules (within 2 cms of the primary) may be found surrounding the lesion which are due to spread through intradermal lymphatics. Such patients will have greatly enlarged, firm, non-tender nodes.
- For Clinical types see Table 11.5

---

1. *Presence of lymphocytes may be an indication of host response 'Fight' against cancer.*

Table 11.5 Clinical types of malignant melanoma

NAME	NATURE	BEHAVIOUR
1. Lentigo Maligna melanoma	Arises from Hutchinson's melanotic freckle	Least common (5-15%)
	Occurs in old people on face and temporal region	Least malignant
2. Superficial spreading	Any part, more in the trunk	Most common (70%)
3. Nodular	Any part, more in the leg	Most malignant, invasive (15-30%)
4. Acral lentigenous	Located on the palm, sole, digits	Presents late, aggressive (4-8%)
5. Amelanotic	Difficult to diagnose	Rare, non-pigmented

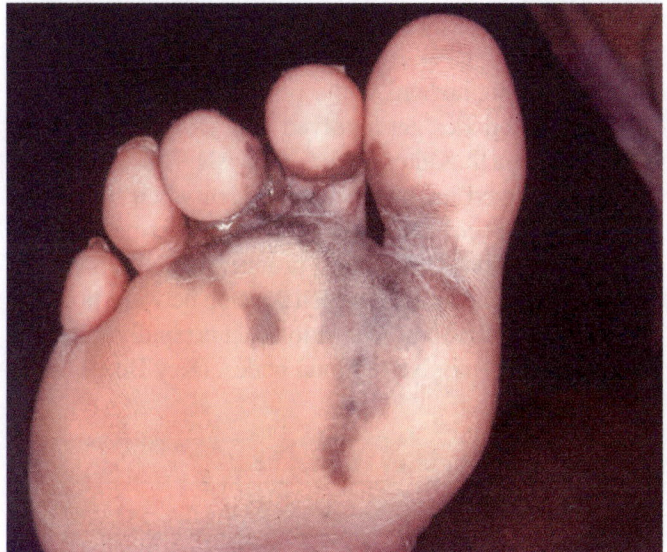

Fig. 11.14 Superficial spreading

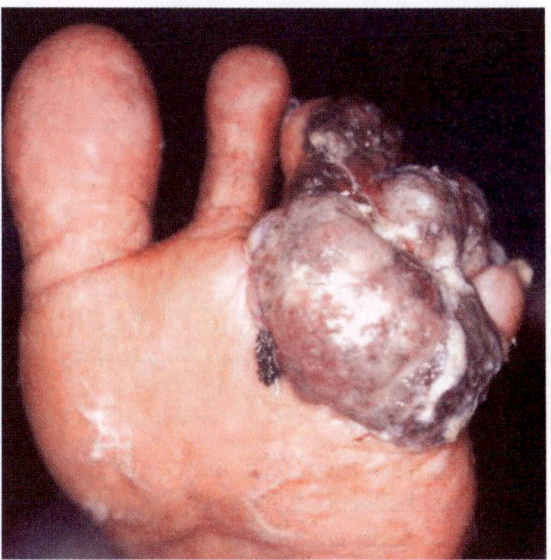

Fig. 11.15 Nodular

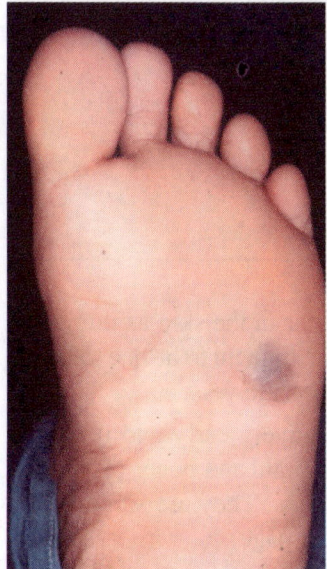

Fig. 11.16 Acral lentigenous variety with early changes- never incise or cauterise such melanomas.

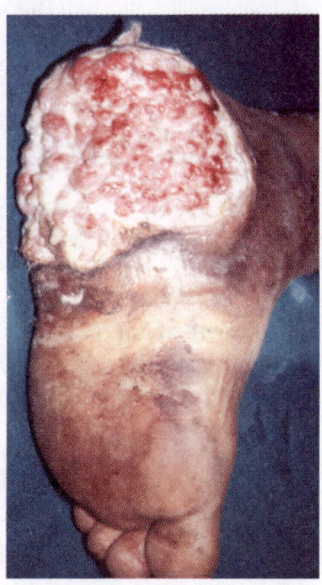

Fig.11.17 The lesion resembles squamous cell carcinoma. Punch biopsy reported as Amelanotic Melanoma

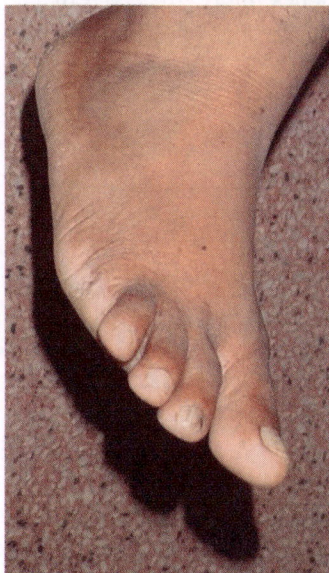

Fig. 11.18 Observe the foot, little toe has been amputated five years back for malignant melanoma

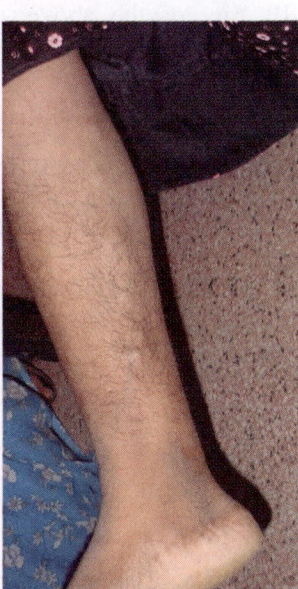

Fig. 11.19 Same patient as in Fig. 11.18 presented to the hospital with in-transit deposits

CLINICAL NOTES

55 year lady presented to the hospital with inguinal lymph nodes. Clinical examination of the leg revealed nodules in the leg with firm to hard enlarged nodes in the inguinal region. On careful observation little toe was missing. On questioning patient admits that the toe has been amputated five years back for a painless blackish lesion elsewhere.

ABCDE OF MELANOMA (Key Box 11.6)

Key Box 11.6
ABCDE OF MELANOMA
A : Asymmetry
B : Border irregular
C : Colour Variegation
D : Diameter >6mm
E : Elevation

STAGING

IA: Thickness less than 0.75 mm
IB: Thickness between 0.76 to 1.5 mm
IIA: Thickness between 1.51 to 4.0 mm
IIB: Thickness more than 4.0 mm
IIIA: Any of the above + nodes less than 3 cm
IIIB: Any of the above + nodes more than 3 cm
IV: Any of the above + any node + M1 (distant spread)

DIFFERENTIAL DIAGNOSIS

Key Box 11.7
DIFFERENTIAL DIAGNOSIS
• Pigmented basal cell carcinoma, Histiocytoma (sclerosing angioma), Naevus
• Kaposi's sarcoma, Cavernous haemangioma

SPREAD

1. **Local spread** occurs mainly by continuity and contiguity. **Satellite nodules** are due to local and lymphatic spread, situated within 2 cms of the primary lesion. Malignant melanoma rarely infiltrates the deep fascia unless and until a 'blunder biopsy' is done. **Inadequate local excision can result in local recurrence later.**

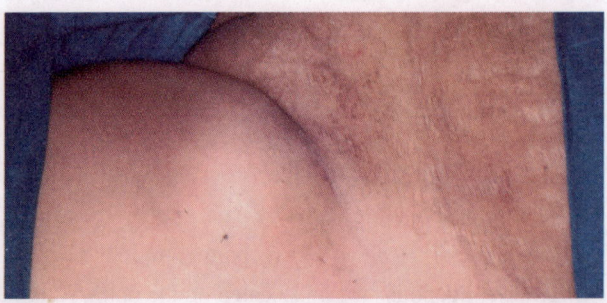

Fig. 11.20 Hugely enlarged inguinal lymph nodes - the nodes can be firm to hard. Sometimes they are soft due to degeneration

2. **Lymphatic spread** is the principal mode of spread. Regional nodes get involved very early in malignant melanoma thus altering the prognosis. Thus, nodes can get enlarged to a large extent even when the lesion looks innocent. Spread occurs both by permeation and embolisation. Permeation produces satellite nodules and in-transit nodules which develop between primary and secondaries. Embolisation occurs rapidly and early producing massive regional nodes. (Key Box 11.8)

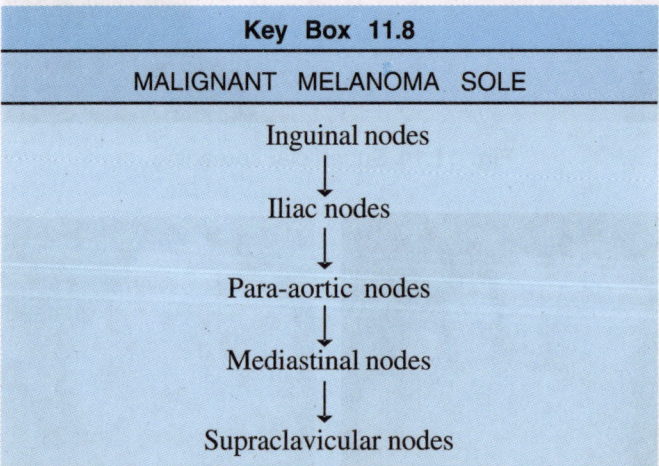

Key Box 11.8
MALIGNANT MELANOMA SOLE
Inguinal nodes
↓
Iliac nodes
↓
Para-aortic nodes
↓
Mediastinal nodes
↓
Supraclavicular nodes

Intransit metastasis appear in the skin as intracutaneous metastasis. They are thought to be due to melanoma cells trapped in lymphatic vessels.

3. **Blood spread** occurs relatively early and it causes secondaries in liver, lung, brain and bones producing miserable, pathetic situations. They are summarised in Table 11.6 (See the next page).

INVESTIGATIONS

1. There is no specific investigation except an **excision biopsy of** the lesion. Excision with 1 cm of the

Table 11.6 Spread of malignant melanoma

SPREAD	DIAGNOSIS	PROBLEMS
1. Metastasis in lung	Cannon ball appearance, pleural effusion	Respiratory failure
2. Metastasis in liver	Massive hepatomegaly, ascites	Abdominal discomfort
3. Metastasis in brain	Raised intracranial tension	Coma
4. Metastasis in bone	Bony pains, pathological fractures	Paraplegia, quadriplegia
5. Metastasis in bowel	Bleeding	Anaemia

margin is all that is required. Incisional biopsy is avoided because of following reasons :

- It may injure the deep fascia and it may open up a new plane of spread.
- It does not allow the pathologist to perform a detailed histological examination.

2. **Nonspecific investigations** to look for metastasis are :

- Chest X-ray - Cannon ball secondary
- Ultrasound abdomen-Secondaries in liver
- X-ray of involved bone-Osteolytic lesions

3. **FNAC** of the regional lymph nodes

- Fine needle aspiration of groin nodes is helpful in detecting the spread and to stage the disease.

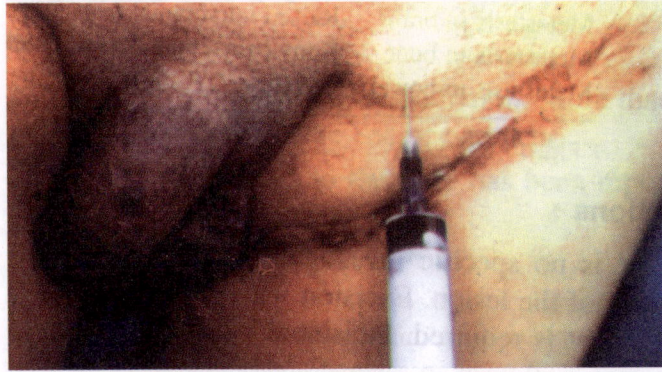

Fig. 11.21 FNAC of the recurrent inguinal node secondaries, bluish black aspirate

4. In advanced cases (as shown in Fig.11.21) punch biopsy can also be taken.

5. Chest X-ray and ultrasound abdomen are other relevant investigations.

TREATMENT

Surgery is the main modality of the treatment available for malignant melanoma. All other modalities of treatment are only palliative and supportive.

Types of surgery possible are as follows

1. **Excision biopsy-wide excision**: A small lesion of 2-4 cm can be excised even under local anaesthesia with 1 cm of healthy margin around (narrow excision). Defect can be closed by primary suturing. While excising the tumour, it is better not to handle the tumour. It is possible to remove the tumour by strictly adhering to the principle of 'No Touch' technique. (Fig. 11.23 and 11.24)

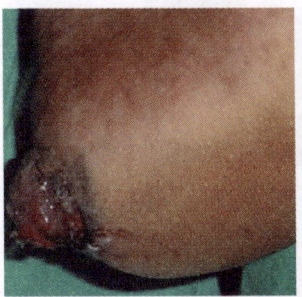 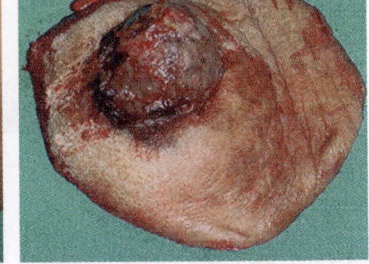

Fig. 11.22 Ulcerated melanoma over the heal   **Fig. 11.23** Wide excision (Minimum 2 cm.) specimen

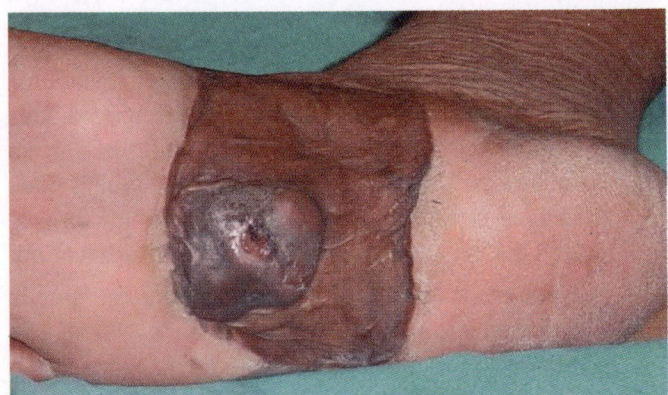

Fig. 11.24 Local recurrence after 2 years probably because of inadequate local excision – You can see the previous skin graft

2. **Clarke's level II lesions** are managed by a wider excision along with 2 cm of healthy margin around. Resulting defect is closed by split skin grafting.

3. **Subungual malignant melanoma** is treated by amputation of the digit.

4. **Malignant melanoma of the choroid** has good prognosis. It is treated by enucleation of the eye.

5. Amputations (advanced and large lesions). (Fig. 11.25)

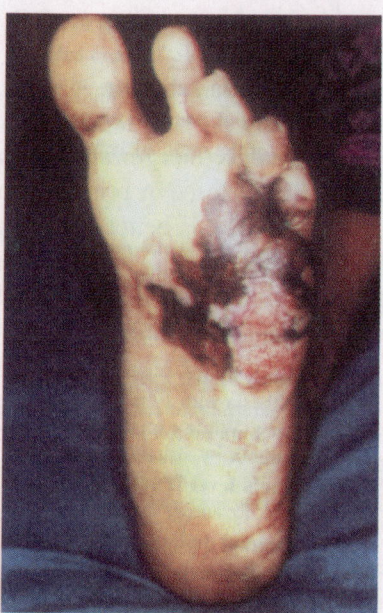

Fig. 11.25 Malignant melanoma foot required amputation

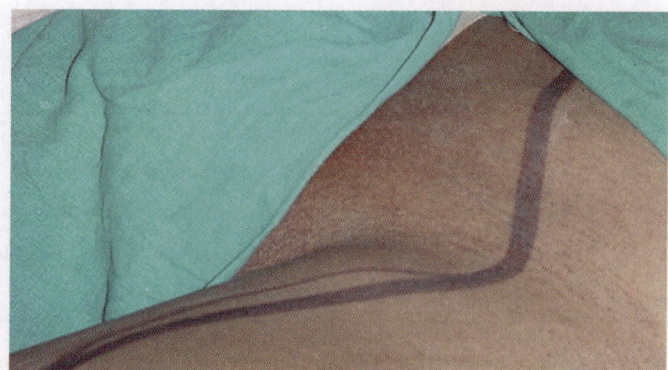

Fig. 11.26 Lazy S incision is given for inguinal block dissection - this incision decreases incidence of flap necrosis

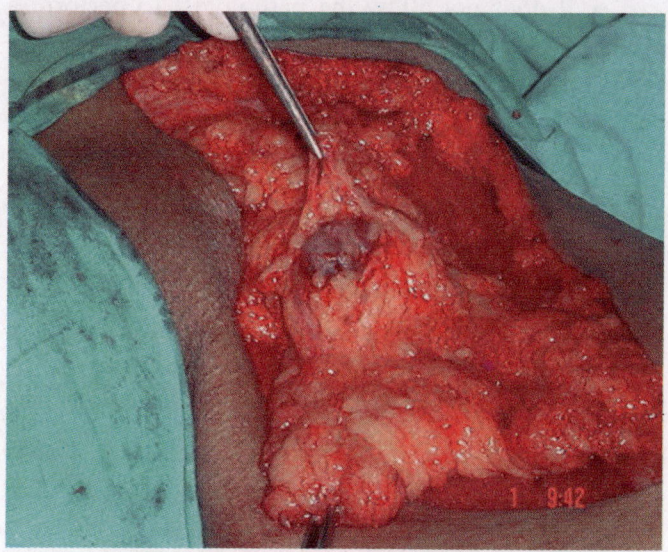

Fig. 11.27 Observe pigmented lymph nodes

MANAGEMENT OF LYMPH NODES

1. If lymph nodes are situated adjacent to the primary lesion, block dissection is done along with primary lesion in continuity so as to include 'in-transit' deposits also.

2. If lymph nodes are away, radical block dissection is done. Example: for a lower limb malignant melanoma inguinal nodes along with iliac nodes are removed. This is called **Ilioinguinal Block** dissection. If these group of nodes are positive at frozen section, lymph node clearance should include lymph nodes of obturator vessels. This is called **Ilio-obturator block dissection**.

   • **Sentinel lymphnode mapping**: Isosulfan Blue is injected intradermally and the node which gets stained is identified and sent for frozen section (Haematoxylin and Eosin stains and immunohistochemical technique). **If the node is positive regional lymphadenectomy is done even when nodes are clinically not palpable.**

Atleast 20-30% of the patients who are in Stage I will go to Stage III after sentinel node biopsy. Also there is a **definite survival advantage in patients** who undergo sentinel node biopsy and regional lymphadenectomy when the nodes are not palpable.

• Otherwise prophylactic block dissection is indicated only if melanoma has poor prognostic histological factors.

3. If lymph nodes are enlarged, hard and fixed, palliative radiotherapy is given.

MANAGEMENT OF ADVANCED MALIGNANT MELANOMA

• The aim of treating this group of patients is only to afford a reasonable palliation. More than 50% of patients, who have metastasis in the regional nodes are dead by the end of one year.

- **Choroid has no lymphatics**, hence good prognosis. However, blood spread, metastasis to the liver has been reported even 15-20 years later.

Modes of treatment

1. **Radiotherapy** for bone, brain and skin metastasis

2. **Systemic chemotherapy** - DTIC (Diethyl Triamine Imidazole Carboxamide) is the standard agent. The response rate is around 20-30%. Cisplastin, Vinblastine, Bleomycin are also used in combination. The addition of immunomodulators like BCG or Levamisole to chemotherapy has been tried. Intralesional injection of BCG has caused regression of the cutaneous nodules in some patients.

3. **Immunotherapy**
   - Alpha-interferon
   - Interleukin-2 (IL-2), interferon
   - **Monoclonal antibodies**: These are directed against antigen, expressed on the surface of melanoma cells. These antibodies like IgG3 activates the immune system.

- Cutaneous nodules can be managed by surgery or CO_2 laser excision.

4. **Hormone treatment**: Antioestrogens like tamoxifen have been tried in the systemic disease with 15-20% response rate.

5. **Isolated limb perfusion**: This is tried when there are extensive intransit deposits in the limb or recurrent disease in the limb. Melphalan is the drug of choice. A tourniquet is applied first, femoral vein and artery are cannulated, the blood which comes out is passed through a pump and **oxygenetor**, into which high dose of Melphalan or DTIC is given. Input temperature is kept at 41°C. Therapy is aimed at controlling local disease in the limb and to give a better functional limb even in presence of metastasis.

Complications of isolated limb perfusion

- Deep vein thrombosis
- Pulmonary emboli
- Complications of Anticoagulants
- Damage to the vessels

SUMMARY OF SKIN TUMOURS (Table 11.7)

Table 11.7 Summary of the skin tumours

	SQUAMOUS CELL CARCINOMA	BASAL CELL CARCINOMA	MALIGNANT MELANOMA
1. Incidence	Common (20-30%)	Most common (60-70%)	Less common (10-20%)
2. Origin	Prickle cell layer	Basal layer	Melanoblasts
3. Aetiology	Chronic irritation	Ultraviolet rays, fair skin	Ultraviolet rays, fair skin, pre-existing mole
4. Site	Trunk, leg, hand, oral cavity	Tear cancer	Head and neck, face, digits, palm and sole
5. Types	Ulcerative or cauliflower	Nodular or ulcerative	Nodular or ulcerative
6. Edge	Everted	Rolled out and beaded	Irregular
7. Induration	Maximum	Moderate	Minimum
8. Scab	Never occurs	Occurs	Never occurs
9. Pigmentation	Absent	Absent	Present in 90% of cases
10. Spread	Mainly by lymphatics Blood spread is rare and late	Does not spread by lymphatics. Blood spread is very, very late. Spreads by local spread. Hence the name, rodent ulcer.	Mainly by lymphatics, also by blood spread, does not infiltrate like rodent ulcer

OTHER MALIGNANT SKIN TUMOURS

DERMATOFIBROSARCOMA PROTUBERANS

- This is a locally malignant tumour arising from the dermis (Page 170)
- Common sites are – Trunk, flexor region of limbs. It presents as nodular (Bossellated) ulcerative lesion of 'many years' duration.
- Regional lymph node involvement is uncommon.
- It is less aggressive, hence curable.
- Treatment is by local wide excision followed by primary closure or skin grafting.

KAPOSI'S ANGIOSARCOMA (Key Box 11.9. 11.10)

- Common in **Black population**
- This neoplasm arises from **proliferating capillary vessels** and perivascular connective tissue cells.
- **Multiple, purplish nodules** appear in the limb, which ulcerates with bleeding is characteristic feature.
- Regional lymph node involvement can occur
- Increasing incidence due to AIDS

Differential diagnosis

1. Malignant melanoma
2. Soft tissue sarcoma
3. Multiple cutaneous metastasis
4. T Cell lymphoma

Key Box 11.9

DISEASES ASSOCIATED WITH KAPOSI'S SARCOMA

- Diabetes mellitus
- Lymphoma
- Following renal transplantation
- Acute and chronic immunosuppression (HIV)

Key Box 11.10

TYPES OF KAPOSI'S SARCOMA

• European	: Elderly males
• African	: Young and children
• Transplant	: Due to immunosuppression
• AIDS	: Homosexuals

OTHER SKIN LESIONS

They arise from sebaceous glands, sweat glands, hair follicles etc. See Key Box 11.11 for types of exocrine glands.

Key Box 11.11

TYPES OF EXOCRINE GLANDS

- **Holocrine**: Entire cell dies or disintegrates to liberate secretion. E.g.: **Sebaceous gland**
- **Apocrine**: Only the luminal part of the cell disintegrates, cell regeneration takes place from the nucleus and basal portion. E.g.: **Mammary gland**
- **Merocrine**: Without destruction of the cells, secretion is discharged – Most of the glands belongs to this type

---

- Few examples are syringoma, hidradenoma, trichoepithelioma, etc.
- They present as localised swelling treated by excision.
- **They have to be kept in mind as a differential diagnosis for malignant skin tumours**. Details of few skin leisons are given below:

KERATOACANTHOMA – Molluscum Sebaceum, Molluscum Pseudo - carcinomatosum

- Self limiting benign neoplasm of viral origin (probably)
- Arises due to overgrowth of hair follicle and subsequent spontaneous regression is characteristic.
- It is painless swelling in the skin with central dark brown core. After initial rapid growth of 2-4 weeks, spontaneous regression occurs in 24 hours. After separation of the central core, lump diminishes in size leaving a deep indrawn scar.
- Usually single, face is the commonest site
- Like sebaceous cyst, it presents as hemispherical swelling.
- Treated by excision

TURBAN TUMOUR

It is the **blanket term** used to describe a tumour occupying the whole of the scalp thus resembling a **turban**.

- Most often used to describe multiple cylindromata
- They produce **pink nodular masses**

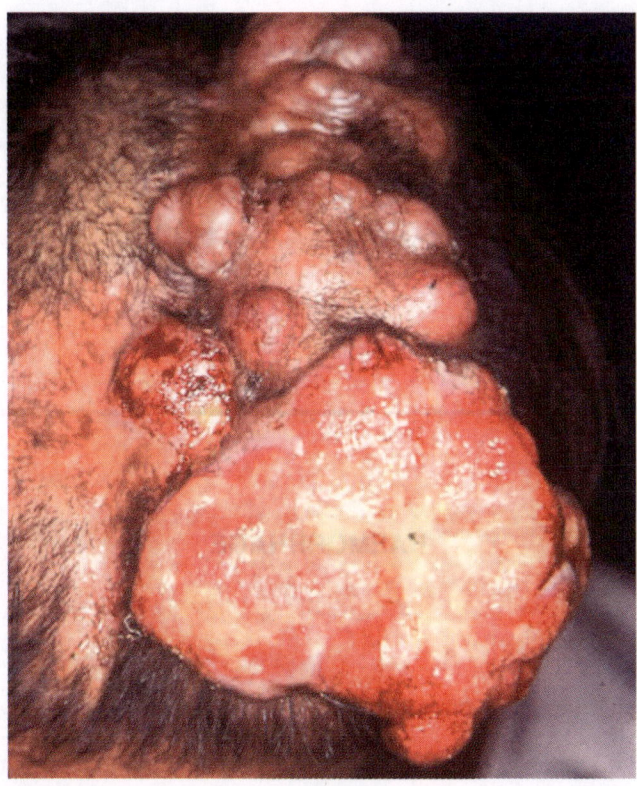

Fig. 11.29 Turbon tumour due to squamous cell carcinoma scalp

- Diagnosis confirmed by biopsy
- For differential diagnosis see the Key Box 11.12 below (Fig. 11.29)
- Treatment includes excision and reconstruction by skin grafting or rotational flaps

Key Box 11.12
TURBAN TUMOUR
• Very very rare
TYPES
• Multiple cylindromata
• Multiple nodular basal cell carcinoma
• Hidradenomata
• Plexiform neurofibromatosa of scalp

CORN

It is a **popular painful lesion in the plantar surface of the foot. (sole of the foot)**

- It affects the plantar surface of toes and sole of the feet.
- Corn develops due to intermittent pressure over a limited area.
  - Basically it is a localized hyperkeratinisation of the skin with a hard central core.
  - It will be a 'CONE' shaped lesion with broad surface and narrow at deeper plane.
- They are **painful and very tender.**
- Most of these are **hard corns**
- **Soft corn** can occur in between the toes.

Treatment

- Diabetic patients have to be carefully explained the consequences of a 'mistreated' corn. Sensations and pulsation have to be checked in those patients.
- Symptomatic corns have to be excised , one has to **take out a good 'CONE'** shaped tissue for the permanent cure. Otherwise **recurrence can occur.**

WART

- A wart is a rough excrescence on the skin
- Papilloma viruses are responsible for this
- They are pigmented, keratinized, irregular lesions
- Common in young adults
- Common sites: Fingers, feet, genitalia, beard area etc.
- **Veneral Warts** : They are also called as **papilloma accuminata**. They can occur in the anal region, perineum and in the coronal sulcus of the penis. Some of the warts may regress spontaneously. **Fulguration** with diathermy is the treatment.

MERKEL CELL CARCINOMA

- It is derived from neuroendocrine cells which function as touch receptors.
- **Highly malignant tumour**
- Elderly white males are affected.
- Sun affected areas such as head and neck region are involved probably due to **ultra violet rays**.
- Surgery, radiation and chemotherapy has been tried
- Histopathological report resemble **metastatic oat cell carcinoma**

12

Haemorrhage, Shock, Blood Transfusion

Haemorrhage
- Classification
- Pathophysiology
- Management

Shock
- Classification
- Pathophysiology
- Management

Acute adrenal insufficiency

Hyperbaric oxygen

Central venous pressure

Pulmonary capillary wedge pressure

Blood transfusion

Blood products

Plasma substitutes

CLINICAL NOTES

A patient who underwent subtotal thyroidectomy for toxic goitre was shifted to the postoperative intensive care unit. Within 10 minutes, the nurse came to inform the surgeon that 450 ml of blood was collected in the "Redivac" suction bottle. The dressing was opened and there was no large collection of blood in the surgical wound. The presence of a large haematoma requiring drainage was thus ruled out. The blood pressure (BP) which was previously under control had shot up to 210/110 mmHg postoperatively, possibly due to pain. Careful monitoring and treatment reduced the BP to 140/90 mmHg. After 24 hours, the drainage was only 100 ml. The incision did not need re-exploration. This case illustrates reactionary haemorrhage due to hypertension.

HAEMORRHAGE

Classification

I. Depending on nature of the vessel involved

A. Arterial haemorrhage: Bright red in colour, jets out. Pulsation of the artery can be seen. It can be easily controlled, as it is visible.

B. Venous haemorrhage: Dark red in colour. It never jets out but oozes out. Difficult to control because vein gets retracted, nonpulsatile.

C. Capillary haemorrhage: Red colour, never jets out, slowly oozes out. It becomes significant if there are bleeding tendencies

II. Depending on the timing of haemorrhage

A. Primary haemorrhage: Occurs at the time of surgery

B. Reactionary haemorrhage: Occurs after 6-12 hours of surgery. Hypertension in postoperative period, violent sneezing, coughing or retching, are the usual causes.

e.g. Superior thyroid artery can bleed postoperatively, if ligature slips. Hence, it is better to **ligate it twice**.

C. Secondary haemorrhage: Occurs after 5 – 7 days of surgery. It is due to infection which eats away the suture material, causing sloughing of vessel wall. e.g. bleeding after 5-7 days of surgery for haemorrhoids.

III. Depending on the duration of haemorrhage

A. *Acute haemorrhage* : Occurs suddenly. e.g. oesophageal variceal bleeding due to portal hypertension.

B. *Chronic haemorrhage* : Occurs over a period of time. e.g. haemorrhoids/piles or chronic duodenal ulcer, tuberculous ulcer of the ileum, diverticular disease of the colon.

IV. Depending on the nature of bleeding

A. *External haemorrhage/*Revealed haemorrhage e.g. Epistaxis, haematemesis

B. *Internal haemorrhage/*Concealed haemorrhage e.g. splenic rupture following injury, ruptured ectopic gestation, liver laceration following injury.

PATHOPHYSIOLOGY OF HAEMORRHAGIC SHOCK

A loss of more than 30-40% blood volume results in a fall in blood pressure and gross hypoperfusion of the tissues leading to haemorrhagic shock. **The evolution of haemorrhagic shock can be classified into four stages**:

1. Class I

When blood loss is less than 750 ml (<15 % of blood volume), it can be called mild haemorrhage

60-70% of blood volume is present in the low-pressure venous system (capacitance vessels). 10% of the blood volume is present in the splanchnic circulation.

When there is blood loss, peripheral venoconstriction takes place and compensates for the loss of blood volume by shifting some blood into the central circulation. Some amount of correction of blood volume also occurs due to withdrawal of fluid from the interstitial spaces.

Apart from a mild tachycardia and thirst, there may be no other symptom or sign suggesting hypovolaemia. The blood pressure, urine output and mentation are all normal in Class I shock.

2. Class II

Loss of 800-1500 ml (15 – 30% of blood volume) results in moderate (Class II) shock.

Peripheral venoconstriction may not be sufficient to maintain the circulation. Hence, adrenaline and noradrenaline (catecholamines) released from the sympatho-adrenal system cause powerful vasoconstriction of both arteries and veins.

Increased secretion of ADH causes retention of water and salt. Thirst increases.

Clinically, the patient shows a heart rate of 100 – 120 beats/minute and an elevated diastolic pressure. The systolic pressure may remain normal. Urine output is reduced to about 0.5 ml/kg/h and the capillary refill is more than the normal 2 seconds. Extremities may look pale and the patient is confused and thirsty.

3. Class III

Loss of 1500 – 2000 ml (30 – 40% of blood volume) produces Class III shock. All the signs and symptoms of Class II haemorrhage get worse.

The patient's systolic and diastolic blood pressures fall, and the heart rate increases to around 120 beats/minute. The pulse is thready.

The respiratory rate increases to more than 20/minute. Urine output drops to 10 to 20 ml/hour. The patient appears pale and is aggressive, drowsy or confused.

4. Class IV

A blood loss of more than 2000 ml (> 40% of blood volume) results in Class IV shock. The peripheries are cold and ashen.

The pulse is thready and more than 120/minute. The blood pressures are very low or unrecordable.

There may be **renal shut down** and the patient may be moribund.

If persistent, can damage other organs, e.g.

GIT : **Mucosal ulcerations** → upper GI bleeding, absorption of bacteria and toxins, **bacterial translocation** and bacteraemia

Liver : Reduced clearance of toxins

Kidney : Acute renal failure

Heart : Myocardial ischaemia, depression

Lungs : Loss of surfactant, increased alveolocapillary permeability, interstitial oedema, increased arteriovenous shunting → Acute lung injury

These result in **multiorgan failure** associated with a high mortality rate.

The only hope of survival is early diagnosis of bleeding and appropriate management.

MANAGEMENT

I. Treatment of the shock - General measures

Hospitalisation

Care of all critically ill patients starts with **A, B and C**
A – Airway, B – Breathing and C – Circulation.

Oxygen should be administered by facemask for all patients who are in shock but are conscious and are able to maintain their airway.

If unconscious, endotracheal intubation and ventilation with oxygen may be necessary.

Intravenous line: Urgent intravenous administration of isotonic saline to restore the blood volume to normal. Colloids such as gelatins or hetastarch have also been used. If there has been massive blood loss as in Class IV shock or the patient is anaemic, blood transfusion is indicated.

Investigations: Blood is collected at the earliest opportunity for routine investigations as well as for blood grouping and cross matching

Cross-matched blood is usually given. If life-threatening, uncross-matched, O^{-ve} packed cells may be transfused into the patient.

Use of inotropes and vasoconstrictors is not indicated as they may harm tissue perfusion.

If started, they should be terminated as soon as the volume status is corrected.

II Treatment of the shock – Specific measures

1. Pressure and packing

To control bleeding from nose, scalp: packing using roller gauze with or without adrenaline to control bleeding from nose.

Bleeding from vein – middle thyroid vein during thyroidectomy, lumbar veins during lumbar sympathectomy can be controlled using pressure pack for a few minutes.

Sengstaken tube is used to control bleeding from oesophageal varices – internal tamponade.

2. Position and rest

Elevation of the leg controls bleeding from varicose veins

Elevation of the head end reduces venous bleeding in thyroidectomy – **Anti-Trendelenberg position**.

Sedation to relieve anxiety – Morphine in titrated doses of 1–2 mg intravenously

3. Tourniquets

Indications

*   Reduction of fractures
*   Repair of tendons
*   Repair of nerves
*   When a bloodless field is desired during surgery

Contraindications

*   Patient with peripheral vascular disease. (The arterial disease may be aggravated due to thrombosis resulting in gangrene).

Types

*   Pneumatic cuffs with pressure gauge
*   Rubber bandage

Precautions

*   *Too loose* a tourniquet does not serve the purpose.
*   *Too tight:* Arterial thrombosis can occur which may result in gangrene.
*   *Too long* (duration of application): Gangrene of the limb. Hence, when a tourniquet is applied, the time of inflation should be noted down and at the end of 45 minutes to an hour, deflated at least for 10 minutes and reinflated only if necessary.

Complications

*   Ischaemia and gangrene
*   Tourniquet nerve palsy[1]

4. Surgical methods to control haemorrhage:

Application of **artery forceps** (Spencer Well's forceps) to control bleeding from veins, arteries and capillaries.

Application of **ligatures** for bleeding vessels

Cauterisation (diathermy)

Application of **bone wax** (Horsley's wax which is bee's wax in almond oil) to control bleeding from cut edges of bones.

Silver clips are used to control bleeding from cerebral vessels (Cushing's clip).

---

1. In M.S. examination, a candidate was asked to examine a case of radial nerve palsy. Patient had an injury to the wrist 4 months back. The cut flexor tendons had been sutured. The candidate could not correlate the radial nerve palsy to the injury at the wrist. He failed! It was a case of tourniquet palsy.

Surgical procedure: **Splenectomy** for splenic rupture, hysterectomy for uncontrollable postpartum haemorrhage, laparotomy for control of bleeding from ruptured ectopic pregnancy etc.

SHOCK

Definition

Shock is defined as an acute clinical syndrome characterised by **hypoperfusion and severe dysfunction of vital organs.** There is a failure of the circulatory system to supply blood in **sufficient quantities** or under **sufficient pressure** necessary for the optimal function of organs vital to survival.

Classification

Hypovolaemic shock
Cardiogenic shock
Distributive shock
Obstructive shock

HYPOVOLAEMIC SHOCK

Loss of blood – haemorrhagic shock
Loss of plasma – as in burns shock
Loss of fluid – dehydration as in gastroenteritis

Features (Key Box 12.1)

The primary problem is a decrease in preload. The decreased preload causes a decrease in stroke volume.

Clinical features depend on the degree of hypovolaemia. Severe (Class III or IV) shock results in tachycardia, low blood pressures and decreased urine output.

The peripheries are cold and the patient may be confused or moribund.

Key Box 12.1

HYPOVOLAEMIC SHOCK

Decreased preload
↓
Decrease in stroke volume
↓
Sympathetic nervous system activation

Treatment

The primary goal is to return the blood volume, tissue perfusion and oxygenation to normal as early as possible.

Replace the lost blood volume

Crystalloids: 2 – 3 times the volume of blood lost must be replaced with isotonic saline (0.9% saline) or Ringer lactate. Large volumes of saline infusion can cause hyperchloraemic metabolic acidosis. 5% dextrose does not produce expansion of intravascular volume as it gets distributed throughout the different fluid compartments.

Colloids: 1 – 1.5 times the blood lost can be replaced with colloid instead of crystalloid (5 % albumin, gelatin or hetastarch).

Blood transfusion may be needed if large amounts of blood is lost (Hb < 8 –10 gm%) or if the patient is anaemic.

CARDIOGENIC SHOCK

The blood flow is reduced because of an intrinsic problem in the heart muscle or its valves. A massive myocardial infarction may damage the cardiac muscle so that there is not much healthy muscle to pump blood effectively. Any damage to the valves, especially acute may also reduce the forward cardiac output resulting in cardiogenic shock.

Features

The primary problem is a decrease in contractility of the heart. The decreased contractility causes a decrease in stroke volume.

Left ventricular pressures are high as forward cardiac output suffers. The sympathetic nervous system is activated and consequently, systemic vascular resistance increases.

Clinically, the patient presents with tachycardia, low blood pressures and decreased urine output.

The jugular venous pulse may be raised, a S_3 or S_4 gallop may be present.

The lung fields may show bilateral extensive crepitations due to pulmonary oedema.

The peripheries are cold and the patient may be confused or moribund.

Treatment

The primary goal is to **improve cardiac muscle function**.

Oxygenation can be improved by administering oxygen, either by facemask or by endotracheal intubation and ventilation as necessary.

Inotropes : improve cardiac muscle contractility.

Vasodilators such as nitroglycerine may dilate the coronary arteries and peripheral vessels to improve tissue perfusion. High systemic vascular resistance increases impedance to forward cardiac output (afterload). However, the patient must be monitored closely to avoid excessive drops in blood pressure due to these drugs.

Intra-aortic balloon pump or ventricular assist devices may be used to help the ventricles.

If unresponsive, revascularisation (surgical or interventional) or valve replacements may be considered on an emergency basis.

DISTRIBUTIVE SHOCK

This occurs when the afterload is excessively reduced. Distributive shock can occur in the following situations.

Septic shock
Anaphylactic shock
Neurogenic shock
Acute adrenal insufficiency

SEPTIC SHOCK

Pathophysiology

Sepsis is the response of the host to bacteraemia/ endotoxaemia.

It may be produced by gram-negative or gram-positive bacteria, viruses, fungi or even protozoal infections.

Severe sepsis can result in persistent hypotension despite adequate fluid resuscitation and is called septic shock.

Local inflammation and substances elaborated from organisms, especially endotoxin, activate neutrophils, monocytes, and tissue macrophages. **This results in a cascade of proinflammatory and anti-inflammatory cytokines and other mediators, such as IL-1, IL-8, IL-10, tumour necrosis factor-alpha, prostaglandin E_1, endogenous corticosteroids, and catecholamines**.

Effects of this complex mediator cascade include cellular chemotaxis, endothelial injury, and activation of the coagulation cascade.

Features

These substances produce **low systemic vascular resistance (peripheral vasodilatation)** and ventricular dysfunction resulting in persistent hypotension.

Generalised tissue hypoperfusion may persist despite adequate fluid resuscitation and improvement in cardiac output and blood pressures. This is due to abnormalities in regional and microcirculatory blood flow. These abnormalities may lead to **cellular dysfunction, lactic acidosis (anaerobic metabolism) and ultimately, multi-organ failure.**

The early phases of septic shock may produce evidence of volume depletion, such as dry mucous membranes, and cool, clammy skin.

After resuscitation with fluids, however, the clinical picture is typically more consistent with **hyperdynamic shock.** This includes tachycardia, bounding pulses with a widened pulse pressure, a hyperdynamic precordium on palpation, and warm extremities.

Signs of possible infection include fever, localized erythema or tenderness, consolidation on chest examination, abdominal tenderness, guarding, rigidity and meningismus.

Signs of **end-organ hypoperfusion** include tachypnoea, cyanosis, mottling of the skin, digital ischaemia, oliguria, abdominal tenderness, and altered mental status.

Often, a definitive diagnosis cannot be made on the basis of initial findings on history taking and physical examination, and treatment for several possible conditions commences simultaneously.

Treatment

Removal of the septic focus is an essential step and a priority in the treatment of septic shock.

e.g., Resection of gangrenous bowels, closure of perforation, appendicectomy.

Appropriate **antibiotics** are necessary to treat the precipitating infection.

Supportive care : Oxygenation and if necessary, endotracheal intubation and mechanical ventilation should be administered.

Intravenous fluids: Restoration of intravascular filling pressures must be done using crystalloids, colloids and blood as necessary. **Crystalloids such as isotonic saline or Ringer's lactate** may be used. Large amounts may be required and may contribute to tissue oedema. Colloids restore intravascular volume faster and remain longer in the central circulation. However, they are expensive and are more often used in patients where there is a high risk of pulmonary oedema due to cardiac dysfunction and may not tolerate large volume of fluids. **Blood transfusions** may be required to maintain the patient's haemoglobin levels to 10 gm%.

Vasoactive agents such as norepinephrine to produce vasoconstriction and raise the systemic vascular resistance to normal. Dopamine, dobutamine or adrenaline to increase myocardial contractility may be necessary. Vasopressin as a vasoconstrictor is under trial. All these potent drugs are given as infusions under careful and continuous monitoring of the blood pressures as well as cardiac filling pressures (central venous pressures, pulmonary capillary wedge pressures).

Role of infusions of sodium bicarbonate and anti-inflammatory mediators have not been found to be helpful.

Activated Protein C shows some promise as it prevents release of inflammatory mediators and also prevents/deactivates the action of these mediators on cellular response to inflammation and activation of coagulation cascade. It is highly expensive and is undergoing trials.

> *No matter what antibiotics you use, unless surgical drainage of pus or resection of gangrene etc is done septic shock patients do not improve.*

Summary of septic shock (Key Box 12.2)

Key Box 12.2
SEPTIC SHOCK
Early diagnosis of septic shock
Empirical antibiotics initially
Appropriate antibiotics after culture
Ultrasonography, CT scan and chest x-ray are key investigations
Treatment of source of infection
- Pneumonia
- Drainage of pus
- Closure of perforation
- Resection of gangrene
Aggressive resuscitation, supportive care and close monitoring in Intensive Care Unit (ICU)

A 54-year-old lady was admitted to the casualty with low blood pressures and dyspnoea since one day. She had a history of fever, vomiting and diarrhoea since 3 – 4 days, was treated in a local nursing home and when she got worse, was referred to our hospital. In spite of fluid therapy, profound hypotension persisted and within half an hour of arrival to the casualty, she suffered a cardiopulmonary arrest.

Her trachea was immediately intubated, cardiopulmonary resuscitation (CPR) given and was shifted to the intensive care unit for further management. She required high doses of dopamine, adrenaline and noradrenaline to maintain blood pressures. A blood gas analysis showed severe metabolic acidosis (pH = 7.02, $PaCO_2$ = 35 mmHg and HCO_3^- = 12 mmol/L).

Considering the history, a diagnosis of septic shock was made when she continued to have hypotension even after her central venous pressures were normal. Peritoneal dialysis was done as she was in oliguric renal failure. Haemodialysis was not possible as she was hypotensive and on inotropes. A search for septic focus was initiated. An ultrasound abdomen showed dilated kidney and obstructed urinary system. A double J stenting of the ureter, which was done to relieve the obstruction, drained pus. Once the pus was drained, appropriate antibiotics given and with continued cardiorespiratory support, she showed steady improvement. She was gradually weaned off the ventilator and inotropes, and was discharged from the hospital five weeks later. At discharge, she was fully conscious, stable, ambulant and very grateful to the medical fraternity. **This case illustrates the importance of removal of septic focus, antibiotics and cardiorespiratory support in the treatment of septic shock.**

ANAPHYLACTIC SHOCK

Features

Occurs on exposure to an allergen the patient is sensitive to. It may be pollen, foodstuffs, preservatives and additives in the food or a medication. The anaphylactic shock that occurs in the hospital is usually due to some drug the patient is allergic to. e.g., penicillin allergy.

The reaction may be in the form of **mild rashes** with or without **bronchospasm** or it may be a full blown anaphylactic shock wherein the patient presents with rashes, **generalized oedema** including laryngeal oedema,

bronchospasm and **hypotension** and if not treated in time, cardiac arrest.

Treatment

Primary :

Oxygen and if necessary, endotracheal intubation and ventilation.

Adrenaline, 0.5 – 1 mg IM or 50 – 100 μg intravenous bolus as necessary to maintain blood pressure.

Intravenous fluids – isotonic saline or Ringer lactate

Leg end elevation of bed

Secondary :

Chlorpheniramine maleate

Hydrocortisone 100 mg intravenously

If facilities exist, take a 10 ml sample of blood to analyse for serum tryptase levels. If raised, they confirm anaphylactic reaction.

NEUROGENIC SHOCK

Causes

High spinal cord injury

Vagolytic shock

Features

Hypotension without tachycardia, may deteriorate to produce shock and cardiac arrest.

Treatment

Intravenous fluids, inotropes and vagolytics as necessary.

ACUTE ADRENAL INSUFFICIENCY

Causes : (Key Box 12.3)

Key Box 12.3
RISK FACTORS FOR ADRENAL CRISIS
• Infection • Trauma or surgery • Adrenal gland or pituitary gland injury • Premature termination of treatment with steroids such as prednisolone or hydrocortisone

Adrenal crisis occurs if the adrenal gland is deteriorating as in :

Primary adrenal insufficiency (Addison's disease)

Secondary adrenal insufficiency (Pituitary gland injury, compression)

Inadequately treated adrenal insufficiency

Features

Headache, profound weakness, fatigue, slow, sluggish, lethargic movement, joint pain

Nausea, vomiting, abdominal pain, high fever and chills

Low blood pressure, dehydration, rapid heart rate and respiratory rate, confusion or coma

Treatment

Care of airway, breathing and circulation

Intravenous fluids

Hydrocortisone 100–300 mg intravenously

Treat the precipitating factor

Antibiotics as necessary

OBSTRUCTIVE SHOCK

It can be due to cardiac tamponade or due to tension pneumothorax.

Cardiac Tamponade

Features

In obstructive shock, there is impedance to either inflow or outflow of blood into or out of the heart.

In **cardiac tamponade**, the pericardium is filled with blood and hampers venous filling as well as outflow.

The filling pressures of the left-sided and right-sided chambers equalise.

The central venous pressure is high and the blood pressure is low.

The patients also have pulsus paradoxus where there is 10% decrease in systolic blood pressure with inspiration.

Treatment

To maintain preload with fluids or blood as indicated.

Relief of obstruction, drain the pericardial cavity as early as possible.

Tension pneumothorax

Causes

Injury to the lung due to trauma

Ventilator induced barotrauma

Rupture of emphysematous bulla in a patient with chronic obstructive pulmonary disease

Features

Profound cyanosis, distended neck veins

Tachypnoea, dyspnoea or respiratory arrest

No air entry on the side of pneumothorax, hyper-resonance to percussion

Tachycardia, hypotension and cardiac arrest

Treatment

A wide (large) bore needle/cannula to be inserted into the pleural cavity to drain the air. The needle is inserted in the midclavicular line in the 2nd intercostal space on the affected side. This is followed by insertion of a tube thoracostomy.

A massive pulmonary embolus is a differential diagnosis for obstructive shock.

HYPERBARIC OXYGEN

Here, O_2 is administered one to two atmospheres above atmospheric pressure in a compression chamber in order to increase the arterial O_2 content, mainly the dissolved O_2.

Indications

1. Carbon monoxide poisoning
2. Infections such as tetanus and gas gangrene
3. Cancer therapy to potentiate radiotherapy
4. Arterial insufficiency
5. Decompression sickness and air embolism

CENTRAL VENOUS PRESSURE (CVP)

One of the essential requirements while treating patients in shock includes monitoring of CVP.

CVP indicates volume of blood in the central veins, distensibility and contractibility of the right heart chamber, intrathoracic pressure and intrapericardial pressure. Thus, in shock, measurement of CVP is essential so as to plan for proper fluid management.

Key Box 12.4
ACCESS TO RIGHT HEART/GREAT VEINS
• Internal jugular vein
• Subclavian vein
• Median cubital vein
• External jugular vein

Method

Right internal jugular vein (IJV) is preferred whenever IJV is chosen (Key Box 12.4).

A 20 cm long I.V. cannula is introduced into IJV with the patient supine, head down and neck rotated to the opposite side. Head down position helps in engorging the IJV. Seldinger's technique is employed and the catheter is advanced up to superior vena cava or right atrium.

The patency of the catheter is confirmed by lowering the saline bottle to check free flow of blood into the connecting tube.

The tube is connected to the saline manometer and readings of saline level are taken with the "ZERO REFERENCE POINT" at the **midaxillary level** in the **supine position** or at the **manubrio-sternal joint** in the semi-reclining position (45^0). An electronic pressure transducer may be used for greater accuracy.

Uses

1. If CVP is low, venous return should be supplemented by IV infusion, as in cases of hypovolaemic shock.
2. When CVP is high, infusion of fluids may result in pulmonary oedema.
3. In cardiogenic shock, CVP may be normal or high

Complications

1. Pneumothrorax, haemothorax
2. Accidental caroid artery puncture
3. Haematoma in the neck
4. Air embolism
5. Infection

PULMONARY CAPILLARY WEDGE PRESSURE (PCWP)

• This is a better indicator of circulatory blood volume and left ventricular funtion.

• It is measured by a pulmonary artery balloon flotation catheter - **SWAN GANZ** catheter.

Uses of PCWP

1. To differentiate between left and right ventricular failure
2. Pulmonary hypertension
3. Septic shock
4. Accurate administration of fluids, inotropic agents and vasodilators

Method of measuring PCWP

Swan-Ganz catheter is introduced into the right atrium. The catheter has a balloon near its tip. The advancement of catheter is monitored by watching the pressure tracing. Pressure tracing becomes flat, when the balloon gets wedged in a small branch to give capillary pressure. When the balloon is deflated, the pulmonary artery pressure is obtained.

Complications

Arrhythmias

Pulmonary infarction

Pulmonary artery rupture

> *Normal values: PCWP: 8-12 mmHg. PAP: systolic 25 mmHg; diastolic 10 mmHg.*

Interpretation in various conditions: CVP and PCWP (Table 12.1)

Table 12.1		
CONDITIONS	**CVP**	**PCWP**
Hypovolaemic shock	Low	Low
Right heart failure	High	Normal
Left heart failure	Normal	High
Cardiogenic shock		
(Rt. and Lt. heart failure)	Normal	High
Cardiac tamponade	High	High
Pulmonary embolism	Normal/ High	High

Note: CVP reflects right atrial pressures only. It may not correlate with left ventricular pressures. **PCWP is better indicator of left ventricular pressures** and is a preferred monitor in cardiogenic shock.

BLOOD TRANSFUSION

Indications for blood transfusion

I. To replace acute and major blood loss as in

- Haemorrhagic shock
- Major surgery — open heart surgery, gastrectomy
- Extensive burns

II. To treat anaemia due to

- Chronic blood loss as in haemorrhoids, bleeding disorders, chronic duodenal ulcer etc.
- Inadequate production as in malignancies, nutritional anaemia.

Although blood transfusion, has several advantages (Key Box. 12.5), it is also associated with a multitude of risks.

Key Box 12.5
ADVANTAGES OF BLOOD TRANSFUSION
• Volume replacement
• $\uparrow$ O_2 carrying capacity
• Replacement of clotting factors

This has led to revised guidelines regarding the threshold for transfusion of blood (Key Box 12.6).

Key Box 12.6
THE REVISED GUIDELINES
1. Blood loss > 20% of blood volume
2. Haemoglobin < 8 g/dL
3. Haemoglobin < 10 g/dL in patients with major cardiovascular disease (e.g., ischaemic heart disease)

In order to conserve the donated blood and to minimise reactions, it is customary to transfuse blood components rather than whole blood. Hence, packed cells are used to replace oxygen carrying capacity, platelet concentrates in thrombocytopaenia and fresh-frozen plasma for replacement of coagulation factors.

The following changes occur in stored blood:

- Reduced pH - as low as 6.7 - 7.0 due to high PCO_2
- Increased $[K^+]$ - upto 30 mmol/L
- Reduced viability of platelets and leucocytes
- Reduced coagulation factors

Key Box 12.7

STORAGE OF BLOOD

Preservative	Red cell survival (days)
ACD (Acid - Citrate - Dextrose)	21
CPD (Citrate - Phosphate - Dextrose)	28
CPDA (Citrate - Phosphate-Dextrose Adenine)	35
SAGM (Saline - Adenine - Glucose Mannitol)	35

COMPLICATIONS OF BLOOD TRANSFUSION

I. IMMUNE COMPLICATIONS

1. Haemolytic reactions

a. Major (ABO) incompatibility reaction

- This is the result of mismatched blood transfusion.
- Majority of cases are due to technical errors like sampling, labelling, dispatching, etc.
- This causes intravascular haemolysis

Clinical features

- Haematuria
- Pain in the loins (bilateral)
- Fever with chills and rigors
- Oliguria is due to the products of mismatched blood transfusion blocking the renal tubules. It results in *acute renal tubular necrosis.*

Treatment

- Stop the blood. Send it to blood bank and recheck.
- Repeat coagulation profile
- I.V. fluids, monitor urine output, check urine for Hb
- Diuresis with Furosemide 20-40 mg I.V. or injection Mannitol 20% 100 ml I.V. to flush the kidney.

b. Minor incompatibility reaction

- Occurs due to extravascular haemolysis
- Usually mild, occurs at 2-21 days
- Occurs due to antibodies to minor antigens
- Malaise, jaundice and fever
- Treatment is supportive

2. Non-haemolytic reactions

a. Febrile reaction

- Occurs due to sensitisation to WBCs or platelets

- Increased temperature - no haemolysis
- Use of 20-40 mm filter or leucocyte - depleted blood avoids it

b. Allergic reaction

- Occur due to allergy to plasma products; manifest as chills, rigors and rashes all over
- They subside with antihistaminics such as chlorphenaramine maleate 10 mg I.V.

c. Transfusion related acute lung injury (TRALI)

- It is a rare complication resembling ARDS
- Anti-leucocyte antibodies cause patient's white cells to aggregate in pulmonary circulation
- Treatment similar to ARDS
- Typically results in 12-48 hours of therapy

d. Congestive cardiac failure (CCF)

- CCF can occur if whole blood is transfused rapidly in patients with chronic anaemia.

Treatment

- Slow transfusion
- Injection Furosemide 20 mg I.V.
- Packed cell transfusion is the choice in these patients.

II. INFECTIOUS COMPLICATIONS

Serum hepatitis, AIDS, malaria, syphilis are dangerous infectious diseases which can be transmitted by blood from one patient to another. The danger is increased in cases of multiple transfusions and in case of emergency situations. *"Prevention is better than cure".* Hence, it is mandatory to screen the blood for these diseases before transfusion.

Key Box 12.8

MASSIVE BLOOD TRANSFUSION

1. > 500 ml over 5 minutes
2. > 1/2 the patient's blood volume in 6 hours.
3. > the whole blood volume in 24 hours.

Problems :

- Citrate toxicity-hypocalcemia
- Thrombocytopaenia
- Clotting factors deficiency

Disseminated Intravascular Coagulation (DIC)

Occurs in massive blood transfusion wherein all factors of coagulation are used up resulting in a bleeding disorder.

It produces a severe afibrinogenemia

It is treated by replacement with fibrinogen (cryoprecipitate) and other clotting factors.

AUTOLOGOUS TRANSFUSION

The concept originated to avoid transfusion reactions which develop when homologous blood is used.

Here patient's own blood is used.

Types of autologous transfusion

1. **Predeposit**: 2-5 units of blood may be donated over 2-3 weeks before elective surgery.

2. **Pre-operative haemodilution**: Cases such as surgery for thyrotoxicosis or abdomino-pelvic resection wherein one can expect 1-2 units of blood loss. Just before surgery, 1-2 units of blood are removed and retransfused at appropriate time.

3. **Blood Salvage**: Blood which was lost during surgery is collected, mixed with anti-coagulant solution, washed and reinfused. This can be done provided surgery does not involve severe infection, bowel resection or malignancy e.g. multinodular goitre.

Advantages

All the risks involved with blood transfusion are avoided.

Disadvantages

May not be acceptable to the patient

Sophisticated equipment required

BLOOD PRODUCTS (Key box 12.9)

After removal of red cells, the following components may be separated from whole blood:

1. **Platelets**
   - Last for 3 to 5 days
   - Used with platelet count < 50,000 cells/mm^3
   - 6 units increase platelet count by 20-30,000 cells/mm^3
   - Do not use filters. Use ordinary I.V. sets

2. **Fresh Frozen Plasma**
   - Indicated in surgeries where patient has severe liver failure.
   - After massive blood transfusion

3. **Cryoprecipitate**
   - Rich source of Factor VIII and fibrinogen
   - Used in fibrinogen deficiency, DIC

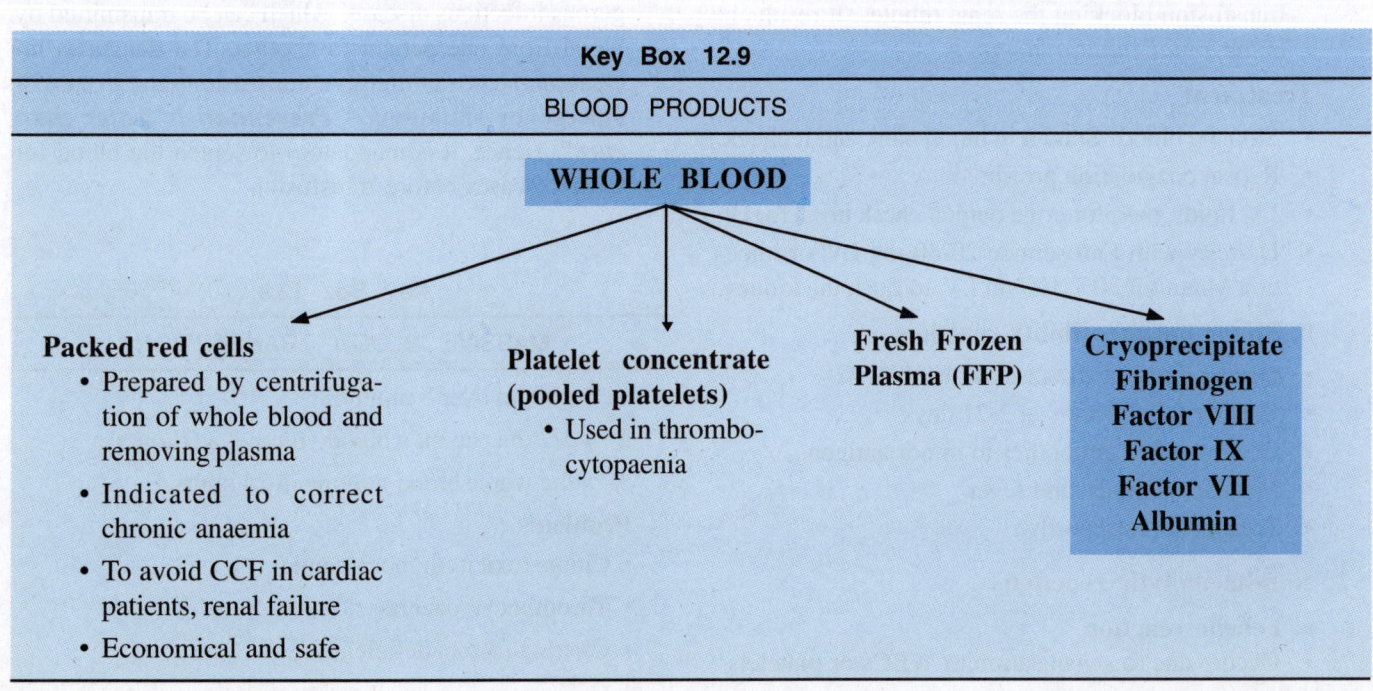

Key Box 12.9

BLOOD PRODUCTS

WHOLE BLOOD

Packed red cells
- Prepared by centrifugation of whole blood and removing plasma
- Indicated to correct chronic anaemia
- To avoid CCF in cardiac patients, renal failure
- Economical and safe

Platelet concentrate (pooled platelets)
- Used in thrombocytopaenia

Fresh Frozen Plasma (FFP)

Cryoprecipitate
Fibrinogen
Factor VIII
Factor IX
Factor VII
Albumin

4. Fibrinogen

- Concentrated from donor pools and rarely used
- High risk of hepatitis

5. Factor VIII and Factor IX concentrates

- Used in haemophilia and Christmas disease respectively

6. Factor VII concentrate

- Used in DIC

PLASMA SUBSTITUTES

These are colloidal solutions used for re-establishment of a normal blood volume in emergency situations.

   e.g. Polytrauma with severe haemorrhage. Massive GI bleed, shock.

1. Albumin

- It is a rich protein but carries no risks of hepatitis.
- It is available as 4.5% and 20%
- Used in severe burns - acute severe hypoalbuminaemia
- Used in nephrotic syndrome

Should not be used in chronic renal disease, chronic liver disease and to treat malnutrition.

2. Gelatins

- Good plasma expander
- Plasma expansion lasts a few hours
- Severe reactions with urea - linked gelatin. e.g., Haemaccel (1:2,000),
- Reactions less with succinylated gelatin. e.g., Gelofusin (1:13,000)

3. Dextrans

- **a.** Low molecular weight Dextran 40,000 - (Dextran 40)
- Reduces viscosity and red cell sludging
- May affect renal function and coagulation

- **b.** High molecular weight dextrans (70,000 and 110,000 – Dextran 70 and 110) - used rarely

4. Hydroxyethyl starch

- Derived from starch
- Plasma expansion lasts for over 24 hours
- Maximum dose - 15 ml/kg
- Large doses may interfere with coagulation
- Incidence of severe reactions (1:16,000)

13

Burns, Skin Grafting, Flaps

- Burns
- Electrical burns
- Flaps
- Skin grafting
- Chemical burns

BURNS

DEFINITION: It is a type of coagulative necrosis caused by *heat,* transferred from source to the body. *Frost bite* which occurs in cold countries is also a coagulative necrosis but it is caused by extreme degrees of cold. Hence it is not a burn. Scald is a burn but caused by moist heat (steam). Burns never occur at temperatures less than 44°C.

TYPES

Thermal: Flame burns and scald burns

Electrical

Chemical

PATHOPHYSIOLOGY OF BURNS SHOCK

Although the exact mechanism of the postburn microvascular changes and hypovolaemia leading to low cardiac output and poor tissue perfusion has not been determined, the following various mechanisms have been proposed.

1. **Increased capillary permeability** leading to fluid and protein leakage from the intravascular space.

2. **Decreased plasma oncotic pressure** due to hypoproteinaemia resulting from loss of protein from the intravascular space.

3. **Increased capillary hydrostatic pressure** due to vasoconstriction or partial blockage of vessels with aggregate of cells and platelets.

4. **Reduced clearance of fluid and protein** from the interstitital space by lymphatic ducts due to blockage with platelet aggregates and fibrin clots.

5. **Intracellular fluid accumulation** due to impaired cell membrane function.

6. **Increase in burned tissue osmotic pressure** leading to further fluid accumulation

7. **Inceased evaporative water loss**.

8. **Depressed myocardial function**.

Chemical mediators released from the site of injury are responsible for the development of typical inflammatory response. This results in rapid and dramatic oedema formation.

The activated complement cascade system facilitates liberation of various permeability factors like Histamine, prostaglandins (PGF-1, PGF-2, PGF-2α) and thromboxane.

Macromolecular leakage into burned areas, catabolism and reduced immunoglobulin synthesis results in a decreased concentration of all individual immunoglobulin levels and triggering of complement cascade.

Inhalation injury: Glottic oedema, necrotising bronchitis, pneumonia are the dangerous events which follow an inhalation injury.

MANAGEMENT OF BURNS PATIENTS

1. **First aid**: cold water bath should be given immediately. This takes away the heat and stabilises mast cell, thus decreasing the release of histamine thereby reducing oedema.

2. Careful history, **duration since the time of injury** with heat source should be recorded.

3. Hospitalization and admission in the burns ward with air conditioning facility.

4. **Assessment of depth of burns**: (Table 13.1)

   Partial thickness burns: Here, superficial layers of the skin are destroyed. Epidermis and variable portion of dermis is involved. Since the nerve endings are exposed, it causes severe degree of pain.

   Full thickness burns: Involvement of full thickness of dermis with epidermis. Since the nerves are destroyed, it is less painful.

5. **Assessment of extent of burns in terms of body surface area (BSA)** : It is calculated by a *RULE OF 9 – RULE OF WALLACE"*

   Burns of head and neck: 9%

   Burns of upper limbs: 9 x 2 = 18%

   Burns of anterior trunk = 18%

   Burns of posterior trunk = 18%

   Burns of the lower limbs: 18 x 2 = 36% (front and back of each limb is 9%)

   Burns of external genitalis : 1%

6. Temperature, pulse, respiration and blood pressure have to be monitored and maintained.

7. An indwelling **urinary catheter** (Foley's catheter) is introduced, and strict intake and output chart has to be maintained.

8. A **Ryle's tube** is passed. Burns patient can develop "acute stress ulcers" called as *Acute peptic ulcers* or *Curling ulcers*. Hence, to prevent bleeding, a cold stomach wash is given through the Ryle's tube and antacids and H_2 receptor blockers such as ranitidine 150 mg twice a day is given.

9. **Replacement of fluid volume**

(a) *Muir* and *Barclay Formula*.

$$1 \text{ ration} = \frac{\% \text{ of burns x body weight}}{2}$$

3 rations in 12 hours, 2 rations in next 12 hours and 1 ration in next 12 hours.

Example : 40% burns patient weighing 60 kg.

$$1 \text{ ration} = \frac{40 \times 60}{2} = 1200 \text{ ml}$$

1st 12 hours : 3600 ml fluid
2nd 12 hours : 2400 ml fluid
3rd 12 hours : 1200 ml fluid

The best solution for replacement is plasma. For fear of transfusion reactions, a crystalloid such as *Ringer's lactate* can be used.

In any patient with burns above 20%, blood to be given in the 2nd ration (after 12 hours).

After 36 hours, depending upon the urinary output and depending on the requirements of the body, about 2-3 litres fluid are given in 24 hours.

(b) *Parkland's formula*: 4 ml / % /Kg in the first 24 hours.

1/2 : In 1st 8 hours, 1/4 : Next 8 hours each.

(c) *Modified Brookes formula :*

1st 24 hours : 2ml/% of burns/Kg (deficit) + maintenance (2500ml)
2nd 24 hours : 50% of the deficit in 1st 24 hours + maintenance (2500ml in adults).

	INVOLVED AREA	PAIN	*ADNEXA*	APPEARANCE	HEALING
I° Burn	Only Epidermis	+	+	Erythema/oedema	3-5 days without scar
II° Burn	Varying depth of Dermis	++/-	+	Blister, soft waxy, white, elastic, pain sensation to needle prick present.	10-20 days, with hypertrophic scar.
III° Burn	Involvement of entire depth of epidermis and dermis.	--	Lost	Tough, dry, eschar, thrombosed subcutaneous vein. Pain sensation to needle prick absent.	3-5 weeks, eschar separate. **Always needs SSG.**

Table 13.1

Rate of administration : 50% in the first 8 hours after injury and 50% in the next 16 hours.

10. **Broad-spectrum antibiotics** are given against gram +ve, gram -ve, and anaerobic organisms.

To treat septic shock, higher antibiotics such as cephalosporins have to be given.

Narcotic analgesics like injection morphine 10-12 mg **IM** or injection pethidine 60-75 mg **IM** is given to relieve the pain. (If the veins are not visible, a "cut down" needs to be done, so that the infusion cannula can be maintaned for a long time.)

TREATMENT OF BURNS WOUND

1. Clean the wound with antiseptic agents like savlon, iodine, etc.

2. **Open method** : Exposure line of management : If facilities available are good, with a fumigated ward, the wound can be left open to the atmosphere after applying *Silver Sulfadiazine* cream.

3. **Closed method** : Alternately, after applying silver sulfadiazine, 1% silver nitrate, Mefenide cotton rolls are applied, over which a bandage is applied. This is called closed method. Advantages of closed method are less pain, reduced infection and sogging and better medication.

4. **Tangential excision** followed by grafting is done after about 48-72 hours in which the burn wound is excised *tangentially* till fresh bleeding occurs. This is followed by skin grafting. Skin is taken from rest of normal area, or can be obtained from skin bank. A mesh expander and cell culture are also used.

Advantages of tangential excision

1. It prevents secondary infection and septicaemia.

2. Decreases the hospital stay. (2-5 weeks is the usual time taken for eschar of III° burn to separate. This is cut short by tangential excision.)

3. Decrease of the incidence of contractures and hypertrophic scar.

4. Cost of the treatment is reduced.

CAUSES OF DEATH IN BURNS PATIENT

1. Uncontrolled hypovolaemic shock (Refractory hypervolaemia).

2. Choking, suffocation due to respiratory burns especially burns of head and neck.

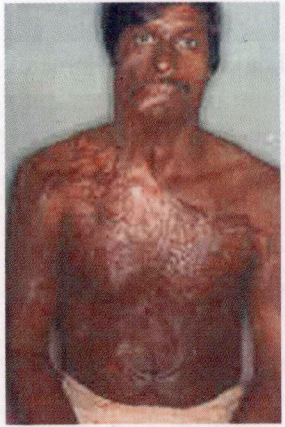
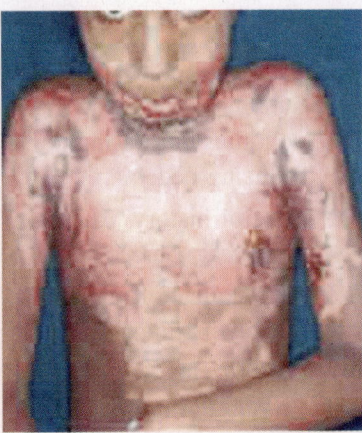

Fig. 13.1 Post burn contracture in an adult

Fig. 13.2 Post burn neck contracture in a child

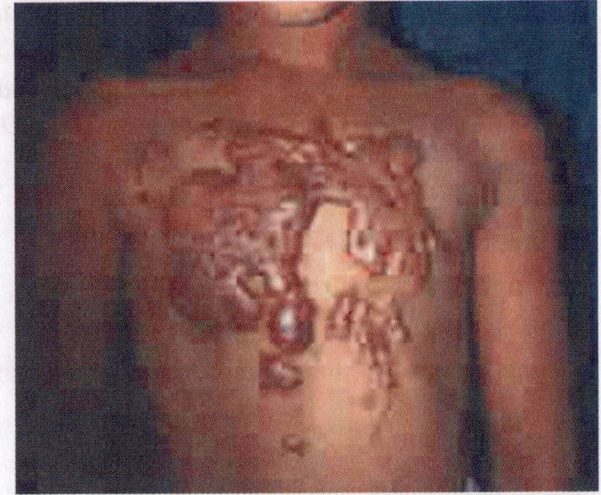

Fig. 13.3 Hypertrophic scar in a deep dermal burns

3. *Septicaemic shock* is the most common cause of death.

PROGNOSIS

It depends upon several factors (Key Box 13.1) - The most important being percentage of burns and facilities of treatment.

Key Box 13.1
FACTORS AFFECTING OUTCOME
• Extremes of age
• Depth of burns
• Inhalation of noxious fumes
• Cardiopulmonary disease

FREE SKIN GRAFTING

Skin grafting is the commonest method of achieving wound cover.

TYPES

1. Split skin graft (SSG – Thiersch graft)

Also called as partial thickness graft

Consists of epidermis and a variable portion of dermis. (Fig. 13.4, 13.6)

Split skin graft is usually harvested using **Humby's knife**, (Fig. 13.5) one can also use Drum Dermatome or power dermatome.

Preferred donor area is thigh

2. Full thickness graft (Wolf graft)

Consists of epidermis and full thickness of dermis

Harvested using ordinary scalpel

Needs excellent vascularity of the recipient wound for graft survival

Used for small uncontaminated wounds produced after excision of skin lesions or after release of skin contractures (lower eyelids, fingers)

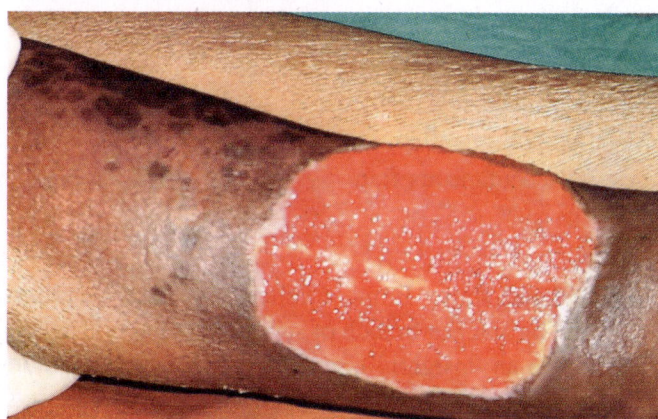

Fig. 13.4 Wound is ready for skin grafting observe red granulation tissue

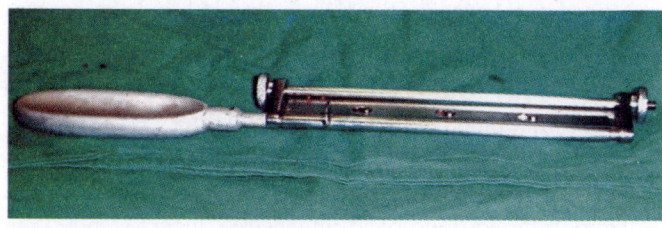

Fig. 13.5 Skin graft is taken from thigh using Humby's knife

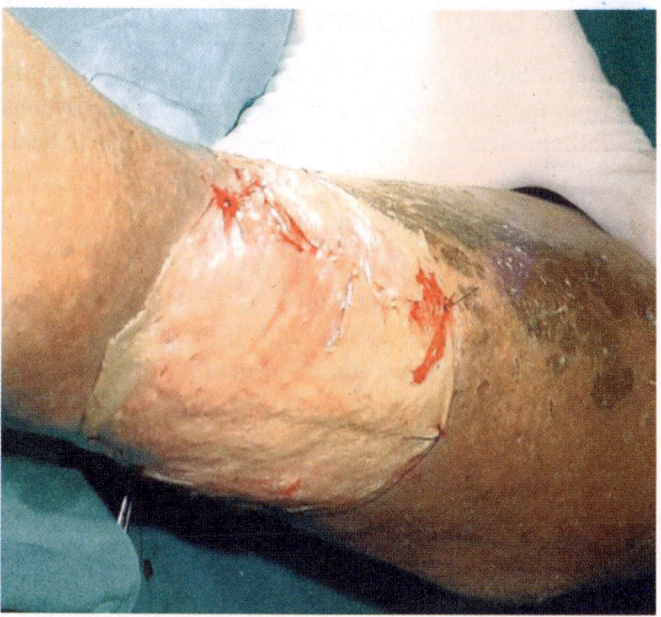

Fig. 13.6 Skin graft is applied over the recipient area

Donor area needs primary suturing or split skin graft for healing and hence limits the size of the graft.

Unlike split skin grafts, full thickness grafts doesn't contract and retains it's colour and hence it is cosmetically superior.

INDICATIONS OF SKIN GRAFT

1. Skin loss

Post traumatic (eg. Avulsion and degloving injury)

Post surgical (eg. Excision of tumours, excision of burn wound)

As a result of **pathological process**. (eg. Venous ulcer, Diabetic ulcer)

2. Mucosa loss

After **excision** of lesions of oral cavity, tongue.

For **resurfacing** reconstructed vagina in cases of vaginal agenesis.

CONTRAINDICATIONS FOR SKIN GRAFT

Infection by **beta hemolytic streptococcus,** which produces fibrinolysin which dissolves fibrin.

Any nearby **infected wound** with copious discharge.

Avascular wounds: with exposed bare bone without periosteum, exposed tendon without **paratenon** and exposed cartilage without perichondrium.

HEALING OF THE DONOR AREA

Donor area of split skin graft heals by epithelization from the adnexal remnants of dermis, pilosebaceous follicles and/or sweat gland apparatus. Complete healing of donor area occurs by 8-10 days.

THE PROCESS OF GRAFT TAKE

The processes which result in **reattachment** and **revascularization** of the graft to the bed are collectively referred to as **"take" of graft.**

The graft initially adhere to it's new bed by fibrin, and the revascularization which starts by 48 hours and gets completed by 4-5 days is achieved by the out growth of capillary buds from the recipient area to unite with those on the deep surface of graft. For the first 2 days after grafting , the skin graft derives its nutrition from the wound by the process of serum imbibition/plasmatic circulation.

Key Box 13.2

IDEAL REQUIREMENTS FOR FREE SKIN GRAFT

1. Wound should be free from infections like streptococcus and pseudomonas

2. Vascular wounds. eg. Wounds with healthy granulation tissue

3. Wound should be thoroughly debrided

4. To achieve haemostasis before placing the graft

5. To have close and immobile contact between the graft and the wound

6. Recipient area should be immobilized with **POP** slab

FLAPS

Flap is a block of tissue transferred from donor to recipient area with it's integrated vascularity.

COMMON INDICATIONS OF THE FLAP SURGERY

To cover defects/wounds **where free skin graft can not be used. Eg : Exposed bare bones, bare tendons, bare cartilage.**

Wounds with exposed joints, exposed major vessels and nerves.

Implant exposure following orthopedic procedures.

In wounds with **soft tissue loss**, where future reconstructive surgery is contemplated.

Defects which need better contour to improve cosmesis. Breast reconstruction following mastectomy.

CLASSIFICATION OF FLAPS

I. Broadly classified into Pedicled flaps and Free flaps

PEDICLED FLAPS: Pedicle or the base remains attached to the donor site during its transfer to the recipient area. Pedicled flaps may be of following types

1. Local flaps eg : Rotation, Transposition, Limberg and bilobed

2. Regional flap eg : PMMC, DP for head and neck defects, TRAM for breast reconstruction

3. Distant flaps eg: Groin flap, sub axillary flap for hand defects.

FREE FLAPS: These are completely detached from the donor area before being transferred to the recipient area. The vascularity of the flap at the recipient site is immediately restored by anastomosing the vessels of the flap with the vessels at the recipient area using microvascular techniques.

II. Based on the composition, the flaps may be classified as:

Skin flap

Fasciocutaneous flap

Muscle flap

Myocutaneous flap

Adipofascial flap

Osteocutaneous flap

SOME OF THE COMMONLY PERFORMED FLAPS

Forehead flap : Entire forehead skin can be raised based on anterior branch of superficial temporal artery. It bears an unsightly scar of the donor site. **Median (Indian) forehead flap** based on supratrochlear vessels is a very useful flap in reconstructing defects over nose.

Deltopectoral flap (DP) : It is supplied by upper 4 perforating branches of internal mammary artery, used to reconstruct the defects of neck and lower face. After about 4 weeks, the flap is divided and the base is returned to the chest wall.

Pectoralis Major MyoCutaneous Flap (PMMC): Pectoral branch of thoracoacromial artery is the pedicle of the flap. It is the ideal pedicled flap for reconstruction of head and neck defects following ablative surgeries for various head and neck cancers. Hence it is described as workhorse among the flaps.

Osteomyocutaneous PMMC **flap by including 5th or 6th rib can be used for mandibular reconstruction.**

Latissimus Dorsi Flap (LDF): As a myocutaneous flap, based on thoracodorsal vessels can be used for reconstruction of the lower half of face, neck, breast, chestwall, axilla and upper arm.

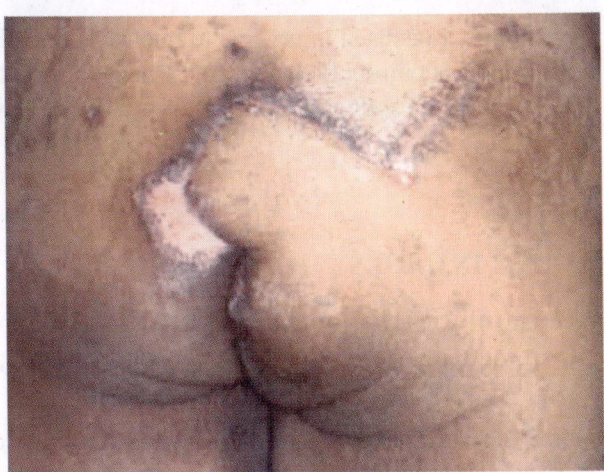

Fig. 13.9 Bed sore covered with local advancement flap

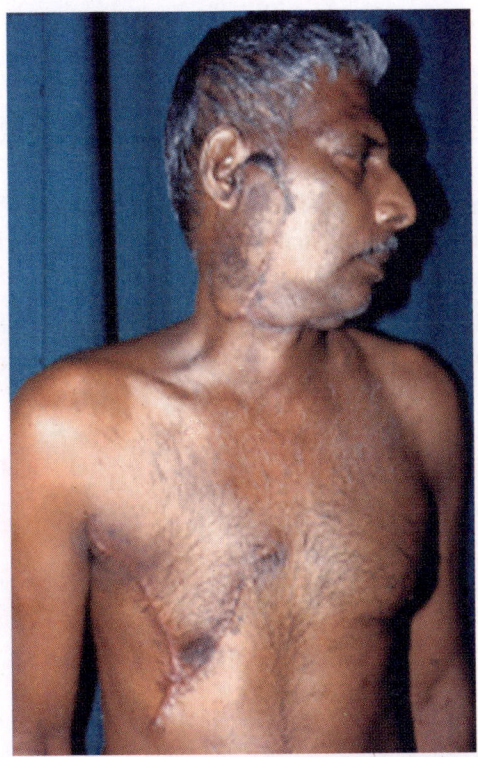

Fig. 13.7 PMMC Flap following radical parotidectomy

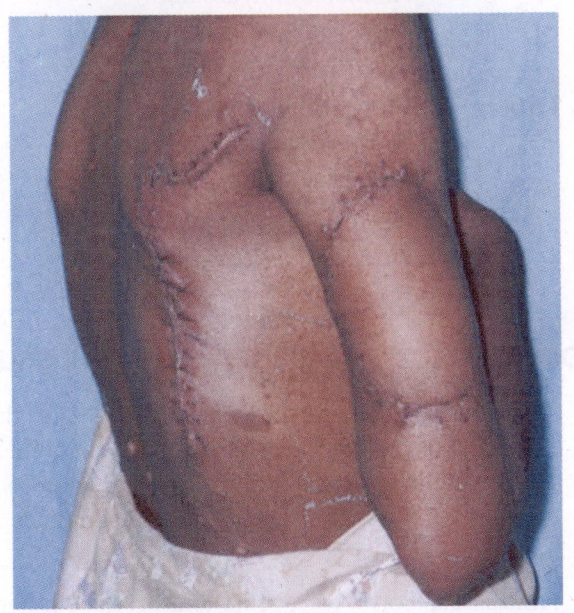

Fig. 13.8 Latissimus dorsi flap used to cover the defect in the arm following radical excision of a sarcoma

FREE (MICROVASCULAR) FLAPS

Using operating microscope and microvascular techniques, it is possible to do a free tissue transfer of tissues like skin muscle, bone, intestine, omentum etc. Procedure involves anastomosis of vessels of the flap to the vessels at the donor site. Eg: Latissimus dorsi muscle myocutaneous flap, radial artery forearm flap, gracilis flap, free fibula flap etc.

ELECTRICAL BURNS

The most important factors taken into consideration while assessing the damage caused by the passage of electrical current through the body are – **the nature of electric current and the resistance of body tissues through which the electric current is passing.**

When a portion of body comes in contact with a live electric wire, the actual point where the electric current enters the body is known as point of entry or is grounded as the point of exit. The most important factor which decides the severity of injury is the **"voltage"** of current.

The resistance offered by the tissues to the flow of current leads to the **conversion of electrical energy to thermal injury** and hence tissue damage.

TYPES OF INJURIES

True electrical injury : Damage is as a result of heat generated due to the passage of current.

Flame burns : Due to an electrical flash or spark.

Arc burns: Localised injury due to intense heat at the termination of current flow. It occurs when it jumps the gap between the source and the conductor. Eg : Flexor aspect of joints

CLASSIFICATION

A. ACUTE INJURIES

I) Burn injuries due to electric current itself

    a. Low voltage injuries (Less than 1000 volts of current) (i) Flash burns (ii) Contact burn.

    b. High voltage injuries (More than 1000 volts of current) (i) Flash (ii) Arc or contact

      1. Punctate

      2. Extensive

      3. Extensive with vascular impairment of extremities.
         Compartment syndrome

         Dry gangrene

II) Other associated injuries

    a. Thermal burns due to ignited cloth

    b. Acute CNS problems

    c. Acute peripheral neuropathy

    d. Cardiac/Respiratory arrest

    e. Injuries to other internal organs due to fall or electric current.

Key Box 13.3

SUMMARY OF MANAGEMENT OF ELECTRICAL INJURY

Initial resuscitation as in thermal burns

Low voltage injury

Superficial - conservative
Deep dermal - tangential excision and split skin graft
Contact burns - excision with SSG/flap

High voltage injury

Flash burns: Superficial – conservative
Deep dermal-Tangential excision and split skin graft
Arc or Contact burns: Vascular compromise – immediate fasciotomy, amputation

Punctate wounds : Excision and grafting

Extensive injury without vascular compromise:
Wider excision with split skin graft or flap cover

Recipient area should be immobilized with **POP** slab

(B) DELAYED INJURIES

    1. Delayed spinal cord injury

    2. Delayed peripheral neuropathy

    3. Optic nerve atrophy

    4. Cataract

Summary (Key Box 13.3)

CHEMICAL BURNS

Chemicals are a relatively uncommon cause of burns. The chemicals used in industry, science laboratories and home are the usual agents.

The tissue damage in chemical burns is mainly due to the prolonged contact period and the effects of systemic absorption.

CLASSIFICATION OF AGENTS THAT CAUSE INJURY

1. **Acids** : Hydrochloric acid,
            Sulphuric acid
            Nitric acid
            Hydrofluoric acid
            Phenol (carbolic acid)
            Oxalic acid

2. **Alkalis** : Sodium hydroxide
            Potassium hydroxide
            Ammonium hydroxide
            Lithium, barium and
            Calcium hydroxide

3. **Others** : **Inorganic substances**:
            Phosphorus, wet cement
            lime, potassium permanganate

            Organic substances:
            Kerosene, petrol, turpentine
            Naphthalene etc.

MODES OF ACTION OF CHEMICALS ON TISSUES

Acid causes coagulative necrosis of the skin due to rapid conversion of protein to coagulum salt of the acid. The coagulated eschar prevents these acids to penetrate deeply. Activity in the tissues continues for a long time.

Alkalis are corrosive agents and produce extensive denaturation of tissue proteins. These produce more tissue destruction than acids.

FIRST AID

Early irrigation of injured area with large volume of water or running water (with few exceptions) is the main focus in the first aid management of chemical injuries. Hydrotherapy mechanically cleans the area reducing the concentration of chemicals and duration of contact. Earlier the hydrotherapy started, more is the benefit obtained.

Since the absorption of phenol increases with dilution, surface phenol is removed by solvent **polyethylene glycol before hydrotherapy** is started.

DEFINITIVE WOUND CLOSURE

Achieved in a similar way as in any other thermal injury
Primary excision and split skin grafting, of all acid and alkali burns, if done before 10 days.

Grafting of granulating wound, if the patient comes late, with wound infection. This takes much longer (1-½ month) compared to thermal burns (3 weeks):

OCULAR INJURIES

Very common in acid and alkali burns. Severe blepherospasm and forceful rubbing increases the severity of injury. Various sequences of events are

Sloughing of corneal epithelium

Stromal oedema

Corneal ulceration

Perforation

Panophthalmitis

If perforation doesn't occur, corneal opacity and heavy vascularization occurs. Quick, thorough and prolonged lavage of cornea with water is the most important measure in the first aid treatment. Systemic and topical steroids minimizes inflammation and scarring of cornea.

---

* *All photographs and the entire text in this chapter are contributed by Prof. Pramod Kumar, Head of the Dept. and Dr. Bhaskar K.G., Associate Professor, Dept. of Plastic Surgery, KMC, Manipal.*

Acid-Base Balance

14

- Basic definitions
- Henderson–Hasselbach equation
- Regulation of acid–base balance
- Acid–base disorders
- Rapid interpretation of an ABG Report

Human blood has a hydrogen ion concentration [H$^+$] of 35 to 45 nmol/L and it is essential that its concentration be maintained within this narrow range. Hydrogen ions are nothing but protons which can bind to proteins and alter their characteristics. All the enzymes present in the body are proteins and an alteration in these enzyme systems can change the homeostatic mechanisms of the body. Hence, a disturbance in acid-base balance can result in malfunction of the various organ systems.

BASIC DEFINITIONS

What is pH?

pH notation is a more common method of expressing the hydrogen ion concentration. It is defined as the negative logarithm to base 10 of the [H$^+$] expressed in mol/L.

Pure water contains a [H$^+$] of 10^{-7} mol/L.

$Log_{10}10^{-7} = -7;$ $-log_{10}10^{-7} = 7;$

The negative logarithm to base 10 of [H$^+$] is called as pH. Hence, pH of pure water is 7.

Similarly, human blood has an average hydrogen ion concentration of 40 nmol/L.

40 nmol/L = 10$^{-7.4}$ mol/L; $Log_{10}10^{-7.4} = -7.4;$
$-log_{10}10^{-7.4} = 7.4;$ pH of blood = 7.4

What is an acid? What is a base? What is a buffer?

An **acid** is a substance that dissociates in water to produce H$^+$.

A **base** is a substance that accepts H$^+$.

A **buffer** is a combination of a weak acid and its conjugate base. By combining with a strong acid or strong base, they produce the corresponding salt and a weak acid or a weak base respectively.

e.g.: A weak acid such as carbonic acid with its conjugate base, sodium bicarbonate is called the bicarbonate/carbonic acid buffer system. When it combines with a strong acid such as hydrochloric acid, it produces sodium chloride and carbonic acid. When it combines with a strong base such as sodium hydroxide, it produces sodium carbonate and water.

The hydrogen ion concentration of blood is maintained within narrow limits because of the presence of buffers in the body. **These natural buffers are of two types; extracellular and   intracellular**.

The extracellular buffers are bicarbonate/ carbonic acid buffer system, phosphate buffer system and plasma proteins. The intracellular buffers are haemoglobin and other proteins.

The most important buffer system in the body is the bicarbonate - carbonic acid buffer system. This is because of the ability of the body to maintain or alter the concentrations of its two components separately. The concentration of carbonic acid is regulated by respiration wherein the excess carbonic acid is eliminated as carbon dioxide by the lungs. The bicarbonate concentrations are independently regulated by the kidneys.

The Henderson and Henderson-Hasselbach equations

It is evident from above that the hydrogen ion concentration is proportional to the concentration of the buffer systems of the body. The hydrogen ion concentration, carbonic acid levels and the bicarbonate levels of blood are related according to the following equation :

$$[H^+] \ (nmol/L) = K \ x \ \frac{H_2CO_3 \ (mmol/L)}{HCO_3^- \ (mmol/L)}$$

Where K = constant. This equation is called the Henderson equation.

The amount of carbonic acid in the blood is directly proportional to the partial pressure of carbon dioxide in the blood. Thus, the carbonic acid concentration is a product of the partial pressure of carbon dioxide in blood times its solubility coefficient.

$[H_2CO_3] = \alpha \ PCO_2$, where α = solubility coefficient of carbon dioxide in blood and $PaCO_2$ is the partial pressure of carbon dioxide in blood.

α = 0.03 ml/mmHg/100 ml blood and normal PCO_2 = 40 mmHg

$[H_2CO_3] = \alpha \ PCO_2 = 0.03 \ x \ 40 = 1.2$ ml/dL.

K = 800 for the carbonic acid/bicarbonate buffer system. The normal bicarbonate level of blood is 24 mmol/L.

$$[H^+] \ (nmol/L) = \frac{800 \ x \ 1.2}{24} = 40 \ nmol/L$$

The Henderson equation can also be written as follows:

$$[H^+] \ (nmol/L) = K \ x \ \frac{\alpha \ PCO_2 \ (mmHg)}{HCO_3^- \ (mmol/L)}$$

From this equation, it is evident that the hydrogen ion concentration increases when the $PaCO_2$ increases or when the $[HCO_3^-]$ levels decrease. Similarly, a decrease in hydrogen ion concentration occurs when the $PaCO_2$ decreases or when the $[HCO_3^-]$ levels increase.

When expressed in logarithmic form, the Henderson equation becomes as shown in the next line:

$$pH = pK_a + log \ \frac{[HCO_3^-]}{[H_2CO_3]}$$

This logarithmic version of Henderson equation is called the Henderson-Hasselbach equation. The pK_a (negative logarithm of the constant K) of the carbonic acid/bicarbonate buffer system is 6.1.

$$pH = 6.1 + log \ 24/1.2 = 6.1 + log \ 20$$
$$= 6.1 + 1.3 = 7.4$$

It is important to appreciate that the $[H^+]$ and pH are inversely related. When the $[H^+]$ rises, the pH decreases and vice versa.

REGULATION OF ACID - BASE BALANCE

The normal pH of blood is 7.35 – 7.45. Acidosis is defined as a pH less than 7.35. Conversely, when the pH is more than 7.45, alkalosis is said to exist. Acidosis and alkalosis are of two types each: respiratory and metabolic.

An increase in carbon dioxide (CO_2) levels increases the plasma $[H^+]$ or decreases the pH (respiratory acidosis). Similarly, a decrease in plasma carbon dioxide levels reduces the $[H^+]$ or increases the pH (respiratory alkalosis). A decrease in $[HCO_3^-]$ reduces the pH and is called metabolic acidosis. Similarly, an increase in $[HCO_3^-]$ increases the pH and produces metabolic alkalosis.

The pH is regulated in the human body by mainly two organs : the **respiratory system** and the **renal system**.

The arterial carbon dioxide levels are regulated by the respiratory system. Any increase in carbon dioxide levels stimulates the respiratory centre in the medulla thus augmenting respiration, alveolar ventilation and elimination of extra CO_2 levels. A decrease in CO_2 levels may reduce the stimulus to breathe. Hypoventilation is limited by hypoxia in patients due to hypoxic drive to maintain respiration. Respiratory response to changes in CO_2 level occurs very fast.

The plasma bicarbonate levels are regulated by the kidneys. Any decrease in $[HCO_3^-]$ stimulates the kidney to retain and synthesise bicarbonate. High [HCO$_3^-$] result in elimination of more bicarbonate in urine. In general, the pulmonary response to a change in acid-base status is faster and occurs immediately. However, the renal regulation takes time, a few hours to days. The kidneys filter and reabsorb all the bicarbonate in the urine. When necessary, the kidneys can also produce extra bicarbonate through the glutamine pathway.

ACID-BASE DISORDERS (Key Box 14.1)

When an acid base disorder occurs, the initial disturbance that occurs is termed the primary disorder. The body attempts to normalise the pH by certain compensatory mechanisms resulting in a secondary disorder, e.g., primary metabolic acidosis results in a decrease in bicarbonate ions and a consequent increase in hydrogen ions. To compensate for this, the patient hyperventilates and reduces the arterial carbon dioxide levels, thus moving the pH back to normal (compensatory respiratory alkalosis).

Thus, there are four primary disorders and four secondary disorders.

Key Box 14.1	
PRIMARY DISORDER	SECONDARY DISORDER
Metabolic acidosis	Respiratory alkalosis
Metabolic alkalosis	Respiratory acidosis
Respiratory acidosis	Metabolic alkalosis
Respiratory alkalosis	Metabolic acidosis

RESPIRATORY ACIDOSIS

Causes

This disorder occurs when the patient's ability to maintain minute ventilation is compromised. This may be acute or chronic in origin. The causes may be classified as follows:

Central nervous system: Central nervous system depression due to trauma, tumour, infections, ischaemia or drug overdose. Spinal cord injuries, especially cervical or high thoracic can cause respiratory muscle paralysis.

Peripheral nervous and muscular system: Guillian Barre syndrome, tetanus, organophosphorus poisoning, poliomyelitis, myasthenia gravis.

Primary pulmonary disease : Asthma, chronic obstructive pulmonary disease, acute respiratory distress syndrome, pneumonia.

Loss of mechanical integrity : Flail chest.

Clinical features

The features of the underlying problem predominate the clinical picture.

If acute, hypoxia and hypercarbia result in tachycardia, hypertension, arrhythmias, confusion, drowsiness and coma. If untreated, can be fatal.

If gradual in onset, as in chronic obstructive pulmonary disease (COPD), the patient's kidneys may compensate by retaining bicarbonate resulting in compensatory metabolic alkalosis. Arterial blood gas analysis typically shows low PaO$_2$, high PaCO$_2$, high bicarbonate levels and a near-normal pH.

Treatment

Treat the cause

Maintenance of oxygenation and ventilation using mechanical ventilatory support till recovery of the primary problem occurs.

RESPIRATORY ALKALOSIS

This occurs due to an increase in minute ventilation. This increase can be sustained only in abnormal conditions. This may be acute or chronic in origin.

Causes : (Key Box 14.2)

Supratentorial lesions: Head injury

Cirrhosis of liver

Pain

Anxiety, hysterical hyperventilation

High altitudes

It may also occur secondarily as a compensation to primary metabolic acidosis

Key Box 14.2
HYPERVENTILATION
• High altitudes
• Hyperpyrexia
• Hypothalamic lesion
• Hysteria

Features

Usually features of the underlying disease predominate the picture.

Acute severe hypocarbia ($PaCO_2$ < 20 mmHg) may cause cerebral vasoconstriction, reduced cerebral blood flow, confusion, seizures and tetany.

The alkalosis and consequent hypokalaemia can also cause cardiac arrhythmias.

METABOLIC ACIDOSIS

Causes

This is associated with a decrease in bicarbonate ions due to one of two reasons:

1. *Overproduction or retention of non-volatile acids in the body,* e.g.,
   - Diabetic ketoacidosis
   - Lactic acidosis
   - Salicylate poisoning, methanol poisoning
   - Renal failure

2. *Loss of bicarbonate ions from the body*
   - Diarrhoea
   - Intestinal fistulae

Features

Usually features of the underlying disease predominate the picture.

Hypotension, reduced cardiac output

Hyperventilation – rapid, deep respirations

Deep, gasping type of respiration seen in diabetic ketoacidosis is called Kussmaul's respiration

Hyperkalaemia, arrhythmias

Lethargy, coma

Treatment

Identify the cause and treat

Adequate ventilation must always be ensured in all these critically ill patients

If pH < 7.2 and the patient is unstable, may administer sodium bicarbonate. The chances of life-threatening arrhythmias are less with a pH > 7.2.

Bicarbonate requirement (mmol) = Body weight (kg) x base deficit (mmol/L) x 0.3

(P.S. : Each ml of 8.4% $NaHCO_3$ solution contains 1 mmol of HCO_3^-.
Each ml of 7.5% $NaHCO_3$ solution contains 0.9 mmol of HCO_3^-)

Half the calculated dose of bicarbonate should be given slowly and should be followed up with repeat blood pH measurements as required.

Anion gap

The law of electroneutrality states that the total number of positive charges must equal the total number of negative charges in the body fluids. Thus, cations (positively charged ions such as sodium and potassium) must produce a charge exactly balanced by anions. However, the concentrations of only sodium, potassium, chloride and bicarbonate ions are routinely measured in clinical practice. The sum of the cations (sodium, potassium) exceeds the sum of anions (chloride and bicarbonate) producing a 'deficit' called the "anion gap". The normal anion gap is 9 – 14 mmol/L. This gap is due to the presence of unmeasured anions in the body. Since the extracellular concentrations of potassium is small, it is often ignored in the calculation of anion gap. The equation may be rewritten as follows:

$$\text{Anion gap} = ([Na^+] + [K^+]) - ([Cl^-] + [HCO_3^-])$$

Anion gap may be used to distinguish the cause of metabolic acidosis.

Anion gap is increased (> 14 mmol/L) in metabolic acidosis associated with an increase in fixed acid load. These acids react with the bicarbonate ions in the plasma lowering its concentration. The anion portion of the fixed acid is not measured in the laboratory and contributes to the 'unmeasured anion' concentration, thus increasing the anion gap.

Anion gap remains unchanged in metabolic acidosis associated with loss of bicarbonate ions as the lost bicarbonate ions are replaced by chloride ions. This type of metabolic acidosis is also called **"hyperchloraemic acidosis"**.

METABOLIC ALKALOSIS

Causes

This may be either due to loss of acid from the body or retention of bicarbonate.

Loss of gastric hydrochloric acid as in vomiting, prolonged nasogastric drainage

When H$^+$ are lost in excess, as in severe hypokalaemia in exchange of [K$^+$] from kidneys.

Primary or secondary hyperaldosteronism

Excessive exogenous administration of alkali, e.g. indiscriminate use of NaHCO$_3$, antacid abuse.

Retention of bicarbonate in exchange for loss of chloride ions as in diarrhoea.

Features

It is one of the common acid-base disorders in the intensive care unit. The underlying problem gives a clue to the cause of metabolic alkalosis. When severe, can cause hypoventilation and seizures. Associated hypokalaemia can cause arrhythmias and contribute to difficulty in weaning patients off a ventilator.

Treatment

Treat the primary problem

Most of the metabolic alkaloses are "chloride-responsive". Administration of saline and correction of potassium deficits reduce the alkalosis.

In life-threatening metabolic alkalosis (pH > 7.7), rapid correction may be necessary and may be achieved by administration of H$^+$ in the form of dilute hydrochloric acid or ammonium chloride.

RAPID INTERPRETATION OF AN ABG REPORT

Analysis and conclusion of arterial blood gas (**ABG**) report must always be done in conjunction with a history and clinical examination. ABG analysis is done to assess:

1. **Oxygenation status**
2. **Ventilatory status**
3. **Acid-base status**

1) Oxygenation

The PaO$_2$ of a normal, healthy, young adult is usually 90-100 mmHg. An increase in inspired oxygen concentration (FIO$_2$) is expected to increase the PaO$_2$. The expected PaO$_2$ of a normal person may be estimated rapidly using the following formula:

$$\text{Expected PaO}_2 = \text{FIO}_2\ (\%) \times 5$$

e.g. A person breathing 40% oxygen is expected to have a PaO$_2$ of 40 x 5 = 200 mmHg.

In patients with diseased lungs and increased shunt fraction (unventilated but perfused alveoli – "wasted perfusion"), the PaO$_2$ will not rise at the same rate as in a normal person. As the shunt fraction increases, the rate of rise in PaO$_2$ reduces and when it exceeds 40 – 50%, there may not be any rise in the PaO$_2$ at all. Since the PaO$_2$ depends on the FIO$_2$, it is important to remember to relate the PaO$_2$ to the inspired oxygen concentration whenever oxygenation status of an individual is to be assessed.

Low PaO$_2$ responds to simple oxygen therapy if shunt fraction is 30% or less. If large shunts are present, measures must be taken to improve ventilation of the lungs, if necessary using endotracheal intubation and mechanical ventilation so that the shunt fraction is reduced.

A PaO$_2$ less than 60 mmHg is life-threatening (corresponding to an arterial oxygen saturation, SpO$_2$ of **90% as measured by a pulse oximeter** and an attempt should always be made to keep a patient's PaO$_2$ (SpO$_2$) above this level. Exceptions to this may be an individual acclimatised to low PaO$_2$ such as at high altitudes, cyanotic congenital heart disease or chronic obstructive pulmonary disease.

Nomograms are available to calculate the shunt fraction but an easy bedside assessment of oxygenation can be made using a PaO$_2$/FIO$_2$ ratio (Key Box 14.3). The ratio can be used for assessment of oxygenation and to evaluate the response to therapy. **A pulse oximeter is helpful** to assess whether the patient's oxygenation is life-threatening or not. A saturation of 98–100% may be reassuring. However, subtle changes in the oxygenation status may be missed if the patient is breathing high concentrations of oxygen. This is because of the sigmoid shape of the oxygen dissociation curve where the SaO$_2$ will be 99–100%, whether the PaO$_2$ is 100 mmHg or 500 mmHg. **Hence, an arterial blood gas analysis must always be obtained whenever a doubt exists about the oxygenation status of the patient.**

Key Box 14.3	
PAO$_2$/FIO$_2$	**STATUS OF OXYGENATION**
5	Good
2.5 – 5	Acceptable
1 – 2.5	Poor
< 1	Critical

2) Ventilation

The **normal PaCO$_2$ is 35 – 45 mmHg**. The PaCO$_2$ must always be related to the alveolar ventilation of the patient. The minute volume of a normal healthy adult at rest would be 100 ml/kg/min. 60-65% of this actually ventilates the alveoli, the rest being dead space ventilation.

If the alveolar ventilation decreases (either due to a decrease in minute volume or an increase in dead space ventilation), the arterial $PaCO_2$ will rise. On the other hand, the arterial $PaCO_2$ may remain normal but the patient's minute volume may have increased.

Do not assume that the patient must be well when the $PaCO_2$ is normal. A clinical examination of the patient is necessary to rule out respiratory distress (dyspnoea, tachypnoea, active accessory muscles of respiration, tracheal tug, flaring of alae nasi etc). The patient may not be able to sustain this increased levels of ventilation for a prolonged period of time, is likely to get exhausted and may require mechanical ventilatory support.

3) Acid-base status

The assessment of acid-base status must be done in three steps and in the following order.

a) *Assess the pH first :* Normal pH – 7.35 to 7.45. If the pH is less than 7.35, the patient has acidosis and if it is more than 7.45, the patient is alkalotic. The direction of change in pH shows the primary disorder. This is because the compensatory mechanisms never overshoot the requirement of reaching the normal pH.

b) *Assess the $PaCO_2$ next :* Is the $PaCO_2$ normal? The normal $PaCO_2$ is 35 – 45 mmHg. If the pH is abnormal but the $PaCO_2$ normal, it suggests a metabolic disorder. However, the body usually tries to compensate for a change in pH. The respiratory compensation is early and fast.

If the change in pH and $PaCO_2$ are in opposite directions (one is increased and the other decreased), the primary disorder is respiratory. If the change in pH

and $PaCO_2$ are in the same direction (both are increased or decreased), the primary disorder must be metabolic.

e.g. **if the pH is 7.2 and the $PaCO_2$ is 60 mmHg**, the decrease in pH suggests acidosis. The $PaCO_2$ has moved in the opposite direction (increased) and suggests respiratory acidosis. Since the direction of change of pH is towards acidosis and there is respiratory acidosis, it must be a primary respiratory disorder. Similarly, if the pH is alkalotic and the $PaCO_2$ is low, it suggests primary respiratory alkalosis.

c) *Assess the bicarbonate level last :* The normal plasma bicarbonate level is 22-26 mmol/L. An examination of the bicarbonate level after assessment of pH and $PaCO_2$ confirms the acid-base disorder. If the change in pH and the bicarbonate level is in the same direction, the disorder is primarily metabolic and vice versa. If the bicarbonate level is normal but the pH is acidotic, the disorder is of respiratory origin.

It must be remembered that these are general guidelines applicable to patients who are breathing spontaneously. These are useful for rapid bedside assessment of acid-base status. Occasionally, the patients can present with different combinations of acid-base disorders such as a mixed respiratory and metabolic alkalosis, or a mixed respiratory and metabolic acidosis. Such disorders are common in patients who are receiving mechanical ventilation in the intensive care unit.

Various nomograms (Key Box 14.4) and formulae are available to evaluate these situations. One example is given below. The pH changes with change in $PaCO_2$, the extent of which depends on whether the change is acute or chronic.

When the **serum bicarbonate levels change**, there is a change in the arterial carbon dioxide levels also (Key Box 14.5).

Any change either in the pH or $PaCO_2$ beyond these

Key Box 14.4	
RESPIRATORY DISORDER	EXCEPTED pH
Respiratory acidosis	
Acute	$7.4 - [($Observed $PaCO_2 - 40) \times 0.008]$
Chronic	$7.4 - [($Observed $PaCO_2 - 40) \times 0.003]$
Respiratory alkalosis	
Acute	$7.4 + [(40 - $Observed $PaCO_2) \times 0.008]$
Chronic	$7.4 + [(40 - $Observed $PaCO_2) \times 0.001]$

Key Box 14.5	
Metabolic disorder	**Expected $PaCO_2$(mmHg)**
Metabolic acidosis	$(1.5 \times [HCO_3] + 8) \pm 2$
Metabolic alkalosis	$(0.7 \times [HCO_3] + 20) \pm 1.5$

values will point towards the presence of an additional disorder. e.g. Suppose a patient with shock has an ABG showing a pH of 7.1 and the $PaCO_2$ is 60 mmHg. **If the patient had pure respiratory acidosis, the expected pH would have been** :

$7.4 - [(\text{Observed } PaCO_2 - 40) \times 0.008] = 7.4 - [(60 - 40) \times 0.008]$

$7.4 - (20 \times 0.008) = 7.4 - 0.16 = 7.24.$

Since the measured pH is 7.1, the patient must be having a co-existent metabolic acidosis. Other disorders can also be analysed in a similar manner. Whether a process is acute or chronic may be deduced from the history and physical examination of the patient.

CLINICAL NOTES

1) A 30-year old man was admitted to the ICU with history of consumption of organophosphorus poisoning 4 hours ago. On admission, he is drowsy, breathing 60% oxygen by face mask and has a bradycardia. A blood gas analysis taken half an hour later shows a $PaO_2 = 100$ mmHg, $PaCO_2 = 60$ mmHg and a pH of 7.24.

Analysis

Oxygenation : The PaO_2 on 60% oxygen should have been about 300 mmHg. The PaO_2/FiO_2 ratio in this patient is 100/60 = 1.67. Thus, although the PaO_2 is adequate to sustain life, the patient's oxygenation status is poor.

Ventilation: Raised $PaCO_2$ suggests respiratory acidosis.

Acid-base status: The pH shows acidosis. The pH has decreased whereas the $PaCO_2$ has increased. Hence, the patient has primary, uncompensated respiratory acidosis.

2) A 60 year old man, a known diabetic since the last 15 years is admitted with diabetic ketoacidosis. He required endotracheal intubation and ventilation with 60%

oxygen. An arterial blood gas analysis shows the following: $PaO_2 = 60$ mmHg, $PaCO_2 = 28$ mmHg, pH = 7.14 and a $[HCO_3^-] = 12$ mmol/L

Analysis

Oxygenation: The PaO_2 on 60% oxygen should have been about 300 mmHg. The PaO_2/FiO_2 ratio in this patient is 60/60 = 1. Thus, although the PaO_2 is just adequate to sustain life, the patient's oxygenation is poor.

Ventilation : Low $PaCO_2$ suggests respiratory alkalosis.

Acid-base status: The pH shows acidosis. The pH has decreased whereas the $PaCO_2$ has also decreased. Hence, it is not respiratory acidosis and must be metabolic. The bicarbonate levels are far below normal and suggests a primary metabolic acidosis. The low $PaCO_2$ suggests secondary respiratory alkalosis. The patient has primary metabolic acidosis with partial compensation.

3) A 65-year old man with a 40-year history of smoking, posted for elective herniorrhaphy was sent to the pre-anaesthetic clinic for evaluation. Since he gave history of poor exercise tolerance as evidenced by breathlessness even on mild exertion, and clinical examination revealed presence of COPD, an arterial blood gas analysis was done while the patient breathed room air. The report showed a $PaO_2 = 55$ mmHg, $PaCO_2 = 60$ mmHg, pH = 7.34 and a $[HCO_3^-] = 30$ mmol/L.

Analysis

Oxygenation : The PaO_2/FiO_2 ratio is 55/21 = 2.62. Thus, although the PaO_2/FiO_2 ratio seems adequate, the actual PaO_2 is less than 60 mmHg and suggests hypoxaemia.

Ventilation : High $PaCO_2$ suggests respiratory acidosis.

Acid-base status : The pH shows acidosis. The pH has decreased whereas the $PaCO_2$ is high. Hence, it is respiratory acidosis. The bicarbonate levels are high and suggests metabolic alkalosis. Since the pH is acidotic but near normal, the patient must be having primary respiratory acidosis with compensatory metabolic alkalosis. He has fully compensated respiratory acidosis. This picture of chronic hypoxaemia and hypercarbia is typical of patients suffering from severe chronic obstructive pulmonary disease.

Fluids, Electrolytes, Nutrition

15

- Normal physiology
- Water regulation
- Disturbances of volume
- Regulation of sodium concentration
- Disturbances in concentration
- Disturbances in composition of body fluids
- Clinical notes
- Perioperative fluid therapy
- Special purpose solutions
- Nutrition

A good understanding of the physiology of fluids and electrolytes is fundamental to the practice of surgery. Most surgical conditions are associated with changes in this balance and it is only appropriate that these are identified and treated effectively.

NORMAL PHYSIOLOGY

The human body consists of about 50 – 70% liquids and 30 – 50% solids by weight. The liquid portion varies with age, sex and body habitus. The variation is the result of individual differences in the fat content of the body which contains very little water. Hence, thin individuals have greater total body water (TBW) content as compared to obese individuals. Similarly, the TBW is about 50% in women and 60% in men. Neonates have upto 80% TBW.

Of this total body water, intracellular water constitutes 40% of body weight (2/3 of TBW) and the extracellular portion, 20% of body weight (1/3 of TBW). The interstitial fluid and plasma portions of extracellular fluid constitute 15% and 5% of body weight respectively (Figure 15.1).

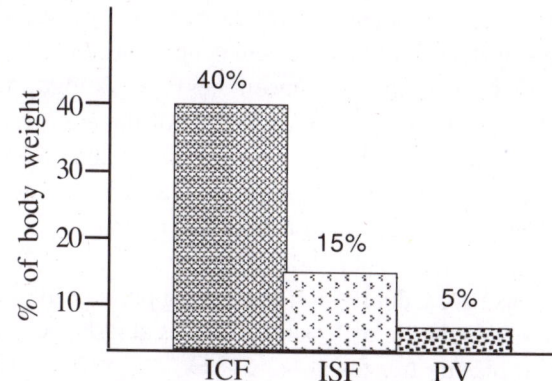

Fig.15.1 Relation of various fluid compartments to body weight.
ICF : Intracellular fluid; ISF : Interstitial fluid; PV : Plasma volume.

COMPOSITION OF BODY FLUIDS

These fluid compartments are separated by semipermeable membranes allowing their fluid composition to be maintained within distinct limits. Table 15.1 shows the composition of the intracellular and extracellular fluid compartments. The composition of the intracellular compartments may vary according to the tissue, *e.g.,* fat contains very little water.

The tonicity of plasma is determined by the solutes, sodium and its corresponding anions, chlorides and

Table 15.1

COMPOSITION	INTRACELLULAR (mmol/L)	EXTRACELLULAR (mmol/L)
Cations		
Sodium	10	140
Potassium	150	4
Calcium	2	2.5
Magnesium	20	1.5
Anions		
Chlorides	10	111
Bicarbonate	10	27
Sulphate	70	1.5
Phosphates	45	1

bicarbonate, together with substances such as glucose, urea and proteins. These particles are osmotically active and hence, tonicity is described in terms of **Osmolality** (mOsm/kg H_2O).

Osmolarity is concentration of a solution in terms of osmoles (or mosmoles) of solute per litre of solution (solute + water). Osmolality is concentration of a solution in terms of osmoles (or mosmoles) per kilogram of solvent. The osmolality is independent of the temperature of the solution and the volume of the solute. Hence, osmolality is the preferred term in clinical practice.

Osmolality of a solution can be measured in two ways:

1) By using the depression of freezing point of the solution: A solution of 1 osm/kg freezes at -1.86° C. Normal plasma freezes at – 0.54° C.

$$\text{Plasma osmolality} = \frac{0.54}{1.86} \times 10^3 \text{ mOsm/kg } H_2O$$

$$= 290 \text{ mosm/kg } H_2O$$

2) By estimating from the solute concentration: Osmolality can be estimated from the concentration of major solutes of plasma.

$$\text{Osmolality} = 2 \times [Na] + \frac{[\text{Glucose (mg\%)}]}{18}$$

$$+ \frac{[\text{Blood urea (mg\%)}]}{6}$$

Example: If a patient's sodium concentration is 140 mmol/L, blood glucose concentration is 180 mg% and blood urea is 30 mg%, his plasma osmolality can be calculated as follows:

$$\text{Osmolality} = 2 \times [Na] + \frac{180}{18} + \frac{30}{6}$$

$$= 280 + 10 + 5 = 295 \text{ mOsm/kg } H_2O$$

From the equation, it is evident that sodium contributes most to the osmolality of plasma.

A change in osmolality is usually due to changes in sodium. The normal range of plasma osmolality is 285 – 300 mOsm/kg H_2O.

Plasma colloidal osmotic pressure

The plasma proteins normally do not pass out of the capillaries into the interstitium. These raise the plasma osmotic pressure above that of the interstitial fluid by an amount referred to as colloidal osmotic pressure (plasma oncotic pressure). The normal plasma colloidal osmotic pressure is 25 mmHg. Albumin is responsible for 75% of this oncotic pressure.

The body has mechanisms to regulate and maintain the volume of fluids, their concentration and composition within narrow limits to maintain homeostasis. Hence, a systematic assessment of fluid status of a patient involves the assessment of body fluid volume, its concentration and its composition in that order.

WATER REGULATION (Regulation of volume)

The primary methods of body water regulation are:

1) *Regulating the volume of liquid ingested* – When the extracellular fluid volume reduces, the thirst centre in the hypothalamus is stimulated which encourages the person to ingest more water.

2) *Regulating the volume of urine excreted* – This is regulated by plasma Antidiuretic hormone (ADH). A reduction in plasma volume releases ADH from the posterior pituitary which in turn acts on the ADH re-

ceptors in the collecting tubules of the kidney, resulting in increased reabsorption of water and reduced production of urine. ADH release may also be stimulated by plasma osmolality and angiotensin.

DISTURBANCES OF VOLUME

A decrease in the circulating volume is called hypovolaemia and an increase, hypervolaemia.

HYPOVOLAEMIA

This is common in surgical patients. The assessment of acute loss of blood volume is detailed in Chapter 12. The reduction in blood volume due to loss of water can be in the following ways:

a) Gut – vomiting, diarrhoea, fistulae

b) Skin and lungs – 0.5 ml/kg/h normally, increases by 12% for every °C rise in temperature

c) Sequestration of fluid in third space

Assessment of dehydration

This is a clinical assessment based upon
1) History: Severity and duration of loss of fluid
2) Examination: Thirst, dryness of mucosa, loss of skin turgor, orthostatic hypotension, tachycardia, reduced jugular venous pressures and decreased urine output in the presence of normal renal function. Dehydration can be classified as follows: (Table 15.2)

Laboratory assessment

Haemoconcentration leads to falsely elevated haemoglobin, packed cell volume estimations and increased blood urea concentration. The kidneys reabsorb more water than usual leading to increased urine osmolality (> 650 mOsm/kg).

HYPERVOLAEMIA

Causes

1. Excessive infusion of intravenous fluids
2. Retention of water in abnormal conditions such as cardiac, renal and hepatic failure
3. Absorption of water as during transurethral resection of prostate using distilled water

Diagnosis

History and physical examination can lead to the cause.

Physical examination – Distended neck veins, pedal oedema, body weight gain

Circulatory overload –

hypertension, tachycardia, pulmonary oedema

confusion, restlessness, convulsions and coma

The development of these signs depends on the rate and volume of fluid overload, renal function and cardiovascular reserve.

Management

1. Treat the cause
2. Restriction of water and salt
3. Diuretics (or dialysis, if necessary) to remove excess water

REGULATION OF SODIUM CONCENTRATION

Water constitutes the major component of all body fluids but the composition varies with the fluid compartment. The most abundant cation of extracellular fluid is sodium and is the prime determinant of ECF volume. 90% of the ECF osmolality is due to sodium.

The human body has no known mechanism to regulate sodium intake.

Table 15.2		
DEGREE OF DEHYDRATION	LOSS OF BODY WEIGHT (%)	CLINICAL FEATURES
Mild	5	Skin turgor, sunken eyes, dry mucous membranes
Moderate	10	Oliguria, hypotension and tachycardia in addition to the above.
Severe	15	Profound oliguria and compromised cardiovascular function

The body regulates sodium output by:

Regulating glomerular filtration rate

Regulating plasma aldosterone levels

Addition or loss of water produces a change in the concentration of the solute. The quantity of solute relative to the volume of water is thereby increased (ECF is concentrated) or decreased (ECF is diluted) with loss or addition of water respectively. Changes in concentration are generally changes in water balance rather than changes in sodium regulation. Since the changes in volume and concentration are interdependent and the changes in water content are not easily measured, an estimate of the fluid volume and concentration is usually made using the measured sodium levels and serum osmolality.

DISTURBANCES IN CONCENTRATION

HYPONATRAEMIA

Hyponatraemia is defined as a sodium level less than 135 mmol/L. It may occur as a result of water retention, sodium loss or both. True hyponatraemia is always associated with low plasma osmolality. It may be associated with expanded, contracted or a normal extracellular volume.

Causes

Assessment of hypovolaemia should begin with an estimation of the extracellular fluid volume (clinically and if necessary, using central venous catheters). Thus, true hyponatraemia can be of three types: hypervolaemic hyponatraemia, hypovolaemic hyponatraemia and normovolaemic hyponatraemia (Figure 15.2).

Hypervolaemic hyponatraemia

Hypervolaemic hyponatraemia may be associated with clinical features of hypervolaemia such as oedema. Acute hypervolaemia (e.g., TURP syndrome – acute absorption of hypotonic fluids into the intravascular compartment) may result in cerebral oedema and pulmonary oedema. As plasma osmolality decreases, water moves from the extracellular space into the cells leading to oedema. The expansion of brain cells is responsible for the symptomatology of water intoxication: nausea, vomiting, lethargy, confusion, restlessness etc. If severe ([Na+] < 100 mmol/L), it can result in seizures and coma. Chronic hypervolaemia as in congestive cardiac failure,

cirrhosis and nephrotic syndrome may manifest with pedal oedema and elevated jugular venous pressures till decompensation occurs. The urinary sodium concentration is less than 15 mmol/L.

Treatment

Acute hyponatraemia (duration <72 h) can be safely corrected more quickly than chronic hyponatraemia. The following factors must be evaluated: patient's volume status, duration and magnitude of the hyponatraemia and the degree and severity of clinical symptoms.

Fluid restriction, diuretics, and correction of the underlying condition may be adequate in most cases. A combination of intravenous normal saline and diuresis with a loop diuretic (e.g. frusemide) also elevates the serum sodium concentration.

Acute symptomatic hyponatraemia is a medical emergency. It should be treated with hypertonic saline (1.6% or 3%). Concomitant use of loop diuretics increases free water excretion and also decreases the risks of fluid overload.

The sodium concentration must be corrected to relieve symptoms and to a concentration of 125 mmol/L. With patients who are acutely symptomatic, the treatment goal is to increase the serum sodium by approximately 1-2 mEq/L/h until the neurologic symptoms subside. The correction should be slow and over a period of 12 – 24 hours with frequent checks of sodium concentration (every 2-4 h) to avoid overcorrection.

Avoid an absolute increase of serum sodium of more than 15-20 mEq/L in a 24-hour period. If sodium correction is undertaken too rapidly, the resulting osmolality changes in the extracellular fluid can cause central pontine myelinolysis. This condition is serious and can be irreversible.

The following equation can aid in the estimation of a sodium deficit to help determine the rate of saline infusion :

Calculated sodium deficit = (125 – current serum Na+) x (body weight in kg) x 0.6

A litre of normal saline contains 154 mEq sodium chloride (NaCl) and 3% saline 500 mEq NaCl. In chronic severe hyponatremia (i.e., serum sodium <115 mEq/L), the rate of correction should be slow and should not exceed 0.5-1 mEq/L/h, with a total increase not to exceed 10 mEq/L/day.

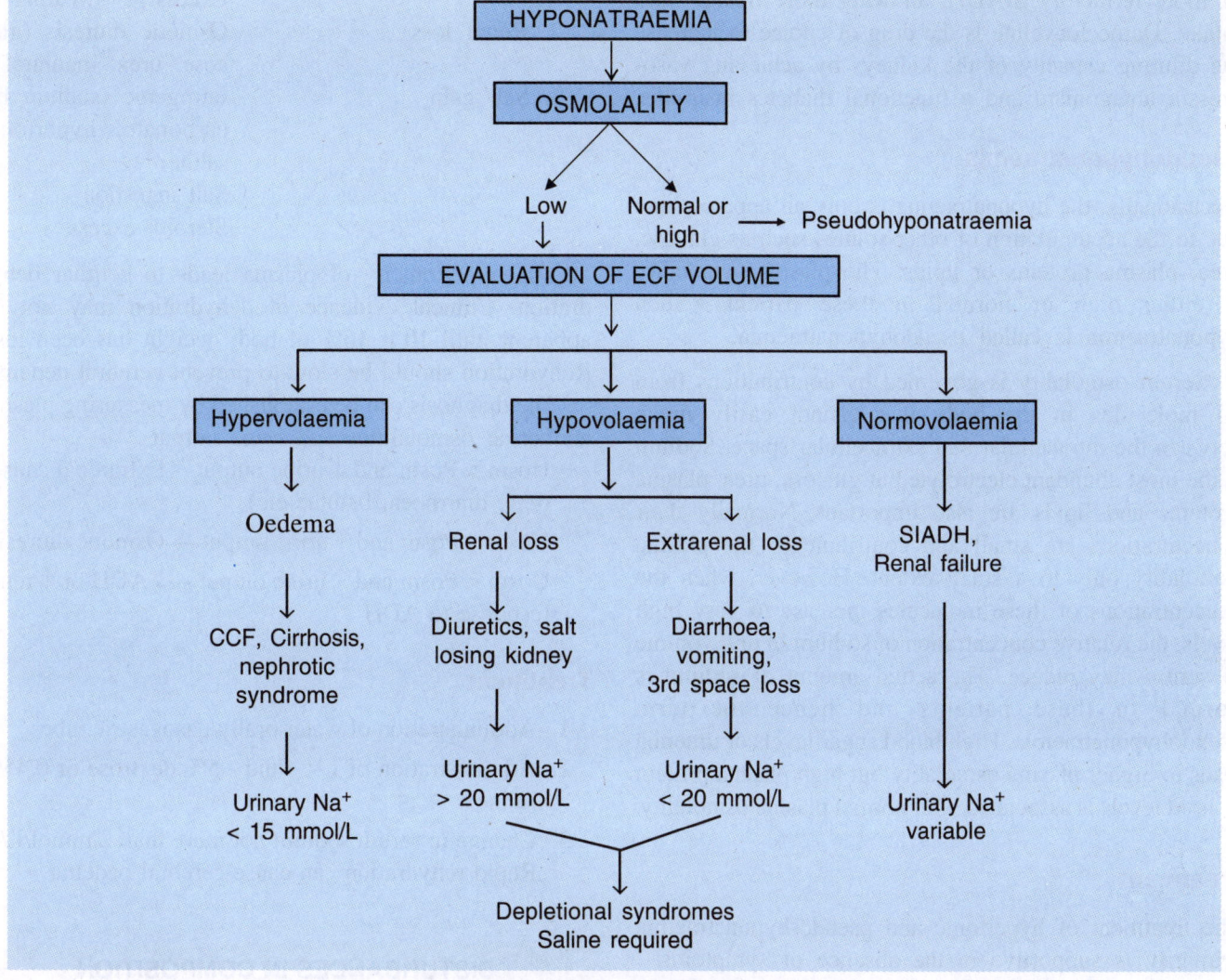

Fig. 15.2 Evaluation of hyponatraemia

Hypovolaemic hyponatraemia

Hypovolaemia with inappropriate correction with hypotonic fluids such as 5% dextrose may result in hyponatraemia. The hypovolaemia may be due to renal causes such as diuresis or a salt-losing kidney. The urinary concentration of sodium is more than 20 mmol/L in these patients. Extrarenal loss of volume as in diarrhoea, vomiting or 3rd space loss may result in urinary concentration less than 20 mmol/L. All these are termed depletional syndromes and require saline infusion.

Treatment

Based upon the volume status, administer isotonic saline to patients with hypotonic hyponatremia who are hypovolaemic to replace the contracted intravascular volume.

Normovolaemic hyponatraemia

Occasionally, hyponatraemia may exist with normovolaemia. In such situations, the plasma osmolality must be estimated. If it is low, renal failure or the syndrome of inappropriate ADH secretion (SIADH) may be considered.

Treatment

For patients who have hypotonic hyponatraemia and are normovolaemic (euvolaemic), asymptomatic, and mildly hyponatraemic, water restriction (1 L/day) is generally the treatment of choice. For instance, a fluid restriction to 1 L/day is enough to raise the serum sodium in most patients. This approach is recommended for patients with asymptomatic SIADH.

Pharmacological agents can be used in some cases

of more refractory SIADH, allowing more liberal fluid intake. Demeclocycline is the drug of choice to increase the diluting capacity of the kidneys by achieving vasopressin antagonism and a functional diabetes insipidus.

Pseudohyponatraemia

Occasionally, the hyponatraemia is only an apparent one due to the accumulation of other solutes such as glucose, urea, plasma proteins or lipids. The plasma osmolality is either high or normal in these patients. Such hyponatraemia is called pseudohyponatraemia.

Serum osmolality is governed by contributions from all molecules in the body that cannot easily move between the intracellular and extracellular space. Sodium is the most abundant electrolyte but glucose, urea, plasma proteins and lipids are also important. Normally their concentrations are small and contribute to the plasma osmolality only to a small extent. However, when the concentrations of these molecules increase to very high levels, the relative concentration of sodium in unit volume of serum may reduce. The actual amount of sodium is normal in these patients and hence the term pseudohyponatraemia. High blood sugar levels or uraemia leads to higher plasma osmolality but high plasma protein or lipid levels is associated with normal plasma osmolality.

Treatment

The treatment of hypertonic and pseudo-hyponatraemia primarily is supportive in the absence of symptoms.

HYPERNATRAEMIA

Hypernatraemia is defined as a plasma sodium concentration of more than 150 mmol/L and may result from pure water loss, hypotonic fluid loss or salt gain.

Causes of hypernatraemia

I. Pure water depletion

1. Extrarenal loss	Failure of water intake (coma, elderly, post operative patients) Mucocutaneous loss – Fever
2. Renal loss	Diabetes insipidus Chronic renal failure

II. Hypotonic fluid loss

1. Extrarenal loss	Gastrointestinal (vomiting, diarrhoea)
2. Renal loss	Excessive sweating Osmotic diuresis (glucose, urea, mannitol)
3. Salt gain	Iatrogenic (sodium bicarbonate, hypertonic saline) Salt ingestion Steroid excess

The hypertonicity of plasma leads to cellular dehydration. Clinical evidence of dehydration may not be apparent until 10 – 15% of body weight has been lost. Rehydration should be slow to prevent cerebral oedema.

The diagnosis can be established by measuring plasma and urine osmolalities and urine output.

Uosm > Posm and ↓ urine output →Extrarenal causes (*e.g.,* diarrhoea, fistulae etc)

Uosm > Posm and ↑ urine output → Osmotic diuresis

Uosm < Posm and ↑ urine output →↓ ADH or ↓ renal response to ADH

Treatment

1. Administration of water orally/nasogastric tube

2. Administration of I.V. fluid - 5% dextrose or 0.45% saline

3. Change in serum sodium not more than 2 mmol/L/h. Rapid rehydration can cause cerebral oedema

DISTURBANCES IN COMPOSITION OF BODY FLUIDS

POTASSIUM BALANCE

The normal potassium level is 3.5 – 5.5 mmol/L. Hypokalaemia and hyperkalaemia are the two important disturbances.

HYPOKALAEMIA

This is defined as a plasma concentration of potassium less than 3.5 mmol/L.

Causes

Reduced intake

Tissue redistribution: Insulin therapy, alkalaemia, β adrenergic agonists, familial periodic paralysis.

Increased loss: Gastro-intestinal losses – diarrhoea, vomiting, fistulae

- Renal causes: Diuretics, renal artery stenosis, diuretic phase of renal failure

Symptoms

- Anorexia, nausea
- Muscle weakness, paralytic ileus
- Altered cardiac conduction: Delayed repolarisation, reduced height of 'T' wave, presence of 'U' wave, wide QRS complexes and arrhythmias.

Management

- Diagnosis and treatment of the cause
- Repletion of body stores
- Potassium supplements, in the form of milk, fruit juice, tender coconut water.
- Syrup potassium chloride orally – 15 ml contains 20 mmol of potassium
- If the patient cannot take orally or the hypokalaemia is severe, intravenous potassium chloride can be given at a rate not exceeding 0.5 mmol/kg/h under electrocardiographic monitoring. A maximum of 200 mmol/day should not be exceeded in a 70 kg individual.

HYPERKALAEMIA

- This is defined as a plasma concentration of potassium more than 5 mmol/L.

Causes (Key Box 15.1)

Clinical features

- Vague muscle weakness, flaccid paralysis

Electrocardiographic changes

- Tall, peaked 'T' waves with shortened QT interval (6 – 7 mmol/L)
- Wide QRS complex, widening and then loss of 'P' wave (8 – 10 mmol/L)
- Wide QRS complex, merge into 'T' waves (sine wave pattern)
- Ventricular fibrillation ($K^+ > 10$ mmol/L)

Treatment of hyperkalaemia

1. Calcium gluconate (10%) → 10–30 ml.
2. Sodium bicarbonate → 1–2 mmol/kg over 10–15 minutes.
3. 100 ml of 50 % dextrose with 10–12 units of insulin over 15–20 minutes.

Key Box 15.1

CAUSES

1. Pseudohyperkalaemia	In vitro haemolysis Thrombocytosis Tourniquet Exercise
2. Impaired excretion	Renal failure Hyperaldosteronism K^+ sparing diuretics
3. Tissue redistribution	Tissue damage (burns, trauma) Acidosis Rhabdomyolysis Tumour necrosis Suxamethonium Familial hyperkalaemic periodic paralysis Massive intravascular haemolysis
4. Excessive input	Stored blood transfusion Excessive intravenous potassium supplementation

4. Hyperventilation
5. Salbutamol nebulisation
6. Calcium exchange resins
7. Peritoneal or haemodialysis

CLINICAL NOTES

A 21-year old lady was found to be collapsed as she was feeding her 15-day old baby in the nephrology ward. On arrival, the cardiac arrest response team found her to have ventricular tachycardia without pulse. Cardiopulmonary resuscitation was given and she was shifted to the intensive care unit after return of spontaneous circulation. Investigations showed that her potassium level was 1.6 mmol/L. She had been admitted to the nephrology unit for postpartum acute renal failure. She had been dialysed three times following which she had gone into the diuretic phase of recovery from acute renal failure. She was putting out about 5 litres of urine per day in the last two days. Her hypokalaemia was corrected over 2 -3 days. She recovered completely and could be discharged from the ward in 5 days' time.

MAGNESIUM

Magnesium is the second most abundant intracellular ion. The normal intracellular concentration of magnesium is about 26 mEq/L and extracellular concentration is 1.5 – 2.5 mEq/L. Almost 60% of the magnesium is deposited in the skeleton. Magnesium is required as a cofactor for several important enzymatic reactions, including the phosphorylation of glucose within cells and the use of ATP by contracting muscle fibres.

A daily dietary intake of 0.3–0.4 g (approximately 20 – 30 mEq) is required. The proximal convoluted tubule reabsorbs magnesium very effectively.

CALCIUM

Calcium is the most abundant mineral in the body. 99 percent is deposited in the skeleton. In addition, calcium ions are important for the control of muscular and neural activities, in blood clotting, as cofactors for enzymatic reactions, and as second messengers.

Calcium homeostasis reflects a balance between reserves in the bone, rate of absorption across the digestive tract, and rate of loss at the kidneys. The hormones parathyroid hormone (PTH), vitamin D and calcitonin maintain calcium homeostasis in the ECF. Parathyroid hormone and Vitamin D raise Ca^{++} concentrations and calcitonin lowers it.

Calcium absorption at the digestive tract and reabsorption along the distal convoluted tubule are stimulated by PTH from the parathyroid glands and calcitriol from the kidneys. The average daily requirement of calcium in an adult is 0.8–1.2 g/day.

Hypercalcaemia (Key Box 15.2)

Hypercalcemia exists when the Ca^{2+} concentration of the ECF is above 11 mEq/L.

Key Box 15.2
CAUSES OF HYPERCALCAEMIA
• Hyperparathyroidism • Malignant cancers of the breast, lung, kidney, or bone marrow

Features

Severe hypercalcaemia (12–13 mEq/L) causes such symptoms as fatigue, confusion, cardiac arrhythmias, and calcification of the kidneys and soft tissues throughout the body.

Hypocalcaemia (Key Box 15.3)

Hypocalcemia exists when calcium level is less than 9 mEq/L. However, the serum calcium level should be related to the albumin levels. Half the serum calcium is bound to albumin and as albumin levels become low, this bound fraction is lower leading to a low total serum calcium concentration. Free calcium ionic concentration is important for the electrical activity of the nerves and muscles and is the ideal parameter to measure but is not easily available.

Key Box 15.3
CAUSES OF HYPOCALCAEMIA
• Hypoparathyroidism • Vitamin D deficiency • Chronic renal failure

Features

Muscle spasms, sometimes including generalised convulsions, myocardial depression, cardiac arrhythmias, and osteoporosis.

PERIOPERATIVE FLUID THERAPY

Normal maintenance needs

The average daily requirement of water for an average sized adult is 2000 ml. In general, a volume of 35 - 40 ml/kg/day meets the daily maintenance needs.

Fluid requirements in a surgical patient whose body homeostasis is normal

Patients awaiting anaesthesia and surgery need to be kept fasting for a few hours prior to and after the surgery. Except in very minor surgery, fluid lost during this period needs to be replaced.

The replacement is as follows

1. Fluid requirement during starvation – 2 ml/kg/h of starvation. This volume is calculated for hours of fasting and then replaced over 2-3 h.

2. Maintenance requirement – 2 ml/kg/h of surgery

3. Third space losses –

   4 ml/kg/h for surgery with minimal dissection – e.g., herniorrhaphy

   6 ml/kg/h for surgery associated with moderate dissection. E.g., gastro-jejunostomy and vagotomy

   8 ml/kg/h – for surgery associated with large amount of dissection – e.g., Whipple's procedure.

4. Blood loss is replaced by compatible blood transfusion (homologous or autologous), if the haematocrit falls below 25%. Blood loss is replaced with an equal amount of colloids or three times the volume with crystalloids if the haematocrit is > 25% in an otherwise healthy individual. Crystalloids are electrolyte solutions and distribute themselves throughout the body water and hence, a larger volume needs to be given.

A patient undergoing surgery should receive fluid deficit due to starvation + maintenance fluids + third space losses + replacement of blood loss (as detaied above). Adequacy of fluid replacement should be checked with haemodynamic stability and urine output in major procedures. When very large fluid shifts are expected (oncologic surgeries), and the patient has compromised cardiac status or has renal insufficiency, it may be necessary to monitor fluid status using central venous pressure monitoring.

WHAT TO GIVE?

The starvation losses are usually replaced by an infusion of 5% dextrose or 5% dextrose in isotonic saline.

The maintenance and third space losses are replaced by Ringer lactate solution.

TYPES OF INTRAVENOUS FLUIDS

These can be broadly divided into three groups – crystalloids, colloids and special purpose solutions.

Crystalloids are essentially solutions of electrolytes in water: e.g. Ringer lactate. Some also contain dextrose, e.g., dextrose saline, 5% dextrose, Isolyte P, Isolyte M. They vary in the content of different electrolytes.

Colloids are solutions of large molecules which tend to remain in the intravascular compartment, *e.g.*, gelatine, hetastarch, pentastarch, dextran 40, dextran 70. They are all plasma expanders since the molecules tend to exert osmotic forces and draw fluid from the interstitial compartment into the intravascular space. The colloids

vary in their magnitude of volume expansion and duration of action. Dextran 40 reduces viscosity of blood and maintains blood rheology better. Hence, it is used as continuous infusion after microvascular surgery. It can also interfere with coagulation which along with reduced viscosity helps in maintaining blood supply to free flaps and vascular grafts.

SPECIAL PURPOSE SOLUTIONS

I. **SODIUM BICARBONATE**: It is available as 7.5% (0.9 mEq/ml) and 8.4% (1 mEq/ml) of sodium bicarbonate. It is used as an alkalinising agent (in metabolic acidosis, hyperkalaemia and forced alkaline diuresis).

The disadvantages of indiscriminate sodium bicarbonate therapy are:

Increased sodium load

Alkalosis with a shift of oxygen dissociation curve to the left (increased affinity of haemoglobin to O_2, reducing its unloading)

Increased intracranial pressure and intraventricular haemorrhages in neonates

Circulatory overload leading to cardiac failure

Carbon dioxide load leading to respiratory failure

II. **MANNITOL** (10% and 20%) – is an osmotic diuretic. Its main use is to reduce intracranial pressure by producing diuresis. It is also used to reduce intraocular pressure. Mannitol expands intravascular volume initially by drawing fluid from the interstitium. This is followed by diuresis. It should be used with caution in patients with cardiac failure, renal failure *etc.*

III. **HYPERTONIC SALINE** (1.6, 3 and 5%): These solutions are available to treat hyponatraemia. 7.5% hypertonic saline is used in rapid expansion of intravascular volume after major trauma.

IV. **ALBUMIN** : 4.5% albumin is used as a plasma expander. 20% albumin can be used to replace lost albumin in severe hypoalbuminaemia in addition to plasma expansion.

PERIOPERATIVE FLUID THERAPY IN PATIENTS WITH DISTURBED FLUID BALANCE

Derangements of fluid therapy can be classified as: (a) Disturbances of volume (b) Disturbances of concentration and (c) Disturbances of composition

In the evaluation of a patient with a suspected problem in fluid and electrolyte or acid-base balance, careful sequential analysis of the volume, concentration and composition (in that order) followed by appropriate therapy protects the patient from severe, perhaps fatal errors in management.

NUTRITION

The value of nutrition is an important but often neglected aspect in the care of a surgical or a critically ill patient. Malnutrition leads to death by starvation. During starvation, the body uses up its reserves and undergoes a process called self-cannibalisation.

The breakdown of body proteins leads to reduced muscle mass and muscle strength, poor wound healing, reduced immunity, coagulation disorders etc. Loss of weight in excess of 30% of the initial body weight can be fatal.

Nutritional requirements

An average human being requires 30 – 35 kcal/kg/day. Thus, an average man requires 2200 – 2500 kcal/day and an average woman, 1800 – 2000 kcal/kg/day. Of this total requirement, at least 500 kcal need to be provided in the form of carbohydrates. This is because red blood cells, brain cells and renal medulla need glucose for their metabolism. Protein requirements amount to 1 g/kg/day. The rest of the diet must consist of fat, vitamins and minerals.

Nutrition can be administered by either the enteral or parenteral route.

ENTERAL NUTRITION

Nutrition can be administered via the gastro-intestinal tract and is called enteral nutrition. It is essential to attempt enteral nutrition at the earliest opportunity. The most optimal route of administering nutrition is by the enteral route for the following reasons :

1) **The integrity of gut mucosa depends on provision of nutrients into the gut lumen.** If the fasting period exceeds more than a few hours, the gut mucosal cells start disintegrating and the villi get destroyed. This may permit the intestinal bacteria to enter the circulation leading to sepsis. Translocation of bacteria from the intestines into the circulation has been identified as the **'motor of multiorgan failure'**.

2) Use of natural route of nutrition requires less nursing supervision.

3) Infection rate is lower with enteral nutrition.

4) Greater insulin response is seen with enteral nutrition.

5) There is a lower tendency to retain salt and water.

6) Enteral nutrition is cheaper.

Administration

Enteral nutrition can be administered through a nasogastric tube or a nasojejunal tube. Alternatively, a feeding gastrostomy or a feeding jejunostomy can be used.

Tube feeds are started initially at a rate of 50 ml every 2 hours on the first day. If tolerated, this can be increased gradually to 200 ml every 2 hours. Clear fluids are given on the first day. Milk and other feeds are added from 2nd day onwards.

The feeds can be given as liquidised food (a mixture of cooked rice, dal and vegetables can be blended in a mixer, diluted and strained). Alternately, commercially available tube feeds can be used. The latter are slightly more expensive but have the advantage of easy preparation containing well-balanced nutrients.

When gastric emptying is delayed, absorption of feeds can be encouraged using prokinetic agents such as metoclopramide (10 mg, three times a day) or erythromycin (250 mg, three times a day).

Enteral nutrition is better tolerated when given as an infusion. Enteral feeds are available commercially in bags which can be given by 'drip' method into the nasoenteric tube using infusion pumps.

Immunonutrition

Glutamine is an essential nutrient for the maintenance of integrity of intestinal cells and there is evidence to show that its inclusion in enteral feeds enhances patient immunity.

Complications of enteral nutrition

1) Intolerance to the feeds: Vomiting, diarrhoea, bowel distention

2) Mechanical problems: Feeding tube block, leak, erosions, sinusitis

3) Nutritional deficiencies – if proper attention to all components is not given.

Table 15.3 Feeding methods (Also refer Fig. 15.3 and 15.4)		
RYLE'S TUBE (RT) FEEDING	**GASTROSTOMY**	**FEEDING JEJUNOSTOMY**
Easy, quick, cheap method Indicated in stroke, comatose patients etc Chances of aspiration are high. Hence, always 30° propped up position is recommended	Indicated when RT cannot be passed e.g., inoperable carcinoma oesophagus, stricture. Malecot's catheter is introduced into the stomach after a purse string suture (Stamm's gastrostomy).	Indicated after major oesophageal surgeries, high duodenal fistulae A Ryles' tube is introduced into the jejunum under vision (during surgery) using a purse string suture.

FEEDING

Different methods of feeding are given in Table 15.3, Fig. 15.3, 15.4.

Percutaneous Endoscopic Gastrostomy (PEG) is more popular now (Details below):

Percutaneous Endoscopic Gastrostomy (PEG)

With the help of an endoscope, a gastrostomy tube is placed in a retrograde manner and brought out through a skin incision.

Technically very easy, can be done under local anaesthesia

It has replaced feeding gastrostomies (open method). It is popular nowadays (Fig. 15.5)

Complications include – colonic perforation, sepsis, bleeding, wound infection etc.

TOTAL PARENTERAL NUTRITION (TPN)

When enteral nutrition is not possible for more than a few days, parenteral nutrition may need to be considered. When all nutrition is done by the parenteral route, it is termed total parenteral nutrition (TPN).

A central venous access is mandatory for the administration of TPN. These solutions are hypertonic and irritant to the peripheral veins leading to venous thrombosis.

The central venous access should be dedicated to TPN and **should not be used for administration of drugs or other fluids**. The line should be handled with strict asepsis.

Central venous access can be through any of the central veins such as external jugular, internal jugular or subclavian veins. The tip of the catheter is optimally placed in the superior vena cava. The subclavian veins, especially tunnelled for the purpose (Hickman line) are the most popular since they are easy to maintain and rate of infection is less.

Administration of nutrients

Carbohydrates: One gram of glucose provides 4 kCal. The entire energy requirement of the day can be given in the form of glucose. This needs to be administered in a concentration of 50%, so as not to exceed the daily

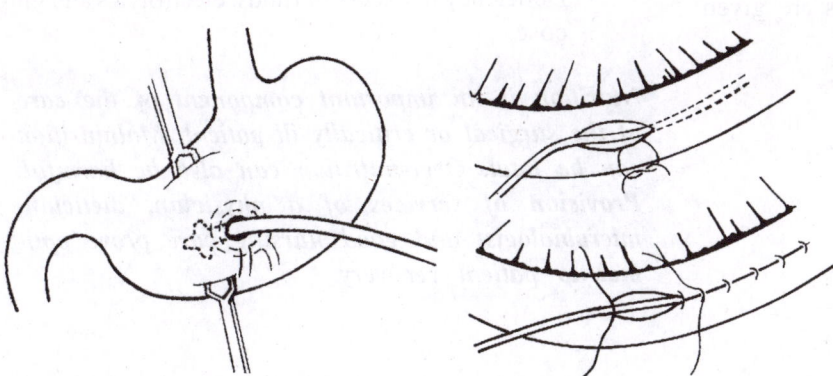

Fig.15.3 Feeding gastrostomy   **Fig.15.4** Feeding jejunostomy

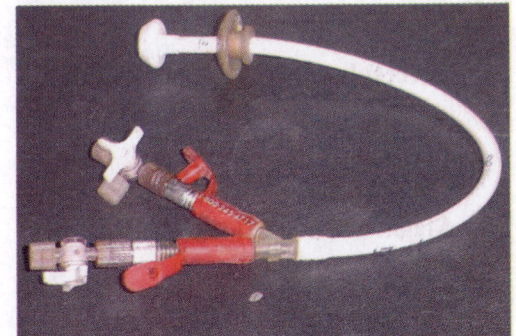

Fig.15.5 Percutaneous Endoscopic Gastrostomy tube

fluid requirement. 1000 ml of 50 % dextrose contains 500 g of dextrose providing 2000 kCal.

Problems

Hyperglycaemia must be prevented by addition of appropriate amounts of insulin.

Potassium supplements to avoid hypo-kalaemia

Increased carbon dioxide production may increase work of breathing and result in difficulty in weaning patients from ventilator.

Hypertonic solutions produce thrombophlebitis

Infusion of dextrose-containing solutions do not take care of daily protein and other nutrient requirements of the body.

Lipids: 1g of fat provides 9 kCals. Since it is a more concentrated form of energy, half the daily caloric requirement can be given using 10 % or 20 % lipid emulsions.

Problems

Occasionally lipid infusion can cause impaired pulmonary diffusing capacity.

Its clearance from plasma may be delayed with impaired liver function

Lipid emulsions are expensive

Proteins: The average protein requirement is 1 g/kg/day. Amino acid replacement solutions are available as 10% and 20% solutions. The calorific value of proteins should not be counted as they are the building blocks of the body. They are not infused to be metabolised for energy.

Electrolyte requirements

The daily requirement of various electrolytes are given below.

Electrolyte	mmol/kg/day
Sodium	1 – 2
Potassium	1
Calcium	5 – 10
Magnesium	5 – 10

One ampule of water-soluble vitamins must be infused daily, over a period of time exceeding 30 minutes to avoid urinary loss. Folic acid, vitamins B_{12}, K, A and D also need to be given once a week. The total volume of TPN should be 2000 – 3000 ml/day. Alternately, commercially available TPN solutions which are well-balanced with all nutrients can be used. Although expensive, good nutrition may reduce the morbidity and duration of hospital stay of the patient thus proving cost-effective.

Monitoring

Aim

1) To identify excess or deficiency of individual nutrients.

2) To identify complications

Daily

Blood sugar, serum electrolytes, blood urea and serum creatinine.

Plasma should be inspected daily for opalescence when lipid emulsions are given. If opalescent, further lipid emulsion should be withheld till the plasma clears.

Biweekly

Liver function tests, coagulation profile, complete haemogram.

Complications

1. **Technical**

   • During catheter placement such as injury to lung and pleura, arteries near to the veins, arrhythmias;

   • During catheter maintenance such as clotted catheter, venous thrombosis; catheter-related infections.

2. **Metabolic problems**:

   • Deficiency or excess of fluids, electrolytes and glucose.

Nutrition is an important component of the care of the surgical or critically ill patient. Malnutrition can be fatal. Over-nutrition can also be harmful. Provision of services of a physician, dietician, microbiologist and good nursing care prove optimal to patient recovery.

Tumours, Cysts, Neck Swellings

16

- Benign tumours
- Neural tumours
- Malignant tumours
- Paraneoplastic syndromes
- Soft tissue sarcoma
- Cystic swellings
- Differential diagnosis of midline swellings
- Swellings in the submandibular triangle
- Swellings in the carotid triangle
- Swellings in the posterior triangle
- AV Fistula
- Secondaries in the neck
- Different types of neck dissections
- Pancoast tumour

Definition

A tumour is a new growth consisting of cells of independent growth arranged atypically and serves no function.

Types: Benign and Malignant.

BENIGN TUMOURS

PAPILLOMA

This is a benign tumour arising from skin or mucous membrane. It is characterised by finger-like projections with a central core of connective tissue, blood vessels, lymphatics and lining epithelium. It can be called Hamartoma or a skin tag. It is an example of overgrowth of fibrous tissue. (Key Box 16.1)

Key Box 16.1

OVERGROWTH OF FIBROUS TISSUE

- Keloid
- Desmoid tumour
- Hypertrophic scar

Types

1. Skin papilloma

a. *Squamous papilloma* occurs in the skin, cheek, tongue, etc.

- **Soft papillomas** are squamous papillomas seen in elderly patients on the eyelid as small, soft, brownish swellings.

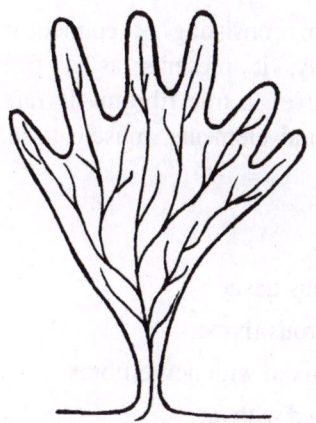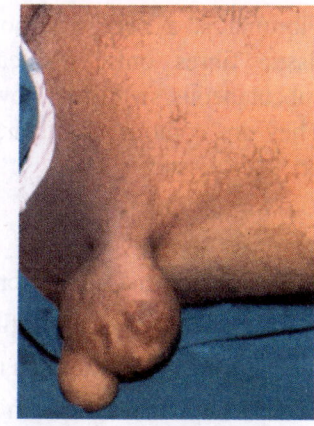

Fig. 16.1 Structure of papilloma

Fig. 16.2 Pedunculated papilloma thigh

157

Squamous papilloma can also be *congenital,* sometimes multiple in number, can be sessile or pedunculated.

b. **Basal cell papilloma** (seborrhoeic keratosis) seen on the trunk of elderly patients as brownish elevated patch of skin, which gives a semitransparent, oily appearance.

2. Arising from mucous membrane of visceral organs:

a. *Transitional cell papilloma* in the urinary bladder as a cause of haematuria.

b. *Columnar cell papilloma* in the rectum as a cause of mucous diarrhoea.

c. *Cuboidal cell papilloma* in the *gall bladder.*

d. *Squamous papilloma* in the larynx can cause *respiratory obstruction.*

e. *Papilloma of breast* **(Duct papilloma) causes bleeding per nipple**.

Treatment

Excision, only if papilloma causes discomfort or if it is symptomatic.

Complications

1. Skin papilloma can get secondarily infected resulting in pain and swelling.
2. Papilloma in the breast, rectum, tongue and gall bladder can undergo malignant change.

FIBROMA[1]

Fibroma is a benign tumour, consisting of connective tissue fibres only. Clinically, it presents as a firm subcutaneous swelling. However, a true fibroma is rare. They are combined with neural elements, muscle tissue or fatty tissue.

Types

1. Soft fibromas-Less fibrous tissue
2. Hard fibromas-More fibrous tissue
   Neurofibroma-Fibroma mixed with nerve fibres
   Fibrolipoma-Fibroma mixed with fat
   Myofibroma-Fibroma mixed with muscle fibres
   Angiofibroma-Fibroma mixed with blood vessels

Treatment

They are treated by excision because of the chance of developing into a sarcoma.

LIPOMA

Lipoma is a benign tumour arising from fat cells of adult type.

Types

1. Single subcutaneous lipoma

This is a single, slow growing, painless swelling (Fig. 16.3).

The swelling is soft, may feel cystic with fluctuation. This is also called pseudofluctuation because fat at body temperature behaves like fluid.

Surface is lobular. Lobulations are better appreciated with firm palpation of the swelling. Due to the pressure, lobules bulge out between the fibrous tissue strands.

Edge slips under the palpating finger which is a pathognomonic sign of lipoma.

Being a subcutaneous swelling, it *is freely mobile.* The flank is the commonest site. Shoulder region, neck, back, upper limbs are the other common sites (refer Table 16.1 for various locations). Few lipomas are also found in the neck.

2. Multiple lipomatosis

Such lipomas are multiple and very often tender because of *nerve elements* mixed with them. Hence, they are called *multiple neurolipomatosis. Dercum's disease* is one example of this variety (*Adiposis dolorosa*) wherein tender, lipomatous swellings are present in the body, mainly the trunk.

3. Uncapsulated lipoma

Diffuse variety is a rare type of lipoma. It is called pseudolipoma. It is an overgrowth of fat without a capsule.

Histological types of lipoma

1. **Fibrolipoma** - Since fibrous tissue is mixed with fat, lipoma feels hard.
2. **Neurolipoma** - *Painful* lipoma, because of nerve elements.
3. **Naevolipoma** - Lipoma is relatively avascular but this variety is vascular.

---

1. Students should not give the diagnosis of fibroma because in majority of cases it is neurofibroma or fibrolipoma.

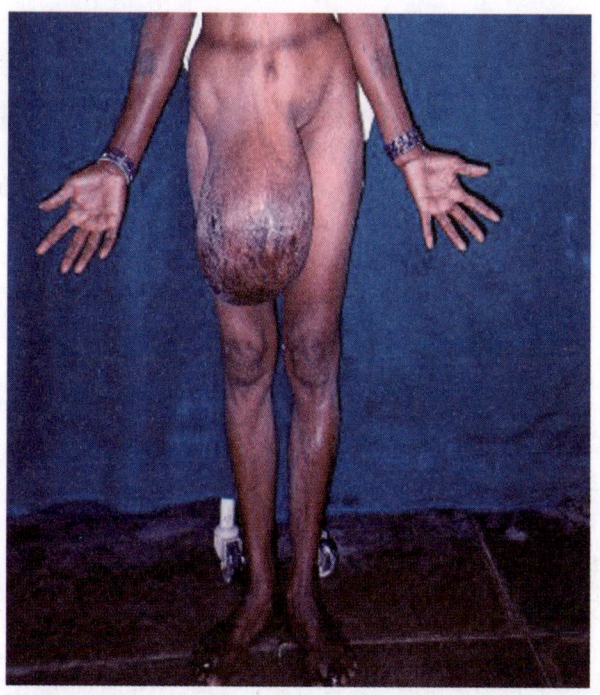
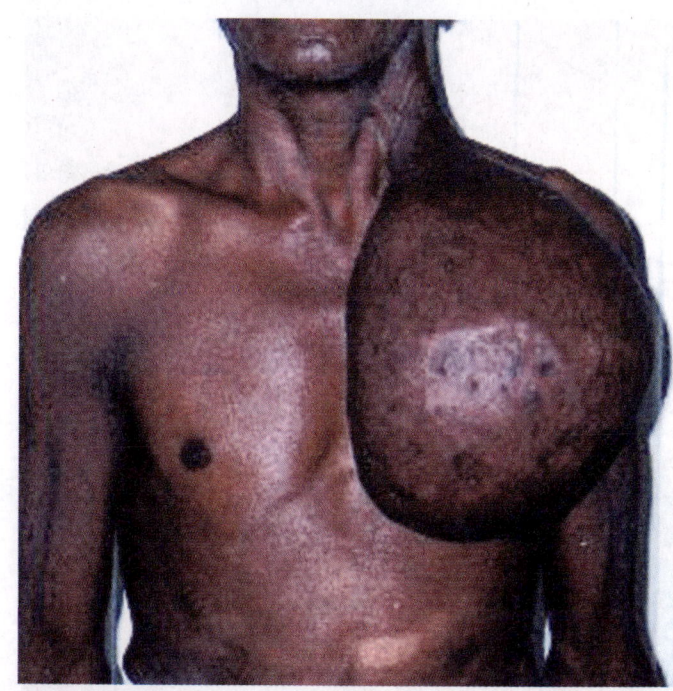

Fig. 16.3 and 16.4 Giant lipoma involving abdominal wall and chest wall. Both these lipomas were of 15 years duration. However, there were no sarcomatous changes. (Contributed by Prof. Rajeev Shetty, Professor of surgery, Bangalore Medical College, Bangalore).

Table 16.1 Various Types of Lipoma

LOCATION	PRESENTATION	DIFFERENTIAL DIAGNOSIS	SIGNIFICANCE
1. **Subcutaneous** Shoulder Flank	Mobile Lobular **Edge slips under palpating fingers.**	Neurofibroma	**The most common variety**
2. **Subfascial** Limbs, Palm, sole	Difficult to appreciate the edge and lobulation	Implantation dermoid, TB tenosynovitis	Subfascial lipoma of the scalp – erodes bone.
3. **Subsynovial, intra-articular** Knee joint, Elbow	Swelling in relation to the knee joint, elbow joint	Bursa Baker's cyst	Intra-articular lipoma is rare.
4. **Intermuscular** Thigh, Shoulder region	Swelling of the thigh. On contraction of the muscles, it is more firm due to transmitted pressure.	Fibrosarcoma Haematoma	Chances of developing liposarcoma are more.
5. **Parosteal**	Under the periosteum of bone, feels hard	Bony tumour	Very, very rare
6. **Submucous** Intestines Larynx	Asymptomatic or stridor	Intestinal tumour Laryngeal tumour	Intussusception
7. **Subserosal** Retroperitoneum	Retroperitoneal swelling	Hydronephrosis Retroperitoneal cyst	Liposarcoma
8. **Extradural**	Very rare	–	–
9. **Intraglandular**	Breast, pancreas	Cystic lesions	Very rare

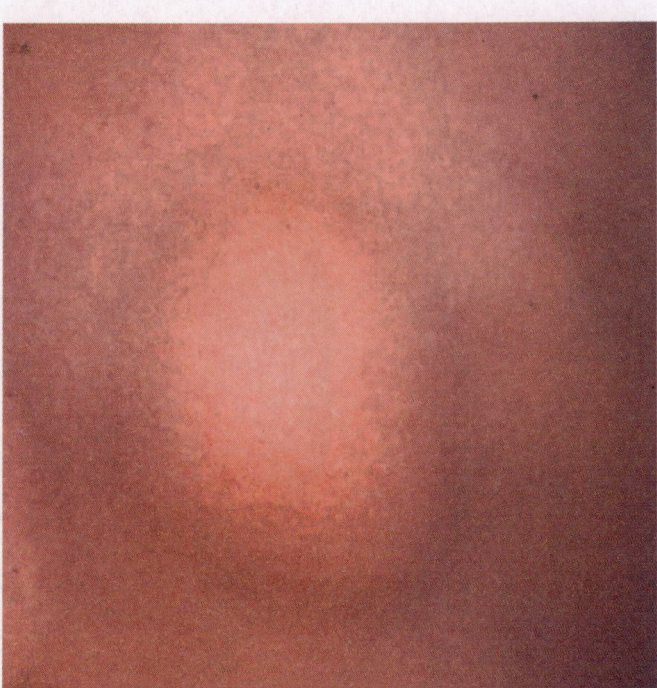

Fig. 16.5 Lipoma in the flank - the most common site

Key Box 16.2
LIPOMA
• Subcutaneous – Commonest type
• Flanks- Commonest site
• Soft, lobular, slipping edge
• Does not occur in the cranial cavity
• **Very few turn into liposarcoma**

Treatment

Excision of lipoma is done by incising the skin followed by squeezing the lipoma out.

Complications

1. **Liposarcoma** : The present view is that benign lipomas do not turn into malignancy. However, a few retro-peritoneal lipomas and lipoma in the thigh can turn into liposarcoma after many years of growth. Malignancy should be suspected when :

   The swelling grows rapidly.

   It becomes painful due to infiltration of nerves.

   The swelling becomes vascular with red colour, dilated veins over the surface.

Surface is warm due to increased vascularity.

Skin fungation or fixation occurs later.

Mobility gets restricted because of infiltration into the deeper plane to the muscle.

The liposarcoma rarely spreads by lymphatics. It spreads by blood. Metastasis in the lung can rarely occur from liposarcoma producing multiple chest secondaries.

Liposarcoma is treated by wide excision followed by reconstruction either by split skin graft or by flaps. In the thigh, sometimes radical surgery may amount to compartmental excision. Chemotherapy and radio-therapy can also be used.

2. Calcification
3. Myxomatous degeneration
4. Intussusception - abdominal emergency
5. Saponification

CLINICAL NOTES

32 year old young man presented with gross swelling of the right leg. He had seen two surgeons earlier wherein he was told to have deep vein thrombosis and nothing was offered. Examination revealed an obvious mass which was palpable in anteromedial and posterior compartment. MRI revealed an intermuscular mass. At exploration, intermuscular lipoma weighing 700 gms. was excised. (Fig. 16.6 and 16.7)

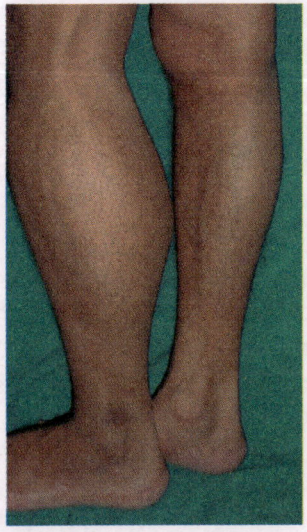

Fig. 16.6 Compare both the legs. Local gigantism can also be caused by extensive lipomatosis involving the leg

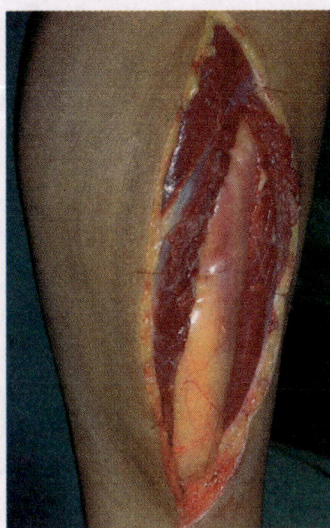

Fig. 16.7 Soleus muscle is cut, lipoma is seen coming out of the deeper plane. Luckily, no major neurovascular bundle was involved in this case

NEURAL TUMOURS

NEUROMA

They are uncommon benign tumours which occur in relationship with sympathetic nervous system or spinal cord. They can be classified into true neuromas and false neuromas.

TRUE NEUROMA

1. **Ganglioneuroma** consists of ganglion cells and nerve fibres of sympathetic chain. They are slow growing tumours. When present in the neck as a *parapharyngeal mass,* it can cause dysphagia. These tumours can occur in the neck, retroperitoneum or mediastinum.

   Excision of the tumour is the treatment.

2. **Neuroblastoma** consists of poorly differentiated cells. It occurs in young children. It is interesting to know that this tumour can undergo spontaneous regression.

3. **Myelinic neuroma** is very rare. It arises in relationship with spinal cord made up of myelinic fibres.

   - Does not contain any ganglion cells.

     All these 3 tumours are called *true neuromas.*

CLINICAL NOTES

18 year old engineering student had backache and was examined by an orthopaedician and refered to general surgery. CT scan of the abdomen revealed, mass in the paraspinal region in the retroperitoneum. Laparotomy and excision of the mass was done, which was reported as ganglioneuroma.

FALSE NEUROMA

These tumours arise from the connective tissue of the sheath of nerve endings. They occur following nerve injuries, lacerations, or after amputation. They are of 2 types.

1. *End neuroma* occurs after amputation due to the proliferation of nerve fibres from the distal cut end of the nerve. This produces a bulbous swelling. If it is caught in the suture line or due to pressure of the prosthesis, it produces severe neuralgic pain. To avoid this, when an amputation is being done, the nerve is pulled downwards and cut as high as possible so that it retracts upwards (Fig. 16.8).

2. *Lateral neuromas* occur due to partial injury to the nerve on the lateral aspect (Fig. 16.9).

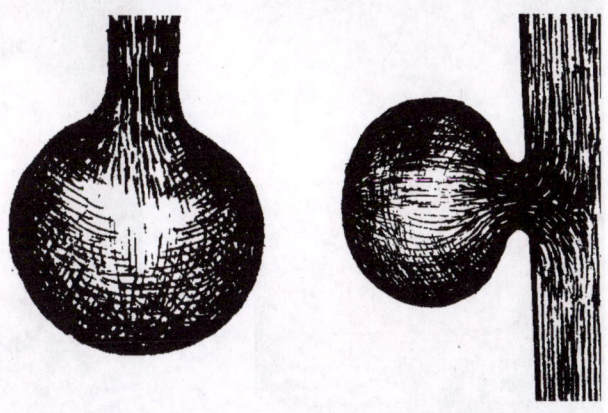

Fig. 16.8 End neuroma   **Fig. 16.9** Lateral neuroma

Treatment

- Excision of the neuroma.

NEUROFIBROMA

It is a benign tumour arising from the connective tissue of the nerve sheath. Typically, it produces a *fusiform swelling* in the direction of the nerve fibres.

Clinical types

1. Single subcutaneous neurofibroma

- Commonly affects the peripheral nerves, like ulnar nerve, vagus nerve or cutaneous nerves.

Clinical features

- Tingling and numbness, paraesthesia in the distribution of the nerve.
- Round to oval swelling in the direction of nerve fibre.
- Smooth surface, with round border. The swelling moves at right angles to the direction of nerve fibres. Vertical mobility is absent.
- Consistency is firm. Sometimes, it is hard.
- Being a subcutaneous swelling, the skin can be lifted up.

Treatment

- It is treated by excision.
- In most of the cases excision is easy as the tumour is well encapsulated.

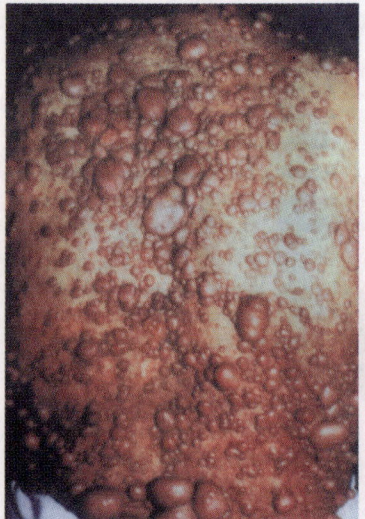

Fig. 16.10 Von Recklinghausen's disease

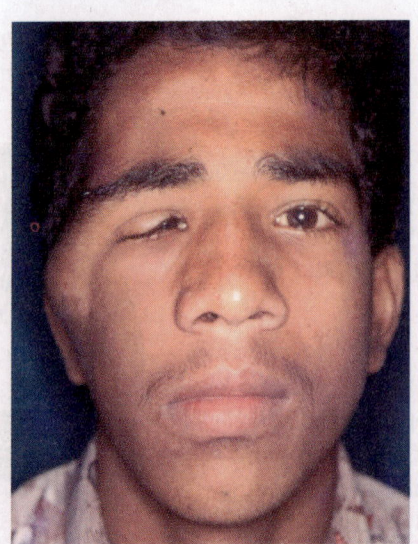

Fig. 16.11 Plexiform neurofibromatosis

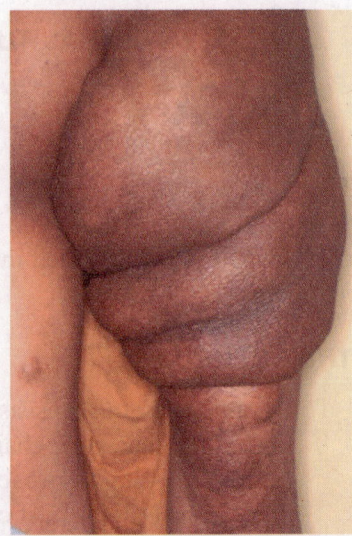

Fig. 16.12 Elephantiasis neuromatosa

2. Generalised neurofibromatosis: Von Recklinghausen's disease (Fig. 16.10)

This is an autosomal dominant disorder transmitted by both sexes. The whole body is studded with cutaneous nodules of varying sizes. They are soft and nontender. The coffee brown pigmentation is characteristic of this condition (Cafe-au-lait spots). Cafe-au-lait spots can be associated with involvement of cranial nerves-VIIIth nerve (auditory nerve) *acoustic neuroma– A Cerebello-pontine angle tumour*.

Fibroepithelial skin tags are often present.

The presence of the skin pigmentation is an indication of the common neuroectodermal origin of nerve sheath cells and melanocytes.

Skeletal deformities such as kyphoscoliosis or osteoporosis are common.

It may be associated with phaeochromocytoma (High blood pressure).

Sarcomatous changes do occur.

3. Plexiform neurofibromatosis (Trigeminal)

In this condition, the branches of 5th cranial nerve are commonly affected. It can also involve the peripheries.

The affected part is grossly thickened due to the **fibro-myxomatous degeneration**.

When it involves the branches of trigeminal nerve, following problems can occur :

- **Tingling paraesthesia** in the distribution of Vth nerve-especially ophthalmic division.

- When it attains a huge size, it can **obstruct the vision**. As it grows bigger in size, it hangs in front of the neck, as a grossly thickened pendulous fold of skin.

Treatment : Very difficult. Excision can be attempted with plastic surgery repair.

4. Elephantiasis neuromatosa

This condition affects the limbs. It represents an advanced stage of plexiform variety. Gross thickening of subcutaneous tissue gives the appearance of elephant's leg. The skin is dry and coarse. (Fig. 16.12)

5. Pachydermatocoele

This refers to the plexiform lesions mainly found in the neck as a thickened, coiled single mass.

Complications of neural tumours (Key Box 16.3)

Key Box 16.3
COMPLICATIONS OF NEUROFIBROMA
• Atrophy of muscles
• Dumb-bell tumours from dorsal spinal nerve root can cause backache or paralysis
• Acoustic neuroma - Deafness
• Cystic degeneration
• Sarcomatous change

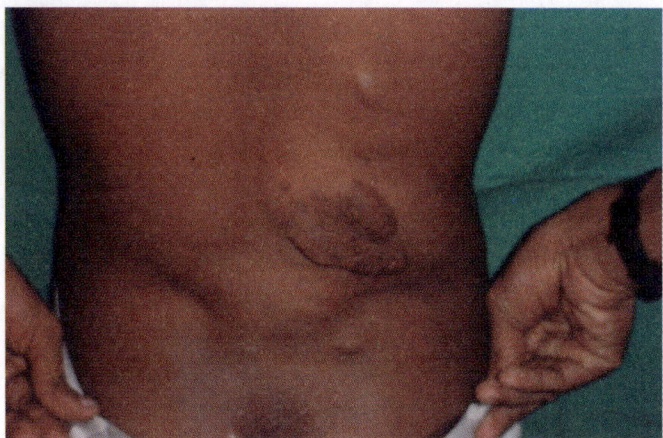

Fig. 16.13 Observe the cafe-au-lait spots - atleast four such spots are necessary for the diagnosis of Von Recklinghausen's disease

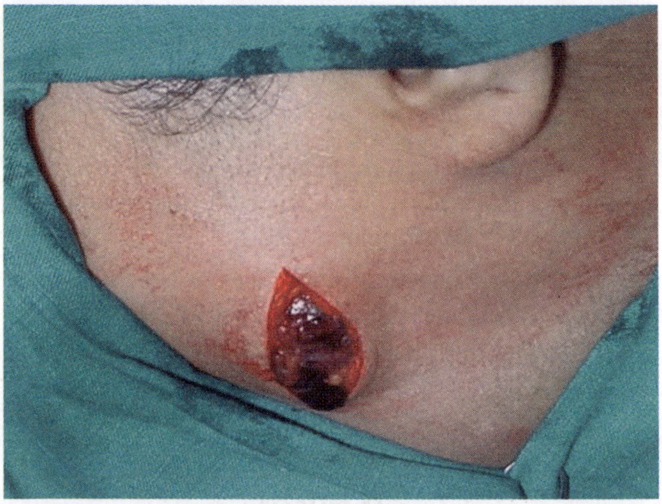

Fig. 16.14 Hamartoma over the face

NEURILEMMOMA (SCHWANNOMA)

This is a benign tumour arising from Schwann cells.

They can be single or multiple and present with a fusiform swelling in relationship with the nerves.

They can occur from cutaneous nerves.

They can also be seen in mediastinum and retroperitoneum.

They are *soft, lobulated, well encapsulated tumours.* They are benign and do not turn into malignancy.

Treatment

Excision of the tumour can be done without sacrificing the nerve because the tumour is well encapsulated and displaces the nerve.

HAMARTOMA[1]

It is a tumour-like developmental malformation of the tissues of a particular part of the body which are arranged haphazardly

Hamartoma is a Greek word which means **fault or misfire.**

Few examples of hamartoma

Haemangioma, Neurofibroma, Glomus tumour, Benign naevus, Lymphangioma

Characteristic features

Being a developmental anomaly, they are seen at birth or in early childhood

In adults there is a long history of swelling

Being a malformation (NOT A TUMOUR), it does not have a capsule.

They can be single or multiple

Some may **regress** as in **strawberry angioma**

They are benign lesions.

Treatment

Excision is not only curative but also gives a correct diagnosis.

Care should be taken when it contains vascular tissue such as haemangioma or neural tissue as in cases of neurofibroma

As shown in the figure above, facial nerve and its branches may be damaged while excising hamartomatous lesions over the face.

CHORDOMA

Rare tumour

Remnant of notochord

Sacrococcygeal region (Common site)

Resection is difficult, chances of neurological deficit and bleeding are high.

Radio-resistant

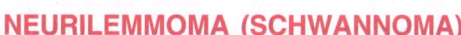

1. *Hamartoma is not a clinical diagnosis.*

MALIGNANT TUMOURS

TYPES OF MALIGNANT TUMOURS (Key Box 16.4)

They are of two types; carcinoma and sarcoma. Carcinoma arises from epithelium-ectodermal, endodermal or mesodermal in origin.

Sarcomas arising from soft tissues or bone which are derived from mesoblast or mesenchymal tissues.

It can be observed that mesoderm can give rise to carcinoma and mesenchymal sarcoma also.

Key Box 16.4
CARCINOMA
ORIGIN
• Ectodermal- Skin cancer
• Endodermal- Gut cancer
• Mesodermal- Renal carcinoma
TYPES
• Squamous cell carcinoma
• Basal cell carcinoma
• Glandular

PATHOLOGY (Table 16.2)

SPREAD

1. **Local spread**: Generally occur into adjacent structures. Few examples are given:

Carcinoma cheek – fixity to mandible, **Significance** : May necessitate removal of mandible along with wide excision.

Squamous cell carcinoma - fixed to tibia may necessitate an amputation.

2. **Lymphatic spread**: It is one of the most important features of **carcinoma.** As you complete reading this book, you will come across many cases and many examples of lymphatic spread of malignant tumours. Few sarcomas also spread by lymphatics (Page 170). Different types of lymphatic spread are given below

Permeation: Refers to tumour cells travelling along the lymphatic vessel.

Eg: Carcinoma tongue with submandibular node enlargement

Embolisation: More aggressive tumour means more aggressive spread – by embolisation wherein nodes can be enlarged in a far away station: e.g. Malignant melanoma

Retrograde lymphatic spread : When main lymphatic pathway is blocked retrograde spread can occur and a node in an unusual location may get enlarged. e.g. : **Irish node (Left axillary node enlargement in carcinoma stomach)**

3. **Haematogenous spread:** This is the most important method of spread of **sarcomas**. Also, a few malignancies such as renal cell carcinoma, follicular carcinoma thyroid, carcinoma prostate, carcinoma breast and malignant melanoma commonly spread by blood. Bony metastasis and lung metastasis result from blood spread. Bone metastasis can be a mild form such as bony pains to a severe form such as **quadriplegia/ pathological fracture** etc.

4. **Seeding**

Cancer of lower lip spreading to upper lip. Also called as kiss cancer. Other example: Cancer of vulva.

Table 16.2 Pathology of tumours

TERMINOLOGY	EXPLANATION	EXAMPLES
1. **Well differentiated**	Cells that resemble very closely their normal counterparts	Well differentiated squamous cell carcinoma
2. **Undifferentiated** (Anaplasia)	Loss of structural and functional differentiation	Poorly differentiated carcinoma (Anaplasia)
3. **Dysplasia**	Loss in the uniformity, Loss in the architectural orientation	Barrett's columnar cell lined oesophagus
4. **Carcinoma in-situ**	Dysplastic changes involving **entire thickness of the epithelium**	Cheek, tongue, breast etc.
5. **Apoptosis**	Programmed cell death	Seen in malignant tumours

Incision and 'port' site metastasis - (port refers to Laparoscopic port)

5) **Transcoelomic spread:** Spread through peritoneal cavity by dislodgement of malignant cells. Eg: Ca. stomach with Krukenberg tumour – Bilateral bulky ovarian metastases, commonly seen in pre-menopausal patients.

Comparison of benign tumours and malignant tumours (Table 16.3)

PARANEOPLASTIC SYNDROMES (PNS)

Certain cancers produce some specific clinical syndromes (symptom complexes other than Cachexia) which cannot be explained by their local or distant spread or by the hormones produced by the tissue of origin of these tumours. These are called as Paraneoplastic syndromes. (Table 16.4 and Key Box 16.4)

Just to give an example : Hypercalcaemia due to skeletal metastasis from carcinoma breast is not considered as PNS, but if it occurs without skeletal metastasis, it is considered as PNS.

Table 16.3 Comparison of benign tumours and malignant tumours

FEATURE	BENIGN	MALIGNANT
• Growth	Very slow	Rapid
• Duration	Long	Short
• Pain	Usually not a feature	Pain can be present due to local infiltration
• Mobility	Present	Restricted
• Fixity	No	Can be present
• Consistency	Firm/Soft	Hard, irregular
• Spread	No	Spreads
• Capsule	Capsulated	Uncapsulated
• Recurrence after surgery	Does not occur	Can occur if wide excision is **not** done

Table 16.4 Paraneoplastic syndromes

CLINICAL SYNDROME	MAJOR UNDERLYING CANCER	MECHANISM
1. **Endocrinopathies**		
• Cushing's syndrome	Small cell Ca. lung, Ca pancreas	ACTH or ACTH-like substance
• Hyponatraemia	Small cell Ca lung	ADH or Atrial natriuretic factor
• Hypoglycaemia	Hepatoma	Insulin or Insulin-like substance
• Hypercalcaemia	Squamous cell Ca lung Ca breast, Ca kidney	PTH-like substance
• Carcinoid syndrome	Bronchial Carcinoid, Ca pancreas, Ca stomach	Serotonin, bradykinin
• Polycythemia	Renal Cell Ca Cerebellar haemangioma	Erythropoietin
2. **Muscle syndrome**		
• Myasthenia gravis	Thymoma	Immunologic
3. **Bone & Soft tissues**		
• Hypertrophic osteo-arthropathy and clubbing of finger	Adenocarcinoma lung	Unknown
4. **Vascular**		
• Venous thrombosis	Carcinoma pancreas	Hypercoagulability

Ca = Carcinoma

Key Box 16.5

IMPORTANT FEATURES OF PNS

- Incidence : 10-15% of patients with cancer
- It may be the earliest manifestation (primary can be occult)
- **Bronchogenic cancer and breast cancer are most commonly associated with PNS.**
- **Hypercalcaemia and Cushing's syndrome are the most common clinical syndromes associated with PNS.**
- PNS can be a major clinical problem and can be treated

AETIOLOGY OF CARCINOMA IN GENERAL

1. **Tobacco** is the most important factor in the development of **lung cancer, upper respiratory tract cancer, gastrointestinal tract cancer and genitourinary tract cancer.** Carcinoma pancreas is found more commonly in smokers. Passive smokers also have increased incidence of development of cancers.

2. **Alcohol**: Smoking with alcohol increases the permeability of the upper digestive tract mucosa and respiratory mucosa to the carcinogens. Thus, they increase the incidence of cancer. Hepatocellular cancer is commonly found in alcoholic cirrhotic liver.

3. **Ionising radiation**: Atomic bomb blasts in Japan have definitely resulted in increased number of cases of breast cancer in premenopausal women and leukaemia in children.

4. **Ultraviolet radiation: Causes all types of skin cancers.**

5. **Genetic causes**: (Key Box 16.6)

Key Box 16.6

GENETIC / DEFECTIVE DNA REPAIR

1. **Xeroderma pigmentosum**– Skin cancer
2. **Bloom's syndrome** – Acute leukaemia, various cancers
3. **Fanconi's anaemia** – Acute leukaemia, squamous cell carcinoma, hepatoma
4. **Ataxia telangiectesia** – Acute leukaemia, lymphoma, breast cancer

---

6. **Hereditary causes**

   MEN syndrome: Medullary carcinoma thyroid.
   (**M**ultiple **E**ndocrine **N**eoplasia)
   FPC : Colonic cancer (Multiple)
   (**F**amilial **P**olyposis **C**oli)
   Li – Fraumeni syndrome - Familial breast cancer.
   Retinoblastoma.

7. **Dietary factors**

   Red meat : Carcinoma colon, carcinoma breast.
   Fat : Carcinoma breast, carcinoma colon.
   Smoked, charred fish : Carcinoma oesophagus, carcinoma stomach.

8. **Chemicals**

   Benzanthracenes-Skin cancer when painted on the skin
   Benzopyrenes - Lung cancer
   β-naphthylamine - Bladder cancer
   Nitrosamines and amides - Cancer stomach
   Aflatoxin B - Hepatocellular carcinoma
   Asbestos – Lung cancer

9. **Viral factors**

   Human T-cell leukaemia virus type 1 (HTLV-1) – T cell leukaemia/lymphoma. (RNA virus)
   Human papilloma virus (HPV)
   Cancer cervix, cancer urogenital region
   Epstein-Barr virus-Burkitt's lymphoma

SOFT TISSUE SARCOMAS

These are the malignant tumours arising from soft tissues. Thus they can occur in any part of the body. Examples are given in the Table 16.6.

INTRODUCTION

These are malignant tumours which are fatal if untreated or mistreated.

Most of them occur in young patients as painless lumps

CT scan, MRI, incision biopsy (details later) are the key investigations.

Early diagnosis and curative resection has major role in the management of soft tissue sarcomas.

Staging: In addition to the TNM staging, pathological grading of the tumour has been included - GTNM staging

Table 16.5 Soft Tissue Sarcoma	
TISSUE OF ORIGIN	**NAME**
• Mesenchymal tissue	• **M**alignant **F**ibrous **H**istiocytoma (MFH)
• Adipose	• Liposarcoma
• Smooth muscle	• Leiomyosarcoma (GIST)
• Striated muscle	• Rhabdomyosarcoma
• Synovial tissue	• Synovial sarcoma
• Neural tissue	• Malignant schwannoma
• Uncertain	• Epitheloid sarcoma
• Blood vessels	• Angiosarcoma
• Lymph vessels	• Lymphangiosarcoma

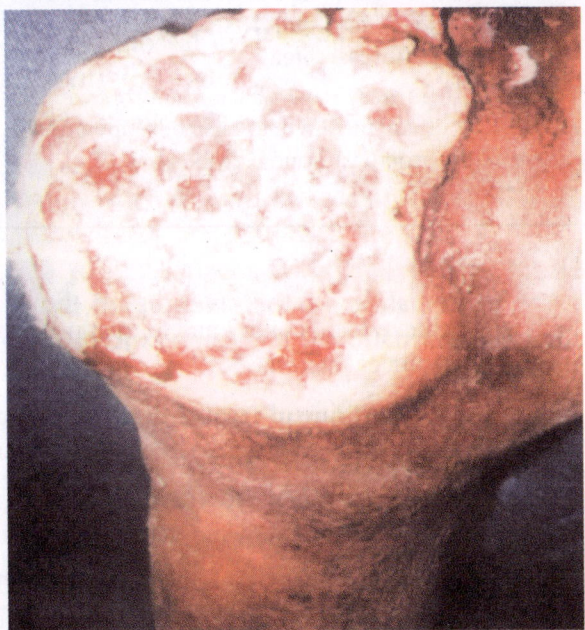

Fig. 16.15 Squamous cell carcinoma leg. Typical everted edge

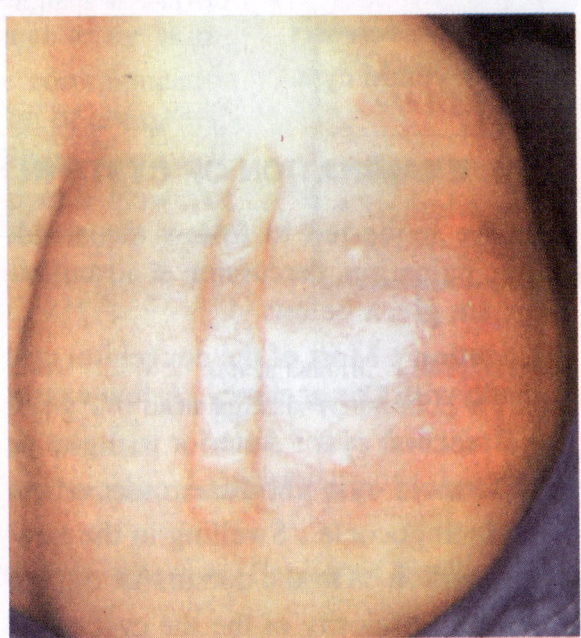

Fig. 16.16 Rhabdomyosarcoma - incomplete excision. See the vascularity

AETIOLOGY OF SARCOMA

1. **Lymphangiosarcoma** can develop from **post-mastectomy lymphoedema** of the upper limb, a few years later. This is called **Stewart- Treves syndrome.** It can occur in any chronic lymphoedematous tissue.

2. **Angiosarcoma** and other soft tissue sarcomas : Polyvinyl chloride, thorium dioxide, arsenic, etc.

3. **Osteogenic sarcoma:** Paget's disease of the bone, exposure to radium (Watch dials).

4. **Fibrosarcoma:** Paget's disease of the bone, post-irradiation.

5. **Kaposi's sarcoma : Cytomegalovirus and human immunodeficiency virus (HIV).** (See next page for comparison of Carcinoma with Sarcoma).

TYPES OF BIOPSY

FNAC   – **Grading not possible**
Core biopsy – Grading may be difficult
Incision biopsy – Adequate sample
Excision biopsy– The Best

Clinical features (Compare Fig. 16.15 and 16.16 and Table 16.6)

Table 16.6 Comparison of Carcinoma and Sarcoma

		CARCINOMA	SARCOMA
1.	Cell of origin	Ectodermal or endodermal	Mesodermal
2.	Age group	Elderly, 40-60 years	Young, 10-30 years
3.	Rate of growth	Slow	Fast
4.	Presentation	**Non-healing ulcer,** cauliflower-like growth with everted edges and induration.	**Fleshy mass, red and vascular, dilated veins** over the surface, local rise of temperature.
5.	Spread	**Lymphatic spread** is very common, both by emboli and permeation. Blood spread does occur as in renal cell carcinoma, thyroid carcinoma, breast carcinoma, etc.	**Blood spread** occurs very early and results in cannon ball secondaries in lung. Rhabdomyosarcoma, synovial sarcoma, epitheloid sarcoma spread by lymphatics. (So also, malignant fibrous histiocytoma, angiosarcoma)
6.	Microscopy	**Cell nests or epithelial pearls** are seen in well differentiated cancers.	Malignant cells resemble their cell of origin. Thus, **spindle-shaped cells** are found in **fibrosarcoma**.
7.	Treatment	**Surgery** is the main treatment of endodermal cancers, surgery or radiotherapy for ectodemal lesions. Chemotherapy is not very useful.	**Surgery** is the main modality of treatment. Radiotherapy and chemotherapy are also beneficial (sandwich therapy)

STAGING OF SOFT TISSUE SARCOMA

1. Grade (G):

G1 – Well differentiated
G2 – Moderately differentiated
G3 – Poorly differentiated
G4 – Undifferentiated

2. Primary Tumour (T):

T_1 Tumour $\leq$ 4-5 cms in greatest dimension

T_2 Tumour $\geq$ 5 cms in greatest dimension

3. Regional lymph Nodes (N):

N0 : No nodal metastasis

N1 : Regional lymph node metastasis present.

4. Distant metastasis (M):

M0 : No distant metastasis

M1 : Distant metastasis present

G – TNM Staging System

STAGE GROUPING

I	G_1	$T_1 - T_2$	N0	M0
II	G_2	$T_1 - T_2$	N0	M0
III	G_3	$T_1 - T_2$	N0	M0
IV	$G_1 - G_3$	$T_1 - T_2$	N1	M0
	$G_1 - G_3$	$T_1 - T_2$	N1	M1

TREATMENT

Aim is to achieve local control and to treat metastasis including subclinical metastasis.

Surgery is the first line of treatment varying from a wide excision to amputation or disarticulation, when it occurs in the extremities.

Tumours do respond to radiotherapy and chemotherapy.

If amputation can be avoided by giving pre-operative radiotherapy, it is preferred first followed by wide excision / compartmental excision followed by postoperative RT.

Low grade tumours can be treated on 1 cm wide excision with 1 cm margin and **high grade tumours by 4cm margin.**

Role of chemotherapy

The high-grade tumours have high potential of metastasis. Hence combination chemotherapy is to be considered before or after surgery.

The most favoured combination chemotherapy drugs include – Mesna, Adriamycin, Ifosfamide and Dacarbazine (**MAID**)

The success rate is around 10-20%

DIFFERENTIAL DIAGNOSIS OF SOFT TISSUE SARCOMA

LIPOSARCOMA

It is a malignant fatty tumour.

Common sites : proximal extremity, trunk or retroperitoneum.

They are generally large at the time of diagnosis eg: retroperitoneum. It results in gross swelling, which is firm to hard.

The compression on blood vessels may result in oedema of the limbs when it occurs in retroperitoneum.

Well differentiated myxoid liposarcomas **are notorious for recurring** many times before spreading to lungs. **Hence prognosis is good.**

Pleomorphic and lipoblastic liposarcomas tend to be of higher grade and often present with metastasis.

They do respond well to radiotherapy.

MALIGNANT FIBROUS HISTIOCYTOMA (MFH)

Malignant tumour of mesenchymal tissue (Fibrous tissue). This is the recent nomenclature of sarcoma. Fibrosarcoma or pleomorphic rhabdomyosarcomas are included under this.

These are high grade tumours which lack differentiation.

It can also arise from bone

The most of the so called fibrosarcomas are today included under MFH.

The MFH – Superficial type rarely metastasise and carries good prognosis.

Locations: Retroperitoneum, trunks and limbs (intermuscular septa of adductors, scapulo-humeral and pectoral muscles).

Clinical features

Common in elderly patients (50 years). But can occur at any age.

Slow growing firm to hard mass with restricted mobility.

Common locations (as mentioned above)

As the tumour is locally invasive, it infiltrates the muscles and adjacent structures, thus can cause muscle weakness or pain etc.

Spread : Local spread is common. Distant metastasis by blood is late (Lungs). Lymph node metastasis is rare.

Like other sarcomas, dilated veins, local rise of temperature, restricted mobility and hardness will clinch the diagnosis.

SYNOVIAL SARCOMA

Any rapidly growing tumour in the region of joint / or near the tendons in young patients (20-40 years), Synovial sarcoma is to be considered.

Common Site: Shoulder, wrist, knee etc.

Age: Young between 20-40 years.

Clinical features are similar to the other sarcomas – hard, painful mass.

In addition to the local and blood spread, **it also spreads by lymphatic route.**

Plain X-ray: may show characteristic calcification

It is aggressive, with high rates of recurrence.

In the G-TNM staging system, they are grade 3.

ANGIOSARCOMA

1 to 2% of soft tissue sarcomas.

Affects elderly patients

They are high grade and aggressive tumours.

They arise from skin and subcutaneous tissue rather than deeper tissues.

Most of them occur in the **head and neck, breast and liver.**

Surgery (excision) followed by radiotherapy/combination chemotherapy may have to be given.

RHABDOMYOSARCOMA

The most common soft tissue sarcoma seen in children, even though they are rare.

It arises from striated muscle.

Resection/Chemotherapy/Radiotherapy (combination) is tried depending on location.

Sites: Head and neck 70%, genitalia (15-20%)

All 3 varieties – Embryonal, alveolar, pleomorphic are considered as Grade 3 in GTNM staging.

Hence, prognosis is not good.

KAPOSI'S SARCOMA

Vulnerable section of people include – Jews, Immunocompromised patients such as transplant recipients and AIDS patients.

Typical Sites: Legs. Other sites include: Chest, arm, neck in epidemic form (Africa)

It presents as **multiple pigmented sarcoma nodules in the leg**.

It is interesting to note that **Kaposi's Sarcoma is "NOT SEEN" in transfusion related 'AIDS'**.

Purplish to red subcutaneous nodules in the leg followed by ulceration with bleeding is the manifestation.

Combination chemotherapy with doxorubicin and etoposide and interferon has been used to control the disease.

Sarcomas that metastasise to lymph nodes

- Rhabdomyosarcoma
- Synovial Sarcoma
- Epitheloid Sarcoma

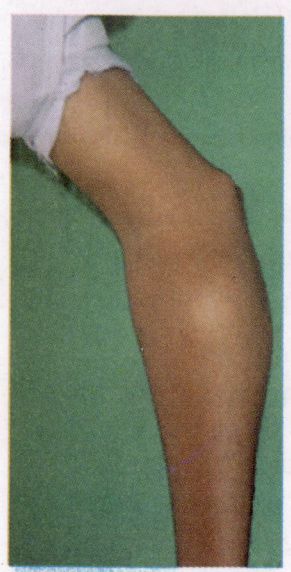

Fig. 16.17 Early stage of liposarcoma - this swelling had local rise of temperature and restricted mobility

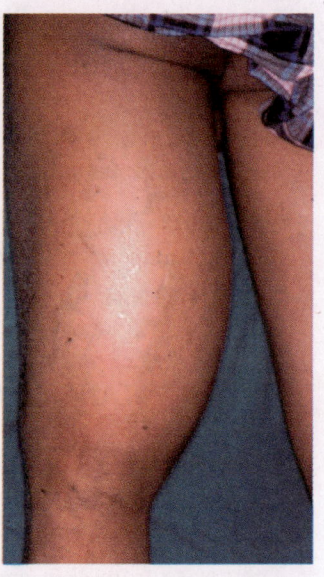

Fig. 16.18 Advanced case of liposarcoma - the swelling was hard and fixed. Dilated veins over the surface and location were characteristic

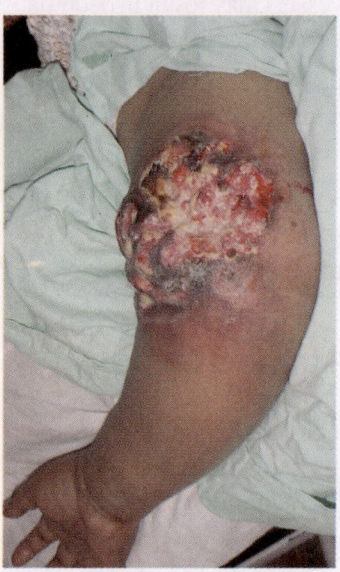

Fig. 16.19 Swelling in the elbow region for two years duration presented to the hospital with bleeding and fungation - advanced case of epitheloid sarcoma

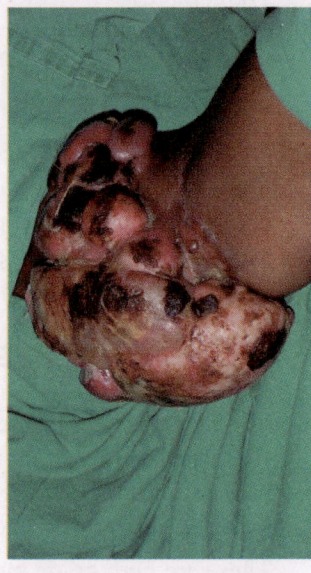

Fig. 16.20 Ulcerated lesion in the elbow region for two years duration presented to the hospital with bleeding - case of dermatofibroma protuberans

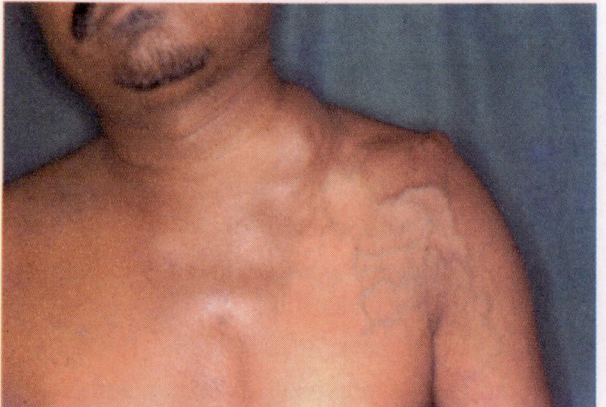

Fig. 16.21 Synovial sarcoma left shoulder region. See the secondary varicosity due to pressure effects

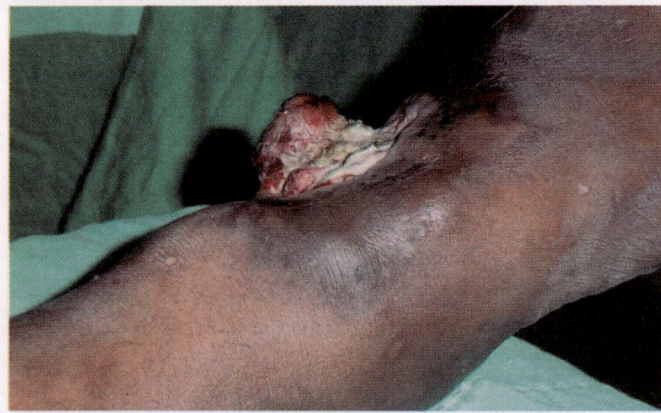

Fig. 16.22 Bleeding vascular lesion ankle region - angiosarcoma

USEFUL TIPS IN A CASE OF SOFT TISSUE SARCOMA

In undergraduate clinical examination, students are adviced to offer soft tissue sarcoma as the diagnosis. When asked the possible type, then only give a possible histological type based on various clinical features mentioned above. ASK FOLLOWING QUESTIONS TO YOURSELF to get ready for the clinical examas.

1. **Is it soft tissue sarcoma?** - Tumour arising from soft tissue, dilated veins, reddish skin, increase in local temperature, firm to hard, rapidly growing swelling, with late involvement of skin. (Carcinoma starts in the skin)

2. **What is the age of the patient?**

- In children – Rhabdomyosarcoma
  Undifferentiated sarcomas

- In 20-40 years – Liposarcoma
  Synovial sarcoma
  Kaposi's sarcoma

- In elderly patients : Angiosarcoma
  Chondrosarcoma (Bone)
  Fibrosarcoma (Fig. 16.23)

3. **Which site has it occurred ?**

- **Head and neck**: Angiosarcoma
  Rhabdomyosarcoma
  Osteogenic sarcoma (jaw)
- **Distal extremity** Synovial sarcoma (Fig. 16.25)
  (limbs) Epitheloid sarcoma

Clear cell sarcoma

- **Retroperitoneum** Liposarcoma (Fig. 16.24)
  and Mesentery MFH
  Leiomyosarcoma

4. **Has it spread to lymph nodes ?**

Rhabdomyosarcoma
Synovial Sarcoma
Epitheloid sarcoma

5. **Has it spread to lungs or liver ?**

Chest X-ray
Ultrasound

6. **Can I preserve the limb ?**

Wide excision
Compartmental excision
Pre-operative radiotherapy combined with surgery and post-operative radiotherapy.

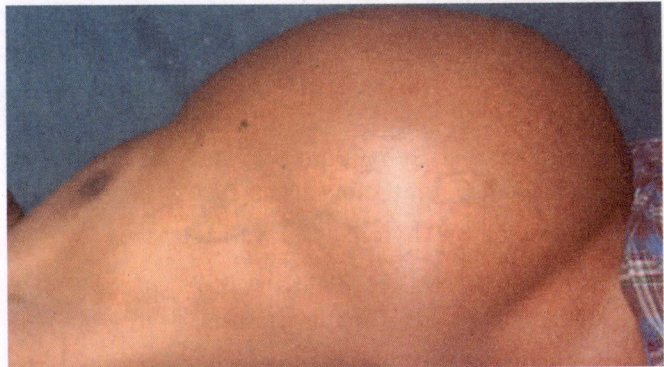

Fig. 16.24 Retroperitoneal liposarcoma

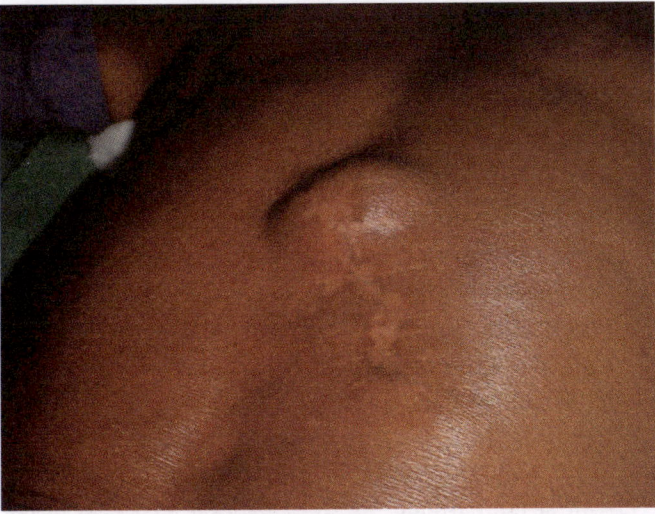

Fig. 16.23 Recurrent fibrosarcoma (MFH)

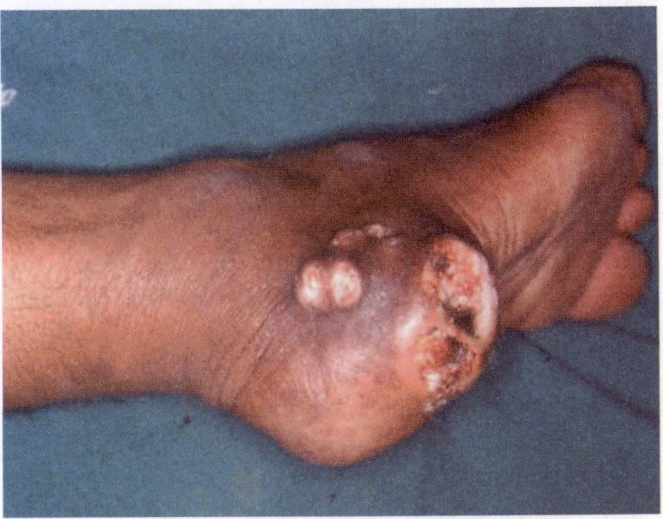

Fig. 16.25 Synovial sarcoma ankle region

CYSTIC SWELLINGS

A cyst is a swelling containing fluid. **True cysts** are lined by endothelium or epithelium. They contain clear serous fluid, mucoid material, pus, blood, lymph or toothpaste like material.

The **false cysts** do not have lining epithelium. They can be *degenerative cysts* as in the case of tumours which undergo tumour necrosis or tumour degeneration, or merely a *collection* of fluid which is walled off by coils of bowel as in tuberculous encysted ascites or an *exudation cyst* as in pseudopancreatic cyst.

CLASSIFICATION OF CYST

I. *Congenital cyst*

Sequestration dermoid cyst

Branchial cyst

Thyroglossal cyst

Lymphangioma

Cysts of embryonic remnants: Cyst of urachus, vitellointestinal duct cyst

II. *Acquired cyst*

Retention cyst-Sebaceous cyst, galactocoele, spermatocoele, Bartholin's gland cyst

Distension cyst-Thyroid cyst, ovarian cyst

Exudation cyst-Hydrocoele

Degenerative cysts-Tumour necrosis

Traumatic cyst-Haematoma, implantation dermoid cyst

Cystic tumours-Cystadenoma of pancreas, cystadenoma of the ovary

III. *Parasitic cyst*

Cysticercosis

Hydatid cyst

CLINICAL EXAMINATION OF CYSTS IN GENERAL

Students are requested to follow the standard practice of examination of the swelling in the form of inspection, palpation, percussion & auscultation in the clinical examination. Some important tests for cystic swellings are given below.

1. **Location**: Most of the congenital cystic swellings have a typical location wherein diagnosis can be made with fair accuracy. A few examples are as follows:

    Branchial cyst: Anterior triangle, partly covered by upper one-third of sternomastoid

    Dermoid cyst: Midline, outer or inner canthus of the eye

    Meningocoele: Swelling in the newborn at lumbosacral region

    Ganglion: On the dorsum of the hand

2. **Shape** : Majority of the the cystic swellings are round or oval

    Subhyoid bursitis: Transverse oval cystic swelling in the midline of the neck

    Thyroglossal cyst: Vertically placed oval swelling in the midline of the neck

    Sebaceous cyst: Hemispherical swelling

3. **Surface** : Almost all the cystic swellings in the skin and subcutaneous tissue have smooth surface

4. **Consistency** : Fluctuation is positive in all cystic swellings. However, depending on the contents the fluctuation may be different, which an experienced surgeon can diagnose

    Soft cystic: Thyroglossal cyst, meningocoele, lymph cyst

    Tensely cystic : Ganglion. Tensely cystic swellings in the neck may feel firm or solid. E.g.: Tense thyroid cyst, Deep seated abscess

    Yielding : Lipoma, as fat at body temperature behaves like fluid (pseudofluctuation)

    Soft with firm thickened periphery: Cold abscess

    Half filled like a rubber hot water bottle: Branchial cyst

    Putty or tooth paste: Sebaceous cyst (true fluctuation is not found)

Rules of fluctuation elicitation

Mobile swelling has to be fixed.

Both hands should be used.

With the index finger and thumb of one hand the swelling is pressed-these are active fingers and the impulse is received by the thumb and index finger of the other hand (passive fingers).

Fluctuation should be elicited in both directions, as fleshy muscle in the thigh can be fluctuant across but not in the longitudinal direction.

When swelling is smaller than 2 cm in size, *Paget's test* is done. Cystic swellings feel soft in the center and firm at the periphery. Solid swellings feel firm at the center than periphery.

Cross fluctuation for swellings having 2 components connected to each other. Eg.: Plunging ranula.

5. **Transillumination test** : Cystic swellings which contain clear fluid show positive transillumination.

6. **Mobility** : Almost all the cystic swellings in the skin, subcutaneous tissue or in the deeper plane are benign and as a rule they should have free mobility. However, this is not true due to various anatomical factors.

Branchial cyst: Restricted mobility is due to its adherence to the sternomastoid muscle.

Thyroglossal cyst : Transverse mobility is absent because the cyst is tethered by remnant of the thyroglossal duct.

Sebaceous cyst : Limited mobility due to the adherence to the skin.

7. **Sign of compressibility:** The swellings which have communication with a cavity or with tissue spaces give the positive sign of compressibility. Thus, a steady pressure is applied over the swellings. The swelling may disappear completely or may partially disappear. However, when pressure is released the swelling fills up slowly. Hence, it is also called the sign of refilling. (Key Box 16.7)

Key Box 16.7

COMPRESSIBLE SWELLINGS

- Haemangioma
- Lymphangioma
- Meningocoele

---

8. **Plane of the swelling**

Almost all significant cystic swellings in the neck are deep to deep fascia. Thus, contracting sternomastoid for laterally placed swellings and bending the chin against resistance for centrally placed swellings has to be done to define the plane of swelling.

The subcutaneous swellings become more prominent when the underlying muscles are contracted as in limbs.

The swellings due to semimembranous bursitis, almost disappear on flexion of knee and become more prominent on extension of the knee (Page 180)

Sebaceous cysts are attached to the skin at the site of punctum.

9. **Pulsations**: (Key Box 16.8)

A. Expansile: Aneurysms are characterised by expansile pulsations. When two fingers are placed over the swelling on the sides, the fingers are not only elevated but are also separated. Popliteal aneurysms typically give this sign.

B. Transmitted: When the swelling is situated over a vessel, the fingers are raised but not separated, e.g. pseudopancreatic cysts. When the swelling pushes the vessel anterior, transmitted pulsation can be obtained, e.g. cervical rib pushing the subclavian artery (Key Box 16.8).

Pulsation can also be present in tumours such as osteogenic sarcoma or secondaries from carcinoma thyroid, etc.

Key Box 16.8

ANEURYSM-TESTS

- Expansile pulsations - Finger separation sign
- Proximal compression test - Size ↓
- Distal compression test - Size may ↑
- Thrill and bruit are present
- Distal pulses may be weak

Effects of aneurysm

Some useful **TIPS**

1. **Thrombosis** : It is one of the common effects of aneurysm particularly aortic and popliteal resulting in ischaemia in the distal territory.

2. **Ischaemia** : Distal parts may become gangrenous and/or can have ischaemic ulcers or claudication.

3. **Pressure effects**

A. **Effect on bone** : Erosion of the vertebral body as in aortic aneurysm (This does not happen in TB spine)

B. **Effect on nerves**: Popliteal aneurysm can give rise to foot drop due to pressure on lateral popliteal nerve.

Key Box 16.9

EFFECTS OF ANEURYSM-TIPS

- **T**hrombosis
- **I**schaemia
- **P**ressure
- **S**kin changes

C. **Effect on the veins**: Results in congestion and oedema of the leg

D. **On the oesophagus**: Dysphagia as in aortic aneurysm.

4. **Skin Changes** may be in the form of oedema and redness.

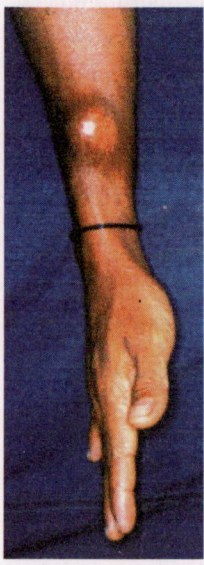

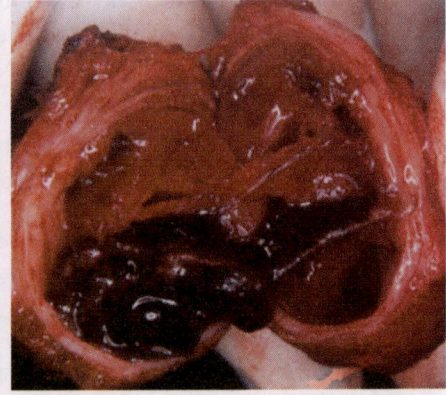

Fig. 16.26b Radial artery aneurysm - with clot - Excised specimen. (Contributed by Prof. L. Ramachandra, Professor of Surgery, KMC, Manipal)

Fig. 16.26a Radial artery aneurysm

Complications of cysts in general

1. **Infection. Eg.: Sebaceous cyst**
2. **Calcification,** e.g. Haematoma, multinodular goitre with cyst, hydatid cyst
3. **Pressure effects**-Ovarian cyst pressing the iliac veins
4. **Haemorrhage** within thyroid cyst
5. **Torsion** – Qvarian dermoid
6. **Transformation** into malignancy
7. **Ovarian cachexia**-Large ovarian tumour with pedal oedema, anorexia, loss of weight, lordosis

DERMOID CYST

This is a cyst lined by squamous epithelium containing desquamated cells. The contents are thick and sometimes tooth paste-like which is a mixture of sweat, sebum and desquamated epithelial cells and sometimes even hair.

Clinical types of dermoid cyst

I. **Congenital/sequestration dermoid** (Key Box 16.10, Fig. 16.27)

They occur along the line of embryonic fusion, due to dermal cells being buried in deeper plane.

The cells which are sequestrated in the subcutaneous plane proliferate and liquify to form a cyst. As it grows, it indents the mesoderm (future bone) which explains the bony defects caused by dermoid cyst in the skull or facial bones.

Thus, they can occur anywhere in the midline of the body or the face.

1. Median nasal dermoid cyst: At the root of the nose at the fusion lines of frontal process.
2. External and internal angular dermoid cyst: At the fusion lines of frontonasal and maxillary processes.
3. In the suprasternal space of *Burns*
4. Sublingual dermoid cyst
5. Pre-auricular dermoid cyst-in front of the auricle
6. Post-auricular dermoid cyst behind the auricle (Fig.16.30).

Pinna is formed by 6 cutaneous tubercles. Both (5 and 6) occur because of failure of fusion of one of the tubercles with the other as they form pinna.

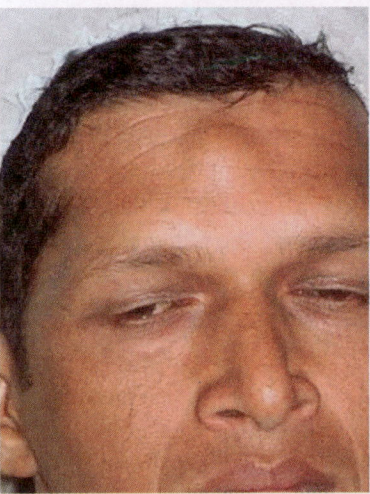

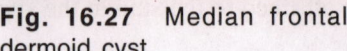

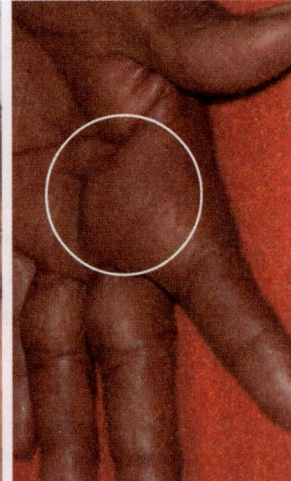

Fig. 16.27 Median frontal dermoid cyst

Fig. 16.28 Implantation dermoid cyst - foot and hand are common sites

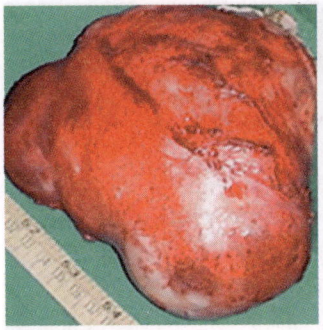
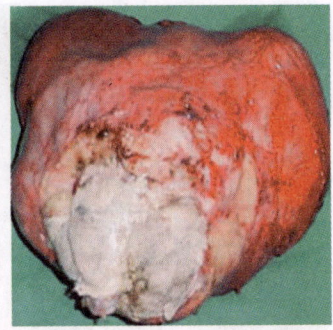

Fig. 16.29a Teratomatous dermoid cyst

Fig. 16.29b Cut open specimen showing cheesy material

Clinical features

1. Though congenital, the cyst manifests in childhood or during adolescence. A few cases also manifest in 30-40 years age group.
2. Typically, patient presents with a painless, slow-growing swelling.
3. Soft, cystic and fluctuant, transillumination is negative.
4. Rarely, it may be putty in consistency.
5. **The underlying *bony* defect gives the clue to the diagnosis**.
6. Classical location of the cyst (along the line of fusion) is a feature of sequestration dermoid cyst (Fig. 16.30)

II. Implantation dermoid cyst (Fig. 16.28)

This is common in women, tailors, agriculturists who sustain repeated minor sharp injuries.

Following a **sharp injury,** few epidermal cells get implanted into the subcutaneous plane. There, they develop into an implantation dermoid cyst. Hence, it is typically found in fingers, palm and sole of the foot. As the cyst develops in the areas where the skin is thick and keratinised, it feels firm to hard in consistency.

III. Teratomatous dermoid cyst (Fig. 16.29)

Teratoma is a tumour arising from *totipotential cells.* Thus, it contains ectodermal, endodermal and mesodermal elements-hair, teeth. cartilage, bone, etc. Common sites are ovary, testis, retroperitoneum, mediastinum.

IV. Tubulo-embryonic dermoid cyst

They arise from ectodermal tubes. A few examples are thyroglossal cyst, post-anal dermoid cyst.

Ependymal cyst of the brain.

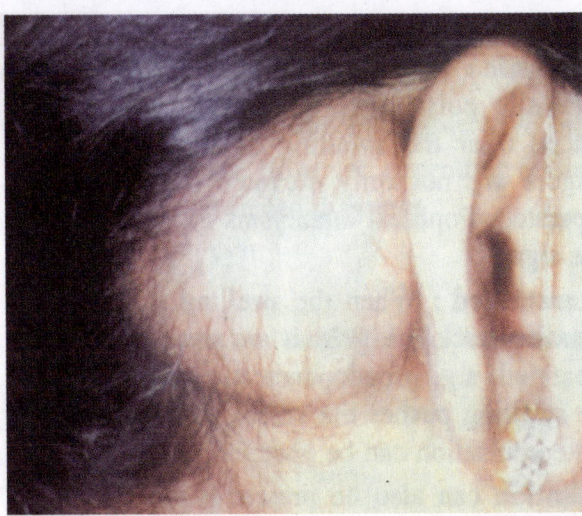

Fig. 16.30 Post-auricular dermoid cyst

Treatment of dermoid cyst

Excision of the cyst

CLINICAL NOTES

A 24 year old female patient was admitted with acute lower abdominal pain of 2 days duration. There was guarding and rigidity of the abdominal wall with rebound tenderness. Per vaginal examination was normal. At exploration, there was a twisted ovarian teratoma on the left side with gangrene. It was excised. The opposite ovary, on careful examination revealed a small teratomatous dermoid cyst which could be enucleated. The significance of this case report lies in the fact that both ovaries should be examined in cases of ovarian dermoid cysts.

EPIDERMOID CYST – (WEN)

This is also called **sebaceous cyst.** This occurs due to obstruction to one of the sebaceous ducts, resulting in accumulation of sebaceous material. Hence, this is an example of **retention cyst.**

Sites : Scalp, face, back, scrotum, etc. *It does not occur in palm and sole,* where sebaceous glands are absent. In the scalp and scrotum (Fig.16.32, 33, 34), multiple cysts are often found.

Clinical features

1. They are slow-growing and appear in early adulthood or middle age.

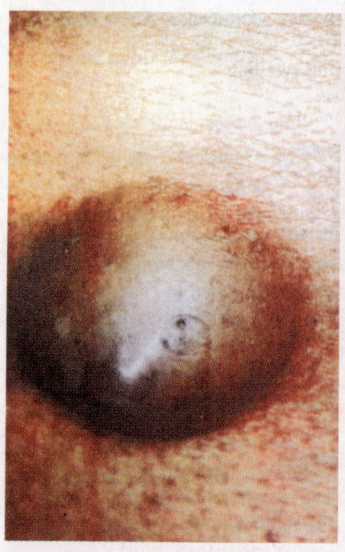

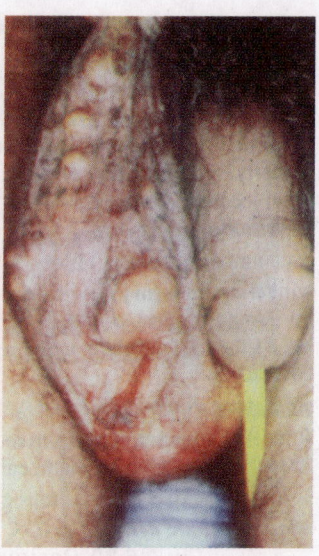

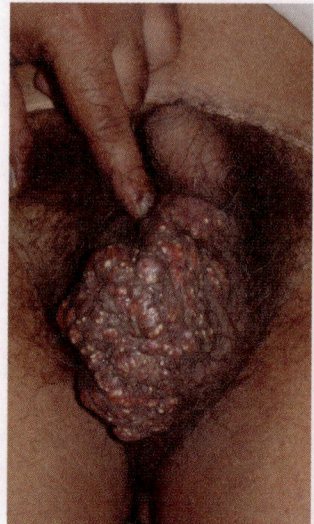

Fig. 16.31 Sebaceous cyst on the back - observe punctum

Fig. 16.32 Multiple sebaceous cysts on the scrotom - common site

Fig. 16.33 Multiple sebaceous cysts on the scrotom - calcified

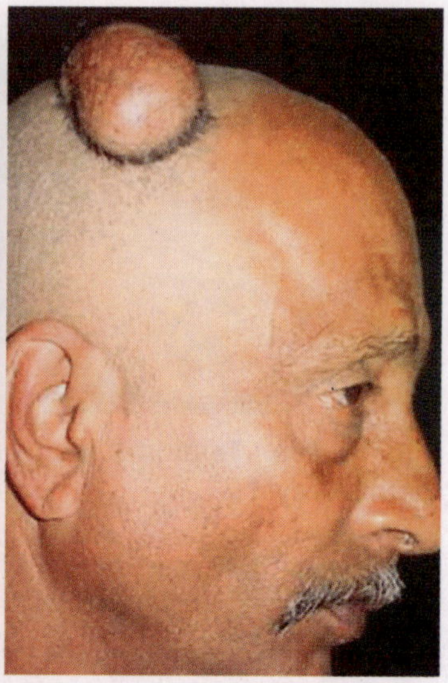

Fig. 16.34 Sebaceous cyst on the scalp - loss of hair is a feature

2. Hemispherical or spherical swelling located in the dermis. The central keratin filled ***punctum*** which is a ***dark spot*** is diagnostic feature of this cyst. The punctum indicates blockage of the duct (16.31)

3. In 20-30% of cases instead of opening into the skin, sebaceous duct opens into the hair follicle, hence punctum is not seen.

4. Smooth surface, round borders, soft and putty in consistency, non-tender.

5. The cyst can be moulded into different shapes which is described as ***sign of moulding.***

6. ***Sign of indentation*** refers to pitting on pressure over the swelling (refer Table 16.7).

7. The swelling is mobile over the deep structures, and the skin is free all around except an area of adherence at the site of punctum.

8. In the scalp, loss of hair is a feature over the swelling because of constant slow expansion of the cyst.

Treatment

Incision and avulsion of cyst with the wall. Very often, during dissection, the cyst wall ruptures. Care should be taken to excise the entire cyst wall. If not, recurrence can occur.

When it is small it can be excised along with the skin.

Table 16.7 Comparison of congenital dermoid cyst and sebaceous cyst

	CONGENITAL DERMOID CYST	SEBACEOUS CYST
• Aetiology	Congenital – Sequestration of the dermal cells in the subcutaneous plane	Acquired – Retention cyst due to accumulation of sebaceous contents
• Location	Midline of the body, along the line of fusion	Face, scalp, scrotum, back
• Sign of indentation, moulding	Uncommon	Very common
• Punctum	Absent	Present in 50% of cases – diagnostic
• Skin fixation	Absent	Skin is fixed at the site of punctum
• Bony defect	Present in majority of cases	Absent
• Intracranial communication	Rare, can be diagnosed by cough impulse test	Absent
• Treatment	Excision	Excision or avulsion

Complications

1. **Infection** can occur due to injury or scratch resulting in an abscess. The cyst will be tender, red and hot. It should be treated like an abscess by incision and drainage. After one to two months, the cyst can be excised.

2. **Sebaceous horn** results due to slow drying of the contents which are squeezed out, specially if a patient does not wash the affected part. Thus, it is not common to find a large sebaceous horn nowadays because of better ways of living and sanitation (Fig. 16.35).

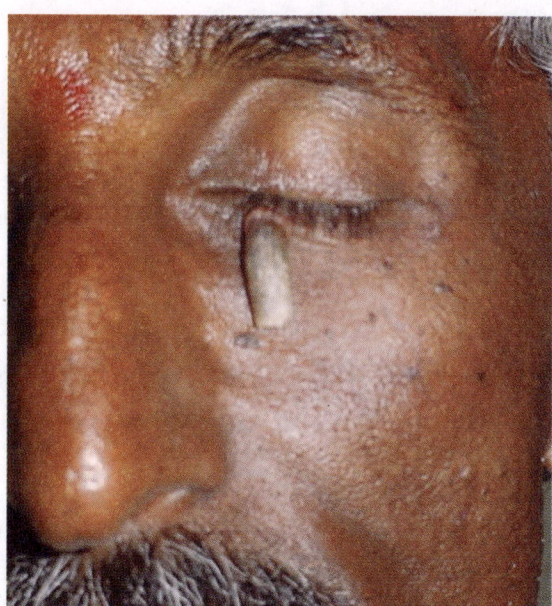

Fig. 16.35 Sebaceous horn

3. **Calcification**
4. **Cock's peculiar tumour**[1] refers to infected, ulcerated cyst of scalp with pouting granulation tissue with everted edge resembling epithelioma (Key Box 16.11)
5. **Rarely, basal cell carcinoma** can arise in a longstanding sebaceous cyst.

Key Box 16.11
SEBACEOUS CYST
• Syndrome - Gardner's syndrome
• Tumour - Cock's peculiar tumour
• Parasitic worm - Demodex folliculorum

GANGLION

It is a tense, cystic, swelling and occurs due to myxomatous degeneration of the synovial sheath lining the joint or tendon sheath. They are common around joints because of abundant fibrous tissue. They contain gelatinous fluid.

Common sites

The dorsum of the hand is the common site, at the **scapholunate** articulation.

In the foot, dorsal or lateral aspect.

Small ganglion in relation to flexor aspect of fingers.

Clinical features

1. Majority of patients are between 20 to 50 years.
2. A round to oval swelling in the dorsum of the hand, with smooth surface and round borders. Skin over swelling is normal.
3. The swelling is tensely cystic, fluctuant and transillumination is negative. It is mobile in the transverse direction.
4. When the tendons are put into contraction, the mobility of the swelling gets restricted.
5. Ganglion is not connected with the joint space. Sometimes, it gives an impression of becoming small due to slipping away between bones.

Treatment

1. The symptomless ganglion is better left alone.
2. Aspiration of the ganglion and injection of sclerosants may reduce the size of ganglion.
3. Sometimes, rupture of the cyst due to trauma may result in permanent cure.
4. Surgical excision can be done. However, recurrence rate is high.

Differential diagnosis

1. Implantation dermoid cyst, when it occurs in the feet or hand.
2. Exostosis of the bone, has to be considered if *swelling is very hard.*
3. Bursa (Vide infra)

---

1. *Pott's puffy tumour refers to osteomyeitis of the frontal bone with oedema of scalp secondary to frontal sinusitis. This and Cock's peculiar tumour are favourite viva questions.*

COMPOUND PALMAR GANGLION

Aetiology

Tuberculous tenosynovitis of the tendon sheaths affecting the flexor tendons. This is a common cause in India (Key Box 16.12)

Rheumatoid arthritis with involvement of multiple joints causing thickening of synovial membrane-common cause in western countries.

Pathology

As a result of tuberculous tenosynovitis, typical caseous material collects within the flexor tendon sheaths. The tendons get matted, a swelling develops in the palm and another swelling develops in lower aspect of forearm. The thickening of synovial membrane, fibrin particles in the fluid and **melon seeds**, are characteristic of this condition.

Clinical features

1. Majority of patients are below 40 years of age.
2. Concavity of the palm is obliterated.
3. Soft, cystic, fluctuant, transillumination-negative swelling situated above and below the flexor retinaculum.
4. **Cross fluctuation test** between these two swellings is positive, which is diagnostic of compound palmar ganglion.
5. Restricted mobility of the fingers due to matting of the tendons.
6. **Wasting of the small muscles** of the hand.
7. Paraesthesia due to compression on median nerve.

Investigations

1. The ESR may be increased if it is due to tuberculosis.
2. Aspiration of the swelling and fluid can be sent for acid-fast bacilli.
3. Synovial biopsy

Key Box 16.12

COMPOUND PALMAR GANGLION

- Tuberculosis and rheumatoid arthritis-common causes
- Synovial thickening
- Cross fluctuation test
- ATT, decompression or synovectomy

Treatment

1. **Antituberculous treatment** (ATT) in case of tubercular pathology. If the response rate is not satisfactory - exploration, decompression, synovectomy and release of matted tendons is the treatment.
2. **Control of rheumatoid arthritis**, with complete excision of the synovial sheath.

GLOMUS TUMOUR

This is also called glomangioma or angioneuromyoma. Glomus is a specialised organ.

Structure of glomus: (Glomus body)

Abundant arteriovenous anastomosis surrounded by large clear cells (Glomus cells) and medullated and non-medullated nerve fibres inbetween the cells is characteristic of glomus.

Clinical features of glomus tumour

1. Typical site: Under the nail beds of hands and feet.
2. It is purple-red in colour, usually single, the size does not exceed 1 cm in diameter.
3. Glomus tumour is usually seen in the 5th decade.
4. Excruciating pain either at rest or on movement of the finger or on pressure is pathognomonic feature of this tumour. Pain is due to compression of the nerve fibres by dilated glomus vessels.
5. The tumour is compressible (Key Box 16.13)

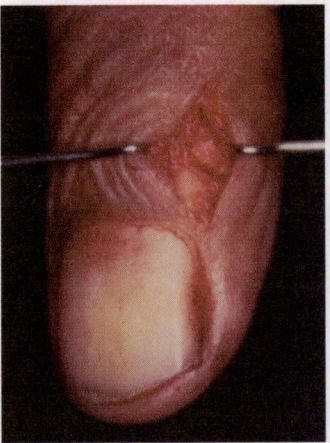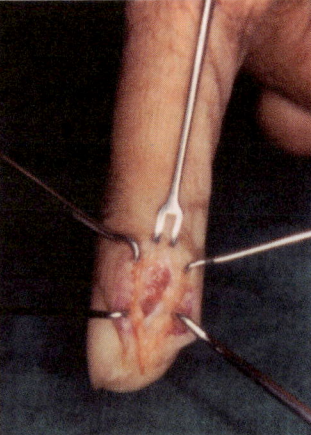

Fig. 16.36 Glomus tumour - the most painful condition in the finger (Contributed by Prof. Bhaskarananda Kumar and Dr. Anil Bhat, Dept. of Orthopaedics, KMC, Manipal)

Key Box 16.13

GLOMUS TUMOUR

- The most painful tumour
- The smallest benign tumour, **does not turn malignant**.
- Nail bed is the commonest site
- Histologically, it is an angioneuromyoma
- Excision gives permanent cure

Treatment

Surgical excision results in *permanent cure*.

Differential diagnosis

1. Subungual melanoma: Painless and pigmented
2. Granuloma pyogenicum : Mild pain, bleeds on touch and evidence of infection is present.

BURSA

Bursa means a sac or a sac-like cavity containing fluid lined by endothelium. It is meant to reduce the friction between the tendons of the muscle with the bone.

Bursitis refers to inflammation of a bursa resulting in accumulation of excessive fluid inside the bursa. This results in a swelling in the anatomical sites of normal bursae.

The causes of chronic bursitis includes constant pressure, constant irritation or minor injuries.

Some examples of bursitis are given in Table 16.8.

Clinical features

A cystic swelling in a known anatomical site of a bursa is a chronic bursitis unless proved otherwise.

Bursitis produces a soft, cystic circumscribed or oval swelling with fluctuation.

As majority of bursitis contains inflammatory fluid, they do not show transillumination.

In a few cases, signs of inflammation may be present

Complications

1. Secondary infection may result in an abscess.
2. Frequent friction may result in ulceration.
3. Cosmetic deformity.

Treatment

Excision is indicated only in the presence of symptoms such as pain or complications mentioned above.

Chances of recurrence are high.

SEMIMEMBRANOSUS BURSA (Fig. 16.37)

This is the commonest swelling in the popliteal space. It presents as a tensely cystic swelling when the knee is extended and it becomes flaccid on flexion of the knee. It is not compressible as it does not communicate with the joint.

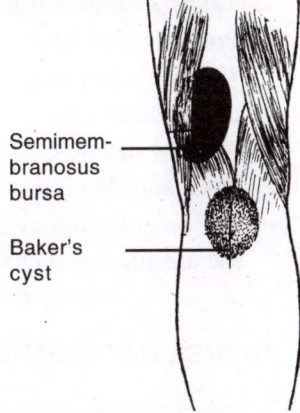

Semimembranosus bursa

Baker's cyst

The differential diagnosis for semimembranosus bursitis is Morrant Baker's cyst, which is a herniation of the synovial membrane.

Fig. 16.37 Popliteal fossa swelling

Table 16.8 Bursae and Bursitis

ANATOMICAL SITE	POPULAR NOMENCLATURE
1. Prepatellar bursa	Housemaid's knee
2. In front of patellar tendon (infrapatellar)	Clergyman's knee
3. Olecranon bursa	Student's elbow
4. Under the insertion of tendons of sartorius, gracilis and semitendinosus muscle	Bursa anserina (extension of the bursa along the sides of tendon-resembles goose's foot)
5. Between the tendon of the semimembranosus and the medial condyle of tibia	Semimembranosus bursitis

Table 16.9 Comparison of semimembranosus bursa and Baker's cyst

	SEMIMEMBRANOSUS BURSA	BAKER'S CYST
1. Aetiology	Friction or pressure	Rheumatoid or osteoarthrosis of knee joint
2. Age	Young patients	Middle aged
3. Location in the popliteal fossa	Higher up and more medial	Below and midline
4. On flexion of the knee	Disappears	Increases
5. On extension of the knee	Appears and is tense	Diminishes
6. Patellar tap	Absent	Present
7. Compressibility	Absent	Present partially
8. Knee movements	Normal	Restricted

The differences between these two swellings are given in Table 16.9.

Adventitious bursae

This refers to a cyst which develops in an anatomical area where no bursa is present. These also occur due to constant pressure or friction. They are summarised below:

1. **Tailor's ankle** - Above the lateral malleolus
2. **Porter's shoulder** - Between clavicle and skin
3. **Weaver's bottom** - Between gluteus maximus and ischial tuberosity
4. **Bunion -** Between prominent head of the first metatarsal and skin due to hallux valgus
- The complications and treatment of adventitious bursae are similar to chronic bursitis.

TRANSILLUMINANT SWELLINGS IN THE BODY

These are the cystic swellings containing clear fluid characterised by **fluctuation and transillumination**.

1. Lymphangioma
2. Ranula
3. Meningocoele
4. Epididymal cyst
5. Scrotal hydrocoele

LYMPHANGIOMA
(Lymphangioma Circumscriptum)

Failure of one of the lymphatics to join the major lymph sac of the body results in a lymphangioma. Hence, it occurs in places where lymphatics are abundant.

The common sites: Posterior triangle of the neck, axilla, mediastinum, groin, etc.

In the neck, it is called cystic hygroma of the neck. As the sac has no communication with lymphatics by the time swelling appears, the lymph is absorbed and is replaced by thin watery fluid (mucous) secreted by endothelium. Hence, it is also called hydrocoele of the neck.

When it is largely confined to subcutaneous plane, it is called as **Cystic Hygroma**.

Clinical features

1. Usually, cystic hygroma presents during infancy or early childhood. Occasionally present since birth and rarely before birth. They can also present as small vesicles.

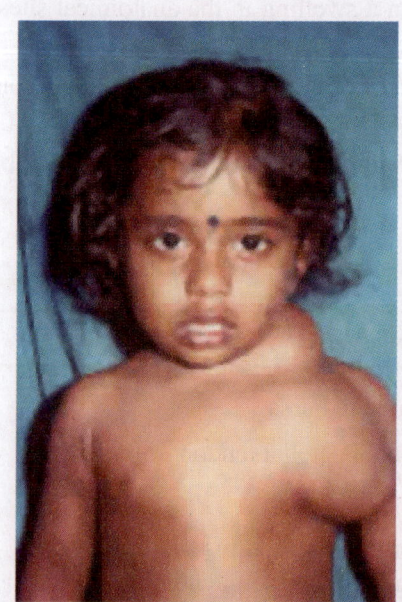

Fig. 16.38 Lymphangioma involving chest wall, neck and axilla

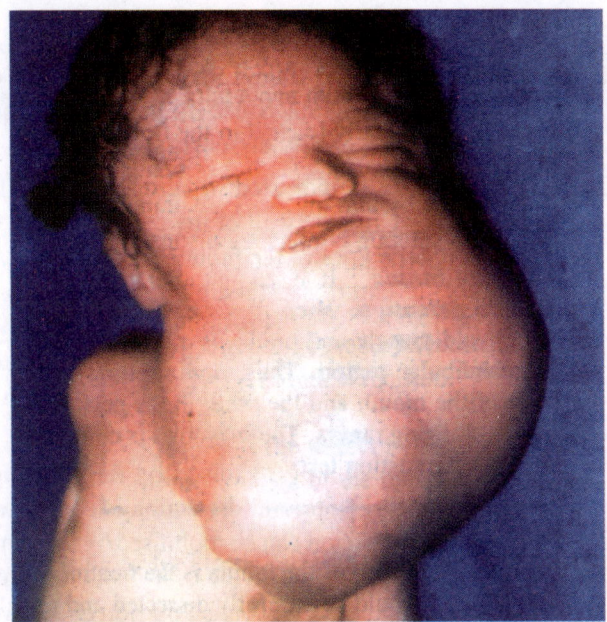

Fig. 16.39 Lymphangioma neck (Prof. P.L.N.G. Rao, K.M.C., Manipal)

2. When the child cries or strains the swelling increases in size and become prominent due to increased intra-thoracic pressure which is transmitted through root of the neck.

3. Typical locations -Lateral aspect of neck (Posterior triangle), groin, buttocks.

Key Box 16.14	
LYMPHANGIOMA - SITES	
• Jugular lymph sac	Neck
• Posterior lymph sac	Groin
• Cisterna chyli	Retroperitoneum

4. Soft, cystic, fluctuant, partially compressible swelling. Lymphangioma is a multilocular swelling consisting of aggregation of multiple cysts. These cysts may inter-communicate and sometimes may insinuate between muscle planes. Hence, it gives the sign of compressibility! However, **complete reducibility is not a feature**.

5. The swelling is **brilliantly transilluminant** because it contains clear fluid (Watery lymph). Key Box 16.15.

Treatment

Surgical excision is the treatment of choice. **All the loculi or cysts should be removed.** Careful search

Key Box 16.15
TRANSILLUMINATION TEST
• Should be done in a dark room
• Avoid surface transillumination
• Transillumination may be negative because of infection, sclerotherapy and haemorrhage

has to be made for the extension of lymphangioma through the **muscle planes** so as to avoid **recurrence**. Sclerotherapy was being used earlier for lymphangioma. But tissue planes are distorted because of sclerosants. Hence, dissection becomes difficult. **Thus, injection type of treatment is not favoured at present**.

Differential diagnosis

1. **Haemangioma** : Posterior triangle of the neck is one of the common sites for haemangioma. Haemangioma is soft, cystic and fluctuant, but transillumination is negative and the sign of compressibility is positive.

2. **Lipoma** : This is a soft lobular swelling with fluctua-tion because the fat behaves like fluid at body tem-perature. However, the edge slips under the palpating fingers. Both transillumination and compressibility tests are negative with lipoma.

3. **Cold abscess** (details follow later).

Complications

1. In neonates and infants, lymphangioma can cause dif-ficulty in breathing due to the large size.

2. Occasionally, secondary infection can occur.

3. Lymphangioma in the mediastinum can give rise to dyspnoea, dysphagia due to compression on the tra-chea/oesophagus.

RANULA

Ranula is a cystic swelling arising from sublingual salivary gland and from accessory salivary glands which are present in the floor of the mouth called **glands of Blandin and Nuhn.**

The word ranula is derived from the resemblance of the swelling to the **belly of frog - Rana Hexadactyla.**

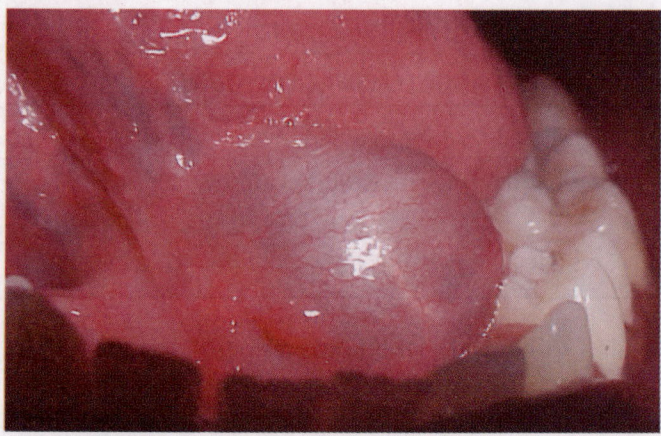

Fig. 16.40 Ranula in the floor of the mouth

Aetiology

1. Ranula occurs due to obstruction to the ducts, secreting mucus. Hence, an example for retention cyst.

2. Some surgeons consider it as an extravasation cyst.

Clinical features

1. Seen in young children and adults.

2. Swelling is typically located in the floor of the mouth or **under surface of the tongue,** to one side of the midline. (Fig. 16.36)

3. Soft, cystic, fluctuant swelling, which gives **brilliant transillumination.**

4. It is covered by thin mucosa containing clear, serous fluid. Hence, it is **bluish in colour.**

5. Surface is smooth, borders are diffuse, non-tender swelling.

6. *Plunging ranula* : It is an intraoral ranula with cervical extension, when it passes on the side of mylohyoid muscle and produces a swelling in the submandibular region. Thus, one swelling in the floor of the mouth and the other in the neck gives rise to plunging ranula. The diagnosis is confirmed by cross fluctuation test. (Key Box 16.16)

Key Box 16.16

CROSS FLUCTUATION TEST

- Indicated when a cyst has two components **interconnected**

- Gentle pressure on one component, **impulse on the other component**.

- Demonstrated by **bidigital palpation**

Treatment

1. **Complete excision** of the ranula is the treatment of choice in plunging ranula. Since the cyst wall is very thin, it should be carefully dissected and removed.

2. *Marsupialization* is indicated in simple ranula. The ranula is incised and the wall of the cyst is sutured to the mucosa of the floor of the mouth, so as to leave an opening to the exterior (Marsupials = Kangaroos). After 5-10 days, the cyst gets collapsed, fibrosis occurs and the entire cavity gets obliterated. Marsupialisation. avoids surgical dissection and chances of injury to the submandibular duct.

   Plunging ranula can be excised by intraoral approach. Once the intraoral dissection is completed the cervical extension can be mobilised by the same incision dissecting close to the cyst wall. However, rupture and chances of leaving a portion of the cyst wall are high.

Differential diagnosis

Sublingual dermoid cyst is a thick walled cyst, whitish in colour and *not transilluminant.*

Complications

1. Rupture of the cyst decreases the size but it can reappear at a later date.

2. When the swelling is big, the tongue is pushed upwards and may cause difficulty in speech or swallowing.

MENINGOCOELE

Meningocoele is a herniation of the meninges through the weak point in the spine (neural arch) where the bony fusion has not taken place effectively (Key Box 16.17). The swelling is covered by piamater and arachnoid mater without a dural covering. The swelling contains cerebrospinal fluid (CSF). Meningocoele is an example of spina bifida cystica.

Clinical features

1. The swelling is present **since birth.**

2. Soft, cystic, **fluctuant with brilliant transillumination** are the typical features of the swelling.

3. Sign of **compressibility** is present due to displacement of CSF.

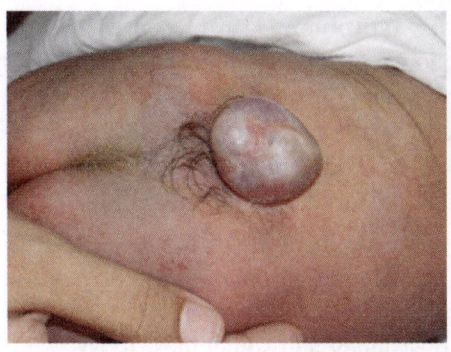 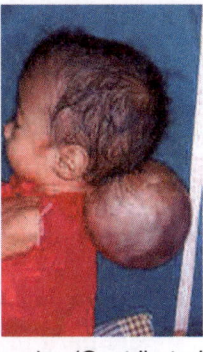

Fig. 16.41 Meningocoele **16.42** Encephalocoele - (Contributed by Dr. Vijaykumar, Paediatric Surgeon, KMC, Manipal)

Key Box 16.18

EXCISION OF MENINGOCOELE

- Surgery: **As early as possible** after birth
- **Early closure** prevents infection
- Transverse elliptical incision
- **Excision** of the sac
- **Closure of the defect** by plication
- Approximation of the muscles

Key Box 16.17

MENINGOCOELE—SITES

- Lumbosacral - The commonest
- Occipitocervical - Second most common
- Root of the nose - Rare

4. When the child cries or when asked to cough, an **expansile impulse** is present.
5. On palpating the edge of the swelling, a bony defect is usually found.

Treatment: (Key Box 16.18)

CT scan is done to look for hydrocephalus. If it is present, a ventriculo-peritoneal shunt is done which will reduce the meningocoele.

Excision of the meningocoele should be done as early as possible to prevent rupture and secondary infection.

Complications

1. Skin covering the swelling is very thin and so, is prone for ulceration. Due to ulceration, secondary infection and meningoencephalitis can occur.
2. Haemorrhage

SPINA BIFIDA OCCULTA

In this condition, the neural arch is defective posteriorly. There is no visible swelling.

It can be suspected when there is a tuft of hair, lipoma, naevus, pigmented patch of skin overlying the lumbosacral region.

Child is normal at birth. Neurological symptoms such as weakness, sciatica-like pain may start appearing at puberty.(neurogenic talipes equinus -Club foot)

During this time because of growth there may be traction on the spinal cord by a ligament called *membrane reuniens*.

X-ray can demonstrate the bifid spine.

Surgical excision of the membrane gives permanent cure to the patient, if there are symptoms.

Types of spina bifida cystica

1. **Menigocoele.**
2. **Meningomyelocoele**

See Table 16.10 for comparison

Protrusion of meninges, with *nerve root of* **spinal cord or disordered spinal cord** results in meningomyelocoele.

Table 16.10 Comparison of meningocoele and meningomyelocoele

	MENINGOCOELE	MENINGOMYELOCOELE
Contents	Membranes	Membranes with nerve roots
Consistency	Soft and cystic	Soft to firm
Transillumination	Brilliant	Partially transilluminant
Longitudinal furrow	Absent	Present due to adherence of the nerve roots to the skin
Neurological deficit	Absent	Trophic ulcers, bladder and bowel incontinence, locomotor problems are present.
Prognosis after repair	Good	Residual neurological deficit is present

Neurological deficit like **foot drop, talipes, trophic ulcer** of the foot (S$_1$ root) may be present (Page 47).

Surgical excision may be followed by residual neurological deficit.

3. **Syringomeningomyelocoele**

In this condition, in addition to the meninges the central canal of spinal cord is also herniated out.

Most of the children are stillborn.

Very difficult to treat, if the child survives.

DIFFERENTIAL DIAGNOSIS OF MIDLINE SWELLING IN THE NECK

Midline swellings : From above downwards

1. Ludwig's angina
2. Enlarged submental lymph nodes
3. Sublingual dermoid cyst
4. Subhyoid bursitis
5. Thyroglossal cyst
6. Enlarged isthmus of thyroid gland
7. Pretracheal and prelaryngeal lymph nodes
8. Retrosternal goitre
9. Thymic swelling
10. Enlarged lymph nodes or lipoma in the suprasternal space of burns

LUDWIG'S ANGINA

This is an inflammatory oedema of the floor of the mouth. It spreads to the submandibular region and submental region.

Tense, tender, brawny oedematous swelling in the submental region with putrid halitosis is characteristic of this condition (Page 11).

ENLARGED SUBMENTAL LYMPH NODES

The three important causes of enlargement:

1. **Tuberculosis**: **Matted submental nodes,** firm in consistency, with enlarged upper deep cervical lymph nodes, with or without evening rise of temperature are suggestive of tuberculosis.

2. **Non-Hodgkin's lymphoma** can present with submental nodes along with other lymph nodes in the horizontal group of nodes such as submandibular, upper deep cervical, pre-auricular, post auricular and occipital lymph nodes (external Waldeyer's ring). Nodes are *firm or rubbery,* **discrete without matting.**

3. **Secondaries** in the submental lymph nodes can arise from carcinoma of the *tip of the tongue, floor of the mouth, central portion of the lower lip.* The nodes are **hard** in consistency and sometimes, **fixed.**

SUBLINGUAL DERMOID CYST (Fig. 16.39)

It is a type of **sequestration dermoid cyst** which occurs due to sequestration of the surface-ectoderm at the site of fusion of the two mandibular arches. Hence, such a cyst occurs in the midline, in the floor of the mouth.

When they arise from **2nd branchial cleft,** they are found lateral to the midline. Hence, **lateral variety**.

The cyst is lined by squamous epithelium and contains hair follicles, sebaceous glands and sweat glands. **It does not contain hair.**

Clinical features

1. Young children or patients between the age of 10-20 years present with painless swelling in the **floor of mouth**.

2. Swelling is **soft and cystic. Fluctuation** test is positive. **Bidigital palpation** gives a better idea about fluctuation with one finger over the swelling in the oral cavity and the other finger in the submental region.

Key Box 16.19
SUBLINGUAL DERMOID CYST

- Origin: At the site of fusion of 2nd branchial arches
- Site : **Midline-Common;** Lateral -Uncommon
- **Supraomohyoid** variety is common
- **Bidigital palpation** for demonstration of fluctuation
- Soft, cystic, fluctuant, transillumination negative swelling

Differential diagnosis

- Ranula-transillumination is positive
- Thyroglossal cyst-moves with deglutition

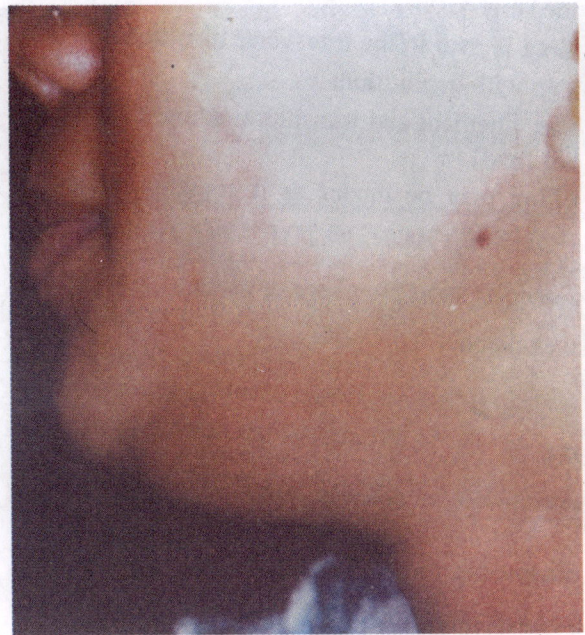

Fig. 16.43 Sublingual dermoid cyst

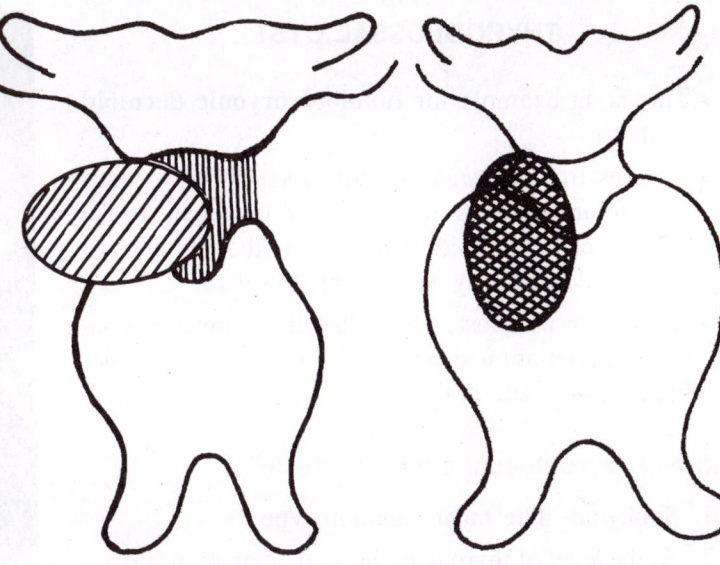

Fig. 16.44 Subhyoid bursits - transversely placed oval swelling

Fig.16.45 Thyroglossal cyst - vertically placed oval swelling

3. **Transillumination test is negative** as it contains thick, cheesy, sebaceous material.

Differential diagnosis

1. **Ranula**: When a sublingual dermoid cyst is in the midline in the floor of the mouth and above the mylohyoid muscle, ranula is considered as differential diagnosis. However, **ranula is bluish in colour, brilliantly transilluminant.**

2. **Thyroglossal cyst** should be considered as differential diagnosis when the sublingual dermoid cyst is below the mylohyoid muscle. Thyroglossal cyst **moves up with deglutition** whereas **a sublingual dermoid cyst does not.**

Treatment

- Through intraoral approach, excision can be done for both types of sublingual dermoid cyst.

SUBHYOID BURSITIS

- Accumulation of inflammatory fluid in the subhyoid bursa results in a swelling and is described as subhyoid bursitis.

- The bursa is located below the hyoid bone and in front of thyrohyoid membrane.

Clinical features

1. The swelling in front of the neck, in the midline below the hyoid bone (Fig. 16.44).

2. The swelling is oval in the transverse direction.

3. It moves up with deglutition.

4. Soft, cystic, fluctuant and transillumination negative swelling (turbid fluid).

5. The swelling may be tender as it contains inflammatory fluid.

Treatment

- Complete excision

Complication

- It can develop into an abscess

Differential diagnosis

1. Thyroglossal cyst is a vertically placed oval swelling whereas **subhyoid bursitis** is transversely placed oval swelling.

   - Thyroglossal cyst moves on protrusion of the tongue outside (subhyoid bursitis does not).

2. Pretracheal lymphnode swelling

3. Ectopic thyroid enlargement

THYROGLOSSAL CYST

- This is an example for **tubuloembryonic dermoid cyst.**

- It arises from *thyroglossal tract/duct* which extends from foramen caecum at the base of the tongue to the isthmus of the thyroid gland. Hence, the thyroglossal cyst can develop any where along this duct.

- It is lined by pseudostratified, ciliated, columnar or squamous epithelium which produces desquamated epithelial cells or mucus at times.

Sites of thyroglossal cyst (Fig. 16.46)

1. Subhyoid- **The most common type**

2. At the level of thyroid cartilage-2nd common site

3. Suprahyoid-Double chin appearance

4. At the foramen caecum-Rare

5. At the level of cricoid cartilage-Rare

6. In the floor of the mouth

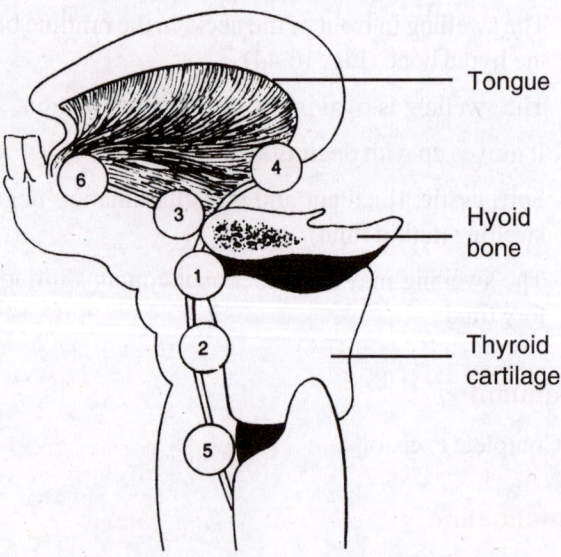

Fig. 16.46 Sites of thyroglossal cyst

Clinical features

1. Even though congenital, thyroglossal cyst appears around the age of 15-30 years.

2. They are more common in females who present with painless, midline swelling. However, in the region of thyroid cartilage, the swelling is slightly deviated to the left side (Fig. 16.47).

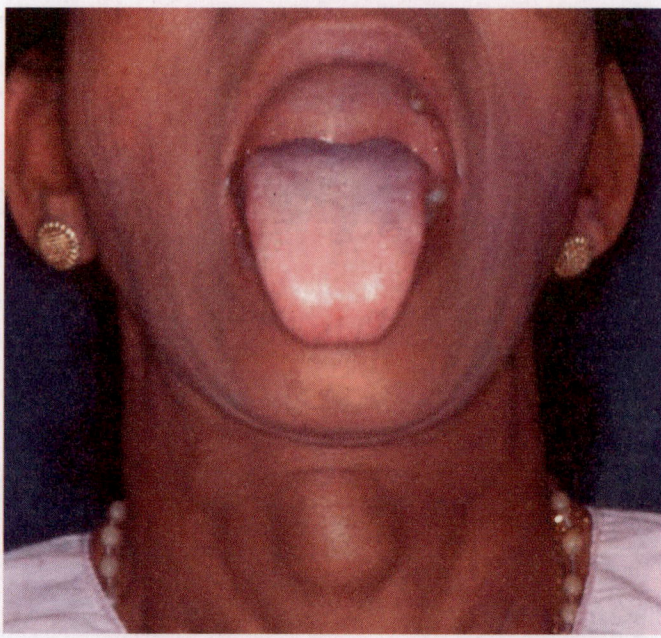

Fig. 16.47 Thyroglossal cyst - moves upwards with deglutition

3. The cyst is soft, cystic, fluctuant, transillumination - negative swelling (very rarely, it can give rise to transillumination). It can be firm if the tension within the cyst is high.

4. Mobility: Thyroglossal cysts exhibit 3 types of mobility which are characteristic of this condition :

- The cyst moves with deglutition.

- **Moves with protrusion of tongue**: Hold the thyroglossal cyst with the finger and thumb and ask the patient to protrude the tongue outside. **The movement of the cyst upwards is described as a tug because of its attachment with the hyoid bone**.

Key Box 16.20
MOVEMENT ON PROTRUSION OF THE TONGUE
• The cyst is attached to the hyoid bone. Hence, it gives a classical TUG
• Not always present, cyst below the thyroid cartilage-tug is absent
• Better appreciated on holding the swelling
EXAMINATION OF THYROGLOSSAL CYST
• Cyst proper, mobility
• Base of the tongue to rule out lingual thyroid and lymph nodes

The swelling moves sideways but not vertically as it is tethered by the thyroglossal duct.

Treatment

Before excision of cyst, a thyroid scan is mandatory since it may be the only functioning thyroid tissue.

Sistrunk operation: Excision of the cyst along with the entire thyroglossal tract which may **include part of the hyoid bone**, is the recommended treatment. The intimate relationship of hyoid bone can be explained by its development from 2nd and 3rd branchial arches.

Complication

The wall of the thyroglossal cyst sometimes contains **lymphoid tissue** which can get infected, resulting in an **abscess**. If it ruptures or is incised it results in **thyroglossal fistula**.

Rarely, a **papillary carcinoma** can occur in the **thyroglossal cyst**.

THYROGLOSSAL FISTULA

Thyroglossal fistula is **never congenital.** It is always acquired due to following reasons:

1. Infected thyroglossal cyst rupturing into the skin
2. Inadequately drained infected thyroglossal cyst
3. Incompletely excised thyroglossal cyst

The track is lined by columnar epithelium

Clinical features

1. Previous history of swelling in front of the neck, which

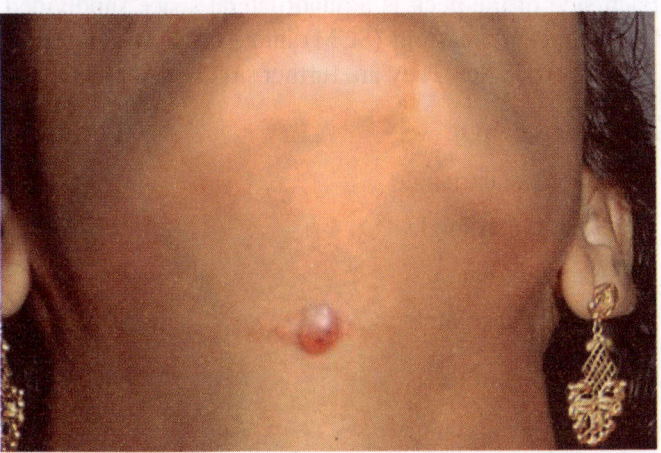

Fig. 16.48 Thyroglossal Fistula

is now painful, red and ruptured resulting in discharging pus. Once the pus is drained, the opening closes. However, after an interval of time, the 'pain and discharge reappear.

Key Box 16.21

RECURRENT ABSCESS – RUPTURE FISTULA OR SINUS

- Thyroglossal fistula
- Pilonidal sinus
- Median mental sinus
- Cold abscess

---

2. When there is no infection, the fistula discharges only mucus and the surrounding skin is normal. Infected fistulae are tender, discharging pus and skin is red hot.

3. Majority of the patients presenting are young in the age group of 10 to 20 years.

4. A fistulous opening in the centre of neck which is covered by a hood of skin can occur due to the increased growth of the neck, when compared to that of fistula. This is described as *semilunar sign or hood sign.*

Key Box 16.22

THYROGLOSSAL FISTULA

- Always acquired
- Fistulous opening is in the midline
- Semilunar sign or hood sign
- It gets pulled up with protrusion of the tongue

Treatment

Infection is controlled with antibiotics

Surgical excision should include the fistula with removal of the entire tract upto the foramen caecum. Otherwise, recurrence will occur.

The central portion of the hyoid bone is removed due to close proximity of the fistula.

An elliptical incision is preferred as it gives a neat scar.

This operation is called **Sistrunk's** operation.

Kindly refer next page for details about Sistrunk's operation (Key Box 16.23).

Key Box 16.23

SISTRUNK'S OPERATION

- Fistula with **entire thyroglossal tract** is excised.

- **Central portion of the hyoid bone** and lingual muscle are removed.

- Removal is facilitated by **pressing the posterior 1/3 of the tongue.**

- **Do not perforate** thyrohyoid membrane.

- **Incomplete removal results in recurrence**

ANOMALIES OF THYROGLOSSAL DUCT

Thyroglossal duct extends from foramen caecum to thyroid cartilage.

Various anamolies have been given in the Key Box below.

However, thyroglossal cyst is common and lingual thyroid and ectopic thyroid tissue are uncommon swellings.

They have to be kept in mind as a differential diagnosis of the swellings in the midline of the neck.

Key Box 16.24

THYROGLOSSAL DUCT ANOMALIES

- Lingual thyroid
- Levator glandulae thyroidae
- Ectopic thyroid tissue
- Thyroglossal cyst

SWELLING ARISING FROM ISTHMUS OF THE THYROID GLAND

Almost all the diseases of the thyroid gland result in enlargement of the isthmus. However, a solitary nodule and cysts can occur in relation to isthmus. The swelling moves with deglutition. However, it does not move on protrusion of the tongue.

PRETRACHEAL AND PRELARYNGEAL LYMPH NODES

These lymph nodes produce nodular swelling in the midline. One or two discrete nodes are palpable. They can enlarge due to following conditions.

1. **Acute laryngitis**: The nodes are tender, soft.
2. **Papillary carcinoma** of thyroid: The nodes are firm without matting, with or without evidence of thyroid nodule.
3. **Carcinoma of the larynx**: The nodes are hard in consistency.
4. In India **tuberculosis** should be considered as a possible diagnosis when the other diseases are ruled out.

SWELLINGS IN THE SUPRASTERNAL SPACE OF BURNS

1. **Lipoma** : Soft and lobular, edge slips under the palpating finger.
2. **Sequestration dermoid cyst** is a midline, soft, cystic, fluctuant swelling.
3. **Gumma** produces a firm swelling with evidence of syphilis elsewhere in the body.
4. **Thymic swellings, an aneurysm** of innominate or subclavian artery are the other causes.

DIFFERENTIAL DIAGNOSIS OF LATERAL SWELLINGS IN THE NECK

Before we discuss the swellings in the lateral side of the neck, it is essential to know the various triangles in the neck. These are discussed below:

TRIANGLES OF THE NECK

Each side of the neck is a quadrilateral space subdivided by Sternocleidomastoid (SCM) into Anterior triangle and Posterior triangle. They are further subdivided as follows:

Anterior triangle

1. Submental triangle
2. Digastric triangle
3. Carotid triangle
4. Muscular triangle

Posterior triangle

1. Occipital triangle
2. Supraclavicular triangle

Refer Fig. 16.49 in the next page

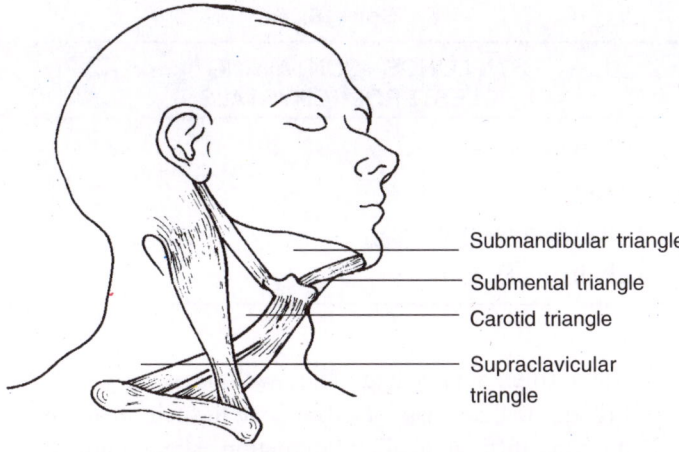

Fig. 16.49 Triangles of the neck

- Submandibular triangle
- Submental triangle
- Carotid triangle
- Supraclavicular triangle

SWELLINGS IN SUBMANDIBULAR TRIANGLE

- The submandibular triangle is a part of anterior triangle
- This is bounded **inferiorly** by anterior and posterior belly of digastric muscles with their tendon, **superiorly** by the attachment of deep fascia to the mandible and to the whole length of hyoid bone.
- This triangle is covered by deep fascia.
- The floor is formed by mylohyoid muscle which arises from mylohyoid line of the mandible, thus closing the space.
- Following are the swellings in the submandibular triangle:
  1. Enlarged submandibular lymph nodes-Common
  2. Submandibular salivary gland enlargement-Common
  3. Plunging ranula - Not uncommon
  4. Ludwig's angina - Not uncommon
  5. Lateral sublingual dermoid cyst - Rare
  6. Tumours of the mandible - Rare

ENLARGED SUBMANDIBULAR LYMPH NODES

They form a nodular swelling which is deep to deep fascia. They are palpable only in the neck (Not intraorally). The nodes can get enlarged due to following conditions.

1. **Acute lymphadenitis**: Very often, poor oral **hygiene** or a **caries tooth** produces painful, tender, soft enlargement of these lymph nodes. Extraction of the tooth or with improvement of oral hygiene, lymph nodes regress.
2. **Chronic tuberculous lymphadenitis** can affect these nodes along with upper deep cervical nodes. The nodes are firm and matted.

3. **Secondaries** in the submandibular lymph nodes arise from carcinoma of the cheek, tongue, palate. The nodes are **hard** with or without **fixity**.
4. **Non-Hodgkin's lymphoma** can involve submandibular lymph nodes along with horizontal group of nodes in the neck. The nodes are **firm** or **rubbery** in consistency.

SUBMANDIBULAR SALIVARY GLAND ENLARGEMENT (Key Box 16.25)

The various causes of submandibular salivary gland enlargement have been discussed under the salivary gland chapter. The common causes are chronic sialadenitis with or without a stone, tumours of the salivary gland or enlargement due to autoimmune diseases. They form irregular or nodular swelling. The diagnosis is confirmed by bidigital palpation of the gland. *Enlarged submandibular gland is bidigitally palpable because the deep lobe is deep to mylohyoid muscle.*

Key Box 16.25
SUBMANDIBULAR SALIVARY GLAND ENLARGEMENT
• Calculus   • Chronic sialadenitis   • Cancer   • Chronic diseases - Autoimmune

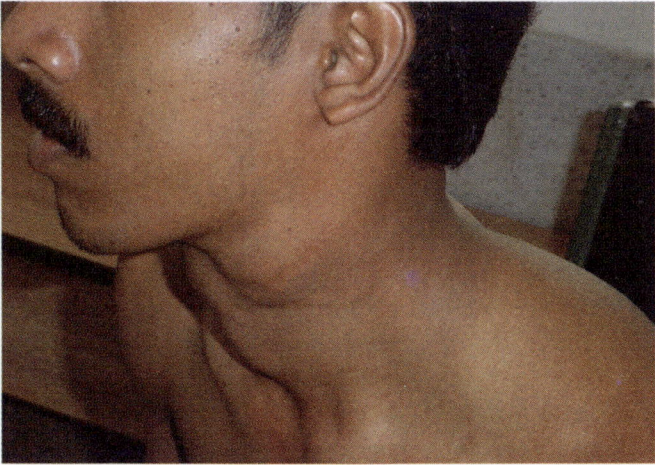

Fig. 16.50 This swelling in the submandibular triangle was bidigitally not palpable. However, it exhibited a doubtful sign of movement with the deglutition. It turned out to be an ectopic thyroid swelling (Contributed by Prof. Sampath Kumar, KMC, Manipal)

DIFFERENTIAL DIAGNOSIS OF SWELLINGS IN THE CAROTID TRIANGLE

The carotid triangle has following boundaries.

Laterally by sternomastoid muscle, superomedially by digastric muscle and stylohyoid muscle and inferomedially by omohyoid muscle.

Few important swellings in this triangle are as follows:

1. Branchial cyst.

2. Lymph node swelling (cold abscess).

3. Aneurysm of the carotid artery.

4. Enlargement of the thyroid gland.

5. Carotid body tumour-Rare.

6. Laryngocoele-Rare.

7. Sternomastoid tumour-Rare.

8. Neurofibroma vagus (Fig. 16.63)

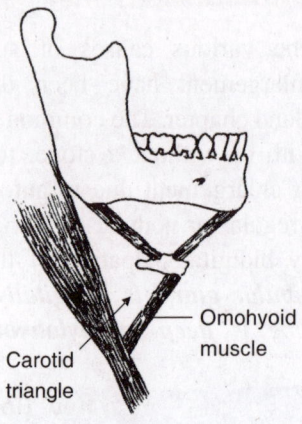

Carotid triangle

Omohyoid muscle

Fig. 16.51 Carotid triangle

BRANCHIAL CYST

Aetiology

Branchial cyst arises from vestigeal remnants of 2nd branchial arch.

The cyst is lined by squamous epithelium and contains desquamated epithelial cells which slowly form a tooth paste like material.

Clinical features

1. Even though congenital, majority of patients are young between the age group 15-25 years.

2. The swelling is typically located in the **anterior triangle of the neck partly under cover of the upper 1/3 of anterior border of sternomastoid**. This can be explained because of the development of *sternomastoid muscle from the myotome in the ridge of second branchial arch* (Fig. 16.52).

3. The swelling has smooth surface, round borders. It is **soft, cystic, fluctuant and transillumination-negative[1]**. Otherwise consistency is that of half

---

1. *Branchial cyst and thyroglossal cyst rarely give rise to transillumination if contents are clear.*

water filled rubber bag. The swelling is very often firm due to thick inspissated content. In such situations, it is very difficult to elicit fluctuation. The mobility of the swelling is also restricted because of its adherence to the sternomastoid muscle.

4. Sternomastoid contraction test: The swelling becomes less prominent.

5. If contents are aspirated, it contains **cholesterol crystals.** (Key Box 16.26)

6. No other lesion is found in the neck (lymph nodes).

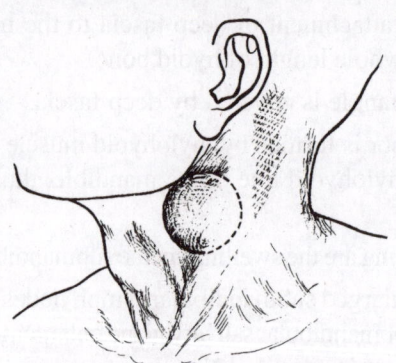

Fig. 16.52 Branchial cyst

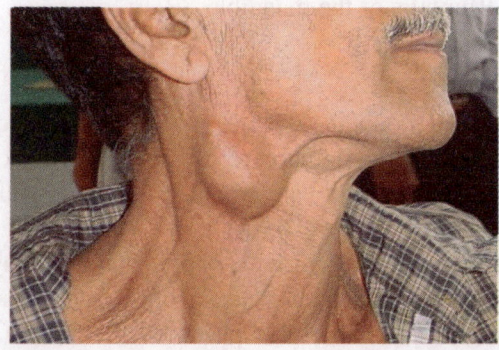

Fig. 16.53 Swelling mimicked branchial cyst. However, it was subcutaneous swelling with lobularity - it turned out to be lipoma

Treatment

- **Excision** of the cyst with *entire epithelial lining* with a curved incision centered over the swelling. One must ensure that epithelial lining should be removed completely or else recurrence will occur.

Complications

- Since the wall is rich in lymphatic tissue, it can undergo secondary infection with pain and swelling. Hence, the swelling has to be excised.

Differential diagnosis

There is no differential diagnosis in a classical case of branchial cyst. However, a few swellings have to be considered as differential diagnosis.

1. **Cold abscess** occurs in young patients due to tuberculosis of jugulodigastric nodes. Presence of multiple lymph nodes in the neck with or without fever gives the clue to the diagnosis.

2. **Lymphangioma** is a brilliantly transilluminant partially compressible swelling. However, anterior triangle is not a common site for lymphangioma.

3. **Lipoma** can also occur in the neck, though it is an uncommon site.

BRANCHIAL FISTULA

- This is always congenital and occurs due to persistent *2nd branchial cleft[1]*.

- External opening is situated at the junction of middle 1/3 and lower 1/3 of sternomastoid.

- The tract from the skin passes through the *fork of common carotid artery* deep to the accessory and hypoglossal nerves and opens in the *anterior aspect of posterior pillars of tonsils* (Fig.16.55). The tract is lined by squamous epithelium and discharges serous or mucous fluid. Sometimes the upper end is obliterated, resulting in a sinus.

- Patient may complain of a **dimple, discharging mucus** and the dimple becomes more obvious when the patient is asked to swallow.

- Usually seen in growing adults

- Can be unilateral or bilateral, equally common in males and females

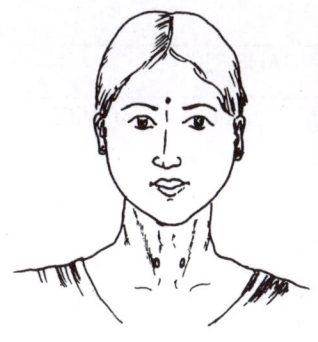 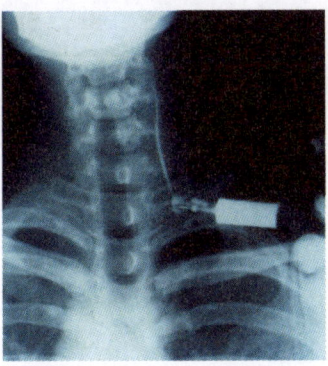

Fig. 16.54 Sites of Branchial fistula - commonly bilateral

Fig. 16.55 Contrast study demonstrating fistulous tract

- It is also called as **lateral fistula of the neck**. (Thyroglossal fistula is called as median fistula of the neck).

Treatment

- **Fistulogram** can be done by injecting methylene blue into the external opening and the tract is defined. This is followed by exploration of the tract. At surgery it should be carefully dissected up to the internal opening and then excised.

Complication

- Recurrent infection of the fistula.

COLD ABSCESS DUE TO TUBERCULOSIS

- In India, this is the commonest cystic swelling in the carotid triangle. The cold abscess results due to caseation necrosis of the lymph nodes. This forms a soft, cystic, fluctuant swelling with negative transillumination. Presence of other lymph nodes in the neck, sinuses in the neck gives the clue to the diagnosis (Page 15).

- Loss of appetite, weakness and fever may be the other features.

ANEURYSM OF THE COMMON CAROTID ARTERY

- Atherosclerosis is the most common cause of aneurysm. This weakens the vessel walls uniformly and produces fusiform dilatation of the blood vessel. Hypertension is another factor which adds to the aneurysm.

- Abdominal aorta is the commonest of aneurysms followed by popliteal artery.

---

1. *Persistant first branchial cleft results in external auditory meatus.*

Key Box 16.27

ANEURYSM – CAUSES

- **Congenital:** Berry aneurysm in the circle of Willis
- **Traumatic**
- **Degenerative:** Atherosclerosis
- **Rare causes:**

  Syphilis – Endarteritis obliterans

  Mycotic – Infective emboli

  Subacute bacterial endocarditis

  Marfans syndrome

  Polyarteritis

Types (Fig. 16.56)

A. Fusiform-Atherosclerosis, hypertension.

B. Saccular-Due to injury.

C. False-In this condition there is a sac lined by cellular tissue which communicates with artery through an opening in its wall

Causes: Refer Key Box 16.27

Clinical features of aneurysm

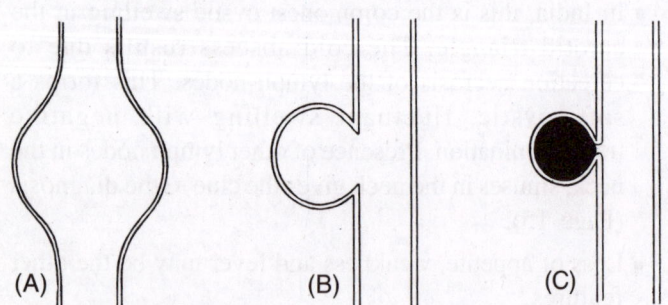

Fig. 16.56 Fusiform, saccular, false aneurysm.

1. Elderly patients are commonly affected.
2. Evidence of atherosclerosis in the form of thick walled vessel is present.
3. Tensely cystic (feels firm), fluctuant, transillumination negative swelling with *expansile pulsation.* (When the fingers are kept over the aneurysm *they are not only elevated but they are separated.*).

4. Compressibility is positive
5. On exerting pressure proximally the swelling diminishes in size - classically it happens in a case of popliteal aneurysms on compression of the femoral artery.
6. Bruit/thrill is characteristic of this condition

Treatment of aneurysm

- Angiography to confirm the diagnosis followed by repair of aneurysm with graft-PTFE graft (polytetrafluoro-ethylene graft - Fig. 16.57).

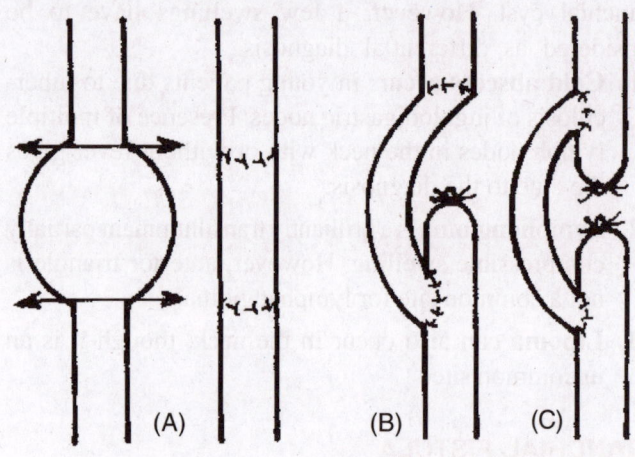

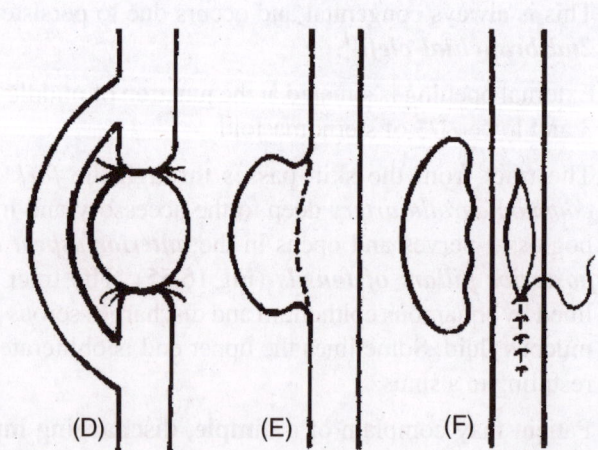

Fig. 16.57 Different methods of operation for aneurysm

A) Excision and end to end graft

B) Excision and end to side graft

C) Excision and side to side graft

D) Excision and bypass grafting

E & F) Matas aneurysmorrhaphy

CAROTID BODY TUMOUR (CHEMODECTOMA)

- This is a benign tumour arising from chemoreceptors in the carotid body. They are situated in the tunica adventitia at the bifurcation of common carotid artery.
- Hence, such a tumour is called chemodectoma.
- Function of the carotid body is regulation of pH.

Key Box 16.28
CHEMORECEPTORS : SITES
• The carotid body • The aortic body • Brain stem • Pulmonary receptors • Myocardial receptors

Clinical features

1. Middle aged or elderly patients are affected.
2. Patient gives the history of painless slow growing swelling for many years.
3. **Typical location** : At the level of the hyoid bone, in the upper part of the anterior triangle of the neck beneath the anterior edge of the sternomastoid muscle. (Fig. 16.58)
4. Surface is smooth or lobulated, borders are round, and is an oval, vertically placed swelling. Consistency is firm to hard. Hence, called **classical potato tumour.**

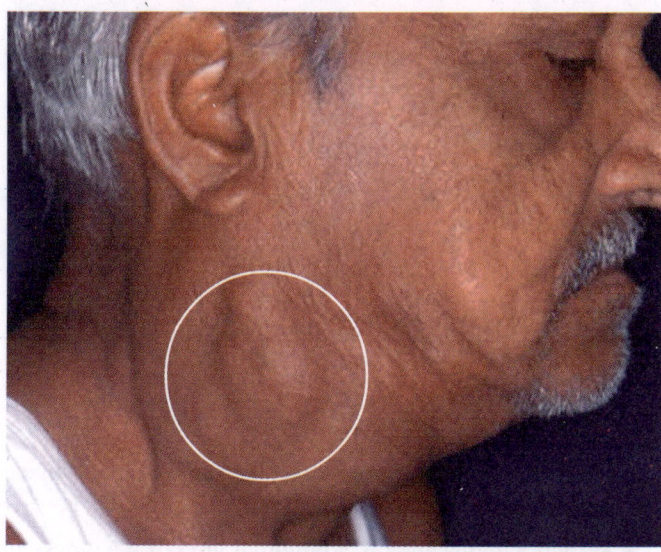

Fig. 16.58 Carotid body tumour – Classical site

5. Horner's syndrome, unilateral vocal cord paralysis can occur due to involvement of the nerves.
6. Pressure on tumour gives rise to syncopal attack due to decrease in the pulse rate (**Carotid body syndrome**).
7. Moves in the transverse direction.
8. Carotid artery is stretched over the swelling and so, transmitted pulsations are felt (Fig. 16.59).
9. Intra-oral examination shows prolapse of ipsilateral tonsil.

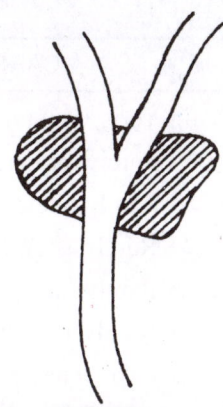

Fig.16.59 Section through carotid body tumour

Diagnosis

- Carotid angiography (Fig. 16.60) should be done if there are neurological symptoms such as syncopal attack. It may demonstrate separation of the carotid bifurcation.
- Splaying of carotid artery can be seen - **Lyre sign** (Fig. 16.60)
- Incision biopsy is dangerous.

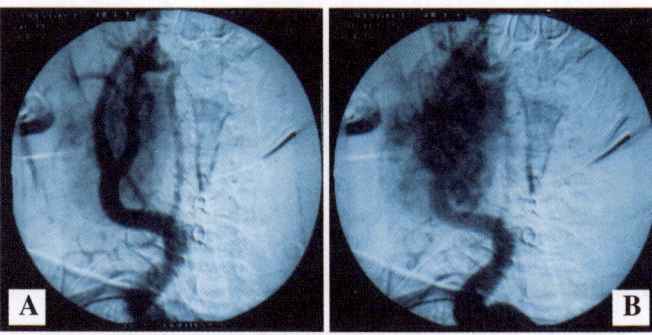

Fig. 16.60 Carotid Angiography - observe separation of internal and external carotid artery by the tumour (A) and vascular blush (B)

Treatment

- Excision of the tumour with reconstruction

It is important to preserve cerebral circulation during surgery. Vascular surgeons help is necessary.

Complication

- Very rarely, it can turn into a malignant carotid body tumour with lymph nodal metastasis.

Key Box 16.29

CAROTID BODY TUMOUR

- Very, very rare tumour
- Rarely malignant
- Rarely bilateral
- Rarely grows fast
- Rarely patient comes early
- Rarely metastasizes
- Experience of a surgeon with this tumour is very, very rare - **RAREST OF RARE TUMOURS.**

STERNOMASTOID TUMOUR

- This is not a tumour, it is a **misnomer**.
- Injury to the sternomastoid during birth causing rupture of few fibres and haematoma. Later, healing occurs with fibrosis, resulting in a swelling in the middle of sternomastoid muscle.
- The other possible theory is that this is a congenital anomaly-short sternomastoid muscle.

Clinical features

1. This is seen in infants or children. Firm to hard, 1-2 cm swelling in the middle of the sternomastoid muscle.
2. Tender, mobile sideways, medial and lateral borders are distinct. But superior and inferior borders are continuous with the muscle.
3. Many cases are associated with torticollis.

Treatment

- Gentle manipulation of child's head.
- Physiotherapy to stretch the shortened sternomastoid muscle.
- Division of lower attachment of sternomastoid from clavicle and sternum with or without removal of lump is the surgical treatment.

LARYNGOCOELE

- It results due to herniation of the laryngeal mucosa. (Fig. 16.61)
- When it enlarges within the larynx, it may displace vocal cord, produces hoarseness and is called **internal laryngocoele.**

Causes

- Glass blowers, musicians, wind instruments and trumpet players are commonly affected.
- Chronic cough may be one of the predisposing factors.

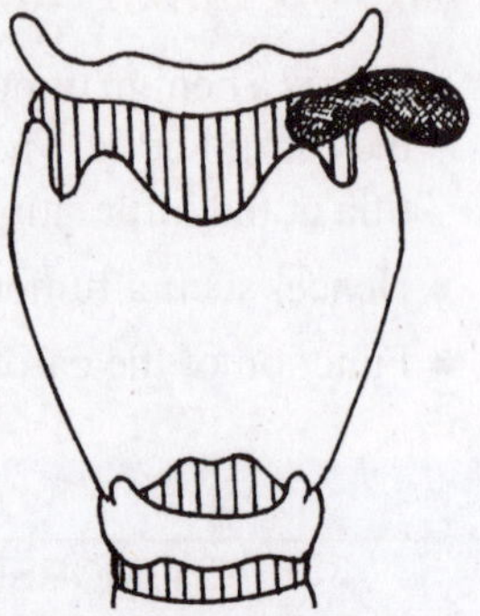

Fig. 16.61 Laryngocoele

Clinical features

1. Smooth, oval, boggy swelling which moves upwards on swallowing.
2. Swelling becomes prominent when the patient is asked to cough or blow.
3. Expansile cough impulse is present.
4. Tympanitic note on percussion (resonant)

Treatment

- Excision of the sac

Differential diagnosis

- Other cystic swellings such as branchial cyst, lymphangioma should be ruled out.

Complications

- Secondary infection results in laryngo-pyocoele. The opening in thyrohyoid membrane may be blocked by mucopus in such cases.

Key Box 16.30

LARYNGOCOELE

- Very rare
- Increased laryngeal pressure
- Expansile impulse on cough
- Ligation of its neck and division of the whole sac is the treatment.

PHARYNGEAL POUCH

- Herniation or protrusion of the mucosa of the pharyngeal wall through the Killian's dehiscence.
- Killian's dehiscence is a potential area of weakness in between the two parts of the inferior constrictor - Upper

oblique fibres (thyropharyngeus) and lower horizontal fibers (cricopharyngeus).

Etiopathogenesis

Due to increase in the intrapharyngeal pressure, in between the parts of inferior constrictor muscles, mucous membrane bulges due to neuromuscular imbalance, hence it is a pulsion diverticulum.

Course of the diverticulum

Pulsion diverticulum deviates to one side mostly to the left because of the rigid vertebral column in the midline posteriorly.

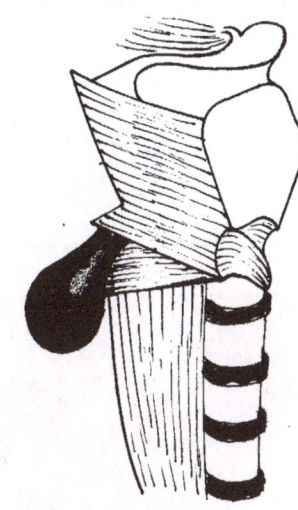

Fig. 16.62 Pharyngeal pouch

Diagnosis

Initially foreign body sensation is present in the throat, later regurgitation of food on turning to one side, sense of suffocation, cough or dysphagia is present.

Gurgling sound and aspiration may cause dyspnoea later.

> *Swelling is behind sternocleidomastoid below the level of thyroid cartilage – soft swelling which can be emptied.*

Treatment

Barium swallow followed by excision of the pouch

Cricopharyngeal myotomy is also given.

NEUROFIBROMA OF THE VAGUS NERVE

This condition produces swelling in the carotid triangle in the region of thyroid swelling.

It is a vertically placed oval swelling

It is firm to hard in consistency

On pressure over the swelling dry cough and in some cases bradycardia may occur.

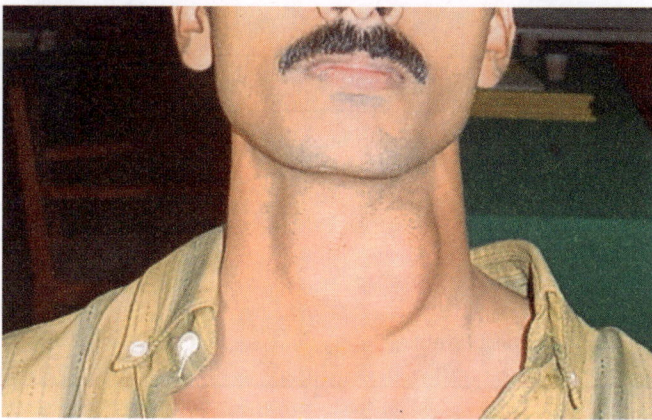

Fig. 16.63 Neurofibroma of the vagus nerve - Contributed by Prof. P. Rajan, Calicut Medical College, Kerala. This swelling was not moving with deglutition

DIFFERENTIAL DIAGNOSIS OF SWELLING IN THE POSTERIOR TRIANGLE

The posterior triangle (Key Box 16.31) is an interesting area as far as swellings are concerned. It is the commonest area of metastasis in lymph nodes from occult primary. Lymphangiomas, haemangiomas, cold abscess, lymphomas commonly occur here. Interesting cases of cervical rib, Pancoast tumour, aneurysms also occur here.

Most of the swellings have been discussed under appropriate chapters. Haemangioma, metastasis in the cervical lymph nodes and pancoast tumour have been discussed below.

Key Box 16.31
BOUNDARIES OF POSTERIOR TRIANGLE

- Anteriorly : Sternomastoid (posterior border)
- Laterally : Trapezius (anterior border)
- Above : Mastoid process
- Below : Clavicle

Classification (Table 16.11)

Common swellings in the location are given below

HAEMANGIOMA

Definition: This is a swelling due to congenital malformation of blood vessels. It is an example of Hamartoma. They are classified into three types: 1. Capillary 2. Cavernous 3. Arterial

Table 16.11 Swellings in the posterior triangle

1. SOLID SWELLINGS	II. CYSTIC SWELLINGS	III. PULSATILE SWELLINGS
1. Metastasis in the lymph nodes	1. Lymphangioma	1. Subclavian artery aneurysm
2. Tuberculosis	2. Haemangioma	2. Vertebral artery aneurysm
3. Lymphoma	3. Cold abscess	
4. Lipoma		
5. Cervical rib		
6. Pancoast tumour		

CAPILLARY HAEMANGIOMA

This arises from capillary tissue. Hence, it commonly occurs in the skin, They can be of the following types:

1. **Salmon patch** is a bluish patch over the forehead, in the midline, present at birth and disappears by 1 year of age. Hence, no treatment is required.

2. **Port wine stain** (Naevus flammeus) is an extensive intradermal haemangioma. This is bluish purple in colour, commonly affects the face or other parts of the skin, is present at birth and usually does not progress.

   Port wine stains are common on the shoulder region, neck and buttocks. These areas represent junction between the limbs and the trunk.

   As the child grows, by 5-6 years of age the swelling regresses.

3. **Strawberry angiomas** produce swelling which protrude from the skin surface. Child is normal at birth. After a month, a bright red swelling appears over the head and neck region, which exhibits **sign of compressibility**. The lesion consists of immature vascular tissue. Even though the lesion grows initially, by 5-7 years of age, swelling regresses and colour fades. Hence, no specific treatment is necessary. The treatment is indicated only when the swelling persists (Fig. 16.64).

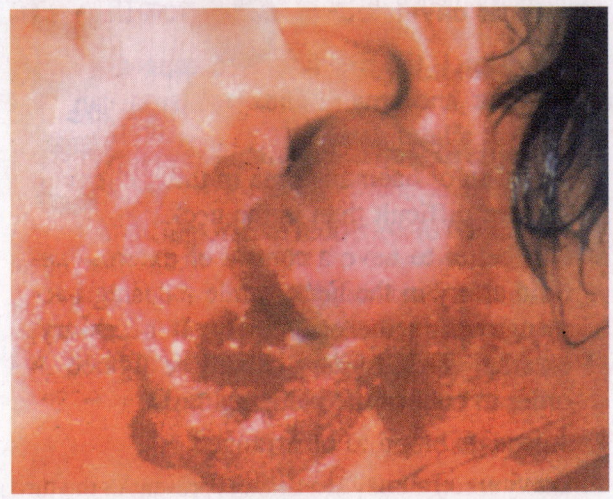

Fig. 16.64 Capillary haemangioma - contributed by Prof. Pramod Kumar, KMC, Manipal

---

Key Box 16.32

CAPILLARY HAEMANGIOMA

- Skin and soft tissue involvement
- Salmon patch: Midline-Forehead
- Port wine stain: Head and neck
- Strawberry angioma: Compressible
- Wait and watch policy is the best.

VENOUS HAEMANGIOMA - CAVERNOUS HEMANGIOMA

This occurs in place where venous space is abundant, e.g. lip, cheek, tongue, posterior triangle of the neck.

Clinical features

1. History of a swelling in the neck of long duration. History of bleeding is present when it occurs in the oral cavity.

2. The swelling is warm and bluish in colour but, not pulsatile.

3. Soft, fluctuant, transillumination is negative.

4. **Compressibility** is present. This sign is also called 'sign of emptying' or 'sign of refilling'. When the swelling is compressed between the fingers, blood diffuses under the vascular spaces and when pressure is released, it slowly fills up. Compressibility is a diagnostic sign of haemangioma.

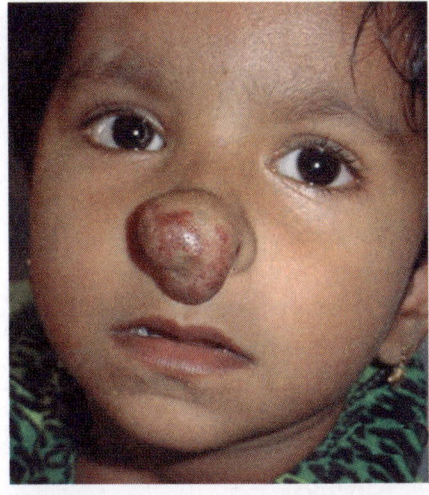

Fig. 16.65 Capillary haemangioma of the nose

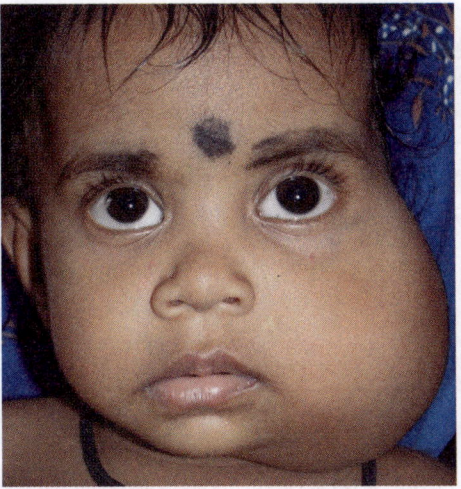

Fig. 16.66 Cavernous haemangioma of the cheek

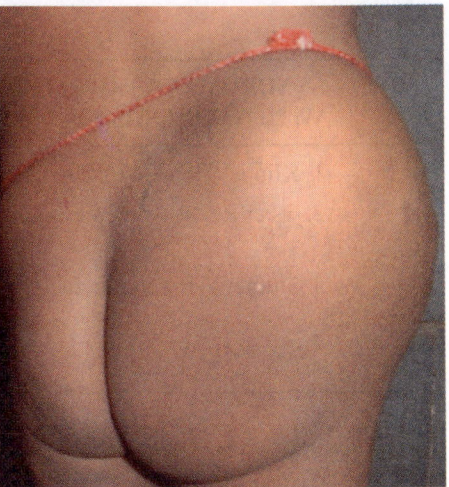

Fig. 16.67 Local gigantism due to haemangioma involving gluteal region

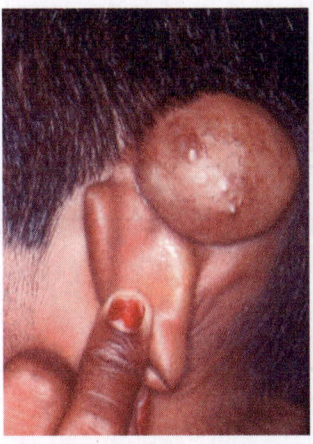
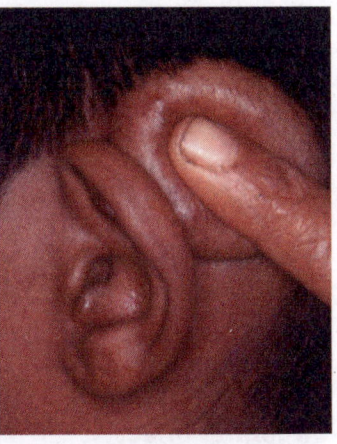

Fig. 16.68 Sign of compressibility was positive in this case. It was initially diagnosed as post-auricular dermoid cyst

---

Key Box 16.33

CAVERNOUS HAEMANGIOMA

- Compressible swelling
- Bluish warm, non-tender swelling
- Associated with arteriovenous communication
- Associated with lipoma-Naevo lipoma

Differential diagnosis

1. Lymphangioma is brilliantly transilluminant. If a lymphangioma is infected or has been treated with preliminary injections, it may not show transillumination.
2. Lipoma is not compressible.
3. Other cystic swellings - cold abscess

TREATMENT OF CAVERNOUS HAEMANGIOMA

Principles

1. **Injection** is the first line of treatment of cavernous haemangioma. It makes the swelling fibrotic, less vascular and small. Thus, excision can be done at a later date (Key Box 16.34, 16.35).

Key Box 16.34

INJECTION LINE OF TREATMENT

- Boiling water or hypertonic saline
- Sodium tetradecyl sulphate (S.T.D. solution)
- In multiple spaces, in multiple sittings
- Aseptic thrombosis and fibrosis occur

Key Box 16.35

SWELLINGS – TREATED WITH SCLEROSANTS

- Haemangioma
- Haemorrhoids
- Prolapse rectum
- Oesophageal varices
- Varicose veins

---

2. **Excision** of haemangioma in the oral cavity is more difficult than in the neck.
3. It is better to have a control of external carotid artery in the neck, while excising haemangioma in the oral cavity. If necessary, external carotid artery should be ligated in order to control the bleeding.

Table 16.12	
SYNDROMES ASSOCIATED WITH HAEMANGIOMA	**FINDINGS**
1. Klippel Trenauny Weber Syndrome	1. Naevus flammeus, Osteohypertrophy of extremities, AV fistula
2. Osler Rendu – Weber Syndrome	2. Haemangioma of lip associated with GI tract Haemangioma
3. Sturge Weber Syndrome	3. Haemangioma of brain, mental retardation, Jacksonian epilepsy, Glaucoma

4. Adequate blood to be arranged

5. **Previous embolisation** into the feeding artery decreases the size of the haemangioma (Therapeutic Embolization).

6. Large haemangiomas in the oral cavity should be excised only after preliminary sclerotherapy and taking all the precautions mentioned above.

Syndromes associated with haemangioma (Table 16.12 and Fig. 16.69, 70)

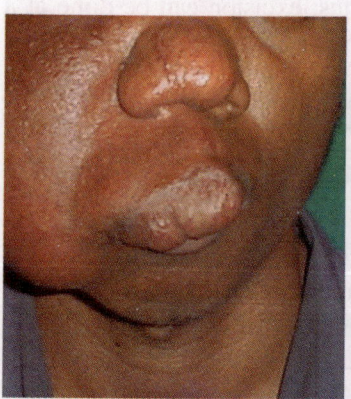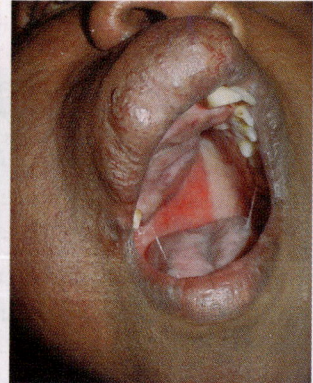

Fig. 16.69 and 16.70 Large haemangioma involving cheek, lip and palate - He also had haemangioma of the liver

Complications of Haemangioma (Key Box 16.36)

Key Box 16.36
COMPLICATIONS OF HAEMANGIOMA
• Ulceration and Bleeding : Commonly occurs with capillary haemangioma
• Infection: Septicaemia usually precipitated by a small ulcer
• High output cardiac failure

CONGENITAL ARTERIOVENOUS FISTULA (ARTERIAL HAEMANGIOMA)

An abnormal communication between artery and vein, results in AV fistula.

Such AV fistula have got structural and functional effects.

Key Box 16.37
ARTERIOVENOUS FISTULA – TYPES
1. Congenital
2. Traumatic
3. Iatrogenic-Done in cases of renal failure

Structural effect

Since high pressure blood from an artery flows into the vein, the veins get dilated, tortuous and elongated-arterialisation of the vein, results in secondary varicose veins.

Physiological effect

Increased pulse rate, increased cardiac output, increased pulse pressure result due to increased venous pressure and arteriovenous shunt.

Functional effect

1. Soft, cystic, fluctuant, transillumination-negative, **pulsatile swelling.**

2. A continuous bruit/murmur is characteristic.

3. **Nicoladoni sign or Branham sign**

   On compressing the feeding artery, the venous return to the heart diminishes, resulting in fall in pulse rate and pulse pressure.

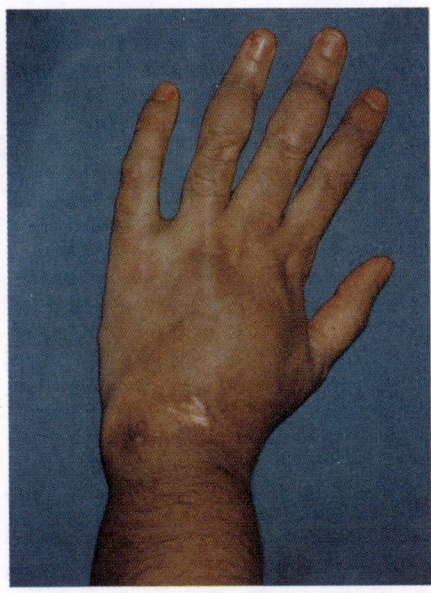

Fig. 16.71 Traumatic AV fistula affecting wrist and hand. Kindly observe prominent veins and swollen fingers

Also, on compressing feeding artery, pulsation or **continuous murmur** may also disappear and swelling will diminish in size.

4. If the AV fistula is big, a high output cardiac failure can occur.

5. The affected part is swollen (because of high pressure) - **local gigantism**. Thus, overgrowth of the limb or toe can occur.

6. Distal to the AV fistula, there are **ischaemic ulcers**, due to comparative reduction in the blood supply.

Investigations

Angiography with **DSA** pictures (Digital Subtraction Angiography) are essential before treating these patients.

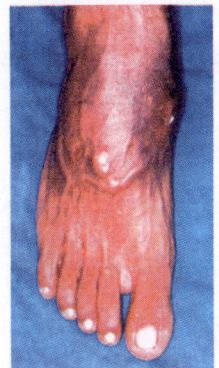 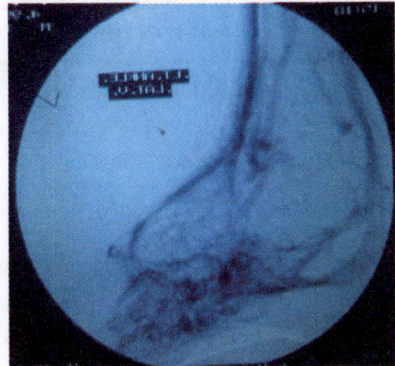

Fig. 16.72A A - Traumatic AV fistula see the arterialisation of the vein **Fig. 16.72B** DSA picture

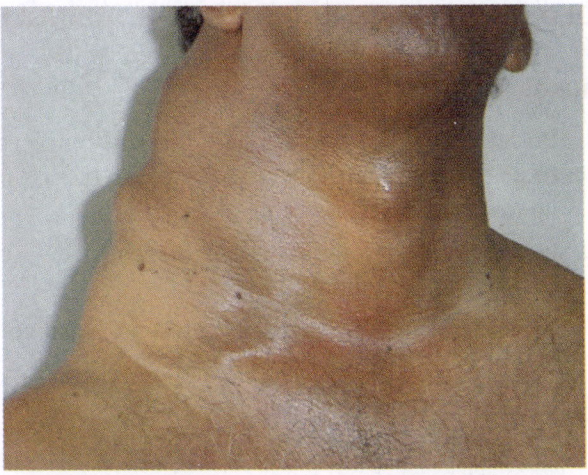

Fig. 16.73 Congenital AV fistula of 25 years duration

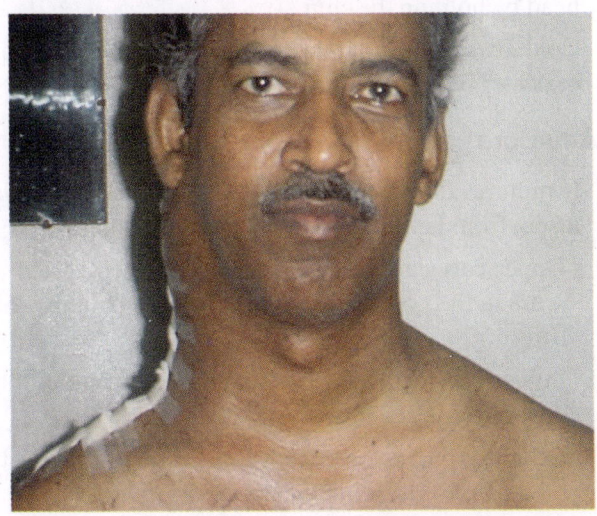

Fig. 16.74 After therapeautic embolisation it has regressed over 70%. Patient is waiting for another course of embolisation (Contributed by Dr. Umesh Bhat, Surgeon, Kundapur and Dr. Subhaschandra, Interventional cardialogist, Manipal Hospital, Bangalore)

Treatment

Therapeutic embolisation is the treatment of choice for arteriovenous fistula, in congenital cases.

Acquired lesion need to be observed or to be treated by quadruple ligation.

CIRSOID ANEURYSM

Not an aneurysm.

But is an AV fistula occurring in older people affecting the temporal region.

The arteries and the veins are dilated and tortuous and are compared to pulsating bag of worms.

COLD ABSCESS IN THE POSTERIOR TRIANGLE

Causes

1. Posterior cervical lymph nodes primarily involved - route of infection from adenoids or with other lymph nodes in the anterior triangle.
2. Lower posterior lymph nodes or Scalene node - route of infection from lungs.
3. **From tuberculous cervical spine - Caries spine.**

CARIES CERVICAL SPINE

Clinically it presents as pain in the back, cold abscess and neurological presentation.

Rust's Sign : Child with caries spine will support the head by holding the chin.

Cold abscess from caries spine can rupture anteriorly or posteriorly.

Anterior rupture

It ruptures deep to prevertebral layer of deep cervical fascia from here it can take following routes.

1. Upper cervical region – presents as deep seated abscess in the posterior wall of the pharynx in the **midline**.
2. Lower cervical region – Pus will press on oesophagus and trachea forwards.
3. Laterally pus passes deep to prevertebral fascia behind carotid sheath in the posterior triangle.

Posterior rupture

Pus may enter spinal canal and then can travel along anterior primary division of the cervical spinal nerves.

Diagnosis

Cervical spine x-ray to rule out spinal tuberculosis

Chest X-ray to rule out pulmonary tuberculosis

Non-dependent aspiration of the cold abscess followed by AFB staining

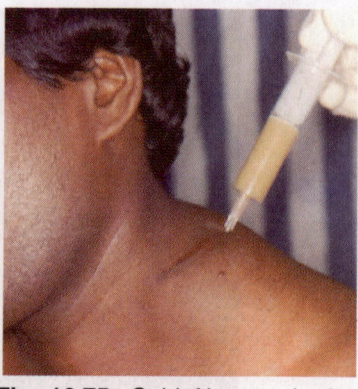

Fig. 16.75 Cold Abscess in the posterior triangle

Treatment

- Anti-tuberculosis treatment
- Non-dependant aspiration if cold abscess is present.
- Please refer orthopaedic books for specific treatment of TB spine.

Differential diagnosis

- Haemangioma, lymphangioma

SECONDARIES IN THE LYMPH NODES OR LYMPH NODE METASTASIS IN HEAD AND NECK

Very often, the patients present to the surgeon with lymph node swelling in the neck with or without any complaints. If there is an obvious lesion in the oral cavity, the diagnosis is easy. On the other hand, difficulty arises in locating the primary malignancy, which is hidden or occult. It is important to know the anatomical location of the lymph nodes in the neck and the drainage area, so that drainage areas can be investigated.

Classification: They can be divided into horizontal (Table 16.12) and vertical group of lymph nodes.

LOCATION	DRAINAGE AREA	COMMON DISEASES
1. Submental	Central part of the lower lip, floor of the mouth, tip of the tongue	Infections, metastasis
2. Submandibular	Cheek, tongue, whole of the upper lip, outer part of the lower lip, gums, angle of mouth, side of nose, inner angle of the eye	Infections, carcinoma
3. Parotid	Nasopharynx, back of nose, eyelids, front of scalp, enamel, auditory meatus, tympanic cavity	Eyelid tumours, parotid tumours, tuberculosis
4. Preauricular	Outer surface of pinna, side of scalp	Scalp infection, tuberculosis
5. Postauricular	Temporal region of scalp, back of pinna	Scalp infection
6. Occipital	Back of the scalp	Scalp infection, secondary syphilis

Table 16.12. Horizontal group of lymph nodes

Table 16.13 Vertical group of lymph nodes

LOCATION	DRAINAGE AREA	COMMON DISEASES
1. Prelaryngeal (on the cricothyroid ligament)	Larynx	Laryngeal carcinoma
2. Pretracheal, paratracheal (in front of trachea)	Trachea, thyroid	Papillary carinoma thyroid, tuberculosis
3. Upper anterior deep (jugulodigastric)	Tonsil, posterior 1/3 tongue, oropharynx, pyriform recess	Tonsillitis, carcinoma posterior 1/3 tongue, oropharyngeal carcinoma, tuberculosis
4. Upper posterior deep	Adenoids, posterior pharynx, retropharyngeal region	Tuberculosis, nasopharyngeal carcinoma
5. Middle group of lymp nodes	Thyroid	Papillary carinoma thyroid
6. Lower anterior (juguloomohyoid)	Tongue, thyroid, mediastinum	Carcinoma tongue, carcinoma thyroid
7. Lower posterior (supraclavicular)	Thyroid, post-cricoid, oesophagus, lungs. breast, etc.	Bronchogenic carcinoma, intra-abdominal malignancy, lymphoma

Interestingly, very often circular group of nodes are enlarged in non-Hodgkin's lymphoma on both sides.

VERTICAL GROUP OF LYMPH NODES (Fig. 16.76)

They can be classified into central and lateral group of lymph nodes. Most of the central group of lymph nodes are in relation to laryngeal cartilages or the trachea. The lateral lymph nodes are the most popular lymph nodes called deep cervical nodes. Majority of them are in close relationship with internal jugular vein. Jugulo-omohyoid and jugulo-digastric lymph nodes belong to this category. The details about the vertical group of lymph nodes are given in Table 16.13.

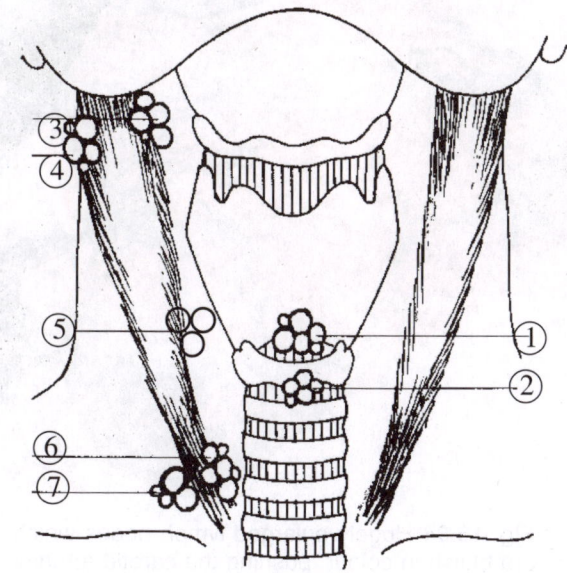

Fig. 16.76 Vertical group of lymph nodes (Refer Table 16.13)

PRESENT NOMENCLATURE OF VARIOUS GROUP OF LYMPH NODES

Level-I : Lymph nodes in the **Submandibular triangle, submental nodes**

Level-II : **Upper jugular nodes** : from posterior belly of digastric superiorly to hyoid bone inferiorly

Level-III : **Middle jugular nodes** : from hyoid superiorly to cricothyroid membrane inferiorly

Level-IV : **Lower jugular nodes** : from crico-thyroid membrane superiorly to clavicle inferiorly

Level-V : **Posterior cervical region** : from anterior border of trapezius posteriorly to posterior border of sternocleidomastoid anteriorly and clavicle inferiorly.

Level-VI : **Anterior compartment nodes**: from hyoid bone superiorly to suprasternal notch inferiorly and laterally by medial border of carotid sheath.

Level-VII : **Upper mediastinal nodes** : inferior to suprasternal notch.

• It is advisable to know these various levels of lymph nodes and their drainage areas.

• When block dissection is being done, you will find the lymph nodes being mentioned in the form of levels.

• Example: In papillary carcinoma thyroid, level III, level IV, level V and level VI lymph nodes are removed. (See next page)

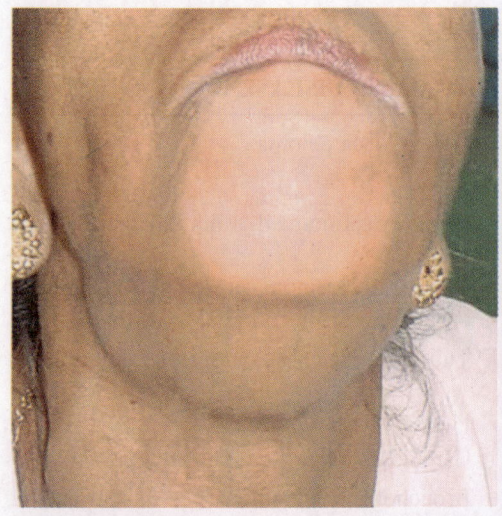

Fig. 16.77 Level I and II nodes. Carcinoma floor of the mouth

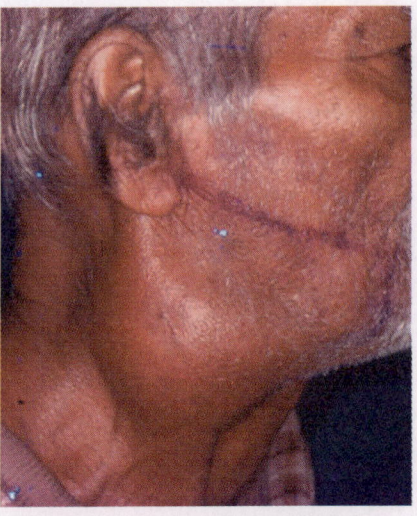

Fig. 16.78 Level II and III nodes - carcinoma alveolus

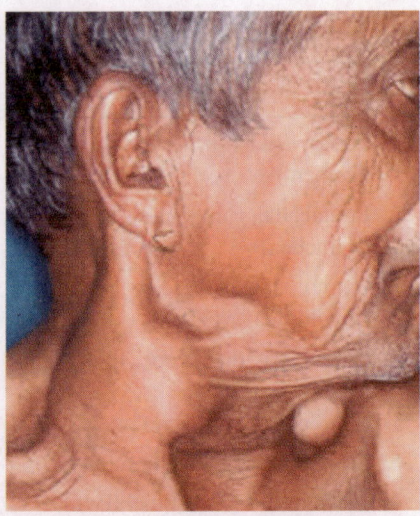

Fig. 16.79 Level III, IV and V nodes - carcinoma posterior 1/3 of tongue

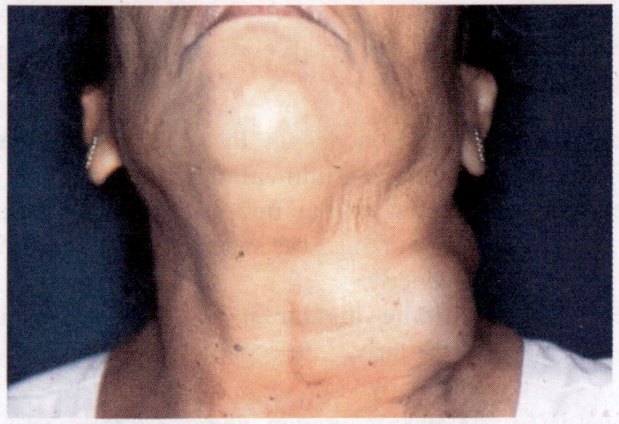

Fig. 16.80 Level V nodes - post-cricoid carcinoma

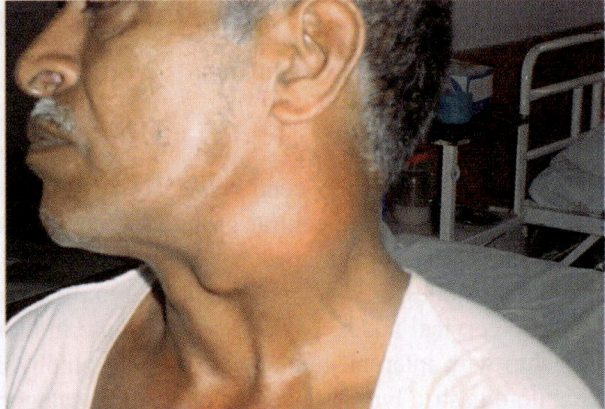

Fig. 16.81 Predominantly Level II, III and V nodes - from nasopharyngeal carcinoma

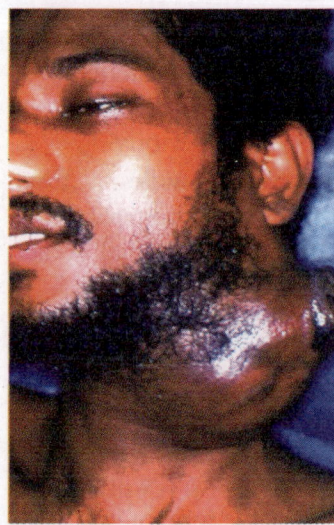

Fig. 16.82 Level I,II,III and V nodes- primary could not be identified- a case of occult primary

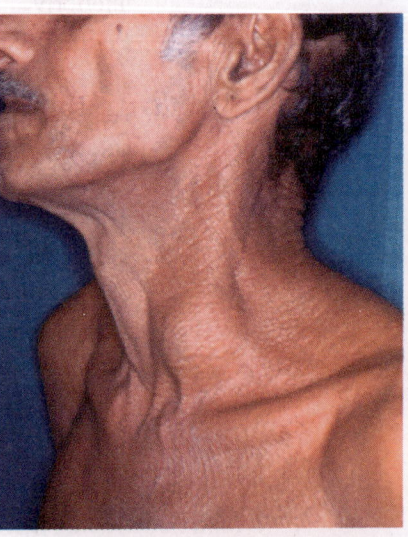

Fig. 16.83 Scalene node - in between the two heads of sternomastoid - a case of bronchogenic carcinoma

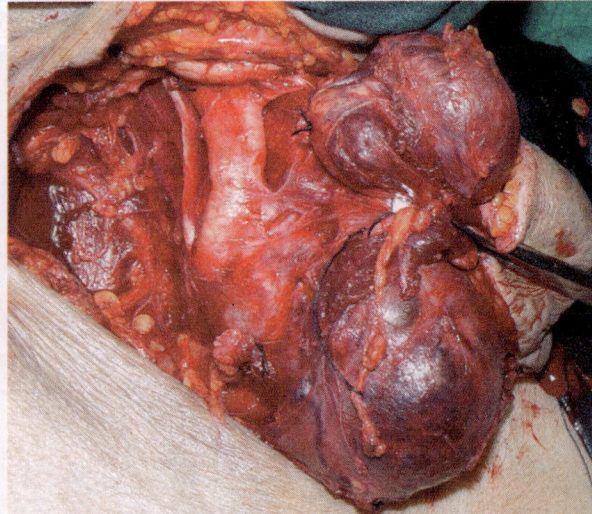

Fig. 16.84 Hugely enlarged lymph nodes which are bluish in colour, pushing the carotid arteries anteriorly - Papillary carcinoma thyroid

CLINICAL PRESENTATION OF METASTATIC DEPOSITS IN THE LYMPH NODES

1. Majority of patients are elderly males (> 50 years), present with painless swelling in the neck of few months duration.

2. The symptoms with which a patient presents to the hospital gives the clue to the site of origin of the primary. Few examples are given below.

   Difficulty in swallowing: Carcinoma posterior 1/3 tongue, oropharyngeal carcinoma or carcinoma oesophagus

   Difficulty in breathing : Laryngeal cancer

   Hoarseness of voice: Larynx or thyroid

   Obvious growth in oral cavity: Carcinoma cheek, alveolus, tongue, etc

   Haemoptysis, difficulty in breathing: Bronchogenic carcinoma

   Epistaxis, ear pain or deafness : Nasopharyngeal carcinoma (Key Box 16.38)

Clinical signs

1. Lymph nodal metastasis appears as a hard, nodular or irregular mass in the anatomical location of the lymph nodes.

2. Early cases may have some mobility. However, in majority of cases nodes get fixed and they attain a huge size. Very often, what appears as one lymph node, is a complex mass of multiple lymph nodes.

3. On sternomastoid contraction test or chin test, these nodal swellings become less prominent. Skin ulceration is a late feature. **A prominent skin fold** is due to infiltration into the platysma - **platysma sign**.

4. The primary malignancy may be evident in the anterior third of tongue, cheek, alveolus, etc.

5. Posterior one third of the tongue should be palpated with gloved finger (Key Box 16.39).

6. Secondaries in the lymph nodes can cause pressure effects or may cause paralysis of nerves. Upper anterior deep cervical lymph nodes can cause **hypoglossal nerve paralysis** (Key Box 16.40). Tongue points towards the side of lesion. **When there is no evidence of the primary lesion clinically, the situation is described as occult primary** with secondaries in the neck. Pain in the distribution of trigeminal nerve (face) suggests nasopharyngeal malignancy infiltrating skull base (foramen lacerum).

Key Box 16.38

NASOPHARYNGEAL CARCINOMA – TROTTER'S TRIAD

1. Conductive deafness
2. Homolateral immobility of soft palate
3. Pain in the side of the head due to involvement of 5th cranial nerve

---

Key Box 16.39

OCCULT PRIMARY SITES

- Posterior 1/3 of the tongue
- Oropharynx
- Nasopharynx
- Sinuses
- Upper oesophagus
- Bronchus
- Thyroid

Key Box 16.40

CLINICAL EXAMINATION IN A CASE OF LYMPH NODES IN THE NECK

- Lymph nodes-all groups
- Drainage areas
- **Pressure effects on** :
- Hypoglossal nerve
- Accessory nerve
- Cervical sympathetic chain

How do you suspect metastasis in the neck?

Any elderly patient presenting with firm to hard lymph node with or without fixity.

Having suspected a metastatic deposits, remember following facts

80% of them are **metastatic** deposits.

Majority of malignant neoplasms are **epithelial** in origin.

Nodes in the **upper half : Level I and II**: can be due to **primary in the oral cavity, tongue, oropharynx, larynx.**

Nodes in the **lower half : Level III and IV**: **can be due to primay in the thyroid, tongue.**

Nodes in the supraclavicular region: Level V: GIT, Genitourinary tract and lungs and in nasopharyngeal carcinoma

Nodes in the pretracheal, suprasternal region: Level VI: papillary carcinoma thyroid.

INVESTIGATIONS

1. Compete blood picture

2. **Chest X-ray** can give following information:

   Secondaries in the lungs with cannon ball appearance as in cases of malignant melanoma of head and neck.

   Bronchogenic carcinoma can be suspected by an irregular dense shadow in the peripheral lung fields.

   Large mediastinal node mass may be made out, with or without tracheal shift.

3. **Biopsy** from the clinically obvious lesion (tongue, cheek, etc.).

4. **Triple endoscopy includes**:

   Direct and indirect laryngoscopy
   Oesophagoscopy
   Bronchoscopy and suspicious area can be biopsied

5. **X-ray base of the skull** may show destruction of the bone by the tumour.

6. **C.T. scan** of the sinuses, or nasopharyngeal area, or skull base to detect a primary growth, its extension, etc.

7. **FNAC** of the lymph nodes can give a diagnosis in more than 90% of the cases. AVOID INCISION BIOPSY **as it will result in tumour recurrence and wound necrosis.**

8. If primary tumour cannot be detected on endoscopy, a **blind biopsy** is taken from **posterior wall of the fossa of Rosenmuller** and of the **pyriform fossa** on the same side.

9. When aspiration cytology is negative, an excision biopsy is advised as a last resort.

TREATMENT

1. When the primary tumour is obvious with enlarged lymph node metastasis, radiotherapy is the preferred line of treatment. However, refer the Chapter 17 on management of oral malignancy.

2. Treatment of occult primary with metastatic lymph nodes :

   If the lymph node or nodes are mobile, radical block dissection is done and if histopathologic report detects poorly differentiated carcinoma, extra-capsular spread, or nodes are large (> 3 cms) radiotherapy is given.

   If there is a large, bulky secondary, bilateral secondaries or fixed secondaries, radiotherapy is given to the neck masses. If the nodes do not completely regress, if the tumour becomes bigger in size after 6-8 weeks of radiotherapy, radical neck dissection would be considered.

DIFFERENT TYPES OF NECK DISSECTIONS

1. **Radical Neck Dissection (RND) – CRILE**:

   Here all the cervical lymph nodes from level 1 to Level VI are removed **along with nonlymphatic structures such as** sternocleidomastoid muscle, internal jugular vein, accessory nerve (XI), the submandibular salivary gland and cervical sympathetic plexus: A few examples wherein radical neck dissection is done are **Carcinoma tongue, oropharyngeal** carcinoma etc.

2. **Modified radical neck dissection or Functional neck dissection (BOCCA).** In this all the lymph nodes from Level I to Level VI are removed but **nonlymphatic structures are preserved**: (mentioned above) : Done for papillary carcinoma thyroid.

3. **Selective neck dissection** : Here any of the lymphatic compartment is preserved (which should have been removed as a part of classic RND). Few examples :

   a) **Supraomohyoid dissection**: removal of nodes in Level I, II and III done for carcinoma oropharynx, carcinoma cheek.

   b) **Lateral neck dissection** : Level II, III, IV are removed as in carcinoma larynx.

   c) **Posterolateral neck dissection** : Level II to V are removed as in cutaneous malignancy of posterior scalp and neck.

4. **Commando's operation: RND, hemimandibulectomy with radical glossectomy : It is a very radical aggressive surgery done for carcinoma tongue.**

Follow up

About 30-40% of treated patients with occult primary with metastatic nodes die with no evidence of the primary later.

In about 30% of patients, the primary will manifest within 1-2 years time.

And about 10% of patients are **cured** but once again primary is not found out.

PANCOAST'S TUMOUR

Pancoast's tumour or superior sulcus tumour is a bronchogenic carcinoma arising from the apex of lung.

Typically patient is an elderly male around 70 years, chronic smoker who presents with cough, weight loss dyspnoea and chest pain

As the tumour grows, it compresses the lower roots of brachial plexus C8 and T1 and results in tingling, pain, paraesthesia in the distribution of ulnar nerve.

The tumour is felt in the posterior triangle, in the lower part. It is hard in consistency, fixed, irregular and sometimes tender. The lower border of the mass cannot be appreciated.

The Pancoast's syndrome refers to following components :

1. Pancoast tumour
2. Erosion of the first rib
3. Paralysis of C8 and T1 nerve roots
4. **Horner's syndrome** due to paralysis of cervical sympathetic chain. The preganglionic sympathetic fibres of the head and neck are given from the 1st and sometimes the 2nd thoracic segments of the spinal cord. These nerve fibers synapse with the cells in the three cervical sympathetic ganglia. They give postganglionic fibres to the head and neck region.

Thus, anywhere along this pathway, disruption, damage or infiltration of the nerve roots results in Horner's syndrome. The causes of Horner's syndrome are depicted above in the box (Key Box 16.41)

Components of Horner's syndrome

Miosis: Small pupil

Anhidrosis: Absence of sweating

Pseudoptosis: Drooping of upper eyelid (Fig.16.85)

Enophthalmos: Regression of the eyeball

Nasal vasodilatation: Nasal congestion

Key Box 16.41

HORNER'S SYNDROME COMMON CAUSES

- Posterior inferior cerebellar artery thrombosis (PICA)
- Cervical sympathectomy
- Pancoast's tumour

UNCOMMON CAUSES

- Syringomyelia
- Injury to lower roots of brachial plexus
- Tumour in the neck
- Aneurysm of carotid artery

INVESTIGATIONS

1. Chest X-ray: May demonstrate a dense mass or collapse of the lobe, etc.
2. C.T. scan may demonstrate infiltration of the tumour into ribs or vertebrae
3. Sputum for malignant cells
4. Flexible bronchoscopy: Tissue biopsy or sputum sample can be collected
5. FNAC of the tumour gives the diagnosis in majority of cases

TREATMENT

Palliative radiotherapy. The response rate is poor.

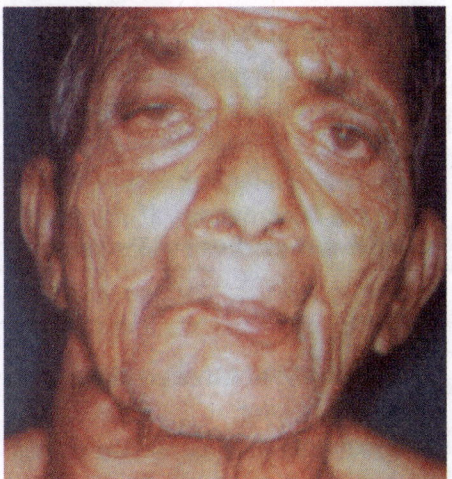

Fig. 16.85 Pseudoptosis due to metastatic deposits in the deep cervical lymph nodes

Oral Cavity, Odontomes, Lip and Palate

17

- Definitions
- Premalignant conditions
- General principles
- Carcinoma cheek
- Carcinoma tongue
- Carcinoma lip
- Carcinoma maxillary antrum
- Ulcers of the tongue
- Odontomes, epulis
- Cleft lip and cleft palate

ORAL CANCER

Oral cavity is bounded by the lips anteriorly, cheek on both sides, tonsils posteriorly, above by the palate and below by the floor of the mouth. It is lined by squamous epithelium. Oral cavity suffers from various ulcers including malignancy because it is insulted by various agents such as alcohol, smoking, tobacco chewing etc. Oral cancer is the commonest malignant neoplasm in the head and neck. Hence, it is discussed first in this chapter. (Key Box 17.1)

Key Box 17.1	
INCIDENCE OF ORAL CANCER	
Tongue	50%
Cheek	20-25%
Floor	10-15%
Gums	10%

DEFINITIONS

- **Hyperkeratosis** refers to increase in keratin layers. It occurs due to **constant irritation**. Once the cause is removed it is **reversible**. It is a microscopic diagnosis.

  e.g. Smokers' hyperkeratosis of the palate and lips. Once the aetiological agent is withdrawn, the lesion returns back to normal.

- **Leukoplakia** appears clinically as a white patch in the mouth and cannot be scraped off. It is irreversible and not attributable to any known diseases. It is important to biopsy leukoplakic portion to rule out malignancy.

1. **Leukoplakia:** The causes for leukoplakia are as follows:
   - **Smoking** results in hyperkeratosis. Nicotine in the form of cigarettes, chewed tobacco[1], powdered snuff produces premalignant changes in the oral cavity.
   - **Spices**
   - **Spirits** have synergistic action with smoking
   - **Sharp** tooth, **sepsis**, poor oral hygiene
   - **Sunlight** - actinic rays
   - **Syphilis** causes endarteritis obliterans and results

---

1. *Tobacco is the starter, accelerator for oral cancer and it is the major killer*

in chronic superficial glossitis of the tongue which is a precancerous condition. (Rare nowadays).

- **Susceptibility**[1] of a person
- **Betel nut**, and slake lime with betel leaf and tobacco (Pan) is eaten and usually kept inside the cheek for many hours. Over the years, it brings about chronic irritation of mucosa of the cheek and causes leukoplakia. Tobacco contains multiple carcinogens including aromatic hydrocarbons.

Stages in the development of leukoplakia

I.   **Keratosis** appears as milky blush on the surface.

II. **Acanthosis** refers to elongation of rete pegs. This appears as a smooth, white, dry patch.

III. **Dyskeratosis** means the formation of keratin cell layer in the deeper aspect of epidermis, before they reach the surface.

IV. **Speckled leukoplakia** appear as multiple, small white patches (Fig. 17.1).

V.   **Carcinoma in situ**

Treatment of leukoplakia

- About 10% of leukoplakia patients develop oral cancer. Hence, superficial excision of the lesion followed by skin grafting should be done.

  Eventhough leukoplakia is irreversible, **Isoretinoin** (13-cis-retinoic acid) can reverse some cases of leukoplakia and possibly reduce the development of squamous cell carcinoma.

2. **Erythroplakia** is a red, velvety lesion with incidence of malignancy around 15% (more malignant than leukoplakia).

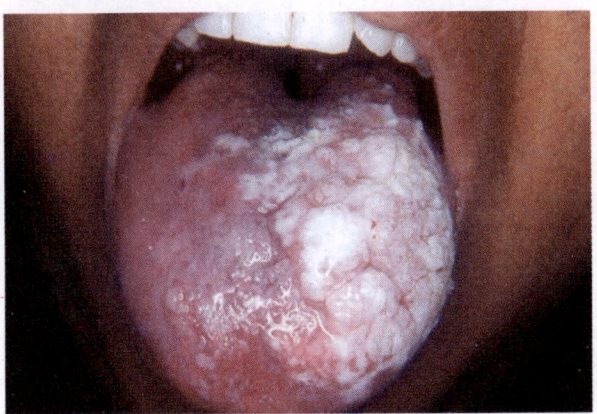

Fig. 17.1 Leukoplakia of the tongue

3. **Submucous fibrosis**

- This is supposedly due to hypersensitivity reaction to chillies, camphor, tobacco or due to vitamin deficiencies.
- Initially it produces ulceration of mucosa of the cheek. These ulcers heal resulting in a dense submucous fibrosis, which appear clinically firm to hard. It can affect the tongue also.
- Chances of malignancy is around 10-15%
- It is treated by excision with reconstruction

4. **Papilloma of the tongue or cheek**

5. **Chronic hyperplastic Candidiasis**

6. **Syphilitic glossitis** : Tertiary syphilis produces chronic superficial glossitis which can lead to carcinoma of the tongue. However, it is rare nowadays.

7. **Discoid lupus erythematosis**.

8. **Dyskeratosis congenita**.

AMERICAN JOINT COMMITTEE STAGING SYSTEM - TNM STAGING (Key Box. 17.2)

PRIMARY TUMOUR (T)

- T_0 : No evidence of primary tumour
- T_{is} : Carcinoma in situ
- T_1 : ≤ 2 cm,
- T2 : >2cm and ≤ 4 cm
- T_3 : > 4 cm
- T_4 : Any cancer invading adjacent structures like cartilage cortical bone, deep (extrinsic) muscles of the tongue, skin or soft tissue of the neck.

Key Box 17.2	
STAGE GROUPING	
Stage I	T1, N0, M0
Stage II	T2, N0, M0
Stage III	T3, N0, M0
	TI-3, N1, M0
Stage IV	T4, N0, M0 ,
	T1, N2-3, M0
	T, N, M1

---

1. 18 year old girl, nonsmoker, nonalcoholic, with good oral hygiene had carcinoma tongue, What was the cause ?

CERVICAL LYMPH NODES (N)

- N_x : Nodes cannot be assessed
- N_0 : No lymph node metastasis
- N_1 : Single positive ipsilateral node less than or equal to 3 cm in diameter
- N_{2A} : Single positive ipsilateral node more than 3 cm but less than or equal to 6 cm..
- N_{2B} : Multiple ipsilateral nodes but all less than 6 cm.
- N_{2c} : Bilateral or contralateral lymph nodes but all less than 6 cm.
- $N3$: Lymph node more than 6 cm.

DISTANT METASTASIS (M)

- M_0: No distant metastasis
- M_1 : Distant metastasis present

GENERAL PRINCIPLES IN THE TREATMENT OF ORAL CANCER

AIM OF THE TREATMENT

1. **Cure of the patient** : Cure of the cancer if possible with wide excision of the tumour which includes removal of the tumour with 2 cms of the normal tissues with or without bone.

2. **Palliation**: If cure is not possible, palliation should be attempted by surgery or radiotherapy.

3. **Preservation of function** such as swallowing, speech, vision, etc.

4. **Cosmetic function**: Following wide excision to maintain the cosmetic function reconstruction with myocutaneous/osteomyocutaneous flap to be done.

5. **Lymph nodes** are treated by radical neck dissection or curative radiotherapy (RT).

6. To achieve **minimal mortality and morbidity**.

7. Treatment of advanced tumours - T3 and T4 lesions:

- These are managed by combination of surgery with postoperative RT. **Surgery is the principle therapeutic modality of the treatment usually followed by post-operative radiotherapy.** The treatment depends upon general condition of the patient, risks of anaesthesia, adequate intensive care management, etc. Chemotherapy also has been tried before surgery or after surgery. However, response rate is improved but it has not affected the survival.

- **The flowchart showing the treatment of primary tumour and metastasis is given in Fig. 17.2.**

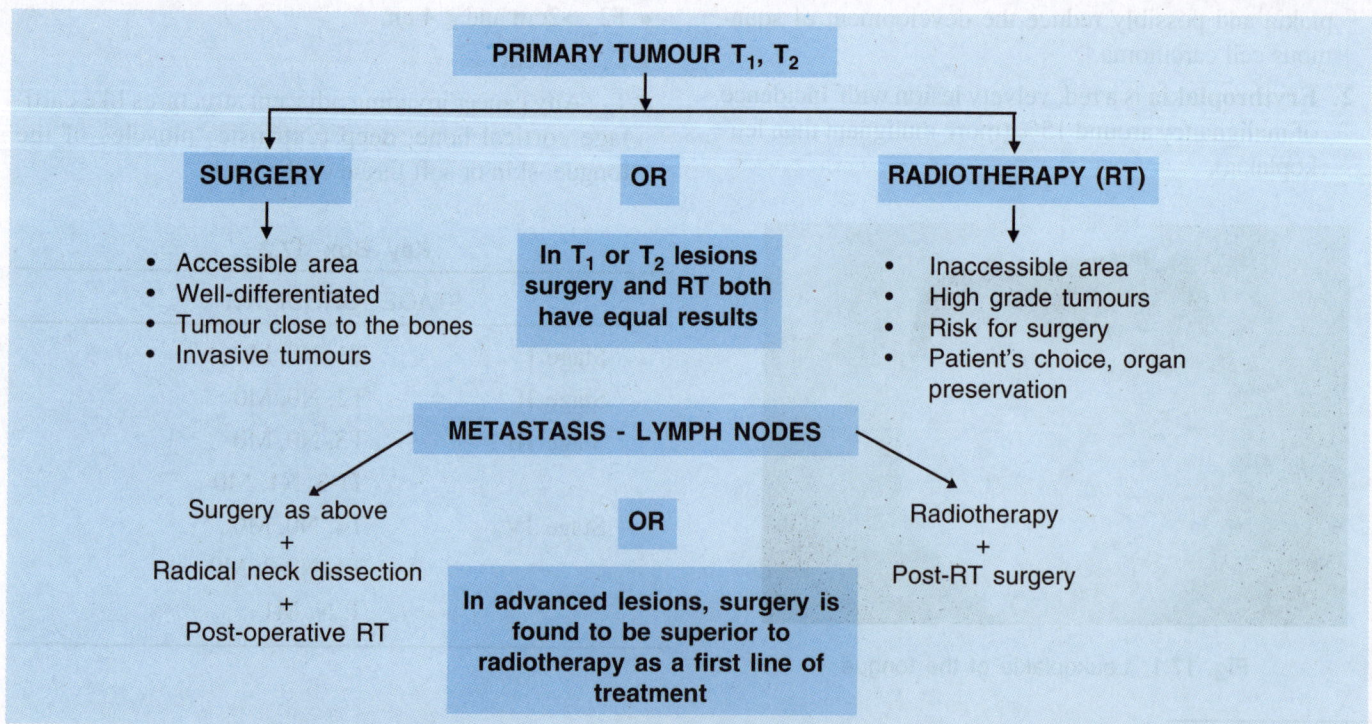

Fig. 17.2 Flowchart showing the treatment of primary tumour and metastasis

ROLE OF CHEMOTHERAPY IN HEAD AND NECK CANCERS

- The most benefit has been in the treatment of laryngeal and nasopharyngeal carcinomas.

- **Cisplatin** is clearly the most effective drug. Other drugs such as carboplatin, 5-flurouracil (5-FU) bleomycin, gemcitabine etc. are also used.

- **Induction chemotherapy**: In advanced cases, chemotherapy is given before surgery or RT. In more than 80% of cases, tumour regression can occur.

- **Concurrent chemoradiotherapy** (CCRT): It improves both local and regional control, specially in those patients with high risk cancers.

  Examples: Locally advanced cancers of the oral cavity, larynx, oropharynx etc. Drug used in CCRT can be high dose cisplatin - 100mg/m^2 IV for 3 cycles every 21 days concomitantly with RT. (For other dosage, kindly refer oncology manual). Side effects include severe mucositis, xerostomia. Gastrostomy may be necessary.

RADIOTHERAPY (Key Box 17.4)

- Irradiation of the oral cancers achieves a cure in about 80-90% of patients. It preserves anatomical part and also preserves the function.

- The dose of RT : 6500-7500 cGy units is required to eradicate squamous cell carcinoma of head and neck. It is usually given in the daily dose of 180-200 cGy units.

- Radiotherapy is given in T_1 and T_2 lesions as first line of treatment and postoperatively in T_3 and T_4 lesions after surgery.

Key Box 17.4

RT: ADVANTAGES

- Easy, safe with minimal mortality
- Preservation of an organ
- Function of the part is preserved
- Cure rate is around 80 to 90%
- First line in early cases

RT: DISADVANTAGES

- Long stay in the hospital
- Tumour cure cannot be assesed by pathology
- Soft tissue fibrosis resulting in ankylostomia
- Adverse effects on skin, loss of hair, mucositis of oral cavity, xerostomia, etc

---

ROLE OF SURGERY (Key Box 17.5)

- Surgery is done in all stages of oral cancers. It may be in the form of wide excision or wide excision with removal of the bone (Composite resection). In advanced stages it may be a palliative surgery such as excision of a fungating, ulcerating, bleeding mass. Surgery is also done for the lymph nodes in the form of radical neck dissection (RND), or modified RND.

- The pectoralis major myocutaneous flap (PMMC Flap): It is the most widely used flap for the reconstruction of oral cancers.

Key Box 17.5

SURGERY: ADVANTAGES

- It removes a fungating, ulcerating, bleeding lesion
- It relieves the pain
- The specimen is available for histopathological examination for the cancer clearance
- 80-90% cure is possible

SURGERY: DISADVANTAGES

- Loss of an organ-total glossectomy
- Functional and cosmetic disability
- Significant morbidity
- Mortality-8-10%

CARCINOMA OF CHEEK

Carcinoma of the cheek is very common in India due to the habit of keeping the **tobacco quid** in the cheek pouch.

PATHOLOGICAL TYPES

1. A **non-healing** ulcer, with slough in the centre of the lesion
2. An **exophytic growth**, or a proliferative growth verrucous carcinoma
3. An **infiltrative lesion** slowly involves the adjacent structures like tongue, mandible, floor of the mouth, skin, etc.

CLINICAL FEATURES

1. A **non-healing ulcer** or cauliflower like growth. Verrucous carcinoma is an exophytic growth.

2. **Edges are everted** (Fig. 17.3) with induration at the base as well as at the edge. **Induration** clinically presents as a hard feeling. Pathologically, it is due to fibrosis, caused by malignancy (carcinomatous fibrosis). It is a diagnostic feature of a squamous cell carcinoma. Possibly, it is a host reaction indicating a good immunity. Due to fibrosis, some lymphatics get obliterated. This delays spread of the disease thereby improving the prognosis.

• Proliferative lesions are often verrucous carcinoma (Key Box 17.6).

Key Box 17.6

PECULIARITIES OF VERRUCOUS CARCINOMA

• Very slow growing
• Growth is exophytic (than infiltrative)
• Rarely spreads by lymphatics
• Well-differentiated carcinoma
• Surgery is the treatment of choice

---

3. Ulcer **bleeds on touch**. Due to secondary infection most of the oral cancers are tender to touch.

4. **Fixity** to the underlying structures such as mandible may be present.

5. **Surrounding area** may also show **induration**.

6. Evidence of **leukoplakia** may be present in the oral cavity.

7. **Trismus** is due to involvement of pterygoid muscles and masseter. This occurs when carcinoma cheek **extends into the retromolar trigone**. Trismus can also be due to soft tissue fibrosis caused by radiation.

8. **Halitosis** is very characteristic.

9. Assessment of fixity to mandible : Severe pain over the jaw indicates periostitis.

• **Bidigital palpation of mandible** is done "by examining with index finger on the outer aspect of the mandible and the thumb on the under surface of the mandible. This test should be done on the opposite side first. Only then, the thickening of the mandible can be appreciated.

SPREAD

1. **Local spread** : Once it involves the entire thickness of the cheek it results in oro-cutaneous fistula (Fig. 17.4 and 17.5). Involvement of mandible results in sinus.

2. **Lymphatic spread** : Submandibular nodes and upper deep cervical nodes get enlarged (Level I and Level II). In 50% of the cases lymph node enlargement is due to infection and remaining 50% it is due to metastasis. Metastatic deposits are hard in consistency, indurated and with or without fixity.

3. **Blood spread** is very rare and it occurs late.

INVESTIGATIONS

1. **Wedge biopsy from the edge of the ulcer** is taken because of the following reasons:

• Tumour cells are concentrated more in the growing edge.

• Comparison with the normal tissues is possible.

• Centre has slough.

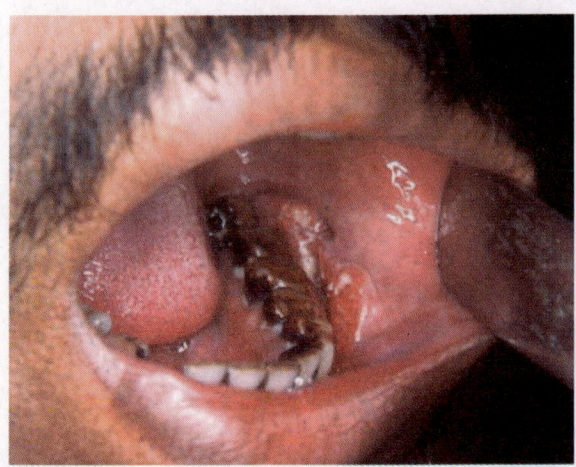

Fig. 17.3 Carcinoma alveolar margin

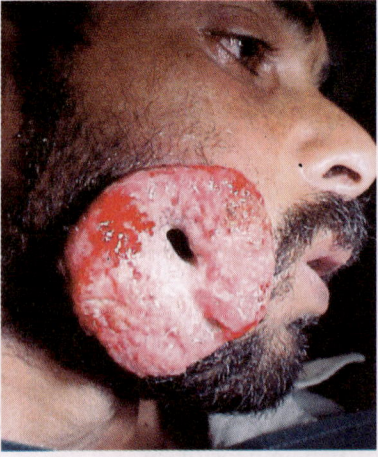

Fig. 17.4 Carcinoma cheek with oro-cutaneous fistula

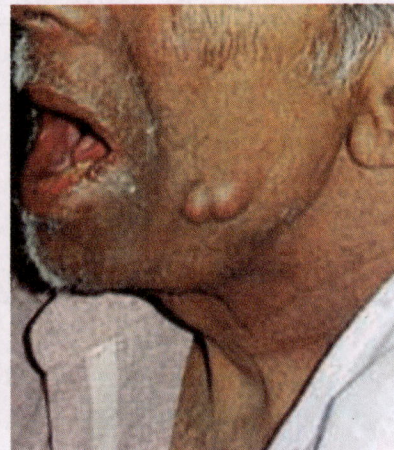

Fig. 17.5 Carcinoma cheek with infiltration into the skin

Histopathological **report** is squamous cell carcinoma and in majority of the cases it is well differentiated.

2. **Orthopantomography**: X-ray of mandible to rule out mandibular involvement

3. **Chest X-ray** to detect inhalation pneumonia

4. **FNAC** of the lymph node

TREATMENT OF CARCINOMA CHEEK

EARLY DISEASE (Key Box. 17.7)

Surgery

1. A small **superficial ulcer** (T_1, T_2) is treated by wide excision followed by split skin graft (SSG).

2. A small **infiltrative ulcer** is treated by wide excision followed by a flap reconstruction. Following flaps can be used.

- **In males,** forehead flap based on anterior branch of superficial temporal artery can be used. Flap is raised, an incision is made above zygoma, flap is brought inside the cheek and sutured to cheek mucosa. After 3-4 weeks, the proximal portion of flap is returned to its original place, after dividing it. This is called as return of the flap (Fig. 17.6).

- In females, deltopectoral flap based on perforating branches of internal mammary artery is used, which gives better cosmetic appearance (Fig. 17.7).

> *Both these flaps have been replaced by pectoralis major myocutaneous flap now (PMMC flap).*

Radiotherapy : As mentioned earlier, early lesions can be managed with radiotherapy.

Key Box 17.7
EARLY CARCINOMA CHEEK
• T_1, T_2 lesions – Surgery/RT
• T_1 lesion and near commissure – RT
• T_2 – Exophytic and superficial – RT
• T_2 – Deep – Surgery is better
• Early disease – No nodes – Surgery is better – No other treatment is necessary.
• Early disease – Positive lymphnodes – **Same modality to be used for primary and secondary**.

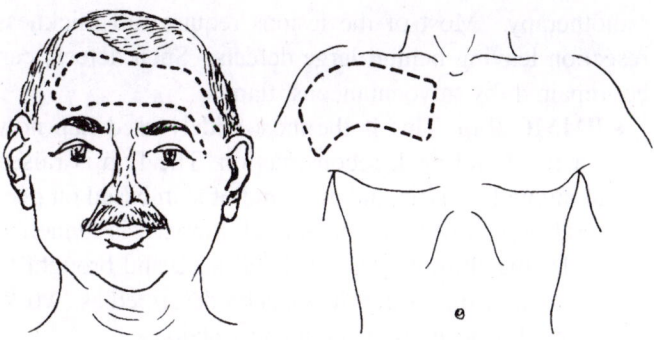

Fig. 17.6 and 17.7 Forehead and Deltopectoral flap

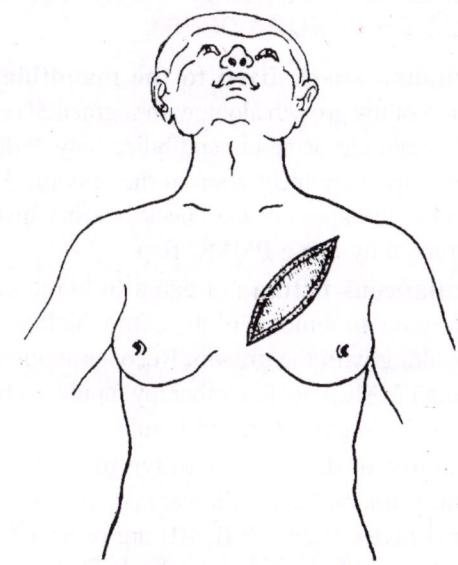

Fig. 17.8 PMMC Flap

Indications for radiotherapy

1. Patient not willing for surgery
2. Patient not fit for surgery
3. T_1 and T_2 lesions
4. Lesion near the commisure

Types

1. **External radiotherapy** Large total dose of 6000-8000 cGy units are given; 200 cGy units/day.

2. **Interstitial radiotherapy** is indicated in infiltrative small lesions. Caesium 137 or Iridium wires are placed within the tumour. Advantage of this method is minimal tissue reaction.

ADVANCED CARCINOMA CHEEK

Surgery : T_3 and T_4 lesions require surgery as the main modality of the treatment followed by post-operative radiotherapy. Most of the lesions require full thickness resection leaving behind large defects. Such defects can be repaired by myocutaneous flap.

- **PMMC flap**: This is the most widely used flap now for head and neck reconstruction. The flap is raised along with muscle and an island of skin based on pectoral branch of thoracoacromial artery. It is tunnelled under the skin of chest wall and neck and brought to the area of the defect. It has been described as 'work-horse' for head and neck reconstruction.

EXAMPLES OF VARIOUS SURGERY FOR ADVANCED CARCINOMA CHEEK

1. **Carcinoma cheek fixed to the mandible**: Wide excision of the growth along with segmental resection of the mandible or hemimandibulectomy is done depending upon the infiltration of the tumour. Very often whole thickness of the cheek is lost which is reconstructed by using PMMC flap.

2. **Orocutaneous fistula** is treated by wide excision which refers to removal of the entire thickness of the cheek along with the growth. Reconstruction is done by using PMMC flap. Radiotherapy should not be given as it results in persistence of fistula.

3. **Carcinoma of the cheek with lymph nodes**: Along with the primary, submandibular nodes and upper deep cervical nodes (Level I, II, III) are removed, along with submandibular salivary gland. This is called as supraomohyoid block dissection. If surgery has been used to treat the primary, the lymph nodes also should be treated by surgery in the form of neck dissection.

4. **Carcinoma of cheek with fixed lymph nodes: Both primary lesion and lymph nodes should be treated by radiotherapy** and reassessment done after 3-4 weeks. If residual glands persist or if the glands become mobile, neck dissection can be done at a later date. Fixity to internal jugular vein, sternocleido mastoid muscle are not contraindications for radical block dissection. Those structures can be removed. However, when the lymph nodes are fixed to the carotid artery, radiotherapy is preferred.

Prophylactic neck dissection

- It is advocated in T_3 and T_4 lesions irrespective of nodal status. This amounts to minimal of supraomohyoid neck dissection with removal of Level I, II and III lymphnodes. It has shown survival benefits.

PATHOLOGICAL TYPES

1. Non-healing ulcer, commonly on lateral border of tongue in 60% of cases, with slough (Fig. 17.10)

2. A proliferative growth, with everted edge

3. Frozen tongue or indurated variety (Fig. 17.11)
   - In this variety, there is maximum induration and sometimes it is more than the size of tumour. The tongue is converted into a hard woody "mass".

4. Fissure variety: The tongue is indurated with deep fissure.

CLINICAL PRESENTATION

1. A bleeding ulcer

2. Pain in the tongue is due to involvement of lingual nerve. In such cases, pain from the tongue can be referred to the ear and lower temporal region[1].

3. **Ankyloglossia** is restricted mobility of the tongue. It is due to infiltration of the floor of the mouth or mandible, or due to an advanced lesion.

4. **Dysarticulation** – difficulty in talking is due to inability of the tongue to move freely.

5. **Dysphagia** is a common presentation from carcinoma of posterior 1/3 (in 20% cases). Elderly gentleman sitting in the out-patient department spitting blood-stained saliva is suggestive of carcinoma posterior 1/3 of the tongue.

6. **Foetor oris** is due to infected necrotic growth.

7. **Bilateral massive enlargement** of lower deep cervical nodes in an elderly patient is suggestive of carcinoma of posterior 1/3. The patient may not be aware of growth at all (Fig. 17.12).
   - **Please note** : Tongue cancers tend to be more rapid in their onset than other cancers in the oral cavity. Compared with other cancers within the oral cavity tongue cancers have greater potential of lymph node metastasis.

CLINICAL EXAMINATION

1. Inspection and palpation of the growth or the ulcer should be described in the same manner as that of carcinoma cheek. Typically, the ulcer bleeds on touch

---

1. Auriculotemporal nerve and lingual nerve are posterior branches of mandibular division of trigeminal nerve.

with central slough. The edge, base and surrounding area are indurated. The carcinoma of the tongue and carcinoma of the penis are the two places in the body wherein induration can be much more extensive than the primary growth or an ulcer. In some cases, induration may be the only finding.

2. Digital palpation of posterior 1/3 of tongue should be done with a glove.

3. Test for mobility of the tongue
   - Forward protrusion-genioglossus. This is the muscle commonly involved.
   - Backward movement-styloglossus
   - Elevation-palatoglossus
   - Depression-hyoglossus

All these muscles are supplied by hypoglossal nerve except palatoglossus which is supplied by glosso-pharyngeal nerve.

4. Bidigital palpation of the mandible should be done which may show thickening.

LYMPHATIC SPREAD (Fig. 17.9)

1. **Apical vessels** drain the tip of the tongue into submental lymph nodes, bilaterally.

2. **Lateral vessels** drain into submandibular lymph nodes, from here to the lower deep cervical lymph nodes jugulo-omohyoid nodes – Level IV.

3. **Central vessels** drain into submandibular nodes

4. **Basal vessels** drain the posterior 1/3 of the tongue. There is criss-crossing of the lymphatics on both sides. Hence, they drain into bilateral lower deep cervical lymph nodes. (Some lymphatics on their way to the nodes, pass through the mandible which explains the frequent involvement of mandible in carcinoma tongue. This is a debatable issue now.)
   - In 50% of cases, the lymph nodes enlargement is due to secondary infection. Such nodes are tender and firm, respond to antibiotics. In remaining cases, they are hard and fixed and hence, significant.

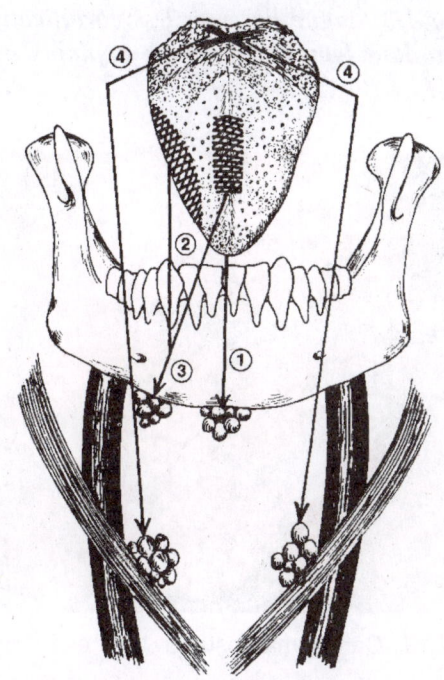
Fig. 17.9 Lymphatic drainage of the tongue - refer text for numbers

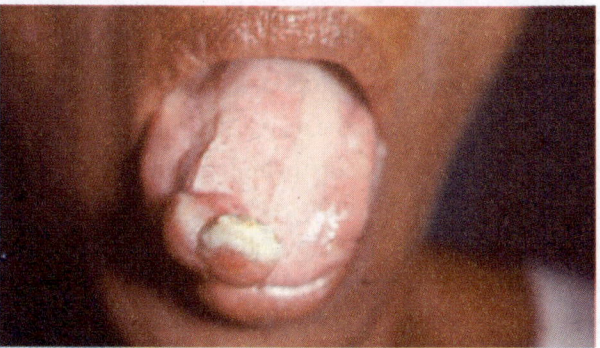
Fig. 17.11 Frozen tongue

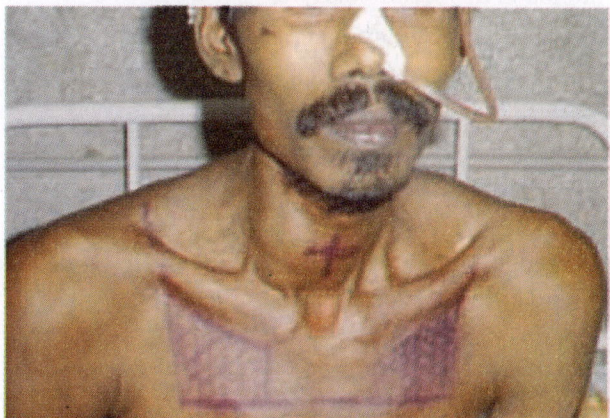
Fig. 17.12 Carcinoma tongue with absolute dysphagia, fixed lymph nodes in the neck and involvement of mediastinal lymph nodes - receiving radiotherapy

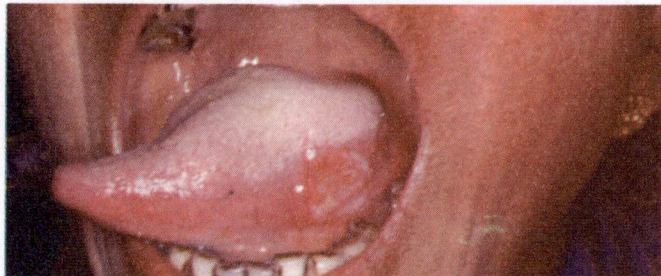
Fig. 17.10 Carcinoma lateral border- the most common site

Posterior 1/3 tongue has very less cornification but has abundant lymphatics which explains massive nodes. (Key Box 17.8)

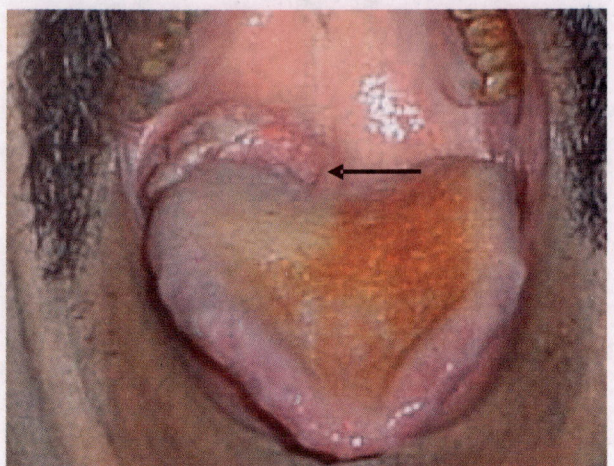

Fig. 17.13 Carcinoma posterior 1/3 - easily missed

Key Box 17.8

CARCINOMA POSTERIOR 1/3

- It presents as **dysphagia** or **change of voice**
- **Easily missed** in a clinical examination
- **Palpation** will give the diagnosis-**Induration**
- It is one of the **occult primaries** for lymph node secondaries in the neck.
- **Criss crossing** of the lymphatics explain bilateral lymph nodes in the neck.
- **Blood spread** is more common.
- Prognosis is bad because **well differentiated** carcinoma in this location is rare.
- **Lymphoepithelioma** can occur.
- **Transitional cell carcinoma (rare)** with undifferentiated epithelial cells can also occur.

INVESTIGATIONS

1. **Wedge biopsy from edge of the ulcer** can be taken under local anaesthesia. In cases of proliferative growths, punch biopsy is recommended. In cases of growth arising from posterior 1/3 of the tongue, biopsy can be taken under general anaesthesia. It also provides an opportunity to examine in detail the posterior spread of the disease into tonsils, pharynx, etc.

2. **Orthopantomogram** : X-ray of the mandible can demonstrate an irregular defect due to invasion, erosion or pathological fracture.

3. Chest X-ray is taken to rule out aspiration or inhalation pneumonia.

4. Routine investigations such as complete blood picture, fasting and postprandial sugar estimation to rule out diabetes, electrocardiography to assess cardiovascular function, should be done.

TREATMENT

- Carcinoma of the tongue is managed similar to a cancer in the oral cavity. However, preserving the function of the tongue, widespread disease in the posterior one-third tumours, general health of patient (elderly with bad bronchopneumonia) may decide the treatment in favour of radiotherapy. However, results of surgery or radiotherapy for early carcinoma of tongue are equivalent.

Various types of surgery

1. **Carcinoma in situ:** This type is uncommon in our country. Wide excision with 1 cm margin and a depth of 1 cm is sufficient. The reconstruction of the tongue is not necessary.

2. **Partial glossectomy** is indicated when the lesion is less than 2 cm (T_1) and confined to the lateral border of the tongue. About 1/3 of the anterior 2/3 of the tongue is removed. The wide excision should include at least 2 cm of tissue away from the palpable indurated edge of the tumour (Fig. 17.14).

   - Alternatively, radiotherapy can be given.

3. **Hemiglossectomy** refers to removal of around 50% of the tongue. This is indicated in a radio-residual tumour, radio-recurrent tumour or where radiotherapy facilities are not available (Fig. 17.15). Reconstruction of the tongue can be done by using PMMC flap.

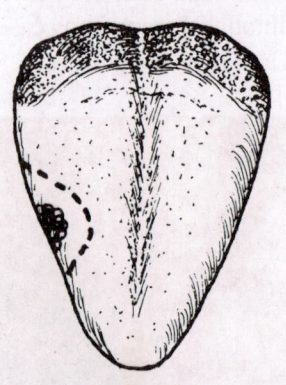 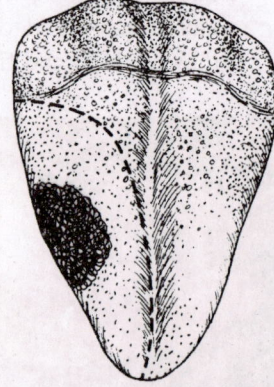

Fig.17.14 Partial glossectomy   **Fig. 17.15 Hemiglossectomy**

4. **Total glossectomy**: Indications are similar to those mentioned above. However, very extensive growths involving the entire tongue are given radiotherapy initially, to reduce the size of the tumour. Surgery can then be undertaken. Total glossectomy carries significant mortality and morbidity.

5. **Commando's operation**: This is indicated when carcinoma of tongue is fixed to the mandible with infiltration of the floor of the mouth. Hemiglossectomy with hemimandibulectomy and removal of the floor of the mouth and radical neck dissection is described as Commando's operation. (Key Box 17.9).

   - However, in a few selected cases, removal of the **hemimandible is not necessary**. Growths which are close to the margin of the mandible without infiltration (confirmed by X-ray) needs to be treated by **marginal excision**. Carcinoma of the tongue with involvement of only a small portion of mandible can be managed by **segmental excision**. Advantage of this method is that it is not only cosmetic but also **preserves the function of the tongue by preserving genioglossus**. Hence, the tongue may not fall backwards after surgery.

TREATMENT OF LYMPH NODES

Lymph node metastasis in the neck from squamous cell carcinoma can be managed both by surgery as well as radiotherapy. Radiotherapy can be given in all stages of secondaries in the neck. However, its main indication is a large primary tumour with neck nodes. In such situations both the primary and secondary can be managed with radiotherapy alone which carries minimal morbidity and mortality.

Key Box 17.9

STRUCTURES REMOVED IN RADICAL BLOCK DISSECTION OF THE NECK

- The fat, fascia, lymphatics from midline to the anterior border of trapezius, from mandible to clavicle below.
- The lymph nodes - submental, submandibular, upper and lower deep cervical nodes, posterior group of nodes (Level I – V).
- Submandibular salivary gland, sternomastoid
- Internal Jugular Vein (IJV)
- Spinal accessory nerve

- If the general condition of the patient is good and the lymph nodes are hard and mobile, hemiglossectomy with excision of the floor of the mouth with radical dissection of the neck is done (commando's operation).
- If radical neck dissection has to be done on both sides, the IJV should be preserved at least on one side to prevent cerebral oedema. In such cases, radiotherapy is a very good alternative.

CAUSES OF DEATH IN CARCINOMA TONGUE

1. Recurrent aspirational pneumonia
2. Gross local recurrence, fungation, ulceration, cachexia.
3. Uncontrolled haemorrhage from growth: In such cases ligation of external carotid artery above superior thyroid branch should be done (Fig. 17.18). If ligature is applied below the origin of superior thyroid artery it results in eddying currents and thrombus at bifurcation of common carotid artery.

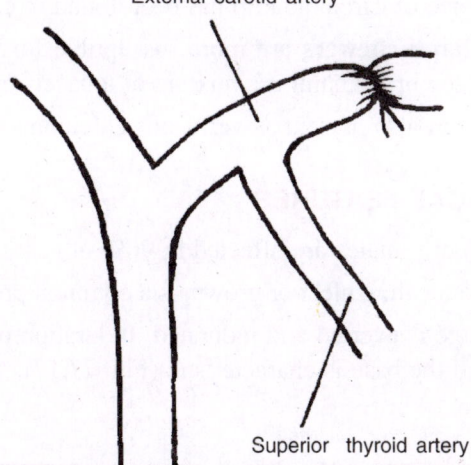

External carotid artery

Superior thyroid artery

Fig. 17.16 Ligation of external carotid artery

CARCINOMA OF THE LIP

- Incidence of carcinoma of the lip is about 10 to 12%. It is common in the western, elderly, white people, specially those exposed to sunlight. The actinic rays produces actinic cheilitis-inflammation of lip, especially lower lip, which over a period of years turns into malignancy.
- Since this is common in agriculturists, who are constantly exposed to sunlight, it is called as **Countryman's lip.** (Key Box 17.10)
- Carcinoma lip includes - growth arising from vermilion surfaces and mucosa.

Key Box 17.10

COUNTRYMAN'S LIP

SUNLIGHT
↓
ACTINIC RAYS
↓
CHEILITIS
↓
ERYTHEMA
↓
CRACKS

- **Leukoplakia** is also responsible for squamous cell carcinoma. Smoking, spirits. spices are the common precipitating factors.
- **Genetic factors** may also play a role. Negroes are less susceptible. On the other hand, increased incidence of carcinoma lip has been found in caucasians.
- **Khaini chewers** are more susceptible for carcinoma of the lip. (Khaini is a mixture of tobacco and lime.)
- It can also present as verrucous carcinoma of lip.

CLINICAL FEATURES

- Elderly males are affected in 90% of cases.
- Nonhealing ulcer or growth is a common presentation.
- Edge is everted and indurated. Induration of the edge and the base is characteristic (Fig. 17.17).

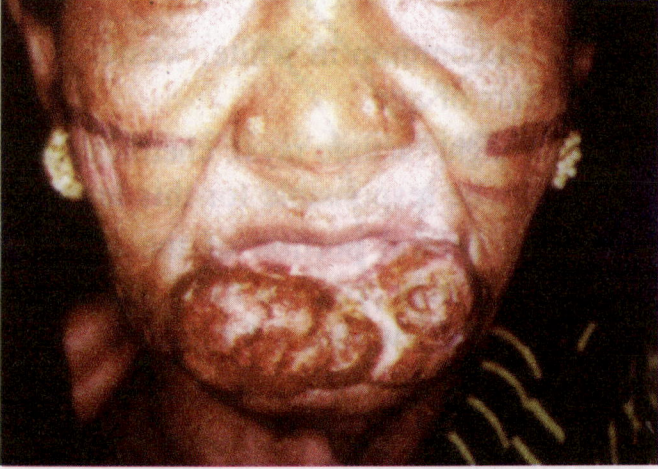

Fig. 17.17 Advanced carcinoma lip - a proliferative lesion, treated with radiation

- Floor is covered with slough. Bleeding spots may be visible.
- Mobility: Ulcer or the growth moves with the lip, it is fixed to the subcutaneous structures of the lip.
- The entire upper lip, lateral portions of lower lip drain into upper deep cervical nodes. Central portion of lower lip drains to submental nodes and submandibular nodes. Like elsewhere in the oral cavity, in 50% of the cases. nodes are enlarged due to secondary infections. In remaining 50% of the cases, they are enlarged due to metastasis. Such nodes are hard, with or without fixity. Blood spread is uncommon.

DIFFERENTIAL DIAGNOSIS (Key Box 17.11)

- In a classical case of carcinoma of the lip with everted edges, with induration there is no differential diagnosis. However, following are the few conditions to be remembered.

1. Keratoacanthoma

- It is a cutaneous tumour arising from hair follicles on the lips.
- It is common in white, western, males between 50-70 years of age.
- Sunlight (actinic rays), chemical carcinogen, viral factors may be responsible for this lesion.
- The central portion of the nodule may ulcerate. The lesion may progress for 6 weeks and may resolve spontaneously within 4-6 months.

2. Ectopic salivary gland tumour

- The lip is one of the common sites of malignant salivary gland tumours. This presents with submucous nodules which slowly grow and ulcerate and may mimic squamous cell carcinoma.
- They are also indurated lesions.
- However, the characteristic everted edge may not be seen.
- These are adenocarcinomas which are treated by surgery.

Key Box 17.11

DIFFERENTIAL DIAGNOSIS OF CARCINOMA LIP

- Keratoacanthoma
- Ectopic salivary gland tumour
- Pyogenic granuloma
- Leukoplakia

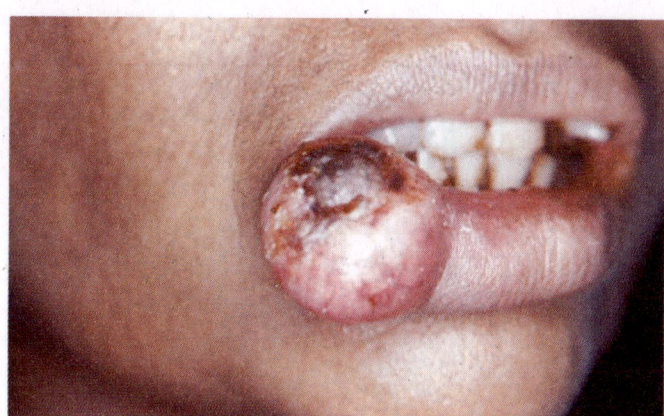

Fig. 17.18 This lesion was diagnosed as carcinoma lip. However, it did not have everted edges. It was indurated. Biopsy reported as ectopic salivary gland tumour

3. Pyogenic granuloma

- Recurrent infections or trauma produces a polypoidal mass with significant bleeding.
- It is rich in granulation tissue and resembles a polyp.
- It is devoid of epithelium
- Histologically, it is a capillary haemangioma
- Absence of induration gives the diagnosis

4. Leukoplakia

- A slow developing leukoplakia presents as whitish nodule or an ulcer. However, biopsy confirms the diagnosis.

TREATMENT

- Surgery and radiotherapy are the two modalities available for the treatment of carcinoma of the lip.

Surgery

- T1 and T2 lesions can be excised followed by direct suturing without much functional problems. This is described as "V" excision which includes removal of growth with 1 cm healthy margin. Care should be taken to excise the full thickness of the lip.
- When removal of more than 1/3 of the lip is required flap reconstruction may be necessary. The primary goal in lip reconstruction surgery is oral competence.

Examples :

1. Abbe flap : Based on upper labial artery – a pedicled flap is rotated down and sutured to the defect at the lower lip.

2. Estlander's flap : Wedge-shaped flap is used to reconstruct carcinoma of lower lip, when it involves the angle.

- **Larger tumours** : T3 and T4 lesions are irradiated first. If the tumour persists after radiotherapy excision of the entire lip may be necessary followed by PMMC flap reconstruction.
- Significant lymph nodes can be removed along with the primary tumour - **supraomohyoid block dissection**.

Radiotherapy

- It is indicated in all stages of carcinoma of the lip. Radiotherapy produces tumour necrosis resulting in a slow healing rate. Treatment lasts for several weeks and it delays the wound healing. Elderly patients who are not fit for surgery and carcinoma lip with fixed nodes are treated by irradiation.
- Commissure involvement is treated with RT than surgery.
- Dose: 4000-6000 centigray (cGy) units

CARCINOMA MAXILLARY ANTRUM

It is rare in western countries but common in Asia. The workers in the furniture industries, chromic and the nickel industries are more prone for the development of carcinoma maxillary antrum.

CLINICAL PRESENTATION (Table 17.1)

1. Growth originating on the **floor of antrum** may result in bulge of the hard palate. This results in pain in the teeth and they may become loose.
2. When **medial wall** is involved, nasal obstruction and epiphora occurs due to obstruction of the lacrimal duct. Bleeding from the nose can also occur, if there is ulceration.
3. If **anterolateral wall** is involved, asymmetry of the face results in pain in the cheek. Anaesthesia over the skin of the cheek including upper lip results due to involvement of infraorbital nerve, a branch of maxillary division of the trigeminal nerve.
4. If the **roof** is invaded proptosis and diplopia occurs.
5. Posterior extension of the growth is difficult to assess clinically. When it involves the pterygoid muscles, it results in trismus. Paraesthesia over the cheek, gums, lower lip, post nasal discharge are the other features of these tumours. They carry poor prognosis because of late presentation.

Table 17.1

CLINICAL EXAMINATION OF A CASE OF CARCINOMA MAXILLARY ANTRUM

• Palatine bulge	→	Growth in the floor
• Unilateral nasal obstruction (He is asked to breathe, closing the nostrils one by one)	→	Growth in the medial wall
• Asymmetry of the face	→	Growth expanding anteriorly superficial surface
• Change in the level and sharpness of inferior orbital margin, proptosis	→	Growth on the roof (orbital surface)
• Swelling (indurated) temporal region	→	Posterior extension into infratemporal region and then into temporal region.
• Hard, fixed or mobile submandibular nodes	→	Metastasis

LYMPHATIC SPREAD

About 50% of the tumours present with enlargement of submandibular lymph nodes and upper deep cervical lymph nodes - jugulodigastric nodes.

INVESTIGATIONS

1. **Computed tomography** (C.T. scan) can define a lesion, its extent, bony destruction, posterior extension, etc. - hence it is the first investigation of choice.

2. **Sinoscopy** : Fenestration will provide tissue for biopsy followed by curettage to reduce the tumour bulk and to drain necrotic contents outside.

TREATMENT

• **Radiotherapy is the main modality** of treatment in carcinoma maxillary antrum. Curative rate is around 70% in early cases. In advanced cases, radiotherapy is given first. This reduces the tumour bulk so that an unresectable lesion becomes resectable and maxillectomy can be done.

• Surgery can be done in the form of **total maxillectomy** when the growth involves entire maxilla or it is of **high grade** followed by postoperative radiotherapy.

• Tumours of the **lower half** of the antrum are treated by **partial maxillectomy**. It includes removal of the entire hard palate, the alveolus and medial wall of the antrum upto and including middle turbinate.

• Indications and contraindications for surgery and radiotherapy are in similar lines as discussed earlier in this chapter.

BENIGN LESIONS IN THE ORAL CAVITY

DIFFERENTIAL DIAGNOSIS OF ULCER IN THE TONGUE (Fig. 17.19, Key Box 17.12, 13)

1. **Aphthous ulcer**

   • Small, multiple, very painful ulcers, can occur at any age group, more common in females at the time of menstruation. These are called as minor aphthous ulcers.

   • When they are larger, deeper, painful, they are called as major aphthous ulcers.

   • They are due to viral infection. These ulcers are superficial ulcers with erythematous margin.

   • They subside within a few days. Temporary relief can be obtained by applying salicylate gel.

Key Box 17.12

PAINFUL ULCERS IN THE TONGUE

• Aphthous ulcers
• Dental ulcers
• Tubercular ulcers

Key Box 17.13

PAINLESS ULCERS IN THE TONGUE

• Carcinomatous ulcers
• Gummatous ulcers
• Systemic diseases

- +Vitamin B complex is usually given for the satisfaction of the patients.

2. Dental ulcer

- These ulcers occur due to broken tooth, sharp tooth, ill-fitting dentures, prosthesis, etc. They are very painful ulcers.
- Such ulcers are common on the lateral margin and they heal when the tooth is removed. This is an example of traumatic ulcer. It should not be confused with carcinomatous ulcer which commonly occurs on the lateral margin.

3. Tubercular ulcer of tongue

- Tuberculosis affects tip of the tongue. These ulcers are very painful with enlargement of regional nodes.
- It occurs in patients with fulminating pulmonary tuberculosis.
- Ulcers have undermined edges. These ulcers are sometimes multiple with serous discharge.

4. Gummatous ulcer

- Gumma is a complication of tertiary syphilis resulting in a firm swelling in the midline in the anterior 2/3 of the tongue. Induration is absent. Ulcer is non tender. Severe endarteritis obliterans results in the necrosis of gumma giving rise to gummatous ulcer. It has punched out edges and wash leather slough on the floor. Other sites of gumma include testis, palate, clavicle and liver. These ulcers are rare nowadays.

5. Systemic diseases

- Pemphigus

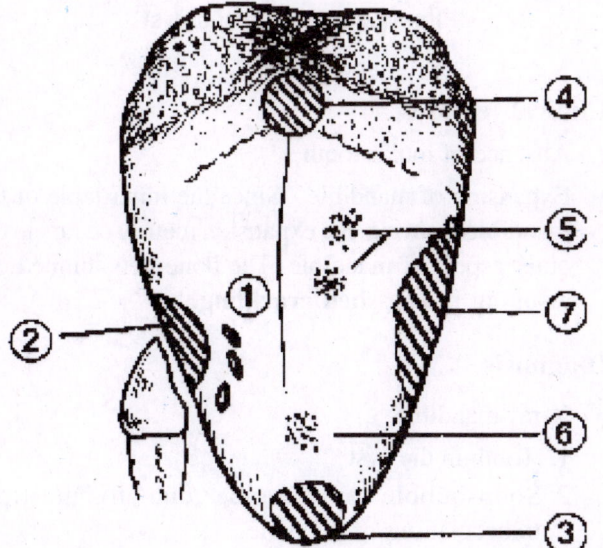

Fig. 17.19 Ulcers of the tongue - refer the text for numbers

- Systemic lupus erythematosis (SLE)
- Lichen planus

6. Post-pertussis ulcer

- It occurs in children due to repeated coughing. Typical location of the ulcer on the under surface of the tongue and on the frenulum clinches the diagnosis.

7. Carcinomatous ulcer

- Lateral margin
- Non-healing ulcer
- Everted edge
- Edge and base are indurated
- Bleeds on touch
- Fixity
- Significant lymph nodes in the neck

MACROGLOSSIA

- Diffuse painless enlargement of the tongue is described as macroglossia. It is a rare condition and can occur due to various causes.

1. **Lymphangioma**: In this condition, the tongue diffusely enlarges. Sometimes, it is a localised swelling. It may be associated with lymphangiomas elsewere in the body like cheek mucosa, lips etc. The tongue becomes larger, indurated and gives rise to severe discomfort to the patients. Due to repeated trauma, the surface becomes ulcerated. It is treated by injecting sclerosants like ethanolamine oleate, hypertonic saline, etc. Partial excision may be necessary in cases of large lymphangioma.

2. **Haemangioma**: Cavernous haemangiomas occur in the tongue, lips etc. It is present since birth but manifests during childhood. It presents with soft, cystic, fluctuant swelling, at times pulsatile. Trauma due to teeth or food results in bleeding. Haemangioma of the tongue is treated on the same lines as lymphangioma. It is much more difficult to excise it, especially a large haemangioma. Preoperative angiography and ligation of lingual artery on both sides is necessary.

3. **Neurofibroma**: It may be associated with Von Recklinghausen's disease. It is treated by hemiglossectomy.

4. **Muscular macroglossia**: This condition, though rare, is seen in cretins. The tongue is thickened and cannot be held in place. Hence, it protrudes outside. It is treated by partial excision.

SYPHILITIC LESIONS OF THE TONGUE

The tongue is involved in all stages of syphilis.

1. **Primary syphilis** : Primary chancre that occurs in the tongue is highly contagious. It affects the tip of the tongue. It produces a painful ulcer with large significant enlargement of regional lymph nodes.

2. **Secondary syphilis** produces white patch in the tongue, lips and on the anterior pillars of fauces. In the tongue, these are multiple which coalesce to form **snail track ulcers**. The ulcers heal with **fine tissue paper scar**. In some cases syphilitic organisms produce a flat, hypertrophied epithelium which is described as **condyloma.** This is called as **Hutchinson's wart.**

3. **Tertiary syphilis** : It produces gumma. Syphilis also produces **chronic superficial glossitis**, which is characterised by bald tongue with loss of papilla and fissured tongue. **It is a precancerous condition**.

ODONTOMES

- **Definition**: Odontomes are the cysts, malformations arising from epithelial or mesothelial elements of tooth resulting in swelling of the jaw. As a developmental anomaly, few epithelial cells proliferate, persisting as **epithelial debris of Mallasuez**.

DENTAL CYST: RADICULAR CYST/ PERIAPICAL CYST

Pathogenesis

- This arises from a normally erupted, chronically infected, pulpless caries tooth. The caries tooth produces a low grade, chronic inflammation which stimulates epithelial debris to proliferate. Later this brings about degeneration of epithelial and mesothelial cells resulting in a cyst within the maxilla.

Clinical features

- Common in women around 3rd-4th decade
- Commonly affects the upper jaw (maxilla)
- It present as a slow-growing swelling in the maxillary region resulting in deformity of the face.

Diagnosis

- Presence of caries tooth with expansion of maxilla
- X-ray – large, unilocular cyst in maxilla or orthopantomogram showing cyst in the mandible
- Aspiration of the cyst demonstrates cholesterol crystals

Treatment

- Excision of cyst with its epithelial lining through intra-oral approach. After excision of the epithelium the cyst wall should be curretted, followed by soft tissue 'push-in' to obliterate dead space.

DENTIGEROUS CYST-FOLLICULAR ODONTOME

- Common in lower jaw (mandible) in women 30-40 years (Fig. 17.20).

- It occurs in relation to unerupted, permanent, molar tooth, most commonly an upper or lower third molar tooth.

- This unerupted tooth constantly irritates the cells, produce degeneration of the cells resulting in a dentigerous cyst. The cyst is lined by squamous epithelium surrounded by connective tissue. Within the cyst, the tooth lies obliquely or sometimes is embedded in the wall of the cyst. As it grows further, the cyst displaces the teeth to which it is attached. Thus, the tooth is displaced deeper and deeper and prevented from eruption.

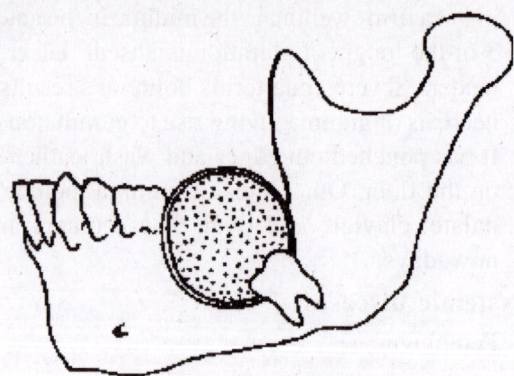

Fig. 17.20 Dentigerous cyst

Clinical features

- Absence of molar tooth

- Expansion of mandible - Since the inner table of the mandible is strong, the expansion mainly occurs in the outer aspect of mandible. The bone gets thinned out resulting in **egg-shell crackling.**

Diagnosis

- X-ray mandible
  1. Tooth in the cyst
  2. Soap-bubble appearance due to multiple trabeculations of the bone
  3. Radiolucent well-defined swelling

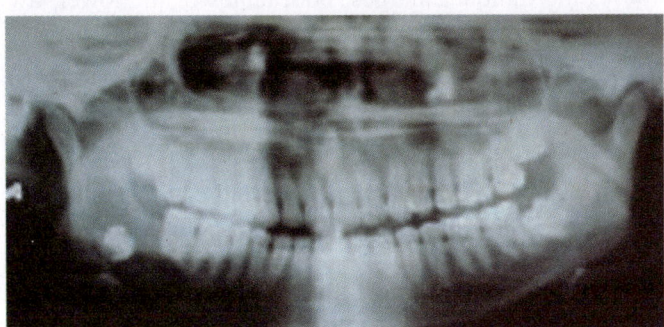

Fig. 17.21 Orthopantomogram showing unerupted tooth

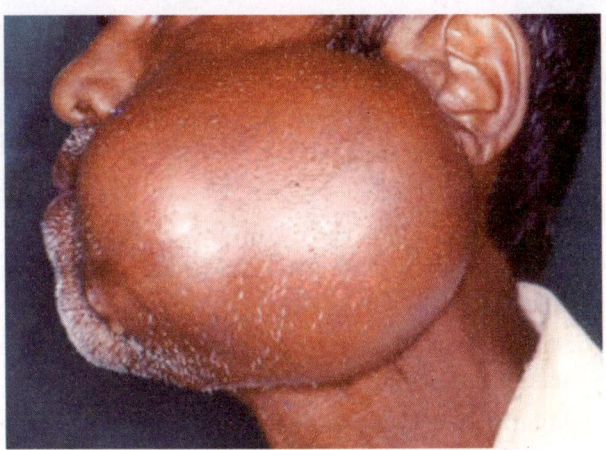

Fig. 17.22 Adamantinoma left jaw

Treatment

*   Small cyst - excision of the cyst by intraoral approach.
*   Large cysts - managed by marsupialisation.

ADAMANTINOMA (Fig. 17.22)

*   It is also called multilocular cystic disease, ameloblastoma, Eve's disease.
*   This tumour arises from ameloblasts (Enamel forming cells).
*   It is a benign tumour, very slow growing, behaves like a basal cell carcinoma. Inadequate treatment results in local recurrence and later metastasis, Hence, even though the tumour is benign, it has to be treated like malignant tumour.

Sites

*   **Mandible** is the most common site
*   **Tibia**-2nd common site. It can be explained by inclusion of abnormal embryonic epithelium.
*   **Pituitary** is another common site where adamantinoma can occur. **Both pituitary stalk and enamel arise from oral epithelium.**

Clinical features

*   Patients in 4th or 5th decades are commonly affected.
*   This is a slow growing jaw tumour in the region of angle of mandible and horizontal ramus of the mandible.
*   As tumour grows, it undergoes cystic degeneration resulting in multiple cystic spaces. Hence, it is called multilocular cystic disease.

*   As it grows it causes expansion of the outer table of the mandible and causes fracture mandible.
*   Patient may present with complaints of falling teeth.

Diagnosis

*   X-ray : A large cyst and small multiple cysts due to the trabeculations called honeycomb appearance.

Surgical treatment of adamantinoma

*   Even though it is **benign, simple currettage or enucleation may result in recurrence** and chances of recurrent adamantinoma turning into malignancy are high. Hence, wide excision with 1 cm of healthy normal tissue should be removed. It may amount to **segmental excision of the mandible or hemimandibulectomy** (Key Box 17.14).

Key Box 17.14
ADAMANTINOMA
<ul><li>Locally invasive solid tumour</li><li>Spreads within the medullary bone</li><li>Invades soft tissues</li><li>Should not fragment the tumour cells</li><li>Subperiosteal excision should not be done as it may result in recurrence</li><li>Incomplete excision results in recurrence and metastasis to the lung</li><li>Hence, even though it is a benign tumour it is treated by wide excision or hemimandibulectomy</li></ul>

DIFFERENTIAL DIAGNOSIS (see also Table 17.2)

1. Giant celled reparative granuloma (Jaffe tumour)

• It is a benign tumour which occurs due to haemorrhage within the bone marrow.

Pathology

• It affects antral part of maxilla or mandible causing enlargement of the jaw.

• Stroma is vascular consisting of thin-walled blood vessels, scanty collagen, connective tissue cells.

• Microscopic features mimic giant cell epulis or brown tumour of hyperparathyroidism.

Clinical features

• Unlike an adamantinoma, this tumour affects females in the age group of 10-25 years.

• Painless enlargement of jaw is the presenting feature. X-ray demonstrates radiolucent artery.

Treatment

• Calcitonin 0.5 mg (100 units) daily subcutaneous injection over a period of one year has been recommended as a first line of treatment. It has shown resolution of the tumour.

• Currettage is the surgical line of treatment.

2. Osteoclastoma

• This is a rare tumour seen in the lower jaw.

• Males between the age of 25-40 years are commonly affected

• Unlike adamantinoma, it is a rapid growing tumour.

• As the tumour enlarges, both tables of the lower jaw are thinned out.

• X-ray may show a large, radiolucent cyst with pseudotrabeculation.

• Even though benign, it is radiosensitive.

• However, recurrence can occur and can turn into malignancy like that of adamantinoma.

Comparison of common three odontomes are given in Table 17.2

EPULIS (Key Box 17.15)

• Epulis means "upon the gum." It refers to solid swelling situated on the gum.

• It arises from alveolar margin of the jaw.

• Very often patients presents with swelling on the gum which is painless.

Key Box 17.15	
EPULIS	
• Soft epulis	– Granulomatous
• Firm epulis	– Fibrous
	– Giant cell
• Hard epulis	– Carcinomatous
• Malignant epulis	– Carcinomatous
• Dangerous epulis	– Fibrosarcomatous

Table 17.2 Comparison of common three odontomes

	DENTAL CYST	DENTIGEROUS CYST	ADAMANTINOMA
1. Aetiology	Caries tooth	Unerupted tooth	True neoplasm-Ameloblasts
2. Site	Maxilla	Mandible	Mandible
3. Age	30-50 years	20-30 years	40-50 years
4. Palpation	Smooth, thin bone-eggshell crackling	Smooth, expansion of the outer table of mandible	Expansion of mandible in the 3rd molar region, cystic areas
5. X-ray	Radiolucent unilocular cyst	Radiolucent unilocular cyst with unerupted teeth	Large radiolucent area with fine honeycombing
6. Treatment	Subperiosteal excision	Subperiosteal excision	Wide excision even though benign
7. Spread	Does not occur	Does not occur	Local spread, recurrence, late spread to the lung are the features

Types (Fig. 17.23 & 17.24)

GRANULOMATOUS EPULIS

- Precipitating factors are – caries tooth, dentures, poor oral hygiene.
- It manifests as a mass of granulation tissue around the teeth on the gums. It is a soft to firm fleshy mass and bleeds on touch.
- Pregnancy epulis refers to this variety. (Gingivitis gravidarum)

FIBROUS EPULIS

- It is the commonest form-A simple fibroma arising from periodontal membrane, presents on the gum. It may undergo sarcomatous change. It is a firm polypoidal mass, slowly growing and nontender.

GIANT CELL EPULIS

- It is also called myeloid epulis.
- It is an osteoclastoma arising in the jaw. It presents as hyperaemic vascular, oedematous, soft to firm gums with indurated underlying mass due to expansion of the bone. It may ulcerate and result in haemorrhage. X-ray shows bone destruction with ridging of walls (pseudo-trabeculation).
- Small tumours are treated by currettage
- Large tumours are treated by radical excision.

CARCINOMATOUS EPULIS

- This is an epithelioma arising from mucous membrane of the alveolar margin.

- Typically, it presents as a nonhealing, painless ulcer. It slowly infiltrates the bone.
- Hard regional lymph nodes are due to metastasis.
- Treated by wide excision which includes removal of segment of the bone.

MEDIAN MENTAL SINUS

- This is a sinus in the midline just beneath the mentum.

Aetiopathogenesis

- It is produced by an apical abscess of lower incisors which penetrate buccal cortical plate below the origin of mentalis muscle. This muscle takes origin from labial surface of alveolar process just above the labial sulcus. Hence, pus discharges through a sinus in the centre of chin.

Clinical presentation (Fig. 17.25)

- Patients present with recurrent swelling in the submental region which bursts open spontaneously discharging at times mucus and sero-purulent fluid.
- Repeated history of swelling, discharge and healing are common presentations.
- Diagnosis is established by examination of the oral cavity which reveals evidence of caries tooth.

Treatment

- Once the caries tooth is extracted, sinus will heal spontaneously.

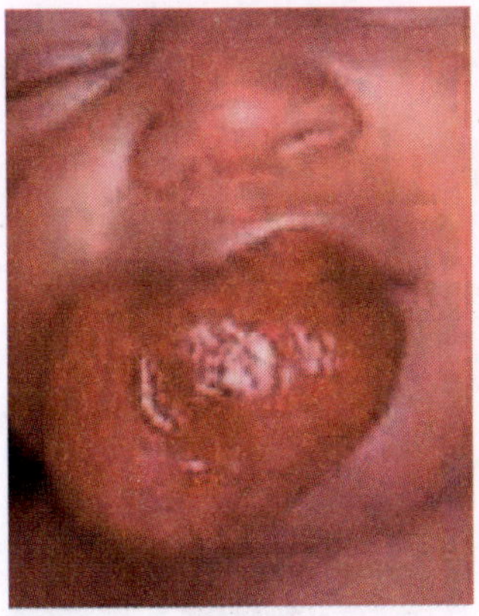

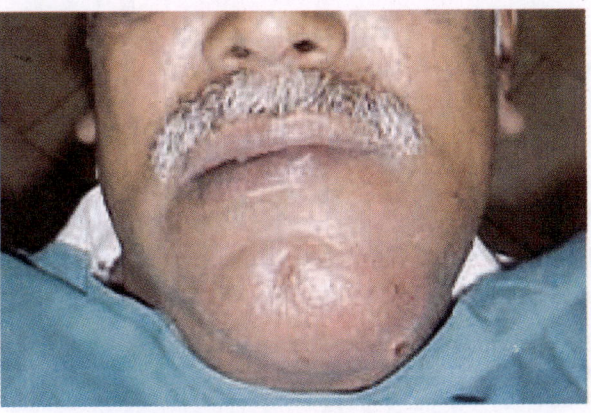

Fig. 17.23 Granulomatous epulis

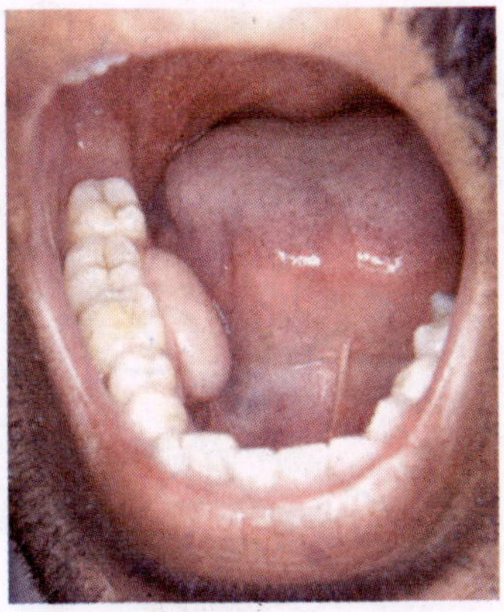

Fig. 17.24 Fibrous epulis

Fig. 17.25 Median mental sinus

CLINICAL NOTES

- We had a patient with discharging sinus in the mental region for 1½ years who had seen many practitioners including a surgeon who curetted the lesion twice. However, the lesion reappeared soon. This case is a classical example of **what the mind does not know, eyes cannot see**.

VINCENT'S ANGINA

It is an acute ulceromembranous stomatitis or acute ulcerative gingivitis and stomatitis. The disease is caused by Vincent's organisms - *Borrelia vincenti*, an anaerobic spirochaete and fusiformis. These are gram negative rods which are the normal pathogens of oral cavity.

Precipitating factors

- Malnutrition, diabetes mellitus, caries tooth, war seasons, winter, etc.

- The disease starts in the intergingival defects as a deep penetrating ulcer which results in a **spontaneous gingival haemorrhage**. There is a thick membrane covering the ulcer.

- Once infection spreads to tonsillar region, it is called as Vincent's angina – very severe painful condition.

Clinical features

- Common in children and young adults between 20-40 years of age.

- It presents with very painful gums with fever, malaise and toxaemia.

- Gums are swollen, red, inflamed with or without slough.

- Difficulty in swallowing, painful swallowing, (Odynophagia) **foetor** oris, features of toxaemia and high grade fever are characteristic of this condition.

Treatment

1. Improve the nutrition; mouth washes with hydrogen peroxide helps in washing away the membrane.

2. Injection penicillin - 10 lakh units, IM 6th hourly for 6-7 days

3. Since they are anaerobic organisms, metronidazole 400 mg thrice/day for 7-10 days, should be given.

CLEFT LIP AND CLEFT PALATE

- Cleft lip results from abnormal development of the median nasal and maxillary process.
- Cleft palate results from a failure of fusion of the two palatine processes.

Types of cleft lip (Fig. 17.26)

I. **Central**: It is very rare and occurs due to failure of fusion of two median nasal processes.

II. **Lateral** : It is the commonest variety wherein there is a cleft between the frenulum and the lateral part of the upper lip. This is due to imperfect fusion of maxillary process with median nasal process. Lateral variety can be unilateral or bilateral.

III. **Complete or incomplete:** In cases of complete variety, cleft lip extends to the floor of the nose. In cases of incomplete variety, the cleft does not extend upto the nostril.

IV. **Simple or compound:** Compound refers to cleft lip associated with a cleft in the alveolus.

Clinical features

1. In 80% of the cases, cleft lip is unilateral and in about 60% of the cases it is associated with cleft palate.

2. In many cases, nostril is widened.

3. Maldevelopment or malalignment of the teeth in relation to the cleft is common.

Functional effect

1. Presence of cleft lip does not interfere much with sucking. However, there may be some difficulty in bottle feeding.

2. Some degree of difficulty in speech (disarticulation) is present.

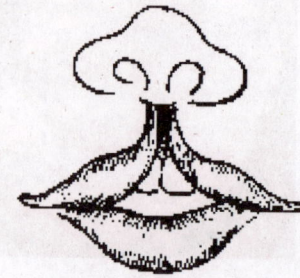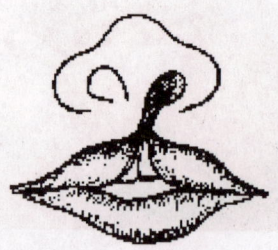

Fig. 17.26 Cleft lip (I and II).

CLEFT PALATE

Development of palate

Palate is developed around 6-8 weeks of life from 3 components.

1. The premaxilla which is developed from the median nasal process.

2 and 3. Maxillary process which contributes one palatine process on each side. The line of fusion of these processes is in the form of a letter Y.

- Imperfect fusion or developmental anomalies results in cleft palate.

Types (Fig. 17.27)

I. **Complete**: Failure of fusion of palatine processes and premaxilla results in complete cleft palate. In such situations, the nasal cavity and mouth are interconnected. When premaxilla is not fused with both palatine processes, it hangs down from the septum of nose. Thus, complete cleft can be of two types as shown below in the diagram.

II. **Incomplete**: When the fusion of three components of palate takes place, it starts from uvula and then backwards. Thus, various types of incomplete fusion results.

(a) Bifid uvula.

(b) The whole length of soft palate is bifid.

(c) The whole length of soft palate and the posterior part of hard palate are involved. On the other hand, anterior part of palate is normally developed. In about 25% of cases, cleft palate alone and in 50% of cases, both cleft palate and cleft lip are encountered.

Effects of cleft palate

1. Presence of cleft palate interferes with swallowing to some extent.

2. They are unable to make the consonant sounds like B, D, K, P, T.

3. Teeth : Upper lateral incisors may be small or even absent. The maxilla tends to be smaller. Teeth are crowded.

4. Nose : Oral organisms contaminate the upper respiratory mucous membrane through cleft palate.

5. Hearing : Even with repair, acute and chronic otitis media and hearing problems can occur.

MANAGEMENT OF CLEFT LIP AND PALATE

- **A multidisciplinary approach** involving plastic surgery, orthodontics, speech pathology, ENT department, Prosthodontics and paediatrics department is needed to rehabilitate the cleft cases. This approach to the problem results in aesthetically acceptable end result without much functional deficiencies.

- **Feeding advice**: Cleft palate babies are unable to suck mothers' milk because intraoral negative pressure cannot be created due to communication between oral and nasal cavity. Thus, expressed mothers milk is given by spoon with head end of baby elevated by 45 degrees. Swallowed air during feeding is released frequently by burping.

CLEFT LIP REPAIR (Key Box 17.16)

- **Timing** : Majority of surgeons follow "RULE OF 10" as a guide for timing of lip and anterior palate repair. At the time of repair, haemoglobin should be more than 10 gm%, age approximately 10 weeks, weight more than 10 Ibs (4.54 kg) and total leukocyte count less than 10,000/cumm (i.e. no infection).

Key Box 17.16
RULE OF 10
• Hb > 10 gm %
• Age approx : 10 weeks
• Weight > 10 lbs
• TC < 10,000/mm^3

Types of cleft lip repair

- For unilateral cleft lip repair most commonly used methods are Millards rotation advancement flap and Tennison - Randall Triangular flap method.

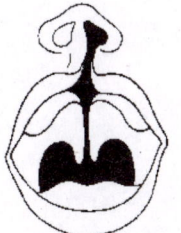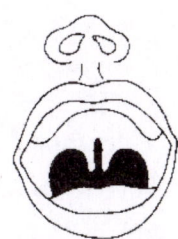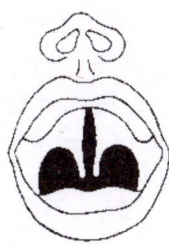

Fig. 17.27 Types of cleft palate (I, IIa and IIb)

- Bilateral cleft lip can be repaired in single stage or in two stages at the interval of 3-6 months. For two stage repair, any one of the methods described for unilateral cleft lip can be used. For bilateral repair in one stage, Veau III method is simple and gives satisfactory results. Other single methods which give good results are **Millard's single stage** procedure and Black procedure.

Basic steps of lip repair

- Markings are made according to the method selected (e.g. Millard's repair-Fig. 17.28A Tennison Randall repair - Fig. 17.28B).

- Adrenaline-saline solution 1 : 2,00,000 is injected in the lip and labial sulcus for haemostasis.

- Full thickness of lip is incised along the marking.

- Lip repair is done in 3 layers-mucosa, muscle and skin. For better aesthetic result, Cupid's bow should become horizontal, **white line** continuity should be repaired and there should be no vermilion notching.

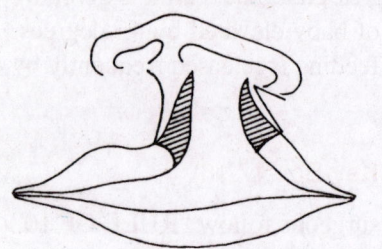 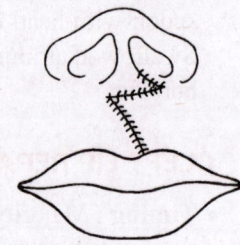

Fig. 17.28 Basic steps of lip repair

CLEFT PALATE REPAIR

Timing

- Early repair results in retarded maxillary growth due to surgical trauma to growth centre and periosteum. Delay in repair results in speech defect. Best balanced result is achieved by repairing between one and a half years.

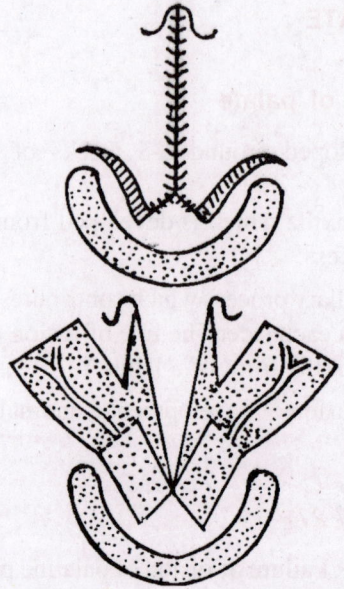

Fig. 17.29 V-Y palatoplasty

Types

- Palate repair: Palate is repaired by palatal shelves. **Mucoperiosteal flaps raised from various methods are available for palate repair**.

- Most commonly used method is V-Y, pushback palatoplasty.

Steps of 'V-Y' pushback palatoplasty (Fig. 17.29)

- Palate is infiltrated with 1: 2 lakhs adrenaline saline solution.

- Two mucoperiosteal flaps are elevated, one from either side of palatal shelves. Then, nasal layers are mobilised.

- Palate is closed in 3 layers-nasal layer, muscle layer, oral layer.

- In V-Y push back palatoplasty, palatal lengthening is achieved by V-Y plasty. Hook of hamulus can be fractured to relieve tension on suture line by relaxing the tensor palati muscle.

Salivary Glands

18

- Surgical anatomy
- Acute parotitis
- Submandibular sialoadenitis
- Salivary gland tumours
- Summary of malignant tumours
- Frey's syndrome
- Sjogren's syndrome
- Mickulicz' disease
- Parotid fistula
- Surgery for facial nerve palsy

There are three pairs of salivary glands-parotid, submandibular and sublingual. In addition to these, there are multiple minor salivary glands located in the cheek mucosa, lips, palate, base of the tongue, etc. The parotid, the "big brother of 3", suffers mainly from 3 diseases-infection, enlargement and tumour. Submandibular salivary gland suffers from mainly 2 diseases-sialoadenitis and tumours. Other salivary glands are of minor importance. However, it should be remembered that the commonest tumour of minor salivary glands is malignancy.

PAROTID GLAND

SURGICAL ANATOMY OF THE PAROTID GLAND

Parotid gland is present on the lateral aspect of the face, divided by the facial nerve into superficial lobe and deep lobe. Superficial lobe overlies the masseter and the mandible. Deep lobe is wedged between the mastoid process and the styloid process, ramus of the mandible and medial pterygoid muscle.

The superficial lobe also receives a duct from the accessory lobe which is in the region of zygomatic arch/ zygomatic process. The **duct of parotid, Stensen's duct**, 2-3 mm in diameter, receives tributaries from superficial, deep and accessory lobes, passes through the buccinator muscle and opens in the

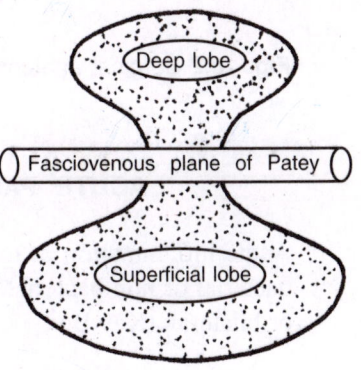

Fig. 18.1 Two lobes of parotid gland

mucosa of the cheek **opposite the upper 2nd molar tooth.** Parotid gland is covered by a true capsule which is a condensation of fibrous stroma of the gland, a **false capsule** and **parotid fascia** which is a part of the deep cervical fascia.

Facial nerve

After emerging from stylomastoid foramen, it hooks around the condyle of mandible, enters the substance of parotid and divides into 2 major branches, **zygomaticotemporal** and **cervicofacial**. Facial nerve along with retro-mandibular vein (which is formed by a branch from superficial temporal vein joining with branches from pterygoid plexus of veins) is present in this plane. This plane is called the **fasciovenous plane of Patey** (Fig. 18.2). Then facial nerve gives rise to 5 branches which are interconnected like the foot of a goose, called **Pes Anserinus.** Following are the branches of facial nerve in the face and the muscles supplied by these nerves (Table 18.1).

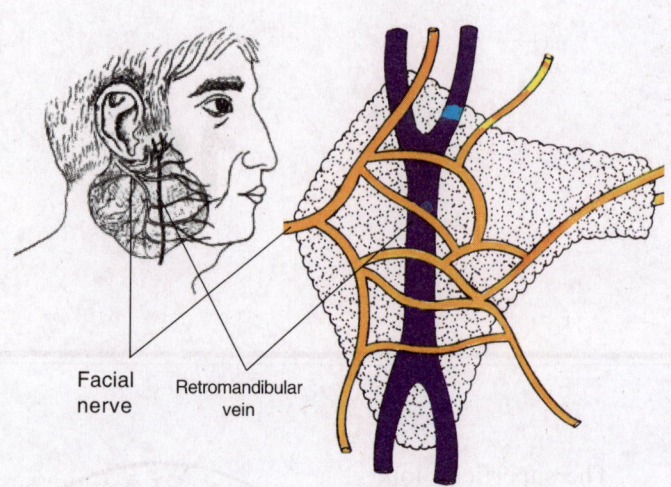

Fig. 18.2 Surgical anatomy of the parotid gland.

ACUTE PAROTITIS

Acute inflammation of the parotid can occur due to bacterial or non-bacterial causes. It can be unilateral or bilateral. (Key Box 18.1)

Causes

1. **Mumps Parotitis** Mumps[1] is an acute generalised viral disease with painful enlargement of salivary glands, chiefly the parotids. The virus belongs to paramyxoviridae family and only one serotype is known. The disease spreads from a human reservoir by direct contact, airborne droplets or fomites contaminated by saliva and possibly by urine.

Key Box 18.1	
CAUSES OF ACUTE PAROTITIS	
1. Viral	: **Mumps** – Commonest Cox Sackie A & B Parainfluenza 1 & 3 ECHO Lymphocytic Choriomeningitis
2. Bacterial	: Usually ascending infection Staphylococcus aureus
3. Recurrent parotitis of childhood	: Recurrent, mistaken for mumps Resolves at puberty
4. Specific infections	: Mycobacterial Cat-scratch disease, Syphilis, Toxoplasmosis
5. Allergic	: Food and drugs
6. Sexual diseases	: HIV related - ↑ incidence
7. Post-irradiation	: Reduction in the salivary juice
8. Post-operative	: Due to dehydration

Clinical manifestation

Incubation period is 10-24 days. Fever, headache, muscular pain are usually found. Both parotids are enlarged with pain and temperature. Swelling starts subsiding by 3-7 days of time.

Treatment

If symptomatic - maintenance of good oral hygiene and hydration is useful. Antibiotics may be given to prevent secondary infection. One episode of infection confers lifelong immunity.

Table 18.1 Facial nerve and its branches

BRANCHES OF FACIAL NERVE		MUSCLES SUPPLIED
1. Temporal	→	Auricularis anterior and superior portion of frontalis
2. Zygomatic		
Upper	→	Frontalis and upper half of orbicularis oculi
Lower	→	Lower half of orbicularis oculi and muscles below the orbit
3. Buccal	→	Buccinator, orbicularis oris and a few fibres of elevators of the lower lip
4. Mandibular	→	Muscles of the lower lip
5. Cervical	→	Platysma

---

1. It causes parotitis, orchitis, pancreatitis

2. **Acute bacterial parotitis** *Staphylococcus aureus* infection of parotid produces serious illness with marked engorgement of parotid. Typically, it produces parotid abscess. Diabetes, malignancy, malnutrition increase the risk. Decreased salivary secretion is an important predisposing factor.

3. **Reduction in salivary juice** can occur due to various factors mentioned in the box. Postoperative parotitis can be prevented by good mouth care and good oral hygiene. Due to poor oral hygiene, ascending infection occurs from the oral cavity resulting in parotitis. (Key Box 18.2)

Key Box 18.2
CAUSES OF ↓ SALIVARY FLOW
• Post-operative
• Poor oral hygiene
• Dehydration
• Enteric fever, septicaemia
• Post-radiotherapy, for oral cancer

Clinical features

Patient who is recovering in the post-operative period may complain of pain and swelling in the parotid region. Presence of severe pain, very sick, toxic look and high grade fever with chills and rigors, indicates parotid abscess. **Diffuse brawny swelling is characteristic**.

The swelling is due to inflammation of parotid and since it is enclosed by parotid fascia, the swelling takes the shape of parotid gland. However, it is not common for a parotid abscess to raise the ear lobule. For the reason mentioned above, fluctuation is a late feature. **If the abscess is not drained, it is likely to rupture into the external auditory canal.** (Key Box 18.3)

Key Box 18.3
SWELLINGS WHEREIN ONE SHOULD NOT WAIT FOR FLUCTUATION
• Parotid abscess
• Breast abscess
• Ischiorectal abscess
• Pulp space infection
• Any deep seated abscess

The opening of the parotid duct may be inflamed and on gentle compression of the parotid gland, pus can be seen coming out of the parotid duct.

Treatment

I. **Conservative line of management** is indicated in a stage of cellulitis with no evidence of abscess.

Maintaining good hydration of the patient in the post operative period.

Improvement in the oral hygiene-mouth washes with potassium permanganate ($KMnO_4$) solution.

Appropriate antibiotics against staphylococci, such as cloxacillin, is administered in the dose of 500 mg, 6th hourly along with metronidazole 400 mg, 8th hourly to treat anaerobic infections.

It takes about 3-5 days for the inflammation to settle down.

II **Surgical treatment** is indicated when there is pus. (Key Box 18.4)

Under general anaesthesia an adequate vertical incision is made in front of the tragus of the ear up to deep fascia. Open the deep fascia in two or three places and drain with blunt haemostat so as to avoid damage to facial nerve. This is described as **Blair's method** of drainage of parotid abscess. The drainage tube has to be kept which can be removed after 3-4 days.

Key Box 18.4
DRAINAGE OF PAROTID ABSCESS
• Should not wait for fluctuation
• High grade fever, toxicity are indications
• Vertical incision
• **Hilton's method** is preferred to break multiple loculi

SURGICAL ANATOMY OF THE SUBMANDIBULAR SALIVARY GLAND (Fig. 18.3)

Submandibular salivary gland is located in the submandibular triangle. It lies partly below and partly above the mandible.

It is in very close contact with the belly of the digastric muscle. At surgery, once the deep fascia is **opened, the intermediate tendon of digastric is located** and when it is retracted downwards, mobilisation of the gland becomes easy.

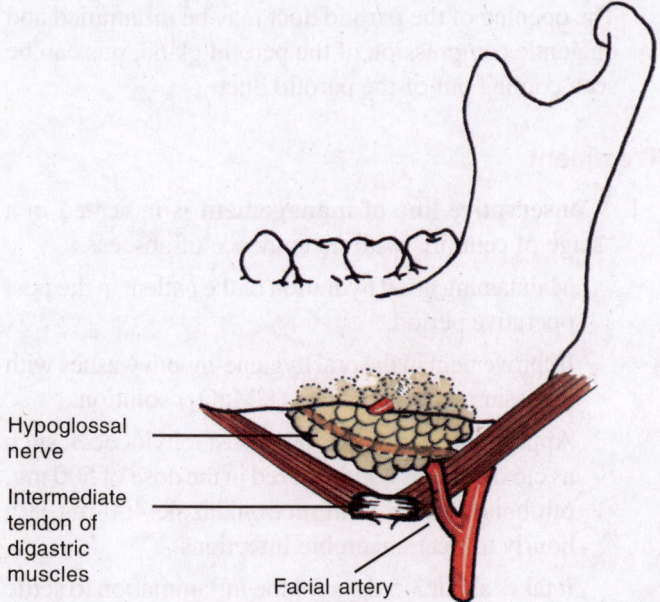

Hypoglossal nerve

Intermediate tendon of digastric muscles

Facial artery

Fig. 18.3 Anatomy of the submandibular salivary gland

Submandibular salivary gland is divided into a superficial and a deep part by the mylohyoid muscle which forms the oral diaphragm. During excision of the gland, a few fibres of mylohyoid are also removed. When submandibular salivary gland enlarges, **it is bidigitally palpable** because the deep portion is deep to mylohyoid and it is in the floor of the mouth.

Facial artery enters the gland from its posterolateral surface and **deeply grooves the gland**. It is ligated at this place first during excision of the gland. After grooving the gland, it ascends laterally and curls the lower border of the mandible to enter the face. At this place it is also ligated.

Main duct of submandibular gland, **Wharton's duct arises** from deep part of gland and opens on a papilla beside the frenulum of the tongue in the oral cavity.

In a deeper plane, the gland is related to **two nerves – lingual and hypoglossal.**

CHRONIC SUBMANDIBULAR SIALOADENITIS

Obstruction is the most important cause of submandibular sialoadenitis. Another cause is trauma to the floor of the mouth.

Obstruction can be due to stone disease, (calculus – most common) stricture of the duct, or fibrosis of the papilla.

The causative organism is *Staphylococcus.*

SIALOADENITIS DUE TO CALCULI

The disease starts with acute bacterial sialoadenitis which occur secondary to obstruction. **The submandibular gland has a poor capacity for recovery following infection**. Despite control of acute symptoms with antibiotics, the gland becomes chronically inflamed.

Calculi (80% of them occur in the submandibular salivary gland) commonly occur in the duct and also within the gland and produce recurrent sialoadenitis. Calculi are more common in the submandibular salivary gland than the parotid gland because of the following reasons.

1. **Higher mucin content** in the submandibular salivary gland secretions.

2. **Calcium and phosphate** content in the secretion is high. (Hence 80% of them are radio-opaque, detected by plain x-ray). (Fig. 18.4)

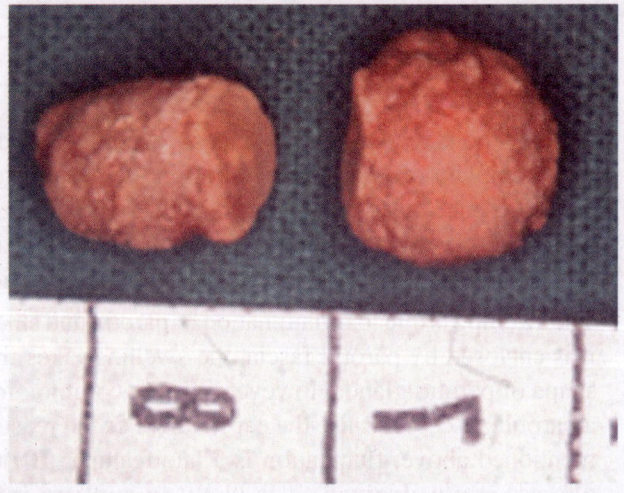

Fig. 18.4 Submandibular calculi in the duct - removed (intraoral approach)

Key Box 18.5
SUBMANDIBULAR SALIVARY GLAND ENLARGEMENT
• Location-Submandibular region
• Lobular, firm swelling
• Bidigitally palpable
• Stone may be palpable within the duct, intraorally

3. **Nondependent drainage** of the secretions. Gland is in the neck and opening of the duct in the oral cavity .

4. **Kinking or hooking** of submandibular duct by lingual nerve.

Clinical features (Key Box 18.5)

Salivary colic It is a severe pricking type of pain which is exaggerated at the. time of meals. Salivary secretions are induced by a meal or lemon (Lemon juice test). As a result of blockage due to a stone, the tension within the gland increases, resulting in pain.

Lingual colic If a calculus is situated within the submandibular duct where it is hooked by lingual nerve, pain can radiate to the tongue as a result of irritation to the lingual nerve.

Enlargement of salivary gland during meals is the characteristic feature of salivary calculus. Classically submandibular salivary gland swelling is located in the submandibular region. It is firm in consistency with a lobular surface. It is tender, and both lobes are enlarged. It is bidigitally palpable, (submandibular lymph node is palpable only in the neck) both inside the oral cavity and in the neck. The swelling will reduce in size once the stimuli are withdrawn (after meals).

The stone may be palpable within the gland (in the neck), within the duct (intra orally), or sometimes it may be seen at the orifice of the submandibular duct on the side of lingual frenulum.

It is not uncommon to get a severe septic sialoadenitis with gross swelling of the gland and inflammatory oedema almost like Ludwig's angina.

Treatment

An oblique lateral or posterior oblique occlusal radiography may demonstrate a stone.

1. **Stone in the submandibular duct** This can be removed by incising the mucosa over the floor of the mouth, after stabilising the stone. Removal of the stone is followed by **gush of old dirty contents** of the submandibular gland.

2. **Chronic sialoadenitis** This requires excision of submandibular salivary gland. Three steps of dissection of the gland include incision, mobilisation and excision (Manipal Rule of 2 - Table 18.2).

Incision It should be a skin crease incision over the lower pole of the gland, the posterior limit of the incision should be at least 2 cm away from the angle of the mandible, to avoid damage to the cervical branch of facial nerve. The incision is deepened till the deep fascia is opened.

Mobilisation of the gland Division of the facial artery twice, once in a deeper plane on the posterolateral aspect and another at the superolateral aspect close to the lower border of the mandible is an important step which gives mobilisation of the gland. Separation of the gland from mylohyoid fibers by dividing small arteries completes the mobilisation.

Excision of the gland It is done by ligating and dividing submandibular duct.

Complications of excision includes damage to lingual nerve, marginal mandibular nerve or even to hypoglossal nerve. Seroma and infection are the other complications.

Table 18.2
SUBMANDIBULAR SALIVARY GLAND EXCISION - **MANIPAL RULE OF 2**

• 2 common indications	→ Stone and as a part of radical neck dissection
• 2" long incision	→ Curved incision over the swelling
• Protect 2 superficial nerves	→ Cervical and marginal mandibular branches of facial nerve
• Protect 2 deep nerves	→ Lingual and hypoglossal nerve
• Ligate facial artery 2 times	→ First at deeper plane and then at superficial plane
• Divide 2 muscles	→ Superficial-Platysma; Deep-Fibres of mylohyoid
• Remove 2 lobes	→ Superficial and deep
• Incision is 2 cm medial to mandible, 2 cms anterior to angle of the mandible	→ To protect 2 superficial nerves

SALIVARY GLAND TUMOURS

INTERNATIONAL CLASSIFICATION

I. Epithelial tumours

II. Non-epithelial tumours

I. Epithelial tumours

A. Adenoma

1. Pleomorphic adenoma

2. Monomorphic adenomas

 Adenolymphoma (Warthin's tumour)

 Oxyphilic adenoma (Oncocytoma)

 Other types

B. Mucoepidermoid tumours

C. Acinic cell tumour

D. Carcinoma

 1. Carcinoma in pleomorphic adenoma

 2. Adenoid cystic carcinoma

 3. Undifferentiated carcinoma

 4. Adenocarcinoma

 5. Epidermoid carcinoma

 6. Acinic cell tumour

 7. Muco epidermoid carcinoma

 8. Malignant mixed tumour

II. Non-epithelial tumours

1. Lipoma

2. Lymphoma

3. Neurofibroma

4. Lymphangioma

5. Sarcoma

Salivary gland tumours are not uncommon. There are dozens of histological types of salivary gland tumours. However, pleomorphic adenoma and adenolymphoma are the common benign types. Carcinoma arising in pleomorphic adenoma, mucoepidermoid tumours and adenoid cystic carcinoma are important malignant tumours.

Incidence 80% of salivary gland tumours are found in parotid gland, out of which 80% are benign and 80% of benign tumours are pleomorphic adenomas.

In the submandibular salivary gland, 50% are benign and 50% are malignant.

In the minor salivary glands, 90% are malignant. Thus, the incidence of malignancy increases from major to minor salivary glands.

PLEOMORPHIC ADENOMA OF PAROTID GLAND (MIXED TUMOUR)

PATHOLOGY

Epithelial cells proliferate in strands, or may be arranged in the form of acini or cords.

There are also myoepithelial cells which proliferate in sheets. They are called spindle-shaped cells.

The tumour produces mucoid material, which displaces and separates the cells resembling cartilage in histological section.

Because of the presence of epithelial cells, myoepithelial cells, mucoid material, pseudocartilage and lymphoid tissue, the tumour is called pleomorphic adenoma.

As the tumour grows, it compresses the normal parotid tissue and the branches of the tumour penetrate the thin capsule and enter the substance of the parotid. Simple enucleation will result in a recurrence. Hence, superficial parotidectomy has to be done.

CLINICAL FEATURES

1. Middle-aged women, around 40 years, are commonly affected (Fig. 18.5).

2. Typically, the history of a very slow growing swelling for a few years is usually present.

3. The swelling is painless. **Any painless swelling near the ear is best assumed to be parotid gland neoplasm unless proved otherwise**.

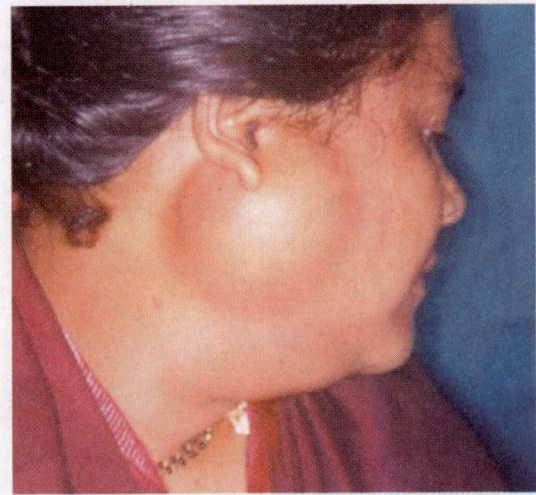

Fig. 18.5 Pleomorphic adenoma – Classical signs

SIGNS (Key Box 18.6)

1. Parotid swelling has the following classical features.

   It presents as a **swelling in front**, below and behind ear.

   Raises ear lobule.

   Retromandibular groove is obliterated.

2. It is rubbery or firm. Soft areas indicate necrosis. In long standing cases, it can be hard. Surface can be nodular or sometimes bosselated. Skin is stretched and shiny. However, being a benign tumour it is neither adherent to the skin nor to the masseter.

3. After a few years, pleomorphic adenoma shows features of transformation into malignancy. (Carcinoma Expleomorphic adenoma).

   It should be suspected when

   It starts growing rapidly

   Skin infiltration occurs

   Facial nerve paralysis

   Gets fixed to masseter muscle

   Red, dilated veins over the surface

   Presence of lymph nodes in the neck

   Tumour feels stony hard

Intraoral examination

Approximately 10% of the parotid tumours are behind the facial nerve in the deep lobe.

This is appreciated by intraoral examination wherein the tumour presents with a parapharyngeal mass which displaces the tonsil or soft palate medially.

Deep lobe tumours present as dysphagia. Such tumours may not show gross swelling on the outer aspect but as they grow, they pass through the stylomandibular tunnel of Patey and push the pharyngeal wall, tonsil and soft palate. These tumours are called as **Dumbell tumours**.

INVESTIGATIONS

Slow growing parotid tumours **should not be subjected to biopsy** for 2 reasons

   Injury to the facial nerve

   Seeding of tumour cells in the subcutaneous plane which causes recurrence in about 40-50% of cases.

1. **Fine needle aspiration cytology** (FNAC) is done to confirm the diagnosis and rule out malignancy.

2. **CT scan** is done when the tumour is arising from the **deep lobe**. It helps to define the **extraglandular spread**, the extent of parapharyngeal disease, and cervical lymph nodes.

3. **FNAC of the lymph nodes** which are palpable in the neck in cases of malignancy of the parotid gland.

4. **X-ray of the bones** (mandible and mastoid process) to see for bony resorption.

5. **MRI is a better investigation however costly – CT Scan and MRI lack specificity for differentiating benign versus malignant lesions.**

TREATMENT

Conservative superficial parotidectomy (Fig. 18.7; Key Box 18.7)

It is the standard surgery done for benign pleomorphic adenoma. It means removal of the entire lobe containing the tumour which is superficial to facial nerve. **Facial nerve should always be preserved**. Enucleation should never be done as it causes recurrence. It is difficult to remove a recurrent tumour.

Key Box 18.6

CLINICAL EXAMINATION OF PAROTID TUMOURS

- Swelling proper
- Facial nerve involvement
  (80-90% cases of malignancy)
- Fixity to mandible and masseter
- Deep cervical nodes
- Opening of parotid duct
- Shift of tonsil and pillar of the fauces
- Other salivary glands (both sides)

Key Box 18.7

CONSERVATIVE SUPERFICIAL PAROTIDECTOMY

- Indicated in pleomorphic adenoma
- Tumour along with the normal lobe is removed
- Preserve the facial nerve, **even in malignant tumours unless grossly involved**.
- Avoid rupture of the gland
- **Enucleation should not be done as it causes recurrence**

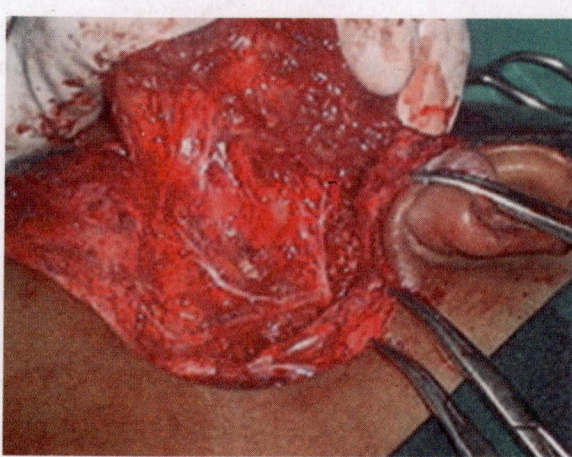
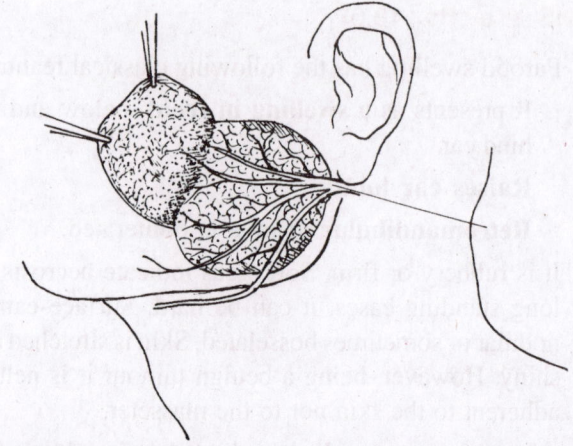

Fig. 18.6, 18.7 Conservative superficial parotidectomy - facial nerve divides the gland into superficial lobe and deep lobe. The entire superficial lobe is removed preserving the facial nerve

A few important steps of superficial parotidectomy

1. **Adequate exposure** by an incision which starts in front of tragus of pinna, vertically descends downwards, curves round the ear lobule up to the mastoid process and is carried downwards in the neck. ('Lazy S' incision)

2. **Recognising the facial nerve at surgery**

   Facial nerve lies **1 cm inferomedial to the pointed end** of the tragal cartilage of the external ear.

   Trace the posterior belly of digastric upto the mastoid process. Facial nerve is in between the muscle and tympanic plate.

   To use **nerve stimulator**.

3. **Developing a plane:** Facial nerve and retromandibular vein divides the parotid gland into superficial and deep lobes. Benign tumours do not invade this **faciovenous plane of Patey**.

4. **Gentle handling**, good suction and perfect haemostasis helps in the clear recognition of the nerve.

5. The tumour along with **the lobe should be removed in toto** to avoid spillage (which is one of the causes of recurrence).

6. **Good suction drainage** of the wound is necessary to avoid haematoma, wound infection, etc.

TREATMENT OF MALIGNANT PLEOMORPHIC ADENOMA

Radical parotidectomy refers to removal of both lobes, facial nerve, parotid duct, fibres of masseter, buccinator, pterygoids and radical block dissection of the neck. If facial nerve is not involved it should be preserved to avoid morbidity. Advanced tumours with fixed nodes in the neck may require radiotherapy even though the response rate is poor.

INDICATIONS FOR POST-OPERATIVE RADIOTHERAPY

If the deep lobe is involved

If the lymph nodes are involved

High grade tumours

If margins are positive

ADENOLYMPHOMA (Warthin's tumour, Papillary Cystadenoma Lymphomatosum)

Adenolymphoma is not a lymphoma. It is a misnomer (vide infra).

It is a benign parotid tumour and next common to pleomorphic adenoma. It constitutes about 10% of parotid tumours (Table 18.3).

Origin of adenolymphoma During development some parotid tissue gets included within lymph nodes (preparotid) which are present within the parotid sheath.

Histology

It is composed of double layered eosinophilic epithelium, **inner cells are columnar.**

Presence of lymphatic tissue in the stroma, and lymph follicles (hence the name) is characteristic of adenolymphoma.

Table 18.3 Comparison between pleomorphic adenoma and adenolymphoma

FEATURES	PLEOMORPHIC ADENOMA	ADENOLYMPHOMA
1. Incidence	70-80%	10%
2. Sex	Common in females	Common in males
3. Number	Single	Sometimes multiple
4. Site	Unilateral	Bilateral
5. Clinical feature	Nodular, firm	Smooth, soft cystic
6. Histology	Pleomorphism	Double layer epithelium and lymphoid tissue
7. 99^m Tc-pertechnetate scan	Cold spot	Hot spot
8. Treatment	Superficial parotidectomy	Enucleation

Clinical features (Table 18.3)

1. Middle aged or elderly males are commonly affected – usually **they are smokers**.
2. Can be **bilateral**, in some cases (10%).
3. It has smooth surface, round border with soft, cystic consistency (Fig. 18.8).
4. Classically, situated at the lower pole of parotid elevating the ear lobule.
5. May be **multicentric**
6. **This tumour affects only parotid gland.** (Very very rarely other glands may be affected).

Treatment

It has got a well-defined capsule. Hence, enucleation can be done.

MUCOEPIDERMOID TUMOUR

As the name itself suggests, it consists of sheets of epidermoid cells and cystic spaces lined by mucus secreting cells (Fig. 18.9).

In childhood, it is the commonest parotid tumour

They are benign, slow-growing but hard in consistency. (Adenolymphoma and mixed tumours are firm, but mucoepidermoid tumour is hard.) Parotid is the commonest site. In cases of minor salivary glands, palate is the commonest site.

Mucoepidermoid tumours can infiltrate local tissues, lymph nodes or skin. Hence, a few consider that **mucoepidermoid tumours are always carcinomatous.**

Well-differentiated tumours behave like benign, intermediate ones are aggressive and undifferentiated

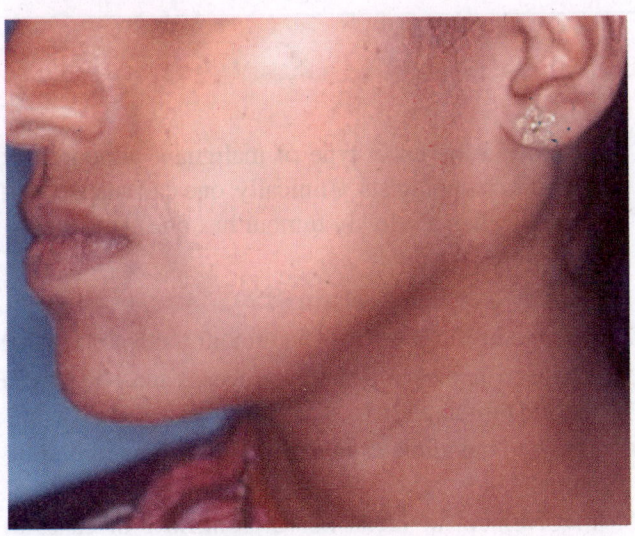
Fig. 18.8 Adenolymphoma

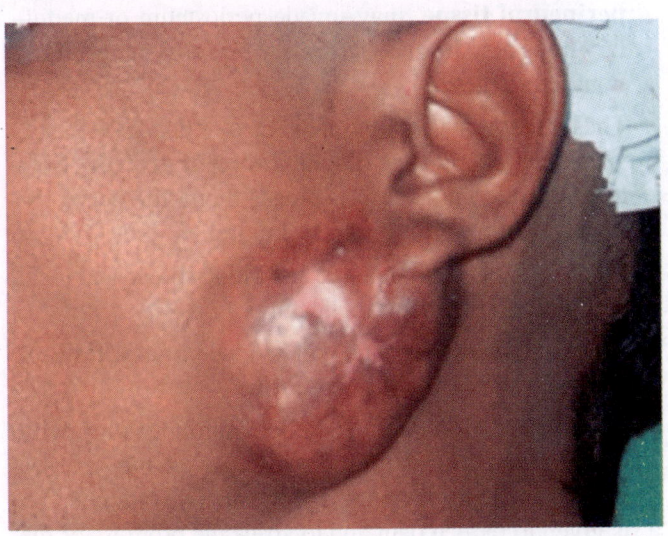
Fig. 18.9 Mucoepidermoid carcinoma

tumours metastasize early. Mucoepidermoid carcinoma is the most common malignant epithelial neoplasm of salivary gland.

The **low grade** tumours are composed of predominantly **mucous secreting cells**. **High grade tumours** have predominantly **epidermoid cells**.

Benign tumours need excision and malignant tumours need radical parotidectomy.

ACINIC CELL TUMOUR

These are the uncommon parotid tumours. Commonly occur in women.

The cells resemble those of serous acini and this tumour also has properties of invasion like mucoepidermoid tumour. It tends to be soft and sometimes cystic.

OXYPHIL ADENOMA

Also called as Oncocytoma. It occurs exclusively in the parotid gland. It is a solid tumour, occurs in the sixth decade of life.

ADENOID CYSTIC CARCINOMA

It is a highly malignant tumour consisting of cords of dark staining cells with cystic spaces containing mucin. It also consists of myoepithelial cells and duct epithelium.

Even though **slow growing**, it spreads along the **perineural tissue,** may invade periosteum or medullary bone at a distance. This bone resorption results in bony tenderness.

These tumours have high incidence of distant metastasis but in general **they display indolent growth.** Skip lesions are common as it spreads along the nerve tissue, which leads to treatment failure.

Local infiltration, lymphatic and blood spread and local recurrence are important features.

It is **hard and fixed** and can produce **anaesthesia of the skin overlying the tumour.**

Early cases are treated by radical parotidectomy with block dissection of the neck. However, many cases present late to the hospital. Thus, palliative radiotherapy is given to reduce pain and to arrest the progress of the disease.

Complications of parotidectomy

Key Box 18.8
COMPLICATIONS OF PAROTIDECTOMY

- **Flap necrosis** – Avoid acute bending of the incision and to use gentle retraction.
- **Facial nerve palsy** – Careful identification.
- **Fluid collection** – Blood or seroma – perfect haemostasis and drain should be used.
- **Salivary Fistula** – Duct should be ligated
- **Frey's syndrome** – Occur in 10% cases.

Observe 5 'F's

Interesting most common for salivary glands

Key Box 18.9
MOST COMMON FOR SALIVARY GLANDS

- Most common benign parotid tumour in adults – Pleomorphic adenoma
- Most common benign parotid tumour in children – Haemangioma
- Most common malignant tumour in submandibular gland – adenoid cystic carcinoma
- Most common minor salivary gland tumour is adenocarcinoma
- Most common site of squamous cell carcinoma is submandibular salivary gland
- Most common response to radiotherapy among the malignant tumours is adenoid cystic carcinoma

Summary of Malignant salivary gland tumours (Fig. 18.10 to 18.16)

To find out the exact type of malignant tumour is of interest to pathologists. Clinically, one can suspect malignancy when a salivary tumour has one of the following features

1. Rapidly growing neoplasm
2. Change in consistency (The tumour tends to be hard)
3. Fixity to underlying muscle such as masseter as in parotid tumours
4. Fixity to mandible as in parotid or submandibular tumour
5. Involvement of facial nerve as in 80% of cases of malignant parotid tumours

MALIGNANT PAROTID TUMOURS

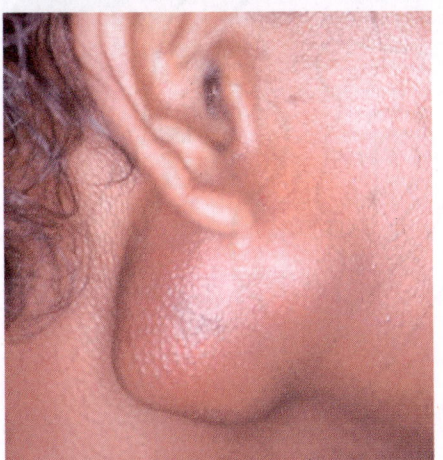

Fig. 18.10 Low grade mucoepidermoid carcinoma - had restricted mobility

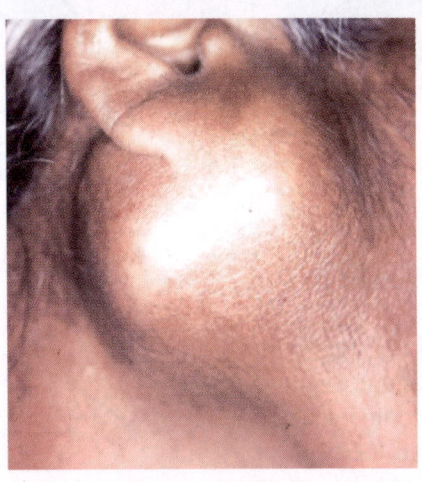

Fig. 18.11 Adenoid cystic carcinoma - perineural spread

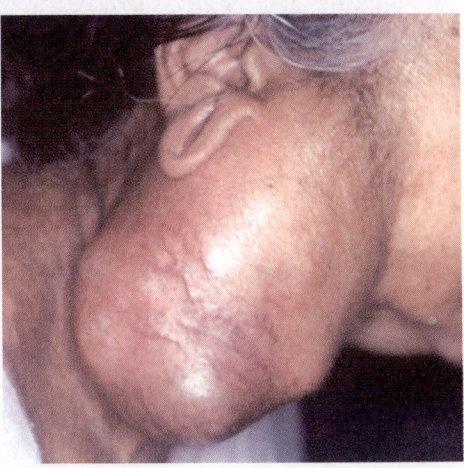

Fig. 18.12 High grade mucoepidermoid carcinoma - rapidly growing and dilated veins over the surface

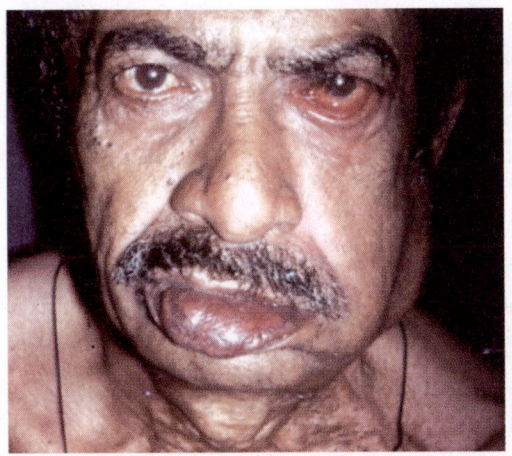

Fig. 18.13 Facial nerve paralysis - one of the strong clinical signs of malignancy in a parotid tumour

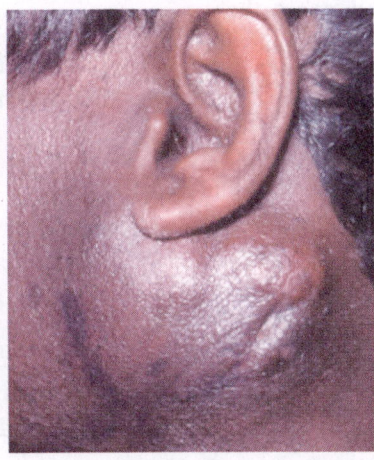

Fig. 18.14 Adenoid cystic carcinoma - hard and fixed receiving radiotherapy

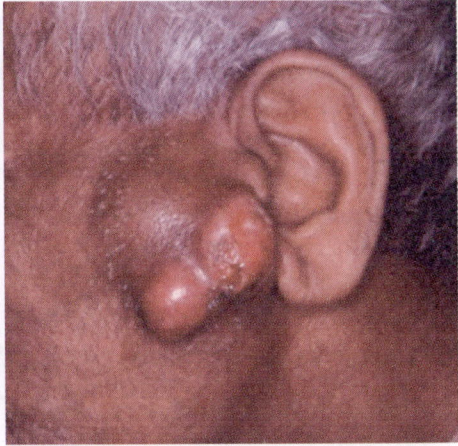

Fig. 18.15 Malignant mixed tumour ulcerated

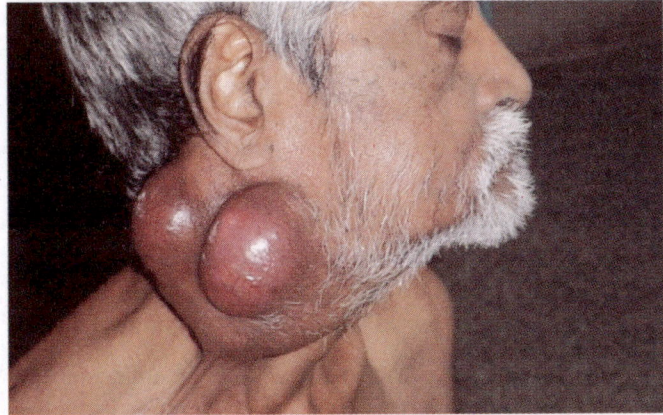

Fig. 18.16 Carcinoma parotid - late stage with involvement of platysma - **platysma sign**

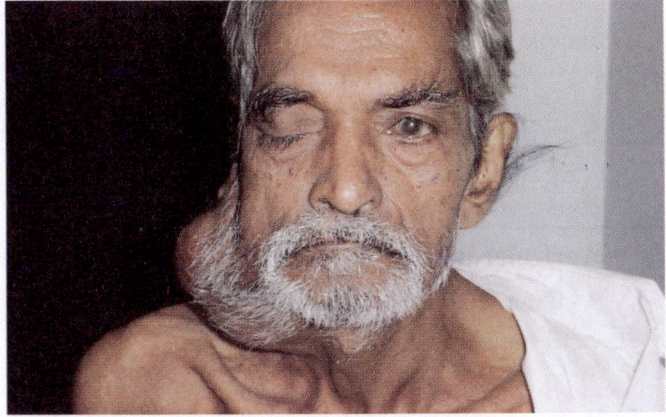

Fig. 18.17 Same patient in Fig. 18.16 also had facial nerve paralysis

6. Resorption of adjacent bone such as mastoid, tenderness as in adenoid cystic carcinoma.

7. Significant hard nodes in the neck.

They are treated by radical sialadenectomy with radical block dissection of the neck. Radiotherapy is used as a palliative treatment.

MISCELLANEOUS

FREY'S SYNDROME – Gustatory sweating

It occurs after surgery for parotid tumours, surgery in the region of temporomandibular joint, or due to injury to the parotid gland. Injury to the auriculotemporal nerve can occur at a site where it turns around the neck of the mandible. The injury is manifested at a later date (2-3 months).

Because of the injury, post-ganglionic parasympathetic fibers from otic ganglion are united with sympathetic fibres of superior cervical ganglion which supplies the vessels and sweat glands over the skin overlying parotid region (Key Box 18.10).

As a result of this, whenever the act of chewing or mastication is started, there is increased sweating and hyperaesthesia in the region supplied by auriculotemporal nerve (cutaneous branch of mandibular division of trigeminal nerve). Hence, it is called "auriculotemporal syndrome".

Diagnosis Starch Iodine Test Paint the affected area with iodine which is allowed to dry, before applying the dry starch.

The starch turns blue on exposure to iodine in the presence of sweat.

Prevention

Principle is to provide a barrier between the skin and

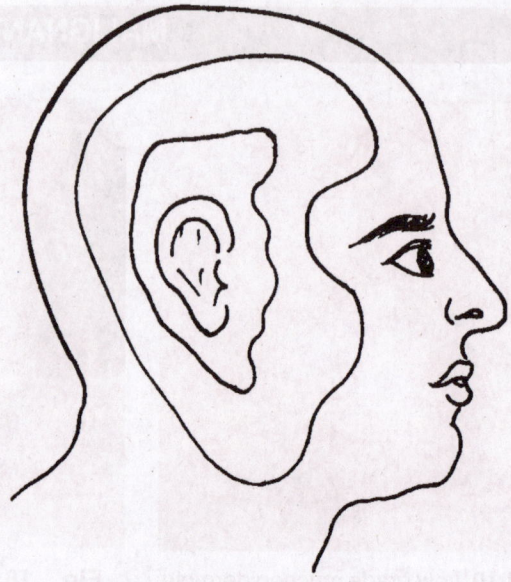

Fig. 18.18 Frey's syndrome

parotid bed by using temporalis facial flap or sternomastoid muscle flap.

Treatment

1. Reassurance

2. Aluminium chloride – antiperspirant which is a useful astringent

3. Denervation by tympanic neurectomy

4. **Latest treatment includes injection of botulinum toxin into the affected skin**

RARE CAUSES OF SALIVARY GLAND ENLARGEMENT

1. SJOGREN'S SYNDROME

The diffuse infiltration of salivary and lacrimal glands with lymphocytes resulting in enlargement of glands and slow destruction of acini. Thus, clinical features include dry eyes (kerato-conjunctivitis sicca) and dry mouth (xerostomia). These along with a third component rheumatoid arthritis, form the triad of **Sjogren's syndrome. (Primary)**

30% of patients with systemic lupus erythematosus and all patients with primary biliary cirrhosis develop Sjogren's syndrome. This is termed as **secondary Sjogren's syndrome.**

Key Box 18.10

PARTS SUPPLIED BY AURICULOTEMPORAL NERVE

- **Auricular part:**
    External acoustic meatus
    Tympanic membrane surface
    Skin of auricle above external acoustic meatus
- **Temporal part:**
    Hairy skin of the temple

Other features include – disease is 10 times more common in females and presents with painful enlargement of the glands.

Complications

1. Lymphomatous transformation (High in primary)
2. Oral candidiasis

2. MIKULICZ'S DISEASE

Due to autoimmune mechanism, symmetrical enlargement of all salivary glands and lacrimal gland enlargement occur. Dry mouth and narrow palpebral fissures are diagnostic of this condition.

3. DRUGS

Carbimazole, thiouracil can cause enlargement of salivary glands.

4. METABOLIC DISORDERS

Diabetes and acromegaly are the other causes.

PAROTID FISTULA

It is a uncommon condition which commonly occurs after surgery on the parotid gland. (Key Box 18.11)

Key Box 18.11

PAROTID FISTULA

- Any surgery on the parotid gland – Superficial parotidectomy, drainage of abscess, surgery for carcinoma cheek, faciomaxillary trauma are the causes.
- Discharging watery fluid, exaggerated by keeping lime in the mouth
- Fistulogram confirms the diagnosis
- Exploration and excision of fistula and ligation of duct is required

---

SURGERY FOR FACIAL NERVE PALSY

Indications for different types of surgery

1. Early immediate nerve repair, in case of injury to the nerve.
2. Late nerve crossing by suturing peripheral branches of facial nerve to one of the following nerves.

   Hypoglossal nerve, Spinal accessory nerve
   Phrenic nerve

3. Surgery to achieve movement in long standing facial palsy (usually after 1 year)

A. Static procedures

Suspension of lips, cheek and angle of mouth to zygomatic bone or temporal fascia using fascia lata, palmaris longus tendon or other alloplastic materials.

Medial canthoplasty to reduce epiphora

Lateral tarsorrhaphy (canthoplasty) to prevent exposure keratitis due to widened palpebral fissure.

B. Dynamic procedures

Muscle transfer with carefully preserved muscle nerve and vessel eg. Temporalis muscle transfer, masseter muscle transfer.

Cross face nerve transplantation using sural nerve Using microscope, sural nerve is sutured to the two or three relatively insignificant branches of facial nerve (selected by intraoperative electric stimulation) on normal side. Other end of the sural nerve is sutured to distal end of the divided facial nerve on paralysed side.

Free neurovascular gracilis muscle graft using microvascular techniques.

19

The Thyroid Gland

- Surgical anatomy
- Physiology
- Thyroid function tests
- Clinical examination
- Goitre
- Multinodular goitre
- Retrosternal goitre
- Grave's disease
- Neoplastic goitre
- Solitary nodule
- Thyroiditis
- Lingual thyroid
- Complications of thyroidectomy

SURGICAL ANATOMY OF THYROID GLAND

- Thyroid gland is present in the neck, enclosed by pretracheal fascia which is a part of deep cervical fascia. It has a right and left lobe joined by isthmus which is in front of 2nd, 3rd and 4th tracheal rings. It weighs about 20-25 gm. A projection from the isthmus usually on the left side is called pyramidal lobe. It is attached to the hyoid bone by a fibrous band or muscle fibers called levator glandulae thyroideae.

- **Suspensory ligament of Berry** This pair of strong condensed connective tissue binds the gland firmly to each side of cricoid cartilage.

- **Pretracheal fascia**, which is a part of deep cervical fascia splits to invest the gland. These few structures are responsible for thyroid moving with deglutition.

Development

- It develops from **median down growth** (midline diverticulum) of a column of cells from the pharyngeal floor between first and second pharyngeal pouches.

- By 6 weeks of time the **central column,** which becomes **thyroglossal duct,** gets reabsorbed.

- The duct bifurcates to form thyroid lobes.

- **Pyramidal lobe** is formed by a portion of the duct.

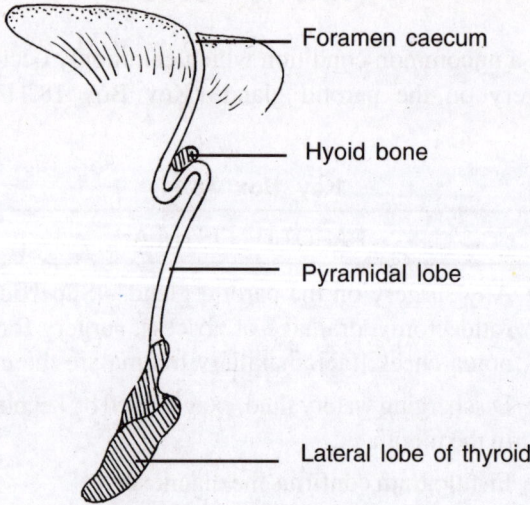

Foramen caecum

Hyoid bone

Pyramidal lobe

Lateral lobe of thyroid

Fig. 19.1 Development

Arterial supply

- Superior thyroid artery is a branch of external carotid artery, enters the upper pole of the gland, divides into anterior and posterior branches and anastomoses with ascending branch of inferior thyroid artery. Upper pole is narrow, hence ligation is easy.

- **Inferior thyroid artery** is a branch of thyro-cervical trunk[1] and enters the posterior aspect of the gland. It supplies the gland by dividing into 4 to 5 branches which enter the gland at various levels (not truly lower pole).

- **Thyroidea ima** artery is a branch of either brachio-cephalic trunk or direct branch of arch of aorta and enters the lower part of the isthmus in about 2 to 3% of the cases.

Venous drainage

- **Superior thyroid vein** drains the upper pole and enters the internal jugular vein. The vein follows the artery.

- **Middle thyroid vein** is single[2], short and wide and drains into internal jugular vein.

- **Inferior thyroid veins** form a plexus which drain into innominate vein. They do not accompany the artery.

- **Kocher's vein** is rarely found (vein in between middle and inferior thyroid vein).

NERVES IN RELATIONSHIP WITH THYROID GLAND

1. **External laryngeal nerve** Vagus gives rise to superior laryngeal nerve, which separates from vagus at skull base and divides into two branches. The large, **internal laryngeal** nerve is sensory to the larynx. The small **external laryngeal** nerve runs close to the superior thyroid vessels and supplies **cricothyroid**

muscle (tensor of the vocal cord) and is sensory to upper half of the larynx.

- This nerve is away from the vessels near the upper pole. Hence, in thyroidectomy, the *upper pedicle should be ligated as close to the thyroid as possible*.

2. **Recurrent Laryngeal Nerve (RLN)** is a branch of vagus, hooks around ligamentum arteriosum on the left and subclavian artery on the right, runs in tracheo, oesophageal groove near the posteromedial surface. Close to the gland, the nerve lies in between (anterior or posterior) the branches of inferior thyroid artery. Hence, **inferior thyroid artery should be ligated away from the gland, to avoid damage to RLN.**

- On right side it is 1 cm within the tracheo- oesophageal groove.(Refer key box 19.1)

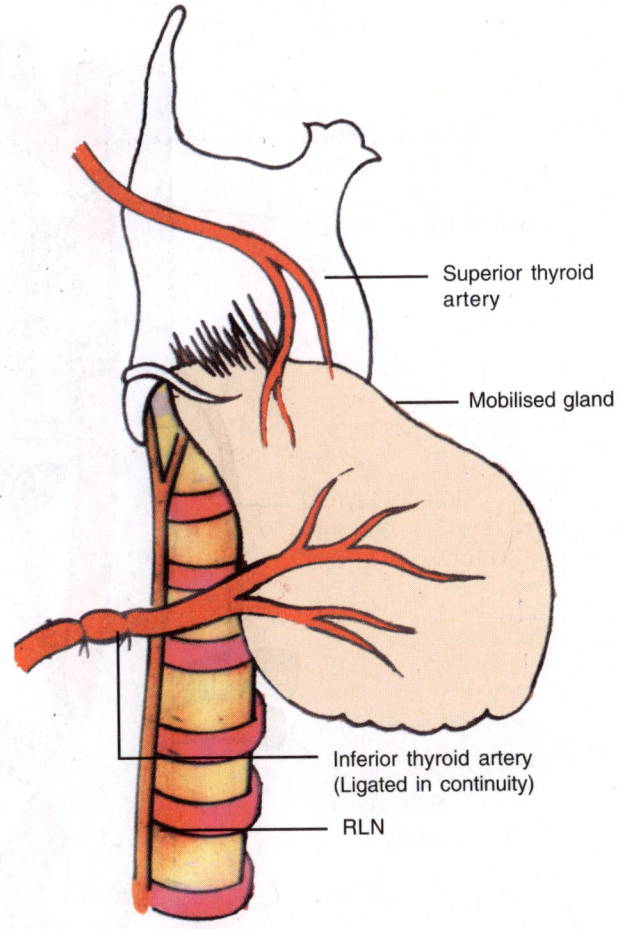

Fig. 19.2 Course of recurrent laryngeal nerve

Key Box 19.1

RECURRENT LARYNGEAL NERVE ANOMALIES

- The nerve **traverses through the gland** in about 5-8% of cases.

- The nerve may be **very closely adherent** to the posteromedial aspect of the gland.

- Nerve not seen-may be **far away** in the tracheo-oesophageal groove.

- **Non recurrent-recurrent laryngeal nerve** is found in about 1 in 1,000 cases. Nerve has a horizontal course.

- In 25% of the cases it is within the ligament of Berry.

---

1. Branches of thyrocervical trunk can be remembered as SIT-suprascapular, inferior thyroid and transverse cervical artery.
2. Superior thyroid artery and vein are like newly married couple, they go together hand in hand, middle thyroid vein is single, a bachelor and inferior thyroid artery and vein are divorced couple.

LYMPHATIC DRAINAGE OF THYROID

- **Subcapsular lymphatic plexus** drains into pretracheal nodes (**Delphic nodes** means uncertain) and prelaryngeal nodes which ultimately drain into *lower deep cervical nodes and mediastinal nodes.*

- The chief lymph nodes are middle and lower deep cervical lymph nodes. (Level III & IV).

- Supraclavicular nodes and nodes in the posterior triangle can also be involved in malignancies of the thyroid gland specially papillary carcinoma thyroid.

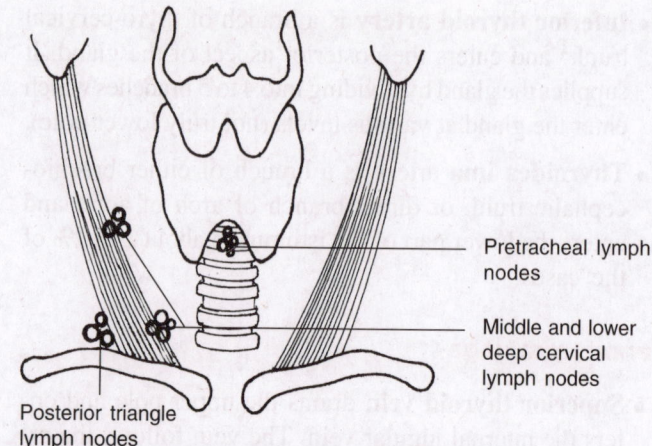

Pretracheal lymph nodes

Middle and lower deep cervical lymph nodes

Posterior triangle lymph nodes

Fig. 19.3 Lymphatic drainage

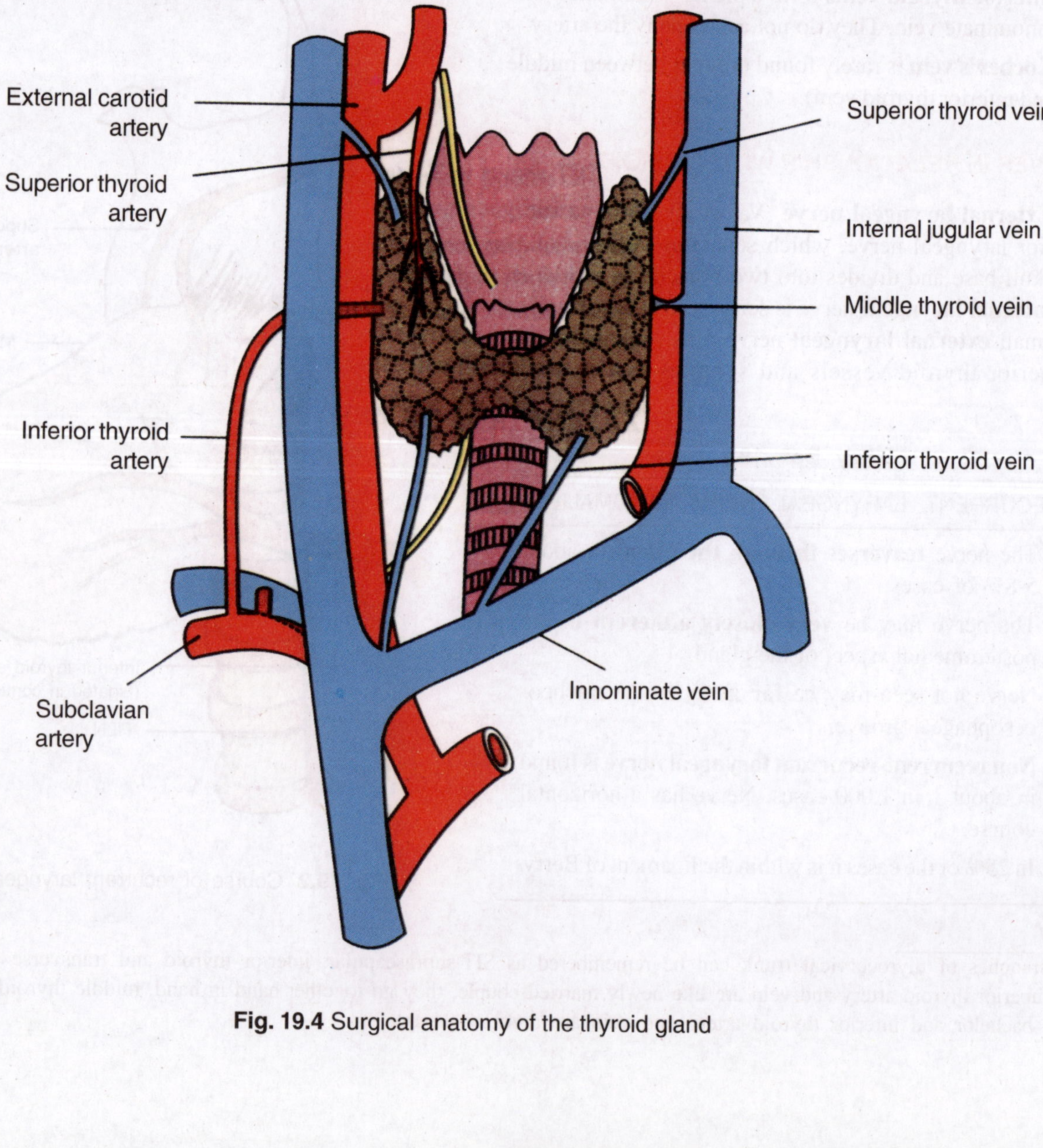

External carotid artery

Superior thyroid artery

Inferior thyroid artery

Subclavian artery

Superior thyroid vein

Internal jugular vein

Middle thyroid vein

Inferior thyroid vein

Innominate vein

Fig. 19.4 Surgical anatomy of the thyroid gland

PHYSIOLOGY

Tri-iodothyronine (T3) and thyroxine (T4) are the hormones secreted by the thyroid gland.

Dietary requirement of iodine per day is 100-200 micrograms. Sources of iodine are milk, dairy products, and sea food including fish.

Steps involved in the synthesis of these hormones

1. **Iodide trapping** from the blood into the thyroid, is the first step in the formation of T3 and T4.

    Thiocyanates and perchlorates block this step.

2. **Oxidation of iodide to inorganic iodine** This step needs the enzyme peroxidase.

    Drugs which block this stage are Sulfonamide, PAS (para-amino-salicylic acid), carbimazole, propylthiouracil, etc. (thioamides).

3. **Formation of iodotyrosines**

    Iodine + Tyrosine = MIT (Monoiodotyrosine) and Diiodotyrosine (DIT)

    This step is inhibited by thiourea group of drugs- i.e. Carbimazole.

4. **Coupling reactions**

    Coupling of two molecules of DIT results in T4 and one molecule of DIT and MIT results in T3.

    This stage is blocked by carbimazole.

    The hormones combine with globulin to form a colloid-thyroglobulin. They are stored in the thyroid gland and released as and when required.

    T3 is an important physiological hormone and fast acting (few hours). T4 is slow acting hormone and takes about 4-14 days to act.

THYROID FUNCTION TESTS

T$_3$ and T$_4$ estimation is the most commonly performed thyroid function tests. Other tests are not commonly done, some of them are obsolete.

1. **Serum T$_3$** Tri-iodothyronine 1-2 to 3 nmol/Ltr. (0.8 – 2.0 ng/ml)

2. **Serum T$_4$** Tetra-iodothyronine 55 to 150 nmol/Ltr. (4 – 12 μg/dl)

3. **Serum TSH** Thyroid Stimulating Hormone 0-5 I.U/ ml of plasma. (0.3–5) (Table 19.1)

    Following table outlines the levels of T$_3$, T$_4$ and TSH in few common conditions

Table 19.1

DISEASE	T$_3$	T$_4$	TSH
• Thyrotoxicosis	↑	↑	Suppressed
• T$_3$ Toxicosis	↑↑	Normal	Suppressed
• Hypothyroidism	Low or Normal	Low	↑

4. **Serum creatinine** In hyperthyroidism it is increased and it is decreased in hypothyroidism.

5. **Serum cholesterol** It is increased in hypothyroidism and decreased in hyperthyroidism.

6. **Serum calcitonin** Primary role is to decrease the levels of calcium. It is increased in Medullary Carcinoma Thyroid (MCT).

7. **Thyroid autoantibody levels** More than 90% of the patients with Hashimoto's thyroiditis and 80% of patients with Grave's disease have antibodies which are called as **antimicrosomal antibodies** (Earlier called as LATS). The detection of these antibodies help in the diagnosis of such cases and also to suspect these diseases before clinical manifestation.

8. **Thyroid scintigraphy** (Table 19.2, Fig. 19.5): Uptake by both lobes - Details can be referred in radionuclear scan chapter (Page 759).

Table 19.2 Thyroid Scintigraphy

IODINE	DOSE	HALF LIFE	IDEAL CASE
I^{131}	High dose radiation (500 mrad)	Long 8-10 days	Lingual thyroid, retrosternal goitre
I^{123}	Low dose radiation (30 mrad)	Short 12-14 hours	Well differentiated carcinoma for bony metastasis

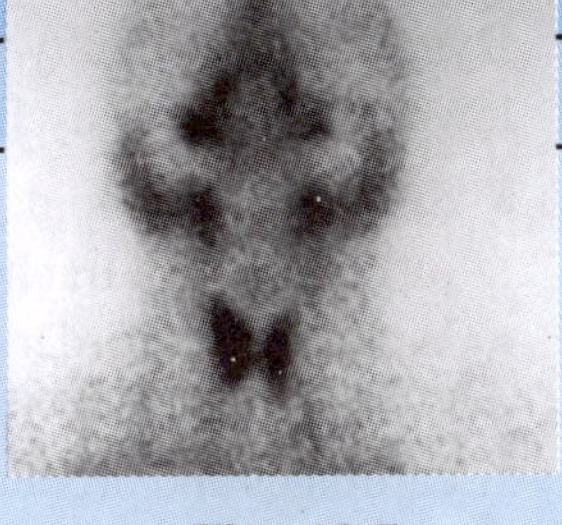

Fig. 19.5

Table 19.3 Nomenclatures of few thyroid diseases

• **Ectopic thyroid** Diagnosis by Isotope scan or CT scan	• Thyroid tissue along the line of descent Example: Floor of the mouth, submental region, mediastinum
• **Lingual thyroid** Diagnosis by Isotope scan or CT scan	• Swelling in the region of foramen caecum (Page 271)
• **Dyshormonogenesis** It is familial.	• Autosomal recessive condition with deficiency of peroxidase or dehalogenase (enzymes)
• **Pendred's syndrome**	• Dyshormonogenesis with congenital deafness
• **Struma Ovarii**	• Malignant ovarian teratoma containing thyroid tissue
• **Jod Basedow's disease** (German word)	• Excessive iodine given for hyperplastic goitre resulting in hyperthyroidism

*Terminology of some thyroid diseases (Table 19.3)

CLINICAL EXAMINATION OF THYROID SWELLING

- Diseases of the thyroid are very common and thyroid swellings are very often common cases in an undergraduate and postgraduate clinical examination. Hence, before discussing the various diseases of the thyroid gland, various aspects of the "CLINICS" are discussed in detail below.

COMPLAINTS

1. **Swelling** Long duration of thyroid swelling indicates benign condition, e.g. multinodular goitre (MNG), colloid goitre, etc.
   - Short duration with rapid growth indicates malignancy, such as anaplastic carcinoma. Majority of thyroid swellings do not produce pain.

2. **Rate of growth** Usually slow growing in benign disease.
   - If it is a rapid growth, it can be denovo malignancy or malignancy developing in a benign lesion, e.g. follicular carcinoma in MNG.
   - Sudden increase in size of swelling with pain indicates haemorrhage in the MNG (Multinodular goitre).

3. **Dyspnoea** Difficulty in breathing can be due to following reasons (Key Box 19.2)
   - Small goitre, rapid growth - anaplastic carcinoma infiltrating the trachea.
   - When lower border is not seen, retrosternal goitre.
   - Long-standing MNG compresses on tracheal cartilages and produces pressure atrophy of tracheal cartilages. This is called tracheomalacia.

Key Box 19.2

DYSPNOEA IN GOITRE - CAUSES

• Infiltration into trachea	**Anaplastic carcinoma**
• Lower border not seen	**Retrosternal goitre**
• Tracheomalacia	**Long standing MNG**
• Cardiac failure	**Secondary thyrotoxicosis**

4. **Dysphagia** is relatively uncommon because *oesophagus is a posterior structure* and it is a fibromuscular tube.

5. **Hoarseness of voice indicates malignancy.** It always occurs in carcinoma thyroid infiltrating the recurrent laryngeal nerve (never in benign diseases of thyroid).

6. **Toxic features suggestive of hyperthyroidism**

   A. CNS symptom are predominantly seen in Graves' disease (primary thyrotoxicosis - Key box 19.3)
   - Tremors of the hand

Key Box 19.3

GRAVES' DISEASE

• **G**oitre • **O**phthalmic symptoms • **I**rritability • **T**remors • **R**estlessness • **E**xcitability	*Students can remember the symptoms of Graves' disease as GOITRE.*

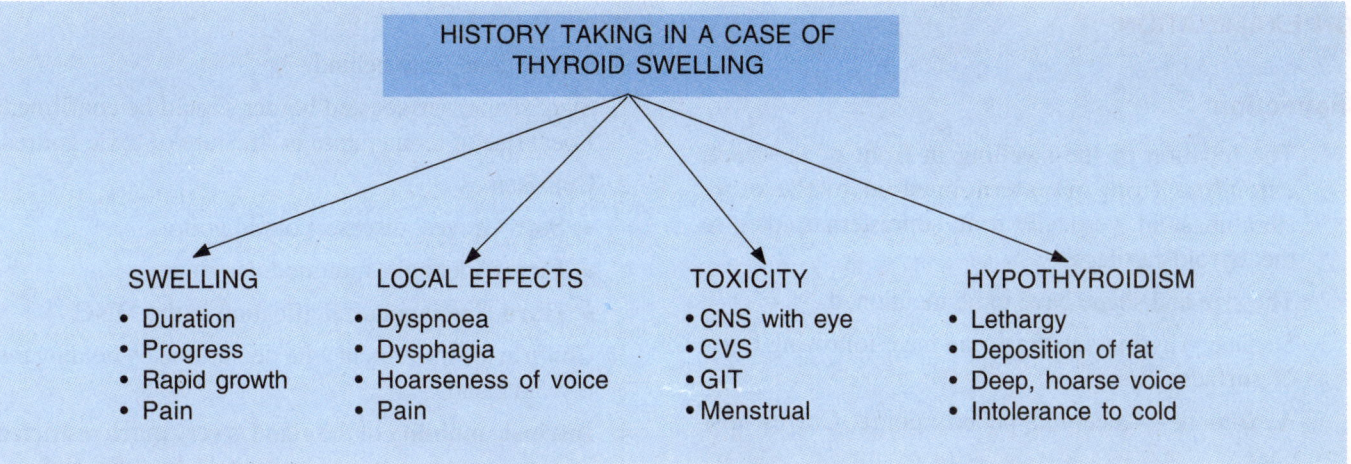

Fig. 19.6 Summary of history taking

- Sweating
- Intolerance to heat
- Preference to cold
- Excitability
- Irritability
- Prominent eyes are observed by other persons. Double vision, oedema of the conjunctiva can be the presenting complaints.

   B. **Cardiovascular symptoms (CVS)** are predominantly seen in secondary thyrotoxicosis. Even though both forms of thyrotoxicosis produce palpitations, it is a significant complaint in multinodular goitre with thyrotoxicosis (secondary thyrotoxicosis). Precordial chest pain, and dyspnoea on exertion are the late manifestations of secondary thyrotoxicosis.

   C. **Gastrointestinal tract (GIT)** symptoms such as increased appetite, diarrhoea, weight loss despite a good appetite are commonly seen in primary thyrotoxicosis. It is mandatory to consider the diagnosis of primary thyrotoxicosis in a young girl who presents with GIT symptoms and a thyroid swelling.

   D. **Menstrual disturbance** Oligomenorrhoea is common. (Page 253)

7. **Symptoms of hypothyroidism** Poor appetite, abnormal deposition of fat in the supraclavicular region, intolerance to cold, failing memory, deep hoarse voice, lethargy are typically seen in myxoedema.

8. **Sudden pain, thyroid swelling** and fever suggest autoimmune thyroiditis. Bacterial thyroiditis is a very rare cause of goitre.

   - Summary of history taking (Fig. 19.6)

Past history

- History of medication in the past is invariably present in toxic goitres. Previous surgery suggests a recurrent goitre.

Family history

- **Pendred syndrome** is a condition where congenital deafness is associated with goitre and hypothyroidism. This is due to the absence of enzyme, peroxidase (dyshormonogenesis). Goitre can also run in families, due to dehalogenase deficiency.

- Medullary carcinoma of the thyroid can run in families.

- In endemic areas many family members may suffer from goitre. It is due to iodine deficiency. Such goiters are called as **endemic goitres.**

General physical examination (Key Box 19.4)

Key Box 19.4
GENERAL PHYSICAL EXAMINATION
• Eye signs: Graves' disease
• Tremors of the tongue and hands: Graves' disease
• Pulse rate: Increased in toxic goitres, decreased in myxoedema
• **Pretibial myxoedema:** Treated Graves' disease
• Bony tenderness: Carcinoma thyroid
• Blood pressure changes: Secondary thyrotoxicosis

ON EXAMINATION

Inspection

1. The location of the swelling in front of the neck, extending from one sternomastoid to the other sternomastoid, vertically from suprasternal notch to the thyroid cartilage.

2. The size and shape have to be mentioned.

3. Surface: Thyroid swellings can have following types of surfaces

   A. Smooth – Adenoma, puberty goitre, Graves' disease

   B. Irregular – Carcinoma of the thyroid

   C. Nodular – Multinodular goitre

4. Borders are usually round

5. **Swelling moves up with deglutition** because of the following reasons

   • Thyroid is enclosed by pretracheal fascia which is condensed to form a ligament posteromedially called **LIGAMENT OF BERRY.** These are pairs of ligaments attached above to cricoid cartilage. During deglutition, the cricoid cartilage moves upwards. Hence, **thyroid gland moves upwards during deglutition**. (Kindly give a glass of water and check for movement with deglutition)

   • **If there is restriction of movement, it can be due to**

     Malignancy with fixity to the trachea

     Retrosternal goitre

     Large goitre because of the size

     Previous surgery.

Key Box 19.5
SWELLINGS WHICH MOVE UPWARDS WITH DEGLUTITION
• Thyroid swellings
• Subhyoid bursitis
• Pretracheal and prelaryngeal lymph nodes
• Thyroglossal cyst

6. **Movement on protrusion** of the tongue suggests **thyroglossal cyst**. This test should be done when there is a nodule or a cyst in the region of isthmus of the thyroid gland. This test has no relevance in cases of MNG or other thyroid swellings.

Palpation (Key Box 19.6)

It should be done from behind.

1. Size, shape, surface and border should be confirmed. Local rise of temperature is a feature of toxic goitres.

2. Consistency
   • **Soft** Graves' disease, colloid goitre.
   • **Firm** Adenoma, multinodular goitre.
   • **Hard** Carcinoma, calcification in the MNG.

3. Confirm the movement with deglutition by holding the thyroid gland.

4. **Intrinsic mobility** of the gland is very much restricted in carcinoma because of infiltration into the trachea.

5. **Sternomastoid contraction test** is done where in only one lobe is enlarged. In this situation the examiner keeps the hand on the side of the chin, opposite the side of the lesion and patient is asked to push the hand against resistance. If the gland becomes less prominent (as with thyroid swellings) it indicates the swelling is deep to the sternomastoid muscle.

6. **Chin test (Neck fixation test)** is classically done in multinodular goitre, where in both lobes are enlarged. The patient is asked to bend the chin downwards against resistance. This produces contraction of both sternomastoids and strap muscles, gland becomes less prominent.

7. Special tests or methods of examination of thyroid gland

   A. **Crile's method** is indicated when there is a doubtful nodule. Keep the thumb over the suspected area of the nodule and and ask the patient to swallow. The nodularity is appreciated better with this test.

Key Box 19.6
PALPATION - TESTS
• Local rise of temperature, size, shape, surface, borders
• Consistency, movement with deglutition
• Intrinsic mobility test
• Sternomastoid contraction test and chin test
• Position of trachea
• Palpation of lymph nodes
• Pulsations of common carotid artery
• Special tests
• Evidence of toxicity

B. **Lahey's method** of examination of thyroid can be done from front as well as behind. In order to palpate the right lobe, push the gland to the right side and feel the nodules in the posteromedial aspect of the gland. The lobe becomes more prominent and thus nodules are appreciated better.

C. **Pizzillo's method is indicated in obese patients especially short-necked individuals.** The patient is asked to clasp her hands and press against her occiput with head extended. Thyroid gland becomes more prominent, thus, palpation becomes better.

D. **Kocher's test** Gentle compression on lateral lobes producing stridor is described as positive. This is due to "SCABBARD" (Narrowed) trachea. Long standing multinodular goitres causing tracheomalacia and carcinoma with infiltration into trachea may give rise to stridor.

8. **Position of trachea** In cases of solitary nodule confined to one lobe, trachea is deviated to the opposite side. However, in cases of multinodular goitres, trachea need not be deviated because of symmetrical enlargement of both lobes.

9. **Palpation of lymph nodes** in the neck If lymph nodes are significant, it indicates papillary carcinoma of the thyroid.

10. **Palpation of common carotid artery** Draw a line from mastoid process to sternoclavicular joint. Then draw a horizontal line from upper border of thyroid cartilage. The point where these two lines meet is the site of bifurcation of common carotid artery. Just below this point this artery should be palpated.

- In large multinodular goitres, the artery may be pushed laterally. Hence, pulsations are felt in the posterior triangle.

- Carcinoma of the thyroid engulfs the carotid sheath, hence, pulsations may be absent. Absent carotid artery pulsation is called **"BERRY SIGN POSITIVE".** Since the lumen is not narrowed, superficial temporal artery pulsations are felt normally.

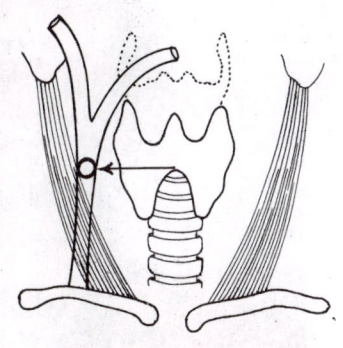

Fig. 19.7 Palpation of common carotid artery

Percussion

- Percussion over the sternum gives a resonant note in normal cases. In retrosternal goitres, it gives a dull note.

Auscultation

- It should be done in the **upper pole** because of following reasons **Superior thyroid artery is a direct branch of external carotid artery. It is more superficial than inferior thyroid artery**.

- Presence of thrill and bruit are the features of toxic goitre.

Systemic examination

- This includes CNS and eye signs, as in Graves' disease, examination of skeletal system to rule out metastasis as in carcinoma of the thyroid, and examination of cardiovascular system in cases of toxic goitre. These have been dealt with in detail in the corresponding topics. Deep tendon reflexes also have to be elicited-there is a slow relaxation phase in hypothyroidism.

Diagnosis

- It is based on following anatomical features. It should be noted that the neural tumours arising from vagus nerve can present in the same location but it will not move with deglutition.

Key Box 19.6
ANATOMICAL FEATURES OF THE THYROID GLAND
1. Thyroid gland is in front of the neck
2. Deep to pretracheal fascia
3. Moves up with deglutition
4. Butterfly-shaped when whole gland is enlarged

Differential diagnosis

- Simple goiter
- Toxic goiter
- Malignant goiter
- Solitary nodule
- Thyroiditis
- Other rare causes of thyroid enlargement

GOITRE

Definition Diffuse enlargement of the thyroid gland is described as goitre. (It is derived from the Latin word, Guttur = the throat.)

CLASSIFICATION OF GOITRE

I. Simple goitre

- Puberty goitre
- Colloid goitre
- Iodine-deficiency goitre
- Multinodular goitre

II. Toxic goitre

- Graves disease
- Secondary thyrotoxicosis in MNG
- Solitary nodule
- Other causes

III. Neoplastic goitre

- Benign adenoma (Follicular adenoma)
- Malignant tumours: They are further classified into

  A. **PRIMARY**

  - **Well-differentiated carcinoma**
    - Papillary carcinoma
    - Follicular carcinoma
  - **Poorly differentiated carcinoma**
    - Anaplastic carcinoma
  - Arising from **parafollicular cells**
    - Medullary carcinoma
  - Arising from **lymphatic tissue**
    - Malignant lymphoma

  B. **SECONDARY (Metastasis)**

  - Malignant melanoma, renal cell carcinoma, breast carcinoma produce secondaries in the thyroid, due to blood spread.

IV. Thyroiditis

- Granulomatous thyroiditis
- Autoimmune thyroiditis
- Riedel's thyroiditis

V. Other rare causes of goitre

- Acute bacterial thyroiditis
- Thyroid cyst
- Thyroid abscess
- Amyloid goitres

However, multinodular goitres, malignant goitres, puberty goitres are common causes of goitre. Bacterial thyroiditis is rare. Riedel's thyroiditis is very very rare.

MULTINODULAR GOITRE

- **A multinodular goitre is the end stage result of diffuse hyperplastic goitre**. Excessive metabolic demands cause an excessive enlargement of the thyroid. Therefore common in women.
- **Metabolic demands increase during puberty**. A goitre appearing during that period is called puberty goitre. A goitre can develop during pregnancy and is called pregnancy goitre. Both of them are physiological but eventually may develop into multinodular goitre (MNG).

AETIOPATHOGENESIS

- Multinodular goitre results due to a continuous stimulation by the TSH which is released from the anterior pituitary.

1. **Puberty goitre, pregnancy goitre**

- Seen in girls at puberty or during pregnancy when the metabolic demands are high and the production of T3, T4 are comparatively normal. Due to feedback mechanism, TSH levels increase, which stimulate thyroid gland and causes diffuse hypertrophy and hyperplasia.
- This is also called physiological goitre and can be treated by giving tablet thyroxine (T4) 0.2 mg/day to suppress TSH.
- Goitre may disappear if treatment is given in the stage of diffuse hypertrophy.

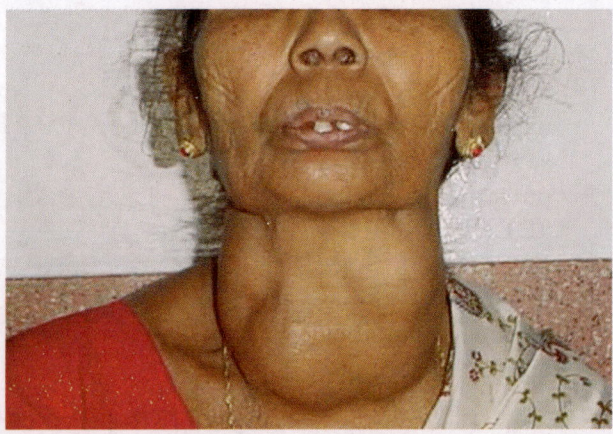

Fig. 19.8 Multinodular goitre

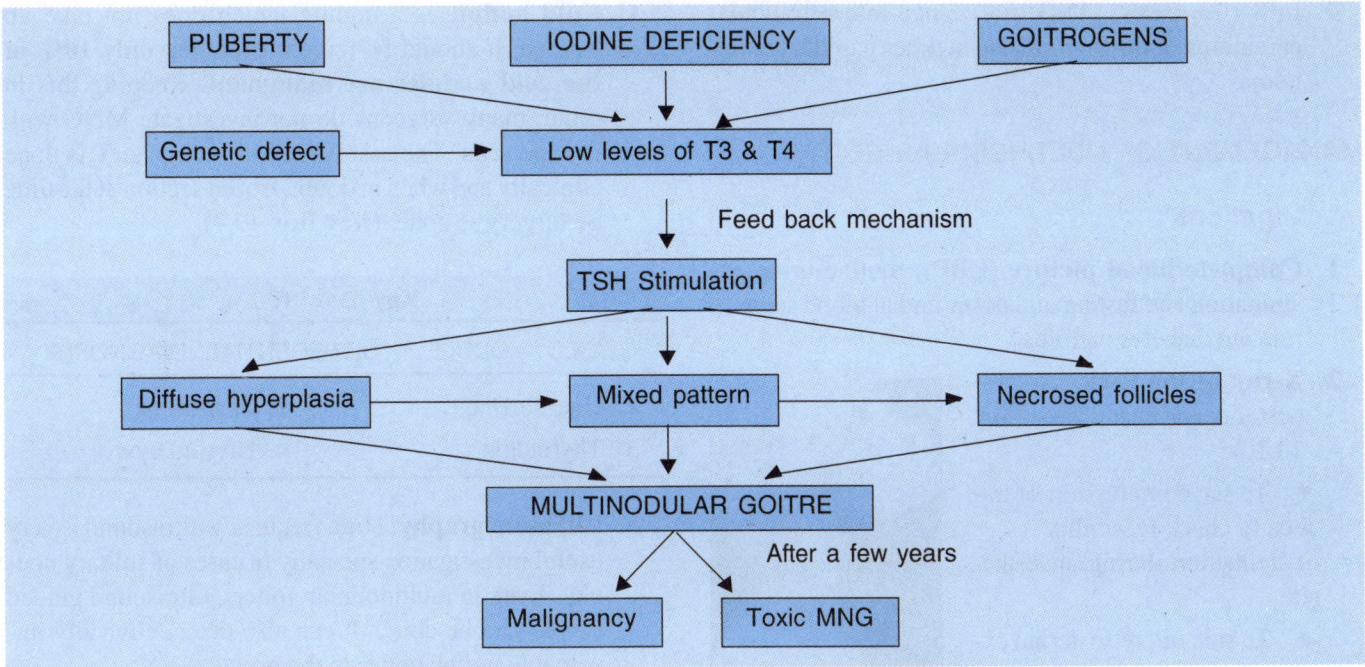

Fig. 19.9 Flowchart showing pathogenesis of MNG

2. **Iodine deficiency goitre**

- Daily iodine requirement is about 100-125 micrograms.
- Common in hill/mountain areas and low-lying areas because of decreased iodide content of water. This causes iodine deficiency goitre, by the same feed back mechanism.
- This is treated by **iodised salt** which is used for food and also iodine-containing preparations.
- If the iodine deficiency status continues for a long time it results in the accumulation of **colloid material** in the gland and causes **colloid goitre**.
- All these 3 types of goitre if left untreated will change to multinodular goitre (Fig. 19.9)

Stage I	Stage of diffuse hypertrophy and hyperplasia of thyroid.
Stage II	Due to fluctuating levels of TSH because of pregnancy, lactation, menstruation, etc., some areas in thyroid are overstimulated and are converted to active follicles.
Stage III	The active follicle ultimately undergoes necrosis and many such necrosed follicles join to form a nodule. Many such nodules form a multinodular goitre. Nodules contain necrosed tissue i.e., inactive tissue. **The internodular tissue is active.**

3. **Goitrogens** such as cabbage, drugs such as PAS and sulfonamides, cause goitre by preventing oxidation of iodide to iodine.

CLINICAL FEATURES

- Common in females. Female Male ratio is - 10:1. Seen in age group of 20-40 years
- Long duration of swelling in front of the neck, dyspnoea due to tracheomalacia and dysphagia are the presenting features. Gland is nodular, firm in consistency and both the lobes are enlarged.
- Hard areas may suggest calcification and soft areas, necrosis.
- Sudden increase in size with pain is mainly due to haemorrhage in a nodule.

The most common site of a nodule is at the junction of isthmus with one lobe.

COMPLICATIONS OF MULTINODULAR GOITRE

1. Calcification in long-standing MNG.
2. Sudden haemorrhage in one of the nodules causes sudden enlargement of gland and even causes dyspnoea.
3. In 10-20% of cases, patients can develop secondary thyrotoxicosis with CVS involvement. **Toxic multinodular goitre is also called as Plummer's disease**.

4. In 8-10% cases, MNG can change into a follicular carcinoma of the thyroid, and at times papillary carcinoma.

MANAGEMENT OF MULTINODULAR GOITRE

Investigations

1. **Complete blood picture (CBP)**, routine urine examination and fasting and postprandial blood sugar to rule out diabetes mellitus.

2. **X-ray of the neck** Antero-posterior and lateral view. (Fig. 19.10)
   - To see compression of trachea to check feasibility of intubation during anaesthesia.
   - To rule out retrosternal extension-soft tissue shadow seen.
   - Calcification in long-standing MNG.

Fig. 19.10 X-ray of the neck - lateral view

3. **Indirect laryngoscopy**[1] is done to see vocal cord mobility.

4. **Isotope scan** by using tracer dose of radio-iodine. It can demonstrate 3 different patterns as follows (Fig. 19.11)

A. **Hot nodule** The gland does not take up isotope but the nodule takes it up, which is a feature of autonomous solitary toxic nodule. Here, the normal thyroid tissue is suppressed.

B. **Warm nodule** Entire gland takes up isotope. This is typical of Graves' disease (primary thyrotoxicosis) wherein each cell is active and equally stimulated.

C. **Cold nodule** is a nodule which does not take up isotope. It should be remembered that **only 10% of the cold nodules are malignant**. Keeping this in mind, many surgeons do not investigate MNG with isotope scan. The assessment of malignancy is done clinically and when in doubt, frozen section at the time of surgery is done. (Key Box 19.7)

Key Box 19.7	
COLD NODULE - DIFFERENTIAL DIAGNOSIS	
1. Haemorrhage	2. Carcinoma
3. Thyroiditis	4. Thyroid cyst

5. **Ultrasonography:** High frequency ultrasound is very useful investigation specially in cases of solitary nodule. Even in multinodular goiters, ultrasound guided FNAC can be done. It can also detect clinically impalpable lymph nodes in the neck.

6. **Fine needle aspiration cytology** (FNAC) should be done in all cases of multinodular goitre even when isotope scan is not done because it is a simple useful investigation which can detect malignancy.

Prevention (Key Box 19.8)

Prevention can be tried in early stages. (Key Box 19.8)

Key Box 19.8
PREVENTION OF MNG
• Puberty goitre: 0.1 mg to 0.2 mg of **thyroxine**
• Iodine deficiency goitre: Use **iodised salt, sea food, milk, egg**, etc.
• Goitrogens : **Avoid cabbage, drugs**

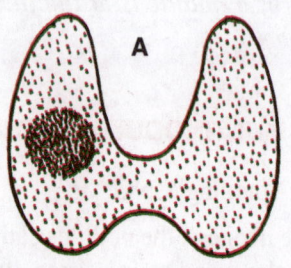 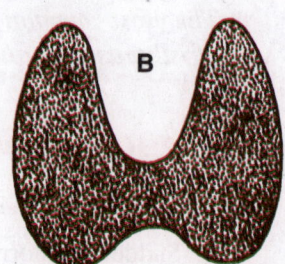 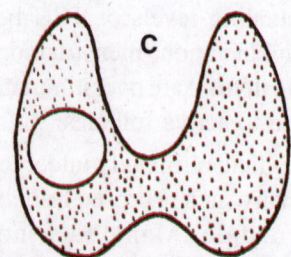

Fig. 19.11A, B, C: Radio isotope scan findings

---

1. Documenting vocal cord paralysis before surgery is for legal purpose. Patient can have normal voice in spite of one vocal cord paralysis due to compensatory movement of the normal vocal cord. Vocal cord paralysis can be due to childhood infections such as mumps. etc.

Classification of investigations

Key Box 19.9

INVESTIGATIONS - GOITRE

1. **Simple goitres**
   - Routine-Blood and urine tests, chest X-ray
   - Indirect laryngoscopy
2. **Toxic goitres**
   - Routine
   - T3, T4, TSH
   - Isotope scan
3. **Malignant goitre**
   - Routine
   - Isotope scan, bone scan
   - FNAC

SURGERY

- **Subtotal thyroidectomy** In this operation, parts of right and left lobes and entire isthmus are removed in flush with tracheal surface leaving behind a little tissue in the tracheo-oesophageal groove to protect recurrent larygeal nerve and parathyroid gland.
- Some surgeons treat these patients with 0.2 mg of thyroxine to suppress the TSH stimulation in the postoperative period, for a period of 2-5 years.

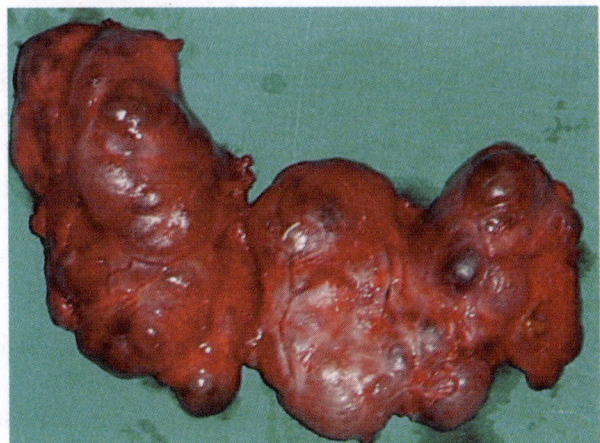

Fig. 19.12 Subtotal thyroidectomy

RETROSTERNAL GOITRE

- Very often, it is a multinodular goitre which develops in the neck and is slowly pulled down behind the sternum due to following reasons
1. Negative intrathoracic pressure

2. Pretracheal muscles are strong in men
3. Short neck, obesity
- Rarely, it arises from an ectopic thyroid tissue

Clinical types

1. **Substernal** the most common type where the lower border of the gland is behind the sternum.
2. **Intrathoracic** No thyroid is seen in the neck, diagnosed by radio-iodine scan.
3. **Plunging goitre** When patient is asked to cough, intrathoracic pressure increases. As the thyroid plunges out, the lower border of gland is clearly seen in the neck.

Clinical features of retrosternal goitre

- It can be suspected when the **lower border of the swelling is not seen.**
- Most of the patients have **difficulty in breathing or even stridor**
- **Dysphagia** is more common
- **Engorgement of neck veins** and superficial veins. These become more prominent when the hands are raised above the head, and the arms touch the ears - **"Pemberton's sign".**

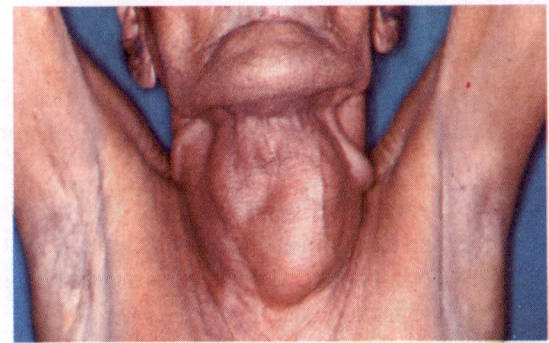

Fig. 19.13 Multinodular goitre

Key Box 19.10

RETROSTERNAL GOITRE

- Very often it is a **MNG with lower border unseen**
- **Rarely** from **ectopic thyroid** tissue
- **Severe breathlessness** even though **small**
- **Drugs should not be given if it is toxic**
- **Pressure effects** diagnosed by **Pemberton's test**
- **Surgical excision is the treatment**

Investigations

- They are similar to MNG. However, isotope scan is very useful in the diagnosis of intrathoracic goitres.

Treatment

- It can be easily explored through the neck incision and removed.
- Very, very, rarely, sternal split may be necessary

TOXIC GOITRE-THYROTOXICOSIS

- It is a complex disorder which occurs due to increased levels of thyroid hormones (Hyperthyroidism) and manifests clinically with various signs and symptoms involving many body systems. Following are the causes of thyrotoxicosis

1. **Primary thyrotoxicosis** (Graves' disease, exophthalmic goitre).

2. **Secondary thyrotoxicosis:** Secondary to multinodular goitre

3. **Solitary toxic nodule** Autonomous nodule which is not under the influence of TSH, but occurs due to hypertrophy and hyperplasia of gland (tertiary thyrotoxicosis).

4. **Other causes of thyrotoxicosis**
   - **Thyrotoxicosis factitia** False thyrotoxicosis occurs due to overdosage of thyroxine, given for puberty goitre.
   - **Jod-Basedow's thyrotoxicosis** Jod means iodine in the German language, Basedow means toxic goitre. Iodine induced thyrotoxicosis (iodine given for hyperplastic endemic goitres)
   - Initial stage of thyroiditis.
   - Very rarely, malignant goitres can be toxic (differentiated carcinoma)
   - **Neonatal thyrotoxicosis** occurs in babies born to thyrotoxic mothers
   - TSH secreting tumours of pituitary
   - Struma **ovarii**
   - Drugs: **Amiodarone** given as anti arrhythmic drug

In the clinical examination, primary thyrotoxicosis and secondary thyrotoxicosis are commonly kept as long cases. Hence, these two have been discussed in detail in the following pages.

GRAVES' DISEASE

AETIOPATHOGENESIS

- The exact aetiological factors responsible for this disease are not clear. Following are considered as possible aetiological factors

1. **Autoimmune** disorder is the first possible cause due to the demonstration of auto-antibodies in the circulation. Example: **TSH Receptor Antibodies**. It can also be associated with other autoimmune disorders like vitiligo.

2. **Familial** The disease can run in families. Familial/Genetic Graves' disease has been documented in identical twins.

3. **Thyroid stimulating immunoglobulins (TSI)** and long-acting thyroid stimulator (LATS) are responsible for pathological changes in the thyroid gland in Graves' disease.

4. **Exophthalmos producing substance (EPS)** is responsible for "ophthalmopathy" which is seen in Graves' disease.

5. **Female sex, emotions, stress, young age** also have been considered as other factors responsible for the disease.

PATHOLOGY

- As a result of continuous stimulation, acinar hypertrophy and hyperplasia take place. The acinar cells which are normally flat, become tall columnar. The normal colloid disappears and the cells are empty, However, rich vascularity is seen. Thus, small follicles with hyperplastic columnar epithelium is characteristic.

CLINICAL NOTES

Following are 3 case reports which highlight the clinical symptomatology of primary thyrotoxicosis.

- An 18 year old girl visited many doctors for her complaint of loss of weight. She was investigated for tuberculosis (common disease in India), malignancy, etc. She was given unnecessary tonics. After nearly 6 months, when eye-signs started developing, it was proved to be Graves' disease.

- A bank clerk's only complaint was that he could not sign the cheque because of excessive sweating. Thyroid gland was not palpable. Pulse rate was very high. Investigations revealed it was a case of primary thyrotoxicosis. On careful questioning, he admitted that he was a "nervous character".

- A 24 year old lady was being asked by her friends every day why her eyes were prominent. Her only complaint was prominent eyes. On careful questioning she admitted having anxiety, tension, excitability.

CLINICAL FEATURES

1. Primary thyrotoxicosis is **8 times more common in females** than in males, aged around 15-25 years.

2. **Symptoms, signs and swelling appear simultaneously**.

3. Very often young women present with unexplained loss of weight in spite of good appetite. Diarrhoea occurs due to increased smooth muscle activity of small intestines. Intolerance to heat, preference to cold, fine tremors, excitability, **hyperkinetic movements**, excessive sweating are the other features. **Free steroid hormone levels decrease in Graves disease, this results in decreased effective oestrogen at the cell level which in turn causes oligomenorrhoea.**

Signs of primary thyrotoxicosis

I. Signs of thyroid gland in Graves' disease

- Uniformly enlarged (mild degree)
- Smooth surface-no nodules
- Gland is soft or firm in consistency
- It is warm-highly vascular (Key Box 19.11)
- Auscultation-a bruit is usually heard.

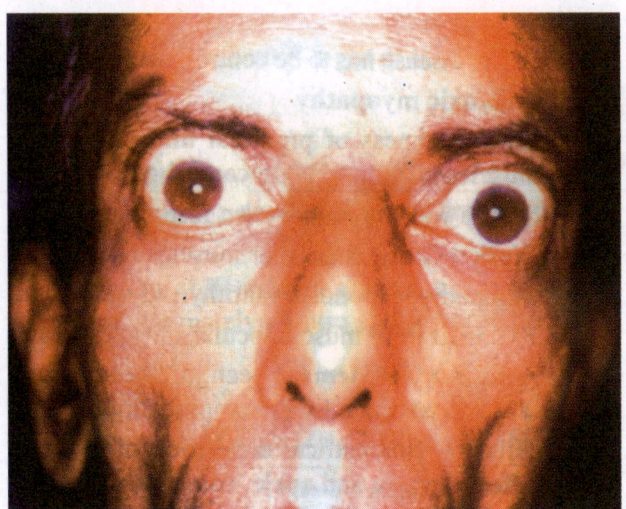

Fig. 19.14 Exophthalmos

Key Box 19.11

PULSATILE THYROID SWELLINGS

- Primary thyrotoxicosis
- Secondary thyrotoxicosis
- Follicular carcinoma
- Vascular malformations

II. Central nervous system (CNS) signs

- Tremors of the tongue **when the tongue is within the oral cavity** and tremors of the outstretched hands are characteristic. A piece of paper may be placed on the fingers in doubtful cases for demonstrating the tremors of the hand. Extensor surface of the hand is used because extensors are weak when compared to flexors.
- Hyperkinetic movements.
- Always a moist, warm hand (shake hands and see).

III. Cardiovascular system (CVS) signs

- Pulse rate is always raised and rapid indicating tachycardia. Depending upon the pulse rate, thyrotoxicosis can be classified as follows **Mild**-90-100/minute, **Moderate**-100-110/minute, **Severe**-more than 110/minute.
- **Palpitation and extrasystoles** can also be found in primary thyrotoxicosis even though other cardiac features such as fibrillation and cardiac failure are rare.

IV. Eye signs

- **Prominent eyeballs** and retraction of the eyelid result in thyrotoxic exophthalmos. This is due to retrobulbar deposition of inflammatory cells, and round cells with venous congestion resulting in oedema.
- **Levator palpebrae superioris** muscle is innervated by oculomotor nerve which also carries sympathetic fibres derived from cavernous plexus for smooth muscle part of the levator. Contraction of this muscle produces **lid spasm**.
- This is aided by **spasm of Muller's muscle**, a sympathetic muscle which lies on the floor of the orbit. This is responsible for keeping the eyeball forwards. All these factors together produce a classical stare.

1. Assessment of exophthalmos

A. When upper sclera is seen above the limbus (upper margin of iris and cornea) - **Dalrymple's sign.**

B. **Naffziger's method** Stand behind the patient and look at the superciliary arch, by tilting the patient's head backwards. In normal cases, eyeball is not seen. In cases of exophthalmos eyeball is protruded outside.

Key Box 19.12

THYROTOXIC EXOPHTHALMOS

- Proptosis and lid retraction result in exophthalmos
- Sclera is visible beyond limbus
- Naffziger's method to examine
- Staring look
- Typically seen in Graves' disease
- Rarely seen in secondary thyrotoxicosis

---

2. Moebius sign

- Loss of convergence of eyeball. Occurs due to muscle paresis as a part of thyrotoxic ophthalmoplegia.

3. Stellwag's sign

- Infrequent blinking and widening of palpebral fissure is due to spasm of sympathetic fibers in the levator palpebrae superioris.

4. Joffroy's sign

- Absence of wrinkling of the forehead when patient is asked to look upwards. This occurs due to increase in the field of vision due to exophthalmos.

5. Von Graefe's sign (Lid lag sign)

- When the patient is asked to look up and down, upper eyelid cannot cope up with the speed of the movement of the finger because of the lid spasm. Hence, the lid lags behind.

Malignant exophthalmos

- This occurs in untreated cases of Graves' disease.
- If the disease continues, infrequent blinking secondary to exophthalmos results in constant exposure of the cornea to the atmosphere. This results in keratitis, corneal ulcer, conjunctivitis, chemosis can occur may even lead to blindness. This is called Malignant Exophthalmos.
- Malignant exophthalmos is probably due to autoimmune disease.
- In late stages **optic nerve damage and blindness** can occur.

Grading of thyroid eye diseases (Key Box 19.13)

Key Box 19.13

GRADING OF THYROID EYE DISEASES

Grade 0	No signs or symptoms
Grade 1	Only signs, no symptoms
Grade 2	Soft tissue involvement
Grade 3	Proptosis
Grade 4	Extraocular muscle involvement
Grade 5	Corneal involvement
Grade 6	Loss of vision with optic nerve atrophy

Comparison of primary thyrotoxicosis and secondary thyrotoxicosis (Table 19.4)

Table 19.4 Differences between primary and secondary thyrotoxicosis

	PRIMARY THYROTOXICOSIS	SECONDARY THYROTOXICOSIS
1. Age	15-25 years	25-40 years
2. Symptoms and signs	Appear simultaneously; duration is short	Long duration of a swelling and short duration of symptoms
3. Skin over the swelling	Warm	Not warm
4. Consistency	Soft or firm	Firm or hard
5. Surface	Smooth	Nodular
6. Auscultation	Bruit is common	Bruit uncommon
7. Eye signs	Commonly found	Rarely found
8. Predominant symptoms	CNS	CVS

Treatment of thyrotoxic ophthalmopathy

1. Massive doses of steroids – oral prednisolone and metronidazole

2. Lateral tarsorrhaphy

3. Orbital decompression may be necessary in late cases.

4. Guanethidine eye drops are useful to decrease lid spasm and lid retraction

5. Primary disease has to be controlled

6. Head end elevation

V. Thyrotoxic myopathy

- Mild weakness of proximal limb muscles is common. On careful questioning, patient may admit difficulty in climbing steps.

- Weakness of extraocular muscles results in double vision (Diplopia)

- Myopathy responds to antithyroid treatment.

- **Proximal limb muscles**, ocular muscles, frontalis are commonly involved (weakness of muscle).

- Features suggestive of **Myasthenia gravis, periodic paralysis** can be found.

VI. Pretibial myxoedema is seen in thyrotoxicosis patients treated with surgery or antithyroid drugs. It is always associated with exophthalmos. (It is a misnomer Key Box 19.15).

- **Bilateral symmetrical deposition** of myxomatous tissue mainly in the pretibial region, may also affect the foot and ankle, sometimes the entire leg below knee. Skin is dry and coarse (thickening of skin by mucin - like deposits).

- Pretibial myxoedema is non-pitting in nature and may be associated with clubbing of fingers and toes- called **thyroid acropachy**. (Key Box 19.14)

Key Box 19.14

SKIN CHANGES

- Pretibial myxoedema
- Pruritis
- Palmar erythema
- Thinning of hair

Key Box 19.15

FEW MISNOMERS

- Pretibial myxoedema — Not seen in myxoedema
- Mycosis fungoides — Not a fungal infection
- White bile — Not white, not bile
- Adenolymphoma — Not a lymphoma
- Sternomastoid tumour — Not a tumour
- Malignant hydatid — Not malignant

MANAGEMENT OF PRIMARY THYROTOXICOSIS

Investigations

1. Routine investigations such as complete blood picture, fasting and post-prandial blood sugar estimation, urine examination, chest X-ray including neck and indirect laryngoscopy are done.

2. Thyroid scan will show warm gland (findings are already discussed)

3. Serum **T3, T4 and TSH** estimation is done. The T3 or T4 levels are high with low levels of TSH. The normal level of T3 is 1.3-3.5 nanomols/litre and normal level of T4 is 55-150 nanomols/litre.

4. **Thyroid antibodies** are elevated.

5. *Sleeping pulse rate is counted after the patient is sedated with 30 mg of phenobarbitone.* In a case of toxic goitre the pulse rate remains high even during sleep because of increased metabolism. **This is a simple bedside investigation in cases of toxic goitre.** In anxiety states, pulse rate may be high in the morning hours and it comes back to normal during sleep.

TREATMENT OF PRIMARY THYROTOXICOSIS

Aim of treatment

I. To **restore** the patients to a **euthyroid state**.

II. To **reduce the functioning thyroid mass** to a very critical level (about 6-8 gm of thyroid tissue).

III. To **minimise complications**

I. To restore the patient to euthyroid state (TABLE 19.5 next page)

- Other drugs such as potassium perchlorate are given in the dose of 200 mg three times a day. Maintenance dose is 200 to 400 mg daily. Propyl thiouracil

Table 19.5 Antithyroid drugs: Routine preoperative preparation

DRUGS AND MODE OF ACTION	DOSE	PRECAUTION/SIDE EFFECTS
Carbimazole: It blocks oxidation of iodide to iodine and coupling reactions, thus reducing T3 and T4 levels. It is metabolised to methimazole after ingestion.	• **10 mg, 6th hourly** and maintenance dose of 10 mg two to three times a day.	• Takes 2-3 weeks for its action. • It should be given at 6 to 8 hourly interval. **Dangerous agranulocytosis** can manifest as sore throat.
Propranolol is a β-blocker, reduces tachycardia.	• **10-20 mg, two or three times a day** depending on the pulse rate.	• **Congestive cardiac failure**. Can precipitate bronchial asthma. T3 and T4 levels are not decreased.
Lugol's iodine is given to reduce vascularity of the gland before surgery.	• 10-12 drops (minims) three times a day for 10 days before surgery.	• It is bitter, has to be used with orange juice.

in the dose of 200 mg three times a day can also be given in patients who develop neutropenia due to carbimazole.

Please note

- Iodine containing antiarrhythmic drug **amiodarone** may worsen thyrotoxicosis.
- Propyl thiouracil is **safe in pregnancy** with Grave's disease
- Role of Lugol's iodine is **doubtful**.
- Antithyroid drugs will not cure the disease. In selected patients (30 to 40%) remission is possible with regular intake of drugs. **They may be continued for maximum period of 2 years.** If by this time toxicity persists or if it recurrs on stopping drugs, surgery is recommended. However, majority of the patients ultimately require surgery or radio-iodine.

Block and replace treatment

- If a small dose of T_3 (20 µg upto 4 times/day) or T_4 (0.1mg/day) is given along with antithyroid drugs, there is less incidence of **Hypothyroidism** development and increase in the size of goitre.

II.To reduce the functioning thyroid mass

1. **Subtotal thyroidectomy** In this procedure, the thyroid gland is removed as for non-toxic multinodular goitre. However, being a toxic goitre, very little gland should be left behind so as to avoid persistent toxicity in the postoperative period. It is recommended that at least 6-8 gm of thyroid tissue be left behind. This is difficult to measure.

Hence, some surgeons advocate leaving thyroid tissue as small as the tip of the little finger, on both sides.

2. **Radio-iodine therapy** This is a suitable alternative to surgery in cases of primary thyrotoxicosis in patients above the age of 40.

III. To minimise complications

- **Good preoperative preparation** of the patient, good anaesthetic and surgical techniques and good postoperative care will reduce the complications of surgery.

Thus, antithyroid drugs, subtotal thyroidectomy and radio-iodine therapy are the three different modalities available for the treatment of primary thyrotoxicosis. The indications, merits, demerits of each treatment are given in the flowchart in Fig. 19.15.

TREATMENT OF SECONDARY THYROTOXICOSIS

- Patients with severe cardiac damage entirely or partly due to hyperthyroidism are middle-aged or elderly with secondary thyrotoxicosis and the hyperthyroidism is not very severe. These patients develop atrial fibrillation and cardiac failure, if left untreated. In elderly patients, when the operative risk is unacceptable, radio-iodine is given. Treatment with antithyroid drugs is started 48 hours later and continued until radio-iodine has had its effect (6 weeks).

- If the cardiac symptoms are controlled well and anaesthesia risk is acceptable, subtotal thyroidectomy is done. However, the gland that is left behind should be equal to the terminal phalanx of the thumb of the patient.

TREATMENT OF GRAVE'S DISEASE

I. Continuation of anti-thyroid drugs

Advantages

1. Avoids surgery
2. No risk to life
3. Economical

Disadvantages

1. Long duration of treatment **1-2 years**
2. Agranulocytosis, fever, skin rash
3. Missed doses
4. Relapses common - 50%

Indications

1. Patient not willing for surgery.
2. Postponement of surgery
3. Recurrence after surgery

II. Surgery - sub-total thyroidectomy

Advantages

1. In good hands, permanent cure to the patient
2. Cure rate is high

Disadvantages

1. Carries mortality and morbidity
2. Side effects of thyroidectomy
3. Recurrence

Indications

1. Young patients aged 25-35 years who are fit for surgery
2. Toxicosis with large goitre
3. Retrosternal goitre
4. Pregnant patients

III. Radio-iodine150 microcuries per gram (10-15 mCi)

Advantages

1. No surgery
2. No drugs
3. Easy, more cost effective
4. No RLN palsy

Disadvantages

1. Contraindicated in pregnancy, lactating women.
2. Permanent hypothyroidism in 10-15% patients.
3. Exacerbation of cardiac arrhythmias.

Indications

1. **Any age group**
2. Recurrent thyrotoxicosis after surgery
3. Patients with cardiac symptoms
4. Small to moderate enlargement.

Fig. 19.15 Indications, merits and demerits of different modalities of treatments for primary thyrotoxicosis

Key Box 19.16
RADIO IODINE THERAPY

- Today there is 'NO RESTRICTION OF AGE AND SEX'.
- **Absolute contraindication is pregnancy**.
- To **avoid conception** for a period of 4 months after radioiodine therapy.

Key Box 19.17
SECONDARY THYROTOXICOSIS EFFECT ON CVS

- Tachycardia
- Wide pulse pressure
- Extrasystoles
- Atrial fibrillation
- Cardiac failure

SOME SPECIFIC TOXIC THYROID CONDITIONS

Thyrotoxicosis in children: Initially anti thyroid drugs are given for 10-15 years followed by surgery.

- Radioiodine is absolutely contraindicated as there is a fear of carcinoma developing at a later date (Key Box 19.16)

Thyrocardiac It refers to a condition wherein cardiac damage has resulted due to hyperthyroidism (Key Box 19.17).

- Classically it happens in secondary thyrotoxicosis usually seen in middle aged or old aged patients.
- Propranolol controls the disease very well.
- Radioiodine therapy is the treatment of choice.

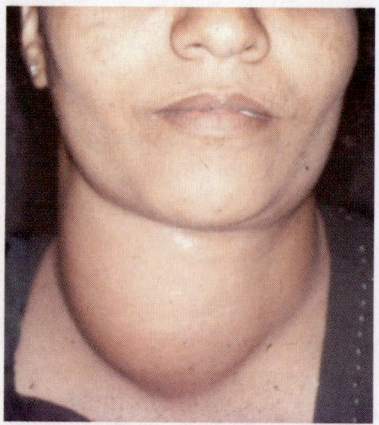

Fig. 19.16 Colloid goitre - smooth surface and round borders

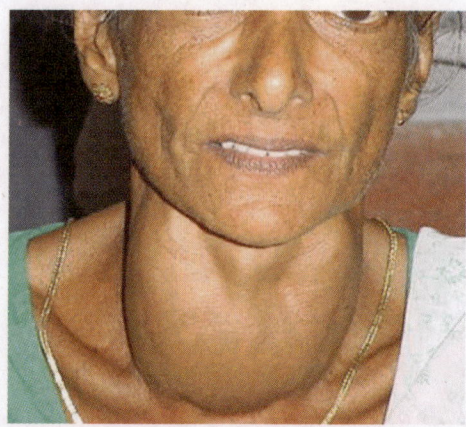

Fig. 19.17 Toxic multinodular goitre - nodular surface and vascular

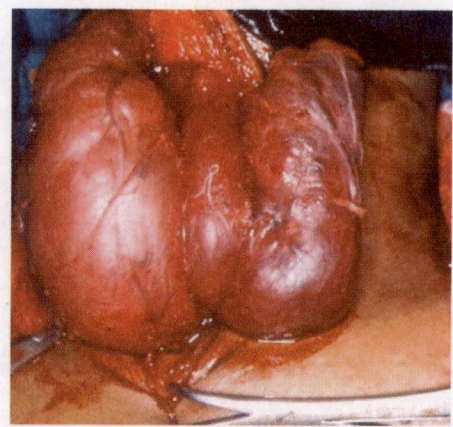

Fig. 19.18 Same patient as in Fig.19.17 at surgery

Hyperthyroidism in pregnancy

- Invariably it is Grave's disease.
- **In the first trimester surgery and radioiodine are contraindicated**. Smallest dose of carbimazole or propyl thiouracil can be used with fetal monitoring (Both TSH and Antithyroid drugs cross the placenta).
- **Surgery, if necessary can be done in 2nd trimester.**

Apathetic thyrotoxicosis

- Thyrotoxicosis in elderly wherein pulse rate is low, they appear hypothyroid rather than hyperthyroid patients.

NEOPLASTIC GOITRE

ADENOMA

- The benign tumours of the thyroid gland are not uncommon. They present as a soiitary nodule, thus causing a worry to the clinician. Adenomas are of follicular type.
- The diagnosis is established by histological examination.
- Adenomas are treated by hemithyroidectomy/lobectomy.
- However FNAC cannot distinguish between a follicular adenoma and follicular carcinoma. Hence a frozen section has to be arranged.

MALIGNANT TUMOURS[1]

- Thyroid is the only endocrine gland wherein malignant tumours are easily accessible to clinical examination.
- Thyroid is the only endocrine gland wherein malignant tumours occur in children, young age, middle age, old age and in both sexes.
- Thyroid is the only endocrine gland wherein malignant tumours spread by all possible routes-local, lymphatic and blood spread.
- Thyroid is the only endocrine gland wherein malignant tumours are usually non-functional.

Malignant tumours of the thyroid are common. They are interesting tumours, having good prognosis if diagnosed early. Papillary and follicular carcinoma are well differentiated, medullary carcinoma are moderately differentiated and anaplastic carcinomas are poorly differentiated.

PAPILLARY CARCINOMA

AETIOLOGY

1. Irradiation to the neck during childhood.

Radiotherapy given for benign conditions such as acne in teenagers or enlarged tonsils or thymus gland in children increases the risk.

2. It can be a complication of Hashimoto's thyroiditis.

---

1. *These were the teachings or sayings of Late Prof. Sharath Chandra. FRCS, Professor of Surgery, Madras Medical College, Chennai. (Conveyed to me by Late Prof Subbu, MMC, Chennai, when for the first and last time, I sat with Prof. Subbu as a co-examiner at Govt. Medical College, Coimbatore, 1998.*

Neck radiation increases risk not only for carcinoma thyroid but also for parotid gland tumours and hyperparathyroidism.

PATHOLOGY

- It is made up of colloid-filled follicles with papillary projections. In some cases, calcified lesions are found which are called **psammoma** bodies. These are diagnostic of papillary carcinoma of thyroid. Characteristic pale, empty, nuclei are present in a few cases which are described as **Orphan Annie eyed nuclei.** (Fig. 19.19) Thyroid gland has very rich intra thyroidal lymphatic plexus. Papillary carcinoma can be unifocal or multifocal.

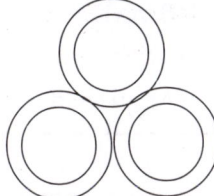
Fig. 19.19 Orphan Annie eyed-nuclei

- **Papillary micro carcinoma**: They measure 1 cm or less in diameter. Distant metastasis are extremely rare. Hence, a simple hemithyroidectomy is the treatment of choice.

- **Follicular variant of papillary cancer**: This is a mixed lesion with a predominance of follicles over papillae. They are treated by near total thyroidectomy.

- **Tall cell papillary cancer:** This is an aggressive tumour, rapidly growing, occurs in elderly patients should be treated by near total thyroidectomy.

CLINICAL PRESENTATION

1. Young females are commonly affected (in the age of 20-40 years).
2. It can present as a solitary nodule.
3. Very often, the lymph nodes in the lower deep cervical region are involved and thyroid may or may not be palpable. When thyroid gland is not palpable, it is called **occult** (hidden). However, papillary carcinoma less than 1.5 cm in diameter is also called "occult".
4. A few patients present late to the hospital with fixed nodes in the neck, and fixed thyroid to the trachea with or without recurrent laryngeal nerve paralysis.

"It should be noted that papillary carcinoma can be offered as a clinical diagnosis only in the presence of significant lymph nodes in the neck along with a thyroid swelling."

PROGNOSTIC CRITERIA

There are many prognostic criterias that have been used in

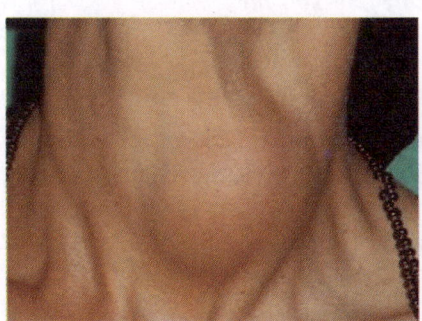
Fig. 19.20 Papillary carcinoma thyroid presenting as solitary nodule. FNAC gave the correct diagnosis

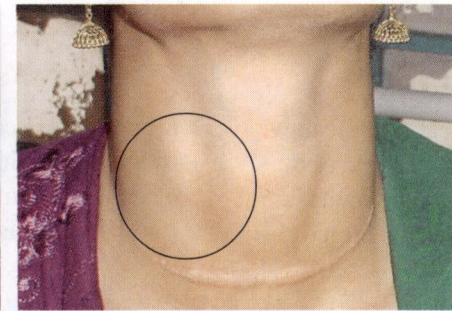
Fig. 19.21 This lady underwent subtotal thyroidectomy for MNG. After one year she presented with a solitary lymph node

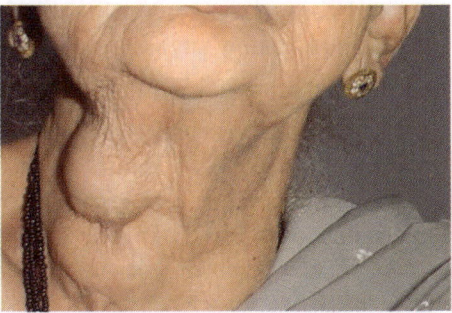
Fig. 19.22 This lady underwent hemithyroidectomy two years back. Now recurrance in the opposite lobe

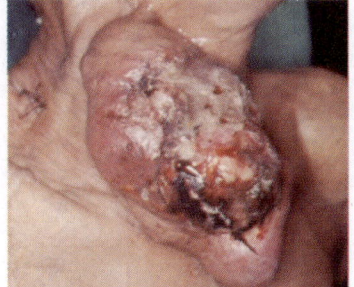
Fig. 19.23 Papillary carcinoma thyroid in a 75 year old lady - it behaves agressively in elderly patients

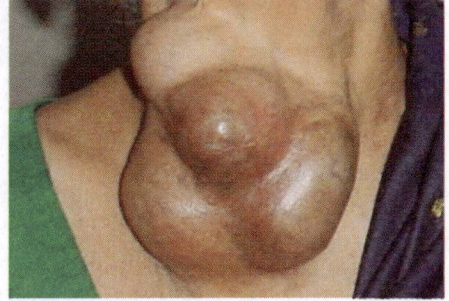
Fig. 19.24 Another case of papillary carcinoma thyroid with huge lymph node secondaries

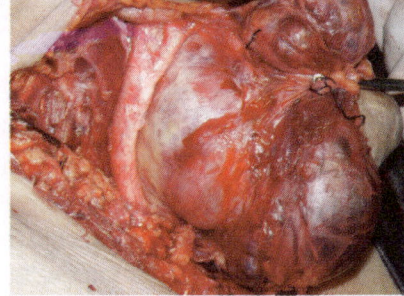
Fig. 19.25 Same patient as in Fig. 19.24 - underwent total thyroidectomy with block dissection of the neck

cases of well differentiated carcinoma. They are helpful in explaining the prognosis to the patient and relatives.

AGES Criteria (Key Box 19.18)

Key Box 19.18		
RISK GROUP STRATIFICATION IN DIFFERENTIATED THYROID CARCINOMAS (AGES)		
	Low Risk	**High risk**
1.**Age**	• Women younger than 50 yrs.	> 50 yrs.
	• Men < 40 yrs.	> 40 Yrs.
2.**Grade**	Well differentiated	Poorly differentiated (Fibrous, insular, mucoid, tall variant)
3.**Extent**	Confined to thyroid	Invasive to adjacent tissues or distant metatasis.
4.**Size**	Diameter < 4 cm.	> 4cm. diameter

INVESTIGATIONS

1. All routine investigations such as blood examination, chest X-ray, laryngoscopy have to be done. Large mediastinal shadow suggests mediastinal nodes.

2. Thyroid scan may demonstrate a cold nodule.

3. **Fine Needle Aspiration Cytology** (FNAC) can demonstrate colloid filled follicles with papillary process. Thus, preoperative diagnosis of papillary carcinoma is possible with FNAC. If the lymph nodes are enlarged, FNAC can be taken from the lymph nodes.

TREATMENT

• It can be discussed under 3 headings. Treatment of the primary, treatment of the secondaries in the lymph nodes and suppression of TSH.

I. Treatment of the primary/near-total thyroidectomy

• Total lobectomy on the side of the lesion and a subtotal on the opposite side is planned if a preoperative diagnosis is available. The purpose of the surgery is to preserve **at least one recurrent laryngeal nerve** and one parathyroid gland and at the same time, remove the primary. (Ref. Fig. 19.22)

• **If FNAC is inconclusive,** hemithyroidectomy specimen or a good portion of the diseased lobe is sent for frozen

Key Box 19.19	
PAPILLARY CARCINOMA NEAR TOTAL THYROIDECTOMY	

REASONS
• Rich intrathyroidal lymphatic spread
• Multicentric origin

section. If frozen section is reported as malignant, near-total thyroidectomy is completed (Key Box 19.19).

• **Histological surprise** If a subtotal thyroidectomy is reported as papillary carcinoma of the thyroid, many surgeons **wait and watch** the patient in low risk group and follow up the patient with thyroxine 0.2-0.3 mg/day. The argument in favour of this method is **papillary carcinoma is very slow growing.** Attempting a completion thyroidectomy has high risks of recurrent laryngeal nerve palsy. However, in all high risk patients it is better to do completion thyroidectomy.

After near total thyroidectomy, thyroxine is not given for a period of 6 weeks so that thyroid remnants can be ablated with radioiodine.

• *Dose of radioiodine 30-100 mCi*

II. Treatment of secondaries in the lymph nodes

• Lymph node secondaries are treated by **functional block dissection.** (**Berry picking** means removal of enlarged lymph nodes only. **It is no longer followed**) - Key Box 19.20.

Key Box 19.20	
PAPILLARY CARCINOMA - LYMPH NODE METASTASIS - PECULIARITIES	

1. They can be palpable even when thyroid gland is *not palpable*-**occult primary**

2. *Very slow growing*

3. Very often, they are **intracapsular**

4. They **need not be hard,** are often cystic and firm in consistency

5. At operation they are *bluish* in colour because of **rupture of the papillae**

6. Presence of lymph node metastasis does not affect the prognosis

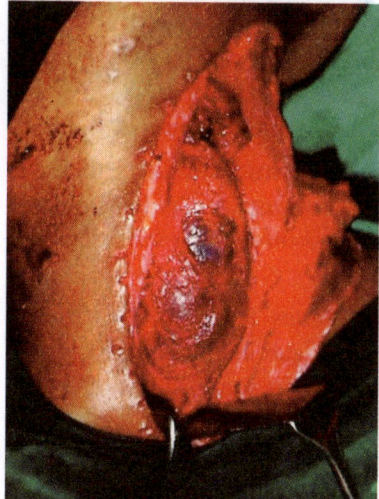

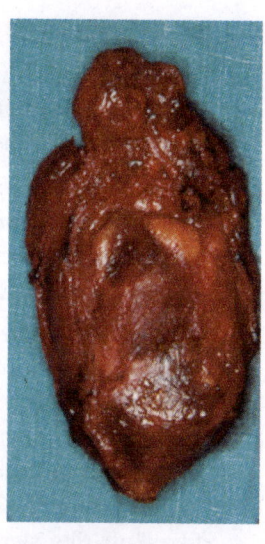

Fig. 19.26 Observe blue lymph nodes at surgery

Fig. 19.27 Completion of functional block dissection

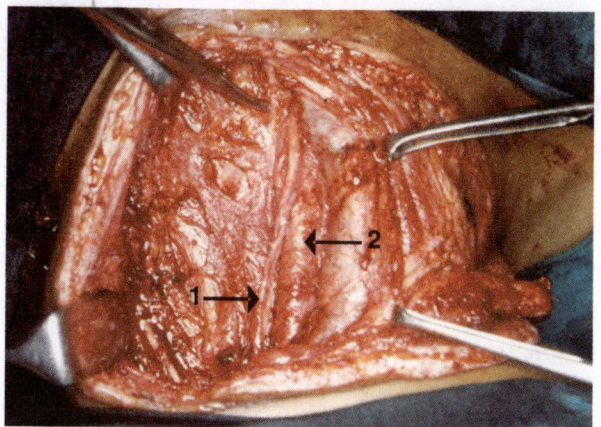

Fig. 19.28 After functional block dissection structures seen - 1. vagus nerve and 2. common carotid artery

- Other structures such as internal jugular vein, sternomastoid muscle etc are not removed because lymph nodes are slow growing and they rarely spread/outside the capsule of the lymph node.

- **Lateral aberrant thyroid** Initially thought as thyroid tissue, however it is metastasis into Level 3 and 4 lymph nodes from papillary carcinoma thyroid.

- No role for prophylactic neck dissection except in children.

III. Suppression of the TSH

- **This** is an important aspect in the postoperative period because papillary carcinoma is a TSH dependent tumour. **To prevent the patient developing hypothyroidism** in the postoperative period and to suppress **TSH, thyroxine** 0.3 mg/day is given (Summary - Fig. 19.29).

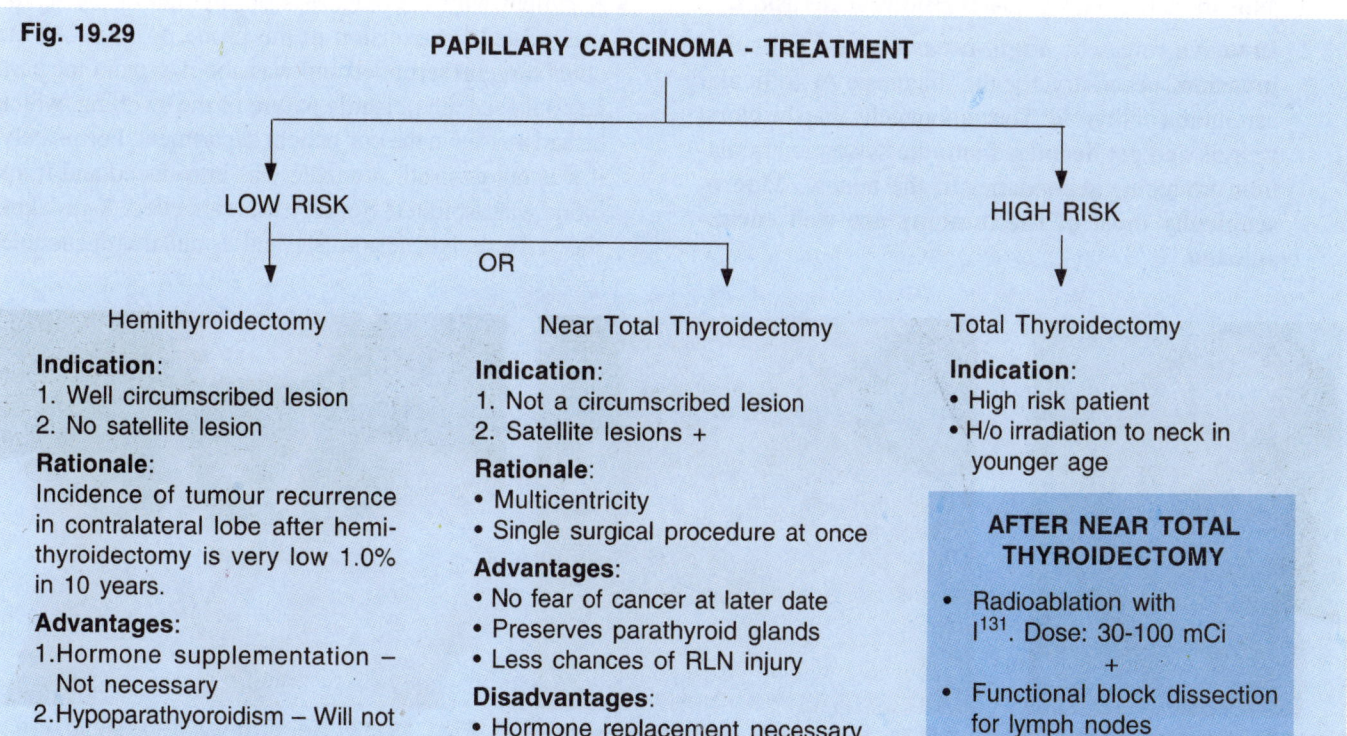

Fig. 19.29

PAPILLARY CARCINOMA - TREATMENT

LOW RISK

OR

HIGH RISK

Hemithyroidectomy

Indication:
1. Well circumscribed lesion
2. No satellite lesion

Rationale:
Incidence of tumour recurrence in contralateral lobe after hemithyroidectomy is very low 1.0% in 10 years.

Advantages:
1. Hormone supplementation – Not necessary
2. Hypoparathyoroidism – Will not occur
3. Thyroid function tests need not be measured frequently

Near Total Thyroidectomy

Indication:
1. Not a circumscribed lesion
2. Satellite lesions +

Rationale:
- Multicentricity
- Single surgical procedure at once

Advantages:
- No fear of cancer at later date
- Preserves parathyroid glands
- Less chances of RLN injury

Disadvantages:
- Hormone replacement necessary
- Ablation is necessary but effective

Total Thyroidectomy

Indication:
- High risk patient
- H/o irradiation to neck in younger age

AFTER NEAR TOTAL THYROIDECTOMY

- Radioablation with I^{131}. Dose: 30-100 mCi
  +
- Functional block dissection for lymph nodes
  +
- Thyroxine 0.3 mg/day

FOLLICULAR CARCINOMA

- Incidence: Constitutes 17% of cases. (Key Box 19.21)
- **Follicular adenoma   20% are malignant** and 80% are benign

Key Box 19.21	
THYROID MALIGNANCY INCIDENCE	
Papillary carcinoma	60-65%
Follicular carcinoma	15-20%
Anaplastic carcinoma	10-12%
Medullary carcinoma	5-10%
Others	10%

AETIOLOGY

- **Follicular carcinoma usually arises in a multinodular goitre,** especially in cases of endemic goitre. It should be suspected when MNG starts growing rapidly.

PATHOLOGY

- Depending upon the property of invasion it is classified into:
1. **Non-invasive** which means **minimal invasion.**
2. **Invasive** refers to **angio-invasion and capsular invasion,** necessary for the diagnosis of follicular carcinoma of thyroid. The tumour cells line the blood vessels and get dislodged into the systemic circulation producing secondaries in the bones. **Macroscopically most of the tumours are well encapsulated.**

CLINICAL PRESENTATION

1. It can present as a **solitary nodule.** The diagnosis is considered only after a thyroid scan in which it appears cold. The peak age group is around 40 years.
2. In cases of **long-standing multinodular goitres, if the goitre is rapidly growing,** if it is hard or it is present with restricted mobility, follicular carcinoma can be considered.
3. **Metastasis in the flat bones** The only clinical situation wherein a follicular carcinoma can be considered as the diagnosis is when a patient with the thyroid swelling presents with metastasis in the bone in the form of pathological fractures or a pulsatile swelling. Commonly, secondaries develop in the flat bones like skull, ribs, sternum, vertebral column, etc., because the flat bones retain red marrow for a longer time.

The clinical features of secondary in the skull are

1. They are rapidly growing
2. They are warm
3. Vascular and pulsatile
4. Underlying bony erosion may be present

CLINICAL NOTES

- A patient with the diagnosis of "lipoma of the scalp" was posted for excision in the prone position. As the chief surgeon scrubbed and was about to paint the part, he could see the pulsatile nature of the swelling, which he had missed in the out-patient department. Fortunately, it was not excised. A needle was introduced and frank blood was aspirated. Surgery was cancelled. X-ray skull showed osteolytic lesion. She had a small thyroid nodule.

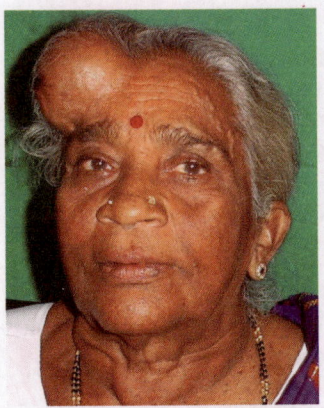

Fig.19.30 Ulcerated secondary in the scalp bone from follicular carcinoma thyroid. See the dilated veins in the neck

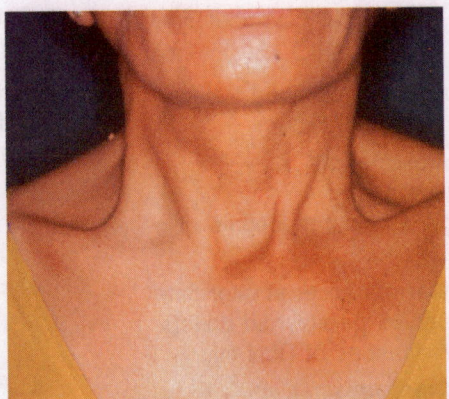

19.31 This lady presented with secondary in the left second rib. She did not have thyroid swelling. A case of occult follicular carcinoma thyroid

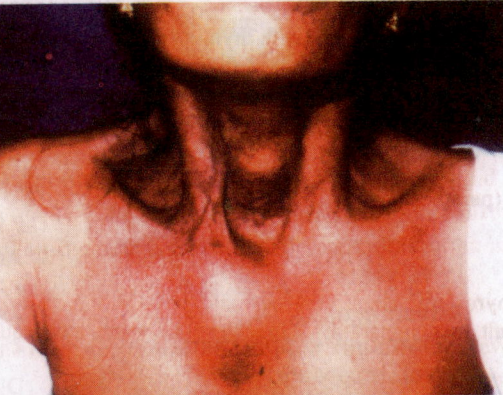

Fig. 19.32 Secondary deposit in the sternum in a patient who underwent near-total thyroidectomy for follicular carcinoma 5 years back

Differential diagnosis of bone secondaries

Key Box 19.22
CAUSES OF SECONDARY IN THE SKULL
1. Follicular carcinoma of thyroid
2. Carcinoma breast
3. Renal cell carcinoma
4. Prostatic carcinoma
5. Bronchogenic carcinoma

INVESTIGATIONS

1. Routine investigations

2. **Thyroid scan** is done which can demonstrate cold nodule

3. **FNAC** of the cold nodule It should be remembered that **FNAC cannot differentiate a follicular adenoma from follicular carcinoma.** Hence, if a patient presents with solitary nodule, the only way to get a pre-operative diagnosis of follicular carcinoma is to do an incision biopsy which is NOT ACCEPTABLE. Hence, frozen section is arranged at the time of surgery (Key Box 19.23).

Key Box 19.23
MALIGNANT TUMOURS WHEREIN OPEN BIOPSY IS NOT TAKEN
• Thyroid
• Parotid
• Testis

4. Alkaline phosphatase - if increased, bone scan should be done

5. Plain x-ray of the involved bone can reveal osteolytic lesions

6. When primary is not found, bone biopsy from the secondaries

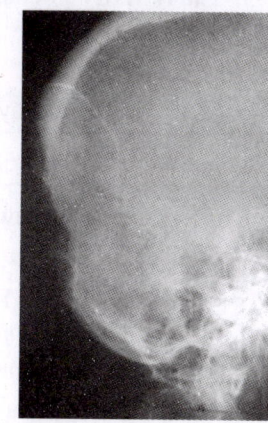

Fig.19.33 Erosion of skull bone

TREATMENT OF FOLLICULAR CARCINOMA OF THYROID

I. **Near-total thyroidectomy** is indicated for following reasons

- The secondaries do not take up the radio isotope (I^{131}) in the presence of primary tumour. Hence, lobectomy or hemithyroidectomy should not be done.

- Patients presenting with solitary nodule should undergo hemithyroidectomy and frozen section examination. If frozen section is positive, then, a near-total thyroidectomy is done.

- If frozen section is negative, in high risk patients it is better to do near total thyroidectomy rather than waiting for histopathological report and subjecting the patient for second surgery.

II. **After near-total thyroidectomy,** a **whole body bone scan** is done to see for metastasis in the bone.

- A single secondary can be treated by radiotherapy followed by oral radio-iodine therapy, so as to suppress the secondary. Multiple secondaries are treated by oral radio-iodine therapy.

III. In the postoperative period, patients should receive **thyroxine** 0.3 mg/day (reasons same as papillary carcinoma).

HURTHLE CELL CARCINOMA

- Hurthle cell carcinoma is a variant of follicular carcinoma. It is more agressive than follicular carcinoma. These tumours are defined by the presence of more than 75% of follicular cells having oncocytic features.

- Does not take up ^{131}I.

- **Secretes thyroglobulin**

- Less likely to respond to ^{131}I ablation

- Even if hurthle cell **adenoma** is well encapsulated it is potentially malignant.

Criteria to diagnose Hurthle cell carcinoma

- Capsular/vascular invasion, distant metastasis

- Higher chance of spread to lymph nodes than follicular thyroid carcinoma.

Treatment

- Total thyroidectomy. In many cases of Hurthle cell carcinoma, lymph nodes are enlarged. Hence, modified radical neck dissection is done (MRND).

- TSH suppression, follow-up are regularly required.

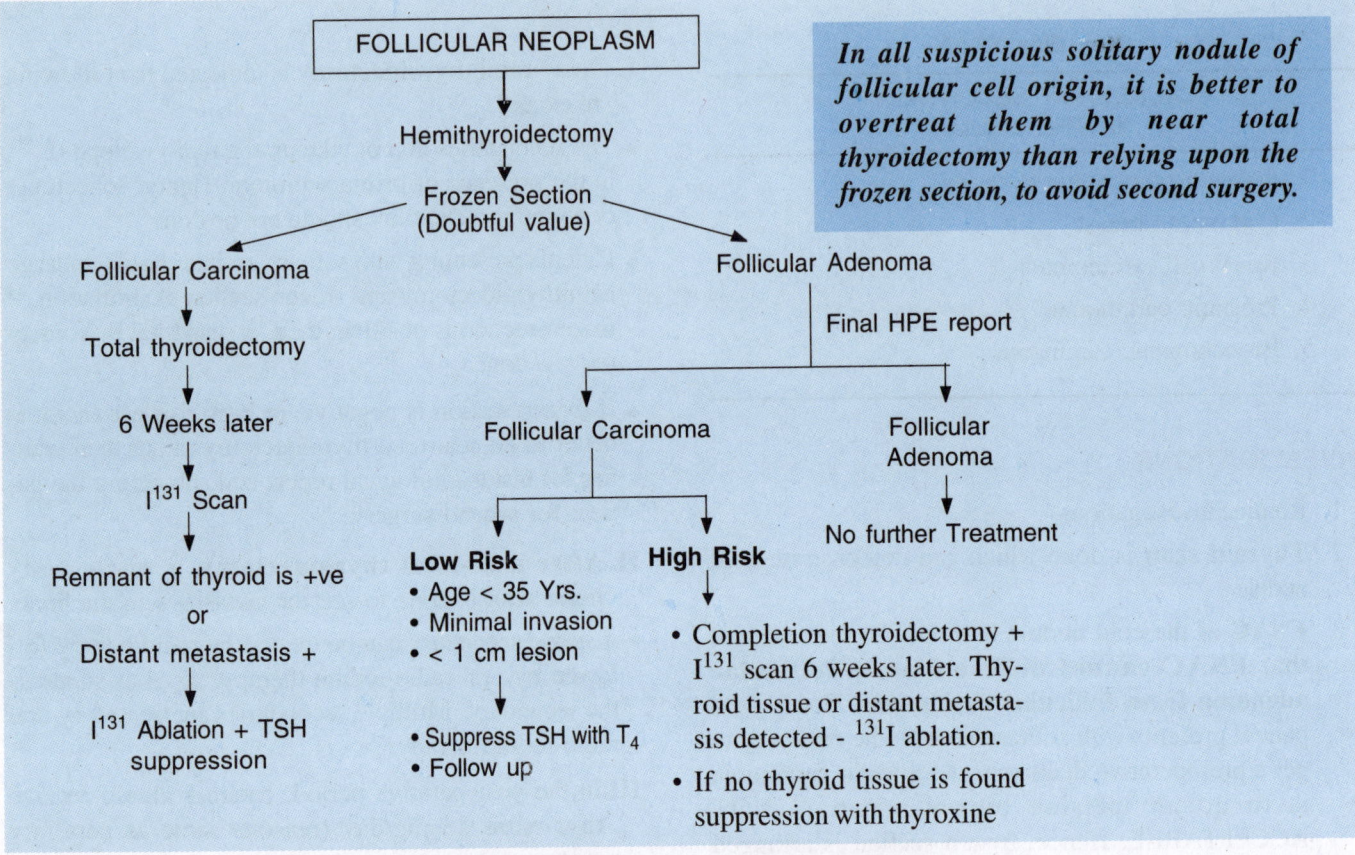

Fig. 19.34 Management of follicular neoplasm

Case of FNAC proved follicular neoplasm. Management is given in Fig. 19.34.

FOLLOW-UP OF PATIENTS WITH PAPILLARY AND FOLLICULAR CARCINOMA THYROID

- Serum **thyroglobulin** (Tg) levels greater than 1 to 2 ng/mL in patients receiving replacement thyroxine therapy indicate presence of metastasis. Hence assess the serum Tg response to injected recombinant human TSH, every year.

- Ultrasonography or MRI scans of the neck for localisation of residual or recurrent tumour

- Regular measurment of **serum calcium** and **thyroid hormones** after near total thyroidectomy

ANAPLASTIC CARCINOMA

Incidence 10-12% of cases

Clinical features (Key Box 19.24)

1. Common in elderly woman around 60-70 years of age

2. Majority of the patients present with rapidly growing thyroid swelling of short duration. The surface is irregular and consistency is hard.

3. **Early infiltration of the trachea** results in stridor (scabbard trachea).

4. **Infiltration of carotid sheath** In such cases, common carotid artery pulsation will not be palpable which is described as **Berry sign positive.**

5. **Early fixity** is characteristic. Thus, the resectability rate is almost nil.

Key Box 19.24

ANAPLASTIC CARCINOMA THYROID

- The most rapidly growing thyroid malignancy
- Advanced age group at presentation
- Advanced nature of presentation
- Gross local infiltration-Berry's sign positive
- No form of treatment is successful
- **Intrinsic carcinoma of larynx** spreading outside and infiltrating the skin should be considered as a differential diagnosis.

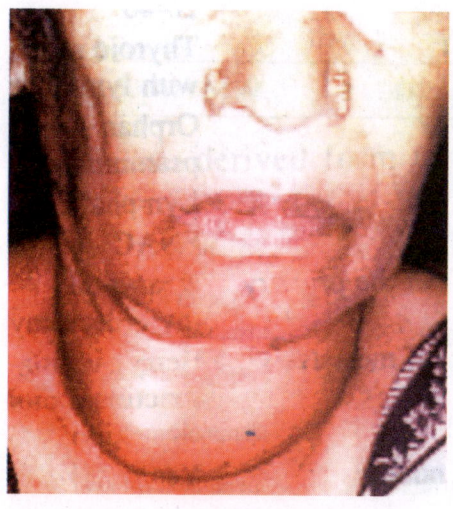

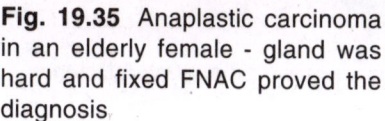

Fig. 19.35 Anaplastic carcinoma in an elderly female - gland was hard and fixed FNAC proved the diagnosis

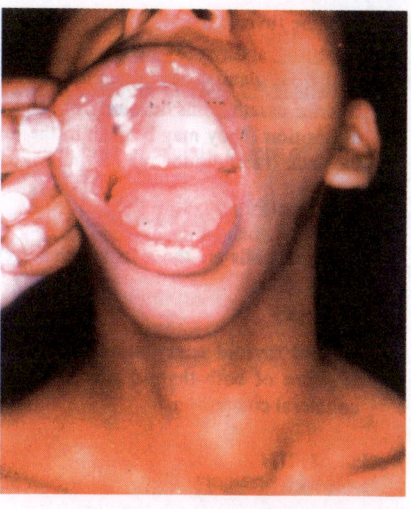

Fig. 19.36 FNAC proved medullary carcinoma with mucocutaneous neuroma - MEN type IIb

Key Box 19.25
CALCITONIN AND MEDULLARY CARCINOMA THYROID
• Not measurable in normal persons
• MCT produces very high levels
• Tumour marker of MCT
• Level decreases after thyroidectomy
• Level increases in case of recurrence
• Prophylactic thyroidectomy in relatives if calcitonin levels are high

Diagnosis

- It is established by FNAC

Treatment

- Due to the gross local infiltration into the vital structures in the neck such as common carotid artery and trachea, the resectability rate is low.
- However, very rarely a surgeon will get an opportunity to excise isthmus so as to relieve compression of the trachea.
- Postoperative radiotherapy is given as a palliative treatment.
- In many cases, death occurs within 6 to 8 months.

MEDULLARY CARCINOMA OF THE THYROID (MCT)

- These tumours arise from **parafollicular 'C' cells** which are derived from ultimobranchial bodies and not from thyroid follicle.
- These tumours present in two different ways.
  1. **Sporadic** is common, seen in about 80-90% of cases.
  2. **Familial** variety presents as a part of Multiple Endocrine Neoplasia (MEN).

MEN Type I

- Pituitary adenoma
- Parathyroid adenoma
- Pancreatic adenoma

MEN Type IIa

- Parathyroid adenoma
- Phaeochromocytoma
- Medullary carcinoma of thyroid
- When it is associated with mucocutaneous neuromas involving lips, tongue, eyelids, it is called **Sipple syndrome**, with an occasional marfanoid habitus (MEN type IIb)
- It has got a characteristic **amyloid stroma**.
- These tumours are not hormone dependent and do not take up radioactive iodine.

Hormones produced by MCT

- Calcitonin (Key Box 19.25)
- Prostaglandins
- Serotonin (5-HT)
- ACTH

Spread

- Both by lymphatics and blood, thus, worsening the prognosis.

Treatment

- Before proceeding with surgery, look for an associated phaeochromocytoma.

I.   Near-total thyroidectomy or total thyroidectomy

Table 19.6 Summary of the malignant tumours of thyroid gland

		PAPILLARY	FOLLICULAR	ANAPLASTIC	MEDULLARY
1.	Aetiology	Irradiation	Endemic goitre	Unknown	Sporadic or familial
2.	Incidence	60%	17%	13%	6%
3.	Age (years)	20-40	30-50	50 and above	Middle age
4.	Diagnosis	Thyroid swelling with lymph nodes	Thyroid swelling, metastasis -bone	Thyroid swelling, local fixity, stridor	Difficult to diagnose clinically
5.	Microscopy	Orphan Annie-eyed nuclei, psammoma bodies	Angio invasion, capsular invasion	Poorly differeniated cells	Amyloid stroma-like carcinoid
6.	Spread	Lymphatic	Blood	Local infiltration	Lymphatic, blood
7.	Investigation	FNAC	Frozen section	FNAC, biopsy	FNAC, calcitonin
8.	Treatment of the primary	Near-total thyroidectomy	Near-total thyroidectomy	Isthmusectomy, external RT	Total thyroidectomy
9.	Treatment of metastasis	Functional block dissection	Radio-iodine I^{131} or external RT	Palliative external radiotherapy	Radical block dissection
10.	TSH dependence	Yes	Yes	No	No
11.	Hormone production	Very rare	Very rare	No	Calcitonin, 5HT, ACTH
12.	Prognosis	Excellent	Good	Worst	Bad

II. The lymph nodes are treated by radical block dissection because they are fast growing, when compared to papillary carcinoma.

If there are multiple secondaries in the bone. oral radio-iodine has no role because this tumour does not arise from the thyroid cells. Only palliative radiotherapy can be given.

Summary of malignant tumours of thyroid (Table 19.6)

MALIGNANT LYMPHOMA (Fig. 19.37)

- It is rare. Hashimoto's thyroiditis can predispose to malignant lymphoma.
- Older patients are commonly affected
- The tumour can present as rapidly growing, large thyroid swelling (primary lymphoma).
- Sometimes, they can appear as a part of generalised lymphoma (non-Hodgkin's variety).

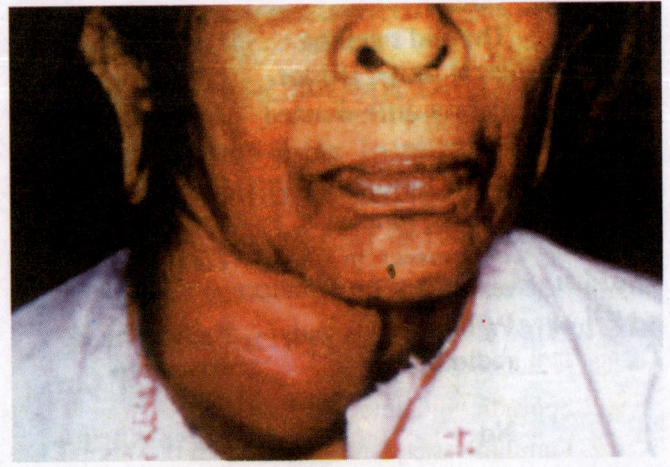

Fig. 19.37 FNAC proved lymphoma thyroid which responded to chemotherapy

- FNAC can give the diagnosis
- It is interesting to note that lymphomas of the thyroid respond very well to chemotherapy or radiotherapy.

CLINICAL CRITERIA FOR THE DIAGNOSIS OF CARCINOMA OF THYROID

1. A thyroid swelling which is rapidly growing
2. Thyroid swelling with **lower deep cervical lymph nodes** and lymph nodes in the posterior triangle (papillary carcinoma thyroid)
3. **Hard gland, fixed to the trachea**-anaplastic carcinoma of the thyroid.
4. Thyroid swelling with a **rapidly growing vascular, pulsatile swelling,** commonly in the skull (follicular carcinoma).
5. Thyroid swelling with **hoarseness of the voice** indicates infiltration of recurrent laryngeal nerve which is a feature of malignancy.
6. Thyroid swelling with **Berry sign positive** (anaplastic carcinoma of the thyroid).
7. **Kocher's test positive** may be an indication of infiltration into trachea.

SOLITARY NODULE THYROID GLAND

- Almost all of the thyroid swellings initially can present as a solitary nodule. However, puberty goitres, colloid goitres, diffuse toxic goitres produce uniform enlargement of the thyroid gland. Multinodular goitre (MNG) presents as multiple nodules. However, very often a solitary nodule on clinical examination, may turn out to be a multinodular goitre at exploration. The solitary nodule has a higher incidence of malignancy when compared to MNG.

Causes of solitary nodule thyroid gland

1. In 50% of the cases, a clinically palpable solitary nodule is a part of multinodular goitre
2. Toxic autonomous nodule
3. Adenoma
4. Carcinoma
5. Cysts

Management (Fig. 19.38)

- The solitary nodules should be investigated with radio-iodine scan. Presence of a cold nodule arises the suspicion of malignancy. However, haemorrhage, thyroiditis, cysts are the other causes of cold nodule.
- Ultrasound of the thyroid gland is an extremely useful

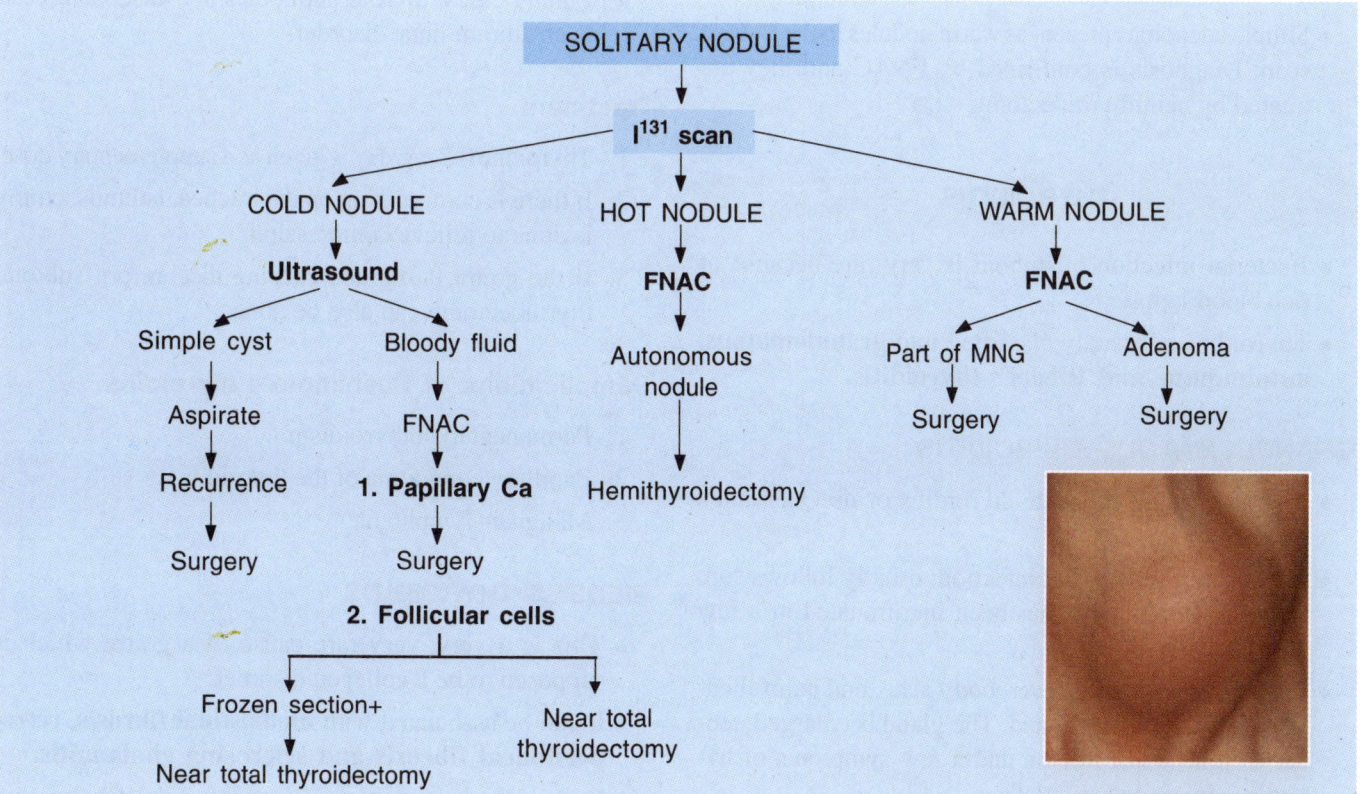

Fig. 19.38 Flowchart showing management of solitary nodule

Key Box 19.26

ULTRASOUND AND SOLITARY NODULE

- It can detect cyst
- Can guide FNAC
- Cyst larger than 3 cm, has 14% chance of malignancy
- Hypoechoic pattern, incomplete peripheral halo, irregular margin and microcalcification are suggestive of carcinoma

investigation in the evaluation of solitary nodule (Key Box 19.26).

- Once the ultrasound is done, they are subjected to a fine needle aspiration cytology (FNAC). If FNAC proves the diagnosis of malignancy as in papillary carcinoma thyroid, near-total thyroidectomy is done. If there is a doubt regarding a follicular neoplasm in FNAC, a frozen section is arranged.
- If there is a toxic goitre diagnosed by high pulse rate and increase in T3, T4 levels, I^{131} scan can demonstrate a hot nodule. Histological diagnosis can be made by FNAC.
- Simple adenomas present as warm nodules in the isotope scan. Diagnosis is confirmed by FNAC and they are treated by hemithyroidectomy.

THYROIDITIS

- Bacterial infection of thyroid is very rare because of rich blood supply.
- Thyroiditis is broadly classified into **granulomatous, autoimmune and Riedel's thyroiditis.**

GRANULOMATOUS THYROIDITIS

- It is also called subacute thyroiditis or de Quervain's disease.
- This occurs due to viral infection; usually follows sore throat. (Mumps virus has been incriminated in a few cases.)
- Patients present with fever, body ache, and painful enlargement of thyroid gland. The gland is enlarged, tender to touch, soft to firm and a few symptoms of hyperthyroidism occur initially.
- ESR is increased

Treatment

- Majority of the patients respond to conservative treatment in the form of analgesics and a short course of prednisolone. There are no permanent sequelae of this condition.

AUTOIMMUNE THYROIDITIS

- **Hashimoto's** thyroiditis is the main component of thyroiditis.
- Autoimmune aetiology is characterised by extensive lymphocytic infiltration resulting in destruction of thyroid follicles with variable degree of fibrosis.
- **Females in perimenopausal group** (40-50 years) commonly affected. Initially, symptoms of mild hyperthyroidism (hashitoxicosis) may be present. Later, extensive intrathyroidal fibrosis results in permanent hypothyroidism.
- The thyroid follicles are destroyed by significant fibrosis. The deep eosinophilic-staining thyroid follicular cell, **Askanazy cell,** is characteristic.
- The gland can be firm to hard and sometimes rubbery in consistency, smooth or irregular and can involve a lobe or the entire gland.
- In many cases, thyroid antibodies are raised, suggesting an autoimmune disorder.

Treatment

1. Thyroxine 0.2 mg/day is given as a supplementary dose.
2. If there is compression on the trachea, isthmusectomy is done to relieve compression.
3. If the goitre is big and causing discomfort, subtotal thyroidectomy can also be done.

Complications of Hashimoto's thyroiditis

1. Permanent hypothyroidism
2. Papillary carcinoma of the thyroid
3. Malignant lymphoma

RIEDEL'S THYROIDITIS

- This is a very, very rare cause of a goitre which is supposed to be a collagen disorder.
- It can be associated with **mediastinal fibrosis, retroperitoneal fibrosis and sclerosing cholangitis.**
- In this condition, there is intrathyroidal fibrosis but **extrathyroidal fibrosis** is more.

Table 19.7 Comparison of three forms of thyroiditis

	GRANULOMATOUS	HASHIMOTO'S	RIEDEL'S
1. Aetiology	Virus	Autoimmune	Collagen disorder
2. Age group	Young	Woman at menopause	Old age
3. Pathology	Inflammatory cells	Lymphocytes, fibrosis	Extensive fibrous tissue
4. Clinical	Painful, tender, smooth, sudden goitre	Irregular or nodular, firm, nontender	Hard, irregular, fixed, nontender
5. Toxicity	Initial toxicity, later normal	Initial toxicity, later hypothyroidism	Hypothyroidism
6. Laboratory tests	ESR is increased	Antithyroid antibodies ↑	No biochemical test
7. Treatment	Symptomatic	Thyroxine, surgery	Thyroxine, surgery
8. Differential diagnosis	Acute bacterial thyroiditis	Multinodular goitre	Anaplastic carcinoma

- Involvement of trachea, oesophagus, internal jugular vein, carotid artery etc., result in dysphagia and dyspnoea.
- As a result of fibrosis, all the thyroid follicles are replaced by fibrous tissue.
- By the time patients present to the hospital, it is an advanced stage and excision is very difficult.

Treatment

- Treatment with thyroxine may be necessary to treat hypothyroidism.
- In selected difficult cases, isthmusectomy can be tried to relieve compression on trachea. Three types of thyroiditis are compared in Table 19.7.

COMPLICATIONS OF THYROIDECTOMY

1. **Haemorrhage** can be a primary haemorrhage which occurs on the table.
   - **Reactionary haemorrhage** is more dangerous and occurs within 6-8 hours after surgery. This is due to slipping of ligature because of straining, coughing, hypertension, etc.
   - It is a **tension haematoma** which develops deep to deep fascia, compressing the larynx. Re-exploration of neck under GA, control of bleeding points and evacuation of haematoma should be done immediately.
   - Without evacuating haematoma, an attempt to intubate the patient may result in cardiac arrest (as such patient will be struggling)

2. **Respiratory obstruction** can be due to tension haematoma resulting in compression of the larynx, collapse, tracheal cartilage softening (tracheomalacia).
   - Endotracheal intubation and a dose of steroid is necessary.

3. **Laryngeal nerve paralysis** -Table : 19.8

   A. **Unilateral recurrent laryngeal nerve(RLN) palsy** produce a whispering voice, the opposite vocal cord compensates. There will not be problems of aspiration or airway obstruction.

   B. **Bilateral recurrent nerve palsy** It is also known as Bilateral abductor paralysis. Both the vocal cords come to be in median or paramedian position, the airway is inadequate causing dyspnoea and stridor but the voice is good.
   - **Treatment:** Tracheostomy is required as an emergency procedure. Following tracheostomy, patient is followed up on out-patient basis for a period of 8-9 months, this period is required for any spontaneous recovery. No recovery after this period requires permanent solution or, the choice is between a permanent tracheostomy with a speaking valve

or a surgical procedure to lateralise the cord which can be done by endoscopic method. The former relieves stridor and preserves good voice but has the disadvantage of a tracheostomy hole in the neck. The latter relieves airway obstruction but at the expense of good voice, however there is no tracheostomy hole in the neck.

C. **Superior laryngeal nerve paralysis:** This results in paralysis of **cricothyroid muscle, the sequence** of which is weak and husky voice and the inability to raise the pitch of voice (this is of particular importance in singers).

D. **Combined (Complete paralysis)**

I. **Unilateral**

This results in paralysis of all muscles of larynx on one side. Vocal cord will be in cadaveric position. The healthy cord is unable to approximate the paralysed cord, thus causing glottic incompetence. This results in horarseness of voice and aspiration of liquids through glottis. Cough is ineffective due to air wastage.

- Treatment includes the procedures to **medialise** the cord and **speech** therapy.

II. **Bilateral:** This is an uncommon condition. This results in paralysis of all the intrinsic muscles of the larynx. Both vocal cords assume cadaveric position. There is also a total anaesthesia of larynx.

4. **Permanent hypothyroidism** can develop slowly after thyroid surgery especially after subtotal thyroidectomy for Graves' disease. It takes 2-3 years for manifestation of hypothyroidism.

5. **Permanent hypoparathyroidism** is managed with calcium tablets or with 1,25-dihydroxy cholecalciferol.

6. **Thyrotoxic crisis (storm)**

- Thyrotoxic storm occurs in patients with primary thyrotoxicosis who are improperly treated or prepared for surgery. At surgery, due to handling of the gland, sudden release of thyroxine into the systemic circulation results in thyrotoxic crisis.

- Hyperpyrexia-above 105°F, severe sweating, gross dehydration, hypovolaemic shock, tachycardia are the diagnostic features.

- It is treated by following measures
  1. Correction of dehydration by rapid I.V. fluids.
  2. Cold tepid sponging, to control the temperature.

Table 19.8 Various positions of vocal cord in laryngeal nerve paralysis

POSITION	INFERENCE	DISTANCE FROM THE MID LINE	FIGURE
1. Median	Seen in phonation	Nil	
2. Paramedian	RLN palsy	Distance: 1-2 mm	
3. Intermediate (cadaveric)	Combined paralysis of RLN and superior laryngel nerve	Distance: 3-4 mm	
4. Full abduction	Forceful inspiration	Distance: 8-9mm	

3. IV propranolol 2-4 mg with ECG monitoring and oral propranalol. In spite of the above treatment, mortality is high.

Key Box 19.27

THYROTOXIC STORM PREVENTION

- Euthyroid before surgery
- β blockers, carbimazole
- Lugol's iodine
- Good anaesthesia
- Perfect haemostasis
- Gentle manipulation

---

7. **Wound infection:** It is not common to get wound infection after thyroid surgery. However, antibiotics are started if there is evidence of local erythema, tenderness and if patient has fever.

8. **Scar hypertrophy and keloid**

9. **Stitch granuloma** May occur with/without sinus formation and is seen after the use of non-absorbable suture material.

   - Absorbable ligatures and sutures (VICRYL) can be used through out thyroid surgery except for skin closure where silk is still appropriate.

Miscellaneous

LINGUAL THYROID

- Occasionally, a patient presents with a small swelling in the middle of the tongue at the **junction of anterior 2/3 and posterior 1/3 of the tongue**.
- It could be lingual thyroid - an **aberrant thyroid tissue** found in the region of foramen caecum on the tongue (Key Box 19.28)
- **Foramen caecum** represents the junction of epithelial floor of the mouth with proximal portion of thyroglossal duct.
- Even though lingual thyroid is rare, it can give rise to significant complications.

Clinical features

- Swelling in the tongue in the classical location, firm in consistency, can be irregular, impairment of the speech, haemorrhage, dysphagia.

Key Box 19.28

ECTOPIC THYROID TISSUE

- Lingual thyroid
- Thyroglossal ectopic thyroid-in the upper part of the neck
- Struma ovarii-malignant ovarian teratoma containing thyroid tissue

---

Treatment

- Lingual thyroid may be the **only thyroid tissue** present in a patient. Hence, a thyroid scan is done to confirm the presence of normal thyroid tissue.
- Small dose of thyroxine may decrease the size of the swelling (similar to a puberty goitre).
- Large swelling with significant symptoms needs to be excised.

ABOUT BERRY

Key Box 19.29

REMEMBER IN THYROID

1. Berry picking (Page 260)
2. Berry sign (Page 247)
3. Berry ligament (Page 240)

20

Parathyroid and Adrenals

- Surgical anatomy
- Physiology - Action of PTH
- Congenital anomaly
- Tetany
- Hyperparathyroidism
- Acute hypercalcaemic crisis
- Neuroblastoma
- Phaeochromocytoma

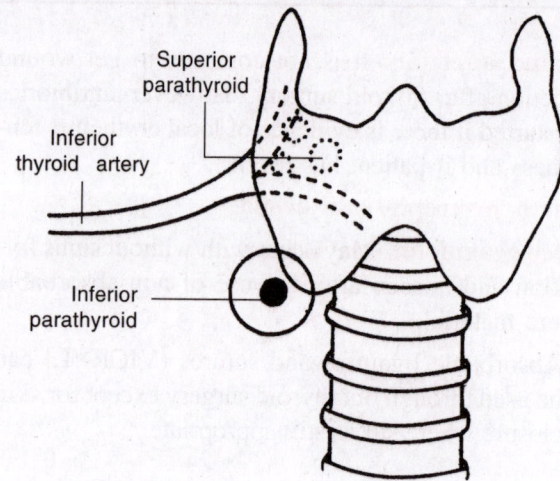

Fig. 20.1 Sites of parathyroid glands

PARATHYROID GLANDS

SURGICAL ANATOMY

- They are the endocrinal glands situated in the neck which secrete the hormone parathormone (PTH). Their secretion is *not dependent on pituitary gland*.
- They are 4 in number; 2 on the right, 2 on the left. It is pinkish in children, and yellow to brown in adults.
- **Superior parathyroids** are derived from endoderm of **4th branchial arch** and thus, they are developed with the thyroid gland.
- Superior parathyroids are found in relation to inferior thyroid artery in the middle of posterior aspect of thyroid gland. They are constant in position. They are smaller (20-40 mg)
- **Inferior parathyroids** develop from endoderm of **3rd branchial arch** (with thymus) and are not constant in position. They may be seen in the lower pole, within fascial sheath of thyroid gland low down in the neck (rarely in the mediastinum), outside the fascial sheath or even within thyroid gland. They are larger (30 to 50 mg)

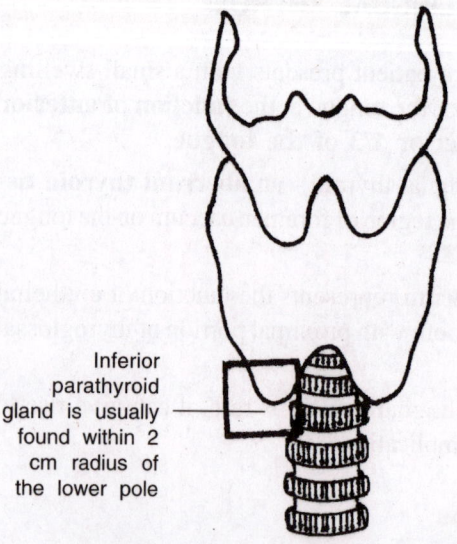

Fig. 20.2 Location of inferior parathyroid gland

Blood supply

Inferior thyroid artery supplies both the parathyroids in about 95% of cases by a leash of vessels. Ligature of both thyroid arteries may not result in hypoparathyroidism because there is adequate collateral circulation.

Histology

Principal cells are the cells which secrete PTH (parathormone). Water clear cells are found in hyperplastic and neoplastic glands.

CONGENITAL ANOMALY AND SYNDROME

Di George's syndrome

Congenital absence of the parathyroid glands and thymus. Neonatal hypoparathyroidism + absence of thymus dependent lymphoid system.

PHYSIOLOGY - ACTION OF PTH

1. Resorption and mobilization of calcium from the bone.
2. Increased reabsorption of calcium from kidney and promoting excretion of phosphate.
3. Enhances absorption of calcium from the gut
   - Thus, PTH increases serum calcium level
   - Normal serum calcium level 9-11 mg/100 ml (total)
   - In normal persons, the PTH is balanced by calcitonin, secreted from *C-cells* of the thyroid glands.

TETANY

Tetany is a condition wherein there is hyperexcitability of peripheral nerves.

Causes of tetany

1. **Hypoparathyroidism**: It results from surgical removal of parathyroids. Subtotal thyroidectomy, near total thyroidectomy are the most common causes of tetany. After thyroidectomy, it may be temporary or permanent if all the 4 parathyroids are removed or deprived of their blood supply. The incidence is around 1-2%.
2. **Severe respiratory alkalosis** can cause tetany as in hyperventilation.

3. The low calcium levels can occur due to dietary factors or due to poor absorption from the gut or due to **acute pancreatitis, chronic renal failure**.
4. **Osteomalacia** and **rickets** due to deficiency of **vitamin D**.
5. **Hypokalaemic alkalosis** of pyloric stenosis.

Signs and symptoms (Key Box 20.1)

1. Tingling and numbness of the fingers, toes, lips (circum oral paraesthesia), at times with circumoral pallor.
2. Cramps of the hands and feet.
3. In severe hypocalcemia, there may be *carpopedal spasm*. Metacarpophalangeal (MP) joints are flexed, extension at interphalangeal joints, adduction of the thumb, *thumb in palm deformity* (**obstetrician's hand**). In the foot, extension in the ankle joints and flexion of the toes.
4. A **stridor** is a dangerous complication of severe tetany due to spasm of muscles of respiration.
5. *Latent tetany* can be diagnosed by:
   - Tap the facial nerve at the angle of jaw. This produces twitching of eyelids, corner of the mouth, etc. It is called *Chvostek sign*. It indicates facial nerve hyperexcitability.
   - **Trousseau's sign**: When a blood pressure cuff is applied to the arm and is inflated above the systolic pressure (200 mm of Hg), the hand goes into spasm (obstetrician's hand).
6. Spasm of intraocular muscles results in blurring of vision.
7. **Convulsions**, even though rare, can occur in infants.

Key Box 20.1
FEATURES OF TETANY
<ul><li>Circumoral paraesthesia</li><li>Carpopedal spasm</li><li>Chovstek sign</li><li>Trousseau's sign</li></ul>

Diagnosis

- This is established by estimating **serum calcium level** which is usually < 7 mg%.

Treatment

1. Oral calcium such as calcium lactate, calcium gluconate may relieve mild symptoms.

2. In **acute cases**, **injection calcium gluconate** 10% (10 ml) should be given *slowly intravenously* over 10 minutes to avoid cardiac arrhythmias.

3. If any precipitating cause is detected, it needs to be corrected.

HYPER PARATHYROIDISM

- Hyperparathyroidism is an uncommon disease and occurs due to an increased activity of parathyroids and manifests as hypercalcemia.

CAUSES

1. Single chief cell adenoma is the most common cause (80%) (Key Box 20.2)

2. It can be due to **diffuse hyperplasia** involving all 4 glands (5 to 10% of cases)

3. Very rarely it can be due to carcinoma arising in the parathyroid glands

- Adenoma can be a part of **multiple endocrine neoplasia** (MEN) syndrome

---

Key Box 20.2

PATHOLOGY

- Adenoma-Reddish brown - Only 1 gland is enlarged
- Chief cell hyperplasia-Reddish brown - > 1 gland is enlarged
- Water cell hyperplasia - Chocolate brown - > 1 gland is enlarged

---

CLINICAL FEATURES   (Key Box 20.3)

- More common in *females,* female/male ratio is 2:1.
- Age: 20-60 years, the most common age group is 5th decade.
- Incidence is 1:1000 patients
- **The most common** presentation is **asymptomatic hypercalcaemia** in about 50% of the patients and **renal stones** in 25% of the patients. The clinical features are as follows:

1. Bone Disease

- Due to increasing levels of PTH, extensive *skeletal decalcification* occurs. This results in bony pains, *pathological fractures* due to brittle bones, *subperiosteal erosions*, cysts in the phalanges, jaw bone (mandible), skull etc. They are called **pseudotumours**. The changes are similar to that seen in *Osteitis fibrosa cystica* (Von Recklinghausen's disease).

2. Renal Disease

- Increased calcium levels result from increased calcium absorption from the kidneys. Hence, patients are prone to develop **renal stone and nephrocalcinosis** (calcification of kidney), renal ischaemia and hypertension.

- Calcium also increases the tone of the vessels which adds to the hypertension. Primary hyperparathyroidism is the cause of stones in 1-3% of all patients with kidney stones and in 10 percent of those who have recurrence of stones.

3. Abdominal groans

- Calcium stimulates **gastrin** which is a powerful stimulator of acid. This may result in pain abdomen due to peptic ulcer. Patient can present with dyspeptic symptoms.

- Calcium can cause **pancreatitis**, resulting in pain radiating to the back.

- Metastatic calcification is also a feature

4. Psychiatric moans

- These patients, more often a woman, mostly of middle age, having bony pains, backaches and behavioural abnormalities are thought to have a psychiatric illness. They are referred to mental institutions, orthopaedic department, gynaecology department and are shunted from doctor to doctor.

Key Box 20.3

HYPERPARATHYROIDISM A DISEASE OF

- Bones
- Stones
- Abdominal groans
- Psychic moans

Other features

- Corneal calcification/band keratopathy may be seen in the eye on **slit lamp examination**.
- Proximal myopathy, muscle wasting is also seen
- Interestingly, clinical examination of the neck *may not reveal* any parathyroid enlargement. Hence, the diagnosis should be suspected by the various symptoms. High index of suspicion is necessary in arriving at a proper diagnosis.

INVESTIGATIONS

It can be classified into –

I. To prove hyperparathyroidism
- Serum Calcium, Phosphate, Albumin
- Serum PTH assay
- Alkaline phosphatase
- X-ray of bones

II. To localise parathyroid glands
- Ultrasound of neck
- Thallium and technetium subtraction scan
- Selective venous sampling with PTH assay, most reliable, but more difficult.
- Sestamibi scanning

I. To prove hyperparathyroidism

1. Serum **calcium** levels are always raised above normal limits (9-11 mg %). There are many causes of hypercalcaemia which are depicted in the Key Box 20.4. Hence, estimation of serum calcium alone will not give the diagnosis.
2. **Albumin is the main calcium binding protein** in the plasma, hence it also should be measured.
3. Serum **PTH** level which is estimated by immunoassay is the *diagnostic investigation*. It is called as **tumour marker** for hyperparathyroidism. Estimation of PTH is difficult, costly and needs sophisticated setup.
4. Serum **phosphorus** levels are decreased.
5. **Alkaline phosphatase** is increased when bones are involved.
6. **X-ray of the hand** may reveal decalcification cysts in the phalanges, telescoping of finger tips, etc. **X-ray of the skull** may reveal subperiosteal erosions, hazy outline of the skull **pepper-pot** appearance (Key Box 20.5)

Key Box 20.4

CAUSES OF HYPERCALCAEMIA

- Multiple bone secondaries[1]
- Multiple myeloma
- Hyperparathyroidism
- Oat cell carcinoma[2]
- Sarcoidosis
- Vitamin D intoxication

1. The common causes are carcinoma breast, prostate, kidney, bronchus, follicular carcinoma thyroid.
2. It produces PTH like polypeptide (pseudo-hyperparathyroidism).

Key Box 20.5

INTERESTING RADIOLOGICAL CHANGES

• Osteopaenia	• Bone density loss
• Bone cysts and brown tumours	• Aggregation of osteoclasts (Osteoclastoma)
• Rugger jersey spine	• Generalised loss of bone density
• Pepper pot skull	• Demineralised bone
• Subperiosteal resorption (**Pathognomonic**)	• Seen in radial aspect of middle phalanges in hand and clavicle etc.

II. To localise parathyroid glands

1. **Ultrasound** of the neck can be very accurate in the hands of an experienced sonologist. It can also detect renal disease, pancreatic disease, etc. It cannot scan behind sternum and cannot pick up lesions less than 0.5 cms.
2. **Thallium-technetium isotope scan**: First outline thyroid with ^{99m}Tc and then isotope ^{201}TiCI (thallium chloride) is administered which is taken up by both thyroid and parathyroid. By computer subtraction of the two and enlargement of images, the parathyroid appears as a hot spot.
3. **Sestamibi scanning**: This test has been proved to be superior to Thallium and technetium subtraction scanning.

- Sestamibi is a protein labelled with technetium – 99m that localises diseased gland.
- It is **very sensitive to identify adenomas** (90%) than Hyperplasia.
- However, it is very expensive, hence it can be used in **'Re-exploration of neck'** for parathyroidectomy.

TREATMENT

- The surgery of the parathyroid glands needs patience, skill and **expertise**. The neck is explored with a collar neck incision similar to subtotal thyroidectomy. Parathyroid gland, when it is enlarged can have dark-brown or chocolate brown colour. Occassionally, the surgeon is lucky to encounter a single adenoma usually located on the posterior surface of the thyroid gland, when it arises from superior parathyroid (Key Box 20.6). Very often, the identification of the parathyroid may be difficult because they may be intrathyroidal or within the mediastinum.
- **Frozen section** of parathyroid glands is essential to confirm whether it is an adenoma or hyperplasia because depending upon the pathological nature of the gland, the treatment has to be carried out.

Following are few examples of types of surgery

- **Single adenoma**: Excision of the gland. **However, one other normal parathyroid gland is also removed for histopathological study.**

Key Box 20.6
UNUSUAL LOCATIONS AT SURGERY
• Behind oesophagus • Within carotid sheath • Intrathyroidal • Upper mediastinum

- **Diffuse hyperplasia**: 3½ or 3¾ parathyroids are removed and a **small piece is auto-transplanted into the forearm muscle tissue.** In case there is hyperactivity of this parathyroid tissue, surgical exploration becomes easy. At the same time, if this functions normally, patient will not develop hypoparathyroidism.
- **Carcinoma**: All four glands should be removed along with thyroid tissue.

FOLLOW UP

- Estimation of calcium should be done in the postoperative period to assess the functioning of the parathyroid tissue. Very often, after surgery for adenoma, there is a sudden drop in the levels of calcium because of absorption of the calcium by the bones. This is described as **'hungry bone syndrome'**. **This is seen in patients who have generalised bone disease.** In one of our patients calcium levels dropped down to 4 mg % with severe tetany. It took 7-10 days for the calcium to return to the normal levels. She required 24 hrs constant calcium drip.

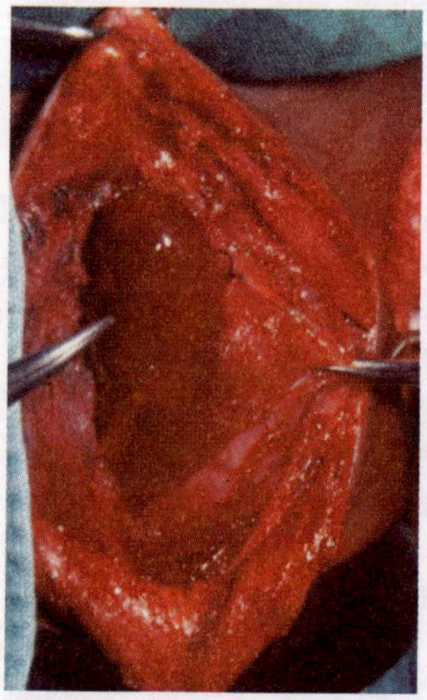

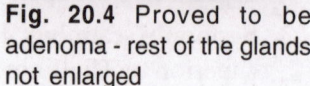

Fig. 20.3 Superior parathyroid found near the upper pole of the thyroid gland

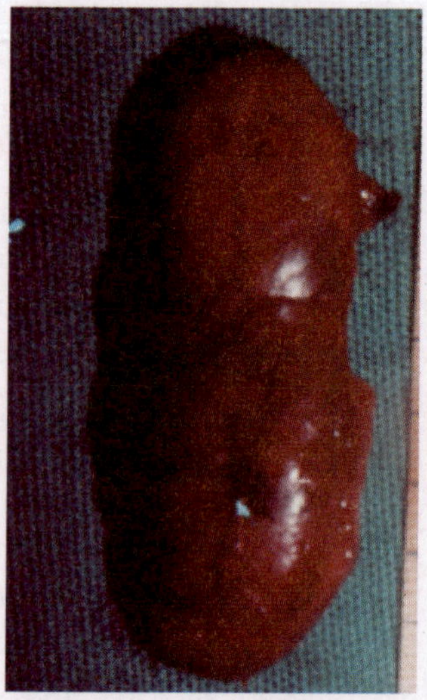

Fig. 20.4 Proved to be adenoma - rest of the glands not enlarged

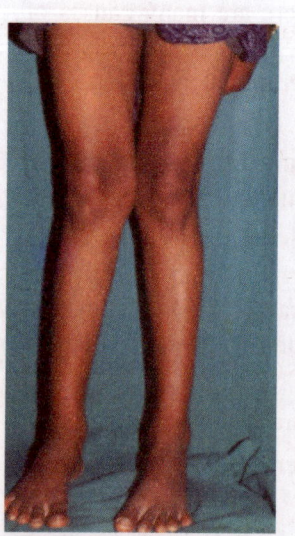

Fig. 20.5 Parathyroid adenoma with genu valgus deformity

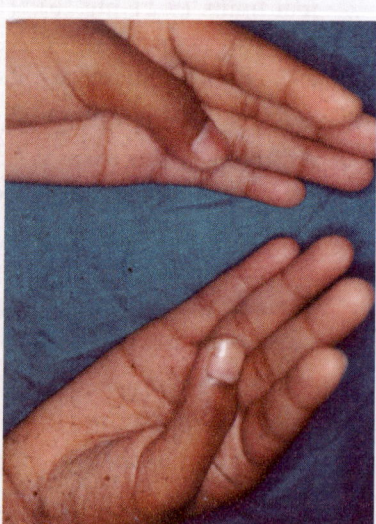

Fig. 20.6 Severe tetany following removal of the parathyroid adenoma required calcium infusion

Contributed by Prof. L. Ramachandra, KMC, Manipal

- Absorption of calcium can be enhanced by **oral administration of 1, 25 - dihydroxycholecalciferol**, which is the metabolite of vitamin D.

CLINICAL NOTES

A 20 year old boy attended dental outpatient department for a loose tooth. He was diagnosed to have a loose tooth and a cyst in the lower jaw as confirmed by X-ray. Patient also had genu valgus deformity with backache. An ortho opinion was sought for. Investigations revealed high calcium levels. An ultrasound neck revealed a parathyroid adenoma of 6 cms. At exploration a single adenoma was found arising from right inferior parathyroid and was excised. Incidentally, X-ray abdomen also revealed bilateral nephrocalcinosis. This case illustration has been given to highlight the various presentations of hyperparathyroidism. High degree of suspicion is necessary for a clinician to consider the possibility of hyperparathyroidism.

ACUTE HYPERCALCAEMIC CRISIS

- It presents with severe abdominal pain and effortless vomiting. Dehydration, oliguria, renal failure follow soon. Untreated cases develop coma and cardiac arrest.

Causes

1. **Hyperparathyroidism**
   - Sudden increase in PTH levels occur due to spontaneous bleeding in a parathyroid tumour or rupture of a cystic parathyroid tumour.
   - Severe dehydration also precipitates a crisis
2. **Disseminated carcinoma** with bony metastasis (usually carcinoma of the breast)

Treatment

1. Restore fluid volume urgently
2. The **biphosphonates** – Disodium pamidronate slow intravenous 15-60 mg single infusion or over 2-4 days. Maximum dose is about 90 mg. This drug stops mobilization of calcium from the bone.
3. Mithramycin
4. Steroids (in cases of vitamin D intoxication and sarcoidosis).

TYPES OF HYPERPARATHYROIDISM

- **Primary hyperparathyroidism**: It refers to hyperactivity of parathyroids due to an adenoma or primary hyperplasia of parathyroid glands.
- **Secondary hyperparathyroidism**: It occurs due to persistently low levels of calcium as in chronic renal failure and malabsorption, which results in decreased levels of calcium which in turn stimulates the parathyroid gland.
- **Tertiary hyperparathyroidism**: This is seen in patients who undergo dialysis and transplantation for chronic renal failure. After a few years, autonomy develops and the secondary hyperparathyroidism changes into tertiary hyperparathyroidism.

ADRENAL GLANDS[1]

Adrenal glands are the important endocrinal glands which are essential for life. The life-saving hormones such as corticosteroids, catecholamines are secreted by the adrenals. The disorders of adrenal cortex include Addison's disease, Cushing's syndrome, Conn's syndrome, etc. These are of great interest to the physicians. Tumours arising from adrenal medulla including neuroblastoma and phaeochromocytoma are of interest to surgeons. In this chapter, only these two topics are discussed.

Classification of tumours of adrenal medulla
I. Neoplasm of the sympathetic neurons
1. Ganglioneuroma: It is a benign neuronal tumour, commonly arises from retroperitoneal lumbar sympathetic trunk. FNAC, ultrasound followed by surgical excision is the management.
2. Neuroblastoma

II. Neoplasm of the chromaffin cells
- Phaeochromocytoma

NEUROBLASTOMA

- It occurs in 1 in 10,000 live births.
- It is the **most common solid tumour** of infancy and childhood.
- It originates from the neural crest. Hence, it can be found from **orbit to pelvis** where sympathetic nerve tissue is found.

---

1 Students are requested to refer Medical Text Books for appropriate topics.

Key Box 20.7

NEUROBLASTOMA

- Most common solid tumour in infancy and childhood.
- Adrenals is the most common site
- Mass abdomen and metastasis are common presenting features
- Surgical excision is the best treatment
- Younger the child, better the prognosis
- Highest incidence of spontaneous remission

- Adrenal gland is **the most common** site of neuroblastoma.
- As the name suggests, the tumour occurs due to **malignant proliferation of the neuroblasts** or failure of maturation of primitive sympathetic nerve cells, the neuroblasts. (Key Box 20.7)

Clinical features

- 50% of children present to the hospital **under the age of one year** and 80-90% are less than 3 years of age.
- An **abdominal mass** is the most common presenting feature. The mass has all features of a renal mass but location is slightly higher. It is firm to hard, nodular and fixed.
- Child is **sick** with weight loss, fever, abdominal distension, anaemia, etc.
- Functional tumours produce diarrhoea and hypokalaemia due to release of **vasoactive intestinal polypeptide** (VIP), sweating and flushing due to release of **catecholamines**.
- **Proptosis** and **periorbital swellings** are due to bony metastasis and subcutaneous nodules are quite common (Key Box 20.8).
- Posterior mediastinal neuroblastomas can produce cord compression and even paraplegia due to protrusion within the spinal canal (**dumb-bell tumours**)

Key Box 20.8

TYPES OF NEUROBLASTOMA

1. Pepper type: Right sided tumours with secondaries in the liver
2. Hutchinson's type: Left sided tumour with metastasis in bones – Orbit and skull

---

Investigations

1. **Vanillyl mandelic acid (VMA)** and homovanillic acid (HVA) are the byproducts of catecholamines passed in the urine. 24 hour urinary excretion of catecholamines and these 2 metabolites will be very high.
2. **Plain X-ray** abdomen shows fine stippled calcification. X-ray chest to rule out cannon-ball secondaries.
3. Abdominal **ultrasound** and **computed tomography (CT)** can define the mass, nature and extent and can detect hepatic metastasis.
4. **Excretory pyelography** is done to rule out renal mass. Displacement of the kidney, laterally and downwards, is also a feature.
5. **Magnetic resonance imaging (MRI)** is better than CT scan in detecting the mass as well as bony metastasis.
6. **Bone marrow aspiration** is positive in around 60-70% of cases.

Treatment

- Early cases respond very well to surgical excision.
- However, many children present with metastasis and, chemotherapy and radiotherapy is given first to control the disease followed by surgical excision. Autologous bone marrow transplantation has improved the outlook for patients with advanced disease.

PHAEOCHROMOCYTOMA

- As the name suggests, phaeochromocytoma is a neoplasm arising from chromaffin cells (Key Box 20.9)
- 90% of the tumour occurs in adrenals
- Extra-adrenal sites include organ of Zuckerkandl (the most common site), urinary bladder, renal hilum, chest, neck, etc. These are the sites of paraganglionic system.

Key Box 20.9

PHAEOCHROMOCYTOMA - RULE OF TEN

10%	Bilateral
10%	Malignant
10%	Extra-adrenal
10%	Multiple
10%	Familial
10%	Children

- In about 5% of cases, the tumour can be a component of multiple endocrine neoplasia (MEN) Type IIa or Type IIb.

- Other syndrome associated with **Phaeochromocytoma is von Hippel-Lindau syndrome** (Key Box 20.10).

- The clinical manifestations are due to release of adrenaline and noradrenaline. When the level of noradrenaline is high, symptoms are severe.

PATHOLOGY

- It is a soft, highly vascular tumour consists of large sympathetic ganglionic cells. Most of the cells are differentiated.

- Usually, it is small in size and well encapsulated.

- Sometimes, it can present as a large abdominal mass.

- Microscopic features are polygonal or spheroidal chromaffin cells within a vascularised fibrous stroma.

CLINICAL FEATURES

- The most common presenting feature is paroxysmal or persistent hypertension. It is associated with palpitation, fever, pallor, tremors, sweating and severe headache.

- The paroxysmal attack may last for few minutes to few hours. (Key Box 20.11)

- **The factors which stimulate an attack are**:
  - Surgery
  - Invasive procedure
  - Late pregnancy
  - Drugs-Histamine, glucagon, etc.
  - Palpation of the mass

- **High index of suspicion is necessary to diagnose phaechromocytoma in a hypertensive patient.**

INVESTIGATIONS

1. Urinary levels of free catecholamines, vanillylmandelic acid (VMA) in excess of 7 mg/24 hours and meta-adrenaline 1-3 mg/24 hours are suggestive of phaeochromocytoma.

2. **Computed tomography** :
   - Non-invasive, safe investigation
   - It has a high degree of accuracy
   - It can pick up lesions of less than 1 cm in size

3. ^{131}I-Meta-Iodo-Benzyl-Guanidine (MIBG) scan
   - Iodine labelled MIBG (Radionuclide) scan is found to be very specific for phaeochromocytoma. This radionuclide scan locates only abnormal adrenal tissue and is **more useful in detecting ectopic sites of phaeochromocytoma.**

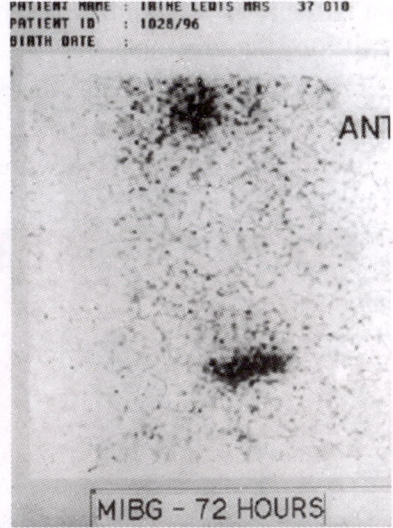

Fig. 20.7 MIBG scan showing extra-adrenal phaeochromocytoma

TREATMENT

- Surgical removal is the treatment. However, a good pre-operative preparation is essential before doing surgery. It includes control of blood pressure and tachycardia, by α and β-blockers. (Key Box 20.12)

- Contraction **of vascular bed which occurs** due to **catecholamines results in hypovolaemia** which is to **be corrected by IV fluids**.

- **First**, alpha-adrenergic blocker such as phenoxybenzamine is given to control hypertension and to permit **re-expansion of intravascular volume. Only after the complete alpha-adrenergic blockade, beta-adrenergic blockade may be added**.

Key Box 20.12

PHAEOCHROMOCYTOMA (PRE-OPERATIVE PREPARATION)

- **Phenoxybenzamine** 20-60 mg/day for 3-4 weeks before surgery to control **hypertension**.
- **Propranolol** 20-60 mg/day for 5-7 days before surgery to control **tachycardia** and **arrhythmias**.
- Plenty of **fluids** before surgery to correct **hypovolaemia**.

Surgery (Key Box 20.19)

Excision is the treatment. Certain steps of excision are as follows: (adrenalectomy)

- **Sodium nitroprusside** to be kept ready to treat hypertension on table as it is a **direct peripheral vasodilator** (0.5 to 10 µg/Kg/minute).

- Thorough search in the abdomen for other sites, due to the possibility of multiple tumours.

- Postoperative hypotension can be a serious problem

Key Box 20.13

PRECAUTIONS DURING SURGERY

- Midline incision for familial cases
- Anterior or posterior approach for sporadic cases
- Careful positioning
- Gentle handling
- Haemodynamic monitoring
- Ligation of adrenal vein first
- Avoid rupture of the tumour to prevent recurrence
- Laparoscopic adrenalectomy is very popular now

---

which needs to be treated with large volume of plasma expanders, blood transfusions, corticosteroids and vasopressors.

CLINICAL NOTES

An 18 year old girl was admitted for tonsillectomy. This girl suffered from occasional headache. She was diagnosed to have migraine. Pre-operative blood pressure showed mild elevations which were thought to be due to anxiety. During tonsillectomy, there was a rise in BP, which was controlled well. However, in the postoperative period, there was severe tachycardia, hypertension, arrhythmias and hypovolaemia. Within 8 hours of surgery, patient died as the diagnosis of phaeochromocytoma was being considered.

INCIDENTALOMAS

- Incidentally detected adrenal masses
- Detected by ultrasound or CT Scan
- Majority of such tumours are **non-functioning cortical adenomas of no clinical significance**

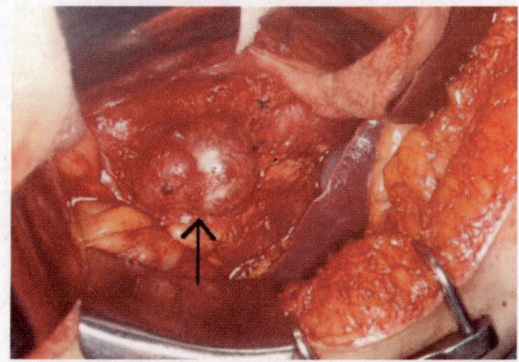

Fig. 20.8 Phaeochromocytoma at surgery

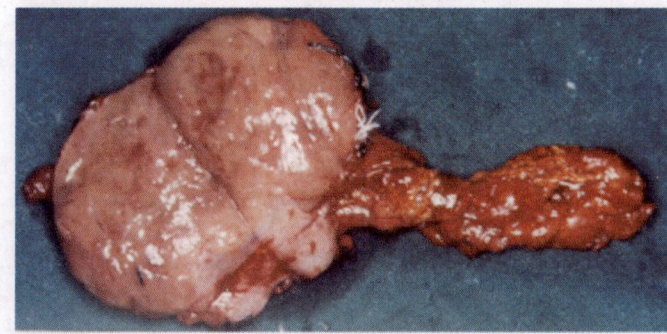

Fig. 20.9 Phaeochromocytoma excised. Contributed by Prof. M.G. Shenoy, Senior Consultant, KMC, Manipal

Breast

21

- Congenital anomalies
- Surgical anatomy
- Cystic swellings of breast - classification
- Acute bacterial mastitis
- Antibioma
- Retromammary abscess
- Phylloides tumour
- Intracystic carcinoma of breast
- Aberrations of normal development and involution
- Macrocysts
- Duct papilloma
- Duct ectasia - plasma cell mastitis
- Fibroadenoma
- Galactocoele
- Carcinoma breast
- Effects of lymphatic obstruction from carcinoma breast
- Breast reconstruction
- Mondor's disease
- Carcinoma male breast
- Angiosarcoma breast

CONGENITAL ANOMALIES OF BREAST

I. **Amazia**: Congenital absence of breast is very very rare. It can be unilateral or bilateral.

II. **Polands syndrome**

Amazia

Absence of sternal portion of pectoralis major

Occurs commonly in males

III. **Polymazia**: Accessory breasts occur along the milk line – axilla (commonest), groin, thigh or buttock.

IV. **Athelia**: Absence of nipple

V. **Supernumerary nipples**: Accessory nipples

VI. **Micromastia**: Due to congenital defects of ovary, lack of hormonal stimulation occurs which results in small breast.

SURGICAL ANATOMY OF BREAST

Breast occupies the pectoral region from the 2nd to the 6th rib vertically, and from the lateral border of sternum to the midaxillary line, horizontally. It is hemispherical, and lies in the superficial fascial planes.

It is composed of fatty tissue and does the function of secreting milk. **The *axillary tail of Spence* is the part of the breast which is in the axilla and is deeper to the deep fascia**, whereas the entire breast is a *subcutaneous structure*.

STRUCTURE OF THE BREAST

1. **Nipple and areola complex**: The **nipple** is located in the 4th intercostal space, in the midclavicular line. It is the erectile structure of the breast, and is directed forwards and laterally for the convenience of feeding the child. **Areola** has modified sweat glands and sebaceous glands, these enlarge during pregnancy and they are called *glands of Montgomery*. Both nipple and areola are pigmented due to melanin deposition which increases during pregnancy. Hair is absent in the areola of women (present in males).

2. **Parenchyma** of breast.

3. **Stroma** gives support to the glandular structure. There-in lie ligaments of Cooper which are cone-

shaped fibrous band. Their apex is attached to overlying skin, and base to the fascia over pectoralis major.

4. **Lobule** is the chief functional and structural unit of breast. Many lobules join to form a lobe. There are **15-20 lobes and** each lobe is drained by a **lactiferous duct**. They are 15-20 in number arranged radially, lined by myoepithelial cells, which converges into the nipple.

LYMPHATIC DRAINAGE OF BREAST (Fig. 21.2)

Superficial lymphatics drain the nipple and areola and form a **subareolar plexus of Sappey**. This is situated beneath the areola and they communicate with the deeper lymphatics within the parenchyma of breast. They drain into following lymph nodes:

1. **Pectoral,** also called the anterior group of lymph nodes.

2. **Central group** of nodes which lie on the medial wall of axilla.

    These 2 groups of lymph nodes are commonly involved in carcinoma breast.

3. **Posterior,** or subscapular lymph nodes.

4. **Lateral**, along 3rd part of axillary vessels in the upper 1/3 of arm.

5. **Apical group** of lymph nodes are situated deep in the axilla and cannot be felt clinically.

6. **Internal mammary** nodes are found in the first three intercostal spaces, 3 cm away from margin of the sternum.

7. **Supraclavicular nodes** are felt in the posterior triangle above the clavicle

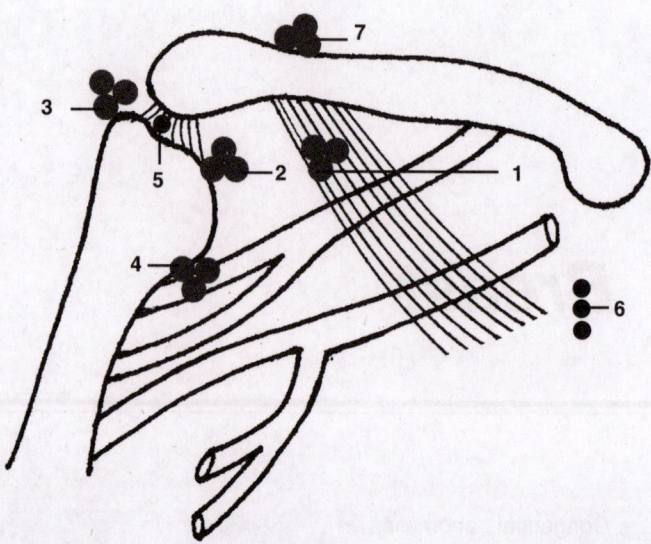

Fig. 21.2 Lymphatic drainage of breast (refer text for numbers)

Cutaneous lymphatics of one breast communicate with cutaneous lymphatics of opposite breast across midline.

For the examination of lymph nodes refer page 296.

BLOOD SUPPLY OF THE BREAST

1. **Lateral thoracic artery** gives many branches which penetrate through the pectoralis major and supply the breast.

2. **Internal mammary artery** gives branches through intercostal spaces.

3. **Pectoral branches of acromiothoracic artery** supplies upper part of the breast. *Venous return follows the artery but drain into large veins which also receives blood from vertebrae and thoracic cage, e.g. posterior intercostal veins joining paravertebral plexus of veins. This explains metastasis in the vertebrae from carcinoma of the breast.*

CYSTIC SWELLINGS OF BREAST - CLASSIFICATION

CLASSIFICATION

I. **Inflammatory:** Acute bacterial mastitis with abscess.

II. **Neoplastic**:

   A. Benign: Phylloides tumour

   B. Malignant: Intracystic carcinoma

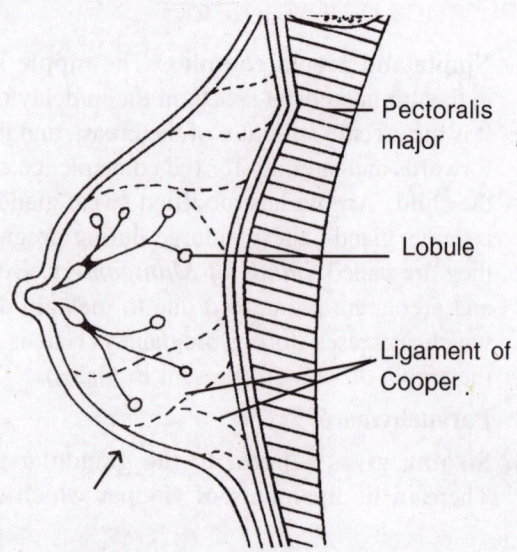

Pectoralis major

Lobule

Ligament of Cooper

Fig. 21.1 Structure of the breast

III. **Non-neoplastic cyst** :

    A. Fibroadenosis – Cyclical mastalgia

    B. Simple cysts of the breast

IV. **Retention cyst of the breast**: Galactocoele

V. **Other rare causes of cysts of the breast**:

    A. Tuberculous mastitis with cold abscess

    B. Lymphatic cyst of the breast (congenital)

    C. Hydatid cyst of the breast

    D. Haematoma of the breast

ACUTE BACTERIAL MASTITIS
(Breast abscess - pyogenic mastitis)

AETIOPATHOGENESIS

1. Most commonly encountered during **lactation** called as lactational mastitis.

   Precipitating factors

   - Crack/fissure in the nipple
   - Retracted nipple. Hence, cleaning of the breast is a problem
   - Oral cavity infection in the child

2. It can be due to an infection of a **haematoma.**

   - In both conditions, the common organism is *Staphylococcus aureus,* which enters through the nipple, proliferates intraductally and produces *clotting of the milk.* Within the clot the organisms multiply, which results in a **cellulitic stage of the breast** (mastitis) and in untreated cases, it may give rise to a breast abscess. Initially, only one lobule and duct get affected, later other lobules, giving rise to an intramammary abscess.

3. **Non lactational breast abscess**

   It occurs in patients with duct ectasia and periductal mastitis. When such an abscess ruptures, it results in a mammary duct fistula. It classically drains at the junction between the areola and breast skin. **Anaerobic bacteria** is the cause in majority of cases.

CLINICAL FEATURES

1. Severe pain in the breast due to spreading inflammatory exudate.

2. Breast is swollen, tense, tender, warm to touch. These are the signs of *cellulitic stage.*

Key Box 21.1

BREAST ABSCESS

- Common organism - *Staphylococcus aureus*
- Commonly seen during lactational period
- Very painful condition
- **Do not wait for fluctuation**
- Cloxacillin is the drug of choice
- Incision and drainage

---

3. Once *breast abscess* develops, there is high grade fever with chills and rigors and a soft, cystic fluctuant swelling can be felt in the breast. In untreated cases, abscess may rupture through the skin resulting in *necrosis of the skin of breast, ulceration and* discharge.

4. In deep seated abscess, it is difficult to elicit fluctuation and often fluctuation is a late sign. Hence, if **throbbing pain, fever with chills and rigors**, are present, immediate drainage is mandatory. If not done, significant amount of breast tissue will be destroyed.

TREATMENT

Stage of cellulitis

1. Not to feed the child on the affected side.

2. Cloxacillin 500 mg, 6th hourly, orally for 7-10 days.

3. Anti-inflammatory drugs such as Ibuprofen 400 mg three times a day

4. Good support to the breast

5. For non-lactational breast abscess, add Metronidazole 400 mg 3 times a day for 5-7 days

Breast abscess

1. The abscess should be drained-Incision and drainage (I & D) under antibiotic cover.

2. If the abscess is situated in any quadrant of breast, other than lower quadrant, it is drained by *radial incision.*

3. Abscess in lower quadrant is drained by *inframammary* incision placed in the inferior aspect of breast (Refer I & D of breast abscess under operative surgery section).

4. When both the breasts have an abscess, the breasts should be emptied and the milk that is expressed *can be boiled and given to the child.*

Complication of acute mastitis (Key Box 21.2)

Key Box 21.2
COMPLICATIONS OF ACUTE MASTITIS
• Abscess
• Toxaemia
• Skin necrosis
• Antibioma

CLINICAL NOTES

An 18 year girl was admitted in a medical ward with the diagnosis of pyrexia of unknown origin (PUO). All investigations were normal except a high total WBC count. After about a week, the duty nurse noticed that the patient's dress was stained with pus. It was a large breast abscess with necrosis of the overlying skin. It was drained later. The girl was so shy that she did not even complain of pain or swelling of the breast. These types of cases are not uncommon in our country.

ANTIBIOMA

- It means antibiotic induced. 'Oma' = Tumour (swelling).
- When an abscess occurs in the breast and antibiotics are given, without draining the abscess, the abscess cavity may become fibrous and it results in **firm to hard lump** in the breast. It gives rise to vague **ill health of the patient**.
- This hard lump can be confused for *malignancy*.
- It is treated by excision

OTHER TYPES OF BREAST ABSCESSES

Retromammary abscess

It is collection of pus behind the *pectoralis major.*

Common causes

1. Haematoma with secondary infection
2. Tuberculosis of ribs with cold abscess
3. Cold abscess arising from lymph node
4. **Empyema necessitans**: Empyema of lung, if left un-

treated, the pus tracks out, collects in the subcutaneous plane posteriorly and retromammary region anteriorly thereby forms retromammary abscess. There may be a tense, tender and cystic, lump palpable which can be confused with breast abscess.

Management

- Chest X-ray to rule out pulmonary tuberculosis.
- It is treated by draining the abscess by means of submammary incision.

Subareolar abscess

It is common in nonlactating women. It communicates with lactiferous duct resulting in mammary fistula. In chronic cases, retraction of the nipple can occur which is partial or slit-like. It can also be due to an infected sebaceous cyst.

PHYLLOIDES TUMOUR

Earlier known as cystosarcoma phylloides and mistakenly labelled as a giant intracanalicular fibroadenoma. It is a benign tumour of the breast, with a predilection to attain massive size, and recurs locally after lumpectomy. (Fig. 21.3, 21.4 and 21.5)

Clinical features (Key Box 21.3)

- Rapid growth
- Stretched, shiny skin
- Red, dilated veins over surface
- Bosselated surface (big nodules) Few cystic areas
- Warm to touch

It is differentiated from carcinoma by

1. No fixity to the skin
2. No fixity to the pectoralis

Key Box 21.3
BOSSELATED SURFACE - CONDITIONS
• Phylloides tumour
• Polycystic kidney
• Polycystic liver
• Large nodular goitre

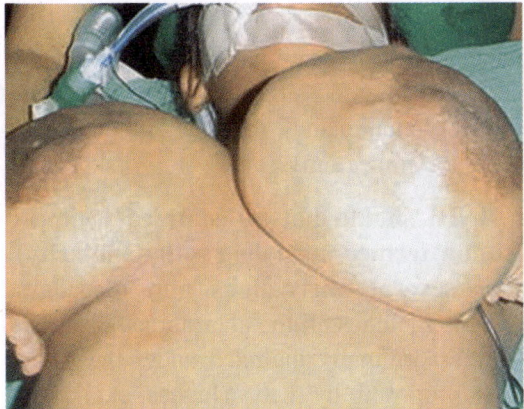
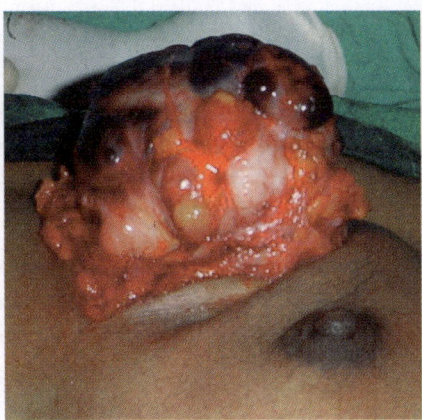
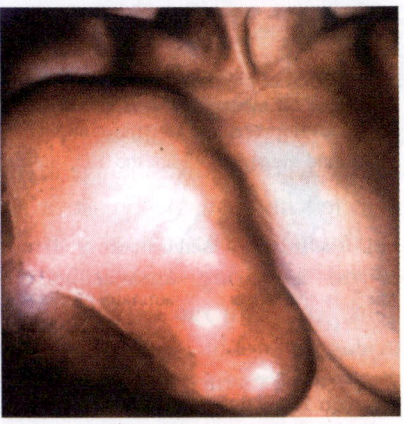

Fig. 21.3 Phylloides tumour of the left breast causing massive enlargement

Fig. 21.4 Phylloides tumour of the left breast at surgery

Fig. 21.5 Malignant phylloides tumour (recurrent)

3. Lymph nodes will not be involved
4. No nipple retraction.

- As the tumour grows very fast, it undergoes necrosis in various places resulting in cystic areas within the breast. It discharges serous fluid. Hence, the name *serocystic disease of Brodie*.
- Histologically, the tumour cells have a branching pattern, penetrating the cystic cavity (*phyllus* means leaf-like pattern). Fibrous stromal proliferation is a feature.

Complications

1. Necrosis of the skin and fungation.
2. It can turn into a *sarcoma* or *carcinoma*.

Treatment

1. **Small** - Wide excision of the lump or even subcutaneous mastectomy. Lumpectomy should not be done as it will lead to recurrence.
2. **Giant cystosarcoma** - Simple mastectomy may be necessary. Lymph nodal dissection is not required as sarcomas do not metastasize to lymph nodes.

INTRACYSTIC CARCINOMA OF BREAST (REECLIN'S DISEASE)

- Rapidly growing carcinoma of the breast can undergo cystic degeneration resulting in a cyst, called intracystic carcinoma of the breast. Aspiration reveals haemorrhagic fluid, containing malignant cells and which refills after aspiration. Other features of carcinoma of the breast may be present.

ABERRATIONS OF NORMAL DEVELOPMENT AND INVOLUTION (ANDI) OF THE BREAST

The concept of Aberrations of Normal Development and Involution (ANDI) of the breast was first published by **L.E. Hughes et.al of Cardiff breast clinic in 1987**. The ANDI classification is based on pathogenesis, and recognizes that a spectrum exists from normal, through mild abnormality, to disease. This has resulted in a radical change in attitude to the understanding and management of breast disorders. Changes previously regarded as disease are so common that they must be regarded as lying within the spectrum of normality.

This concept is of value in dispelling the supposed association between the benign conditions and cancer. Most patients with lumps and mastalgia are concerned that they may be harboring cancer (the result of a successful information campaign!!), and once a definite opinion of the benign nature of the lump is conveyed and the patient is informed that no further treatment is required, most would be reassured.

Normal process

↓

Aberration
(Benign breast disorder)
Conditions considered too common an occurrence and too mild a state to warrant the designation of a diseased state

↓

Disease
(Benign breast disease)

Having noted the above, a word of caution is due here – it is preferable to overtreat a benign breast disease rather than miss or delay treatment of an early carcinoma of the breast. So following the clinical dictum "In a patient who is above the age of 40 years, with a recently detected lump in the breast, it should be considered to be carcinoma breast until proved otherwise" may prove to be a wrong answer in many but the correct management in most. From the above, it follows that, in case of doubt (where there is a high risk patient or doubtful signs of malignancy) it would be prudent on the part of the treating surgeon to rule out malignancy by triple assessment (physical examination, mammography and cytology). If it is not possible to conclusively rule out the possibility of malignancy then the patient would be best adviced a lumpectomy.

The term ANDI should not be confined to imply fibroadenosis (now termed mastalgia with nodularity). ANDI includes several aberrations and disorders. The following table includes all the aberrations, disorders and disease entities originally included under the ANDI classification as proposed by L.E. Hughes et.al.

Table 21.1 Aberration of the Normal Development and Involution of the breast

| STAGE (Peak age in years) | NORMAL PROCESS | ABERRATION | | DISEASE STATE |
		UNDERLYING CONDITION	CLINICAL PRESENTATION	
EARLY REPRODUCTIVE PERIOD (15-25 Years)	Lobule formation	Fibroadenoma	Discrete lump	Giant fibroadenoma (more than 5 cms.)
	Stroma formation	Juvenile hypertrophy	Excessive breast development	Multiple fibroadenoma
MATURE REPRODUCTIVE PERIOD (25-40 Years)	Cyclical hormonal effects on glandular tissue and stroma	Exaggerated cyclical effects	generalized or discrete lump	Cyclical mastalgia and nodularity
INVOLUTION (35-55 years)	Lobular involution (including microcysts, apocrine changes, fibrosis, adenosis)	Macrocysts	Discrete lumps	Cystic diseases
		Sclerosing lesions	X-ray abnormalities	
	Ductal involution (including periductal round cell infiltrates)	Duct dilatation	Nipple discharge	Periductal mastitis with bacterial infection and non lactational breast abscess - leading to mammary duct fistula
		Periductal fibrosis	Nipple retraction	
	Epithelial turnover	Mild epithelial hyperplasia	Histological report	Epithelial hyperplasia with atypia

Terms to be avoided: Fibroadenosis – replace with mastalgia and nodularity.
Cystosarcoma phylloides – replace with phylloides tumour.

Note: Fibroadenoma is an **AND** (Aberration of Normal Development) of a lobule. Cyst (macrocyst) is an **ANI** (Aberration of Normal Involution) of a lobule.

Instructions to the students: Carefully go through the Table 21.1 and Fig. 21.6

References: British Medical Bulletin: Volume 47, Number 2, April 1991

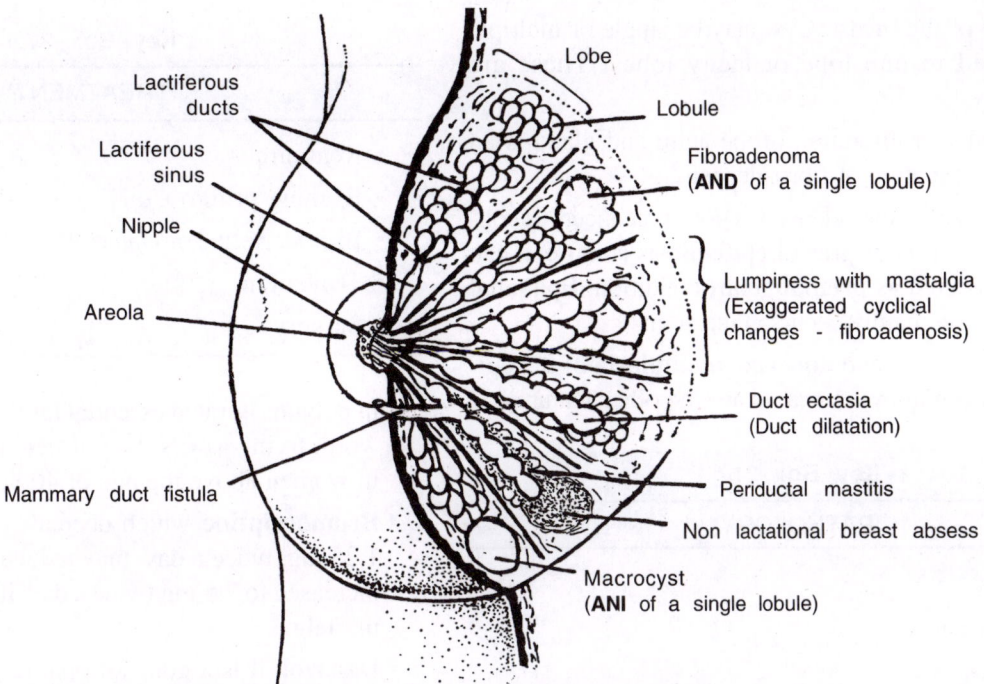

Fig. 21.6 Benign breast disorders and diseases

Table 21.2

MASTALGIA

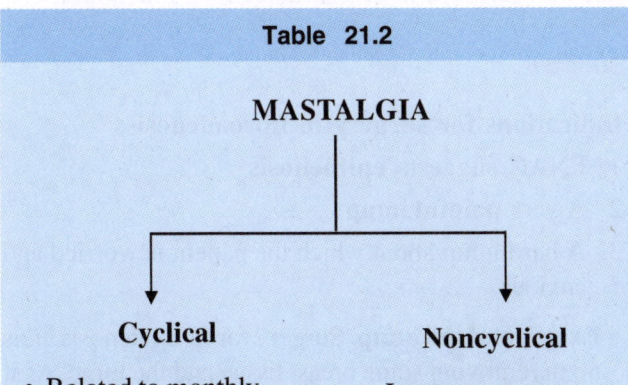

Cyclical

- Related to monthly cycles
- Associated with premenstrual nodularity and breast discomfort
- Excessive prolactin release from pituitary gland may be the cause
- Young woman are affected
- Reassurance
- Drugs
- Excision - last resort

Noncyclical

- Less common
- Pain can be due to periductal mastitis or costochondritis (Tietze's disease)
- Simple measures such as well supported bra
- Analgesics may be beneficial
- Injection with local anaesthetic on a trigger spot

CYCLICAL MASTALGIA WITH NODULARITY

Also called as **mammary dysplasia**, fibrocystic disease, Schimmel Busch's disease, hormonal mastopathy, or fibroadenosis.

The term ANDI should not be confined to imply fibroadenosis (Now termed as mastalgia and nodularity). In fact Fibroadenoma is an AND of a lobule and cyst (macrocyst) is an ANI of a lobule.

DEFINITION

- It is an aberration of physiological changes that occur in the breast from menarche till menopause. It is an ANDI (Aberration in Normal Development and Involution).
- Women around the age of 40 are the usual sufferers.

PATHOLOGY (Key Box 21.4)

1. **Fibrosis** results in increased connective tissue growth. Fat and elastic tissue become less, and chronic inflammatory cells such as plasma cells, can be present.

2. **Cyst formation**: Fibrosis compresses the ductules, which is responsible for cyst formation. Hence, it is a retention cyst. The cyst contains dark mucoid material and it may discharge serous fluid or green coloured fluid through the nipple. Hence, it is called *fibrocystic*

disease of the breast. Cyst may be single or multiple confined to one lobe or many lobes. These are microcysts.

3. **Adenosis:** Proliferation of the acini and gland is an important feature of fibroadenosis.

4. **Epitheliosis:** Fibroadenosis is not a precancerous condition but if the degree of **epitheliosis** is more, it can be considered as **premalignant** condition. Epithelial hyperplasia mainly occurs in the acini.

5. **Papillomatosis** and **apocrine metaplasia** of the epithelium lining cystic spaces are the other features.

Key Box 21.4

PATHOLOGY

- Fibrosis
- Cyst formation
- Adenosis
- Epitheliosis
- Papillomatosis
- Apocrine metaplasia

CLINICAL FEATURES

- Females around the age of 30-40 are the victims - Spinsters, married childless women and women who have not suckled their babies are the usual sufferers.

- Severe pain in the breast in the premenstrual period and during menstruation. **It is called cyclical mastalgia.** Upper outer quadrant, bilaterally is affected.

- Clinical examination of the breast reveals a coarse, nodular, tender, lumpiness which is better felt with the finger and the thumb. Often, there are multiple, irregular, firm, nodularity palpable bilaterally, especially in the upper outer quadrants.

- Nipple discharge which is serous or green coloured may occur.

TREATMENT (Key Box 21.5)

I. Conservative line of management

Evening primrose oil in adequate doses for 3 to 4 months are beneficial in few patients. These patients have abnormal fatty acid profiles and decreased levels of metabolites of linolenic acid. Treatment with primrose oil improves essential fatty acids because it is rich

---

Key Box 21.5

TREATMENT

- **Reassure**
- **Evening primrose oil**
- **Bromocriptine or Danazol**
- **Tamoxifen**
- **Surgery**

---

in polyunsaturated essential fatty acids. Costly but still worth trying as first line of treatment, specially useful in women above the age of 40 years.

- **Bromocriptine** which decreases the prolactin levels, 1.25 mg, twice a day, may reduce the pain and may be increased to 2.5 mg twice a day. It is useful for cyclical mastalgia.

- **Danazol**, it is a gonadotrophin releasing hormone inhibitor. 200-400 mg/day, thrice a day is given. It acts by reducing FSH and LH levels.

- **Tamoxifen** 10 mg, twice a day is a better alternative to danazol.

Treatment may have to be continued for some months.

II. Surgery

Indications for surgery in fibroadenosis:

1. FNAC suggests **epitheliosis**

2. A very **painful lump**

3. A hard lump about which the patient is worried and anxious

- **Excision of the lump.** Surgery for fibroadenosis ends up in removing some breast tissue and the lump. As it has no capsule of its own it is a messy surgery unlike fibroadenoma surgery.

- Is there a role for **subcutaneous mastectomy?** In patients with family history of breast carcinoma, if they have lumps in the breast with severe degree of epitheliosis, it may be worth doing subcutaneous mastectomy.

CLINICAL NOTES

A paediatrician's mother, 52 years old, underwent surgery for fibroadenosis. The pathology report was fibroadenosis with severe epithelial dysplasia. She came for follow up after 3 months. There were no fresh changes in the breast. However, after 9 months of surgery she presented with a hard lump with significant nodes in the axilla. She underwent Patey mastectomy. The case illustrates, epitheliosis is undoubtedly premalignant. Should the lady have been advised to undergo subcutaneous mastectomy after the first surgery? (Page 305)

FIBROADENOMA

It is a benign tumour in which the epithelial cells are arranged in a fibrous stroma. It is an **AND** (**A**berration of **N**ormal **D**evelopment) of a single lobule.

Types

1. Pericanalicular type in which fibrosis is more
2. Intracanalicular type in which fibrosis is less

Clinical features

1. Peak age incidence is at 20 years
2. Patients present with painless lump in the breast
3. It is smooth, round bordered, firm to hard in consistency, and freely mobile within the breast. Due to its free movement, it is known as **Breast Mouse**.

Treatment

- Excision of the lump.
1. In **pericanalicular** type, the lump is superficial. It is removed by periareolar incision.
2. In **intracanalicular** type, the lump is deeper and peripheral. It is removed by submammary incision.

Complications

- Very, very rarely after 20-30 years, it can undergo a sarcomatous change.

Fibroadenoma and fibroadenosis are compared in Table 21.3.

DUCT ECTASIA-PLASMA CELL MASTITIS

- Common in middle aged woman.
- There is primary dilatation in one of the lactiferous duct.

Aetiology

- Actual cause is not known. Mild low-grade infection has been considered as one of the factors.
- Increased in smokers

Pathology

- There is dilatation of one of the lactiferous duct
- Due to dilatation, the contents tend to undergo stasis. The epithelial debris, and serous fluid, collectively form a thick paste-like material rich in lipid.
- It may cause discharge per nipple
- There is intense periductal inflammation with lymphocytes and plasma cells. Hence, it is called plasma cell mastitis.
- Fibrosis causes nipple retraction

Clinical features

- Middle-aged woman
- Paste-like material discharge per nipple

Table 21.3 Differences between fibroadenoma and fibroadenosis

	FIBROADENOMA	FIBROADENOSIS
Incidence	Less common	More common
Nature	Benign tumour of one lobule	Aberration of normal changes in the breast
Pain in the breast	Not a feature	Very common, premenstrual
Location	Unilateral	Usually bilateral
Lump	Well-defined, firm, mobile	Irregular, ill-defined, tender lump
Capsule	Well-defined	No capsule
Discharge	No	Serous or green coloured
Malignancy	Rarely-sarcoma	Carcinoma (if epitheliosis is present)
Treatment	Excision	Excision or drugs

Key Box 21.6

PLASMA CELL MASTITIS

- Aseptic, abacterial dilatation of lactiferous ducts
- Peri ductal infiltration of plasma cells and lymphocytes
- Thick creamy or paste like discharge
- Partial retraction of the nipple
- Excision of the lump

- After some time, because of fibrosis, a lump can be felt, which can be confused for carcinoma of breast.
- **Bilateral slit like retraction of nipple** of long duration.

Management

- FNAC and treated by excision

MACROCYSTS

- They occur due to excessive secretion of thin fluid within the lobules which enlarge to produce a cyst. Clinically, they present as soft, cystic, fluctuant, transillumination-positive swelling in the breast. It is an ANI of a single lobule.
- They can be single or multiple. One of them can have huge dimensions having a thin bluish capsule – *Blue domed cyst of Bloodgood.*

Treatment

Excision of cyst in the following situations
1. Recurrence after 2 aspirations
2. Blood stained aspirate
3. Residual lump after aspiration

GALACTOCOELE (Fig. 21.7)

- It is a solitary, subareolar retention cyst filled with milk. It occurs and dates back to the lactational period.
- It occurs due to inadequate drainage of the milk added by epithelial debris which block the lactiferous duct. Once the duct is blocked, proximally, the milky fluid accumulates resulting in a huge enlargement of breast. (Key box 21.7)

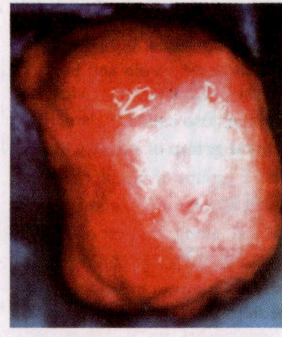

Fig. 21.7 Galactocoele

Key Box 21.7

MASSIVE ENLARGEMENT OF THE BREAST - CAUSES

- Diffuse hypertrophy
- Galactocoele
- Lymphatic cyst
- Cystosarcoma phylloides
- Filariasis of the breast

- Rarely, they undergo calcification.
- It is treated by excision of cyst along with lactiferous duct.

DISCHARGE PER NIPPLE - Table 21.4

Physiological discharge

- Lactation
- In infants, secretion of colostrum can occur for 1-2 days after birth, probably due to influence of maternal hormone.

Table 21.4 Discharge per Nipple	
NATURE OF THE DISCHARGE	**CAUSES**
1. Serous discharge	Fibrocystic disease
2. Greenish discharge	Fibrocystic disease, duct ectasia
3. Yellowish discharge (pus)	Breast abscess
4. Bloody discharge	Duct papilloma, duct carcinoma
5. Milky discharge	Galactocoele, hypothyroidism, pituitary tumours
6. Paste-like material	Duct ectasia

Pathological discharge

- The discharge per nipple is not an uncommon problem encountered in the surgery OPD.
- Majority of the discharge per nipple is due to fibroadenosis – (serous discharge). They respond once the primary disease is controlled.
- Bleeding per nipple can be due to a duct papilloma which is benign (described below) or due to carcinoma of the breast.
- Smear for malignant cells can be taken at the outpatient department from the discharge which can be examined immediately.
- Other causes of discharge per nipple need treatment of the primary problem.

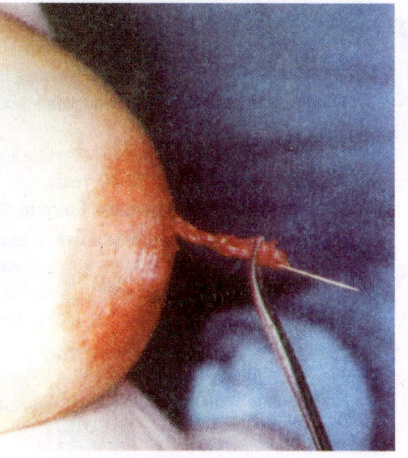
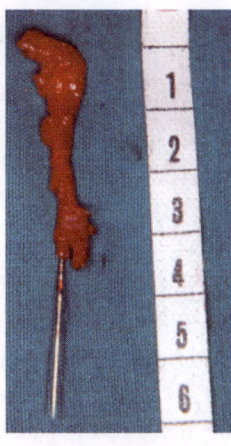

Fig. 21.9 Papilloma excision

Fig. 21.10 Specimen of papilloma

DUCT PAPILLOMA

- It is a benign lesion of the breast, usually single and unilateral, rarely multiple.
- Middle-aged women are affected and present with bleeding per nipple (Fig. 21.15).
- The tumour is situated in one of the larger lactiferous ducts.
- It presents as a small swelling just beneath the areola, palpation of which results in **discharge of blood**.
- Since, it is a *premalignant condition,* it is treated by microdochectomy.
- **Microdochectomy** : The opening of the lactiferous duct discharging blood is identified. It is probed with lacrimal probe or a straight needle. A small triangular piece of skin, along with the needle, and a wedge of breast tissue to a depth of about 5-6 cm is removed (Fig. 21.9).
- **Hadfield's Operation** : Cone excision of the lactiferous ducts.

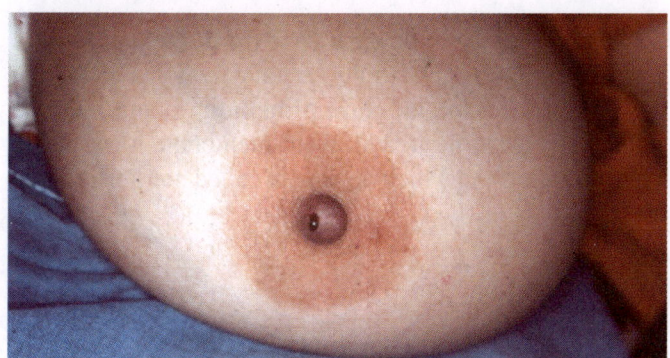

Fig. 21.8 Bleeding per nipple

GYNAECOMASTIA

- This is a painful, unphysiological *enlargement of the male breast.*

Causes

Idiopathic is the most common wherein no cause can be found. However there are many other causes of gynaecomastia which can be summarised as "**MASTIA**".

- **M**alignant tumour : Teratoma, bronchogenic carcinoma.
- **A**norchism: Absent testis
- **S**ex chromosome anomaly : Klinefelter's syndrome (XXY).
- **T**ablets: Cimetidine, stilbesterol, digitalis, spironolactone
- **I**diopathic: No cause is found
- **A**trophy of the testis: Liver cell failure, leprosy, etc.

Clinical features

- In idiopathic variety, gynaecomastia is bilateral. In other cases, it may be unilateral.
- A "disk" like tender lump is palpable, with smooth surface.

Treatment

- Lumpectomy or mastectomy with preservation of nipple and areola.

Complications

- Rarely, gynaecomastia can predispose to male breast carcinoma.

CARCINOMA OF THE BREAST

Carcinoma of the breast is the major killer of middle-aged women in western countries.

CLINICAL NOTES

A 35 years old lady came to the hospital with fracture of the right femur. An intern while taking the history could elicit the history of lump in the breast of 8 months duration. The patient allowed the doctors to examine the breast reluctantly as it was painless. She had carcinoma of the breast with pathological fracture of femur.

"However innocent be the breast lump, it can be malignant, unless proved otherwise."

AETIOLOGLCAL FACTORS

1. **Age** : It is very rare below the age of 20. The highest incidence is found between 40-60 years of age.

2. **Breast cancer and syndromes**:

   a) **Li-Fraumeni syndrome** is a rare disease with familial breast cancer and is associated with inherited mutation suppressor P^{53} gene.

   - It is a rare autosomal dominant disorder.

   - 90% of carriers will develop breast cancer by the age of 50.

   - They also can have other tumours in childhood such as soft tissue sarcoma, osteosarcoma, leukemia.

   b) **Cowden's disease (multiple hamartoma syndrome)**

   - It is associated with tumour suppressor gene PTEN

   - 30-50% of patients will develop breast cancer by 50 years of age.

   - The lesions found in this syndrome are **multiple facial trichilemmoma** (pathognomonic), oral papilloma, bilateral breast cancer, haemangiomas, lipomas, thyroid tumours, etc.

   c) **Ataxia telangiectasia**: It is associated with haemangioma and carcinoma breast.

3. **Chromosomal abnormalities** have been found in short arm of chromosome 17 in women with a family history of carcinoma of the breast. BRCA-1 and BRCA - 2 are the genes associated with increased risk.

Breast cancer with BRCA-1 tend to be ER - negative (ER-)
Breast cancer with BRCA-2 tend to be ER + positive (ER+)

4. **Diet**: Increased risk has been found in postmenopausal obese women and is due to increased synthesis of oestrogen (oestradiol) in the body fat. Alcohol intake is associated with a 1.5 fold increased risk of breast cancer. Vit C may have protective value. Increased intake of saturated fats and reduced intake of phytooestrogens increases risk.

5. **Endocrinal causes**:

   a. Longer the cumulative period of menstruation more the risk (Early menarche and late menopause)

   b. More the cumulative period of lactation better the protection (More children, each child breast fed longer)

   c. More abortions and each occurring later increases risk.

   d. More oestrogen content in OCP and OCP taken early in the reproductive life (before first pregnancy) increases risk.

   e. HRT increases risk if the estrogen content is higher and if taken for more than 5 years.

6. **Female sex** itself is a risk factor as only 1% of patients with breast cancer are males.

7. **Geographical**: Carcinoma of the breast is the disease of WHITE, WESTERN, WOMEN. It is rare in Japan and Taiwan. Genetic predisposition exists in a few cases, especially in bilateral breast carcinoma.

- *Students can remember the aetiological factors as "ABCDEFG".*

PATHOLOGY

- Majority of the tumours arise in the **ductal epithelium** (90%) which is called the ductal carcinoma and about 10% arise within **lobular epithelium** (lobular cancer). Those that infiltrate basement membrane it are called infiltrating and which do not are called non-infiltrating.

Infiltrating carcinomas

Scirrhous carcinoma (Fig. 21.11)

- It is the most common form seen in about 60-75% of patients. In this variety, there is increased fibrotic reac-

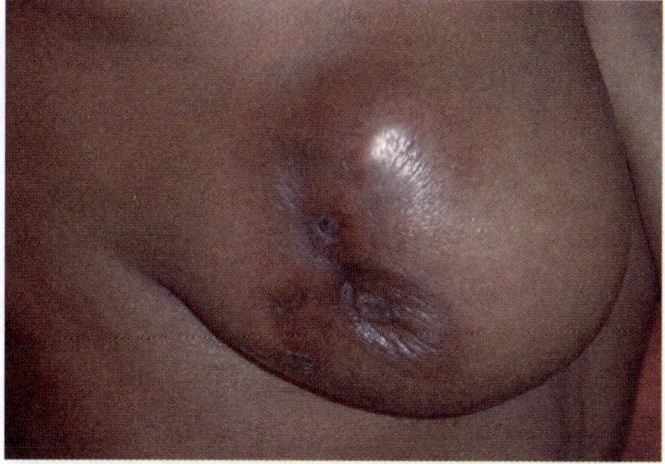

Fig. 21.11 Scirrhous carcinoma

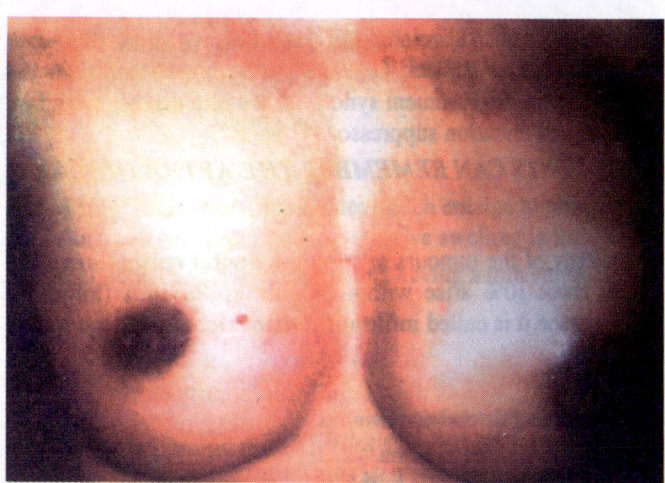

Fig. 21.12 Medullary carcinoma

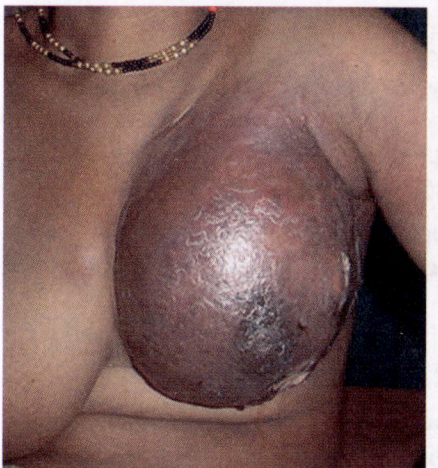

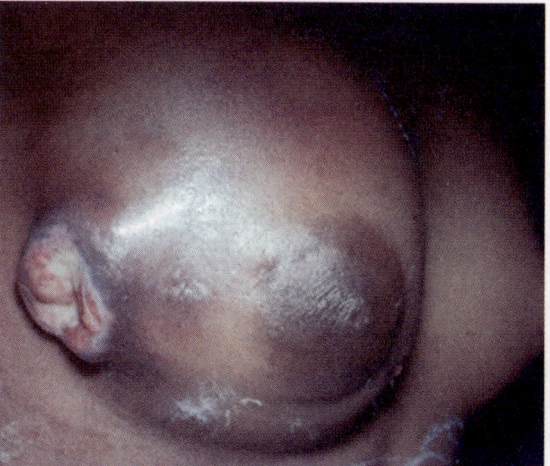

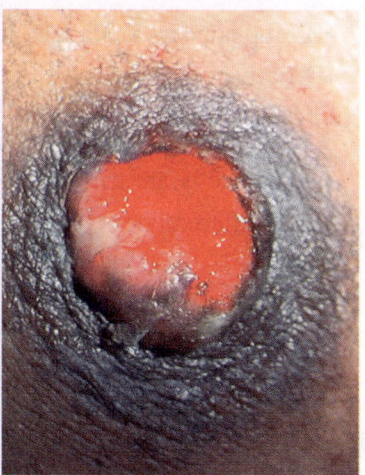

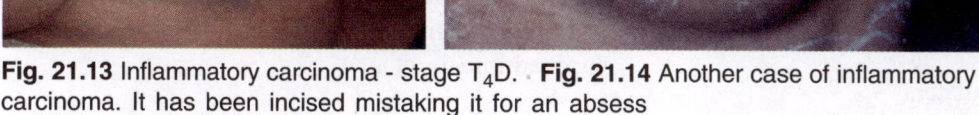

Fig. 21.13 Inflammatory carcinoma - stage T₄D. **Fig. 21.14** Another case of inflammatory carcinoma. It has been incised mistaking it for an absess

Fig. 21.15 Paget's disease of the nipple - totally destroyed nipple

tion and less cellular reaction. It presents as a hard lump. Hence the name, scirrhous carcinoma. It produces grating sound when it is cut. Cut surfaces are concave. The chalky white necrosis and calcification may be visible occasionally. This is the type of lesion which produces retraction of the nipple, infiltration of the skin and fixity to the chest wall.

- Malignant cells are round to polygonal with dark nuclei. Perivascular and perineural space infiltration is common.
- Atrophic scirrhous is an infiltrating duct carcinoma seen in elderly patients when there is atrophy of the breast.

Medullary carcinoma of the breast (Fig. 21.12)

- It is seen in around 15% of cases. It tends to occur in **well formed breasts** in the reproductive age group and it feels more soft than hard. In addition to undiffer-

entiated cells, occasionally well differentiated gland formation is present. Hence the name, medullary adenocarcinoma; Presence of lymphatic infiltration is thought to represent a good host response, thus indicating a good prognosis.

Inflammatory carcinoma (Fig. 21.13, 21.14)

- It constitutes less than 1 % of all cases of carcinoma breast.
- Predominantly seen during pregnancy and lactation.
- Malignancy grows so rapidly to invade more than half of the breast tissue.
- Redness, pain and sudden enlargement appear so suddenly that it is diagnosed as breast abscess. Hence the name, *mastitis carcinomatosa*. It is differentiated from breast abscess by absence of fever and presence of gross peau d'orange due to blockage of subdermal lymphatics.

- Blunder biopsy (incision) should not be done thinking that it is an abscess (Fig. 21.14).
- This variety has the worst prognosis.

It comes under staging T_4D

Paget's disease of the nipple (Fig. 21.15)

- It is a misnomer. It is *not a disease of the nipple* but an intraductal carcinoma involving excretory ducts which infiltrates nipple and areola early.
- Nipple can be ulcerated, fissured, cracked and oozing is present.
- In advanced cases, entire nipple is destroyed (ulcerated).
- Lump appears much later than changes in the nipple.
- Microscopically, large; **hyperchromatic cells** with clear cytoplasm or clear halo which represents intracellular accumulation of mucopolysaccharides is seen. These cells are called **Pagets cells**.
- It is differentiated from eczema by following points:

Key Box 21.8	
ECZEMA	PAGET'S DISEASE
Seen in lactating women	Seen in elderly women
Bilateral	Unilateral
Itching is present	Absent
Responds to antibiotics and local treatment	Does not respond

Colloid carcinoma

- It is diagnosed because of production of mucin, intracellularly and extracellularly. Prognosis of this is better than other infiltrating duct carcinomas.

NON-INFILTRATIVE LESIONS

Carcinoma in situ

- It can be Ductal – Ductal Carcinoma In Situ (DCIS)
- Lobular – Lobular Carcinoma In Situ (LCIS)

  This is a type of **cancer without infiltration** of epithelial basement membrane.

Lobular carcinoma is more dangerous because it is multifocal and bilateral.

- Lobular carcinoma refers to a lesion developing from the acini or terminal ductules of the lobule.
- Most in-situ carcinomas are diagnosed because of mammography and most of the breast conserving surgery is done in this group of patients.

Comedo carcinoma of breast

- Comedos means cast or plug. It is a peripheral carcinoma wherein the tumour cells block the ductules by forming a cast or plug producing a small cystic lesion. It is an example of intracystic carcinoma.

CLINICAL FEATURES OF CARCINOMA BREAST

- Lump in the breast is the most common presentation. It is the breast tissue in the upper and outer quadrant which is most frequently involved (65%). Typically it is hard and irregular but it can also be firm.
- Bleeding per nipple is an uncommon symptom of carcinoma of the breast. **It involves multiple ducts and is unilateral**.
- Fixation to the skin, ulceration, peau d'orange, fixation to pectorals and chest wall occurs late.
- About 5% of patients present with bony metastasis giving rise to bony pains i.e. pathological fractures, paraplegia, quadriplegia, etc.

CLINICAL EXAMINATION OF A CASE OF CARCINOMA OF THE BREAST

Inspection should be done in three positions:

I. Hands by the side of the patient

1. Nipple

- **Bloody discharge** indicates duct carcinoma.
- **Centrally retracted nipple**: Recent retraction indicates malignancy. It is due to fibrosis caused by extension of growth along the lactiferous duct. Remote retraction is either idiopathic or due to recurrent mild infection (mastitis)

Causes of retraction of the nipple

- Carcinoma of the breast
- Chronic mastitis

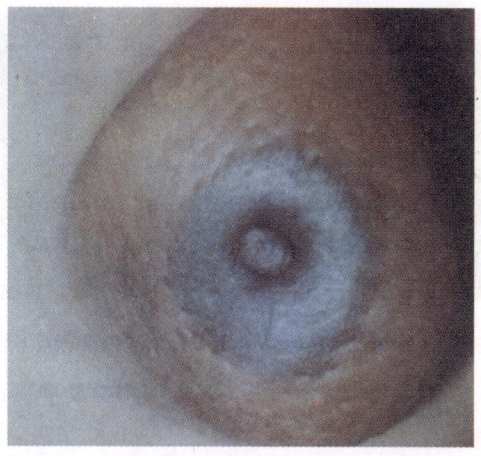

Fig. 21.16 Peau d'orange

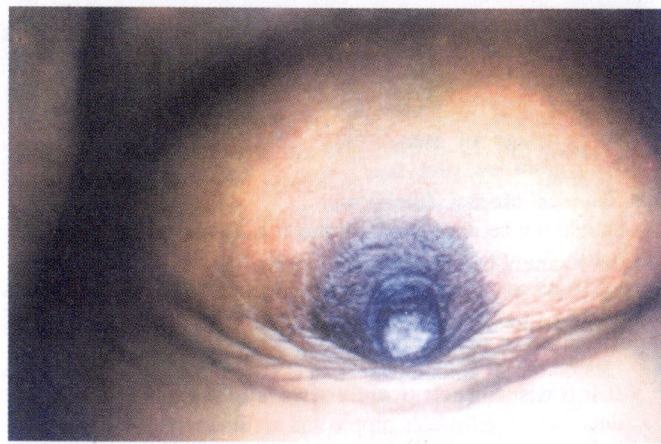

Fig. 21.17 Retraction of the nipple and peau d'orange

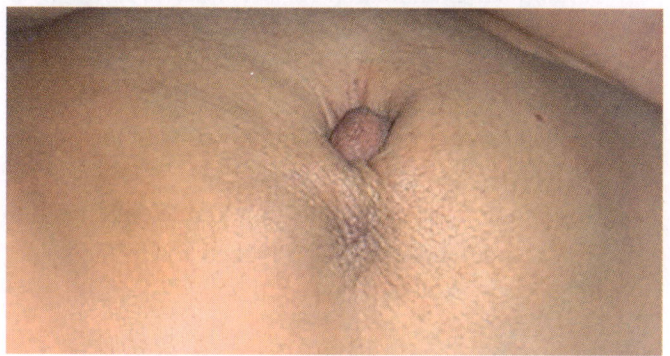

Fig. 21.18 Retraction of the nipple - classical feature of intraductal carcinoma

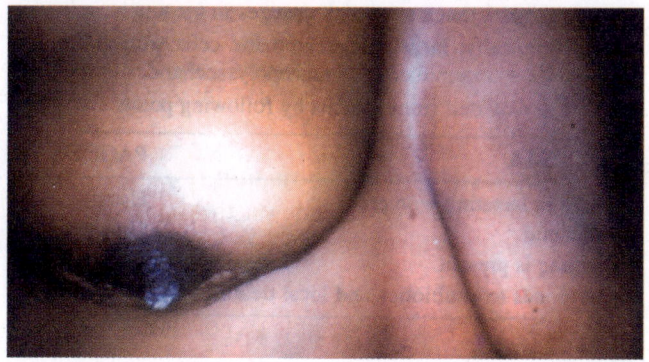

Fig. 21.19 Right nipple is elevated and retracted

- Congenital
- Chronic disease-Tuberculosis

- **Level of the nipples**: The nipple may be elevated (Fig. 21.16) because of fibrosis induced by the growth. Destruction of the nipple is a feature of Paget's disease of the nipple.

2. Areola

- Presence of *peau d'orange* indicates the tumour infiltrating the areola. It has been compared to the orange skin because of following reasons (Fig. 21.16).
- The areola becomes thick because of lymphatic obstruction giving rise to lymphoedema.
- Fixation of hair follicles and sweat glands to the underlying malignancy.

3. Skin over the breast

- **Puckering or dimpling of skin** is due to thin fibrous bands which are embedded in the subcutaneous fat and are attached to the skin and pectoral fascia called **ligaments of Cooper** which are infiltrated by the malignancy. Multiple nodules indicate advanced disease.

4. **Lump** - if visible give details
5. **Oedema** of the arm is due to lymphatic blockage caused by lymph nodes in the axilla.

II. Hands raised above the head

- **Peau d'orange**, (on elevation of hands) become more prominent.

III. Bending forward

- In cases of carcinoma infiltrating the chest wall, on bending, the breast will not fall forward.

PALPATION

1. **Local rise of temperature and tenderness** are usually not found in cases of carcinoma of the breast.

However, rapidly growing carcinoma and inflammatory carcinomas do exhibit local rise of temperature, redness and tenderness.

2. **Describe the lump**: The lump is the commonest presentation of carcinoma of the breast The upper and outer quadrant is the commonest site of carcinoma of the breast. Typically, the lump is hard and irregular. However, very often a firm lump which is removed, thinking it to be benign, is reported as carcinoma of the breast. In mastitis carcinomatosa the lump can be soft due to tumour necrosis.

3. **Intrinsic mobility** may be present but it moves with the breast tissue. (Fibroadenoma moves independent of breast tissue.)

4. **Plane of the swelling**

   - Lift the skin, if it is not possible, it indicates the tumour is fixed to skin.

   - *Pectoralis major contraction test* : Ask the patient to keep the hands on the flanks and press against the hip. If the lump cannot be moved after contraction, it indicates fixity to pectoralis major.

   - Fixity to the chest wall is assessed by 2 methods :

1. A tumour which is fixed to the chest wall will not be mobile when pectoralis major is relaxed.

2. Breast will not fall forwards (Fig. 21.20).

   - *Serratus anterior contraction* test by pressing the hand against the wall. The test has to be done when the tumour is situated in the outer and inferior quadrant.

AXILLARY LYMPH NODE EXAMINATION

- There are 5 groups of nodes in the axilla which are described under lymphatic drainage of the breast. However, very often, central group of nodes and pectoral nodes are enlarged. It is very difficult to feel the apical group of nodes.

- If the *axillary nodes* are *hard,* with or without *fixity,* they are significant.

- Soft to firm nodes need not be malignant but can be due to secondary infection because of fungating, ulcerating growth.

Presence of supraclavicular lymph nodes does not indicates metastatic disease. (Stage IV)

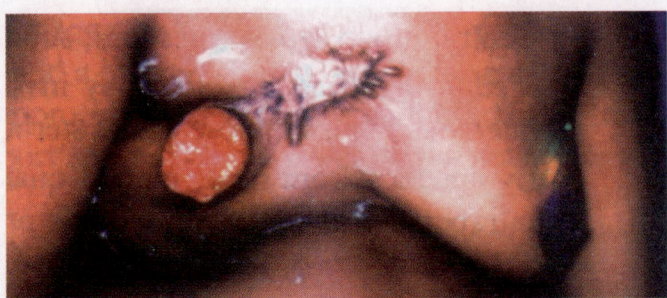

Fig. 21.20 Recurrent carcinoma breast fixed to the chest wall

EXAMINATION FOR DISTANT METASTASIS

1. Opposite axilla and opposite breast

2. Abdominal examination for secondaries in the liver which present as nodular liver, ascites and Krukenberg's tumour – bilateral bulky ovarian metastasis.

3. Rectal examination to rule out deposits in recto-uterine pouch

4. Respiratory system examination to rule out effusion.

5. Bony tenderness should be looked for in the spine, long bones, skull etc.

SPREAD OF CARCINOMA OF THE BREAST

1. **Local spread**

   - As the tumour grows in size, it infiltrates the skin causing ulceration, fungation, bleeding, foul smelling discharge. Later, it involves pectoral muscles, chest wall, etc.

2. **Lymphatic spread**

   - Central group, pectoral, lateral, subscapular and supraclavicular nodes.

   - *Medial quadrant tumours* may involve the internal mammary glands in the upper three or four intercostal spaces, close to the sternum.

   - Lymphatics from inferomedial quadrant of the breast, penetrate the rectus sheath and join the intraperitoneal lymphatics, thus producing ascites, Krukenberg's tumours (in premenopausal patients, ovary is vascular and fertile), rectovesical deposits, secondaries in the liver.

3. **Blood spread**

   - Secondaries in bones-flat bones (vertebral column, femur, ribs, scalp, etc.), secondaries in brain, etc.

   - Malignant pleural effusion is a common cause of death in carcinoma of breast.

TNM STAGING SYSTEM FOR BREAST CANCER

(AJCC cancer staging Manual, Col. 6, New York, 2002, Spinger PP 227-228)

Tumour

Tis Tumour in-situ

T_x Primary tumour cannot be assessed

T_0 No evidence of primary tumour

T_1 Tumour 2 cm or less in greatest dimensions

T_2 Tumour more than 2 cms but not more than 5 cm. in the greatest dimensions

T_3 Tumour more than 5 cm in the greatest dimensions

T_4 Tumour of any size with direct extensions (a) to chest wall or (b) to skin

T_{4a} Extension to chest wall, not including pectoralis muscle.

T_{4b} Involvement of skin in the form of oedema, ulceration or satellite skin nodules.

T_{4c} Both T_{4a} and T_{4b}

T_{4d} Mastitis carcinomatosa

Nodal status

N_x Regional lymph nodes cannot be assessed (eg. previously removed)

N_0 No regional lymph node metastasis

N_1 Mobile ipsilateral axillary lymph nodes

N_{2a} Fixed (either to one another or to other structures)

N_{2b} Metastasis only in clinically apparent ipsilateral internal mammary nodes and in the absence of clinically evident axillary lymphnode metastasis.

N_{3a} Ipsilateral infraclavicular lymph node and axillary lymph nodes.

N_{3b} Ipsilateral internal mammary lymph nodes and axillary lymph nodes.

N_{3c} Ipsilateral supraclavicular lymph nodes.

Metastasis

M_x Distant metastasis cannot be assessed.

M_0 No distant metastasis.

M_1 Distant Metastasis.

a- Clinically apparent means either by imaging or clinical examination.

Table 21.5 Stage grouping

STAGE GROUPING			
Stage 0	Tis	N0	M0
Stage 1	T1	N0	M0
Stage IIA	T0	N1	M0
	T1	N1	M0
	T2	N0	M0
Stage IIB	T2	N1	M0
	T3	N0	M0
Stage IIIA	T0,T1,T2	N2	M0
	T3	N1, N2	M0
Stage IIIB	T4	N0-2	M0
Stage IIIC	Any T	N3	M0
Stage IV	Any T	Any N	M1

MANCHESTER STAGING[1]

Stage 1 Tumour *confined to breast tissue,* not fixed to pectoralis major, not fixed to chest wall, no nodes in the axilla, no metastasis.

Stage 2 Tumour of any size with **peau d'orange** or infiltration of skin *less than the size of the tumour,* tumour not fixed to pectoralis major/ chest wall. Axillary nodes are palpable/mobile (NI), no metastasis.

Stage 3 Involvement of skin or **peau d'orange** more than the size of tumour. Tumour fixed to pectoralis major, axillary nodes are fixed (N2) or supraclavicular nodes are palpable, no metastasis.

Stage 4 Chest wall fixation, involvement of opposite breast and axilla, distant metastasis in the bones, lungs, etc.

INVESTIGATIONS

1. **Complete blood picture**: Hb% may be decreased.

2. ↑ ALP levels in the blood suggests bone metastasis

3. **Chest X-ray** to rule out pulmonary secondaries, or effusion, mediastinal widening

4. **Ultrasound** of the breast to detect solid cystic lesion. It is indicated in patients under 40 years of age.

---

1. Manchester staging is obsolete now. However few examiners may still ask this questions in clinics, hence mentioned here.

5. **Abdominal ultrasonography** is done to rule out secondaries in the liver, ascites, recto-uterine deposits.

6. **FNAC** (Fine Needle Aspiration Cytology) is quick, safe, easy method in which a cytological diagnosis can be made. The accuracy is more than 95% with an experienced cytologist.

   • If FNAC is negative, a trucut biopsy or **vacuum-assisted biopsy** (VAB) using 11 guage biopsy probe can be taken. The advantage of these biopsies is preoperative assessment of hormone receptors can be done.

   • Otherwise the patient is prepared for mastectomy and *frozen* section is arranged. Under anaesthesia, a small incision is made over the lump and a biopsy is taken, which is sent for frozen section. If frozen section report is malignant, an appropriate mastectomy is done. If the frozen section is negative, a lumpectomy is done and if report comes later as malignant, a mastectomy is done.

7. **Mammography** (Fig. 21.21)

   • This has become popular in the recent days

   • Diagnostic accuracy is about 90-95%

   • It should always be combined with a clinical examination

   • Mammography is done when there is a doubt about the diagnosis.

45% of breast cancers can be seen on mammography before they are palpable

Procedure

• A selenium coated X-ray plate is used directly in contact with the breast and the breast is exposed to low voltage and high amperage X-ray.

• 2 views: a. Medio-lateral b. Cranio-caudal

Indication

• Coarsely, nodular breast

• Fibroadenosis

• Woman, aged 40 years with family history of breast cancer

Advantages of mammography

• Non-invasive

• Minimum hazards of radiation

Disadvantages of mammography

• False positive cases are around 5%. Hence,

mammographic positive cases should undergo FNAC to confirm the diagnosis.

• If a lesion is detected by mammography, but if it is impalpable, the following special techniques will help.

Technique of mammography

1. **Double dye technique** of injecting contrast medium and patent blue.

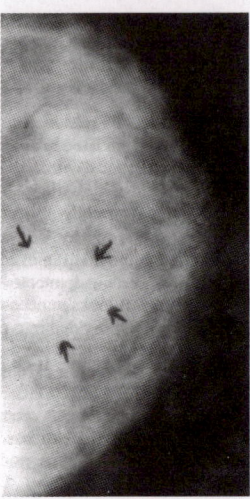

Key Box 21.9

MAMMOGRAPHIC SIGNS OF MALIGNANCY

• Mass with irregular edges- **Spiculation**

• Long tentacles - **Tentaculation**

• Fine scatter calcification - **Microcalcification**

• Distortion of architectural pattern of the breast.

Fig. 21.21 Mammography of the left breast with a cystic lesion

2. **A hooked wire** is pushed down the needle left in the breast tissue which act as a guide to the surgeon.

Thus '**TRIPLE ASSESSMENT**' is the most important method for the diagnosis of carcinoma. It includes:

   • History and clinical examination

   • Imaging : Below 40 years – Ultrasound

   Above 40 years – Mammogram

   • Fine needle aspiration cytology

7. **Bone scan** and radiological evaluation of the liver is considered if patient is symptomatic or is found to have an **elevated alkaline phosphatase**.

8. **Bone marrow aspiration** in cases of unexplained cytopenia or leukoerythroblastic blood smear.

TREATMENT OF CARCINOMA BREAST

• Halsted did the first radical mastectomy for carcinoma breast in 1878. This was the gold standard operation for carcinoma breast for nearly 100 years. However, today carcinoma breast is no longer considered as a local disease but as a systemic disease. Also, the other modalities of treatment like radiotherapy, chemotherapy, hormonal therapy are playing a major role together with surgery. Hence, the current approach is to do minimal local surgery and aggressive approach towards management of lymph nodes or metastasis. Treatment can be classified into early disease (Stage I & II) and advanced disease (Stage III & IV).

TREATMENT OF EARLY DISEASE

Aim of the treatment

- To achieve a cure
- If possible, conserve the breast
- To achieve locoregional control

I. SURGERY (Table 21.6)

1. **Wide local excision (lumpectomy)** is indicated in tumours less than 4 cm in size and with well-differentiated histology. It includes removal of the tumour plus a rim of at least 1 cm of normal breast tissue. If the nodes are palpable and enlarged, this is combined with axillary block dissection, using separate incision. Currently, this procedure has become more popular. It is also called as **Breast Conservative Therapy** (BCT).

Contraindications (Key Box 21.10)

Key Box 21.10
CONTRAINDICATIONS FOR LUMPECTOMY
• Multifocal disease
• Pregnancy
• Central quadrant tumour
• Prior radiotherapy to the breast
• Prior chest irradiation

Radiotherapy to the breast tissue is mandatory in all cases of breast conservation surgery.

2. **Simple mastectomy with axillary clearance** is equally good (good retraction of pectoralis minor facilitates axillary dissection – **Aadimelon** modification).

3. **Patey mastectomy**: This is the most acceptable and most widely practiced surgery. It is also called as modified **radical mastectomy**. In this, the entire breast including nipple and areola (simple mastectomy) are removed with, pectoralis minor, followed by axillary block dissection. A complete axillary block dissection should include node clearance upto Level III (Fig. 21.12).

   - **Level I** : Extends from axillary tail to the lateral border of pectoralis minor.
   - **Level II** : Extends from lateral border of pectoralis minor to medial border of pectoralis minor.
   - **Level III** : Up to the apex of axilla.

4. **Quart therapy by Veronasi**: It includes **Q**uadrantectomy (the entire segment of the breast containing tumour is removed), **A**xillary block dissection and **R**adiotherapy to the breast or axilla.

   - However, quadrantectomy, by removing large amount of breast tissue, gives rise to poorer cosmetic results. It seems unnecessary to remove entire segment of the breast, when in reality breast cannot be strictly divided into quadrants (unlike hepatectomy). Hence, it is not very popular.

Table 21.6 Different types of surgery for carcinoma breast

TYPES OF SURGERY	WHAT IT MEANS	COMMENTS
1. Local wide excision	• Tumour along with 2cm. of normal tissue is removed with an ellipse of the skin over lump	• Most popular breast conservative surgery done in T_1 and T_2 cases
2. Quadrantectomy	• Quadrant containing the tumour is removed	• **Not done**
3. Total mastectomy and axillary clearance	• Entire breast tissue is removed. Both pectoralis minor and major are preserved	• Frequently done – good retraction of pectoralis major and minor are necessary for the axillary clearance
4. Patey mastectomy	• Breast tissue + Pectoralis minor is removed and axillary block dissection	• Mostly done and removal of pectoralis minor helps the axillary dissection
5. Halstead radical mastectomy	• Entire breast tissue and both the pectoral muscles are removed	• **Not necessary** as carcinoma breast is considered as systemic disease today

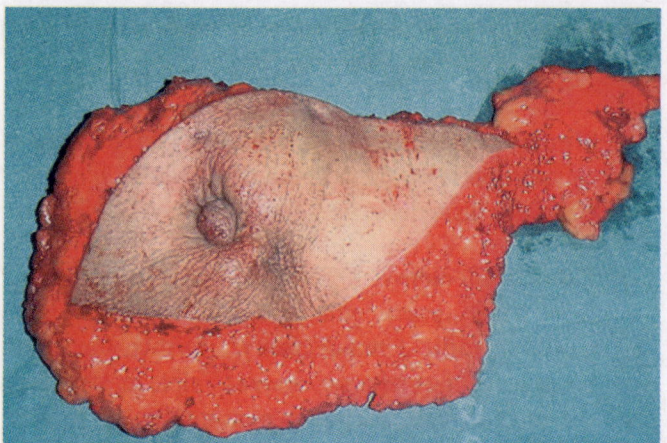

Fig. 21.22 Patey mastectomy specimen

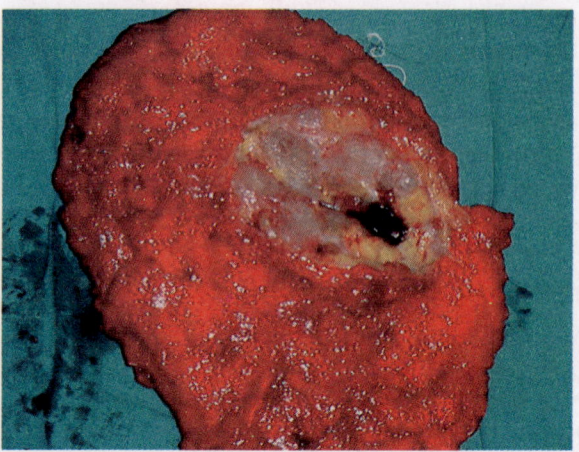

Fig. 21.23 Showing the tumour with degeneration

Advantages of Patey mastectomy over Halstead radical mastectomy

- Cosmetically better accepted as axillary fold is maintained.
- Function of the shoulder is better, and it gives a stronger and more useful arm.
- By preserving pectoralis major, it provides a good vascular bed for skin grafting once the excess skin has been removed.

5. **Radical mastectomy**: In this operation, following structures are removed.

- Entire breast including nipple and areola with skin overlying the tumour along with fat, fascia and lymphatics.
- Axillary block dissection, including complete clearance of axillary fat and up to Level III nodes clearance.
- Sternocostal portion of pectoralis major, entire pectoralis minor, few fibres and aponeurosis of internal oblique, serratus anterior, latissimus dorsi and subscapularis.

Three important structures should be preserved

1. **A**xillary vein
2. **B**ell's nerve (long thoracic nerve which supplies serratus anterior)
3. **C**ephalic vein

Disadvantages of radical mastectomy

1. Mutilating surgery
2. Poor cosmetic results
3. Lymphoedema of arm

Please note: In our country, Patey mastectomy and total mastectomy are more frequently done. However, more and more an early carcinoma is being treated by breast-conserving surgery nowadays.

II. POSTOPERATIVE RADIOTHERAPY

- Breast is irradiated to a dose of 5,000-6,000 cGy units, 200 cGy per day along with axilla when only sampling has been done, 5 days per week for 5 to 6 weeks.
- However, if a level III axillary clearance has been done, it is not necessary to irradiate the axilla because of high chances of lymphoedema. Also, if more than 10 nodes are removed, it is not necessary to irradiate the axilla. Internal mammary and supraclavicular nodes also can be included in the radiating field. (Key Box 21.11)

Key Box 21.11
INDICATIONS FOR POST OPERATIVE RADIOTHERAPY
• Tumour margin is positive • Pectoralis major is involved • Inner quadrant tumour • High grade tumours • Axillary clearance not satisfactory • Breast conservative surgery • Tumour size more than 5 cms

III. ROLE OF HORMONAL THERAPY

- Before starting hormonal therapy steroid hormone receptors have to be checked and measured. Depending

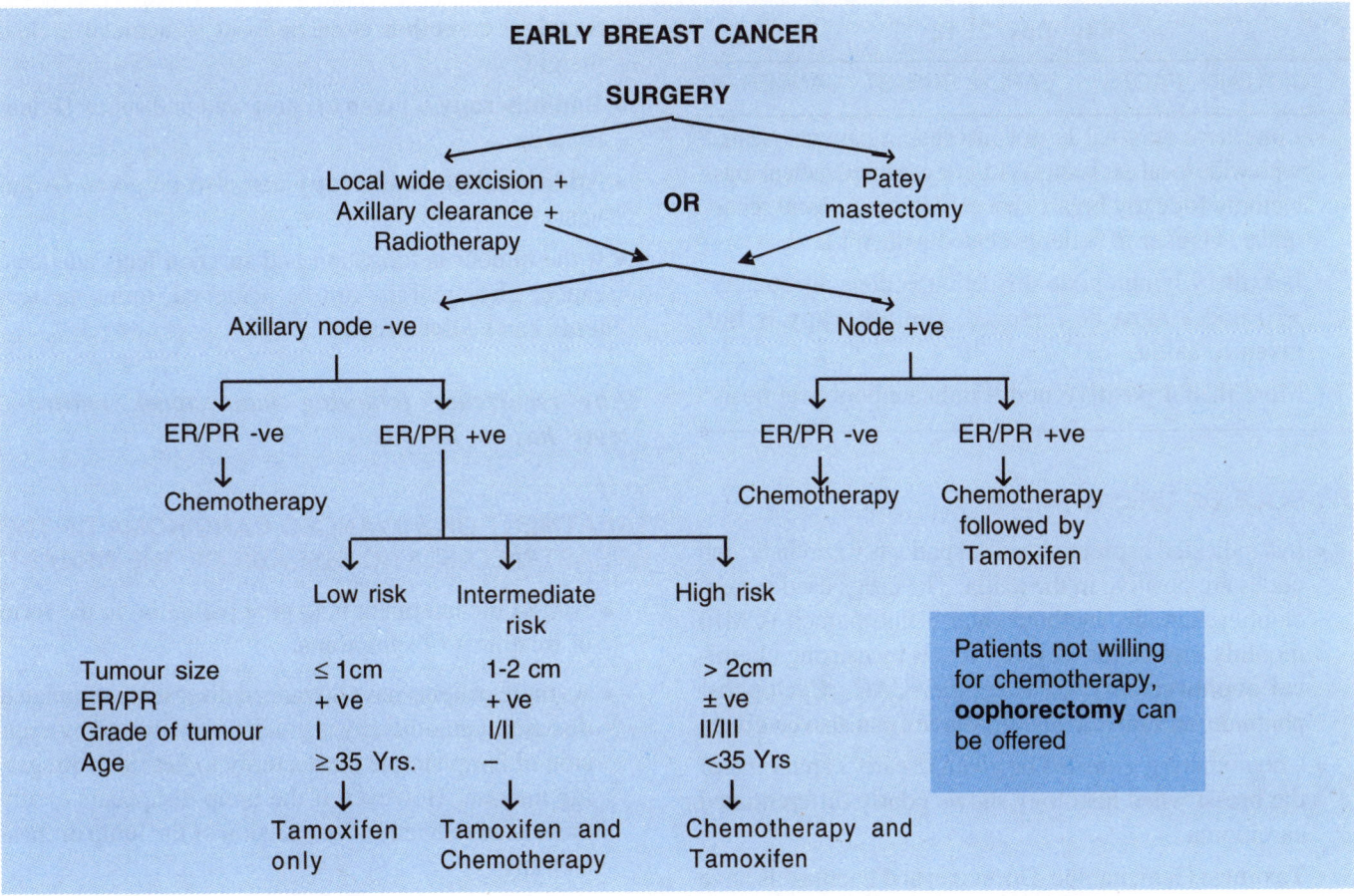

Fig 21.24 Summary of the treatment of early carcinoma of breast

upon the levels, whether positive or negative the hormonal therapy is given. (details below)

STEROID HORMONE RECEPTORS

- Intracellular steroid hormone receptor proteins, primarily ER (Estrogen Receptors) and PR (Progesterone Receptors) have shown to be indicators of prognosis and a guide to hormone and endocrine therapy. About 50% to 85% of invasive breast cancers contain measurable amounts of ER. The **concentration of ER increases with age** with both having their highest levels in postmenopausal patients.

- Normal value of ER is < 10 fmol/mg proteins. It is **considered positive** > 10 fmol/mg proteins. Upper levels as high as 1000 fmol/mg proteins may be there.

- Enzyme immunoassays and immunohistochemical methods are employed to measure levels of ER.

- The presence of ER implies that normal cellular mechanism for processing estrogen has been maintained despite the malignant change. **Patients with ER positive tumours have longer disease-free survival** after primary treatment, superior overall survival and longer survival after recurrence compared with patients with ER-negative tumours.

- The clinical importance of ER relates principally to the fact that its presence identifies hormone sensitive tumours. About 50-60% of patients with significant increase in ER in their tumour respond favourably to endocrine therapy. A higher percentage respond if ER levels are high and if both ER and PR are positive.

Postmenopausal women with positive axillary nodes should receive Tamoxifen 20 mg/day for a period of 5 years as it is known to delay the recurrence

- All other patients may benefit from tamoxifen except premenopausal ER/PR negative patients.

- Tamoxifen is started only after chemotherapy is completed.

- It should be given for 5 years.

Key Box 21.12

CERTAIN FACTS - EARLY BREAST CANCER

- Long term survival is **not altered** in patients treated with wide local excision (WLE) or modified radical mastectomy for early breast cancer. However, local recurrence is higher in patients treated with WLE.
- If axillary lymph node dissection is done adequately, >10 nodes must be removed, **radiotherapy is not given** to axilla.
- More than **4 positive nodes** indicate poor prognosis.

IV. ROLE OF CHEMOTHERAPY

- It is indicated in premenopausal patients wherein lymph nodes are positive in the axilla. The drugs used are cyclophosphamide, methotrexate, 5-fluorouracil (CMF) monthly regime for 6 cycles. It acts by causing **chemical oophorectomy.** CAF regime (CAF : Cyclophosphamide, adriamycin and flurouracil can also be given.
- Chemotherapy can also be given in early carcinoma of the breast when histology shows poorly differentiated carcinoma.
- **Taxanes:** Gemcitabine, Docetaxel and Paclitaxels have been popular and accepted as post anthracycline (Adriamycin and Epirubicin) second line drugs. They are well tolerated with less toxicity. They are much more active than other drugs such as Cisplatin and Cyclophosphamide.

LOCALLY ADVANCED BREAST CANCER (LABC)

Many patients come to the hospital with gross skin involvement, pectoral muscles involvement or chest wall involvement. Eventhough the cure rates are low, with proper planning, a good control of the disease, good palliation in major group of patients and 'cure' in a small group can be achieved.

Aim

- Good locoregional control
- Attempt at 'cure' by chemotherapy

Treatment

- Biopsy is done to confirm the diagnosis followed by **identification of receptor** status.
- Neoadjuvant chemotherapy is given first which will **shrink the tumour.**

- **Surgical resection** is carried out to achieve a clear margin.
- **Radiotherapy** is given to chest wall and supraclavicular area.
- **Additional chemotherapy** can also be given (Adjuvant).
- If the tumour is fungating and surgeon feels adequate cancer clear margin can be achieved, toilet mastectomy can be done first.

Any recurrence following lumpectomy, mastectomy has to be done.

TREATMENT OF ADVANCED CARCINOMA OF THE BREAST/METASTATIC DISEASE OF THE BREAST

- Aim of the treatment is to give palliation in the form of treatment of symptoms.
- As these patients have advanced disease/disseminated disease, chemotherapy is given first followed by excision of lump/simple mastectomy to get rid of fungating tumour. However, if the lump disappears totally there is no indication for excision of the lump or mastectomy.
- Following chemotherapy tamoxifen is given for a period of five years. Repeated courses of second and third line chemotherapeutic drugs may have to be given.

Key Box 21.13

TREATMENT OF METASTATIC DISEASE

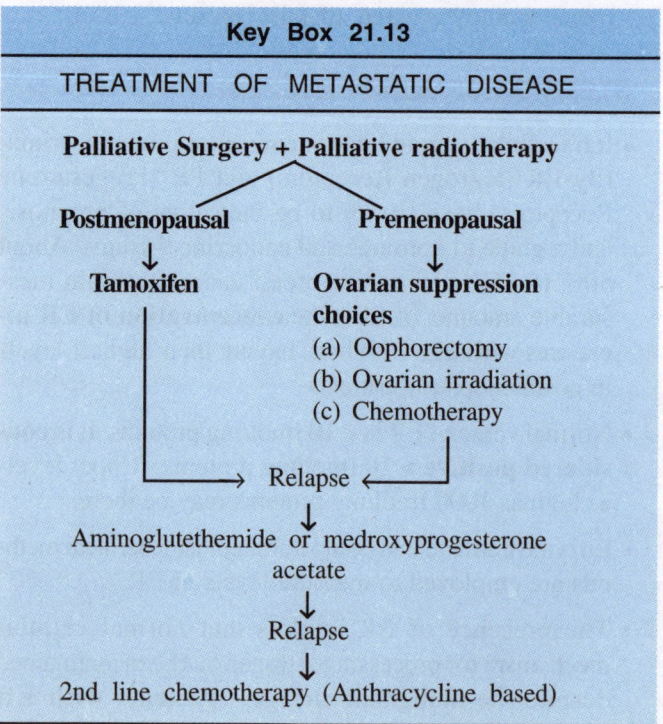

- The treatment of individual organ involvement or system involvement is given below (Key Box 21.13).

Malignant pleural effusion

- Once effusion is confirmed by aspiration and cytology, an intercostal drain is left in place for a few days. Once the drainage is nil or completely dry, talc insufflation is done, to achieve pleurodesis. Talc is the most effective agent, followed by tetracycline or bleomycin, etc. In selected cases, effective pleurodesis has given an asymptomatic period up to 1-2 years.

Bone metastasis

- Eventually 60-70% of patients with carcinoma breast develop bone metastasis. Bone metastasis produces intractable pain, pathological fractures, quadriplegia and paraplegia etc (Key Box 21.14).
- Localised bone lesions are treated by palliative radiotherapy or decompression as in quadriplegia, etc.
- Biphosphonates eg. oral clodronates have been found to arrest progression of bone disease, given at the dose of 1,600 mg/day.

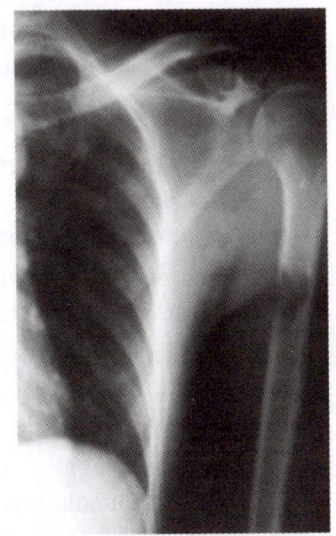

Fig. 21.25 Pathological fracture humerous - treated by internal fixation followed by radiotherapy

Key Box 21.14
BONE METASTASIS
• **P**ain
• **P**athological fractures
• **P**aralysis
• **P**erish – due to hypercalcaemic crisis

Cerebral metastasis

- Patients present with features of raised intracranial pressure such as headache, nausea, vomiting, etc., with papilloedema.
- Treatment includes corticosteroids, cranial radiotherapy, etc. However, treatment is distressing.

Causes of death

- Malignant pleural effusion
- Bony metastasis
- Cerebral metastasis
- Cancer cachexia.

EFFECT OF LYMPHATIC OBSTRUCTION FROM CARCINOMA OF BREAST

1. Peau d'orange.
2. Oedema of the arm is also called *elephantiasis chirurgens*.
   - It is a complication of radical mastectomy when all the nodes in the axilla are removed and especially when postoperative radiotherapy is given in the axilla.
   - It occurs due to destruction of all lymphatics and lymph nodes.
   - It does not pit on pressure. Some amount of infection also plays a role.

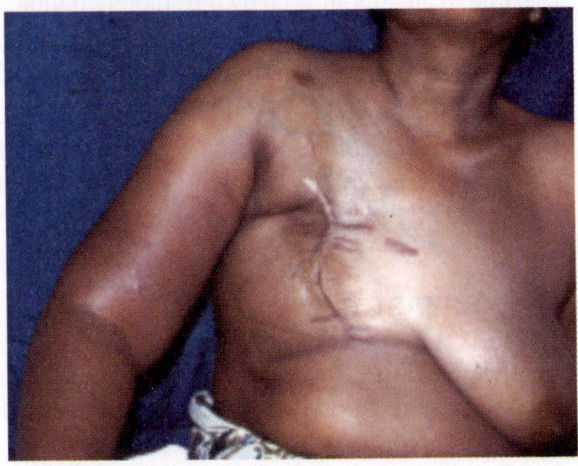

Fig. 21.26 Lymphoedema right upper limb

Treatment

- Difficult. Elastic bandage, exercise, massage, antibiotics may help.

3. **Brawny oedema of the arm**
   - These occur in inoperable carcinoma of breast with fixed nodes in the axilla.
   - Arm is oedematous and does not pit on pressure.
   - It is brawny, indurated, painful.
   - It is treated like above.

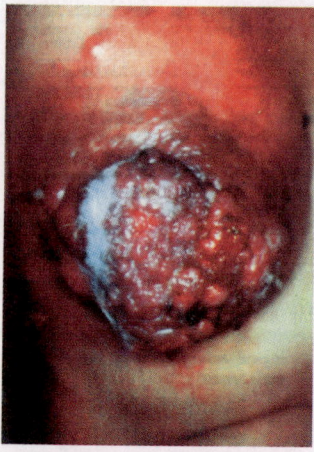

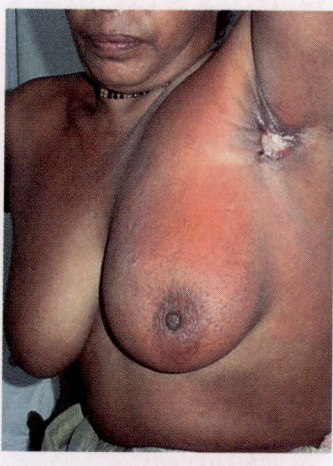

Fig. 21.27 Cancer - en - cuirasse - chest wall studded with cancerous nodules - very painful bleeding lesion

Fig. 21.28 Extensive lymphoedema and lymphangitis due to carcinoma axillary tail of the breast

4. **Cancer-en-cuirasse** (Fig. 21.27)
   - In this, the entire chest wall is studded with cancerous nodules which are hard and fixed to the skin and to the chest wall. The condition has been compared to an armour used by the soldier. It indicates advanced carcinoma of breast. Palliative treatment is given in the form of radiotherapy or chemotherapy and analgesics to relieve the pain.

5. **Lymphangiosarcoma**: It is a rare complication after mastectomy and arises from lymphoedematous limb. It is treated by fore-quarter amputation.

BREAST RECONSTRUCTION

- The ideal candidate for breast reconstruction is a patient who has undergone modified radical mastectomy.

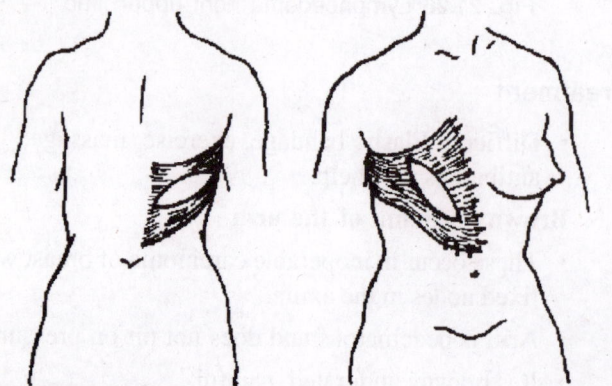

Fig. 21.29 Breast reconstruction with latissimus dorsi myocutaneous flap

Components of breast reconstruction

- **Chest wall reconstruction** : This can be achieved by using latissimus dorsi musculocutaneous flap (Fig. 21.19) or contralateral transversus abdominis muscle (TRAM) flap.
- **Creation of a mould**: A silicone gel implant is inserted under pectoralis major muscle (subpectoral pocket).
- **Reconstruction of nipple and areola**: This can be achieved by skin taken from inner thigh, labia minora or from opposite breast (nipple sharing). However, this reconstruction is done 4-6 weeks later, once the implant settles down.
- **Symmetry with the opposite breast**: It is achieved by doing reduction mammoplasty of the other breast.

MALE BREAST CARCINOMA

- It is very uncommon carcinoma in males
- **Gynaecomastia** and excess oestrogens are responsible for development of carcinoma (Fig. 21.30)
- Since the subcutaneous fat is less in men, breast carcinoma tends to be advanced at the time of presentation due to **early fixity** to the chest wall.
- Investigations and management is more or less similar to female carcinoma breast.
- However, bilateral orchidectomy can be done to control the disease.

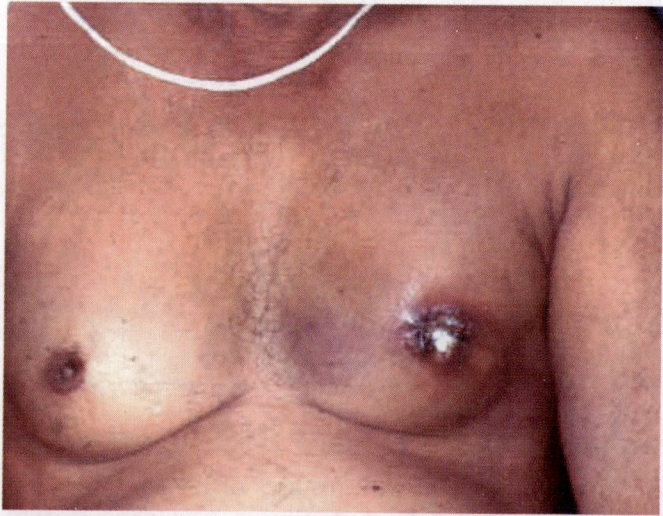

Fig. 21.30 Male breast carcinoma in pre-existing gynecomastia. You can see destruction of the nipple and infiltration into the skin - commonly it is infiltrating ductal carcinoma

Miscellaneous

TRAUMATIC FAT NECROSIS

- As the name itself suggests, it occurs after a trivial trauma. However, fat necrosis can also occur without trauma. As a result of injury to the fat, release of glycerol and fatty acids take place resulting in saponification. Histologically it is characterised by lipid laden macrophages and inflammatory cells.
- Elderly women and women with pendulous breasts are affected. Pain and lump in the breast are the presenting features. The lump is hard, due to extensive fibrosis caused by the tissue reaction. Hence, it is an important differential diagnosis for carcinoma breast.
- Mammography finding of calcification may mimick carcinoma breast.
- Treatment is by excision of the lump

SCLEROSING ADENOSIS

- It is a benign condition now grouped under ANDI
- Histologically, it is composed of proliferation of ductules and acini with stromal tissue.
- It is also confused for carcinoma of the breast.
- FNAC to confirm the diagnosis
- Treatment is by excision of the lump

SUBCUTANEOUS MASTECTOMY

Indications (Pennisi, 1986)

1. Biopsy proved
   - Noninvasive intraductal carcinoma in situ
   - A single focus of lobular carcinoma in situ
   - Florid cystic disease
2. A mammogram that is suspicious of moderate to severe mammary dysplasia
3. Persistent breast nodules that do not vary with menstrual cycles and are of concern to the patient and the physician
4. Familial or heriditary breast carcinoma

Procedure

- Submammary incision is given.
- Breast tissue is dissected from the pectoral muscles.

- Skin flap along with even thickness of subcutaneous fat which is retained under the skin, is raised. (Helps in retaining vascularity of the flap). Haemostasis is obtained. Immediate reconstruction or reconstruction at a later date can be done.

MONDOR'S DISEASE

- Mondor's disease is spontaneous thrombophlebitis of the superficial veins of the breast and anterior chest wall. The common causes of thrombophlebitis such as injury or infection are not found in these cases.

Signs

1. Indurated subcutaneous thrombophlebitic cord about 3 mm diameter of varying length, situated in the subcutaneous plane with an attachment to the skin. Consistency is like that of vas deferens.
2. When the skin over the breast is stretched by raising the arm, a narrow, shallow subcutaneous groove along the side of the cord becomes apparent.

Treatment

- Restricted arm movements (otherwise it is very painful). Spontaneous recovery is expected within few days.

ANGIOSARCOMA OF THE BREAST

- They are uncommon malignant tumours of the breast
- Aetiology is not clear
- Breast is one of the sites of angiosarcoma
- Clinically it presents as rapidly growing lump in the breast with infiltration of the skin producing ulceration.
- On careful observation, the edges are not everted and the lesion is very vascular.

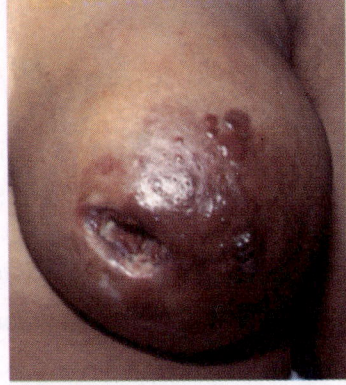

Fig. 21.31 Angiosarcoma left breast

- Confirmation of the diagnosis is by FNAC or by biopsy from the lump.
- Treated by course of chemotherapy followed later by mastectomy.

Oesophagus and Diaphragm

22

- Surgical anatomy
- Physiology
- Reflux oesophagitis
- GORD
- Hiatus hernia
- Plummer-Vinson syndrome
- Achalasia cardia
- Carcinoma
- Stricture
- Perforation
- Diverticulum
- Dysphagia
- Surgical anatomy of the diaphragm
- Diaphragmatic hernia
- Tracheo-oesophageal fistula

SURGICAL ANATOMY

- It is 25 cm in length, extending from the cricopharyngeal sphincter to the cardio-oesophageal junction.

- It runs in the posterior mediastinum as a continuation of pharynx. 2 cm of this tube lies below the diaphragm.

- **Physiological constrictions:** Table 22.1

Muscle layers

- It has inner circular layer and outer longitudinal layer.
- Upper 1/3rd-striated muscle fibres
- Lower 2/3rd-smooth muscle fibres

Mucosa

- The entire oesophagus is lined by squamous epithelium except the last 3 cm which is lined by columnar cells. The columnar cells are similar to gastric mucosa but oxyntic and peptic cells are absent. **Mucosa is the toughest coat of oesophagus.**

Lymphatic drainage

- Upper oesophagus drains into the left and right supra-clavicular nodes.
- Middle oesophagus drains into the tracheobronchial nodes and paraoesophageal nodes.
- Lower oesophagus drains into lymph nodes along the lesser curvature of stomach and then into coeliac nodes.

Nerve supply

- The parasympathetic nerve supply is by vagus nerve through extrinsic and intrinsic plexus. Intrinsic plexus has **no Meissner's network,** and Auerbach's plexus is present only in the lower two-thirds.

Table 22.1 Physiological constrictions

CONSTRICTIONS	DISTANCE FROM INCISOR TEETH	PROBLEMS
1. Cricopharyngeal	15 cm	Foreign body lodgement
2. Aortic and bronchial	25 cm	Perforations during endoscopy
3. Diaphragmatic sphincter	40 cm	Malignancy

PHYSIOLOGY

The main function of the oesophagus is to transfer food from the mouth to the stomach. Voluntary contraction of the oropharynx pushes the food into the upper oesophagus through the relaxed cricopharyngeal sphincter. Then due to primary and secondary peristalsis, the food bolus is transferred to the stomach.

- **Cricopharyngeal sphincter** is closed at rest. It helps in preventing regurgitation of oesophageal contents into the respiratory passage.
- **Lower Oesophageal Sphincter (LOS):** It is a physiological sphincter at the gastrooesophageal junction. It is 3-4 cms long with a resting pressure of 20-25 mm of Hg. Hence it is known as **High Pressure Zone (HPZ)**.
- This HPZ prevents reflux of gastric contents into oesophagus. Cigarette smoking affects this zone, hence smokers have high incidence of reflux oesophagitis.

GASTRO-OESOPHAGEAL REFLUX DISEASE (GORD)

- Loss of competence of LOS leads to gastro-oesophageal reflux disease (GORD). The competence of LOS can be affected by obesity, smoking, excessive eating etc. Sliding hernia is associated with GORD and reflux oesophagitis is a complication of GORD. Hence, reflux oesophagitis and hiatus hernia are included under GORD.

REFLUX OESOPHAGITIS

- Extensive inflammation of the lower oesophagus due to reflux of gastric acid from the stomach to lower end of oesophagus, is described as reflux oesophagitis.

Types

1. Acute: Following alcohol, burns, stress.
2. Chronic: It is associated with hiatus hernia or following oesophagojejunostomy.

Aetiopathogenesis

- Acid refluxes into the lower oesophagus and produces diffuse inflammation with multiple ulcers.

- The symptoms are worse when the patient lies down.
- Due to vagal hyperactivity, the inflammation and ulcers produce severe longitudinal muscle spasm. Consequently, the cardia is drawn up into the thorax, leading to an increase in the oesophago-cardiac angle. This increases the reflux. Later, fibrosis causes shortening of the oesophagus.
- Thus, it becomes a vicious circle of *Oesophagitis - Longitudinal muscle spasm -Displacement of oesophagus -Increased regurgitation.*

Clinical features

1. **Retrosternal pain:** It is burning in nature and becomes worse in the lying down position. Pain is better in the sitting position. The pain is described as *heart burn and can be confused for angina pectoris.* The pain is relieved on taking antacids.
2. **Occult blood in stools** and streak of blood in the vomitus are common.
3. **Anaemia** and weakness are uncommon features.
4. **Dysphagia:** Transient difficulty in swallowing results from spasm due to inflammation of the lower end of oesophagus. Late dysphagia is due to stenosis or stricture of the oesophagus.

Investigations

- Barium swallow[1] in the Trendelenburg's position (head down position) can demonstrate the reverse flow of barium into the lower end of the oesophagus (from the stomach).
- Oesophagoscopy may reveal red, angry looking mucosa in the lower end of the oesophagus.

Treatment

1. Avoid spicy food, smoking and alcohol
2. Small, frequent meals
3. Antacids
4. H_2 receptor antagonists, Proton pump inhibitors
5. Hiatus hernia, if present, should be treated

Complications

1. **Barrett's oesophagus:** In this condition, columnar epithelium is present for more than 3 cm above the

---

1. *Barium swallow: thick paste to see the oesophagus. Barium meal: a thin paste to see the stomach. Both are radio-opaque.*

cardio-oesophageal junction. It occurs in late stages of reflux oesophagitis and it is due to metaplasia.

2. **Stricture** of the lower end of the oesophagus

3. **Barrett's oesophagus** can turn into adenocarcinoma of the oesophagus.

HIATUS HERNIA

Definition: Abnormal protrusion of abdominal viscus through the oesophageal hiatus into the chest.

Types (Key Box 22.1)

1. Sliding hernia or oesophagogastric hernia: It is the commonest type of hiatus hernia, accounting for about 80% of cases (Fig. 22.2). It may be associated with GORD.

2. Rolling or para-oesophageal hernia

3. Mixed hernia

4. Massive herniation

Key Box 22.1
TYPES
I - H^0 - Normal
II - H^1 - Sliding
III - H^2 - Para oesophageal
IV - H^3 - Mixed
V - H^4 - Massive herniation

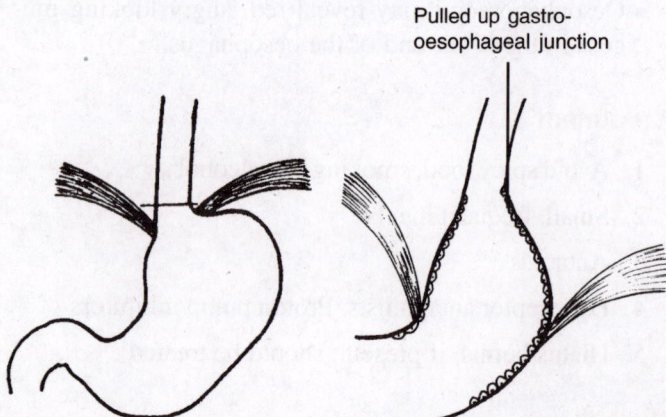

Pulled up gastro-oesophageal junction

Fig. 22.1 Normal position   **Fig. 22.2a** Sliding Hernia

Common symptoms

1. **Symptoms due to reflux:** Regurgitation and heart burn are the two most common symptoms.

2. **Symptoms due to complications:** They are dysphagia, odynophagia, haematemesis and melaena.

3. **Non-oesophageal symptoms:** They are asthma and chest pain.

SLIDING HERNIA

Anatomical factors which prevent sliding hernia:

1. Presence of 2 cm of intra-abdominal oesophagus

2. **The Angle of His,** the oesophago-cardiac angle of about 45° has valvular effect.

3. Mucosal folds at the oesophago-cardiac junction

4. Positive intra-abdominal pressure which closes the abdominal oesophagus.

5. **Lower oesophageal sphincter (LOS):** It is a functional sphincter which increases the pressure during coughing, straining, etc.

Causes of sliding hernia[1]

1. Deposition of **fatty tissue** in the hiatus leads to weakening of the hiatus in obese individuals.

2. Advancing **age** resulting in muscular degeneration can predispose hernia.

3. Raised intra-abdominal pressure due to lower **abdominal tumours**, pregnancy, etc.

4. **Saint's Triad:** Gall stones, diverticulosis and hiatus hernia can occur together in a patient.

Clinical features

- Sliding hernia produces symptoms like reflux oesophagitis - (GORD)
- More common in women, especially if obese

Investigations

- Oesophagoscopy reveals varying degree of inflammation. During oesophagoscopy, when the patient is asked to strain, (Valsalva's manoeuvre) the sphincter is more patulous and herniation of gastric mucosal folds can be seen. **Reflux of the gastric acid is the most valuable sign.** Barium meal demonstrates gastroesophageal reflux in the Trendelenburg position.

---

1. *Causes can be remembered as FATTY. **F** -Fat, **A** -Age, **T** -Tumour, **T** -Triad (Saint's triad), **Y** -Yielding hiatus.*

Treatment

I. Conservative treatment: In all cases of GORD, conservative treatment has to be tried first. The results of surgery are appreciated only when conservative treatment fails and when there are significant symptoms.

Principles

Oh LORD save me from GORD

1. **L**ife style changes
   - Decrease in weight
   - Diet control with increased intake of proteins and decreased consumption of fat and sugar.
   - Decreased alcohol and tobacco consumption.
2. **O**esophageal mucosa protection
   - Antacids - Preparations containing alginates, cytoprotective agents.
   - H_2 blockers : Ranitidine or
   - Proton pump inhibitors: Omeprazole, Esmoprazole.
3. **R**eflux prevention
   - Oesophageal reflux : Cisapride, Metoclopramide
   - Gastric reflux : Domperidone, Metoclopramide, cisapride etc.
4. **D**ecision of surgery

   II. Surgery: Indications
   1. Intractable pain.
   2. Complications such as haemorrhage or stricture
   - The results of antireflux surgery are good with a small mortality rate. (0.1 to 0.5 percent). However careful selection of patient depending upon the symptoms and life style are important factors.

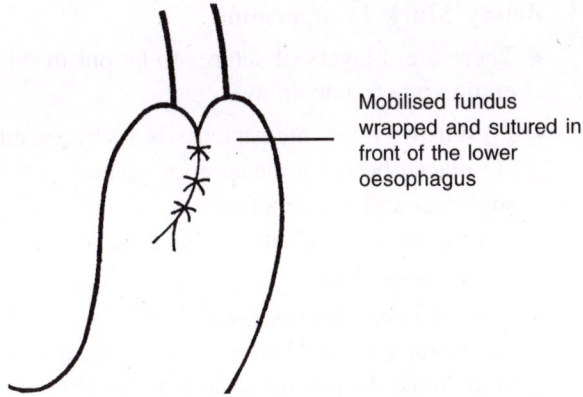

Mobilised fundus wrapped and sutured in front of the lower oesophagus

Fig. 22.3 Nissen's fundoplication

Types of surgery

1. **Nissen's total fundoplication** (Fig. 22.3): Aim is to restore 2 cm of intraabdominal oesophagus by reducing the hernia, followed by repair of the hiatus.
   - In this operation. fundus of the stomach is mobilised by dividing short gastric arteries.
   - Fundus is brought behind the oesophagus and wrapped in front of oesophagus.
   - Diaphragmatic defect is repaired by using nonabsorbable sutures like nylon or silk. This is the operation which serves all aims.

   Complications
   - Too tight plication may result in dysphagia or gas bloat syndrome wherein belching is prevented.
2. **Partial fundoplication (Toupet)** solves the above problem wherein fundus is sutured to side of oesophagus. (Refer Fig 22.4)

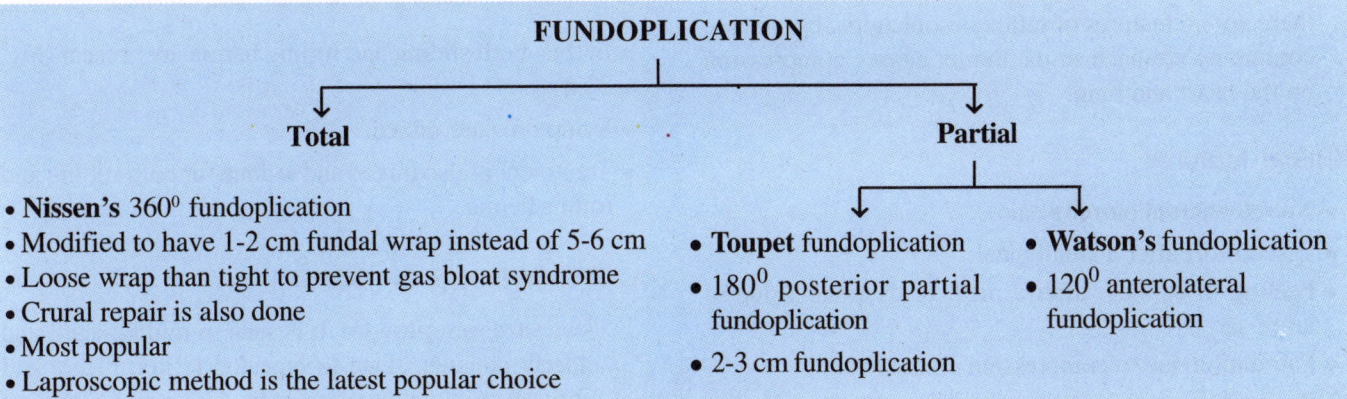

FUNDOPLICATION

Total
- **Nissen's** 360^0 fundoplication
- Modified to have 1-2 cm fundal wrap instead of 5-6 cm
- Loose wrap than tight to prevent gas bloat syndrome
- Crural repair is also done
- Most popular
- Laproscopic method is the latest popular choice

Partial

- **Toupet** fundoplication
- 180^0 posterior partial fundoplication
- 2-3 cm fundoplication

- **Watson's** fundoplication
- 120^0 anterolateral fundoplication

Fig 22.4 Types of fundoplication

3. Belsey Mark IV operation

- There are 3 layers of sutures to be put in this operation, via thoracotomy.
- **First row**: Four interrupted silk mattress sutures are placed between the anterior surface of the oesophagus and adjacent fundus of the stomach so as to wrap the stomach around the anterior two-thirds of the oesophagus.
- **Second row:** Sutures placed between oesophagogastric junction and under surface of the diaphragm to maintain the junction below the diaphragm.
- **Third row:** Posterior crural sutures to tighten the opening.

Key Box 22.2

ADVANTAGES OF BELSEY MARK IV

- Reduces size of the ring
- Creates a valve at the oesophagogastric junction in order to prevent reflux
- Recurrence is low

---

4. **Hill's repair:** Median arcuate ligament repair.

- In this, the long intra-abdominal segment of the oesophagus is firmly fixed below the diaphragm by anchoring the gastro-oesophageal junction to the crura just above **median arcuate ligament.** This is described as **posterior gastropexy.**

ROLLING HERNIA

- In this condition, cardio-oesophageal junction is normal. Greater curvature of the stomach ascends into a preformed sac in the mediastinum (Fig. 22.5). Thus, there are no features of reflux oesophagitis, but the sac containing stomach in the thorax causes compression on the heart and lung.

Clinical features

- No retrosternal burning pain
- Discomfort after a small meal
- Feeling of fullness after a meal or dysphagia due to large sac
- Palpitation due to compression on the heart
- Respiratory tract infection and hiccough due to irritation of phrenic nerve.

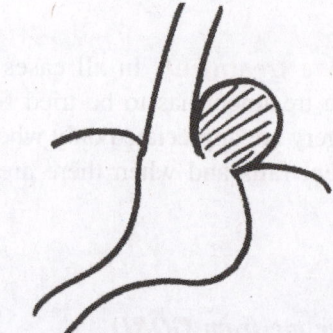

Fig. 22.5 Rolling hernia

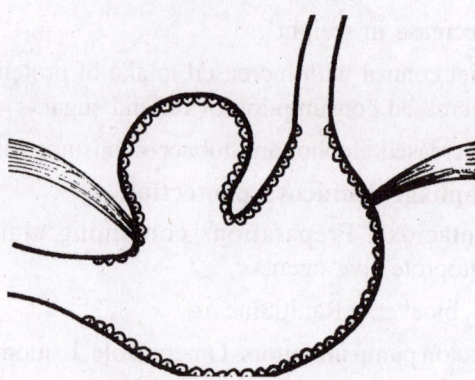

Fig. 22.6 Mixed hernia

Investigation

- Barium meal shows the sac in the thorax containing stomach. Sometimes, it can be upside down.

Treatment

- Reduction of the sac and repair of the hiatus by using non-absorbable suture material to approximate the right crus of the diaphragm.

MIXED HERNIA

- In this, both sliding and rolling hernia are present (Fig. 22.6).
- Symptoms are mixed.
- Treatment is also mixed and is done for both sliding and rolling hernia.

COMPLICATIONS OF GORD

1. **Stricture oesophagus:** It is seen in middle-aged and elderly patients. Due to repeated reflux, ulcers and fibrosis, stricture develops in the lower end of the oesophagus. Early diagnosis by endoscopy followed by

frequent dilatation and **proton pump inhibitors** will help the situation.

- Peptic strictures are difficult to manage surgically.
- Surgery is indicated in refractory cases of dilation, in the form of **gastroplasty**.

2. **Oesophageal shortening** is also treated by Colli's gastroplasty by using stomach.

3. **BARRETT'S OESOPHAGUS:** Also known as columnar lined oesophagus (**CLO**).

Definition

- When metaplastic changes occur in the lining mucosa of the oesophagus, it is described as Barrett's Oesophagus.
- Barrett's CLO is a **pre-malignant lesion and** ulcer in the Barrett's CLO is **Barrett's ulcer.**

Pathogenesis

- Repeated reflux results in shifting of the oesophagogastric junction upwards, which further increases the reflux resulting in intestinal metaplasia of **middle and lower oesophagus.**

Pathological types

1. **Gastric type** with chief and parietal cells.
2. **Intestinal type** with goblet cells is most common. This mucosa is smooth (unlike gastric folds)
3. **Junctional type:** It has mucus glands and resembles gastric cardia.

Clinical types

1. **Long segment :** Metaplastic changes involving more than 3 cms.
2. **Short segment :** Metaplastic changes involving less than 3 cms.

Incidence of malignancy

- 25 times more prone to carcinoma **lower and middle oesophagus** as compared to the general population.

Types of dysplasia

- Low grade: Negligible risk of carcinoma
- High grade: Very high risk of carcinoma

Screening programme

- It is important to screen these patients regularly with repeat endoscopies and multiple biopsies to find dysplasia. (See the box 22.3)

Key Box 22.3

CARCINOMA IN BARRETT'S OESOPHAGUS

- It will be invasive
- It is more proximal
- Carries poor prognosis
- 25 times incresed risk compared to general population

Key Box 22.4

RISK FACTORS FOR CARCINOMA

- CLO > than 8 cm
- Smoking
- Reflux due to previous gastric surgery
- High grade dysplasia

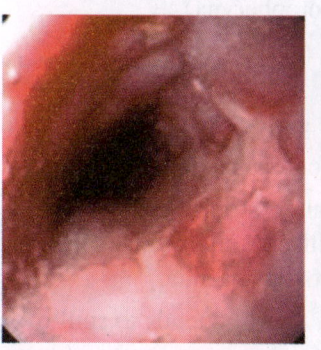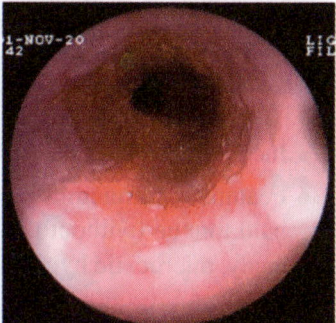

Fig. 22.7 and 22.8 Endoscopic view of reflux oesophagitis and Barrett's oesophagus

Treatment

1. Laser photodynamic therapy
2. Argon beam plasma coagulation
3. High dose proton pump inhibitors for 8 weeks
4. Oesophagectomy in cases of high grade dysplasia

Complications of Barrett's Oesophagus

1. **Oesophageal ulcers:** Barrett's ulcer - pain, bleeding, perforation.
2. **Oesophageal stricture:** Usually located in middle or upper oesophagus.
   - **Peptic stricture occur in the distal oesophagus**.
3. **Dysplasia and Adenocarcinoma.**

LOCALISED MUSCULAR SPASM OF OESOPHAGUS

PLUMMER VINSON SYNDROME

- It is a precancerous condition in which there is a severe spasm of circular muscle fibres at the cricopharyngeal sphincter level or pharyngo-oesophageal junction, and it is associated with **development of postcricoid web.**

Aetiopathogenesis

1. Aetiology is not known
2. It is seen in women who have anxiety and worries
3. As a result of the spasm and web, dysplasia results and leads to features of anemia later. The proximal mucosa is constantly irritated due to stasis. It undergoes hypertrophy, hyperkeratosis and desquamation. This, over a period of years, predisposes to carcinoma oesophagus (carcinoma oropharynx).

Clinical features

- Women in the middle age group are affected
- Increasing **dysphagia** for solids and liquids due to spasm
- Features of **anaemia** - pallor, stomatitis, ulcerations, bald tongue (without papillae), koilonychia, splenomegaly, microcytic hypochromic anaemia.
- As a result of obstruction, the fluid tends to spill over into the larynx giving rise to recurrent aspiration, respiratory tract infection, cyanosis or choking.

Key Box 22.5

PLUMMER-VINSON SYNDROME

- Women
- Dysphagia, anaemia
- Cricopharyngeal spasm
- Dilatation
- Iron supplements
- Precancerous condition

Treatment

- Reassurance
- Improving anaemia-Iron tablets or blood transfusion and correction of nutritional deficiencies.
- Regular dilatation by using gum elastic bougies

ACHALASIA CARDIA

- It is a primary oesophageal motility disorder.
- It is also called cardiospasm because of severe spasm of the circular muscle fibres of the lower end of the oesophagus. The contracted segment does not relax during the act of swallowing (achalasia = failure of relaxation). As a result of this, there is dilatation, tortuosity and hypertrophy of the oesophagus above.
- Incidence : 1 in 1,00,000.

AETIOLOGY

1. **Idiopathic**: This occurs due to absence or degeneration of Auerbach's plexus throughout the body of the oesophagus leading to improper integration of the parasympathetic impulse.
2. **Acquired variety** is seen in South American countries caused by Trypanosoma cruzi[1] (sleeping sickness)-**Chaga's disease.** This organism destroys the ganglion cells of the Auerbach's plexus.
3. Stress and emotional factors and vitamin deficiencies are also associated with this disease.

CLINICAL FEATURES

1. Women around 30-40 years of age are commonly affected. The ratio of female to male is 3:2.
2. **Dysphagia** develops slowly and it is progressive.
- Solids by forming a bolus and aided by gravity, as they touch the contracted segment, may partially open up the sphincter. Thus, there is no dysphagia for solids. Dysphagia for liquids is the important feature and it results in **regurgitation** (oesophageal pseudovomiting). The regurgitant material contains foul-smelling oesophageal contents. Malnourishment, ill health and weight loss follows soon. Dysphagia, regurgitation and weight loss form the triad of achalasia cardia.
3. **Recurrent respiratory tract infection** due to spillage of liquids can also occur.
4. **Features of anaemia**-glossitis, stomatitis, pallor, bald tongue.
5. **Retrosternal discomfort** and radiation of the pain to the interscapular region may be present.
6. **Pseudoachalasia :** Tumours of cardia mimicking achalasia.

Inhalation of amylnitrate leads to sphincter relaxation in achalasia, but not in pseudoachalasia.

---

1. *Trypanosoma cruzi causes megaoesophagus, megaduodenum, megacolon and megaureter. Can we call it "mega" organism?*

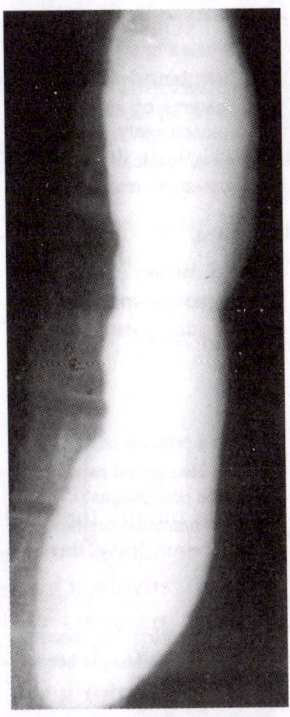

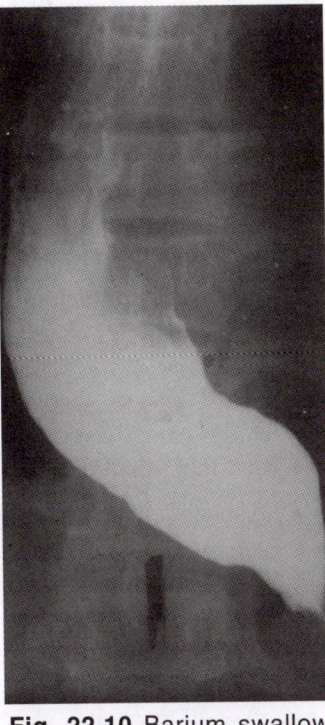

Fig. 22.9 Barium swallow showing dilated oesophagus

Fig. 22.10 Barium swallow showing sigmoid oesophagus

INVESTIGATIONS

1. **Barium swallow**
   - Uniformly dilated oesophagus above, with a smooth tapering segment below - cucumber oesophagus.
   - In chronic cases, it may be sigmoid shaped.

2. **Oesophagoscopy**
   - It reveals a dilated sac containing stagnant food and fluid due to stasis which splashes out with each heart beat and with each respiratory movement.
   - Oesophagoscopy is also done to rule out proximal malignancy.
   - Also done to evaluate oesophagitis, stricture or a tumour at cardia.

3. **Plain X-ray abdomen erect**
   - Fundic air bubble is absent because of the stasis of fluid in the oesophagus.

4. **X-ray chest**
   - Mediastinal mass (pseudotumour)[1] produced by dilated oesophagus can be seen.
   - **Retrocardiac air-fluid level in the lateral view.**
   - Aspiration pneumonitis can be diagnosed.

5. **Oesophageal manometry:** Following features are characteristic of achalasia cardia
   - Hypertensive Lower Oesophageal sphincter (LOS): It does not relax on swallowing.
   - **Aperistalsis in the body**
   - Increased resting pressure in the oesophagus.

6. **Ultrasound :** It may detect subepithelial tumour infiltration in secondary achalasia due to carcinoma distally.

TREATMENT

1. **Heller's cardiomyotomy**: The aim is to reduce outflow resistance at the lower oesophageal sphincter.
   - With a left thoraco-abdominal incision, the oesophagus and the stomach are completely mobilised.
   - The contracted segment is felt between the fingers.
   - A 7 to 10 cm long incision is made through the lower end of the oesophagus and carried over to the stomach. The muscles are cut till the mucosa bulges out. **The myotomy should extend proximally upto the aortic arch and distally up to the stomach to 1 to 2 cm below the junction.** Success rate is around 90%. 3 to 5% of the patients develop reflux oesophagitis which needs to be treated conservatively.

2. **Forceful dilatation -** By using **Pneumatic balloon:** The balloon is positioned under fluroscopic control

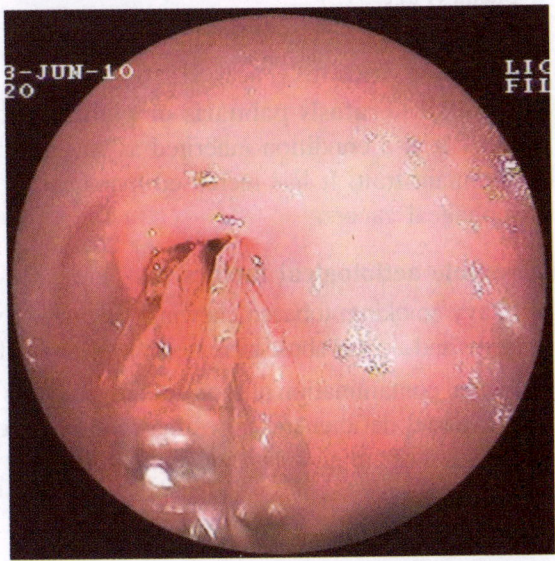

Fig. 22.11 Oesophageal balloon dilators

---

1. Aortic aneurysm, cold abscess (paravertebral), scoliosis are the other pseudotumours in the chest X-ray.

within LOS. It should be rapidly inflated to a pressure of 300 torr for 15 seconds. Success rate is around 70%. 20% chances of reflux are present. Oesophageal perforation can also occur. Recurrences are common.

3. Injection treatment: Inj. **Botulinum toxin** is injected into the lower oesophageal sphincter (LOS) endoscopically. Injection acts by interfering with cholinergic excitatory neural activity at LOS, then blocking acetylcholine release from nerve terminals. It is temporary and repeat injections are necessary.

4. Drugs: Sublingual nifedipine can produce short term relief.

COMPLICATION OF ACHALASIA CARDIA

- Due to prolonged stasis and chronic irritation, it can predispose to **carcinoma** mid and lower oesophagus (due to metaplasia). Hence, it is a precancerous condition.

CARCINOMA OF THE OESOPHAGUS

AETIOPATHOGENESIS

I. Pre-cancerous / predisposing conditions:

- Reflux oesophagitis with Barrett's oesophagus (Page 311)
- Plummer Vinson syndrome with squamous metaplasia (Page 312)
- Achalasia cardia (Page 312)
- Corrosive strictures (Page 318)
- **Familial keratosis palmaris or plantaris (tylosis)** - It is a condition inherited as an autosomal dominant trait. It has increased incidence of oesophageal cancer.

II. Possible aetiological factors

- Heavy smoking, tobacco chewing, spicy food with spirits and alcohol abuse increases risk by 25-100 fold.
- Fungal contamination of food with mycotoxins and nutritional deficiencies is responsible for oesophageal cancer in endemic areas of China.

SITES

- 50% -middle 1/3rd of oesophagus
- 33% -lower 1/3rd of oesophagus
- 17% -upper 1/3rd of oesophagus (Fig. 22.12).

TYPES (SQUAMOUS CELL CARCINOMA)

1. Epitheliomatous ulcer (carcinomatous) with raised edges and flat base.
2. Proliferative growth (cauliflower) with surface ulcer which commonly bleeds.
3. Infiltrative variety or annular stenosing variety with a 5 year survival of 10%, gives rise to early dysphagia due to circumferential and longitudinal spread.
4. Polypoidal lesions (5 year survival 70%)

CLINICAL FEATURES

- Men more than 60 years
- Dysphagia which is progressive and mainly for solids (it takes 18 months for dysphagia to develop). It means ¾ of the circumference of the lumen is involved by the growth. By the time, the patient presents with dysphagia, the disease is fairly advanced. Hence, it has poor prognosis.
- Regurgitation of the food contents. Haematemesis is not very common, vomitus may contain streaks of blood and melaena is rare.
- Loss of appetite, loss of weight and cachexia
- Backache indicates enlarged lymph nodes (coeliac)

SPREAD

1. Local spread or direct spread

- To start with, it is a mucosal ulceration which spreads to the submucosa. Later, it causes fibrosis and the lumen gets narrowed. The spread occurs transversely and longitudinally. Once it spreads to all the layers, the structures in the vicinity are involved.
- When the trachea is involved, tracheo-oesophageal fistula develops from carcinoma upper 1/3 of oesophagus.

Key Box 22.6

FACTORS RESPONSIBLE FOR EARLY SPREAD AND AGGRESSIVE BEHAVIOUR

- Lack of serosal layer
- Proximity of vital structures
- Extensive mediastinal lymphatic drainage

- Broncho-oesophageal fistula from carcinoma middle1/3.

- Oesophagoaortic fistula results in massive bleeding (one of the causes of death).

- All these complications are contraindications for surgery and radiotherapy.

2. **Lymphatic spread** (Page 306)

3. **Blood spread**: It results in secondaries in the liver, which clinically appear as nodular enlarged liver. Later, ascites and rectovesical deposits occur. Palpable left supraclavicular nodes indicate advanced disease. This sign is described as **Troisier's sign.**

INVESTIGATIONS

1. Hb % is low, which is the cause of generalised weakness.

2. Liver function test (LFT) is affected, if secondaries in liver occur (Increased ALP).

3. Ultrasound is done to rule out liver secondaries, lymph nodes in the porta hepatis, coeliac nodes etc.

4. Barium swallow demonstrates irregular, persistent, intrinsic filling defect. (Fig. 22.12)

5. **Oesophagoscopy** to visualise the growth and to take biopsy. (Fig. 22.16)

   - **Multiple biposies** may be necessary. In high risk areas like China, **endoscopic staining with supravital dyes** (indigocarmine) is done to identify dysplastic epithelium. If found, some advocate endoscopic mucosal resection.

Also dysplasia in Barrett's mucosa is a prognostic sign of impending malignant degeneration.

6. Chest X-ray to rule out aspiration pneumonia and mediastinal widening and posterior tracheal indentation etc.

7. Bronchoscopy to rule out involvement of bronchus, as in carcinoma middle 1/3rd.

8. **C.T. scan** of the chest to find out local infiltration. It is very useful investigation before contemplating for total oesophagectomy, to assess the vital structures involvement like bronchus, airway etc.

9. **Endoscopic ultrasound** to know the depth of wall involvement, to detect mediastinal lymph nodes etc.

TREATMENT

I. Carcinoma upper l/3rd of oesophagus

- A growth (squamous cell carcinoma) with the secondaries in lymph nodes or fixity to trachea is treated by external radiotherapy.

  Dose: 5000-6000 cGy units given with linear accelerator.

- **Small, mobile growth**: Total oesophagectomy followed by gastric pull up and pharyngogastric anastomosis in the neck. The anastomosis in the neck is safe. It is a major surgery and carries 5-8% mortality rate.

- Should be attempted in special centres

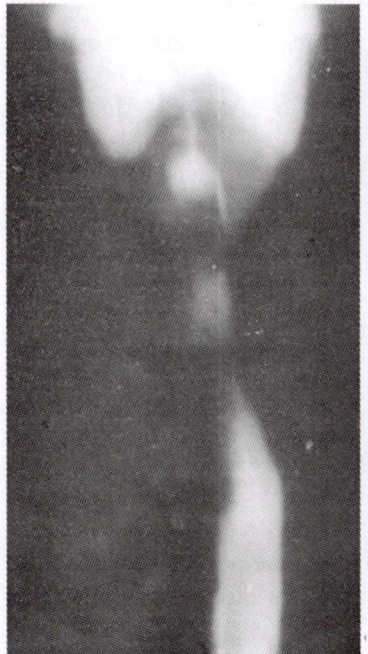

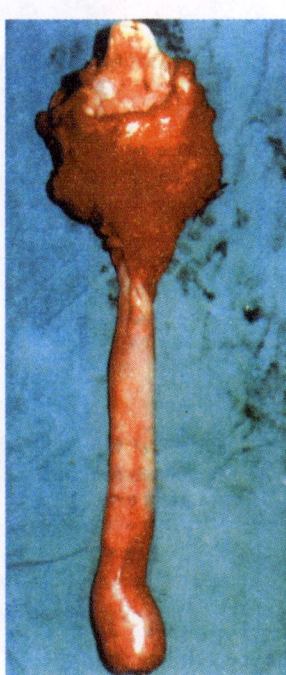

Fig. 22.12 Barium swallow - intrinsic irregular filling defect - Carcinoma upper oesophagus

Fig. 22.13 Total pharyngolaryngo-oesophagectomy

II. Carcinoma middle 1/3 of oesophagus (Fig. 22.14)

- It is squamous cell carcinoma.

- Surgery is difficult due to infiltration of surrounding structures. However total oesophagectomy can still be done if general condition of the patient is good and mediastinal structures adjacent to the growth are not involved.

- Lymph node clearance in the mediastinum has been found to be beneficial in expert hands.

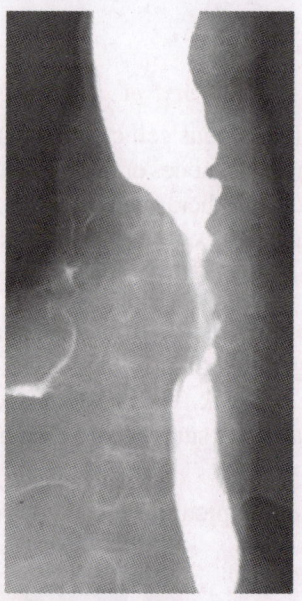

Fig. 22.14 Barium swallow - Carcinoma middle oesophagus

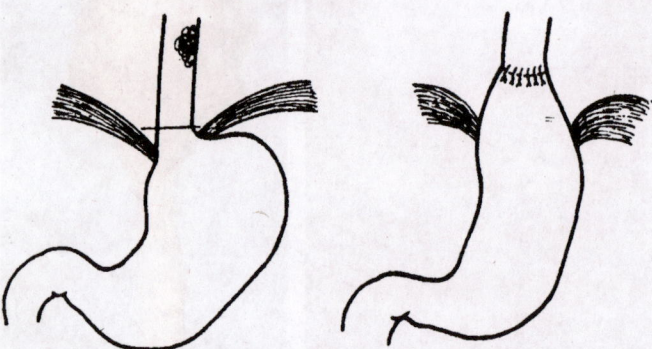

Fig. 22.15a Ivor-Lewis operation

Fig. 22.15b Anastomosis in the thorax

- Radiotherapy is given in the post operative period to prevent recurrence. The dosage is the same as above.
- Due to irradiation, oedema develops causing further narrowing of the lumen.
- Fibrosis develops later in the oesophagus which needs regular dilatation by using gum elastic bougies.

Ivor-Lewis operation

- It is indicated for carcinoma involving lower part of middle 1/3 or upper part of lower 1/3 of oesophagus.
- In this operation, abdomen is opened first, stomach is mobilised and the wound is closed. The patient is put in left lateral position, and right thoracotomy is done through 6th intercostal space. The growth is removed and oesophagogastric anastomosis is done inside the

thorax, above the level of aortic arch. Hence, it is described as a two-stage Ivor-Lewis approach (Fig. 22.15a, 22.15b)

III. Carcinoma lower l/3rd of oesophagus:

1. **A mobile growth**: Trans-hiatal oesophagectomy without thoracotomy (Orringer) - Fig. 22.17.

- Radical oesophagogastrectomy- Oesophagus and upper part of stomach and the involved lymph nodes are removed, followed by gastric pull-up and anastomosis in neck.

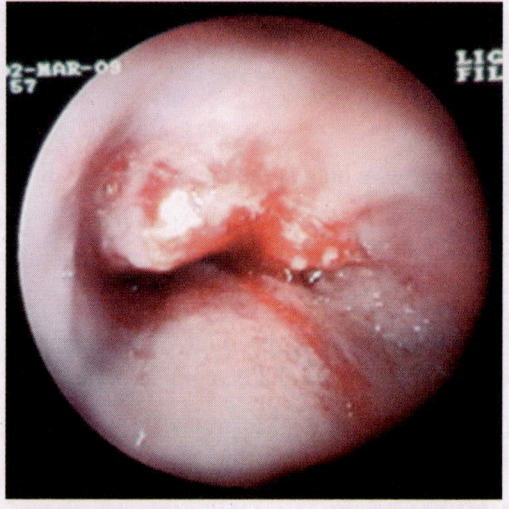

Fig. 22.16 Endoscopic view of Carcinoma lower oesophagus - it is an adenocarcinoma

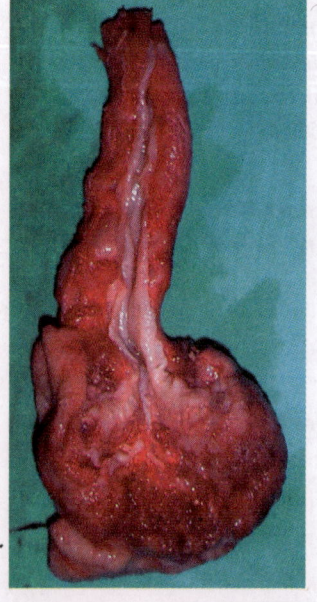

Carcinoma lower end of oesophagus - without opening the thorax by mobilisation from above and below, the oesophagus with the growth can be removed.

Fig. 22.17 Trans-hiatal (Orringer) total oesophagectomy. Contributed by: Dr. Sachidanand, Associate Professor, Karnataka Institute of Medical Sciences, Hubli, Karnataka

2. A fixed growth: Celestin tube or Mousseau-Barbin tube (MB tube) is introduced to reduce dysphagia. This is only a palliative treatment. These tubes give temporary relief but food particles getting struck, regurgitation and a kind of a retrosternal discomfort are the complications.

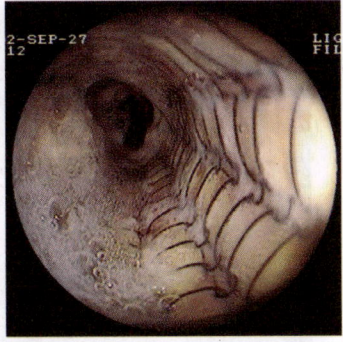

Fig. 22.18 Oesophageal stenting with metallic stent

Metallic self expandable stents are currently the choice of tubes to relieve palliation

3. Palliative oesophagojejunostomy is a better alternative to relieve dysphagia, provided the general condition of the patient permits a major thoraco-abdominal procedure with acceptable mortality and morbidity.

IV. Chemotherapy

Intravenous 5 Fluorouracil 500-750 mg diluted in 500 ml of saline for 5 days per month for about 6 cycles. Its value is doubtful.

CAUSES OF DEATH IN CARCINOMA OESOPHAGUS

* Cancer cachexia
* Complications like bronchopleural fistula, aspiration pneumonia, haematemesis due to erosion of aorta, perforation of the growth and mediastinitis.

SUMMARY OF TREATMENT OF CARCINOMA OESOPHAGUS

* Inspite of endoscopy and other investigations, in more than 95% of cases, the treatment of carcinoma oesophagus is palliative. By the time the first symptom dysphagia appears, it is too advanced. Also, the location of the tumour, adjacent structures in the mediastinum, widespread lymphatic drainage alters the overall prognosis to a very low % of survival.

CERTAIN FACTS

* Majority of oesophageal cancers are advanced at the time of diagnosis.

* 5 year survival rates after curative resections are around 10%.

* The best results are obtained after surgery and endoscopic laser ablation.

* Radiotherapy, chemotherapy, dilatation and stenting also can give better palliation.

* Curative resections are major surgeries and should be undertaken by an experienced surgeon.

* Curative resections can be attempted at all levels of carcinoma oesophagus (upper, middle, lower) provided vital structures are **not involved** (assessment by CT Scan).

* **Chemotherapy never cures the disease** but shrinkage of tumour can occur.

* **Palliation:** As majority of the patients with carcinoma oesophagus have dysphagia, all the methods of palliation are aimed at relieving dysphagia. Endoscopy followed by dilatation using guide wire is a simple procedure with complication such as perforation rate around 2-3%. However the results are only for few weeks. Self expandable metal stents are regularly used nowadays as a palliation. They have two layers. A superalloy monofilament wire with a layer of silicon between them. This prevents the tumour from growing within the stent.

* **Endoscopic laser therapy** relieves obstruction and bleeding . It can be carried out as an outpatient treatment but needs multiple sittings.

* **Radiotherapy** alone has been tried for squamous cell carcinoma of the oesophagus - Dose is 6,000 cGy units. No survival advantage with this method

* **Combination chemotherapy** using Cisplatin and 5-Fluorouracil with radiotherapy has been tried in patients who are not fit candidates for surgery.

* **Palliative oesophago-jejunostomy** or palliative colonic interposition are the other surgical modalities of treatment as palliation.

* **Endoscopic intraluminal brachytherapy** is used in cases of recurrent tumour growing inside the lumen and causing obstruction.

The entire treatment of carcinoma of oesophagus is aimed at 'Cure' in minority of cases and relief of dysphagia in almost all cases.

STRICTURE OESOPHAGUS

CORROSIVE INJURY

These caustics are taken acidentally or in attempted suicide. The agents are sodium hydroxide, sulphuric acid, household bleach.

- The acids affect acidic stomach mucosa
- The squamous epithelium of oesophagus is relatively resistant to acids. (Also due to rapidity of fluids)
- The alkali - sodium hydroxide affects oesophageal mucosa.
- The corrosive injuries may involve oropharynx, the larynx, the oesophagus, the stomach and sometimes intestines also.

Classification of injuries

Superficial: Erythema, oedema, blisters etc. Re-epithelialisation of mucosa is complete by 6th week.

Deep: Circumferential ulcers, produces scarring and contractures. Major injury of stomach produces gastric outlet obstruction.

Clinical features

- Severe pain, drooling of saliva, inability to swallow.
- Retrosternal burning, abdominal guarding and rigidity.
- Hoarseness, stridor, laryngeal oedema, if there is laryngeal injury.
- Dysphagia later due to stricture

- **What should not be done:** Stomach wash or induced vomiting, as it will aggravate oesophageal injury or it may result in aspiration. **No role for corticosteroids in cases of deep injuries or acid injuries**.
- **What should be done:** Verification of the etiologic agent and accurate assessment of depth and extent of injury.

Treatment

- **Acute surgical intervention** should be tried only in selected, referral centres wherein depending upon case, oesophagectomy, pharyngostomy or gastrostomy, may be the choice.
- **Chronic cases** present with **stricture** which needs

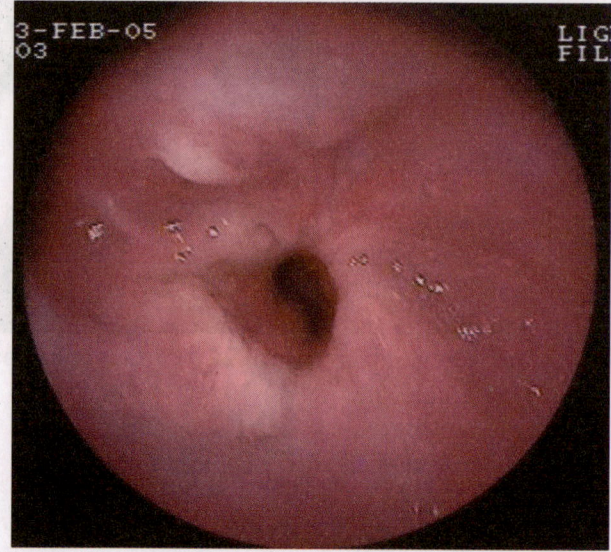

Fig. 22.19 Endoscopic view of corrosive strictures of lower end of oesophagus. Scope could not be negotiated through the oesophagus

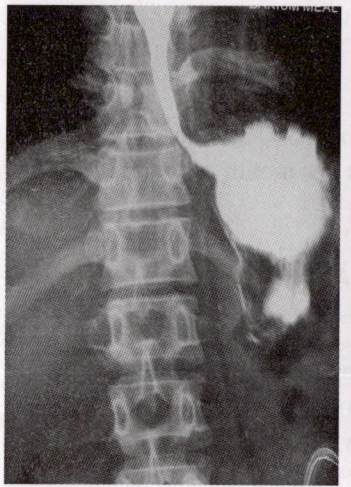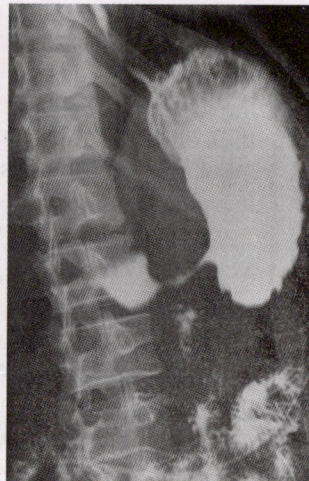

Fig. 22.20, 22.21 Corrosive strictures of lower end of oesophagus and pyloric antrum of stomach. Oesophageal stricture was dilated. However, antral stricture could not be dilated. Hence he underwent vagotomy and gastro-jejunostomy

regular dilatation, which is ideally done after 6 weeks (the time for re-epithelialisation of oesophagus).

- **Colonic pull up** is the choice for impassable strictures, only after adequate nutrition is achieved through feeding jejunostomy.

Complications of stricture

- **Development of malignancy**

Table 22.1 Comparison between corrosive stricture and carcinomatous stricture

CORROSIVE STRICTURE	*CARCINOMATOUS STRICTURE*
History of ingestion of caustics is present	Absent
Age : Young (20-40 years)	Old age (> 50 years)
Number : Multiple	Single
It presents as acute dysphagia	Chronic dysphagia

Comparison of corrosive stricture with carcinomatus stricture - Table 22.1 and **Other causes of stricture** (Key Box 22.7)

Key Box 22.7
CAUSES OF STRICTURE
1. **C**orrosive (caustic) injuries
2. **C**arcinoma
3. **C**olumnar lined oesophagus - Barret's
4. **C**apsules of tetracycline group of antibiotics
5. **C** Vitamins - potassium compounds
6. **C**hronic reflux due to GORD, results in **Schatzki's ring** - a stricture at lower oesophagus at squamocolumnar junction

OESOPHAGEAL PERFORATIONS

- Oesophageal perforation is a serious, acute emergency carrying a very high mortality rate. Fortunately it is not common. The causes are very many and totally different from gastric or duodenal perforations.

Causes

1. **Instrumentation:** Endoscopy, dilatation of strictures, injection sclerotherapy and laser treatment are the common causes.
2. **Operative:** Thyroidectomy, vagotomy, spine surgery, mediastinoscopy.
3. **Traumatic:** Caustic trauma, sharp and blunt
4. **Oesophageal diseases:** Carcinoma, Barrett's Oesophagus
5. **Spontaneous rupture:** Boerhaeve's syndrome

Diagnosis

- Severe pain in the neck, chest or abdomen, stiffness of the neck depending upon the site of perforation.

- Haematemesis, dysphagia, dyspnoea, hypotension, shock and pleural effusion are the other features.
- The investigation of choice is plain chest X-ray which can demonstrate pneumomediastinum, subcutaneous emphysema and mediastinal air fluid levels. When in doubt, CT chest is diagnostic.
- Contrast swallow can also be done

Treatment

- Exploration by thoracic or abdominal route, trimming or suturing or even resection of oesophagus should be done in appropriate cases.
- Conservative treatment has risk of continuing leak, sepsis and mediastinitis etc.

DIVERTICULUM OF OESOPHAGUS

- **Cervical diverticulum** is the commonest type of diverticulum which can present with regurgitation of meals, or aspiration of food contents into the lungs or recurrent respiratory tract infections. It is treated by excision of the sac and repair of the defect with cricopharyngeal myotomy - **posterior midline**. (Refer Table 22.2)

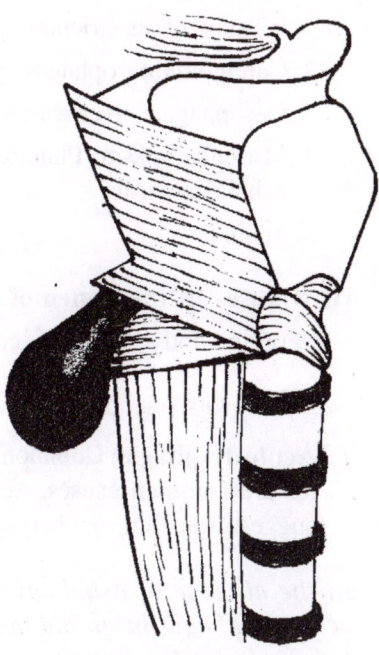

Fig. 22.22 Diverticulum

Table 22.2 Types of diverticulum

NAME	SITUATION	AETIOLOGY
1. Zenker's diverticulum (cervical or pulsion)	Proximal to the upper oesophageal sphincter	Protrusion of oesophageal mucosa between cricopharyngeus muscle inferiorly and thyropharyngeus muscle superiorly
2. Epiphrenic diverticulum	Proximal to the lower oesophageal sphincter	It is due to some kind of motility disturbance, wherein protrusion occurs in the lower end
3. Parabronchial diverticulum	Mid-oesophagus	Tuberculosis, by causing enlargement of mediastinal nodes, fibrosis and adhesions produce traction on the oesophagus, which results in the diverticulum

Types of diverticulum (Table 22.2)

DIFFERENTIAL DIAGNOSIS OF DYSPHAGIA

I. Causes from outside (extraluminal)

1. Thyroid swellings
2. Cardiomegaly
3. Aortic aneurysm
4. Mediastinal nodes-Tuberculosis
   - Lymphoma or Secondaries
5. Rolling hiatus hernia

II. Causes in the wall of oesophagus (luminal)

1. Oesophageal stricture
   - Corrosive acid poisoning
   - Tuberculous stricture
2. Carcinoma oesophagus
3. Oesophageal diverticulum
4. Muscular spasm: Plummer-Vinson syndrome and achalasia cardia
5. Tetanus

III. Causes in the lumen of oesophagus

1. Foreign body: Dentures, coins etc.

History (For investigations refer flowchart-Fig. 22.23)

1. **Acute dysphagia:** Common in children. Foreign bodies are common causes. Acute dysphagia with pain suggests tonsillitis or pharyngitis.

In the absence of usual causes mentioned above, acute dysphagia in an old man may be a manifestation of vertebro-basilar insufficiency.

2. **Chronic dysphagia**
   - Stricture, achalasia, Plummer-Vinson syndrome and carcinomas produce chronic dysphagia. The increasing difficulty to swallow, first to solids and later to liquids is typical of carcinoma oesophagus (in achalasia cardia, it is the reverse).

3. **Age and sex**
   - Achalasia and Plummer-Vinson's syndrome is common in females, carcinoma in men and foreign body in children.

4. Change in the voice or even hoarseness with dysphagia suggests advanced laryngeal carcinoma.

Dysphagia means difficulty in swallowing. Odynophagia means painful swallowing as in Quinsy, retropharyngeal abscess, tonsillitis etc.

CLINICAL NOTES

A 60 year old agriculturist was referred to the department of ENT for dysphagia of 3-4 days duration. A Registrar who saw the case did rigid oesophagoscopy under G.A. The findings were normal. Later in the evening he was called to see this patient who had rigid abdomen. A general surgeon was consulted. He suspected a perforation. An X-ray abdomen (erect) however, was normal. A senior faculty surgeon was consulted who examined the case properly and gave a correct diagnosis. It was a case of tetanus with mild trismus. Patient had injured his left thumb a few days back. Anaesthesiologist acknowledged later that the patient had some difficulty in opening of the mouth.

- Very often, patients undergo gastroscopy for dysphagia which will be normal only to realise later that what he is having is a stroke!!!.

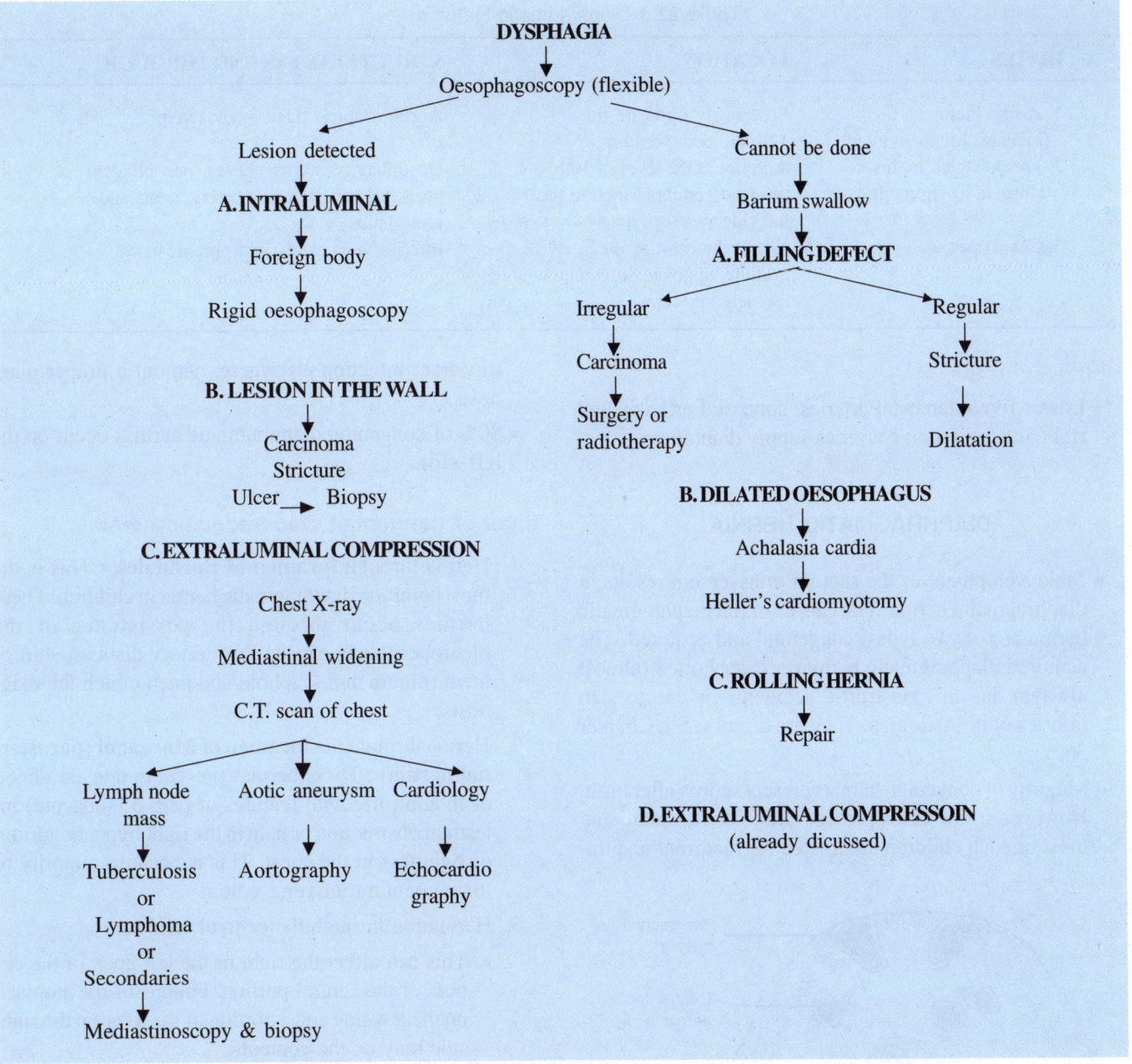

Fig. 22.23 Flowchart showing investigations for a case of dysphagia.

SURGICAL ANATOMY OF THE DIAPHRAGM

- The diaphragm is a dome-shaped thin sheet of muscle which separates the thoracic cavity from the abdominal cavity.
- It is derived from the inner most layer of the muscles of the body. Hence, it arises in continuity with transversus abdominis fibres from within the costal margin.
- It has right and left dome with a central tendon.

Attachments

- Anteriorly : Lower sternum
- Laterally : Costal margin
- Posteriorly (crura) : First three lumbar vertebrae

Nerve supply

- The muscles of the dome on its abdominal surface is supplied by phrenic nerve (C4). The crura are supplied by the lower intercostal nerves.

Table 22.3 Diaphragmatic hiatus		
HIATUS	**LOCATION**	**STRUCTURES PASSING THROUGH**
1. Aortic hiatus (median arcuate ligment)	Posteriorly opposite the 12th thoracic vertebra	Aorta, thoracic duct, azygos vein
2. Oesophageal hiatus (formed by right crus)	Anterior at the level of 10th thoracic vertebra 1inch to the left side	Oesophagus, vagus nerves, oesophageal branches of left gastric artery, veins and lymphatics
3. Caval opening	Just to the right of the midline, opposite 8th thoracic vertebra	Inferior vena cava, right phrenic nerve

Blood supply

- Lower five intercostal arteries, subcostal arteries, and right and left phrenic arteries supply diaphragm.

DIAPHRAGMATIC HERNIA

- Maldevelopment of the septum transversum results in diaphragmatic hernia. The causes of the diaphragmatic hernia are of two types: congenital and acquired. The acquired diaphragmatic hernias are very often (almost always) due to road traffic accidents or due to stab injuries of the abdomen. They are discussed in Chapter 36.
- Majority of congenital hernias present shortly after birth. However, a few cases present late to the hospital, and most of such children are treated for recurrent respira-

tory tract infection elsewhere, without a proper diagnosis.

- 80% of congenital diaphragmatic hernias occur on the **left side.**

Sites of congential diaphragmatic hernia

1. Hernia through **foramen of Bochdalek** : This is the most common diaphragmatic hernia in children. These hernias occur through the persistence of the pleuroperitoneal canals. Respiratory distress, shift of mediastinum and scaphoid abdomen clinch the diagnosis.

2. Hernia through the **foramen of Morgagni (parasternal hernia)** : These hernias present in late childhood or in adult life with features of partial (subacute) intestinal obstruction or pain in the right hypochondrium or tightness in the chest. This is because majority of them contain transverse colon.

3. Herniation through the **central tendon**:
   - This can affect the right or the left apex of the cupola or the central portion. Fundus of the stomach on the left side and a portion of the liver on the right side may be the contents.
   - These cases are very often diagnosed accidentally by routine chest radiograph.

4. **Eventration**: Due to paralysis or atrophy of the muscle fibres, one or both hemidiaphragms are weak and they are, elevated in position. Truly speaking, this is not a hernia, but signs and symptoms are almost like other types of hernia.

Diagnosis

- Chest radiograph: Gas and fluid level is within the chest.
- The thin rim of the diaphragm, as seen in a plain radiograph is broken or shows a defect.

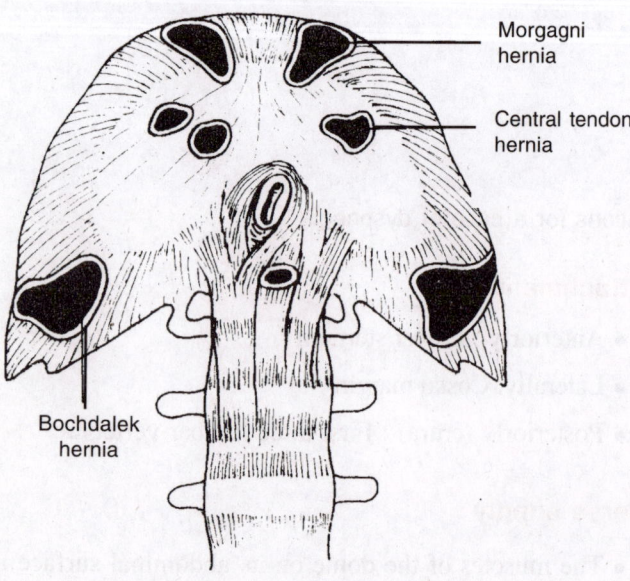

Morgagni hernia

Central tendon hernia

Bochdalek hernia

Fig. 22.24 Diaphragmatic hiatus

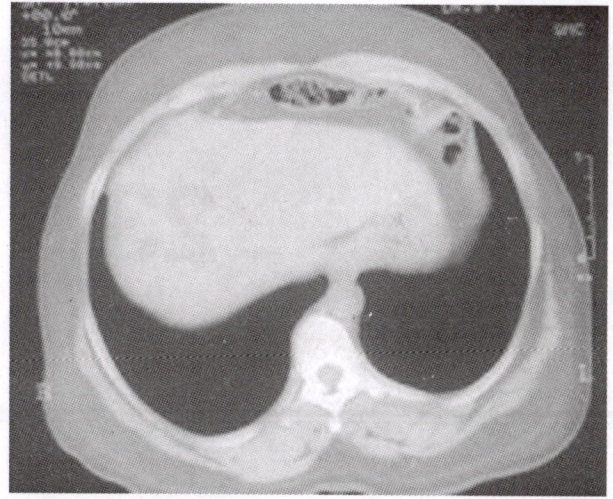

Fig. 22.25 Bochdalek hernia - CT scan showing intestine (colon within the thorax)

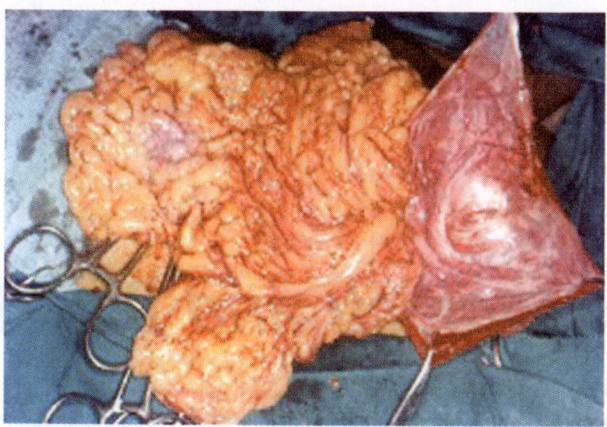

Fig. 22.26 Bochdalek hernia - showing the contents intestine and omentum. The defect was two fingers (5cm in diameter) nonabsorbable sutures were used to close the defect.

Treatment

The repair of the defect is done by using nonabsorbable sutures.

Eventration of the diaphragm is repaired by plicating the redundant diaphragm.

Miscellaneous

TRACHEO-OESOPHAGEAL FISTULA

Types

- In majority of the cases (85%) lower end of oesophagus communicates with the trachea and the upper end is blind (Refer Fig. 22.27).

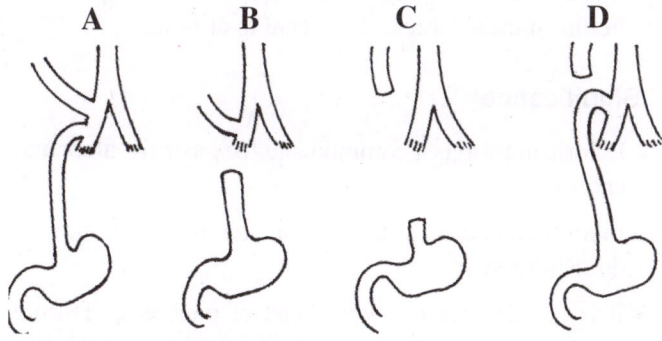

Fig. 22.27 Types of Tracheo-oesophageal fistula A. H type, B. Lower end is blind and upper end is connected to trachea, C. Both ends are blind, D. Upper blind end and lower end are connected to trachea - the most common variety (85 %)

Associated anomalies

Key Box 22.8
ASSOCIATED ANOMALIES
V - Vertebral defects
A - Anorectal malformation
C - Cardiac defect (PDA/VSD)
TE - Tracheo-oesophageal fistula
R - Radial hypoplasia and renal agenesis

Clinical features

- Continuous pouring of saliva from the mouth in the newborn baby is a diagnostic feature.
- New born baby regurgitates all feeds
- Aspiration, cough and cyanosis are other features.
- It is commonly associated with maternal hydramnios (50%).

TOF should be recognised and diagnosed within 24 hours of birth - by introducing a Ryle's tube.

Management

- Right thoracotomy, ligation of TOF and primary anastomosis of oesophageal ends.
- Feeding gastrostomy and oesophagostomy in type III fistula.
- In difficult cases of long atretic segment colonic or gastric transposition is required.

Complications

- Pneumonia, reflux, dysphagia, anastomotic leak.

Stomach and Duodenum

23

- Surgical anatomy
- Physiology
- H. Pylori infection
- Gastritis
- Peptic ulcer disease
- Acute complications of peptic ulcer
- Chronic complications of peptic ulcer
- Carcinoma stomach
- Gastrointestinal stromal tumours (GIST)
- Gastric lymphoma
- Differential diagnosis of haemetemesis
- Idiopathic hypertrophic pyloric stenosis
- Complications of peptic ulcer surgery
- Acid function tests
- Acute dilatation of stomach
- Chronic duodenal ileus

SURGICAL ANATOMY

- Oesophagus continues at oesophago-gastric junction as (OG), a muscular tube - stomach.

PARTS (Fig 23.1)

1. Fundus: Part which projects upwards in contact with left dome of diaphragm. Usually is full of gas

Significance

- To recognise the side (right or left) of the X-ray in a plain X-ray abdomen
- In achalasia cardia, fundic air bubble is absent.
- Fundic **'Wrap'** is used in hiatus hernia.

- During splenectomy or mobilisation of fundus short gastric arteries need to be divided. If ligatures are too close to the stomach on fundus - gastric fistula may occur due to **necrosis of the stomach**.

2. Body: Extends from fundus to incisura angularis. It has a lesser curvature and greater curvature.

Significance

- Ability to have a large meal is due to receptive relaxation of body of the stomach.
- Greater curvature is at the level of umbilicus.
- Classical GJ, anterior or posterior, involves using body of the stomach.
- Posteriorly is the lesser sac and pancreas. Carcinoma body may infiltrate pancreas - necessitates careful dissection to separate from pancreas (sometimes not resectable).

3. Pyloric antrum: It extends from incisura till pylorus. Pylorus is thicker than rest of the stomach. It is a sphincter of circular muscle fibres. It's canal is closed.

Significance

- Pyloric antrum is a common site for gastritis, ulcer and carcinoma.
- Incompetence of pyloric sphincter results in severe duodenogastric reflux.
- It is in close contact with head of pancreas. During gastrectomy extreme care has to be taken to mobilize the antrum to avoid bleeding in the pancreatic head region.

4. **Greater curvature**: It lies in contact with transverse colon, gastrocolic omentum. This has to be divided from transverse colon in gastrectomy done for carcinoma or ulcer.

BLOOD SUPPLY OF THE STOMACH (Fig. 23.2)

It is mainly supplied by coeliac trunk and its branches:

1. **Left gastric artery-** a direct branch of coeliac trunk, ascends up to oesophageal hiatus and turns to the right along the lesser curvature of stomach. It branches and anastomoses with branches of right gastric artery and supplies anterior and posterior wall of the stomach. There is true anastomosis between branches of left gastric artery and branches from other arteries.

2. **Right gastric artery** is a branch of hepatic artery which comes from coeliac trunk. It also supplies lesser curvature and body of stomach, along with left gastric artery.

3. **Left gastro-epiploic artery** arises from splenic artery and supplies greater curvature of stomach and anastomoses with right gastro-epiploic artery.

4. **Right gastro-epiploic artery** is a branch of gastroduodenal artery, which is a branch of hepatic artery.

5. **Short gastric arteries** are the branches of splenic artery. They supply the fundus of the stomach. They are also called the vasa braevia.

Venous drainage

- Veins run with the corresponding arteries. Right and left gastric veins drain into the portal vein directly. Right gastro-epiploic vein joins superior mesenteric vein and left gastro-epiploic and vasa braevia join splenic vein.

Surgical importance

- Because of extensive anastomoses of blood vessels, (extramural and intramural collateral vessels) stomach can survive with right gastric and right gastroepiploic arteries only. This stomach can be used to replace the entire oesophagus after oesophagectomy - gastric pull up.

- The order of ligation of blood vessels in gastrectomy- Left gastroepiploic, Right gastroepiploic, Right gastric (after stomach is divided) and last will be Left gastric artery.

LYMPHATIC DRAINAGE (Fig. 23.3)

- It is an important pathway for spread of carcinoma stomach. Spread occurs both by emboli and permeation.

1. Right gastric nodes/suprapyloric nodes, mainly drain the pyloric antrum.

2. Subpyloric nodes/gastro-epiploic nodes (right) drain the greater curvature of stomach and pyloric antrum.

3. Left gastro-epiploic nodes (splenic nodes) drain the upper portion of stomach, mainly the fundic growths (carcinoma of fundus).

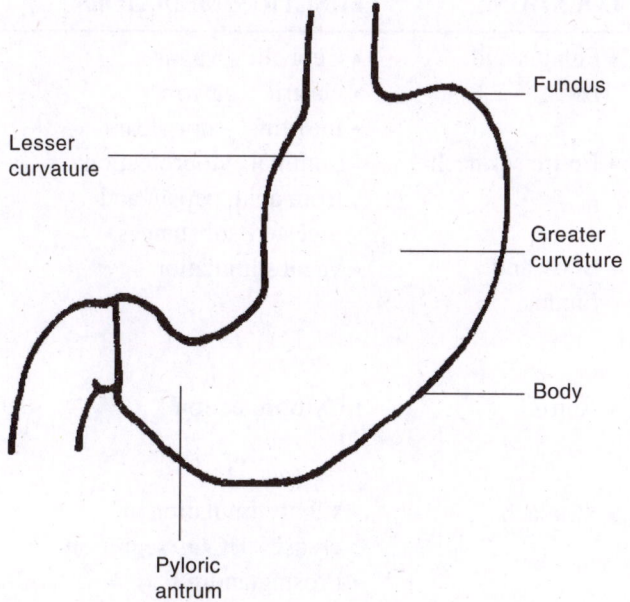

Fig. 23.1 Parts of the stomach

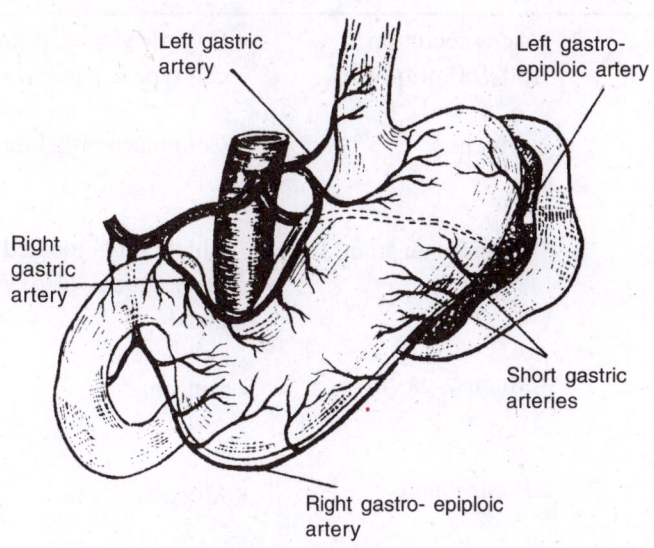

Fig. 23.2 Blood supply of the stomach

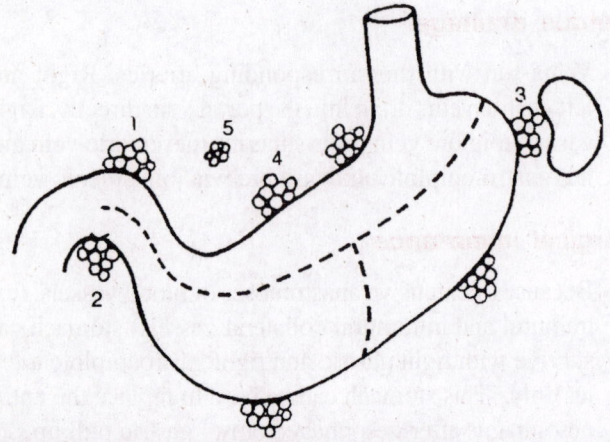

Fig. 23.3 Lymphatic drainage of the stomach - refer the text for the numbers

4. Left gastric nodes drain the lesser curvature and body of the stomach (anterior and posterior wall).

5. Coeliac nodes receive lymph from the entire foregut (including stomach) and drain directly into the cisterna chyli and the thoracic duct. Later, mediastinal nodes and left supraclavicular nodes are involved (**Virchow nodes**).

- **Lymphatic zones are discussed under carcinoma stomach**

GASTRIC PHYSIOLOGY (Table 23.1)

HELICOBACTER PYLORI INFECTION (H. PYLORI INFECTION)

- H. pylori is a gram-negative spiral organism with the stomach being its natural environment
- Produces abundant **urease**
- Most of the infection is **acquired in childhood**
- Route of infection: oro-oral or faeco-oral

Evidences

- Most patients with peptic ulcer are infected with H. pylori.
- After the treatment for H. pylori, the incidence of ulcer recurrence has decreased.

Mechanism of action (Key box 23.1)

- An alteration in mucosal barrier by the various enzymes it produces.
- Increase in the release of gastrin from the antrum.
- Decrease in somatostatin (D cells) in the antrum
- Increase in the pepsinogen I secretion.
- Cytotoxins release: Vac A : Vacuolating Toxin, Cag A : Cytotoxin associated protein.

	CELLS	LOCATION	FUNCTION/MEDIATORS
1. Acid secretion 150-160mEq/litre	• Oxyntic glands, principal cell type is parietal	• Fundus and body	• Cephalic - vagus • Gastric - gastrin • Intestinal - not clear
2. Mucus	• Columnar epithelium	• Entire stomach	• Luminal cytoprotection from acid, pepsin and ingested substances
3. Pepsinogen I and II	• Chief cells - located in deeper areas of oxyntic gland	• Body and fundus	• Vagal stimulation
4. Mucus, gastrin	• Antrum	• Antrum	• Cytoprotection
5. Bicarbonate	• Mucus cells	• Stomach	• Vagal stimulation increases HCO_3 secretion • Prostaglandin E_2
6. Intrinsic factor	• Parietal cells	• Fundus	• Necessary for absorption of B_{12}

Table 23.1 Gastric secretion

Key Box 23.1

MECHANISM

Hypersecretion of acid

↓

Gastric metaplasia of
duodenal bulb

↓ ← H. pylori

Duodenal mucosal injury

↓

ulcer

H.pylori testing

1. **Mucosal biopsy:** Endoscopic mucosal biopsy from the antrum can reveal evidence of H. pylori. The same specimen can be tested for presence of urease with rapid urease test : Biopsy specimen is added to urea solution containing phenol red. Colour change can occur due to increased pH brought by ammonia - as urea is split by urease.

2. **Serologic test** in the initial stages as a screening procedure - IgG antibodies.

3. **Urea breath test**
   - Principle: H. pylori splits urea because of urease. So, urea labelled cells like C^{13} or C^{14} are ingested. Because of urease, labelled CO_2 will be split off and absorbed into circulation which can be detected in the breath.

3. **Polymerase chain reaction**

GASTRITIS

- Various forms of gastritis have been depicted in the Table 23.2 below.

- Type B gastritis and erosive gastritis are common.
- Endoscopy and biopsy are the key investigations in all forms of gastritis.
- The treatment depends upon the type of gastritis.
- Rarer forms of gastritis include granulomatous gastritis, lymphocytic gastritis etc.

PEPTIC ULCER DISEASE

DEFINITION

- Acid peptic digestion of the alimentary mucosa, resulting in an ulcer is called peptic ulcer disease. The corrosive effects of acid with proteolytic effect of pepsin are responsible for peptic ulcer disease. Duodenum and stomach are the common sites of peptic ulcer disease. Rarely, they can occur in the jejunum and in Meckel's diverticulum when it contains ectopic gastric mucosa.

TYPES OF PEPTIC ULCER

I. **Depending on the site**
   A. **Chronic duodenal ulcer:** Typically occurs in the first inch of the first part of the duodenum.
   B. **Chronic gastric ulcer:** Occurs in the lesser curvature adjacent to acid secreting parietal cell mass.
   C. **Combined:** Gastric ulcer type II
      - Zollinger Ellison syndrome
   D. **Anastomotic ulcer**

II. **Depending on the duration**
   A. Chronic peptic ulcer
   B. Acute peptic ulcer (Page 349)

Table 23.2 Gastritis

Type - A	Type - B	Reflux	Erosive
• Autoimmune- antibodies to parietal cell	• H. pylori associated	• After cholecystectomy, gastric surgery.	• It occurs due to NSAID
• Antrum is not affected.	• Antrum is affected	• Antrum is affected	• It affects entire stomach
• Atrophy of parietal cell mass hence hypochlorhydria and decrease intrinsic factor	• Predisposes to peptic ulcer disease	• Usually does not give rise to peptic ulcer disease	• It occurs due to defective gastric mucosal barrier
• Hypochlorhydria stimulates antral gastrin. Predisposes to development of gastric cancer	• Can give rise to intestinal metaplasia, dysplasia and for the development of gastric cancer	• Treated by prokinetic agents or bile chelating agents	• Treated by H_2 blockers or proton pump inhibitors

AETIOLOGY OF CHRONIC PEPTIC ULCER

CHRONIC DUODENAL ULCER (CDU)

- Hyperacidity is the chief cause of duodenal ulcer. **No acid**, **no ulcer** still holds good for CDU.

1. **Neurological causes**: Stimulation of vagus increases secretion of acids. This is brought about by **anxiety, worry, hurry and curry**.

2. **Nonsteroidal anti-inflammatory drugs**
   - They are responsible for gastric ulcer rather than duodenal ulcer by altering mucosal defence.

3. **Genetic causes**
   - Family history of duodenal ulcer may be present in a few cases which suggests a genetic cause.
   - Patients with blood group 'O' are more prone for the development of **CDU** because of increased parietal cell population.

4. **Food habits:** Spicy food, diet poor in vitamins, smoking and alcohol, alone or in combination precipitate the development of chronic duodenal ulcer.

5. **Bacteriological causes:** Helicobacter pylori, a spirochaetal bacteria has been demonstrated in the submucosa of the antrum and duodenum, from the biopsies of the ulcer. It increases pH levels by splitting urea and releasing ammonia. Rise in pH results in proliferation of bacteria.

6. **Endocrinal causes**
   - Zollinger-Ellison's syndrome is a non-β cell tumour of the pancreas with hypergastrinaemia.
   - Hyperparathyroidism causes increased levels of calcium which stimulate the parietal cell mass there by resulting in hyperacidity.

CHRONIC GASTRIC ULCER

- In majority of the patients there is **No Hyperacidity.** Many patients have hypoacidity, or normoacidity. Ulcer occurs due to a defective gastric mucosal barrier. This barrier is a coat of thick mucous which is impermeable to pepsin. Normally present prostaglandins in the gastric mucosa do not allow back diffusion of hydrogen ions from the lumen. Non-steroidal anti-inflammatory drugs inhibit the production of prostaglandins thereby causing loss in protective activity. This can also be damaged by smoking, spicy food, alcohol and reflux of bile into the stomach.

> *A prepyloric gastric ulcer is associated with hyperacidity and it should be treated like a duodenal ulcer.*

Classification of benign gastric ulcers (by Johnson) TYPES (Fig. 23.4 to 23.7)

Acute superficial: Single or multiple (erosions)

Chronic

Type 1: Primary gastric ulcer on the lesser curvature in the antrum near the junction of oxyntic cells and central mucosa.

Type 2 : Gastric ulcer with duodenal ulcer

Type 3 : Prepyloric or channel ulcer

Type 4 : High gastric ulcer (cardia, proximal stomach) < 2 cms from oesophageal junction.

> *Type 2, 3 are to be treated like duodenal ulcer because they are associated with hyperacidity.*

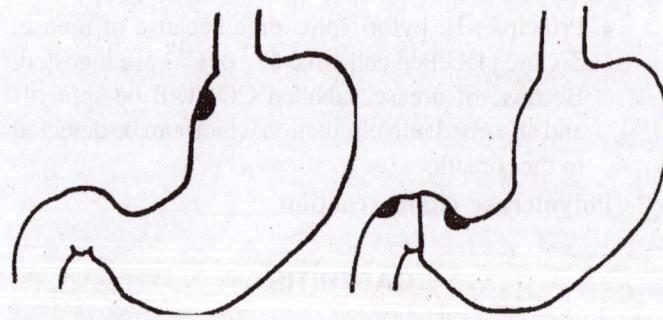

Fig. 23.4 Gastric ulcer - Type 1

Fig. 23.5 Gastric ulcer - Type 2

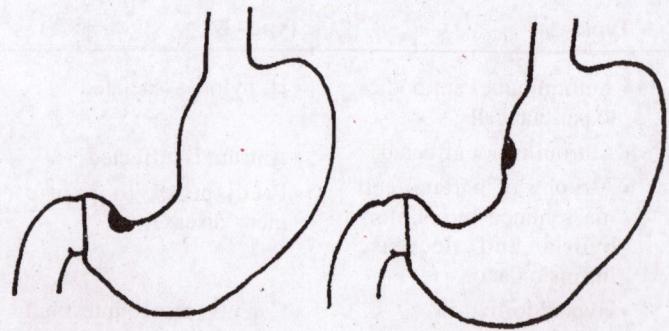

Fig. 23.6 Gastric ulcer - Type 3

Fig. 23.7 Gastric ulcer - Type 4

Table 23.3 Comparison of clinical features

	CHRONIC DUODENAL ULCER	CHRONIC GASTRIC ULCER
1. Incidence	Common	Less common
2. Site	Ist inch of 1st part of duodenum	The lesser curvature or prepyloric region
3. Pain	It is due to the acid irritating the ulcer (hunger pain). It is relieved on taking food. After 1-2 hours of food, the pain becomes severe. It is burning in nature with retrosternal radiation (heart burn) and increased salivation (water brash)	Pain occurs on taking food and it is relieved by induced vomiting. Pain is of burning nature as in duodenal ulcer.
4. Vomiting	Never occurs in duodenal ulcer till the patient develops pyloric stenosis	Frequent and it occurs immediately after patient takes food
5. Weight	Weight gain	Weight loss
6. Periodicity	Common	Less
7. Haematemesis: malaena ratio	40 : 60	60 : 40
8. Incidence of malignancy	Never becomes malignant	0.5-5% (2%)
9. On examination	Tenderness in the right hypochondrium	Tenderness in the epigastrium

CLINICAL FEATURES: (TABLE 23.3)

INVESTIGATIONS

1. **Oesophagogastroduodenoscopy: (OGD)**: Ulcer appears as a crater with/without slough or bleeding in their typical locations. In gastric ulcers, routine biopsy is advised to rule out malignancy. In duodenal ulcers biopsy is done in recurrent cases to rule out Helicobacter pylori.

   - In long-standing duodenal ulcers, there may be narrowing of the pylorus, with stasis of food in the stomach suggestive of pyloric stenosis.
   - Other uses of OGD (Key box 23.2)

2. **Barium meal study** (Fig. 23.8, 23.9)
   - **Duodenal ulcer:** Deformed duodenal cap. Trifoliate deformity is seen when secondary duodenal diverticulum occurs.
   - **Gastric ulcer** appears as a niche in the lesser curvature due to ulcer crater and as a notch on the greater curvature due to the spasm of stomach.
   - To detect **hour glass stomach** and **gastric outlet obstruction.**

Key Box 23.2

OESOPHAGOGASTRODUODENOSCOPY - OGD

Diagnostic (Fig. 23.10, 23.11)

- Peptic ulcers - acute and chronic
- Gastritis
- Carcinoma stomach
- Oesophageal varices, ulcers, oesophagitis
- Biopsy to rule out H. pylori infestation

Therapeutic:

- Injection of adrenaline into the bleeding vessel
- Variceal injection
- Snaring of polyps
- Electrocoagulation of bleeders
- Endoscopic cystogastrostomy
- Foreign body removal
- Percutaneous endoscopic gastrostomy (PEG)

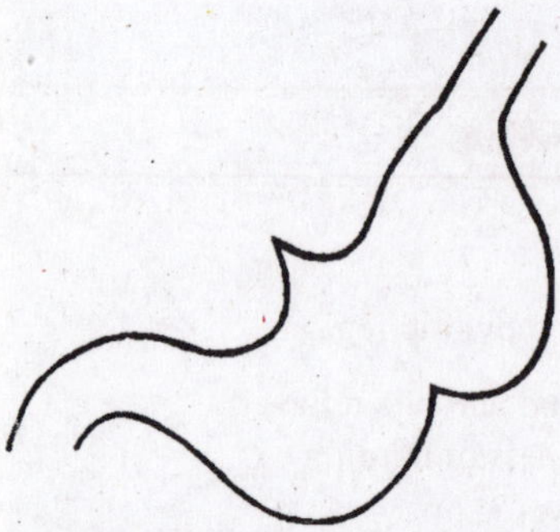

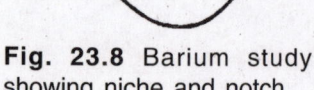
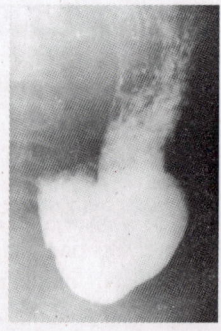
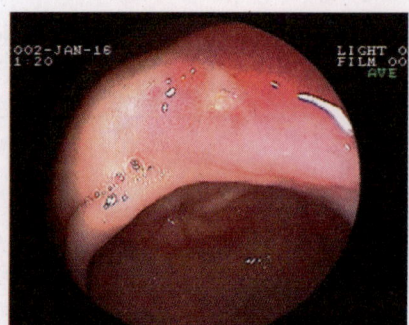
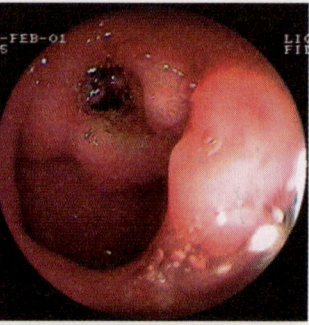

Fig. 23.8 Barium study showing niche and notch

Fig. 23.9 Barium study showing dilated stomach

Fig. 23.10 OGD showing chronic gastric ulcer

Fig. 23.11 OGD showing bleeding duodenal ulcer

3. Test for Helicobacter pylori (already discussed)

TREATMENT OF CHRONIC DUODENAL ULCER (CDU)

Aim is to decrease the pain because of its severity (by reducing acidity) and to prevent relapses.

Key Box 23.3
AIMS OF THE TREATMENT
• To relieve symptoms • To heal the ulcer • To prevent recurrence • To prevent complications

1. MEDICAL LINE OF MANAGEMENT

1. **H$_2$ receptor blockers (Histamine H$_2$-receptors)**
   - **Ranitidine**-150 mg twice a day, for 6 weeks. 90-95% of the healing occurs within 6 weeks. At the end of 6 weeks, 150 mg at bed time is given for a period of 3 months as a maintenance therapy. Re-endoscopy can be done in between, to assess the healing of the ulcer.
   - **Famotidine**-20 mg twice a day is as effective as ranitidine.
   - **Roxatidine**-Can be used along with food, bronchodilators and antacids, unlike the other H$_2$ blockers. The dosage is 75 mg twice a day.

   The problem in H$_2$ blockers is that relapse occurs if they are stopped. 80-90% healing rates occur after 6 weeks of therapy.

2. **Hydrogen ion antagonist (Proton pump inhibitor)**
   - Omeprazole-20 mg once a day for 2 weeks.

   - 95-99% of healing within 2-4 weeks.
   - Today omeprazole is being used as a first line of drug treatment for peptic ulcer disease.
   - Patients who receive omeprazole for one month are put on a maintenance dose of ranitidine for 3 months (150 mg **HS** for 3 months).
   - Other drugs such as Esomeprazole : 40 mg/day, Lansoprazole : 30 mg/day, Pantoprazole : 40 mg/day are also used.

3. **Regular antacids**
   - Given in high doses (120 ml/day) they will neutralize the acid (not practical). Small dose of antacids can be added to H$_2$ blockers. This gives a psychological benefit to the patient.

4. **Diet** should be bland, no spicy food, no alcohol, no smoking

5. **Eradication therapy**
   - If response to the initial treatment is poor or in case of repeated relapses, anti-Helicobacter regime is given.
   - **First regime:**

     2 weeks course of amoxycillin 500 mg 8th hourly, metronidazole 400 mg 8th hourly is given to eradicate H. pylori, along with omeprazole.
   - **Alternative regime**

     Clarithromycin 500 mg twice a day can be given along with metronidazole or with tinidazole (600 mg twice a day) with proton pump inhibitors.
   - **Bismuth compounds**

     They are not palatable hence used in about 10-15% of patients who do not respond to H.pylori eradication treatment. Cure rate with 7-10 days of treatment is 80-90%.

II. SURGICAL LINE OF MANAGEMENT

Key Box 23.4

INDICATIONS FOR SURGERY

---

1. **Intractable pain** in spite of treatment with H_2 receptor blockers, omeprazole and not responding to anti H. Pylori regime
2. **Frequent relapses**, H. pylori negative
3. **Complications** of duodenal ulcer:
   - Gastric outlet obstruction
   - Haemorrhage

SURGERY

1. **Highly selective vagotomy (HSV):** It is also called PCV (parietal cell vagotomy) or PGV (proximal gastric vagotomy) (Fig. 23.12).

   - In this operation, **vagi are not divided at the trunks**. Both anterior and posterior vagus are identified, isolated and preserved. Their branches which run along the lesser curvature are isolated. They are anterior and posterior greater gastric nerves of Latarjet. The branches of the nerves of Latarjet supplying parietal cell mass are divided. Hence, it is called parietal cell vagotomy. The terminal fibers of the nerve of Latarjet which supply pylorus are preserved (5-7 cm of 'Crow foot').

Advantages of HSV

1. More physiological, with minimal **disturbances.**
2. No drainage procedure is required because pyloric functions are preserved.
3. Nerve supply to gall bladder and liver are not disturbed.
4. No diarrhoea which occurs in 5-8% of cases of truncal vagotomy and can be life-threatening.

It is important to note that experience of many surgeons today with HSV is 'minimum'. Hence it is safe to do 'Vagotomy & GJ'.

Disadvantages of HSV

- Complicated procedure-needs an experienced surgeon.
- Recurrence rate: 10-15%.
- Rare chance of lesser curvature necrosis

2. **Total truncal abdominal vagotomy with gastro- jejunostomy - Mayo[1](Fig. 23.13) or pyloroplasty**

   - This is the most popular and most commonly done operation for peptic ulcer disease. However it is important to realise that indications for vagotomy and GJ are becoming less and less today.

Procedure

- Anterior and posterior trunks of vagus are divided just below the diaphragm followed by a drainage procedure like a gastro-jejunostomy (GJ). Vagus is secretomotor

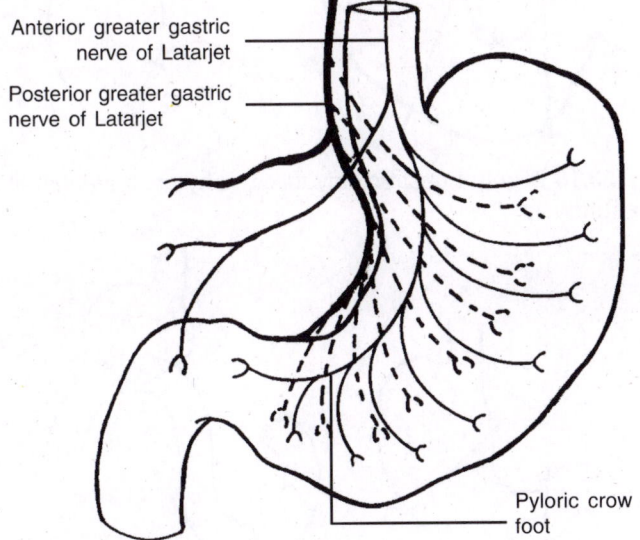

Anterior greater gastric nerve of Latarjet

Posterior greater gastric nerve of Latarjet

Pyloric crow foot

Fig. 23.12 Highly selective vagotomy

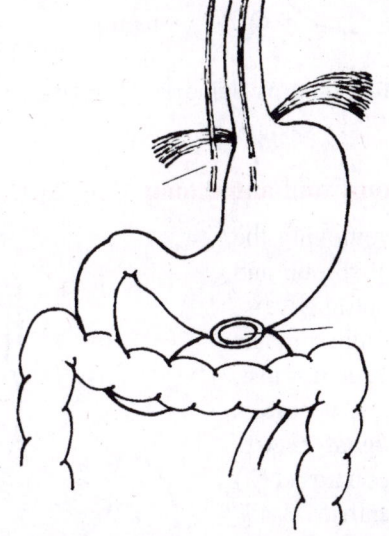

Fig. 23.13 Posterior GJ with vagotomy

---

1. About Mayo - Mayo's scissors, Mayo's GJ, Mayo's umbilical hernia repair to be remembered.

to stomach and after vagotomy the motility of the stomach is lost and gastric stasis occurs. Hence, drainage procedure is done.

- Posterior GJ is preferred because it gives a dependent drainage by gravity, of the food contents due to gravity. Classically, it is described as "Posterior, Vertical, Retrocolic, Isoperistaltic, No loop (short loop), No tension, GJ of Mayo (P.V.R.I.N.G.)".
- Alternatively pyloroplasty is preferred by a few surgeons instead of GJ
- In this operation, pylorus is incised longitudinally and sutured vertically. Thus, the pyloric ring becomes incompetent and wide open. Bile reflux gastritis is a major problem after pyloroplasty.

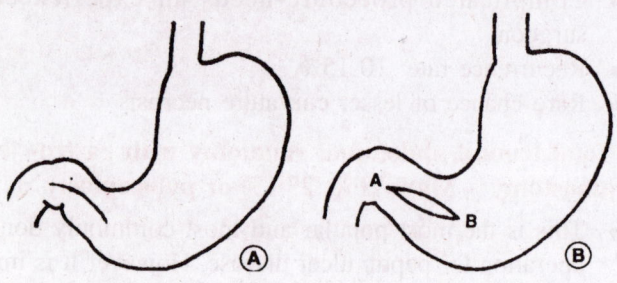

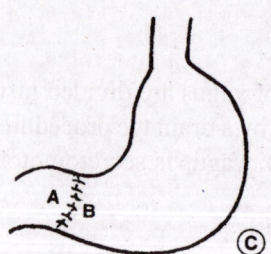

A. Gastroduodenal incision

B. Incision is deepened upto the mucosa

C. Sutured in the vertical direction

Fig. 23.14 Steps of Heinecke-Mickulicz pyloroplasty

4. Vagotomy and antrectomy (Fig. 23.15)

- By removing the vagal stimuli and the antral gastrin, the entire stimulus to the acid is lost. Hence, it carries the **least recurrence rate (1%)** but carries 3-4% mortality rate. Not done routinely.

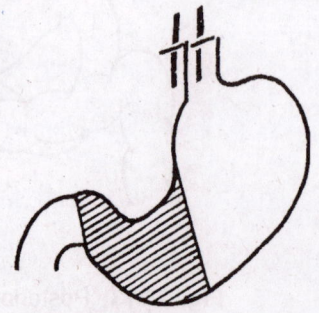

Fig. 23.15 Vagotomy with antrectomy

TREATMENT OF GASTRIC ULCER

- Aim: Healing of the ulcer and relief of symptoms.
- Frequent biopsy is done to rule out malignancy.

I. Medical line of treatment can be given like in duodenal ulcer, in the form of Ranitidine or Omeprazole. Cigarette smoking should be stopped. Drugs such as NSAID e.g., aspirin are to be avoided. If an ulcer persists after 6 weeks, the aim is to eradicate H. pylori **provided malignancy is ruled out.**

II. Surgery is indicated in case of persistent gastric ulcer inspite of medical treatment.

1. **Billroth I partial gastrectomy** (Fig.23.16)

- Partial gastrectomy is done including removal of the ulcer followed by gastroduodenal anastomosis. It has the least recurrence rate of less than 1 % but mortality rate is around 1-2%.

2. **Billorth II gastrectomy** (Fig.23.17)

- It is indicated when the gastric ulcer is located on the lesser curvature. Here the gastrectomy is done below the ulcer and remnant of the stomach is anastomosed to a jejunal loop (gastro-jejunal anastomosis). This is also described as Polya gastrectomy.

3. **HSV with excision of the ulcer** can be done if the experience of surgeon is good.

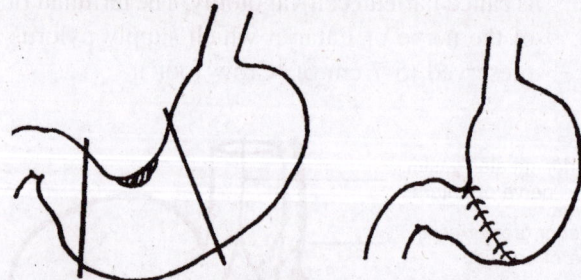

Fig. 23.16 Billroth I gastrectomy followed by gastroduodenal anastomosis

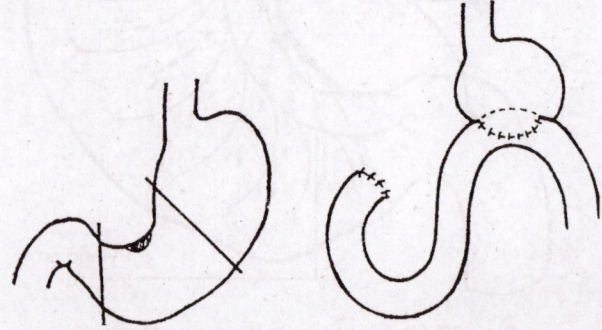

Fig. 23.17 Billroth II gastrectomy followed by gastrojejunal anastomosis

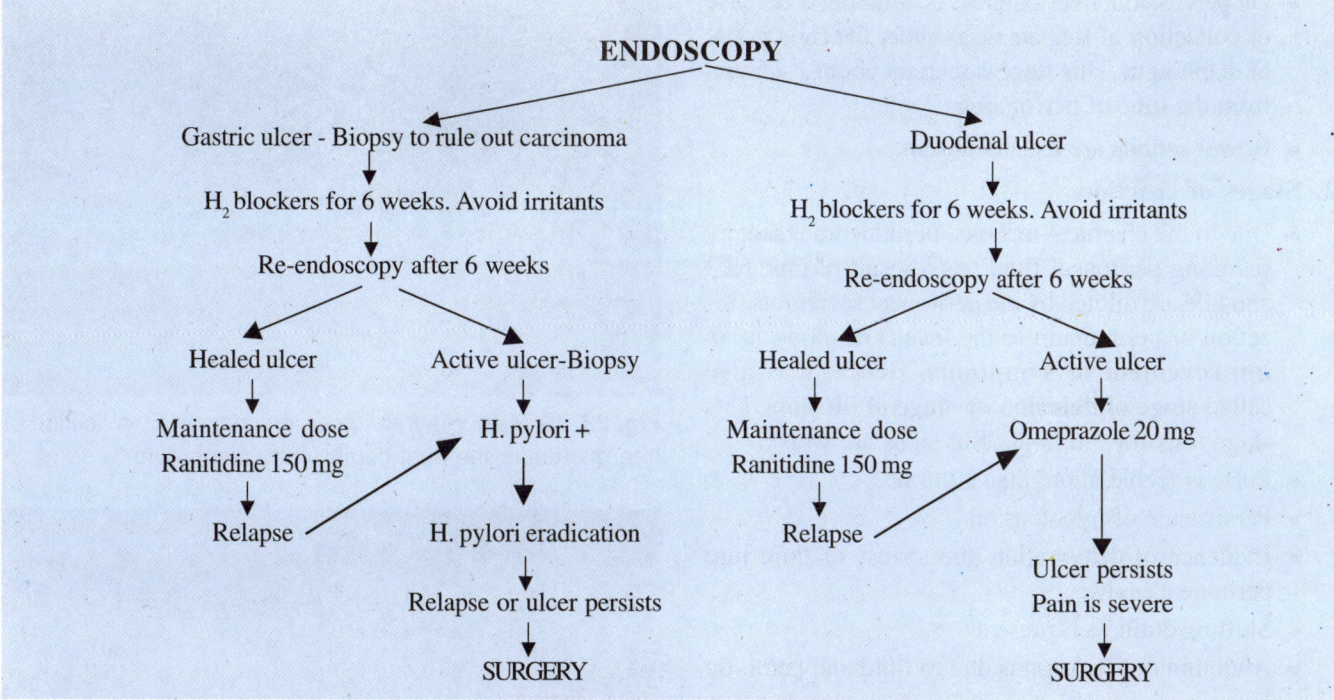

Fig. 23. 18 Flow chart showing management of peptic ulcer

Summary of the management of peptic ulcer is given in Fig. 23.18

COMPLICATIONS OF PEPTIC ULCER

A. Acute
- Perforation
- Haematemesis and/or melaena

B. Subacute - residual abscess

C. Chronic
- Gastric outlet obstruction (Pyloric stenosis)
- Teapot deformity
- Hour glass contracture of the stomach
- Penetration into the pancreas
- Carcinoma of stomach

ACUTE COMPLICATIONS

PERFORATED PEPTIC ULCER

- More common in male. The ratio is 8-10 men to 1 women in India.
- Anterior duodenal ulcer perforates and posterior duodenal ulcer bleeds. Ulcer on the posterior wall of the stomach can perforate into the lesser sac.

- Usually, patients with long history of peptic ulcer, suddenly complain of something that has given way. It may be precipitated by excessive smoking, alcohol or drugs etc. Rarely a 'silent' ulcer can also perforate (especially those patients treated with cortisone).
- Patients taking NSAIDs (elderly) can present less dramatically.

Stages of duodenal ulcer perforation

1. **Stage of chemical peritonitis**
   - Immediately after the perforation, gastric and duodenal contents leak into the peritoneal cavity and produce severe agonizing pain in the right hypochondrium. It is mainly HCl which produces pain.
   - There may be an episode of coffee-ground vomitus, followed by melaena.
   - Pulse rate is increased. The patient is pale and anxious.
   - Blood pressure may be normal in the initial few hours.
   - Per abdomen, there is guarding and rigidity of the abdominal wall.
   - Rebound tenderness is present all over the abdomen – BLUMBERG SIGN.

- On percussion, liver dullness is obliterated because of collection of free air (gas) under the right dome of diaphragm. This stage is seen for about 2-4 hours from the time of perforation.
- Bowel sounds are usually absent.

2. Stages of reaction

- Due to the chemical irritants, peritoneum reacts by secreting peritoneal fluid. As a result of this, HCl and bile are diluted by the peritoneal secretions (reaction of peritoneum to the insult) resulting in an **improvement of symptoms**. Hence, it is also called **stage of delusion or stage of illusion.** This stage lasts for 3-6 hours. But signs are worse:
- Pulse is feeble, more than 120/min.
- Persistence of hypotension
- Evidence of dehydration due to loss of fluid into peritoneal cavity.
- Shifting dullness is present
- Abdominal distension is due to fluid and paralytic ileus[1]
- Bowel sounds are absent
- Guarding and rigidity are worsened

3. Stage of bacterial peritonitis

- The peritoneal contents get contaminated with gram-negative organisms resulting in bacterial peritonitis (the organisms are from the intestine itself and not from the peritoneum).
- Patient is severely ill, dehydrated, toxic with drawn in cheeks. The tongue is dry and coated but with bright eyes (**Hippocratic facies**).
- Features of hypovolaemic and septicaemic shock such as feeble thready pulse, cold peripheries, shallow respiration, high grade fever and persistent hypotension are present. Gross abdominal distension, guarding, rigidity, abdominal tenderness all over suggest generalized peritonitis.

Management of perforated duodenal ulcer

- Complete blood picture and electrolyte study
- Plain X-ray chest or abdomen in **erect position** shows collection of free gas under the right dome of diaphragm, in majority of cases. If patient is unable to stand, left lateral decubitus films are taken. (Fig 23.19, 23.20)

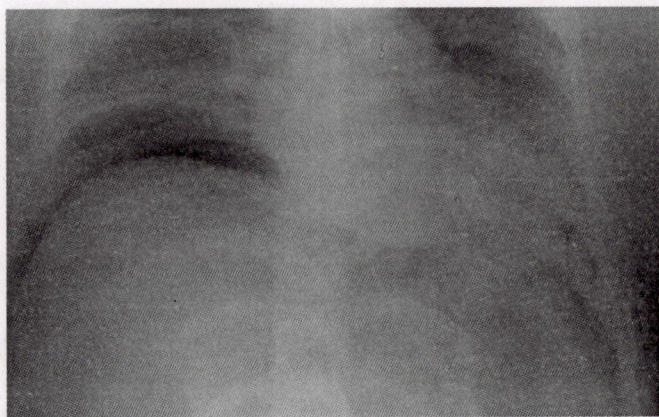

Fig. 23. 19 Plain x-ray abdomen erect showing collection of free gas under the right dome of the diaphragm

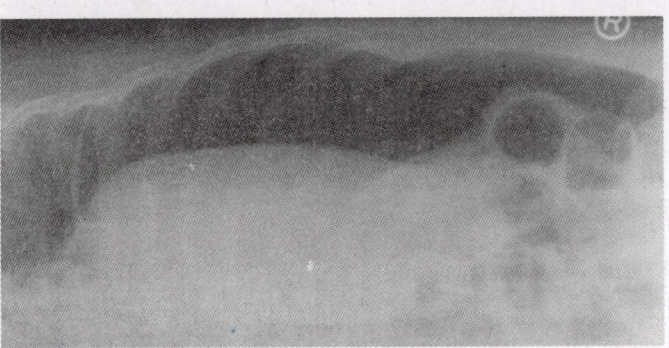

Fig. 23. 20 Plain x-ray abdomen lateral decubitus showing collection of free gas under the abdominal wall

Treatment: (A.B.C.D.E.F.)[2]

A **A**spiration with Ryle's tube of stomach contents to reduce further contamination, to decrease biliary and pancreatic juice.

B **B**lood grouping and cross matching may be necessary for surgery.

C **C**harts: temperature, pulse, BP, respiration, urinary output (A Foley's catheter is introduced).

D **D**rugs:

- Injection ampicillin 500 mg I. V. 6th hourly against gram-positive organisms.
- Injection gentamicin 60-80 mg I. V. 8th hourly against gram negative organisms.
- Injection metronidazole 500 mg I. V. 8th hourly to treat anaerobic organisms.
- Cephalosporins can also be used depending upon the severity of the shock.

---

1. *It resembles a strike by employees paralysing the work of a factory in response to an insult.*
2. *Students should remember that **ABCDEF** are the basic principles of any **ACUTE ABDOMEN**. In majority of cases of acute abdomen, these principles can be applied with minor modifications.*

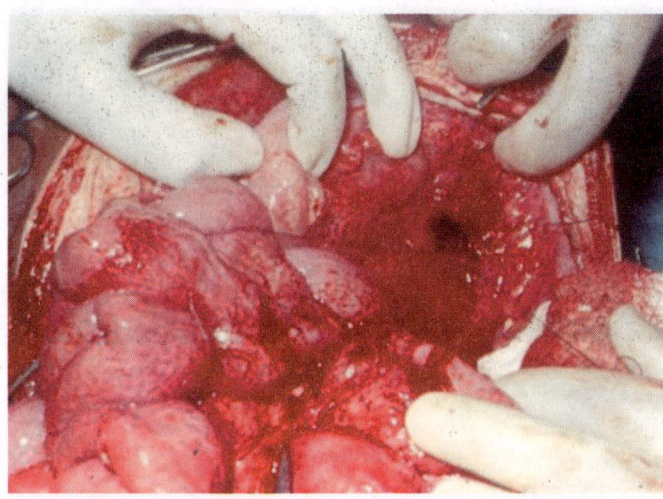

Fig. 23.21 Duodenal ulcer perforation - closure

E Exploratory laparotomy is done through a midline incision. The perforation is identified and closed with interrupted non-absorbable silk sutures, which is strengthened by **placement of omentum** (Fig. 23.11) Peritoneal toilet/wash is given to avoid residual abscess. Abdomen is closed with a drain which is removed after 3-5 days. If it is a large gastric ulcer, it is better to do a gastrectomy, if condition of the patient permits.

- Vagotomy and GJ is not done at this stage as the general condition of the patient is very poor and there is peritoneal sepsis.

- Post-operatively, the patient is put on anti-ulcer drugs.

- An endoscopy is done after 2 months. If the ulcer persists, it is likely to be a chronic ulcer and an elective operation such as vagotomy and GJ is done. Simple suturing cures majority of acute ulcers.

F Fluids are given pre-operatively to treat dehydration and postoperatively for 3-4 days till the paralytic ileus settles down (soft abdomen and bowel sounds +).

Early cases of perforation

- It can also be managed by laparoscopic closure of perforation with peritoneal drainage. In fact a thorough wash is really possible with a laparoscope.

Subacute

- Perforation with abscess. Few patients present late to the hospital with features of sealed perforation.

HAEMORRHAGE FROM PEPTIC ULCER

- Haemorrhage from peptic ulcer can be chronic which causes anaemia or acute resulting in massive haematemesis and melaena.

- It is the **posterior duodenal ulcer which commonly bleeds,** because it erodes the gastroduodenal artery which runs posterior to the duodenum. The lesser curvature gastric ulcer erodes into one of the branches of left or right gastric artery.

Precipitating factors for haemorrhage

1. **Chronicity,** results in destruction of the layers of the stomach, exposing the vessel

2. Sudden, severe acid peptic digestion brought about by **irritants** like alcohol, drugs, etc

3. **Atherosclerosis-**Sclerotic artery does not contract, resulting in massive haemorrhage

Clinical features of bleeding peptic ulcer

1. Previous history of peptic ulcer disease in the form of abdominal pain.

2. History of haematemesis or melaena (black tarry stools), one or more attacks.

3. There may be features of haemorrhagic shock such as thready feeble pulse, hypotension, syncope.

   - Oliguria, due to inadequate renal perfusion.

   - Brain stem hypoxia results in change in rate and depth of respirations.

   - There may not be any abdominal signs. However, due to accumulation of blood in the intestines, and stomach, mild distension may be present. **Perforation produces abdominal signs and haemorrhage produces systemic signs.**

Blead risk classification

- Following few factors are associated with increased morbidity and mortality.

Key Box 23.5
BLEAD RISK CLASSIFICATION
• **BL**ood pressure low
• **E**levated prothrombin time
• **A**ltered mental status
• **D**ysfunction - myocardial, renal, co-morbid disease

Management

Emergency upper OGD is done to confirm the diagnosis. If the source cannot be detected due to large clots or massive bleeding, it can be repeated a few hours after a stomach wash and blood transfusion.

I. Conservative line of management

1. Emergency replacement of blood, after initial resuscitation with plasma expander.
2. Ryle's tube is passed and cold saline stomach wash is given to produce vasoconstriction.
3. Cold antacids are given every 2nd hourly, about 10-20 ml.
4. I.V. ranitidine 50 mg, 8th hourly or I.V. pantoprazole 40mg is given to reduce acidity.
   - Majority of cases respond to conservative line of management within 48 hours.

II. Nonsurgical treatment

1. Laser coagulation

- It can arrest the bleeding without direct tissue contact. Nd: YAG laser has been used more commonly because it can penetrate tissue more deeply compared to argon laser which penetrates very superficial tissues. The success rate of laser coagulation is around 80%.

2. Sclerotherapy (Key Box 23.6, 23.7)

- 1:10,000 epinephrine arrests the bleeding by vasoconstriction. 2% ethanolamine, a sclerosant causes dehydration and shrinkage of surrounding tissues. It also produces inflammation and thrombosis of the bleeding vessel. This is the most popular method.

Key Box 23.6
ENDOTHERAPY
• Bipolar electrocoagulation failure rate 50%
• Inj. sclerotherapy - failure rate 20%
• Haemclip application

Key Box 23.7
ENDOSCOPIC PROGNOSTIC FACTORS
• Visible level : 40-60% rebleeding ulcer > 2 cm
• Adherent clot : 20% rebleeding
• Flat pigmented spot : 10% rebleeding
• Clean ulcer base : Rarely bleeding

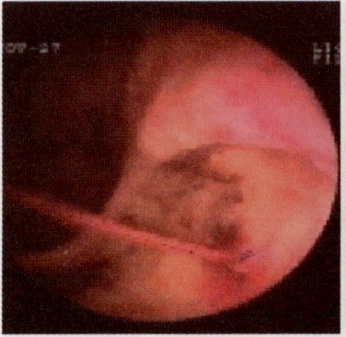 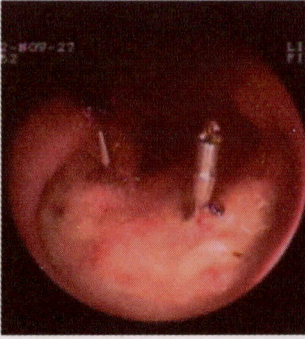

Fig. 23.22a Bleeding vessel   **Fig. 23.22b** Haemclip applied

Success rate is around 80-90%. It is a cheap and easy treatment.

3. Haemclip application (Fig 23.22)

4. Bipolar electrocoagulation - failure rate is 50%

> *Surgical eradication of H. pylori prevents rebleeding*

III Surgical control of bleeding peptic ulcer

Indications

1. Failure of endoscopic haemostasis - prognostic factors are given below. (Key box 23.7)
2. Rebleeding in the hospital (rebleeding is more common in gastric ulcer patients)
3. Bleeding requiring transfusion of more than 2000 ml blood in 24 hours. (6 units)
4. Elderly patients with rebleeding

Types of surgery

1. Surgery for bleeding duodenal ulcer

- Laparotomy **anterior gastroduodenotomy**
- Visualise the bleeding ulcer in the first part of duodenum
- **Underrunning** of the ulcer base by direct suture or 4 quadrant ligation of gastroduodenal artery by using nonabsorbable sutures (Fig. 23.23)
- Gastroduodenotomy incision is converted into a pyloroplasty followed by vagotomy which completes the treatment.

2. Surgery for bleeding gastric ulcer (benign) (Fig. 23.24, 23.25)

- Laparotomy, gastrotomy and visualise the bleeding ulcer.

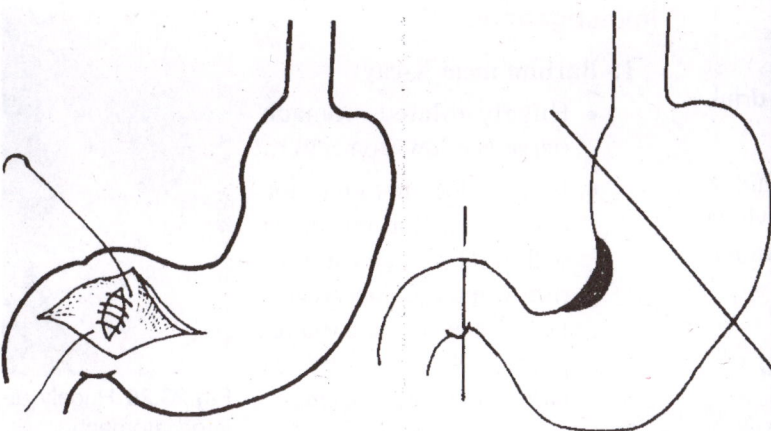

Fig. 23.23 Under-running of the duodenal ulcer

Fig. 23.24 Partial gastrectomy for gastric ulcer

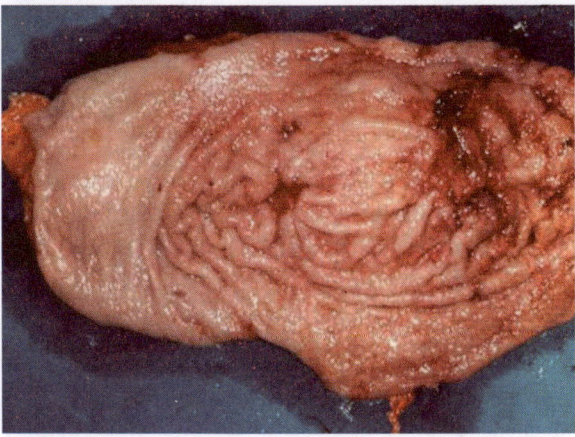

Fig. 23.25 Partial gastrectomy for bleeding gastric ulcer

- Under-running of the ulcer base. There are chances of rebleeding with this method.
- Partial gastrectomy is the best treatment provided general condition of the patient is good. Otherwise, local excision of the ulcer, vagotomy followed by GJ or pyloroplasty can also be done.

SUBACUTE COMPLICATION

A small perforation of peptic ulcer which is sealed off by omentum may result in a residual abscess in one of the subphrenic spaces. It responds to conservative treatment. Otherwise percutaneous drainage can be done with ultrasonographic guidance.

CHRONIC COMPLICATIONS OF PEPTIC ULCER

GASTRIC OUTLET OBSTRUCTION

Earlier it was called as pyloric stenosis. However, gastric outlet obstruction is a better word. Chronic cicatrisation of a duodenal ulcer or juxtapyloric ulcer results in narrowing of pyloric antrum which is described as pyloric stenosis. In India pyloric stenosis is more common in south Indian patients, who usually present with long history of duodenal ulcer with recent history of vomiting (Key Box 23. 28).

Symptoms

- Classical **hunger pain** of duodenal ulcer disappears. It may be replaced by a dull aching pain because of gastric distension. Colicky pain is due to hyperperistalsis of stomach.

Key Box 23.8
PYLORIC STENOSIS

- Pyloric stenosis in CDU - **Misnomer**
- Stenosis is very often found in the **first part of duodenum**
- In cases of pyloric channel ulcer, true pyloric stenosis occurs
- Metabolic changes, like paradoxical aciduria are usually seen in ulcer cases, **NOT IN carcinoma** because of relative achlorhydria in the latter

- **Vomiting** is profuse, projectile, persistent, foul smelling (because of stasis) and non-bilious.
- There may be **distension of upper abdomen** with epigastric fullness.

Signs

1. **Visible gastric peristalsis (VGP)-stomach that you see**

- It is a wave of contraction of the stomach which starts in the left hypochondrium, runs across the umbilicus and ends in the right hypochondrium. These contractions can be felt- **stomach that you feel.** Presence of VGP is diagnostic of pyloric stenosis (Right to left peristalsis is seen in left-sided obstructive colonic tumours). **If VGP is not seen, it can be made prominent by :**
- Asking the patient to drink at least 500-1000 ml of water. (It is difficult. Try and see!)
- Stimulating the abdomen by flicking movement.

2. Succussion splash

- Should be done on 'fasting' stomach. This test should be done before asking the patient to drink water.

- In pyloric stenosis there is always residual fluid in the stomach, which gives a splashing sound which can be heard with/without stethoscope-**stomach that you hear.**

Thus, the stomach which is seen, felt and heard is diagnostic of pyloric stenosis.

3. Auscultopercussion test/ Auscultoscraping test

to find out the greater curvature of the stomach.

Procedure: Keep the "bell" of stethoscope in the centre of epigastrium (ask the patient to hold the bell of steth) and percuss radially. Stomach gives a dull note because of fluid. When the note is changed it indicates the greater curvature of stomach. Mark it on the abdomen (instead of percussion, scraping can be done with finger nail). 3 or 4 such marks, when joined, outlines greater curvature of the stomach.

Electrolyte changes in gastric outlet obstruction

- Hypochloraemic alkalosis
- Hyponatraemia
- Hypokalaemia
- Paradoxical aciduria (Key Box 23.9)

Key Box 23.9

PATHOGENESIS OF PARADOXICAL ACIDURIA

Gastric outlet obstruction (GOO)
due to CDU
↓
Vomiting
↓
Hypochloraemic alkalosis
↓
Excretion of HCL with sodium
↓
Hyponatraemia and dehydration
↓
Sodium retention and potassium and hydrogen excretion
↓
Hypokalaemia and paradoxical aciduria

Investigations

1. Barium meal X-ray

- Hugely dilated stomach (large and low stomach)

- Barium does not enter the duodenum. Barium mixed with food residue can give rise to mosaic appearance. Delay in evacuation (on repeated X-ray study) of barium into the duodenum.

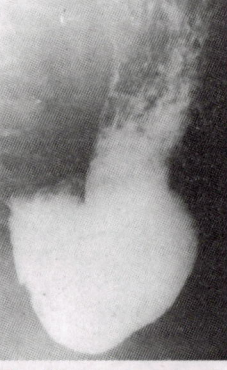

Fig.23.26 Hugely dilated stomach.

2. Gastroscopy

- The scope will not enter the duodenum. Stomach is full of foul smelling food residue.

- Gastroscopy is also done to rule out carcinoma of the stomach.

3. Electrolyte study (vide infra)

Treatment

A. Aspiration with Ryle's tube-good stomach wash, twice a day is given to keep the stomach empty. Saline is used as it decreases oedema of the stomach wall. At least 3-5 days before surgery, a stomach wash is given.

B. Blood is arranged for surgery. Blood may be required pre-operatively to treat anaemia.

C. Charts-Adequate urinary output is maintained by intravenous fluids

D. Drug-Antibiotics are given in the postoperative period

E. Exploratory laparotomy-**vagotomy followed by GJ is done.** Pyloroplasty should not be done because the duodenum is scarred, cicatrised, fibrosed and narrowed.

F Fluids to correct electrolyte abnormalities. Pyloric stenosis patients can develop "Hyponatraemic, Hypochloraemic, Hypokalaemic alkalosis", Ringer lactate is an ideal supplement.

- Post-operatively these patients recover very fast. Dehydration improves and nutritionally they show dramatic improvement. Even the gastric tone may return after few years.

Differential diagnosis of gastric outlet obstruction

- Carcinoma pyloric antrum (refer Table 23.4)

Table 23.4 Differential diagnosis of pyloric stenosis

	CICATRISED CHRONIC DUODENAL ULCER	CARCINOMA PYLORIC ANTRUM
1. Age	20-40 years	> 40-50 years
2. Duration of the symptoms	Long duration of abdominal pain and recent history of vomiting	Pain is usually absent, but vomiting is a feature. Symptoms are of short duration
3. Appetite	Decreased because of vomiting	Severe loss of appetite
4. Weight loss	Present	Significant
5. Anaemia	Not a feature	Present
6. Mass	**NOT PALPABLE**	HARD, IRREGULAR MASS IS PALPABLE

1. The palpable mass is the deciding clinical factor (sign). Other differences cannot truly differentiate between the two conditions. Rarely, carcinoma of the stomach is also seen in young patients at the age of 20. In congenital, hypertrophic pyloric stenosis, the mass is palpable (Page 359).

TEAPOT DEFORMITY - HANDBAG STOMACH (Fig. 23.27)

- A long-standing lesser curve gastric ulcer causes shortening of the lesser curvature due to fibrosis. Such stomach resembles a teapot. As a result of this, the pylorus becomes non-dependent. Hence, stasis occurs.

- **Treatment:**

  Partial gastrectomy followed by Billroth I anastomosis.

HOURGLASS CONTRACTURE (Fig. 23.28)

- When a saddle-shaped ulcer in the lesser curvature gets cicatrised, it involves both surfaces of the stomach resulting in conversion of stomach into two compartments.
- Features of stasis such as fullness, distension, persistent vomiting are present.
- Females are affected more often.
- Weight loss is present. Appetite is decreased.
- It is treated by **Billroth I partial gastrectomy** with removal of 2nd pouch.

PENETRATION INTO PANCREAS

- Posterior gastric ulcer can penetrate into pancreas, resulting in severe referred pain to the back resembling pancreatic pathology. However, this type of pain is relieved on lying down.

CARCINOMA OF THE STOMACH

- It is a complication of benign gastric ulcer. Incidence is around 2%.

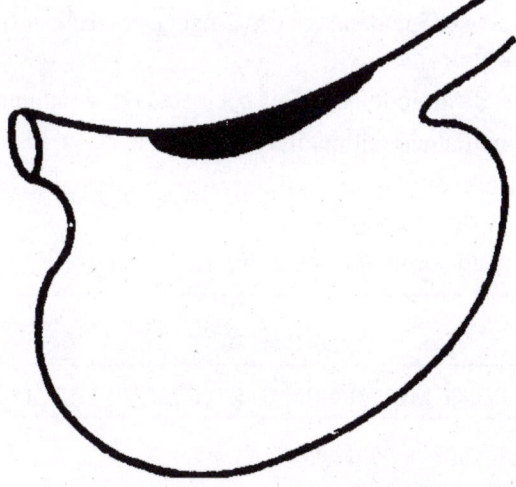

Fig. 23.27 Tea-pot deformity

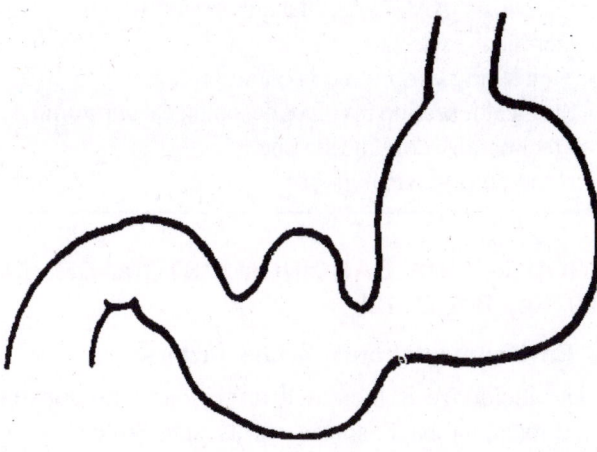

Fig. 23.28 Hourglass contracture of the stomach

CARCINOMA STOMACH

CLINICAL NOTES

A 32 year old male was admitted with loss of appetite of 3 months duration. Endoscopy revealed a growth in the body of the stomach. At exploration, large para-aortic nodes were present. Subtotal gastrectomy was done. The patient died after 6 months due to extensive metastasis. No wonder, carcinoma of the stomach is called **Captain of men of death.**

Certain facts about carcinoma stomach (Key Box 23.10, 23.11)

Key Box 23.10

CERTAIN FACTS ABOUT CARCINOMA STOMACH

- Increased incidence of proximal gastric cancer (OG junction)
- Distal carcinomas in low socioeconomic patients
- Proximal carcinoma in rich patients
- Carcinoma body and antrum is associated with H.Pylori infection
- Overall survival has not improved much

Key Box 23.11

CARCINOMA PROXIMAL STOMACH (CARDIA)

- Incidence is increasing
- More aggressive
- Thin muscularis mucosa hence submucosal invasion early
- Diagnosis may also get delayed as endoscopy needs technical expertise
- Signet ring carcinoma is common here
- Surgical resection involves oesophageal anastomosis - technically demanding one
- Hence prognosis is poor

AETIOLOGY OF CARCINOMA STOMACH (Fig. 23.29, Key Box 23.12)

1. Environmental and Dietary factors

- The incidence is increased in persons who consume red meat, cabbage, spices, spirits, salt-fish etc.
- Smoked salmon fish was responsible for increased in-

Key Box 23.12

FOOD PRODUCTS WHICH MAY BE CARCINOGENIC

- Smoked food
- Spirits
- Smoking
- Salted food
- Contaminated water rich in lead, zinc and nitrosamines (with soil)

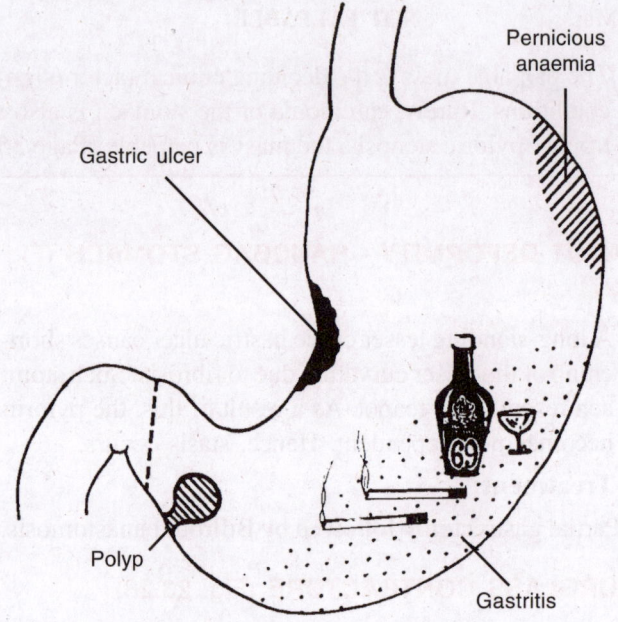

Fig. 23.29 Aetiology of carcinoma stomach

cidence of carcinoma stomach in Japanese population. Probably, it is related to release of polycyclic hydrocarbons and aromatic amino acids. Smoking, spicy food and alcohol taken over a period of many years produce chronic gastritis which may change into carcinoma of stomach.

WHO recommends- Increased fruits and vegetable consumption. VIT-C antioxidant is a protective agent.

2. Precancerous conditions

a) Atrophic gastritis: This may be due to smoking, spicy food, continuous ingestion of drugs, reflux of bile into the stomach etc.

b) Pernicious anaemia patients have increased risk (four to six times) of development of carcinoma when compared to general population.

- It causes atrophic gastritis and precipitates carcinoma of fundus of the stomach.

c) Patients with **hypogammaglobulinaemia** (50 fold increase) are at high risk.

d) H. pylori infection results in atrophic gastritis, followed by the intestinal type of gastric mucosa, then metaplasia, then dysplasia. Eventually it leads to **intestinal type of gastric cancer.** H. pylori also cause proliferation of gastric cancer cells and decrease secretion of vitamin 'C'.

- Also both **type A** and **type B** gastritis can predispose carcinoma stomach. Type A - Proximal stomach, Type B - Distal stomach.

e) Adenomatous polyps which occur in the antrum have highest risk of malignant transformation (Larger more than 2 cm).

f) Menetrier's disease is a protein-losing enteropathy, along with giant hypertrophy of gastric mucosal folds. It is a precancerous condition.

g) Gastric ulcer (benign): Incidence of malignancy is 2% (0.5 to 5%). Carcinoma arising in a gastric ulcer is called as "*Ulcer Cancer of the Stomach*".

h) Previous GJ or gastric resection predisposes to development of carcinoma of the stomach after a period of 15-20 years. Such a carcinoma is described as stump carcinoma. Pathogenesis is related to development of atrophic gastritis, achlorhydria and duodenogastric bile reflux.

3. Genetic and familial factors

- Carcinoma stomach can run in families[1]. However, only 10% of patients give family history of carcinoma stomach.

- Carcinoma stomach is more common in blood group 'A' patients. These patients have different mucopolysaccharide secretion in the stomach and greater susceptibility to ingested carcinogens. These patients develop diffuse type of carcinoma.

PATHOLOGICAL TYPES AND PATHOLOGY

I. Gross types

1. **Cauliflower** like growth with friable tissue. This variety can give rise to melaena or bleeding causing anaemia.

2. **Infiltrative** type of lesion (diffuse) with dense submucosal fibrosis which convert the stomach into a small contracted, functionless stomach - **Linitis Plastica** or **Leather Bottle Stomach**. Mucosa may appear normal.

3. **Ulcerative** variety, with classical everted edges with central slough

4. **Ulcer cancer** refers to carcinoma arising in a preexisting gastric ulcer. In this variety, complete destruction of the muscle coat is present.

5. **Colloid carcinoma**-In this condition, malignant cells are separated by colloid material. This is the type which is common in women and gives rise to Krukenberg's tumour - Bilateral, bulky ovarian metastases common in premenopausal women (signet ring carcinoma produces this).

II. Depending on depth of invasion

1. **Early Gastric Cancer:** Cancer limited to the mucosa and submucosa with or without lymph node involvement (T1 and N). This is represented below as Japanese Classification (Fig. 23.30)

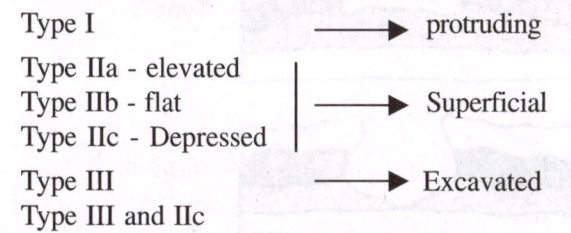

Type I	$\longrightarrow$ protruding
Type IIa - elevated Type IIb - flat Type IIc - Depressed	$\longrightarrow$ Superficial
Type III	$\longrightarrow$ Excavated
Type III and IIc	

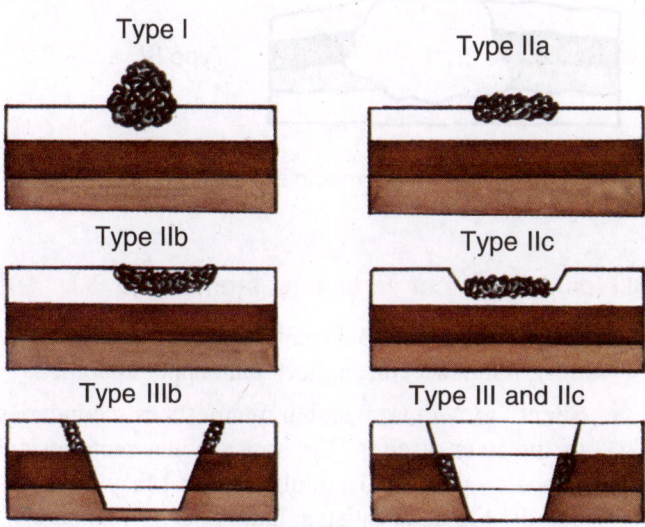

Fig. 23.30 Japanese classification

---

1. Napoleon Bonaparte, his father, brother, grandfather and three sisters died of carcinoma stomach

Criticism for early gastric cancer

- 5 year survival in **node negative** early gastric cancer is more than 95%. However it falls to 70% if nodes are positive. Hence the suggestion - node positive cases should not be included under early gastric cancer.

2. **Advanced gastric cancer:** It refers to involvement of muscularis mucosa and/or serosa with or without involvement of lymphnodes.

Borrmann's classification

- Type I   -   single polypoidal carcinoma
- Type II   -   ulceroproliferative
- Type III   -   ulcerative
- Type IV   -   diffuse carcinoma

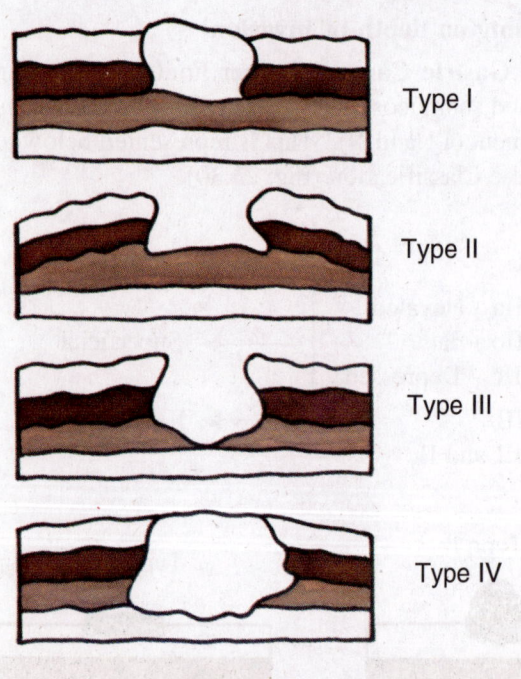

Type I

Type II

Type III

Type IV

Fig. 23.31 Borrmann's classification

Clinical features of carcinoma stomach (S O L I D)[1]

- Very often patients would have vague symptoms - early satiety, flatulence, discomfort, pain upper abdomen.

S - Silent : growth is silent but manifests as secondaries in the liver, ascites, Virchow's node, rectovesical deposits, umbilical nodule (Sister Mary Joseph's nodule- Fig. 23.34), left axillary nodes (Irish nodes).

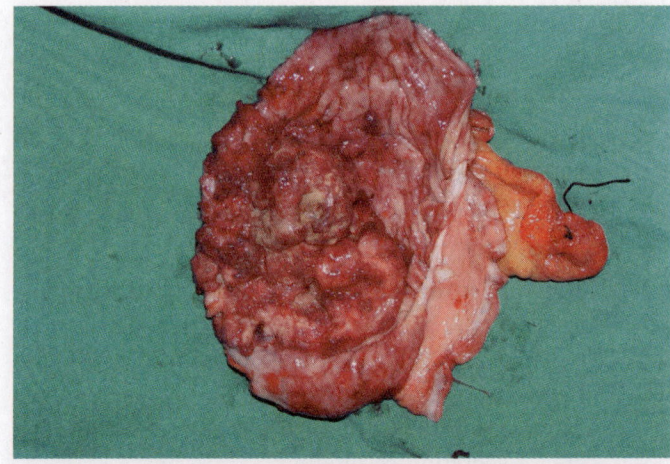

Fig. 23.32 Carcinoma stomach ulcerative variety gives rise to bleeding, hence anaemia

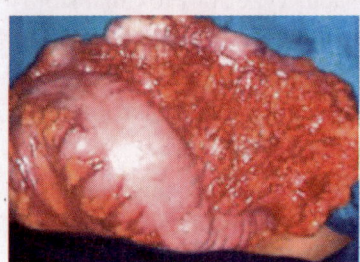

Fig. 23.33 Carcinoma stomach with nodules in the greater omentum

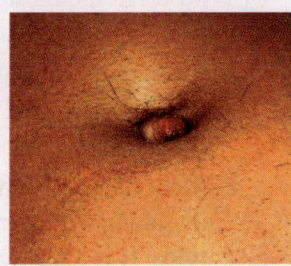

Fig. 23.34 Umbilical nodule -popularly called as Sister Mary Joseph's nodule

O -Obstruction at pylorus (pyloric antrum) with features of vomiting with / without blood. VGP can also be present. Obstruction at cardio-oesophageal junction, producing dysphagia.

L - Lump in the abdomen which is hard and irregular. Clinically, stomach mass is differentiated from liver mass by features mentioned below.

I - Insidious in onset-Anaemia, anorexia, and asthenia of short duration (Fig. 23.32)

D -Dyspepsia in a man over the age of 40, carcinoma stomach should be ruled out. Early gastric cancer presents as dyspepsia.

Features of stomach mass

1. Stomach moves with respiration
2. Upper border of the stomach mass can be made out
3. Anatomical location of the mass-right hypochondrium

---

1. If you know in carcinoma stomach **SOLID**, you will get solid marks!!!

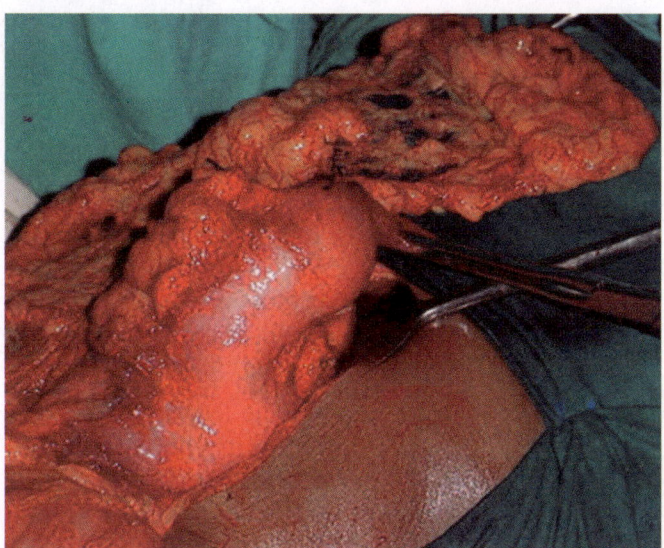

Fig. 23.35 Carcinoma stomach with involvement of serosa

in a pyloric mass, epigastrium and left hypochondrium in a mass arising from body of the stomach.

4. Knee elbow position-The mass does fall forwards, unless fixed

5. The mass may have intrinsic mobility

SPREAD

1. **Penetration of gastric serosa:** This is the most important prognostic indicator. When serosa is NOT penetrated 50% survive for 5 years after resection. When serosa is penetrated this figure drops to 20%.
   - Once serosa is involved adjacent organs - liver, pancreas, spleen, omentum, transverse colon get involved.

2. **Lymphatic spread:** 420 lymphnodes have been identified (Refer Page 345).
   - Lymph node involvement is a poor prognostic indicator.
   - Involvement of 4 or more nodes is less favourable.

Lymphatic zones: Lymphatic drainage from the stomach has been classified into 4 zones.

Zone 1 : In the gastrocolic omentum along the right gastroepiploic vessels. This drains the pyloric antrum and lower half of greater curvature.

Zone 2 : It lies in the gastrocolic omentum and gastrosplenic ligament along the left gastroepiploic vessels. This drains upper half of the greater curvature.

Zone 3: It lies in the lesser omentum draining proximal two thirds of the stomach. From here lymph drains into perioesophageal lymph nodes.

Zone 4: It is from distal portion of the lesser curve and pylorus along hepatic artery and right gastric artery into para aortic nodes.

3. **Blood spread:** Most common sites are liver and lungs. It produces extensive secondaries. They are signs of inoperability.

4. **Transcoelomic spread** results in ascites, Krukenberg Tumour - bilateral bulky ovarian deposits and rectovesical deposits. (Blummer's shelf).

INVESTIGATIONS

1. **Complete blood picture:** 20% of early gastric patients have anaemia, iron deficiency - microcytic. Preoperative blood transfusion may be necessary.

2. Routine examination, fasting and post-prandial sugars, ECG, renal function for fitness before surgery.

3. **Videoendoscopy**
   - To know the extent of the lesion
   - To confirm the diagnosis
   - To take 6 quadrant biopsy

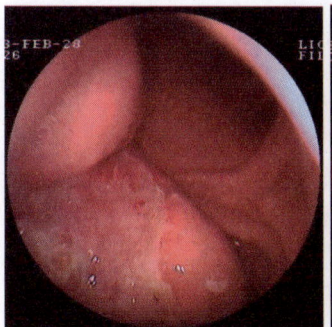 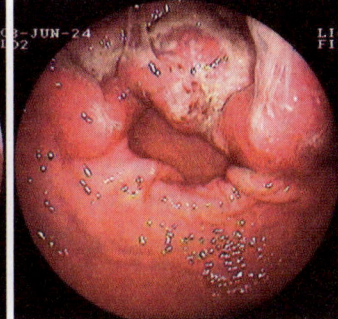

Fig. 23.36 Endoscopy showing superficial ulceration   **Fig. 23.37** Endoscopy showing ulcero-proliferative growth

4. **Ultrasound, C.T. Scan and MRI**
   - To rule out secondaries in liver
   - To look for enlarged coeliac nodes
   - Ascites can also be demonstrated
   - To detect Krukenberg tumour
   - Useful in detecting metastatic disease

5. **Endoscopic ultrasonography** can differentiate early gastric cancer from advanced tumours in 80% of patients.

4. **Barium meal** may show intrinsic, persistent, irregular, filling defect. Double contrast air-barium study is used for mass screening in Japan to detect early cases.

- Barium meal study is useful in cases of linitis plastica wherein mucosa may be normal in early cases.

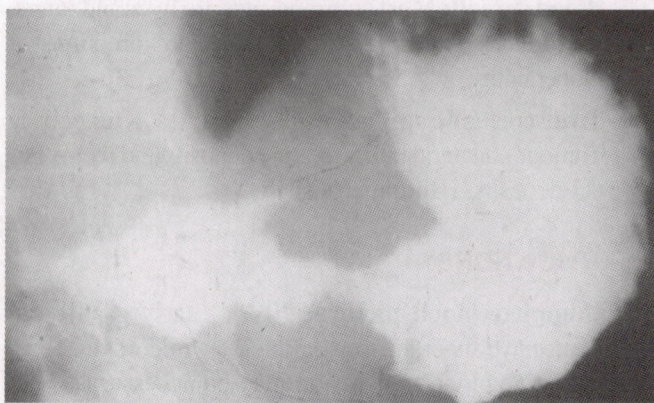

Fig. 23.38 Barium meal study showing filling defect

STAGING[1]

Key Box 23.13
TNM STAGING OF CARCINOMA STOMACH
T : Primary tumor
T_0 : No evidence of primary tumour
Tis : Carcinoma in situ
T_1 : Invasion of lamina-propria or submucosa
T_2 : Invasion of muscularis propria or subserosa
T_3 : Penetration of serosa
T_4 : Invasion of adjacent structures
N : Lymph nodes
N_0 : No regional lymph nodes
N_1 : 1-6 lymph nodes positive for malignancy
N_2 : 7-15 lymph nodes positive for malignancy
N_3 : More than 15 lymph nodes positive for malignancy
M : Metastasis
M_0 : No distant metastasis
M_1 : Distant metastasis present

Please Note: This staging is after surgical resection. Lymph node stations (Key Box 23.15) are **not related to** number of lymph nodes involved by malignancy in TNM staging.

1. It is desirable to know the staging to get more marks.

HISTOPATHOLOGY

- It is an adenocarcinoma of the stomach. There are basically two types of gastric carcinomas as per Lauren's classification. It is also called D.I.O. classification. (Key Box 23.14)

D DIFFUSE is more common in young, females and carries poor prognosis.

I INTESTINAL is more common in elderly males. It shows areas of intestinal metaplasia. It has better prognosis.

O OTHERS (mixed lesions). The leather-bottle stomach or linitis plastica is poorly differentiated with anaplastic cells.

Key Box 23.14
COMPARISON OF INTESTINAL AND DIFFUSE TYPE

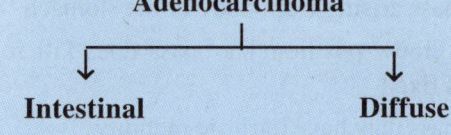

Adenocarcinoma

Intestinal	Diffuse
• Similar to adenocarcinoma colon - gland formation	• No gland formation
• Defined by cellular architecture	• Defined by pattern of growth
• Polypoidal Tumours, superficial spreading, ulcerative are examples.	• Linitis plastica, ulcerative variety
• Synchronous cancers are more common in this type	• Not common
• Duodenal involvement rare	• 25% of diffuse variety involves duodenum
• Good prognosis	• Poor prognosis

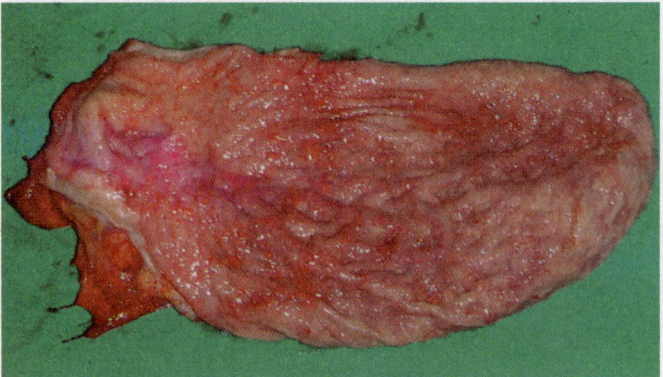

Fig. 23.39 Intestinal type of carcinoma stomach

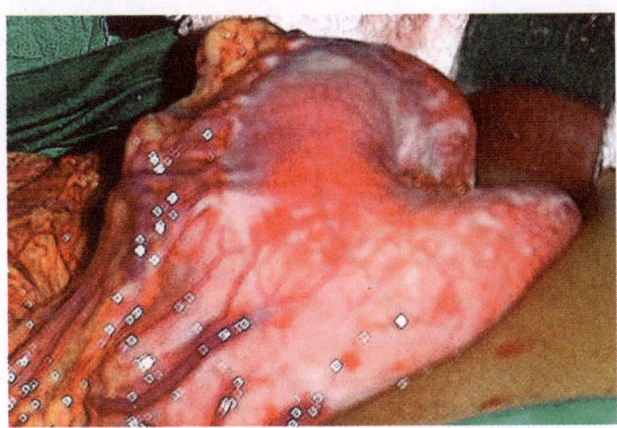

Fig. 23.40 Diffuse type of carcinoma stomach

TREATMENT OF CARCINOMA STOMACH

- **SURGERY** is the main modality of the treatment. Adjuvant chemotherapy has been found to be beneficial in a few patients only.
- Resectable means the growth can be removed.
- Inoperable means there are no chances of cure but growth may be resectable. Operable means cure is possible.

Signs of inoperability

- Growth fixed to pancreas or posterior abdominal wall
- Secondaries in the liver, hard nodular liver
- Rectovesical deposits, due to peritoneal seedlings which are felt on per rectal examination
- Enlarged, fixed coeliac nodes, paraaortic nodes and left supraclavicular nodes
- Krukenberg tumour, malignant ascites
- Sister Mary Joseph's nodule

Aim of surgery

1. Curative resection should be done whenever possible
2. Bypass procedure (GJ) to relieve vomiting in advanced cases or palliative gastrectomy in appropriate cases (bleeding).
3. Palliative gastrectomy can be done to remove a fungating, ulcerative, bleeding mass. It gives better palliation.

CURATIVE RESECTIONS

A resection is considered to be curative if:

- There is no evidence of microscopic or gross residual tumour.

- Serosa is not involved (this means that curative resection is not possible for T3/T4 tumours.
- There is no evidence of metastatic disease
- D resection exceeds the nodal involvement by one

    N0 - D1 resection is curative

    N1 - D2 resection is curative and so on.

- Japanese Research Society for gastric cancer advocates very aggressive resection including lymphadenectomy. Hence more details of lymph node station are given in Key Box 23.15. However the rest of the cancer research groups were not able to produce the same results as the Japanese.
- D_1 resection refers to the removal of primary group of nodes such as nodes along the lesser and greater curvature, juxtapyloric nodes etc.
- D_2 resection refers to the removal of lymph nodes such as left gastric, common hepatic, splenic, retropancreatic nodes, etc.
- D_3 resection refers to the removal of lymph nodes such as para-aortic, porta hepatis nodes, behind the head of the pancreas, etc.
  - In the presence of serosal invasion, the number of

Japanese classification of nodes at surgery

Key Box 23.15
LYMPH NODE STATIONS

Station No.		
1-2	:	Adjacent to cardiac end
3-4	:	Adjacent to lesser and greater curve
5	:	Suprapyloric (Rt. gastric nodes)
6	:	Infrapyloric
7	:	Left gastric artery
8	:	Common hepatic artery
9	:	Coeliac artery
10	:	Hilum of spleen
11	:	Splenic artery
12	:	Hepatoduodenal ligament
13	:	Behind pancreatic head - retropancreatic
14	:	At root of mesentery (SMA)
15	:	Middle colic
16	:	Paraaortic

D_2 refers to the removal of stations 1 to 11 - average 27 nodes

D_3 refers to the removal of stations 1 to 16 - average 43

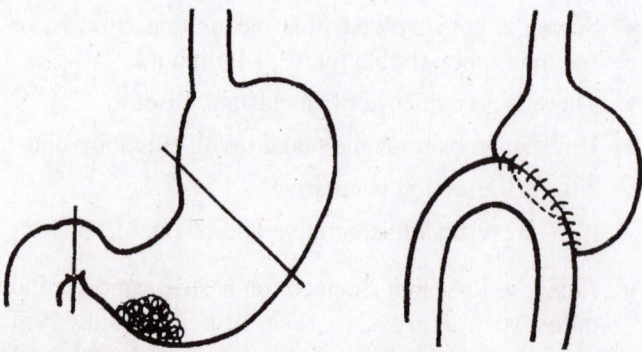

Fig. 23.41 Radical subtotal gastrectomy with Billroth II anastomosis

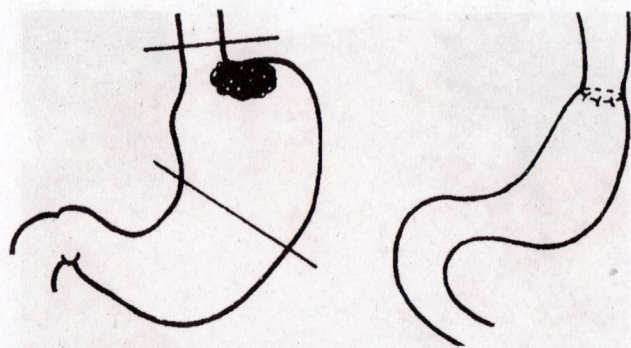

Fig. 23.42 Radical upper gastrectomy with oesophagogastric anastomosis

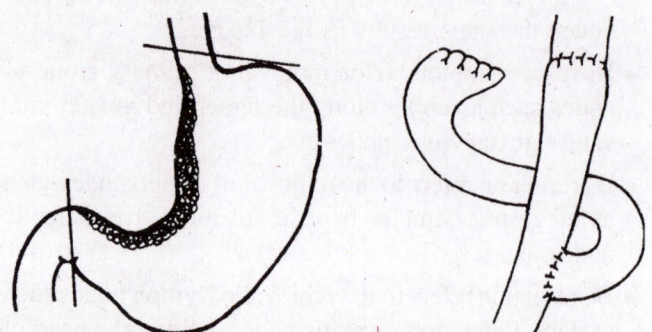

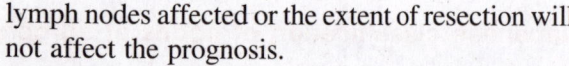

Fig. 23.43 Radical total gastrectomy, with Roux-en-y oesophagojejunostomy

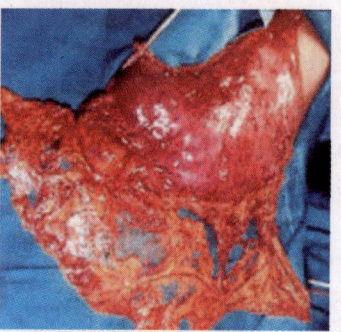

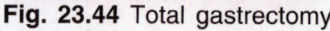

Fig. 23.44 Total gastrectomy

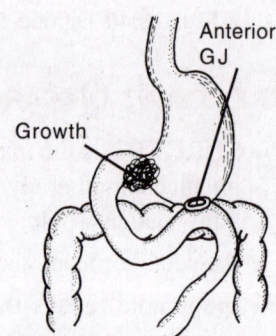

Fig. 23.45 Palliative anterior G.J.

lymph nodes affected or the extent of resection will not affect the prognosis.

1. **Carcinoma of pyloric antrum and body of the stomach.**
   - Radical subtotal gastrectomy which includes the removal of 60- 70% of the stomach, with greater omentum along with enlarged lymph nodes followed by gastrojejunal anastomosis is the treatment of choice.(Fig. 23.42).

2. **Carcinoma of the fundus:** Oesophago-gastrectomy (Fig. 23.42). Removal of the upper part of the stomach, lower end of oesophagus, with regional lymph nodes and spleen, followed by oesophagogastric anastomosis or oesophagojejunal anastomosis.

3. **Diffuse growth (linitis plastica) :** Radical total gastrectomy followed by oesophagojejunostomy.(Fig. 23.43, 23.44)

PALLIATIVE SURGERY (Fig. 23.45)

1. Carcinoma pyloric antrum (inoperable). Palliative anterior GJ is done to relieve vomiting, by anastomosing a jejunal loop to the stomach in the prepyloric region (Fig. 23.39). If posterior GJ is done the growth may involve the GJ stoma early resulting in stomal obstruc-

tion. With anterior G.J entero-enterostomy can be added to prevent bilious vomiting.

2. Palliative gastrectomy to get rid of ulcerated, necrotic or bleeding lesion.

CHEMOTHERAPY FOR CARCINOMA STOMACH

- Now it is understood that gastric cancers partially respond to chemotherapy - in about 30% of cases given at advanced stage (Results are better than cancer colon). Injection 5-FU (Fluorouracil) 500 mg IV daily for five days, every 28 days. It can be given by IV infusion or IV bolus over 15 minutes.

- **Mechanism of action:** It is an antimetabolite and acts by interfering with DNA synthesis. Side effects are myelosuppression, mucositis, excessive lacrimation, nausea, vomiting, etc.

- Combination of 5 FU with adriamycin (Doxorubicin), mitomycin and cisplatin also has been tried. However, toxicity is more with these drugs. FAM (5 fluoruracil, adriamycin and mitomycin C) and ECF (Epirubicin, cisplatinum and 5-FU) are popular agents.

- Intraperitoneal mitomycin and mitomycin C-impregnated charcol also has been used (Target the recurrence site-gastric bed).

Other tumours of the stomach

GASTROINTESTINAL STROMAL TUMOURS (GIST)

- Previously named leiomyoma, leiomyosarcoma are called as GIST, today.
- In gastrointestinal tract, **stomach is the commonest** site of GIST.
- **Bleeding** is the commonest presentation. It occurs due to ulceration of mucosa which on endoscopy gives **Cervix appearance** (Fig 23.46).

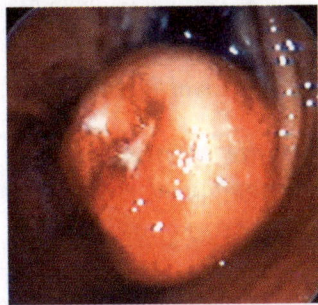

Fig. 23.46 Bleeding ulcer of the stomach

- Larger tumours can present with dysphagia, weight loss, anaemia, palpable mass.

The diagnosis of malignancy is by greater mitotic figures.

- **If mucosa is not ulcerated, biopsy on a biopsy** or well biopsy is necessary.
- Immunohistochemistry is mandatory for diagnosis
- CT scan is useful investigation
- Resection is the best treatment

Chemotherapy for GIST

- Capsule imatinib 100 mg 4 capsules - to a total of 400mg per day is given till toxicity appears or metastasis or residual tumour regresses (Investigated by CT scan). This is a promising new drug.

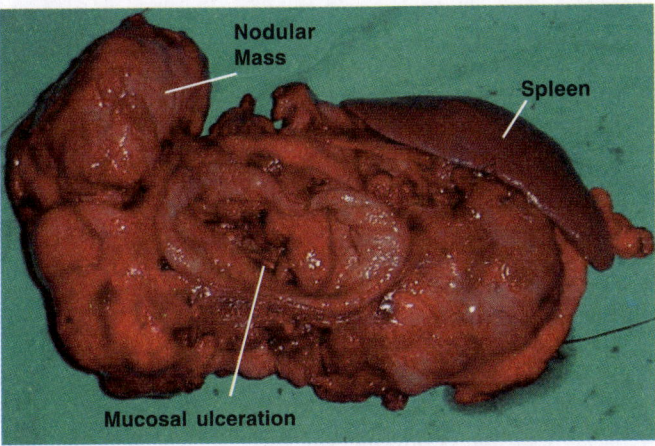

Fig. 23.47 A large GIST arising from the fundus of the stomach presenting as a nodular mass in the left hypochondrium resected successfully with spleen

GASTRIC LYMPHOMA

- Incidence of primary gastric lymphoma is increasing.
- They are B-cell derived - from mucosa associated lymphoid tissue (**MALT**) - **MALTOMA**.
- Pain, weight loss, bleeding are common presentation.
- **6th decade** is the common age group.
- Endoscopic features are not specific but diffuse thickening with or without ulcerations.
- It is important to rule out **generalized process** by CT, ultrasound, bone marrow aspirate.
- Gastrectomy is the best treatment
- Chemotherapy is better for systemic disease

Lymphoma associated with H. pylori infection may regress and totally disappear after eradication treatment for H. pylori.

DIFFERENTIAL DIAGNOSIS OF HAEMATEMESIS (Upper GI tract bleeding)

- Haematemesis refers to vomiting of fresh red blood. Melenemesis refers to vomiting of dark altered blood. However, both are included under upper GI tract bleeding. Small bowel, even though is a midgut structure, some of its lesions can produce haematemesis. Hence, they are also included under this heading.

CAUSES (Fig. 23.48)

1. **Oesophageal causes**
   - Reflux oesophagitis
   - Mallory Weiss syndrome
   - Oesophageal varices
   - Cancer of oesophagus
2. **Gastric and duodenal causes**
   - Gastric ulcer
   - Acute erosive gastritis
   - Gastric cancer
   - Duodenal ulcer
   - Gastric polyp
   - Dieulafoy vascular malformation
3. **Intestinal causes**
   - Peutz-Jegher's syndrome
   - Polyps, Meckel's diverticulum

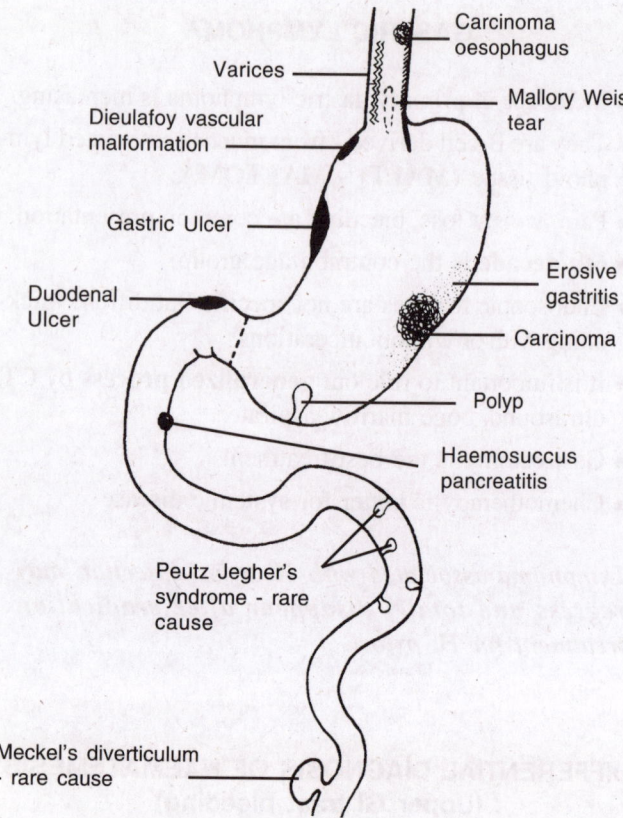

Fig. 23.48 Various causes of haemetemesis

4. Other rare causes

- Purpura
- Haemophilia
- Pernicious anaemia
- A.V. fistula
- Liver diseases

Acute erosive gastritis, chronic peptic ulcer and oesophageal varices constitute almost 90% of the cases.

INITIAL ASSESSMENT: Refer the table 23.5

INVESTIGATIONS

- **Fibreoptic endoscopy** should be done on an emergency basis within 6 to 36 hours of admission. It can diagnose variceal bleeding, erosive gastritis, bleeding peptic ulcer, carcinoma stomach etc.
- Only when endoscopy cannot yield any diagnosis, selective coeliac angiography should be done which can detect uncommon causes such as angiodysplasia of the stomach or bleeding from a rolling hernia etc.

Table 23.5 Initial assessment	
1. History	**Probable causes**
Abuse of drugs and alcohol	Acute erosive gastritis
Previous abdominal pain	Chronic peptic ulcer
H/O jaundice, liver cell failure	Oesophageal varices
Anaemia, loss of weight, loss of appetite	Carcinoma stomach
Violent vomiting-haematemesis	Mallory-Weiss syndrome
2. General physical examination	
Testicular atrophy, gynaecomastia, etc.	Cirrhosis of the liver
Palpable left supraclavicular node	Carcinoma stomach
Arthritis-multiple joint involvement	Acute erosive gastritis (use of NSAID)
Purpuric spots	Bleeding tendencies
3. Abdominal examination	
Palpable spleen, ascites	Portal hypertension
Palpable stomach mass	Carcinoma stomach
Tenderness in the epigastrium	Peptic ulcer disease
4. Assessment of haemorrhage	
Massive haemorrhage (more than 1,000 ml of blood)	Portal hypertension, acute erosive gastritis.
Moderate haemorrhage (500-1000 ml of blood)	Chronic peptic ulcer
Mild haemorrhage (less then 500 ml of blood)	Chronic peptic ulcer
	Other causes

Table 23.6 Surgery for haemetemesis

CAUSES	CONSERVATIVE	SURGICAL METHOD
1. Acute erosive gastritis	Yes	Rare - gastrectomy
2. Chronic duodenal ulcer	Yes	Rare - vagotomy, underrunning, pyloroplasty
3. Chronic gastric ulcer	Yes	Rare - vagotomy + partial gastrectomy
4. Mallory-Weiss syndrome	Yes	Suturing of the tear
5. Cancer of the stomach	No	Gastrectomy
6. Duodenal polyp	Endoscopic snaring	Surgery, if endoscopic facility not available
7. Bleeding Meckel's	No	Diverticulectomy
8. Variceal bleeding	Yes, Sclerotherapy	Devascularisation
9. Haemosuccus pancretitis	Yes, Therapeutic embolisation	Ligation of pseudo aneurysm
10. Dieulafoy leision	Yes, Injection sclerotherapy	Wide excision

Barium study is done to rule out intestinal causes in less urgent cases.

- **Isotope studies:** Intravenous injection of **99^{m} Tc pertechnetate** can demonstrate hypertrophic gastric like mucosa in **Meckel's diverticulum.**

Treatment

- Initial management is to treat the shock in the line discussed for peptic ulcer haemorrhage.

Indication for surgery

1. Elderly patients with re-bleed in the hospital
2. Rarity of blood groups
3. Spurting vessel in an endoscopy

Surgery

- Surgical management of individual case has been discussed along with the chapter. However, summary of the treatment is discussed in Table 23.6.
- Thus, upper GI bleeding can occur due to various causes. However, acute erosive gastritis, chronic peptic ulcer, oesophageal varices are the three important causes of bleeding. Endoscopy is the investigation for the diagnosis of upper GI bleeding. Today, most of the upper GI bleeding is managed either in the form of injection sclerotherapy, laser coagulation or with powerful H2 blockers or with proton pump inhibitors. In appropriate cases, surgery is definitely indicated. Few common conditions which gives rise to haematemesis are discussed in the following pages.

ACUTE PEPTIC ULCER

- They are also called as acute erosive gastritis/acute stress ulcers / acute steroidal ulcers and **Acute Gastric Mucosal Lesions (AGML)**

Aetiology

- Drugs-aspirin, analgin, steroids, phenylbutazone
- Any stress, acute infection which results in sepsis
- Following tetanus
- After burns they are called **Curling's Ulcer**
- After head injury or neurosurgical operations "Cushing's Ulcer
- Following **hypotension** and shock which produces **hypoperfusion,** which results in **mucosal ischaemia**, which results in acute stress ulcers. Example : myocardial infarction.
- Excessive consumption of spirits and smoking
- Respiratory failure can also produce acute erosions

Pathology

- There is a diffuse mucosal damage and disruption of gastric mucosal barrier. Reflux of bile also may be a precipitating factor. This results in acute erosions when they are 1 to 2 mm or acute ulcers when they are 1 to 2 cm in size, shallow, well demarcated. The entire stomach is involved by these ulcers.

Clinical features

- Dyspepsia due to minor bleeding

- Haematemesis - sometimes massive, fresh bleeding can produce hypotension and shock.
- Acute abdominal pain due to acute erosions or perforation of an acute ulcer.
- In ICU: **drop in BP**, nasogastric aspirate of blood and or melaena.

Diagnosis

- Emergency endoscopy to confirm diagnosis

Key Box 23.16

ENDOSCOPIC FINDINGS OF RE-BLEED RISKS

- Pulsatile vessel
- Fresh clot
- Adherent clot
- Visible vessel in the base

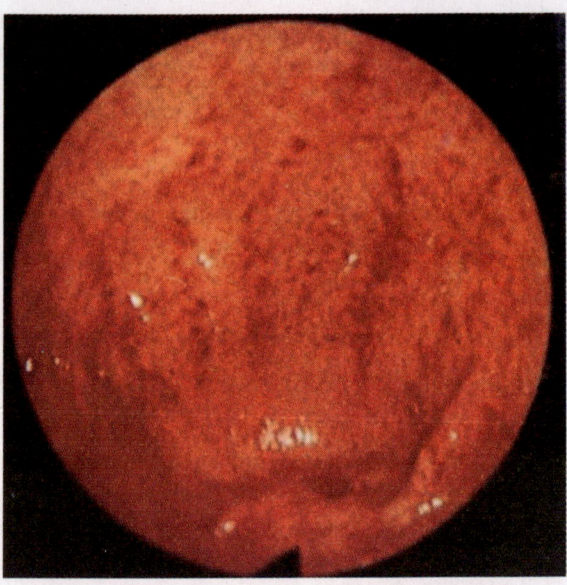

Fig. 23.49 Endoscopy showing erosions

Treatment of acute peptic ulcers with bleeding

1. Admission in intensive care unit (ICU) - Key Box 23.17
2. Ryle's tube, empty the stomach, ice cold water or saline stomach wash (vasoconstriction).
3. Regular antacids 20-30 ml, 2nd hourly, preferably cold antacids.
4. Replacement of blood
5. Injection ranitidine I.V. 50 mg 8th hourly or I.V. pantoprazole 20 mg. Majority of cases respond to conservative line of treatment.

Key Box 23.17

VERY IMPORTANT MEASURES IN ICU

- Correct coagulopathy
- Improve oxygenation
- Blood transfusion, Control sepsis

---

6. **Endotherapy:** If there is solitary bleeding site (Page 336)
7. In spite of above treatment, to save the life of the patient, a total gastrectomy or a subtotal gastrectomy may be necessary (very very rare).

MALLORY-WEISS SYNDROME

Aetiopathogenesis (Key Box 23.18)

- It occurs due to a tear in the gastric mucosa near the oesophagogastric junction (OG).
- Also called as partial thickness mucosal rupture.

Key Box 23.18

CONDITION WHEREIN MALLORY WEISS TEAR IS SEEN

Spirit or alcohol
Pancreatitis
Infarction myocardial
Renal failure
Infection - Cholecystitis
Tumour - pregnancy

* You can remember as **SPIRIT**

Clinical features

- The patient is usually a middle-aged male who, after consumption of alcohol, vomits the food contents first. During the course of vomiting because of straining and retching, a tear develops near the oesophagocardiac junction. Hence, the **second vomitus contains blood**.
- Sometimes, the bleeding can be so massive to produce hypotension and shock. In 90% of cases, bleeding stops spontaneously.

Treatment

1. Urgent resuscitation of haemorrhagic shock
2. Endoscopy to confirm the diagnosis - Tear is seen in the lesser curvature

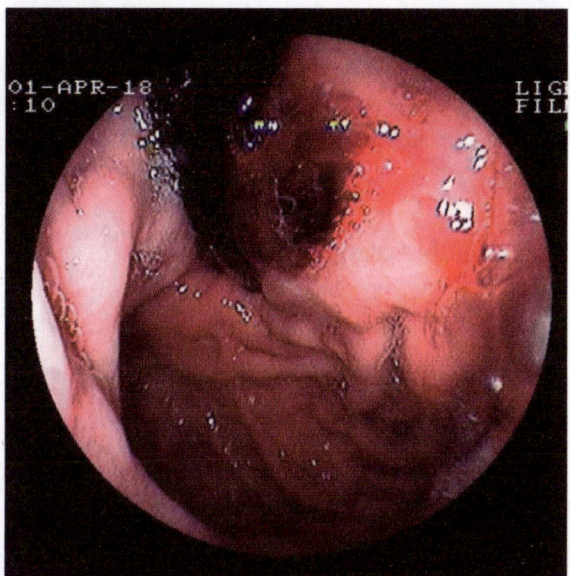

Fig. 23.50 Mallory Weiss tear - with the endotherapy bleeding stopped - Contributed by Dr. Filipe Alvaris, Gastroenterologist, KMC, Manipal

3. Blood transfusion
4. Ryle's tube aspiration for 48-72 hours
5. Endotherapy - injection adrenaline 1:10,000 dilution is effective
6. **High gastrotomy** and under-running is necessary when all other measures fail.

DIEULAFOY VASCULAR MALFORMATION

- In this condition, unusually large artery runs in the submucosa which lies in close contact with mucous membrane.
- Mucosal erosion precipitates the bleeding.
- In more than 80% cases, bleeding occurs within 6 cms from OG junction, at the lesser curvature.
- Endoscopy, endotherapy should be tried, if necessary repeated also.
- Failure to achieve control of the bleeding - **Gastrotomy and wide excision** of the lesion should be done.

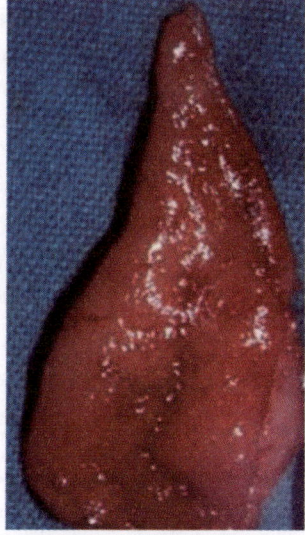

Fig. 23.51 Dieulafoy vascular malformation-excised

COMPLICATIONS OF GASTRIC OPERATIONS

- Can be classified as complications of vagotomy, complications of GJ and complications of gastrectomy.

COMPLICATIONS OF VAGOTOMY

1. Stasis of food in the stomach, resulting in nausea, loss of appetite, distension of upper abdomen, foul eructation, etc.
2. Denervation of gall bladder can cause gall stones
3. Post-vagotomy **diarrhoea**-Can be very troublesome at times (Key Box 23.19).
4. Vagotomy produces hypoacidity which allows bacterial proliferation. Nitrates are reduced to nitrites which are carcinogenic. Such a malignancy which develops at GJ site is called **stump carcinoma**.

Key Box 23.19
CAUSES OF DIARRHOEA

- Vagotomy results in removal of parasympathetic influence on the function of foregut, midgut
- Gastric emptying occuring fast due to GJ or gastrectomy
- Hypoacidity resulting in bacterial proliferation causing enteritis
- Bile salts also play a role

COMPLICATIONS OF GJ

STOMAL OBSTRUCTION

- It is due to oedema as in gastroduodenal anastomosis or non-dependent drainage as in GJ Sometimes, fat in the transverse mesocolon undergoes necrosis resulting in obstruction to the loops. Stomal obstruction also develops if there is narrowing of the lumen. Treatment is conservative. Surgery may also be required later, after confirming obstruction by gastro-grafin studies.

RETROGRADE JEJUNOGASTRIC INTUSSUSCEPTION

- It develops if efferent and afferent loops are not sutured properly. It can appear any time after surgery.

Clinical features

1. Previous history of abdominal surgery (surgery done for peptic ulcer)

2. Acute abdominal pain in upper abdomen

3. Vomiting, sometimes blood stained

4. **Palpable mass** in the upper abdomen

Investigation

- Barium meal X-ray shows filling defect in the stomach. Sometimes, following a barium meal, intussusception is reduced (Fig. 23.52).

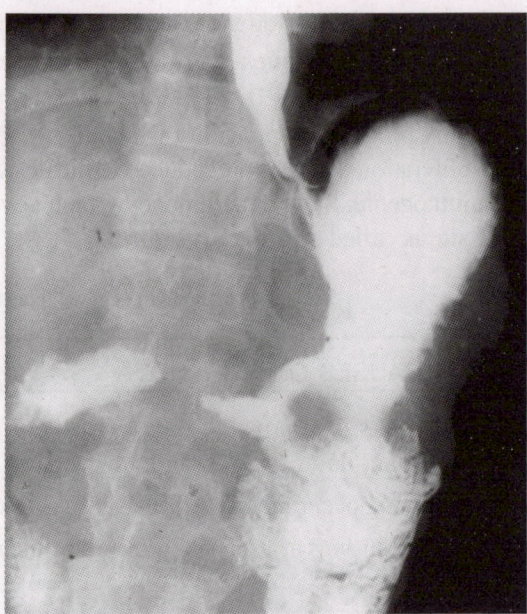

Fig. 23.52 Barium showing filling defect, in a patient who had undergone GJ

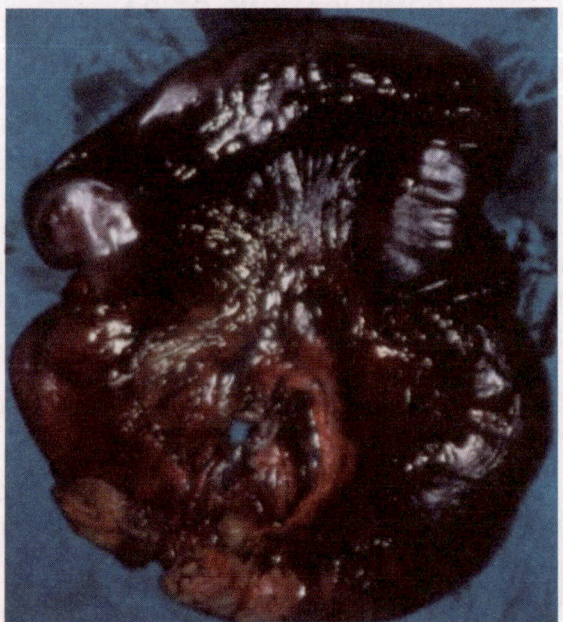

Fig. 23.53 Gangrene of the intestines in a patient who had jejunogastric intussusception

Treatment

- Reduction of the intussusception and suturing of intestinal loops properly. If the loops are gangrenous, resection may be necessary.

Complication

- Gangrene of intestine (Fig. 28.53)

GASTROJEJUNOCOLIC FISTULA

- It is a complication of GJ done for peptic ulcer, more so when vagotomy is not done or incomplete.

- After few years of G.J, a recurrent ulcer can develop at the stoma-GJ site (Fig. 28.54, 28.55).

- This recurrent ulcer slowly invades the adjacent structure such as the transverse colon resulting in gastrojejunocolic fistula.

Clinical features

1. Previous history of vagotomy and GJ

2. Foul eructation and foul vomiting due to colonic contents entering the stomach which is loaded with faecal matter and foul contents.

3. Intense diarrhoea due to severe jejunitis brought about by colonic bacteria entering the jejunum.

4. Rapid deterioration in health-loss of weight, loss of appetite, dehydration and emaciation.

Diarrhoea is not due to food entering the colon. Contents of the colon enter the stomach and then jejunum resulting in jejunitis resulting in diarrhoea.

Diagnosis

- Confirm by barium enema-barium entering the stomach (Because of high pressure in the colon) Barium meal should not be done.

Treatment

- Triple resection (Fig. 23.56, 23.57)

- Pre-operative preparation is necessary in the form of blood transfusion, stomach wash, nutritional supplementation and correction of dehydration.

- Resection of portion of stomach, portion of intestine and portion of colon and end to end anastomosis.

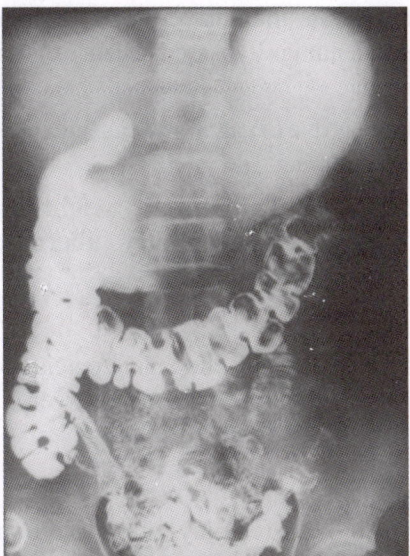

Fig. 23.54 Barium enema - Barium entering into the stomach from colon (Barium meal is not the investigation for Gastrojejunocolic fistula)

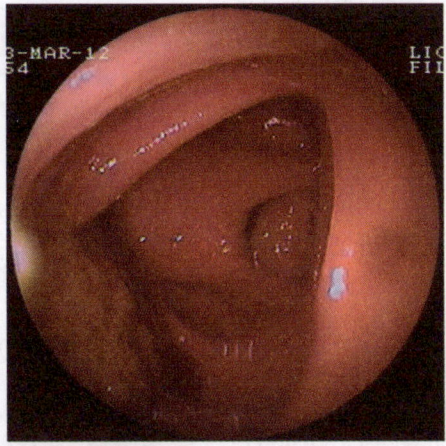

Fig. 23.55 Gastrojejunocolic fistula - Gastroscopy shows faecal matter in the stomach, coming from colon (see the traingular folds of colon)

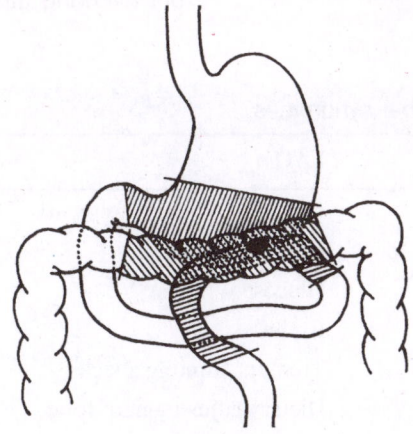

Fig. 23.56 Triple resection

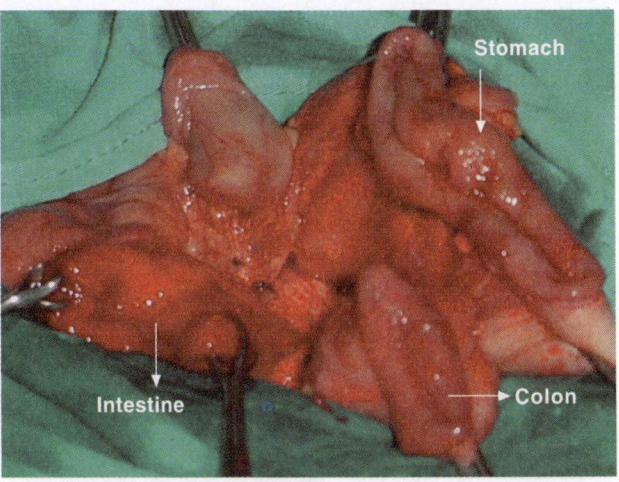

Fig. 23.57 Specimen of triple resection

STUMP CARCINOMA

- It refers to carcinoma developing in the stomach after some surgery on the stomach. Classically it happens after a gastrojejunostomy (GJ) or after a pyloroplasty.

- Reflux of bile, changes in the acidity due to vagotomy are the few factors which precipitate stump carcinoma.

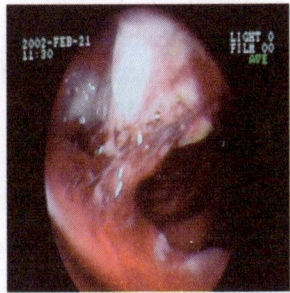

Fig. 23.58 Endoscopy showing stump carcinoma

- Clinical features include sudden loss of appetite, loss of weight with or without mass abdomen.

- Diagnosis is by barium meal or by endoscopy.

- Treated by resection. However, many cases are advanced and they are inoperable (Fig 23.59).

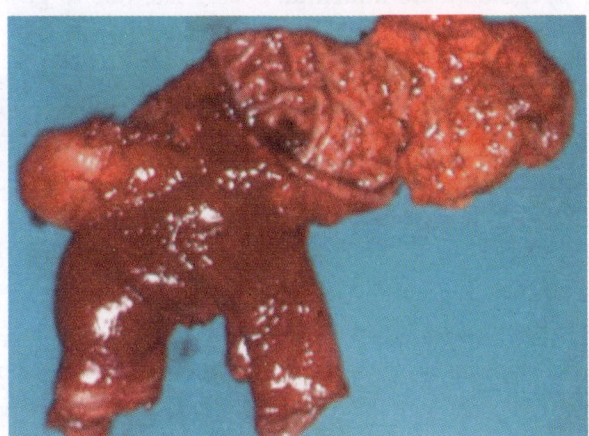

Fig. 23.59 Gastrectomy for stump carcinoma

GASTROILEOSTOMY: Fig 23.60

- It is an avoidable complication.
- Instead of the short loop - jejunum, ileum is anastomosed to the stomach
- There will be severe uncontrolled diarrhoea, loss of weight and emaciation within a short period.
- Barium meal with fluoroscopy should be done which shows rapid flow of barium from stomach into the ileum.
- Laparotomy - undoing of gastroileostomy and fresh gastrojejunostomy should be done.

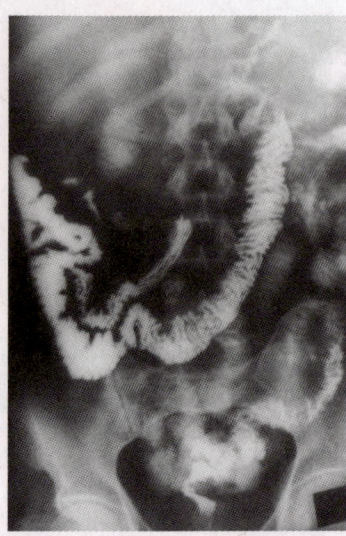

Fig. 23.60 Gastroileostomy - the biggest blunder which surgeon can do can be avoided by identifying the duodenojejunal flexure

POSTCIBAL SYNDROMES (Dumping syndrome)

- This syndrome complex results due to rapid emptying of stomach contents to the distal intestines resulting in various physiological changes like vasomotor symptoms, hypoglycaemia, etc. They are of two types. Their comparison is given in Table 23.7.

COMPLICATIONS OF GASTRECTOMY

1. NUTRITIONAL DISTURBANCES

- **Vitamin B12 and calcium deficiency**
- **Megaloblastic anaemia,** occurs late due to gastric mucosal atrophy.

- **Iron deficiency anaemia,** common after gastrectomy when duodenum is bypassed because of deficient iron absorption.
- **Diarrhoea** is due to vagotomy causing intestinal hurry or due to dumping.
- Due to poor nutrition, there is **weight loss** and they are susceptible for **pulmonary tuberculosis**.

2. DUODENAL FISTULA (DUODENAL BLOWOUT)

- It is the leakage of duodenal contents to the exterior. It commonly occurs after surgery.

Causes (Fig. 23.61)

- After a partial gastrectomy/total gastrectomy, where the closure of duodenum was difficult
- After closure of perforated duodenal ulcer, which gives way once again
- Injuries to duodenum during right hemicolectomy, right nephrectomy, etc.

Precipitating factors

- Faulty technique of closure of duodenal stump
- Severly inflamed duodenum due to an active ulcer
- If there is a distal obstruction, it increases tension in duodenal loop and may result in fistula
- Ischaemia of duodenal stump

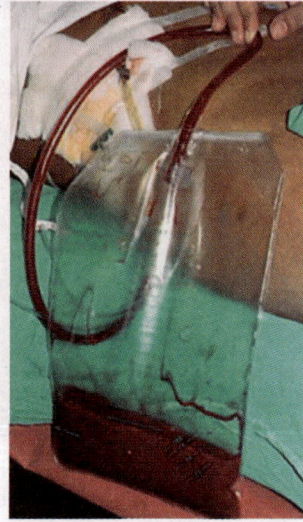

Fig. 23.61 Duodenal blow out following gastrectomy

	Table 23.7 Dumping syndrome - post cibal syndromes	
	EARLY	**LATE**
1. Onset	Immediately after meals	One to two hours afterwards.
2. Causes	Hypovolaemia due to rapid distension of efferent loop	Hypoglycaemia
3. Relief	Lying down	Glucose
4. Aggravating factors	More food	Exercise
5. Symptoms	Epigastric distension, sweating, diarrhoea	Tremors, fainting attacks
6. Treatment	Small, dry food. Over a period of time, symptoms settle down	Dietary adjustment of food

Clinical features

- Signs and symptoms develop usually after 4 to 5 days, at the time when oral fluids are started. These stimulate outpouring of biliary and pancreatic juices.
- Severe upper abdominal pain and guarding, rigidity, hypotension and shock-features of biliary peritonitis develop if there is no drainage tube
- If drainage tube is kept in the first surgery, bile flows to the exterior. In such cases, signs of peritonitis are usually not present. However, severe electrolyte imbalance can occur.

Treatment

- Conservative treatment is successful in majority of the cases. Fistula heals in a few days, provided there is no distal obstruction. During this time hydration, electrolyte care is essential. Appropriate antibiotics are given.
- Surgical-if the fistula persists, laparotomy and closure of the fistula can be done by repairing with non-absorbable sutures.

Complications

- Biliary peritonitis, septicaemia if bile is not drained outside.
- Excoriation of abdominal skin can be prevented by zinc oxide application.

3. RECURRENT ULCER

- It can be true anastomotic ulcer (gastrojejunal, gastroduodenal or jejunal ulcer), or a gastric ulcer in the remnant, or recurrent ulcer following highly selective vagotomy (H.S.V.)

Incidence

- 3% after Billroth II gastrectomy
- 5 to 8% after vagotomy and GJ
- 40% after gastrojejunostomy (GJ)
- 10 to 12% following H.S.V.

Causes of recurrent ulcer (Fig. 23.62)

1. Incomplete vagotomy
2. GJ alone
3. Inadequate gastrectomy
4. Narrow stoma
5. Zollinger-Ellison's syndrome
6. Hyperparathyroidism

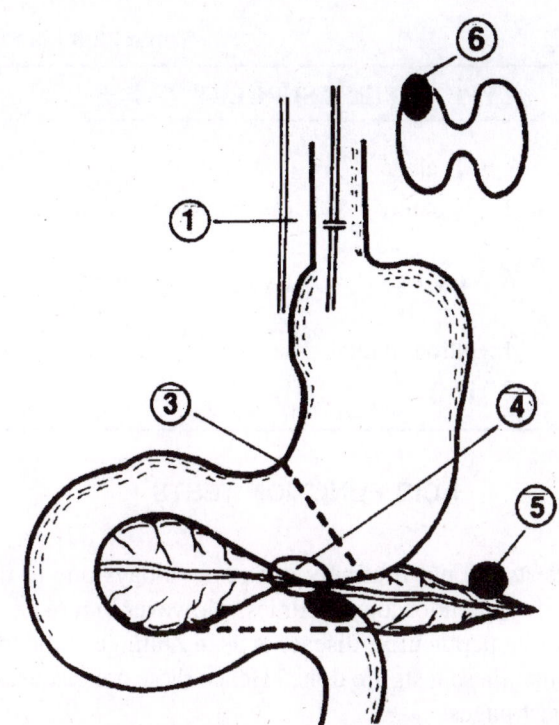

Fig. 23.62 Various causes of recurrent ulcer (See the text for numbers)

Symptoms

- Appears within 1 to 2 years after the operation.
- Severe persistent pain, "boring" type, which gets worse within a few minutes of taking food. Pain is felt on the left side of the abdomen, near the umbilical region and it passes downwards.
- Pain is felt in the lower left chest following ante-colic anastomosis. Pain is not relieved by antacids or milk unlike peptic ulcer. Bleeding is manifested as haematemesis, melaena or anaemia. Perforation can occur, resulting in peritonitis.

Diagnosis

- Gastroscopy gives the correct diagnosis.
- Hypercalcaemia and hypergastrinaemia should be ruled out.

Management (Refer Table 23.8)

- Conservative treatment with H_2 receptor blockers is nearly always effective but relapse occurs if they are stopped. Smoking should be stopped.
- However, definitive surgery is indicated in appropriate cases (Next page).

Table 23.8 Management of recurrent ulcer

TYPE OF FIRST SURGERY		CORRECTIVE SURGERY
1. G.J. alone	→	Vagotomy
2. Vagotomy + G.J. (incomplete vagotomy)	→	Incomplete vagotomy is the cause. Usually posterior vagus is found, and has to be divided it.
3. Vagotomy + G.J. (complete vagotomy)	→	Stoma is not adequate. Partial gastrectomy is the ideal treatment.
4. Billroth partial gastrectomy	→	Vagotomy with or without revision gastrectomy.
5. H.S.V.	→	Vagotomy + partial gastrectomy

ACID FUNCTION TESTS

These tests are not routinely done now-a-days due to the availability of endoscopy facilities. However in rare cases of recurrent peptic ulcer disease or as in Zollinger Ellison's syndrome, these tests are done. Hence these are discussed in the last pages.

PENTAGASTRIN TEST

- It is done to assess peak acid output.

Principle

- Pentagastrin stimulates parietal cell mass resulting in outpouring of gastric acid.

Procedure

- Basal secretion of fasting stomach is measured.
- 6 μg/kg body weight of pentagastrin is administered subcutaneously or intramuscularly.
- 4 samples of stomach secretion are collected for one hour, once every 15 minutes.
- By using suitable formula, peak acid output is measured.

Results

- Very high values are found in Zollinger-Ellison's syndrome.
- Its values are very high in duodenal ulcer patients. Vagotomy and antrectomy may be the treatment of choice.
- It has a role in recurrent ulcer
- In patients with gastrinoma the basal acid output is unusually high and there may be little response to pentagastrin stimulation.

HOLLANDER'S TEST (INSULIN TEST)[1]

- It is done to know the completeness of vagotomy.

Principles

- Insulin produces hypoglycaemia which stimulates vagus which in turn stimulates the parietal cell mass to secrete acid.
- If vagotomy is complete, there is no change in acid output during insulin test-Hollander's test.

Procedure

- Aspirate the fasting stomach contents
- To a fasting patient, 0.2 units /10 kg body weight of insulin is given subcutaneously.
- Blood sugar is estimated at 15 minute intervals and it is maintained between 30-40 mg% after two hours.

Results

- Acid output is measured for one hour. If there is no change in acid output, vagotomy is complete. If there is a rise in concentration of 20 mmol per litre above the basal level in the first hour, it suggests incomplete vagotomy.

Usefulness

- In recurrent ulcers to know whether vagotomy is complete or not.
- To diagnose Zollinger-Ellison's syndrome, where very high values of acid are seen.

Complications

- Hypoglycaemia and coma

---

1. This test should be done very carefully because some deaths have been reported due to hypoglycaemia

NIGHT FASTING SECRETION (DRAGSTEDT)

- The secretions of the stomach in the resting period or interdigestive period for 12 hours in the night are measured.

Procedure

- Introduce a Ryle's tube and aspirate the stomach contents for 12 hours from 9 P.M. to 9 A.M. The volume and HCl in this gastric juice are measured.

Results

- In normal patients the total amount of gastric secretion is around 400 ml. Above this, it suggests vagal hyperactivity.
- In Zollinger-Ellison syndrome the levels may be as high as one litre.
- Free HCl in normal patients is 10-20 mEq, in duodenal ulcer 60-80 mEq, in gastric ulcer 10-20 mEq, and in Zollinger-Ellison's syndrome. it may be around 100-300 mEq.

ACUTE DILATATION OF STOMACH

Aetiopathogenesis

1. Can occur after any operation, particularly splenectomy and pelvic procedures.

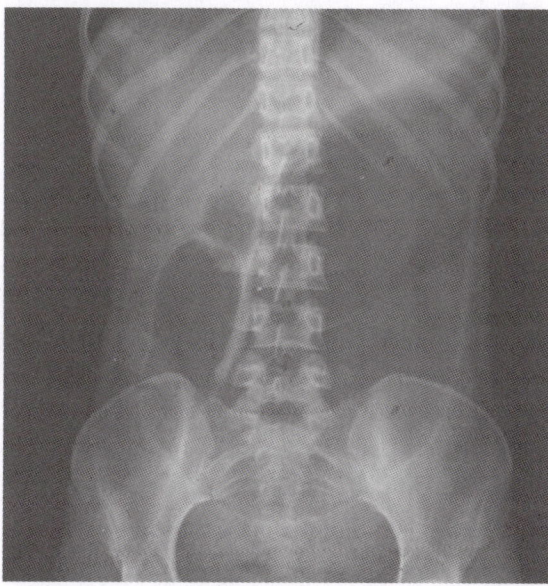

Fig. 23.63 Plain X-ray showing acute dilatation of the stomach. Ryle's tube insertion is a life saving simple procedure in these cases.

2. It can occur following fracture femur. application of plaster of paris, etc. Malnutrition, excessive distension of the stomach due to ventilation, aerophagia are the other precipitating factors.

There is a **sudden loss of sympathetic tone** resulting in massive dilatation of stomach (Fig. 23.63). Improper Ryle's tube aspiration and allowing the fluids orally too early before paralytic ileus settles down are additional factors.

Clinical features

- History of surgery
- **Hiccoughs** -due to irritation of under surface of the diaphragm, by hugely distended stomach
- Abdominal pain, vomiting, distension. Vomiting contains foul smelling dirty fluids and blood and is effortless.
- Features of shock. In untreated cases, can lead to cardiovascular collapse.
- **Effortless vomiting** of litres of dark watery fluid is characteristic of this condition.

Treatment: Urgent resuscitation

- Introduce the Ryle's tube and aspirate the stomach. It is the life saving use of Ryle's tube.
- Rapid I. V. fluid replacement, with normal saline and dextrose saline. Both crystalloids and colloids may be necessary to treat the shock and electrolyte abnormalities.

Complications

- Pulmonary: In debilitated patients, aspiration may result in aspiration pneunonitis (Mendelson syndrome).
- It carries significant mortality.

Miscellaneous

VOLVULUS OF THE STOMACH

- It is a rare condition in which stomach rotates in a horizontal (organoaxial) and vertical (mesentericoaxial) direction resulting in an acute abdomen.
- Many times, volvulus is intermittent.
- In general, initially the colon moves upwards and later greater curvature of the stomach.
- There is associated eventration of the diaphragm which also precipitates this condition.

- Clinical features include epigastric pain, fullness, tenderness.

Diagnosis

- Barium meal can demonstrate twisted stomach
- Inability to pass a Ryle's tube into the stomach

Treatment

- Reduce the volvulus by dividing gastrocolic omentum
- Fix the greater curvature of the stomach to the duodenojejunal flexure or perform a GJ without stoma.
- Repair of eventration

CHRONIC DUODENAL ILEUS

- It is also called **Wilkie's disease or arteriomesenteric compression.** The third part of the duodenum is compressed between vertebral column and superior mesenteric vessels. Acute loss of fat and immobilisation with cast precipitates this. Hence, it is also called cast syndrome.
- In this condition, duodenum is dilated upto the 3rd part with obstruction to the 3rd or 4th part duodenum (Fig. 23.64).
- Patients present with features of gastric outlet obstruction but vomitus contains bile.
- Abdominal pain is not severe as in intestinal obstruc-

tion but on careful questioning history of true nature of spasmodic pain is obtained.

- This condition is often misdiagnosed.
- Barium meal demonstrates the obstruction-dilated stomach and duodenum.
- Duodenojejunostomy is the treatment of choice (Fig. 23.65).

Differential diagnosis

1. **Pyloric stenosis:** In this condition vomitus does not contain bile. Barium meal X-ray shows distended stomach. Duodenum is not seen.

2. **Annular pancreas:** Rarely, it can present in adults with obstruction to the second part of the duodenum. Vomitus may contain bile. Barium meal X-ray shows dilatation of the first part and and also the second part of the duodenum.

3. **Tuberculosis of lymph nodes** can compress the 3rd part of the duodenum and can mimic Wilkie's disease.

IDIOPATHIC HYPERTROPHIC PYLORIC STENOSIS

Aetiopathogenesis

- In this condition there is **hypertrophy** involving the pyloric antral **circular muscle fibres**. Duodenum is normal (Fig. 23.66).
- The lumen is so much narrowed as to give rise to pyloric obstruction.
- Familial history can be obtained in a few patients.

Clinical features

- **Incidence:** 3-5/1000 births. First born male child is affected very often. Child is normal at birth and the symptoms appear around 6-8 weeks.
- First symptom is **vomiting**. It is **projectile**, forcible, does not contain bile. A visible gastric peristalsis (V.G.P.) can be seen especially when the mother feeds the child (Fig. 26.68).
- Loss of weight-dehydration
- Constipation and oliguria are the features
- Per abdomen-Hypertrophied thickened pylorus can be felt as a mass in the right hypochondrium (In adults with pyloric stenosis due to chronic duodenal ulcer, no mass is felt.)

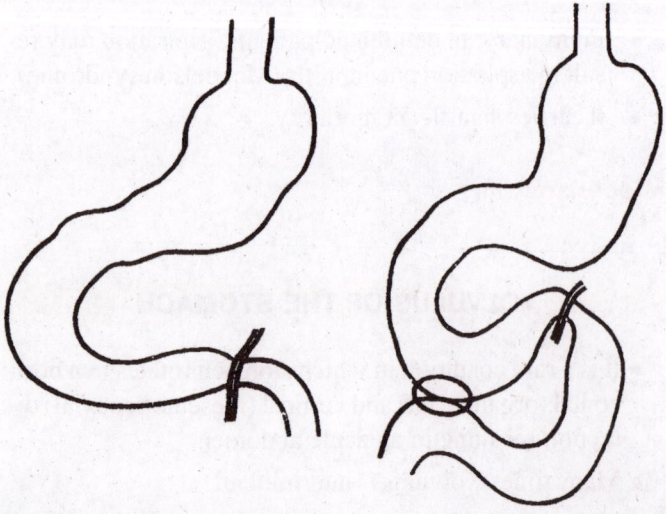

Fig. 23.64 Wilkie's disease - Superior mesenteric artery syndrome

Fig. 23.65 Duodenojejunostomy

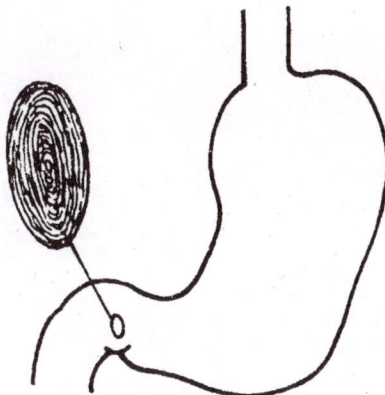

Fig. 23.66 Pyloric mass

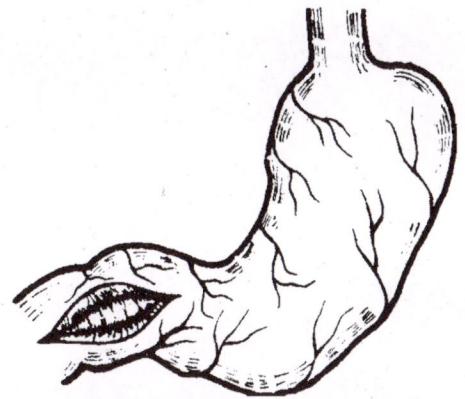

Fig. 23.67 Ramstedt's pyloromyotomy

Treatment

- Correction of dehydration and electrolyte disturbance by intravenous half normal saline must always precede surgery.
- **Ramstedt's pyloromyotomy** is the surgical treatment (Fig. 23.67, 69, 70, 71).

- Laparotomy is done and an incision is made through the serosa. It then cuts through the circular muscle fibres till all the muscle fibres are divided and the mucosa bulges out.
- Avoid injury to the mucosa. If mucosa is opened, it is sutured and reinforced by using omentum.

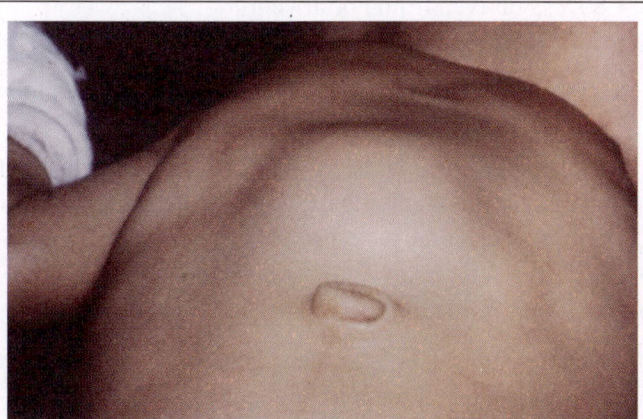

Fig. 23.68 Visible gastric peristalsis

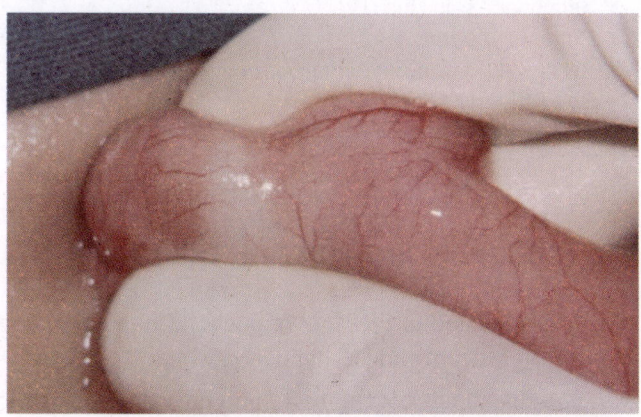

Fig. 23.69 Hypertrophied pylorus

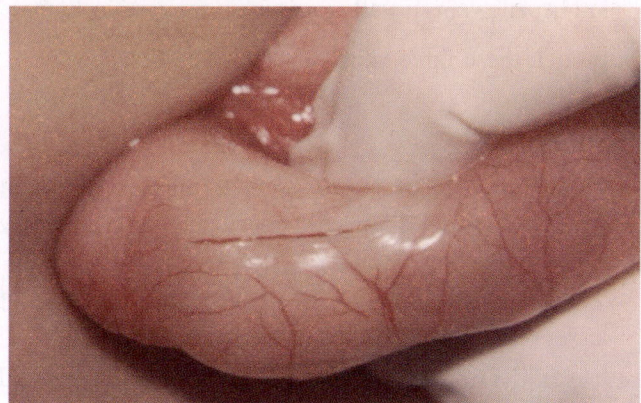

Fig. 23.70 Ramstedt's pyloromyotomy incision

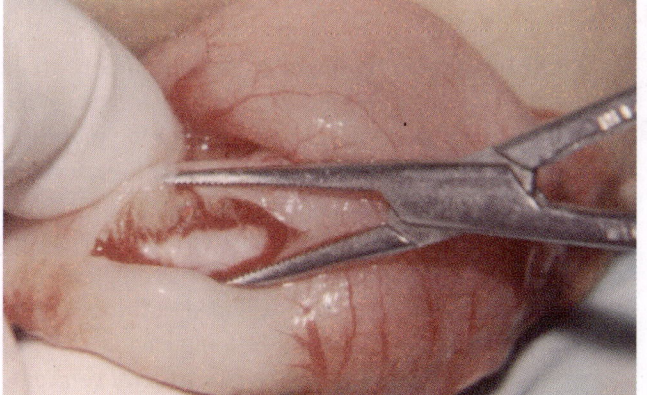

Fig. 23.71 Ramstedt's pyloromyotomy being done

- Contributed by Prof. Vijaykumar, Head of the Dept. of Paediatric surgery, KMC, Manipal

Liver

SURGICAL ANATOMY OF THE LIVER

- Liver is located in the right hypochondrium extending into epigastrium and left hypochondrium.
- It weighs about 1,500 gms - three quarters of it is the right lobe and rest is the left lobe.

Ligaments

1. **Right triangular ligament** fixes the right lobe to the undersurface of the right dome of diaphragm. When this ligament is divided, right lobe can be mobilised and can be turned to left as during right lobectomy or controling bleeding from liver trauma.
2. **Left triangular ligament** fixes the left lobe to the diaphragm in the similar fashion. For a complete vagotomy, when this ligament is divided, left lobe can be easily retracted - vagotomy become easy.
    - Also to get access to retrohepatic inferior vena cava this ligament needs to be divided.

3. **Falciform ligament:** It is the remnant of umbilical vein. It runs from umbilicus to the liver dividing the liver into right and left lobes, passing into interlobar fissure.

Blood supply

- 80% is derived from portal vein
- 20% from hepatic artery
- Right branch of hepatic artery supplies entire right lobe and left branch supplies the left lobe.
- Ligation of hepatic artery may not cause necrosis of liver in normal individuals, however it can cause liver failure in cirrhotic patients.

Venous drainage of the liver

- Major venous drainage is through 3 hepatic veins right middle and left. They join Inferior Vena Cava (IVC) immediately below the diaphragm. Right hepatic vein has a extrahepatic small course. On the other hand middle and left hepatic veins usually join within liver parenchyma.
- In fact, these three veins suspend the liver

Hilum of the liver

- This is also called as porta hepatis. It has most vital structures within it - hepatic artery, bile duct anteriorly and portal vein posteriorly.
- These structures are present within the free edge of lesser omentum - hepatoduodenal ligament.
- It is in the hilum, these stuctures divide into right and left branches. **Left bile duct has a longer**

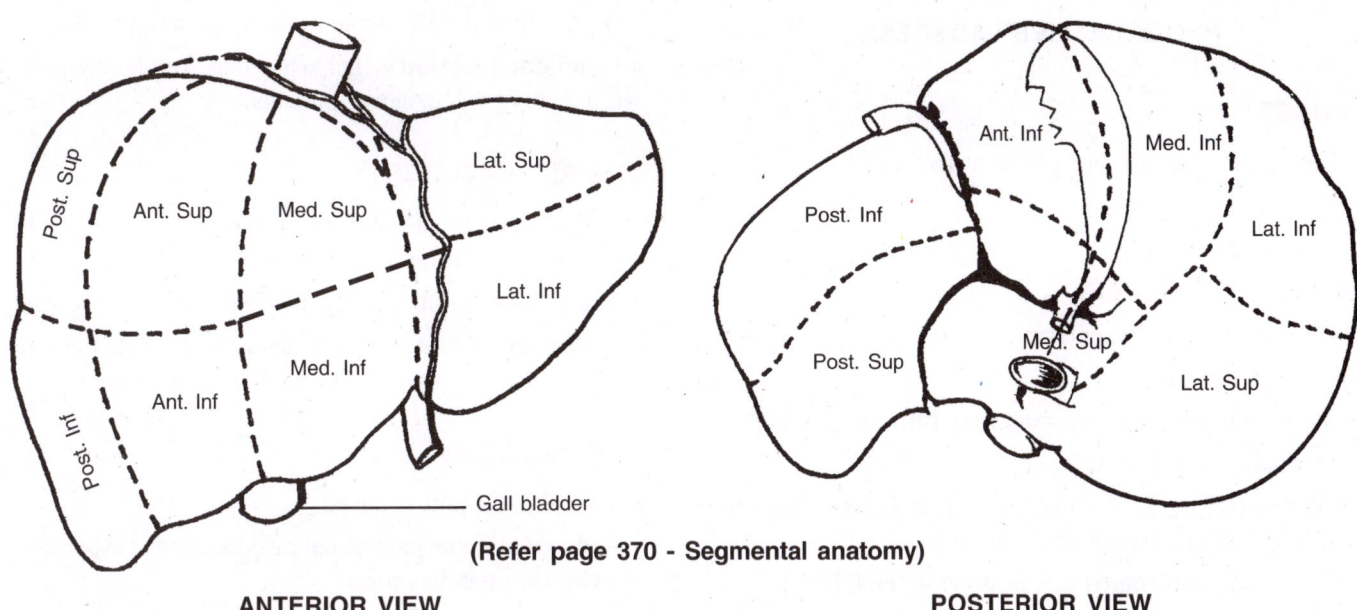

ANTERIOR VIEW　　　　　　　**POSTERIOR VIEW**

(Refer page 370 - Segmental anatomy)

Fig. 24.1 and 24.2 Liver lobes and segments based on the distribution of intrahepatic ducts and blood vessels. Ant. Sup - Anterior superior, Ant. Inf - Anterior inferior, Lat. Inf - Lateral inferior, Lat. Sup - Lateral superior, Med. Inf - Medial inferior, Med. Sup - Medial superior, Post. Inf - Posterior inferior, Post. Sup. - Posterior superior

extrahepatic course of approximately 2 cms. In stricture CBD, this can be used for hepaticojejunostomy (Also see Fig. 24.1, 24.2).

Regeneration

- Liver has an excellent capacity for regeneration after partial resection.
- The **factor released from pancreas** is supposed to be responsible for this.

Hepatic lobules

- The functional unit of the liver are lobules. They consist of sheets of liver cells, separated by hepatic sinusoids, venous channels, which drain blood to central vein, a tributary of the hepatic vein from portal tracts that contain branches of hepatic vein and portal vein.

PHYSIOLOGY : (REFER TABLE 24.1)

Table 24.1 Physiology	
FUNCTIONING OF THE LIVER	**IMPORTANCE**
• Glucose metabolism, Glycolysis and Gluconeogenesis	• Persistent hypoglycaemia is a feature of fulminant hepatic failure (FHF), also seen in hepatoma
• Synthesis of clotting factors	• Bleeding tendencies in chronic liver diease
• Maintaining core body temperature	• Hypothermia in FHF
• Bilirubin formation	• Congenital hyperbilirubinaemia
• Drug and Hormone metabolism	• Hepatitis due to drugs such as rifampicin, anti tuberculous treatment etc.
• Monitoring pH and correcting lactic acidosis	• Severely impaired in FHF
• Removal of endotoxins and foreign antigens	• Severely impaired in FHF
• Urea formation from portein catabolism	• Portocaval shunt, endotoxins bypass the liver, result in encephalopathy

PYOGENIC LIVER ABSCESS

CAUSES

I. Infection through the portal vein
- Acute appendicitis
- Acute diverticulitis
- Acute amoebic colitis
- Acute bacillary dysentery
- Ulcerative colitis

II. Infection through the common bile duct (CBD)
- Stricture of the CBD
- Periampullary carcinoma resulting in stasis of the bile, precipitating infection (cholangitis)
- Recurrent cholangitis due to stone in the CBD
- ERCP

III. Infection through the hepatic artery
- Septicaemia and pyaemia
- Actinomycosis of faciocervical region

IV. Extension abscess
- Subdiaphragmatic abscess
- Empyema thoracis
- Penetrating injuries

V. Infection through umbilicus
- Neonatal umblical sepsis giving rise to pyaemia

CERTAIN FACTS

- Majority of bacteria are derived from gastrointestinal tract (Key Box 24.1).
- In majority of cases it is **polymicrobial** infection
- **E.coli** is the most common facultative organism

Key Box 24.1
BACTERIOLOGY

1. Anaerobic bacteria : 60% (Bacteroides fragilis)
2. Enteric Gram Negative Bacteria
   - Escherichia coli   : 40%
   - Klebsiella pneumoniae : 10-20%
   - Others   : 4 to 40%
3. Gram Positive Bacteria
   - Staphylococcus aureus : 4 to 25%

- Bacteroides fragilis is the most common anaerobe.
- **Candidal infection** is increasing due to chemotherapy, especially for leukaemic patients.

CLINICAL FEATURES

- Alcoholic males, debilitated men suffer more, probably because of poor immunity.
- Acute abscesses are usually multiple, chronic are single.
- Tender hepatomegaly, low grade or high grade pyrexia with abdominal discomfort are the main features.

INVESTIGATIONS

- Total WBC count is raised
- Abdominal ultrasound and ultrasound guided aspiration establishes the diagnosis
- When in doubt, C.T. scan can be done, followed by FNAC which draws frank pus. Pus is sent for Gram's stain, culture and sensitivity. CT also helps in the diagnosis of **associated conditions like diverticulitis**.

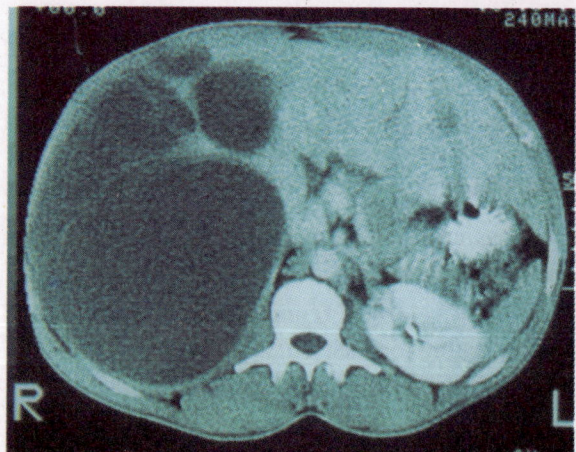

Fig. 24.3 CT scan showing liver abscess

- Further investigations are directed towards the associated conditions. **Examples:**

  Chest X-ray: Air under the diaphragm (perforation of hollow viscus) or diagnosis of empyema thoracis.

  Stool routine examination : Amoebic cysts, culture and sensitivity for Typhoid bacilli.

TREATMENT

1. **Conservative:** Multiple small abscesses may respond to antibiotics. However they have to be given for 4 to 6 weeks.

2. **Percutaneous drainage** (Key Box 24.2)

Key Box 24.2
INDICATIONS
• Superficial abscesses
• Abscess with no intra-abdominal pathology
• Abscess of unknown etiology

Method

- Ultrasound or CT guided aspiration and drainage by using pigtail catheter
- Irrigation of abscess cavity with saline

3. **Open (Surgical) method** (Key Box 24.3)

Key Box 24.3
INDICATIONS
• Abscess with intraabdominal pathology
• Ascites
• Deep seated abscess
• Multiple abscesses

- Laparotomy is required mainly to treat the primary causes e.g. appendicectomy, drainage of appendicular abscess. If liver shows a significant abscess, it is drained or pigtail catheter introduced into the abscess cavity and is brought outside through a separate opening. It helps in longer duration of drainage.

AMOEBIC LIVER ABSCESS

- It is also called as **Tropical Abscess** (Dysenteric Abscess). It is the most common extra intestinal manifestation of amoebiasis.

AETIOPATHOGENESIS

- This disease is caused by Entamoeba histolyticae.
- It is almost always a complication of amoebic dysentery. This can occur in the acute stage or in the chronic carrier stage.
1. **Infection from the caecum** (typhilitis) spreads through the tributary of superior mesenteric vein.

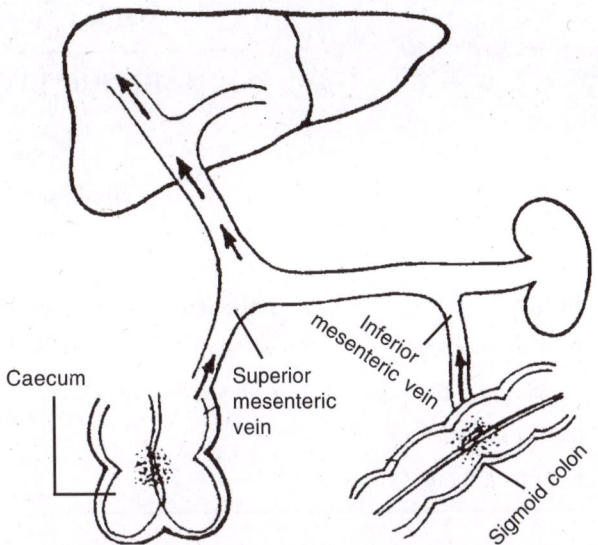

Fig. 24.4 Aetiopathogenesis of amoebic liver abscess

2. **From sigmoid colon**, through the tributary of superior mesenteric vein (Fig. 24.4).
- The right branch of the portal vein is in direct line with the portal vein. Hence, by **stream line phenomenon** organisms reach the right lobe more often than the left lobe. The right lobe is also much bigger than left lobe.
- In the right lobe, it is the postero-superior surface which is involved because it is extraperitoneal (**Bare area of liver**). It has no peritoneal covering.
- After reaching the liver, the organism causes destruction of hepatocytes by releasing powerful **cytolytic enzymes** resulting in **liquefaction necrosis**. Also causes aseptic thrombosis of blood vessels resulting in necrosis of liver tissue.
- At the same time, some RBCs[1] are also broken down. This causes **anchovy sauce pus** chocolate brown in colour, which is the mixture of broken down RBCs[1], hepatocytes, etc.
- **Green pus** is referred to pus mixed with bile, which is seen in a few patients.
- In majority of the cases, pus is sterile. Secondary infection occurs in about 20 to 30% of the cases.
- Amoebae are rarely present in the pus but are present in the wall of the abscess cavity. The wall contains monocytes, plasma cells, lymphocytes and fibroblasts. Abscesses are multiple which fuse to form a single large abscess cavity in about 70% of the cases. Due to perihepatitis, abscess gets fixed to the diaphragm resulting

---

1.Absence of WBC is an important feature. Hence regeneration of abscess cavity is complete without scarring.

Table 24.2 Clinical features

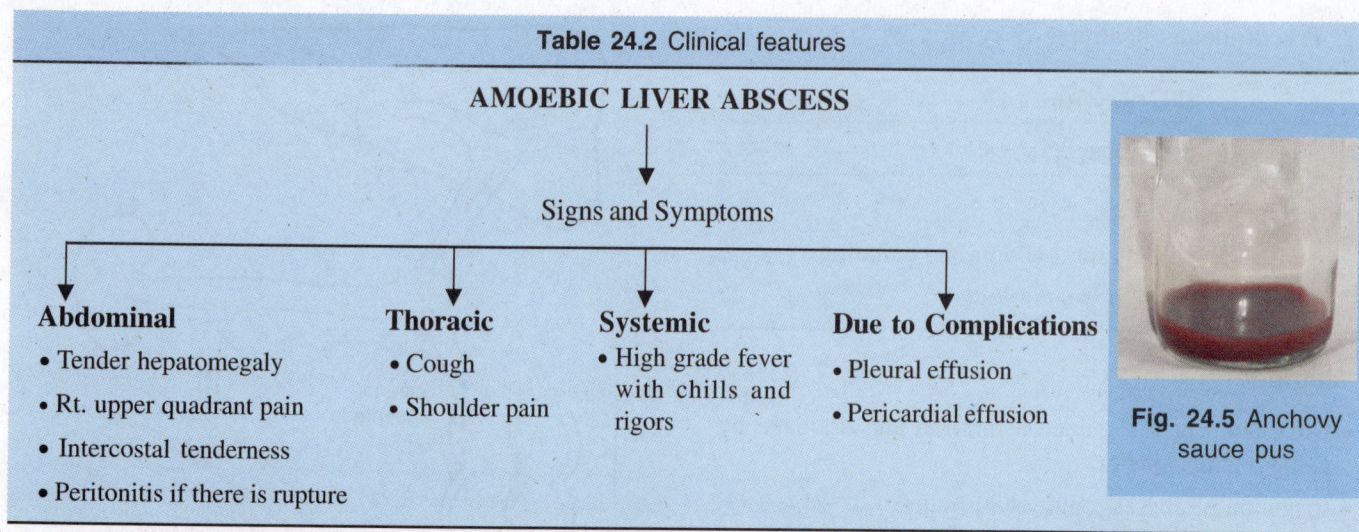

AMOEBIC LIVER ABSCESS

↓

Signs and Symptoms

Abdominal	**Thoracic**	**Systemic**	**Due to Complications**
• Tender hepatomegaly	• Cough	• High grade fever with chills and rigors	• Pleural effusion
• Rt. upper quadrant pain	• Shoulder pain		• Pericardial effusion
• Intercostal tenderness			
• Peritonitis if there is rupture			

Fig. 24.5 Anchovy sauce pus

in immobility of the diaphragm. Left lobe liver abscess gets adhered to anterior abdominal wall.

• It is interesting to note that amoebic infection of gall-bladder and bile does not occur because of **deleterious effect of bile on amoeba**.

CLINICAL FEATURES (Table 24.2)

1. Male alcoholics are commonly affected, in the age group of 20-40 years.

2. Low socio-economic status patient.

3. Severe pain in the right hypochondrium is due to the enlarged liver. This stage is called as stage of **Amoebic Hepatitis**. If USG is done, it may not demonstrate any abscesses but there may be many micro-abscesses. At this stage, there is low grade fever, weakness, anorexia, etc.

4. High grade fever with chills and rigors develop if the stage proceeds to pyogenic liver abscess due to secondary bacterial infection of amoebic abscess.

5. Thoracic symptoms such as nonproductive cough, pleurisy right shoulder pain are common.

Clinical signs

1. Anaemia, emaciation, toxic look and an earthy complexion is present.

2. Jaundice may be present if abscesses are multiple, due to compression of biliary radicles. However it is rare (15%).

3. Liver is enlarged in right hypochondrium, tender and soft (liver enlarges in upward direction) - Key Box 24.4.

4. Intercostal tenderness differentiates it from acute

cholecystitis. Intercostal oedema can also be present.

5. Thoracic symptoms such as nonproductive cough, pleurisy, right shoulder pain are common.

Key Box 24.4

VERY TENDER LIVER

• Amoebic liver abscess
• Hepatoma
• Congestive cardiac failure

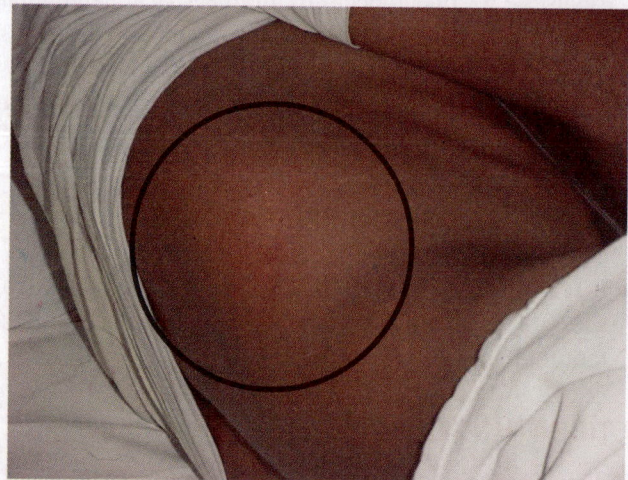

Fig. 24.6 Intercostal bulge and tenderness are important features of amoebic liver abscess of the liver - these signs are not seen in acute cholecystitis

INVESTIGATIONS

1. Total WBC count may be increased if there is secondary infection

2. Stool examination for ova and cysts of Entamoeba histolytica may be positive in 25% of cases.

3. Serologic testing: The indirect haemagglutination test is positive in 90-95% of patients with an amoebic abscess.

4. **Screening chest**: When the patient is asked to take a deep breath, right side of the diaphragm does not move due to inflammatory (**perihepatitis**) adhesions between liver and diaphragm. This is called as **homolateral immobility of the diaphragm**. A small pleural effusion can also be present.

5. **Sigmoidoscopy** may demonstrate large, deep amoebic ulcers.

6. **Abdominal USG:**
   - To locate site of abscess, then to confirm the diagnosis.
   - Ultrasound guided needle aspiration can also be done and biopsy of abscess wall should be taken.
   - Multiple abscesses can be made out.

7. **C.T. scan** can demonstrate an abscess cavity as a low density zone surrounded by peripheral hypo-dense zone due to inflammatory reaction.

TREATMENT

- It can be classified into

I. Conservative

II. Ultrasound guided needle aspiration

III. Surgery - drainage

I. Conservative line of management

- It is indicated in amoebic hepatitis. Tab metronidazole 400-800 mg, 3 times a day is given for 14 days. The only recognizable side effect is metallic taste.

- If the condition does not improve, injection emetine 1mg/kg body weight, a total of 60 mg/day deep 1M for a maximum of 6 days is given.

Side effects and precautions during emetine therapy

- Systolic B.P. should be at least 100 mm of Hg.
- ECG should be recorded before, during and after the therapy.
- Cardiotoxicity in the form of arrhythmias can occur.
- Absolute bed rest during treatment (because of these complications, it is not used nowadays).
- Adequate hydration, rest, analgesics to relieve the pain.

Improvement can be seen within one to two days in the form of disappearance of pain, fever and return of appetite.

II. USG-guided needle aspiration

- It is indicated in cases of amoebic liver abscess.
- Before it is aspirated, BT, CT, PT should be normal and Injection Vitamin K 10 mg, IM should be given for at least 3 days.
- USG-guided aspiration is the treatment of choice where metronidazole is contra indicated. Eg: 1st trimester of pregnancy.
- It is easy can be done under local anaesthesia
- Can be repeated, if pus recollects

Complications

1. Bleeding-rare

2. Incomplete aspiration results in leakage of pus and

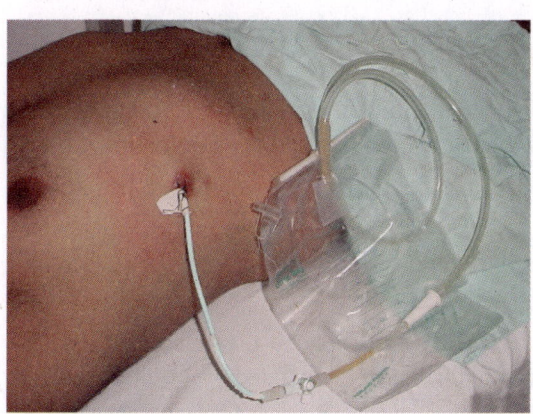

Fig. 24.7 Pig tail catheter drainage of amoebic liver abscess

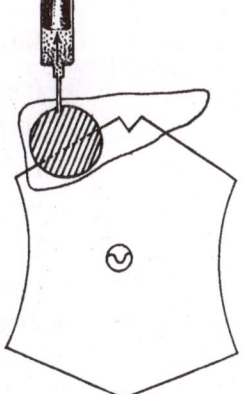

Fig. 24.8 Ultrasound guided aspiration

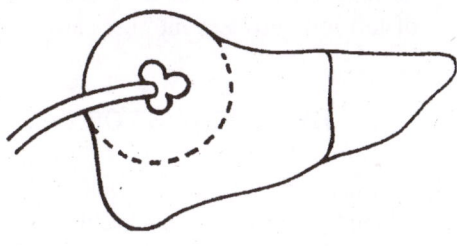

Fig. 24.9 Drainage of liver abscess with Malecot's catheter

bile into peritoneal cavity which may produce peritonitis. Hence, prophylactic antibiotics need to be given before and after the procedure along with metronidazole therapy.

III. Surgery (open drainage)

Indications

1. Failure of USG guided needle aspiration

2. Ruptured amoebic liver abscess with amoebic peritonitis.

Procedure

- Laparotomy is done first. Abscess cavity is identified. Contents are evacuated, a thorough peritoneal wash is given, a self-retaining Malecot's catheter is introduced into the abscess cavity, brought out-side and connected to a bag.

- With the advent of metronidazole, **Amoebiasis Cutis** is rarely seen (not seen), hence catheter can be safely placed inside the cavity and brought out.

- Postoperatively for 3-5 days, necrotic liver tissue, anchovy sauce pus and blood drain outside.

- Once the drainage becomes minimal, Malecot's catheter is pulled out.

COMPLICATIONS OF AMOEBIC LIVER ABSCESS

- **Amoebic peritonitis** resulting in acute abdomen with shock. It has to be treated like any peritonitis. Laparotomy, drainage of pus and drain the abscess cavity to outside (possibility of **amoebiosis cutis** is still present but rare).

- Rupture into pleural space causing **pleural effusion**.

- Rupture into the bronchus resulting in coughing out anchovy sauce (may be a natural cure). **Bronchopleural fistula**.

- **Amoebic pericardial effusion** occurs due to rupture of left lobe abscess into pericardial space.

HYDATID CYST OF THE LIVER

- The disease is caused by Echinococcus granulosus, transmitted by dogs which are the chief mediators (host). and man is the intermediate host. After swallowing the ova, they penetrate the gastric mucosa[1], reach retroperito-

neal structures, penetrate portal vein direclty, then enter liver. Having reached liver, organisms grow and develop their own protective layer and form hydatid cyst.

LAYERS OF HYDATID CYST (Fig. 24.10)

1. The adventitia (pseudocyst)[2]

- This is the fibrous layer derived from the liver tissue. It is the reaction of liver to the parasite. It is adherent to the liver and cannot be separated.

2. The ectocyst (laminated membrane)

- It is white and elastic and is produced by endocyst. It is this layer which gets peeled off at surgery.

3. The endocyst

- This is called as germinal epithelium and it is the innermost part of hydatid cyst. It secretes hydatid fluid inside and ectocyst outside. Within the hydatid fluid, the 'brood capsules', develop within which the scolices of echinococcus granulosus develop (Fig. 24.11).

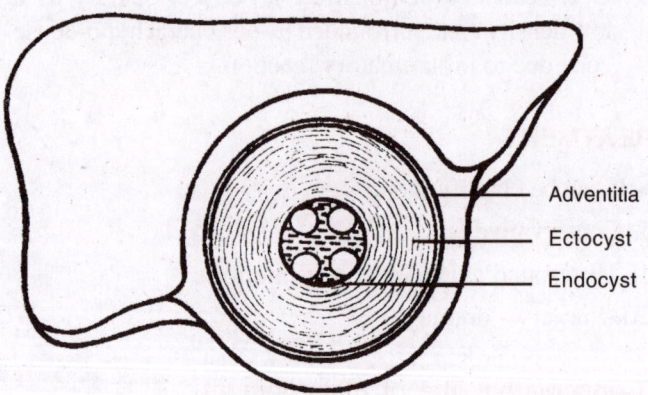

Fig. 24.10 Layers of the hydatid cyst

CLINICAL FEATURES

- It can be silent-without any symptoms throughout life, accidentally discovered on routine examination.

- Dragging pain in the upper abdomen due to hepatomegaly.

- Liver is enlarged, has a smooth surface, round borders and is non-tender.

- **Typical hydatid thrill** can be present in rare occasions. Hydatid thrill is demonstrated by 3 finger method.

---

1. *Probably that is the reason why hydatid ova do not produce lesions in the intestine unlike Entamoebae.*
2. *It is the protective coat given by the host to the ghost.*

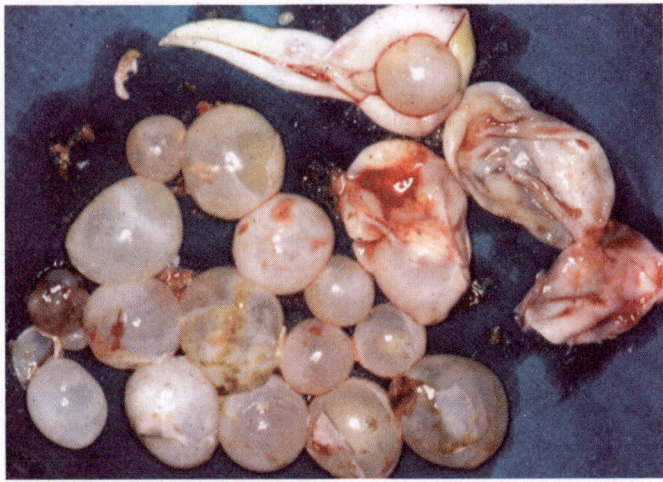

Fig. 24.11 Daughter cysts

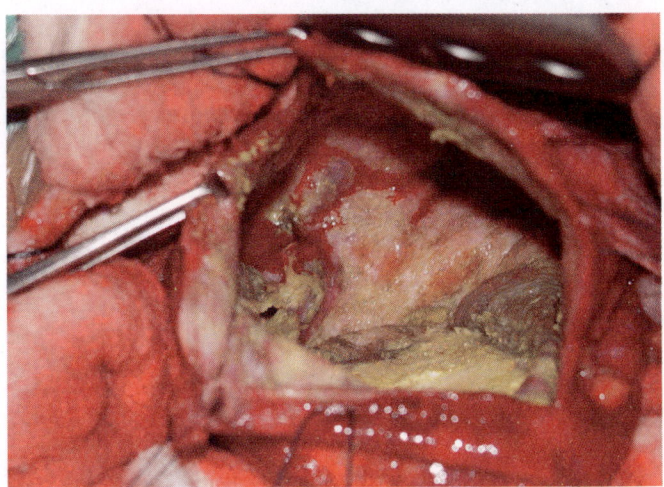

Fig. 24.12 Infected hydatid cyst

Keep 3 fingers over the liver, percuss over the middle finger and get the impulse by other 2 fingers (fluid thrill).

INVESTIGATIONS

1. Casoni's intradermal test, sensitivity and specificity of this test is low, hence no longer used.
2. USG can detect the cyst, localize the cyst and is used for aspiration purposes (details later)
3. Plain X-ray abdomen may demonstrate **speckled** calcification.
4. C.T. scan may be necessary in selected cases (Fig. 24.13). The cyst which is superficial and has reached surface, should be operated upon.
5. **ERCP** if there is obstructive jaundice - in such cases

a wide sphincterotomy should be given so as to allow free drainage of the hydatid contents into the duodenum.

TREATMENT

- It can be discussed under following headings:

I. Conservative

1. Calcified cysts are dead cysts. They are left alone.
2. Symptomless, small hydatid cyst can be left alone. Once symptomatic, or if the size is more than 5 cms they may be treated.

II. Medical treatment

- Trial of albendazole is (400 mg two times a day) given for 6 weeks. If the size becomes small, wait and watch. Repeated courses of albendazole can be given for a period of 6 months. If there is no improvement, surgery is undertaken.
- Watch for neutropaenia (Key box 24.5)

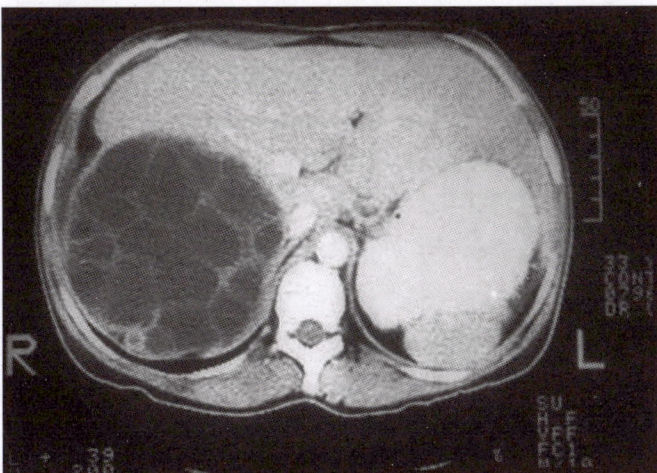

Fig. 24.13 CT scan of the liver showing classical cart wheel pattern

Key Box 24.5
INDICATIONS FOR MEDICAL TREATMENT
• Disseminated hydatid cyst
• Inaccessible for surgery (deep seated, multiple, recurrent)
• Patient unfit for surgery
• Contamination of peritoneal cavity at surgery.

III. SURGERY

- There are different types of surgeries for hydatid disease of the liver which have been summarized below. Indications are given above in the Key Box 24.6.

Key Box 24.6

INDICATIONS FOR SURGERY

- Symptomatic cyst
- Asymptomatic patient with cyst > 5 cm, noncalcified
- Infected cyst (Fig. 24.12)

Principles of surgery

1. **Laparotomy** and **isolation of the cyst** from peritoneal cavity by packs dipped in hypochlorite solution.
2. Aspirate the contents and inject **scolicidal agents** like savlon or hypertonic saline.
3. Incise the cyst, **peel off the laminated membrane** by using sponge-holding forceps.
4. An attempt to remove adventitial layer may result in bleeding. It need not be removed.

Key Box 24.7

SCOLICIDAL AGENTS	SIDE EFFECTS
• Hypertonic saline	Hypernatraemia
• Chlorhexidine	Acidosis
• Alcohol (80%)	Cholangitis
• Sodium hypochlorite	Hypernatraemia

Precautions

1. Albendazole should be given before surgery
2. Avoid spillage into the peritoneal cavity to avoid peritoneal hydatid.
3. **Injection hydrocortisone** 100 mg I.V. before, during and after surgery to avoid anaphylactic shock.

Different types of surgical procedures

- They have been summarised in the Key Box 24.8. However, excision of the cyst leaving the adventitial layer is the most commonly done surgery (Fig. 24.14).

Key Box 24.8

SURGICAL PROCEDURES

- **Excision :** It is most commonly done operation
- **Cystopericystectomy :** Here cyst is excised in a plane outside adventitial layer. It results in excessive bleeding, but it removes cyst completely.
- **Capitonnage :** If omentum is not available for closing the cavity, redundant cyst wall can be infolded into the cyst cavity and sutured.
- **Hepatic resection** in good centers when there are proper indications.

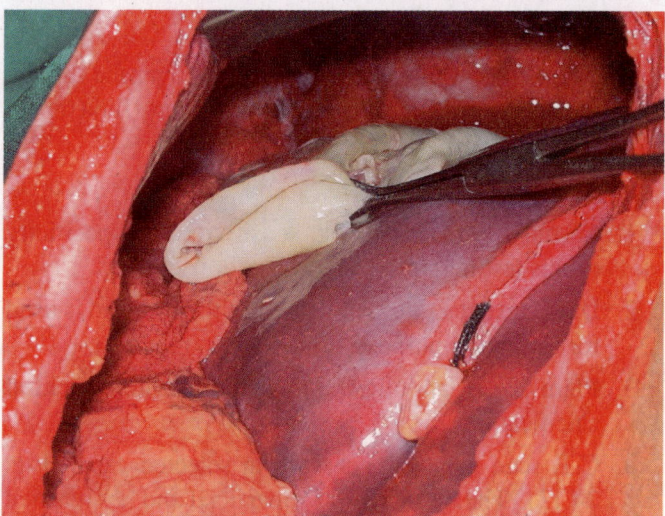

Fig. 24.14 Laminated membrane removed at surgery with sponge holding forceps

---

IV Percutaneous drainage

- It is done after taking all necessary precautions / equipment with all emergency drugs, with the help of CT/ USG guided.
- It is also called as **PAIR** - **P**uncture, **A**spiration, **I**njection and **R**easpiration.

Indications

- Unilocular uncomplicated cyst
- Poor surgical candidate
- Previous multiple abdominal surgeries
- Relapse following surgery

Contraindications to PAIR

- Multiple septal divisions

- Communicating cysts
- Dead or inactive cysts

COMPLICATIONS OF HYDATID CYST

1. **Rupture** of the cyst into the peritoneal cavity can occur due to trauma (rare) and may result in anaphylactic shock. It should be treated accordingly with injection hydrocortisone and laparotomy.

2. **Jaundice** due to cysts within biliary tree or due to a large cyst compressing biliary ducts. ERCP followed by endoscopic removal of hydatid cysts from the common bile duct followed by sphincterotomy should be done.

3. **Suppuration** is rare due to the tough tunica adventitia.

4. **Calcification** of the cyst wall in long-standing cases.

Other type of organism is **Echinococcus multilocularis.** This parasitic infestation is uncommon in our country, but it is more severe. Kindly refer Key box 24.9.

Key Box 24.9
ECHINOCOCCUS MULTILOCULARIS
• Alveolar echinococcosis
• It can cause malignant hydatid disease (misnomer) Difficult to treat hence the name
• Needs resection
• It causes poorly demarcated honeycombing cystic specimen
• It infiltrates liver and invades vascular system

BENIGN TUMOURS OF THE LIVER

- These are not uncommon tumours
- They are more frequently diagnosed now with frequent use of ultrasound. Majority of them are asymptomatic, do not require specific treatment.
- Their removal should be attempted only by an experienced surgeon. Hepatic adenoma and focal nodular hyperplasia are compared in the following table.

HAEMANGIOMA

- Commonest benign tumour of the liver
- It may be associated with cavernous haemangioma in some other sites such as head and neck region. Clinically it is difficult to diagnose as it presents as hepatomegaly.
- Ultrasound / CT scan can diagnose their location, number (single or multiple), or any other complications associated with that (thrombosis, infection). MRI is a better investigation.
- Haemangioma bigger than 8 cm have chances of rupture.
- They can be resected or can be enucleated.

Caution : Before putting a needle into the space occupying lesion in the liver, make sure it is NOT Haemangioma.

Differential diagnosis

- Hepatoma, liver cysts, liver abscess

Other benign tumours are hepatic adenomas and focal nodular hyperplasia. They are given below.(Table 24.3)

Table 24.3	
HEPATIC ADENOMAS	**FOCAL NODULAR HYPERPLASIA**
• Occur in young women	• Occurs in young women
• Occur due to oral contraceptive pills	• Occurs due to oral contraceptive pills
• Usually solitary	• Can be **multiple**
• Haemorrhage, rupture, necrosis can occur	• Haemorrhage, rupture, necrosis does not occur
• Can undergo malignant change	• **Rarely malignant** change can occur
• If it is due to OCPs, it can regress after discontinuing OCPs. Otherwise adenomas need to be resected	• Generally does not regress
• Kupffer cells are **not present** in hepatic adenomas	• In addition to hepatocytes, it also contain Kupffer cells

PRIMARY HEPATOMA OR HEPATOCELLULAR CARCINOMA (HCC)

- Before discussion on HCC, one has to have a knowledge about segmental anatomy of the liver, which forms the basis for hepatic resection.
- Eventhough the details about the hepatic resection may not be required for undergraduate students it is desirable to know about the segmental anatomy to have a better understanding about the hepatic resection.

SEGMENTAL ANATOMY OF THE LIVER

- The liver is divided into two lobes by the main portal fissure, which is also called **CANTLIE'S Line**. This line extends from the gall bladder fossa to the left side of IVC and is inclined at an angle of 75° to the horizontal plane. The main portal fissure is a constant feature. Each lobe is equal in size.
- The right portal fissure divides the right lobe into an anteromedial and posterolateral sector. The right hepatic vein courses along this fissure. This fissure is inclined at an angle of 40° with the horizontal.
- The left portal fissure divides the left lobe into an anterior and posterior sector, and it is in this fissure that the left hepatic vein courses.
- The liver is further divided into segments, which represents the smallest anatomic unit of the organ. In the right lobe, each of the two sectors is divided into two segments. The antero medial section and posterolateral sector. The antero medial section is divided into segment V anteriorly and segment VIII posteriorly, while the posterolateral sector is divided into segment VI anteriorly and segment VII posteriorly.

- In the left lobe, the anterior sector is divided into segment IV (or quadrate lobe) and the segment III. The posterior sector is comprised of only one segment, segment II. The spigelian lobe, or segment I is considered as **autonomous** segment. It is also labelled as **caudate lobe**.
- Each segment has its own identifiable portal vein, hepatic arterial supply, bile duct and hepatic veins. All these segments can be removed individually. However, segment I receives tributaries from both the right and left branches of portal vein and hepatic artery and the hepatic venous drainage is independent and may terminate directly into IVC.

AETIOLOGY OF HCC

1. **Hepatitis B virus (HBV):** High titres of hepatitis B surface antigen (HBSAg) was found in 50 to 60% of patients with HCC. Incidence is more in chronic carriers and it is increased if patients consume alcohol, aflatoxin and smoking.
2. **Cirrhosis:** It is a definite premalignant condition. A palpable hard liver in a cirrhotic patient suggests development of HCC.

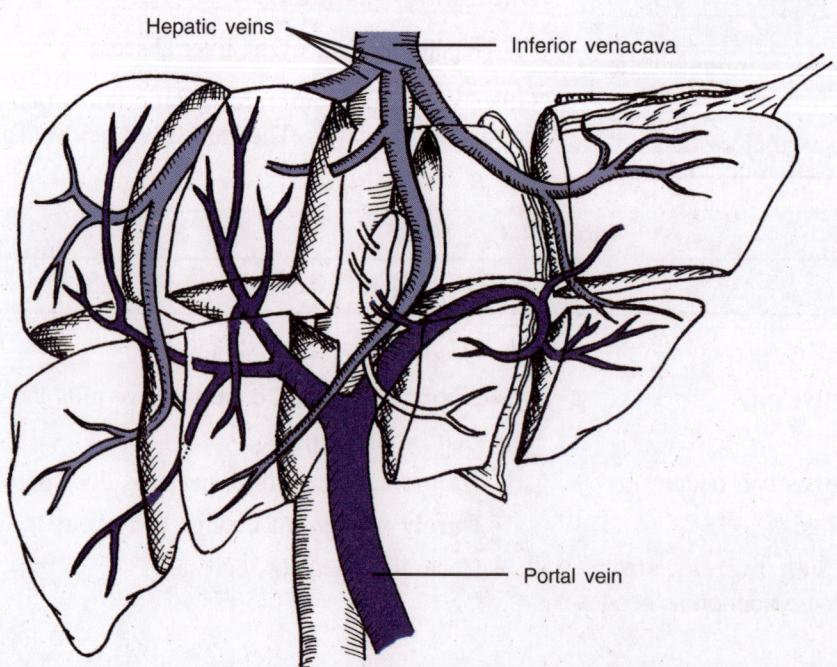

Hepatic veins

Inferior venacava

Portal vein

Fig. 24.15 Segmental anatomy of the liver

Segmental anatomy of the liver with the 8 segments, based on portal vein blood supply and hepatic venous outflow as designated by Couinaud. Segment of the left lobe; segment I is also known as the caudate lobe; segments II and III comprise the lateral segment of the left lobe; segment IV is the medial segment of the left lobe; and segments V to VIII comprise the right lobe (IVC, Inferior vena cava).

3. **Hepatitis C virus (HCV):** HCV infection induces cirrhosis and increases the incidence of development of HCC.
4. **Aflatoxin consumption** (a fungus found in infected butter yellow, bread) is responsible for increased incidence of HCC as in Mozambique.
5. **Oral contraceptive pills** are known to cause adenoma and there is a rare chance of adenoma turning in to HCC.
6. **Other risk factors:** Heavy alcohol consumption, cigarette smoking, diabetes mellitus, haemochromatosis are the other factors responsible for HCC. Wilson's disease is NOT associated with increased risk of HCC.

CLINICAL FEATURES

- **Age group:** Highest incidence is found after 50 years of age. It is rarely seen in children also.
- Sex: **Male alcoholics** are commonly affected
- A **slow growing** mass in the right hypochondrium. It is the enlarged liver with an irregular surface and hard in consistency. Evidence of cirrhosis may be present.
- It can be a **rapidly growing** neoplasm, highly vascular and clinically palpable as a soft to firm pulsatile mass with or without a bruit.
- Rapid development of **anorexia, asthaenia, anaemia and loss of weight**.
- Jaundice is not common unless the tumour arises in a cirrhotic liver in hepatocellular failure.
- **Low grade pyrexia** is common. It is due to tumour necrosis.
- Liver being an important organ of metabolism, **hypoglycaemia** is found in 10% of the patients.

SPREAD OF HEPATOMA

1. **Direct infiltration** of the neighbouring structures such as diaphragm results in hiccoughs due to irritation of phrenic nerve.
2. **Lymphatic spread:** Lymph nodes at the hilum (porta hepatis) are involved first. Later, mediastinal nodes and left supraclavicular nodes (Virchow's node) are involved.
3. **Blood spread** cause massive malignant pleural effusion by dislodgment of tumour emboli into inferior vena cava because of spread through the hepatic veins. Vertebral involvement follows soon.
4. **Haemoperitoneum** due to spread involving peritoneal surface or due to rupture of an enlarging hepatoma may occur.

INVESTIGATIONS

1. CBP: Hb % is usually low
2. **Liver function test** may show hepatocellular failure in the form of high bilirubin, low albumin and high globulin levels.
3. **Abdominal USG**: Findings
   - Diffuse distortion of hepatic parenchyma and a well-circumscribed hyperechogenic mass suggests HCC.
   - **Mosaic pattern** of the tumour with thin halo with lateral shadows and **nodule in nodule pattern** with separating fibrous septa, **posterior echo enhancement**.
   - **Tumour thrombi** in portal vein, hepatic vein or IVC.
4. **Contrast enhanced CT of the abdomen:** It appears as hypodense mass with internal mosaic architecture in early phase, hypodense lesion with enhanced fibrous capsule in late phase. Guided FNAC can be done to confirm the diagnosis. Small fear of tumour embolisation via portal venous radicles.
5. **Alpha-fetoprotein**
   - It is a fetal antigen which disappears after birth. Hence, it is not measurable in normal persons.
   - Levels of alpha-fetoprotein around 100 IU are suggestive of hepatoma.
   - Levels around 1000 IU are diagnostic of hepatoma. Hence, it is the tumour marker of hepatoma. After resection the values come down to normal. If the values start increasing, it indicates recurrence.

Key Box 24.10
INCREASED ALPHA-FETOPROTEIN LEVELS
1. **Hepatoma**
2. Carcinoma stomach
3. Carcinoma pancreas
4. Embryonal cell carcinoma of testis

6. **Selective angiography:** It is done only if hepatic resection is planned. It can demonstrate a highly vascular tumour (tumour blush due to neovascularisation) or involvement of portal vein thrombus in the IVC. Hence, venous phase to be recorded. It can define arterial supply also.
7. **MRI:** It appears as high intensity lesion. (Adenomatous hyperplasia, low intensity)

Table 24.4 Comparison of HCC and fibrolamellar carcinoma

	HEPATOCELLULAR CARCINOMA		FIBROLAMELLAR CARCINOMA
1. Age (years)	50-60		20-30
2. Sex	More common in males		Equal in both sexes
3. Aetiology	Cirrhosis		Does not arise in a cirrhotic liver
4. Involvement of lobe	Right lobe		Left lobe
5. Gross pathology	Solitary or nodular, central necrosis is common		Solitary or nodular, central necrosis is not common
6. Microscopy	Basic structure is trabecular pattern with acidophilic cytoplasm and large nuclei		Deeply eosinophilic hepatocytes, fibrous stroma is arranged in the form of thin hyalinized bands in layers. Hence the name **fibrolamellar**
7. Resectability rate	Less		More
8. Prognosis	Not good		Good

Differential diagnosis

Key Box 24.11
DIFFERENTIAL DIAGNOSIS
• Fibrolamellar carcinoma (Table 24.4)   • Secondaries in liver   • Haemangioma   • Focal nodular hyperplasia   • Polycystic liver

Compare CT scans of hepatoma with secondaries in the liver (Fig. 24.16 and 24.17)

TREATMENT OF HEPATOCELLULAR CARCINOMA

1. **Resection** is the best possible treatment for hepatocellular carcinoma up to 3 segments of the liver can be resected. Rest of the liver will be enough to maintain life provided remaining liver is healthy/non cirrhotic (See next page - Table 24.5, 24.6).
   • Hence in cirrhotic patients, resection is not advisable.

2. **Systemic chemotherapy** by using doxorubicin I. V. has been tried with some success in the post operative period. Also intraarterial 5-F.U.

3. **Transcatheter arterial embolization** by introducing gel foam into the branches of hepatic artery produces some amount of tumour necrosis. If this arterial embolization is combined with chemotherapeutic

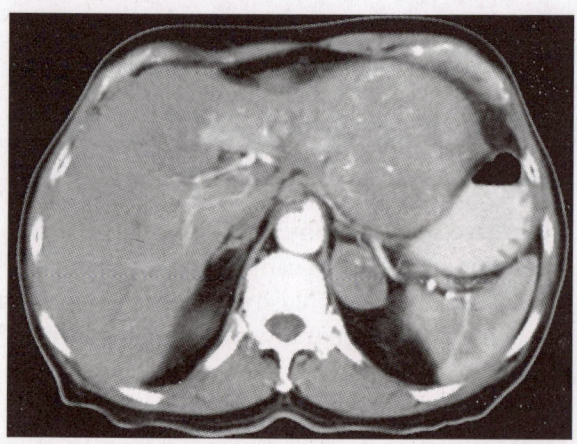

Fig. 24.16 CT scan of hepatoma

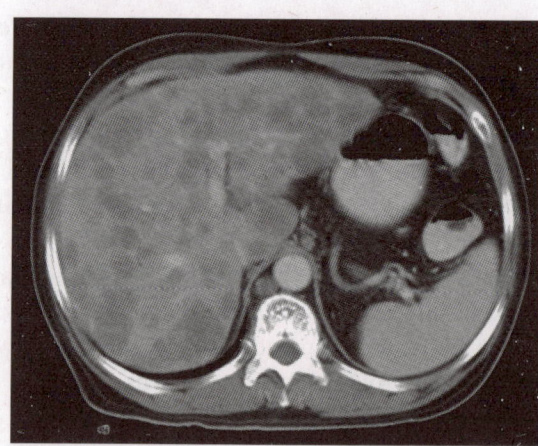

Fig. 24.17 CT scan of secondaries in the liver

Table 24.5 Showing resection of the liver

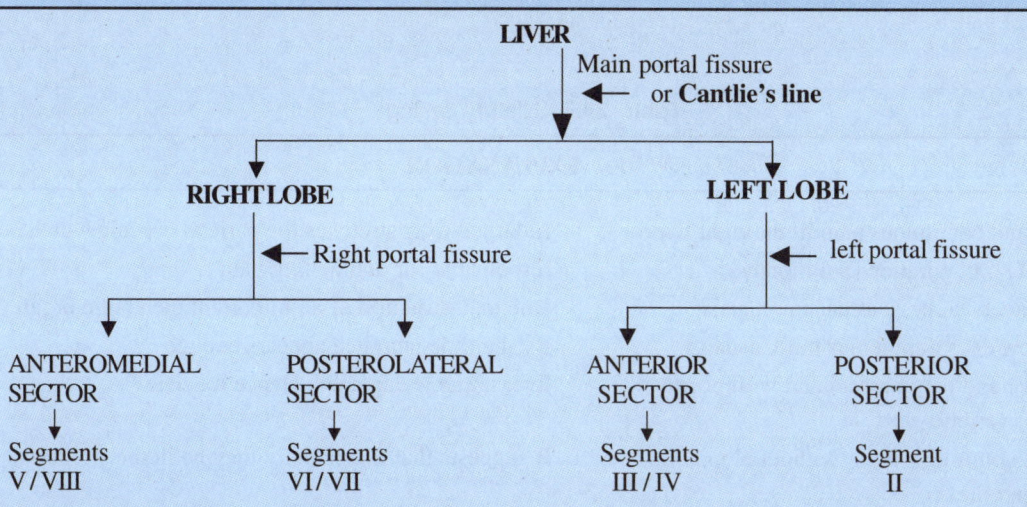

Table 24.6

HEPATIC RESECTION	NOMENCLATURE
1. Resection along the main portal fissure, separating right and left lobes of the liver	• Right or Left lobectomy
2. Resection of entire right lobe and the medial segment of left lobe.	• Right extended lobectomy or trisegmentectomy
3. Removal of segments II and III	• Left lateral segmentectomy
4. Removal of a single segment	• Unisegmentectomy
5. Removal of 2 or more segments	• Plurisegmentectomy
6. Removal of segments VI and VII	• Right lateral sectorectomy
7. Removal of a small portion of liver, entire within a single segment or transfering segmental plane	• Wedge resection

agents like doxorubicin, results are better because the tumour has prolonged exposure to the drug. This is called as chemoembolization. **The method is followed only as a palliative procedure**.

Contraindications
- Serum bilirubin >3 mg/dl
- Tumour thrombus in main portal trunk
- Early HCC

4. Percutaneous ethanol injection

5. Radiofrequency ablation It is being tried now for large inoperable tumours or patients who are not ideal candidates for surgery.

- Electrical energy is deliverd through the needle which is inserted through the skin into the tumour U/S or CT guided. Following few months tumour is destroyed, cells are killed.

- In most cases a tumour can be adequately treated in one session. Procedure can also be repeated. It is done under general anaesthesia

6. Injection octreotide, analogue of somatostatin has been used in advanced cases. It has shown promising results in decreasing the size of the tumour. It also reduces the pain and discomfort. This is combined with chemotherapy such as Gemcitabin and Carboplatin. However, the treatment is costly and the results are temporary (See Page 385).

A CASE OF SECONDARIES IN THE LIVER

HISTORY

Table 24.7 History taking

COMPLAINT	EXPLANATION
1. Dull aching and continuous pain in the right hypochondrium of short duration (3-6 months)	Enlarged liver stretches the parietal capsule which is responsible for dull aching pain
2. Loss of appetite, weakness, asthaenia, malaise	Due to destruction of an important metabolic organ
3. Jaundice of few days duration, is mild, usually nonprogressive and is not associated with pruritis (hepatocellular variety)	By the time jaundice appears enough liver tissue is damaged. Hence it is late
4. H/o persistent vomiting with or without blood, with loss of appetite	It suggests that the primary may be in the stomach
5. H/o severe backache without jaundice, disturbing the sleep at night	Carcinoma body and tail of pancreas infiltrating retroperitoneal nerve plexuses
6. H/o jaundice first and associated with itching	Periampullary carcinoma
7. H/o constipation. bleeding per rectum	Primary may be in the colon or rectum
8. H/o previous surgery such as mastectomy	Probably primary is carcinoma of the breast
9. Amputation of toes or leg or wide excision of mole	Malignant melanoma is the likely cause

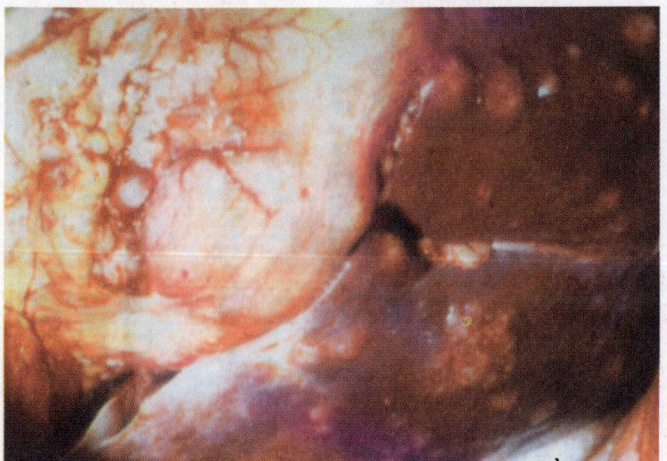

Fig. 24.18 Nodular liver with the stomach mass

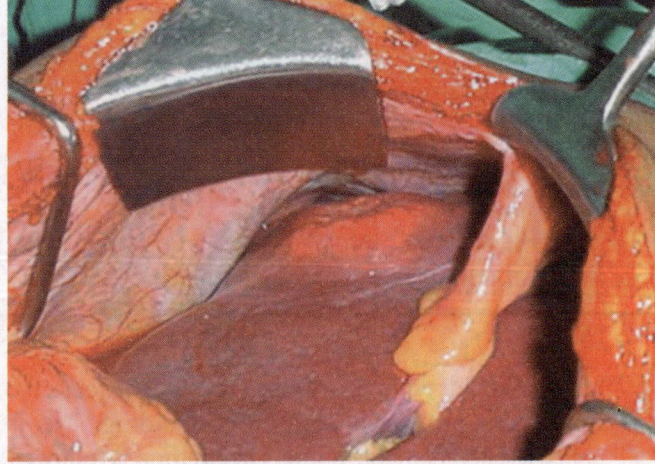

Fig. 24.19 Classical secondary in the liver with umbilication from carcinoma colon

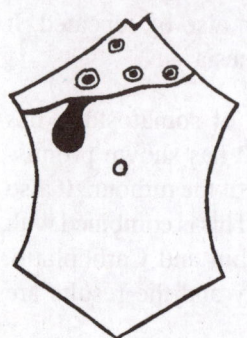

Fig. 24.20 Nodular liver with palpable gall bladder - Carcinoma head of the pancreas.

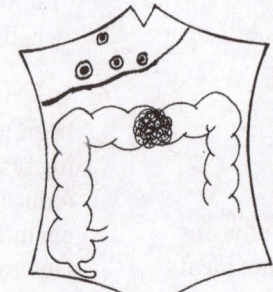

Fig. 24.21 Nodular liver in a case of carcinoma colon

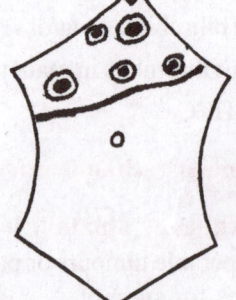

Fig. 24.22 Secondaries in the liver from melanoma

GENERAL PHYSICAL EXAMINATION

1. **Anaemia**	It is a common feature of most of the malignancies. Severe pallor may indicate carcinoma stomach or carcinoma colon
2. **Jaundice**	Deep jaundice is obstructive in nature. Hence, periampullary carcinoma is likely
3. **Bilateral pedal oedema**	Inferior venacaval obstruction due to enlarged liver
4. **Spine tenderness**	Metastasis from breast, prostate, bronchus, kidney etc.
5. **Absent testis in scrotum**	Probably seminoma arising from undescended testis

ABDOMINAL EXAMINATION

I. Criteria of secondaries in the liver

1. Both lobes are enlarged
2. Lower border is sharp
3. Surface is nodular
4. Hard in consistency
5. Umbilication refers to central necrosis in a nodule but difficult to appreciate clinically

II. Evidence of the primary

- **Example 1:** Secondaries in the liver from carcinoma stomach. A distinct stomach mass may be felt.

- **Example 2:** Secondaries in the liver from periampullary carcinoma., A palpable gall bladder gives the clue to the diagnosis.

- **Example 3:** Secondaries in the liver from carcinoma rectum. Distended colon is felt due to loaded faecal matter. Diagnosis is made by rectal examination.

- **Example 4:** Secondaries in the liver from seminoma testis. Many times, deep seated seminoma arising from undescended testis cannot be felt per abdomen.

- **Example 5:** Secondaries in the liver from malignant melanoma of foot or leg. Evidence of amputation with enlarged inguinal nodes is usually present.

Secondaries from neuroendocrine tumours tend to be bulky with huge enlargement of the liver and carry good prognosis.

INVESTIGATIONS[1]

- They depend upon the type of primary which could be detected in a clinical examination. However, when the primary could not be found out, following investigations may have to be done.

1. **Upper gastrointestinal scopy and biopsy:** To detect a growth in the oesophagus or stomach.

2. **Sigmoidoscopy/Colonoscopy:** To rule out carcinoma rectum and colon.

3. **Abdominal ultrasound**

   - It can diagnose secondaries in the liver which can be hypo- or hyperechoeic and multiple with normal hepatic parenchyma in between.

   - It can detect a carcinomatous growth in the periampullary region.

   - It can detect enlarged lymph nodes-portal, coeliac, para-aortic, etc.

   - It can detect deep seated testicular tumour arising from the testis.

   In spite of these investigations, if the primary cannot be found out other investigations may have to be done such as bronchoscopy for bronchogenic carcinoma, acid phosphatase for carcinoma prostate or computed tomography (CT scan), etc.

4. **Liver biopsy:** Laparoscopy and tissue diagnosis is a must if primary cannot be detected. Lymphoma and metastatic endocrinal tumours have better prognosis.

CLINICAL NOTES

38 year old lady came to the hospital with pain in the Rt. hypocondrium. On examination firm to hard nodular liver was paplable upto umbilicus. Before investigations, the treating doctor told the husband and relatives that she has secondaries in liver and she may not live for 6 months. 5 yrs later she came to the hospital. What she is having is **Polycystic Disease of Liver!! -** also refer Table 24.8.

TREATMENT

I. Surgery

- In majority of the cases, treatment is only palliative aiming at relieving symptoms. The following are few examples:

---

1. *Students should remember that there are dozens of investigations available today. At the end of it, one may achieve a diagnosis. However, the ultimate treatment for secondaries is HOPELESS. So. is it worth-doing all the investigations?*

A. Carcinoma stomach with secondaries-Palliative G.J, if vomiting is present.

B. Periampullary carcinoma with secondaries - triple bypass to relieve jaundice.

C. In cases of colonic cancer and carcinoid tumour, the primary can be resected because these primaries are slow growing and they carry good prognosis. Solitary metastasis in the liver is also resected.

II. Chemotherapy

• When the primary is detected to be in gastrointestinal tract, injection 5 FU can be given. The dosage is 500 mg IV for 5 days/28 days for five cycles.

• When the primary is detected outside the gastrointestinal tract, depending on the nature of the malignancy, appropriate chemotherapy is given. (They are discussed in appropriate chapters.)

III. Therapeutic embolization

• A catheter is placed in the hepatic artery and substances like blood clot or gel foam are injected. They produce thrombosis of hepatic artery resulting in liver necrosis and liver regresses in size leading to decrease in pain.

• Gel foam is cheap and easy to manipulate. The effect is temporary.

• Autologous blood clot undergoes lysis within 12-24 hours. Hence, it is not ideal.

• Embolization is an alternative to ligation of hepatic artery.

• Permanent embolizing substances including savlon sponge, steel coils, bicrylate etc.

SOME INTERESTING FEATURES (Key Box 24.13, 24.14, 24.15, 24.16)

Key Box 24.13

DIFFERENTIAL DIAGNOSIS OF NODULAR LIVER

• Secondaries and Hepatoma - hard

• Polycystic disease and Hydatid cyst - firm

Key Box 24.14

COMMON CAUSES OF SECONDARIES IN THE LIVER

• Carcinoma stomach	• Carcinoma pancreas
• Carcinoma rectum	• Carcinoma colon
• Malignant melanoma	• Testicular tumours

Key Box 24.15

CAUSES OF BULKY SECONDARIES

• Malignant melanoma

• Carcinoid tumours

• Colloid carcinoma

Key Box 24.16

SPECIAL TYPES OF SECONDARIES

• **Precocious** metastasis - before primary is suspected, e.g. carcinoid, rectal carcinoma

• **Synchronous** metastasis - primary and metastasis detected at the same time, eg. carcinoma stomach

• **Metachronous** metastasis-metastasis appearing much later than treatment of primary, e.g. melanoma of the choroid

Table 24.8. Liver mass in the surgical ward

HEPATOMA	SECONDARIES IN THE LIVER	HYDATID CYST
1. Not uncommon	Common	Uncommon
2. One lobe is enlarged	Both lobes are enlarged	One lobe is enlarged
3. Consistency is hard or firm	Hard	Firm
4. Surface irregular	Nodular	Smooth
5. Short duration	Short duration	Long duration
6. Tender	Non-tender	Non-tender
7. General condition poor	Poor	Good
8. Vascularity-thrill and bruit may be present	Absent	Absent
9. H/o alcohol intake-Features of cirrhosis are usually present	Evidence of primary like loss of appetite, vomiting, backache	H/o contact with dog may be present

PORTAL HYPERTENSION

- When portal venous pressure is more than 15 mm Hg or 20 cm of saline, it is called as portal hypertension.
- Despite high prevalence of varices in patients with cirrhosis, bleeding occurs in only 1/3 of patients.
- 10-30% of UGI bleed are due to rupture of varices due to cirrhosis.
- Variceal haemorrhage occur in 25-35% of patients with cirrhosis.
- Upto 30% of initial bleeds are fatal and as many as 70% of survivors have recurrent bleed after first variceal bleed.

ANATOMY OF PORTAL VENOUS SYSTEM

- Splenic vein after receiving inferior mesenteric vein, joins behind the neck of pancreas with superior mesenteric vein and forms the portal vein. It runs in the free edge of lesser omentum covered by common bile duct.
- It is 5-8 cm in length in its extrahepatic course and divides at the porta hepatis into right and left branches. Rarely, two branches are given on the right side.
- Potral vein carries 75% of the blood supply to the liver.

Aetiology (Fig. 24.23)

I. Extrahepatic portal hypertension (Prehepatic)

1. Splenic vein thrombosis
2. Portal vein thrombosis
   - It is secondary to umbilical vein sepsis in neonates (Omphalitis). In adults, thrombosed portal vein is surrounded by a leash of vessels 'Cavernoma'. Portal vein thrombosis can also occur due to carcinoma pancreas in elderly patients.
3. Portal vein agenesis

Extrahepatic portal hypertension is seen in 20% to 25% of cases and is common in female children. Liver function is normal in these cases.

II. Intrahepatic portal hypertension (It accounts for nearly 80% of cases)

1. Cirrhosis of the liver
   - The regenerating nodules compress the portal venous radicles within the liver. Liver function is very poor.
2. Schistosomiasis

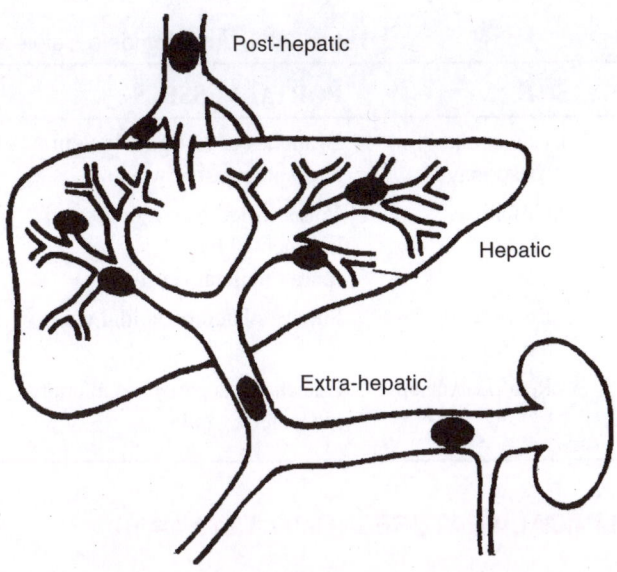

Fig. 24.23 Causes of portal hypotension

- Common in Egypt also a cause of portal hypertension. Schistosoma mansoni and japonicum lay eggs within branches of portal vein and cause hepatic fibrosis resulting in portal hypertension.

III. Post-hepatic portal hypertension (Medical causes of portal hypertension)

1. Tricuspid incompetence
2. Constrictive pericarditis
3. Budd-Chiari syndrome

PATHOPHYSIOLOGY[1] (Table 24.9)

As a result of obstruction to portal vein, in an attempt to reduce portal pressure, the normally present insignificant collaterals open up. They become significant and result in development of portosystemic anastomosis.

- Eventhough, portosystemic shunts develop in many places the important locations and their clinical significance has been outlined in the Table 24.9.
- Specially the lower end of the oesophagus is one of the important areas which gives rise to oesophageal varices. These varices rupture resulting in massive haemetemesis.
- This is exactly the reason why every attempt, newer modalities of treatment - medical or surgical are aimed at controlling oesophageal varices.

---

1. When the main highway is blocked. small insignificant side roads become significant.

	Table 24.9. Anastomosis between the portal and systemic venous system		
SITE	**PORTAL VESSELS**	**SYSTEMIC VESSELS**	**EFFECT**
1. Lower end of oesophagus	Branches of left gastric vein and short gastric vein	Branches from azygos vein	Oesophageal varices
2. Umbilicus	Veins which run in the round ligament of liver (paraumbilical vein)	Anterior abdominal wall veins	Caput medusae[1]
3. Lower end of rectum	Superior haemorrhoidal vein	Inferior and middle haemorrhoidal vein	Piles (very rare), rectal varices
4. Retroperitoneum	Branches of superior and inferior mesenteric veins	Retroperitoneal veins Subdiaphragmatic veins	Retroperitoneal varices (Silent)

CLINICAL FEATURES (Refer Table 24.10)

Table 24.10. Clinical comparison of extrahepatic with intrahepatic portal hypertension		
	EXTRAHEPATIC	**INTRAHEPATIC**
1. Age	10-25 years	> 40 years
2. H/o alcohol	Absent	Strongly positive
3. H/o jaundice	Absent	Present
4. Sex	More in females	More in men
5. Splenomegaly	Moderate to big	Mild to moderate
6. Ascites	Absent	Present
7. Liver cell failure	Absent	Present
8. Encephalopathy	Not a feature	It is common

PREDICTION OF VARICEAL HAEMORRHAGE

1. **Physical factors:** Elastic properties of vessels, intravariceal and intraluminal pressure and variceal wall tension are major factors.
2. **Continued alcohol use**
3. **Poor liver function**
4. **Hepatic venous pressure gradient:** HVPG = (wedged / occluded hepatic venous pressure) - (free hepatic venous pressure). **Normal gradient is 5 mm of Hg.** HVPG > 12 mm of Hg indicates portal hypertension.

INVESTIGATIONS

1. **Complete blood picture**
   - Anaemia is usually present due to bleeding
   - Peripheral smear to rule out hypersplenism-pancytopaenia in the presence of normal bone marrow.

2. **Liver function tests**
   - Serum proteins: Total protein, albumin are low and albumin: globulin ratio is reversed in cirrhosis of the liver.
   - Enzymes SGOT (serum glutamic oxaloacetic transaminase) and SGPT (serum glutamic pyruvic acid transaminase) are increased in hepatocellular failure.
   - Serum bilirubin: Increased levels indicate liver cell failure.
   - Prothrombin time, bleeding time, clotting time are essential before a liver biopsy is done.
   - **Liver biopsy** is done provided BT, PT, CT are normal. However, injection vitamin K 10 mg I.M is given for 3 to 5 days.
   - HBsAg serum hepatitis predisposes to cirrhosis of the liver.
   - Liver functions are usually normal in extrahepatic portal hypertension.

3. **Oesophagogastroduodenoscopy**
   - To confirm oesophageal varices which appear as a bluish red longitudinal column in the lower end of oesophagus. When they extend to the stomach, they are called gastric varices
   - Cherry red spots indicate impending rupture

   For endoscopic pictures (Page 379) and grading Key Box 24.17)

---

1. *Caput medusae is rare because paraumbilical veins are obliterated in newborn, in majority of cases.*

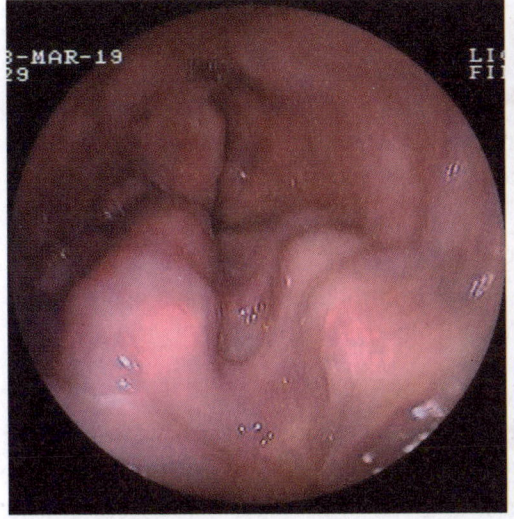

Fig. 24.24 Oesophageal varices

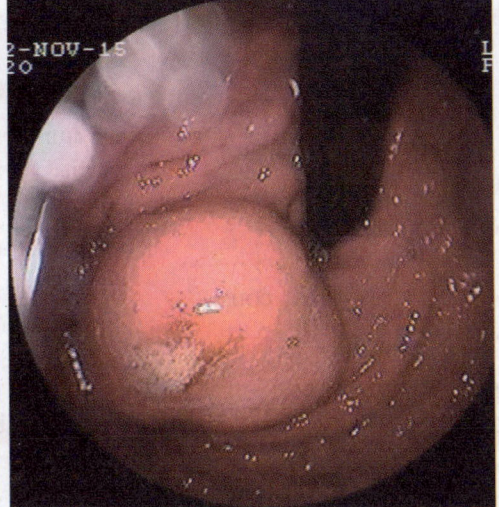

Fig. 24.25 Gastric varices

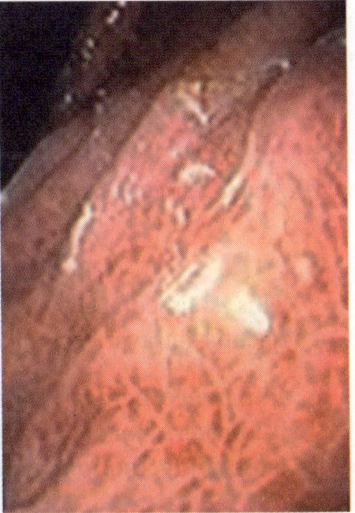

Fig. 24.26 Gastropathy

Key Box 24.17	
ENDOSCOPIC GRADING OF VARICES BASED ON VARIX HEIGHT AT 2CM FROM OG JUNCTION	
Grade	**Bite width 1.7mm forceps = 5mm**
1+	One fourth bite width
2+	One half bite width
3+	Three fourths bite width
4+	One or more bite width(s)

4. Splenoportovenography (SPV)

- A fine lumbar puncture needle is passed through the 9th space in the left mid axillary line into the spleen and a radiopaque dye injected into the splenic pulp which fills up the entire portal system.

Requirement and precautions

- BT, CT, PT should be normal.
- Prophylactic antibiotics are given to avoid pyaemia.

Uses (Fig. 24.27)

- To know the anatomical configuration of portal system, so that a proper shunt operation can be done.
- To locate the exact site of obstruction
- To assess the diameter of splenic vein. When it is more than 1 cm, it is an indication for spleno-renal shunt (lieno-renal shunt).

- If the needle is connected to a manometer, splenic pulp pressure can be recorded.

5. Ultrasonography
- To assess the nature of the liver (**cirrhosis**), to know the portal vein, portal cavernoma, splenic vein diameter, etc. It has become a valuable investigation today.

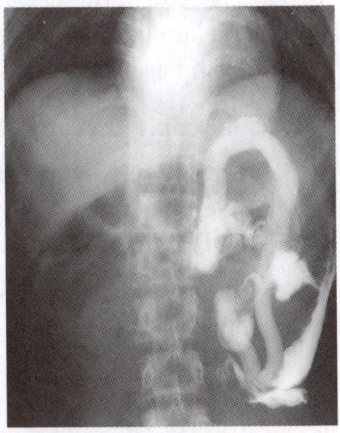

Fig. 24.27 SPV showing dilated splenic vein.

CAUSES OF RUPTURE OF VARICES

- Variceal bleeding can occur even without any specific cause. The bleeding can be very minor in the form of occult blood in the stools to massive bleeding. Following hypothesis has been postulated for massive bleeding from varices.

1. **Eruptive theory:** Due to increased intravariceal pressure.

2. **Erosive theory:** Erosion of mucosa over the the varices.

- Bleeding manifests as haemetemesis or malena. Hemodynamic instability is common.

TREATMENT OF PORTAL HYPERTENSION - GUIDELINES

I.   Primary prophylaxis

II. Secondary prophylaxis

III. Acute variceal haemorrhage

I. Primary phophylaxis (Before bleeding)

This is aimed at reducing portal pressure and consequently intravariceal pressure.

A. Pharmacotherapy: Drugs used are **Nonselective β-blockers** alone (propranalol) or in combination with **isosorbide mononitrate**.

- Reducing portal pressure by at least 20% or HVPG < 12 mms of Hg is associated with significant protection against bleeding.

- The dose of β-blockers are titrated to maintain heart rate around 55 beats / minute or reducing by 25% from baseline rate.

B. Endoscopic therapy: Endotherapy

- **Endoscopic band ligation** of varices is better than sclerotherapy. It is very effective and associated with less side effects.

- Indicated in patients who do not tolerate β-blockers and varices which are large and are associated with red wheal markings.

II. Secondary prophylaxis

- It means prevention of rebleeding following acute variceal haemorrhage.

- The various forms of treatment and their success depends upon the criterias which popularly go in the name of modified Childs criteria. (Refer Table 24.11) Serum albumin, bilirubin, ascites, encephalopathy and prothrombin time are included under this criteria.

III. TREATMENT OF MASSIVE BLEEDING FROM VARICES

1. General measures

- Admission, hospitalization, preferably in an intensive care unit, elevation of foot end of the bed to increase venous return

- Blood transfusion

- Do a cut down or introduce IV cannula and replacement of fluid till blood is ready.

2. Measures to prevent encephalopathy

- Ryle's tube is introduced and stomach wash is given with ice-cold saline.

- Bowel wash is given to decrease blood from gut, to decrease ammonia, uric acid levels so as to prevent encephalopathy.

- Oral neomycin 1gm, 6th hourly as intestinal antiseptic.

- Oral lactulose 30 ml, 8th hourly is given. It also helps in decreasing encephalopathy.

3. Pharmacotherapy for variceal bleeding

- **Injection Vasopressin** 20 units in 200 ml of saline is given intravenously for a period of 20 minutes. This dose avoids coronary vasoconstriction and abdominal vasoconstriction. By causing powerful splanchnic vasoconstriction, it decreases the blood flow to the varices and reduces bleeding in about 50% patients.

- **Injection Somatostatin** 50 mg I.V. bolus followed by an infusion of 50 mg/hour. It is very effective and has no side effects. However, it is costly.

- **Injection Octreotide** and terrapressin are preferred because of their long half life. They act by producing splanchnic vasoconstriction. Thus they decrease the portal pressure. Once started they have to be continued for 2-5 days. Once bleeding stops, they are subjected to **endotherapy** to prevent rebleeding.

Table 24.11 Modified Child's criteria Grade A = 5-6 points, Grade B = 7-9 points, Grade C = above 10 points			
POINTS AWARDED FOR ABNORMALITY			
	1	**2**	**3**
1. Albumin gm/lit	35	28-35	Less than 28
2. Bilirubin mol/lit	15-30	30-45	More than 45
3. Ascites	Absent	Easily controlled	Not controlled
4. Encephalopathy	Absent	Mild	Severe
5. Prothrombin time (prolonged)	1-4	4-6	Above 6

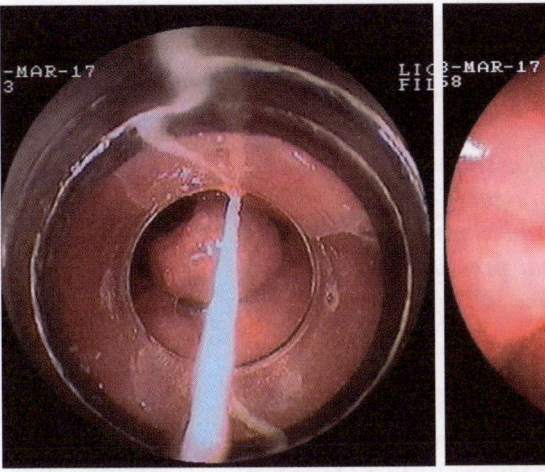

Fig. 24.28 Endoscopic banding

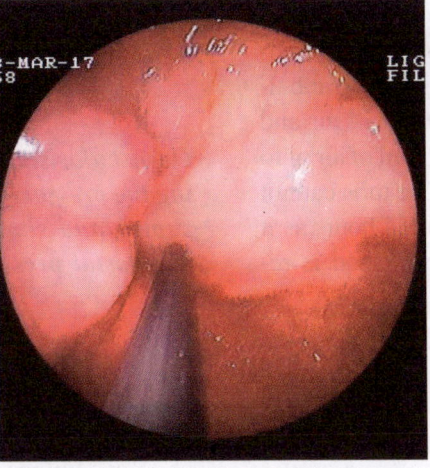

Fig. 24.29 Endoscopic sclerotherapy

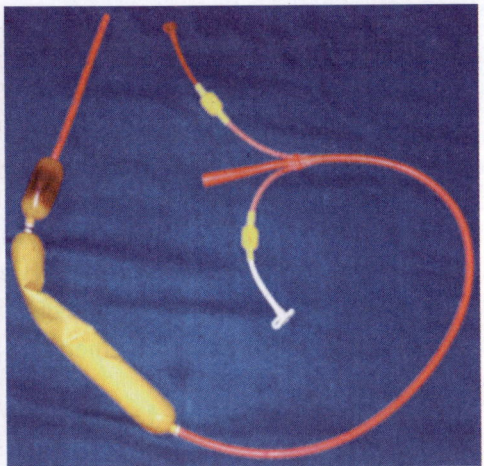

Fig. 24.30 Balloon tamponade

Contributed by: Dr. Filipe Alvaris, Medical Gastroenterologist, KMC, Manipal

- **Metoclopramide** 20 mg I. V. arrests the bleeding by constricting gastro-oesophageal sphincter.

4. Endotherapy - Types

A. Variceal Banding : (Key box 24.18, Fig. 24.28)

- Today variceal banding has become the gold standard for oesophageal varices because of their efficiency with controlling the bleeding and less chances of complication.
- In 10% of the cases rebleeding can occur.

B. Sclerotherapy (Key Box 24.19, Fig. 24.29)

- 2% ethanolamine oleate or sodium tetradecyl sulphate (STD) is used, 3-5 ml into each varices (**intravariceal**) or 0.5 ml into the side of varices (**paravariceal**). Bleeding can be controlled in about 80-90% of patients. If the bleeding continues, repeat injections can be given.

- If the bleeding continues in spite of above measures, balloon tamponade is done.

Disadvantages of endoscopic sclerotherapy

1. Gastric varices cannot be managed by sclerotherapy
2. Multiple oesophageal ulcers can develop at the injection site
3. 10-20% of the patients develop low grade fever
4. It can precipitate massive bleeding
5. It can cause mediastinitis, left pleural effusion
6. Chances of rebleeding are high. Hence, repeated injections are necessary.

C. Balloon tamponade (Fig. 24.30)

- Balloon tamponade must be used as a **rescue procedure** and to bridge more definitive therapy in case of uncontrolled haemorrhage.

Key Box 24.18
VARICEAL BANDING

Advantages

- Controls bleeding in 80-90% of cases
- Less rebleeding rates
- Easy
- Less risk of complication such as perforation or stricture

Disadvantage

- Costly

Key Box 24.19
SCLEROTHERAPY

Advantages

- Cheap
- Easy
- More commonly available

Disadvantages

- Complications such as perforation or stricture and massive bleeding can occur
- More rebleeding rates

- Sengstaken's tube or its modification, the **Minnesota tube** is used. It acts directly by internal tamponade. It is passed through the nose. Gastric balloon is distended with upto 250-300 ml of air and oesophageal balloon with about 50-60ml of air or to get a pressure of 20-30mm of Hg. The tube cannot be kept in place for more than 12 to 24 hours as it can cause **pressure necrosis**. The method is reliable only in experienced hands.

- Recurrent bleeding is common after decompression.

D. TIPSS: Transjugular Intrahepatic Portosystemic Stent Shunt

- Consists of vascular placement of expandable metal stent across the tract created between hepatic vein and major branch of portal system.

- TIPSS helps for small group of patients (5 to 10%) who have refractory bleeding.

- Low morbidity and mortality

- Incidence of encephalopathy is similar to surgical stents (Refer Fig. 24.31).

5. Surgery

- It is of two types - Devascularisation procedures and Shunt procedures.

Devascularisation procedures are aimed at reducing the pressure in the varices by disrupting the blood supply and shunt procedures are aimed at reducing portal pressure.

A. Devascularisation procedures

1. Oesophageal transection

- It is done through left thoracoabdominal route called as 'Milnes Walker Operation'.
- During the transection, varices get disconnected, bleeders are ligated or under-run, followed by oesophagogastric anastomosis.

2. Gastric transection of Tanner

- In this operation the division is made in the stomach through abdominal route.

3. Sugiura and Futugawa operation

- It is an extensive devascularization procedure.

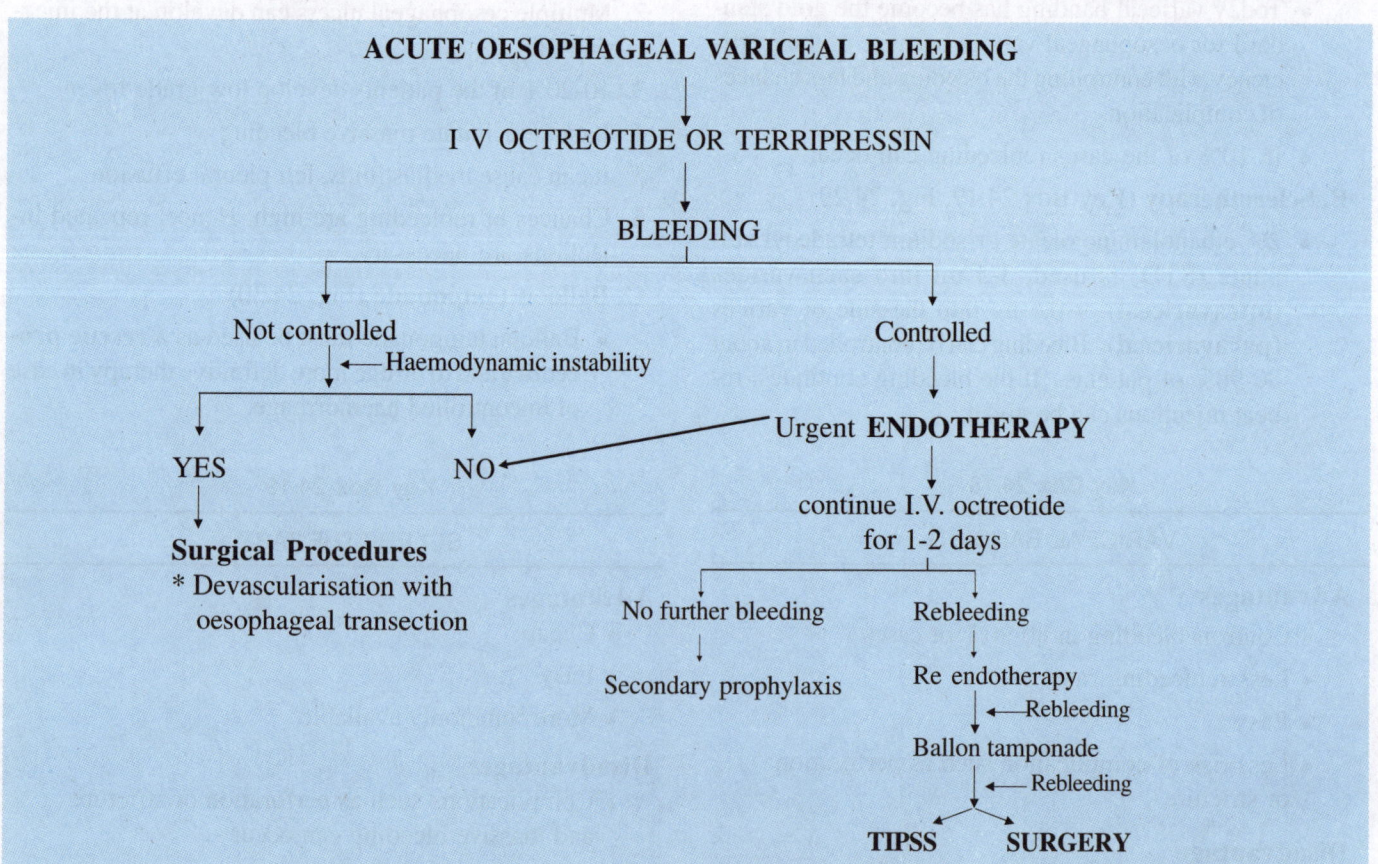

Fig. 24.31 Algorithm showing management of bleeding varices

Aim

- To interrupt the intramural and submucosal veins.

Procedure (Fig. 24.32, 24.33)

- In this operation, following procedures are done:
- Splenectomy
- Devascularization of the greater curvature of the stomach and devascularization of lesser curvature of the stomach as in highly selective vagotomy.
- Oesophagogastric transection and suturing by using EEA (**E**nd to **E**nd **A**nastomosis) staplers. It is a major surgery. Mortality is around 10-15%. It is the most effective devascularization.

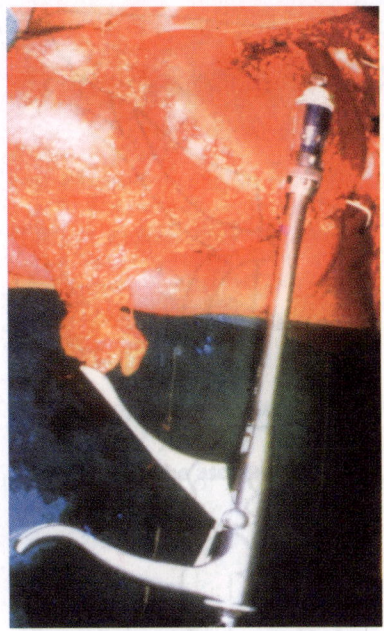

Fig. 24.32 Usage of EEA staplers for devascularisation procedure. Contributed by Prof. U.Santhosh Pai, KMC, Manipal

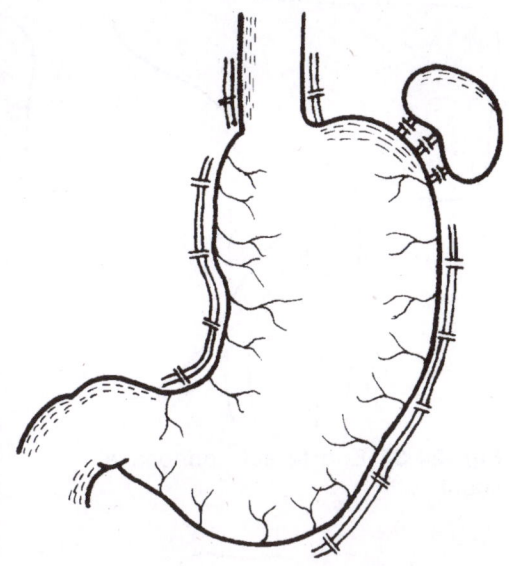

Fig. 24.33 Sugiura and Futugawa operation (Splenectomy with devascularisation). Ideally done through thoraco - abdominal incision

B. Portosystemic shunt procedures

Indications

1. Continuing variceal blceding in spite of sclero-therapy wherein the general condition of the patient is good (Child's A, Child's B).
2. As an elective procedure in patients who had bleeding in the past.
3. The selection of shunt is based on the availability of a good vein. Jaundice, ascites low albumin are contraindications for shunt surgery.

Types

1. End to side portacaval shunt (Fig. 24.34)

- Portal vein is divided from the liver and the end is anastomosed to the side of IVC (inferior venacava).
- This controls the bleeding in 90-95% of patients but chances of encephalopathy is 30% because of sudden deprivation of liver blood supply.

  Indications: Cirrhosis of liver, due to schistosomiasis, provided liver function is reasonably good.

2. Side to side portacaval shunt: Side of portal vein is anastomosed to side of inferior vena cava.(Fig. 24.35).

  Advantage: Incidence of encephalopathy is 10%.

Disadvantage: Control of bleeding is about 50-70%.

3. Proximal splenorenal shunt (Fig. 24.36)

- In this operation, spleen is removed. Then, proximal end of the splenic vein is sutured to the side of renal vein in the retroperitoneum. This is preferred in children.

4. Distal splenorenal shunt (DSRS)-**Warren's shunt** (Fig. 24.37)

Indications

- Extrahepatic portal hypertension with portal vein thrombosis, provided the splenic vein is dilated more than 1cm.
- Can also be done in cirrhosis of liver. Chances of encephalopathy is almost minimal after this procedure.

In this operation, distal end of splenic vein is divided and sutured to the side of renal vein in the retroperitoneum. Post-operatively ascites can occur due to extensive retroperitoneal dissection which damages lymphatics.

5. Mesenterico-caval shunt (Fig. 24.38)

Indications

1. Splenic vein is not dilated or thrombosed.
2. Portal vein is thrombosed.

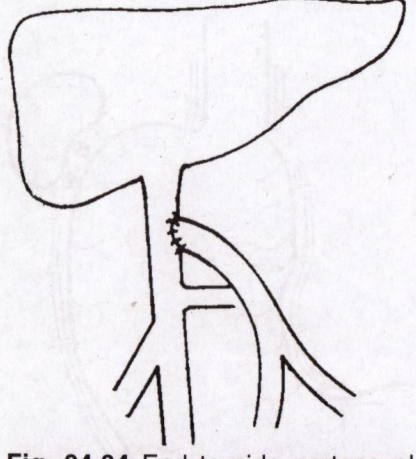

Fig. 24.34 End to side portocaval shunt

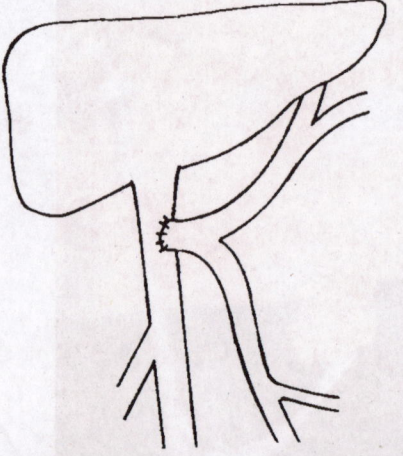

Fig. 24.35 Side to side portocaval shunt

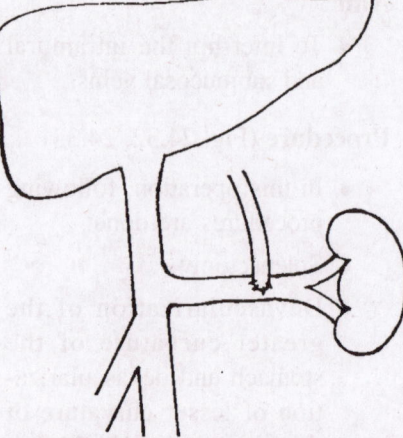

Fig. 24.36 Proximal splenorenal shunt

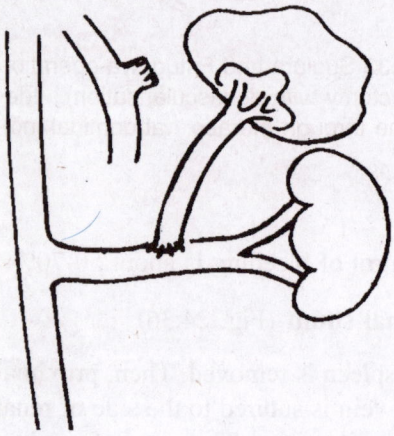

Fig. 24.37 Distal splenorenal shunt

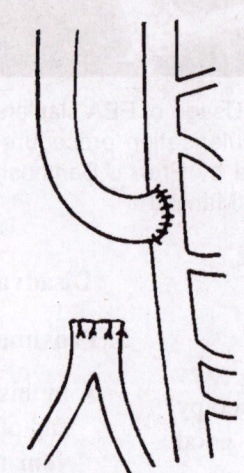

Fig. 24.38 Mesenterico-caval shunt

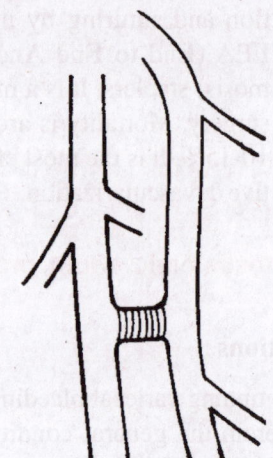

Fig. 24.39 Mesenterico-caval H graft.

Procedure

- **The inferior vena cava is divided** and its proximal end is sutured to the side of superior mesenteric vein (S.M. V.).
- Otherwise, a dacron graft can be placed between I.V.C. and S.M.V. This is described as mesentericocaval H-graft or jump graft (Fig. 24.39).
- In children, I. V .C. can be divided without fear of pedal oedema.

Shunt procedures have to be undertaken only by an experienced surgical gastroenterologist in an institution. These patients have to be carefully monitored in the post-operative period for a possible shunt blockage.

Miscellaneous

CONTROL OF ASCITES IN PORTAL HYPERTENSION

- Ascites in portal hypertension is a slow, insidious accumulation of free peritoneal fluid, a occurrence in advanced liver disease.
- It can be troublesome and refractory to the commonly available treatment.
- Diagnosis is confirmed by ultrasound and aspiration.
- When there is a doubt regarding the diagnosis, **Laparoscopy** is advisable which can not only detect and confirm cirrhosis but also to rule out other intraabdominal pathologies (malignancy, tuberculosis etc).

Causes (Key Box 24.20)

Key Box 24.20
CAUSES OF ASCITES IN PORTAL HYPERTENSION
• Reduction in plasma albumin
• Central hypovolaemia
• Retention of salt and water by kidneys
• Portal hypertension

Treatment (Key Box 24.21)

1. **Diuretics:** K$^+$ sparing diuretics such as spironolactone or frusemide can be given. However hyponatraemia and hypokalaemia should be monitored.
2. **Restriction of salt intake:** 20mg/day is adviced.
3. **Peritoneovenous shunt: Le Veen shunt**

• Le Veen shunt is done by using silastic tube inserted into ascites and it is tunnelled subcutaneously to the neck and inserted under vision into internal jugular veins.

Key Box 24.21
TREATMENT
• **S**alt restriction
• **A**bdominal paracentesis
• **L**iver transplantation
• **T**IPSS
• **I**ntake of diuretics
• **SH**unt - Peritonovenous
* You can remember as **SALTISH**

• **Mode of action:** Because of one way valve, with each respiration, fluid is drawn into systemic circulation.

Complications: Occlusion, displacement, infection

BUDD-CHIARI SYNDROME

• It occurs due to obstruction to the hepatic vein

Causes

1. **Congenital:** It is a potentially curable condition where in a web exists in the suprahepatic portion of inferior vena cava.
2. Clotting disorders-polycythaemia
3. Contraceptive pills
4. Cancerous infiltration of hepatic veins (hepatocellular carcinoma).
5. Crotalaria, a plant extract used in the tea

Clinical features

1. **Acute form** is dangerous, result in rapid enlargement of liver, severe abdominal pain, vomiting, hypotension, etc.
2. **Chronic form** resembles cirrhosis
• Hepatomegaly-firm, can be irregular, dilated veins over the abdominal wall, bilateral pedal oedema which is irritating, signs of liver cell failure, haemetemesis occurs later.

Treatment

• In congenital cases, if web can be proved by venacavography, it can be excised by transatrial meatotomy. However, in general, prognosis is very poor. Peritoneovenous shunt has to be considered as an alternate to drain the ascitic fluid into one of the veins in the neck (internal jugular vein).

ROLE OF OCTREOTIDE IN SURGERY

1. Variceal bleeding
   Acute - 50μg I.V. stat followed by 50μg/hr. infusion for 120 hrs.
   Long term **prophylaxis** is 100μg s/c TDS for 15 days
2. Pancreatic disorders
   ERCP induced pancreatitis
   Acute pancreatitis
   Relapsing pancreatitis
   Chronic pancreatitis
   Pancreatic surgery -100μg s/c TDS 1hr prior to surgery for 7 days
3. Bowel dysfuntion- AIDS related diarrhoea, short bowel syndrome, dumping syndrome, chemotherapy induced diarrhoea
4. Gastro intestinal fistulae
5. Carcinoid and other neuroendocrine tumours
6. Advanced hepatocellular carcinoma, metastatic breast cancer, colonic cancer, pancreatic cancer
7. Acromegaly

Gall bladder and Pancreas

25

- Surgical anatomy
- Bile
- Congenital anomalies
- Acute cholecystitis
- Chronic cholecystitis
- Obstructive jaundice
- Chronic pancreatitis
- Carcinoma pancreas
- Stricture CBD
- Sclerosing cholangitis
- Choledochal cyst
- Caroli's disease
- Cholangiocarcinoma
- Congenital biliary atresia
- Carcinoma gall bladder
- Endocrine tumours
- Acute pancreatitis
- Pseudocyst
- Annular pancreas
- Ectopic pancreas
- Cystic fibrosis
- Pancreatic fistula
- White bile

SURGICAL ANATOMY OF THE GALL BLADDER

- It is a pear or globular shaped organ present in the right hypochondrium on the inferior surface of the liver, situated in the gall bladder fossa. It is about 8-12 cm long.

PARTS OF THE GALL BLADDER

- **Fundus:** It is the dilated portion of gall bladder adherent to undersurface of the liver from which it can be separated easily.
- **Neck:** The narrow angulated distal portion of neck is called **Hartmann's pouch** - common site where stones occur and tend to stay for a long time.
- Gall bladder is connected to common bile duct (CBD) through **cystic duct**, which is 2.5 cm in length. It is lined by cuboidal epithelium. Within the cystic duct, the prominent mucosal folds exist due to prominent circular muscle fibers. It produces a valve called **valve of**

Heister which prevents the migration of stone into the CBD.

BLOOD SUPPLY OF GALL BLADDER

- Cystic artery, a branch of right hepatic artery is given behind the common bile duct. Soon, it branches out over the surface of gall bladder. **Cystic artery is an end artery.** Multiple small veins from the surface of gall bladder join liver surface. There is also a cystic vein, from the neck, draining into portal vein directly. This explains early spread of gall bladder malignancy to the liver.

CHOLECYSTOHEPATIC TRIANGLE OR CALOT'S TRIANGLE: BOUNDARIES

- **Lateral:** Cystic duct and gall bladder
- **Medial:** Common hepatic duct
- **Above:** Inferior surface of right lobe of the liver

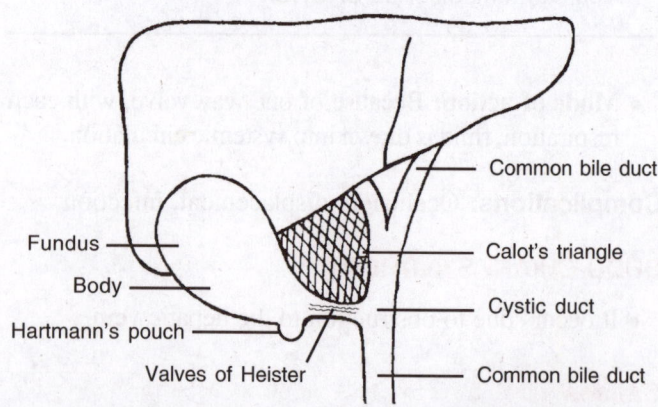

Fig. 25.1 Surgical anatomy of the gall bladder

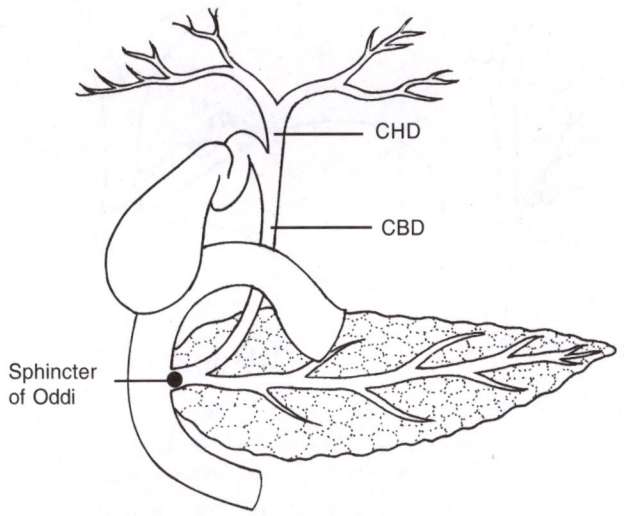

Fig. 25.2 Surgical anatomy of the bile ducts

Contents

- Right hepatic artery and its branch, the cystic artery
- Cystic lymph node of Lund

ANATOMY OF THE BILE DUCTS

- **Common hepatic duct (CHD)** is formed by the union of right and left hepatic ducts. It is 3 cm in length, receives cystic duct and continues as common bile duct (CBD).

- **Common bile duct** is about 8 cms long. It has four parts: supraduodenal, retroduodenal, infraduodenal and intraduodenal. Along with pancreatic duct, it forms ampulla of Vater. Controlled by sphincter of Oddi, it ends by an opening in the second part of duodenum.

BILE

- Secreted from hepatocytes
- 250-1000 ml/day, 98% is water
- Concentrated in gall bladder because of absorption of water
- Fatty food stimulation releases cholecystokinin, which stimulates gall bladder and at the same time sphincter of Oddi relaxes.
- It also has inorganic ions (more than plasma cells) hence severe electrolyte imbalance occurs in biliary fistula.

- Cholesterol, synthesised in the liver gives rise to bile acids - cholic and chenodeoxy cholic acids. They are metabolised in the colon to deoxycholic acid and litho-cholic acids.
- Main function of bile acids in bile is to maintain cholesterol in solution.

CONGENITAL ANOMALIES OF GALL BLADDER
(Fig. 25.3)

A. **Absence** of **gall bladder**-Very, very rare

B. **Floating gall bladder**-Results due to long mesentery. It is more vulnerable to torsion-a rare cause of recurrent upper abdominal pain. Such a gall bladder can be easily removed.

C. **Phrygian cap**-Cap which was worn by people of Phrygia (ancient Asian country, Mongolia). It is an anomaly connected with the fundus of the gall bladder.

D. **Double gall bladder**-The second one is always intrahepatic (rare).

E. **Absence of cystic duct**-Cholecystectomy becomes difficult. There are high chances of injury to the common bile duct.

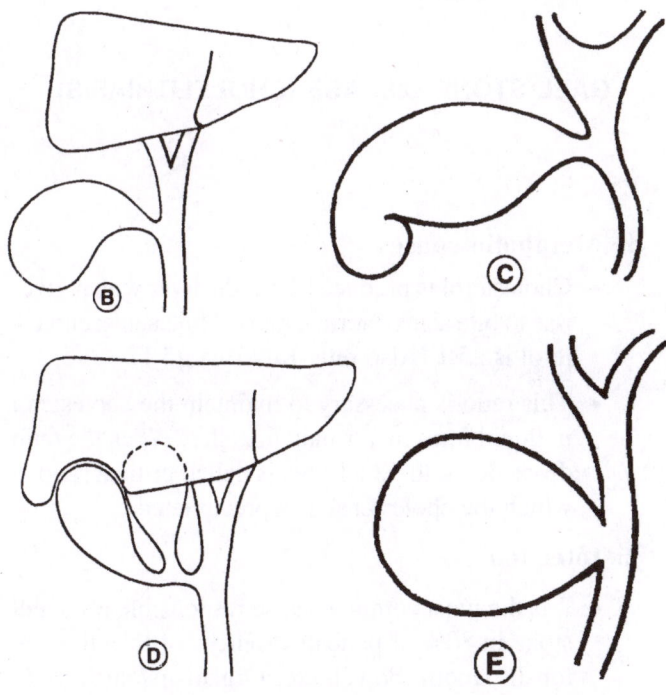

Fig. 25.3 Congenital anomalies of gall bladder

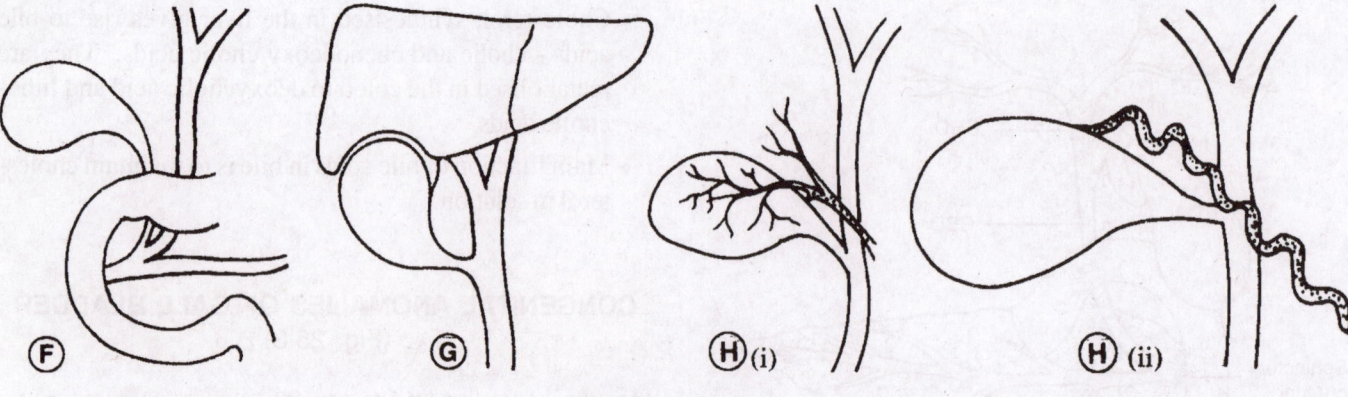

Fig. 25.3 Continued

F. **Low insertion of cystic duct-**Cystic duct opens into the common bile duct near the ampulla. This anomaly should be kept in mind when operating on cases of obstructive jaundice.

G. An **accessory cholecystohepatic duct** is present in about 10% of the patients. It may be the cause of significant bile leakage after cholecystectomy.

H. **Anomalies of blood supply:**

i. Cystic artery is given anteriorly from right hepatic artery.

ii. Very, very tortuous hepatic artery-Caterpillar turn or Moynihan's hump. It runs in front of the origin of cystic duct.

GALL STONE DISEASE (CHOLELITHIASIS)

AETIOLOGY

1. **Metabolic causes**
   - Cholesterol is produced from the liver which gives rise to bile acids. Normal ratio of bile acids: cholesterol is 25:1 (Also refer Key Box 25.1).
   - This ratio is necessary to maintain the cholesterol in liquid form by forming micelles. When the ratio drops down to 13 : 1, this is called critical ratio at which the cholesterol gets precipitated.

2. **Infection**
   - It is the most common cause responsible for a gall stone in 80% of patients. Sources of infection are tonsils, tooth, bowel, etc. Organisms such as *E. coli, Proteus*, anaerobic organisms, Streptococci, etc., through the blood stream reach the gall blad-

---

Key Box 25.1

CAUSES OF DECREASED BILE ACID POOL

1. Cirrhosis of liver
2. Gastrectomy
3. Ileal resection
4. Malabsorption
5. Obesity
6. Hypercholesterolaemia

---

der wall and form a focus/nidus around which cholesterol and bile salts get precipitated.

- Over a period of many years, this results in a mixed stone. They are usually multiple and occur in an infected bile.

"A Gall stone is a tomb stone erected in the memory of organisms within it."-Lord Moynihan

3. **Bile stasis**
   - Pregnancy, oestrogens, following vagotomy and prolonged TPN (Total Parenteral Nutrition).
   - They are prone for mixed stones as a result of bile stasis.

4. **Haemolytic anaemia**
   - Examples: Hereditary spherocytosis, sickle cell anaemia, etc.
   - Because of increased break down of RBC's, the bilirubin production is increased. Since the production is more, they cannot conjugate with glucuronic acid, which is produced at normal levels.

- Such unconjugated bilirubin combines with the calcium and is excreted in the biliary tree resulting in calcium bilirubinate stones (pigment stones) not only in the gall bladder, also in the entire ductal system.

5. Saint's triad

1. Gall stones (can occur along with the other 2 conditions mentioned below).

2. Diverticulosis of colon

3. Hiatus hernia

6. Parasitic infestation

- In oriental countries, Clonorchis sinensis (Chinese liver fluke) infestations can cause stone in biliary tree.

- Ascaris lumbricoides in the biliary tree may produce stones in our country (India).

7. Due to abnormal mucus

- It is produced in congenital cystic fibrosis, gall stones occur in these children due to impairment of bile flow.

OTHER DISEASES ASSOCIATED WITH GALL STONE DISEASE

- Diabetes mellitus
- Type IV Hyperlipoproteinaemia
- Cirrhosis of liver
- Fistulae on treatment with total parenteral nutrition
- Gastric surgery

RISK FACTORS FOR GALL STONE DISEASE

Key Box 25.2
RISK FACTORS
• Female sex • Obesity • Maturity onset diabetes • Age > 40 years

TYPES OF GALL STONES

1. Cholesterol stones (Fig. 25.4)

- Constitutes about 10% of the gall stones
- Occur in patients with increased cholesterol levels
- Fatty women are commonly affected

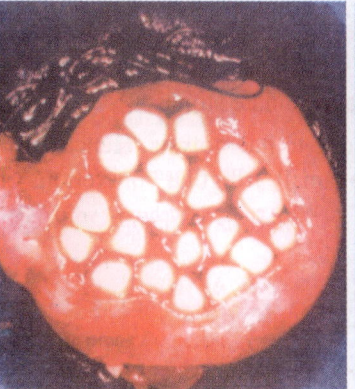
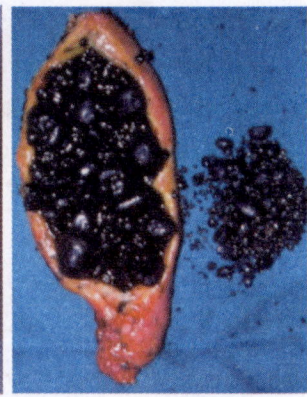

Fig. 25.4 Cholesterol stone   **Fig. 25.5** Pigment stones - case of heriditary spherocytosis

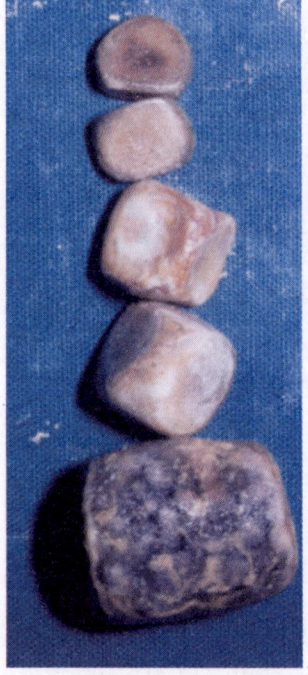
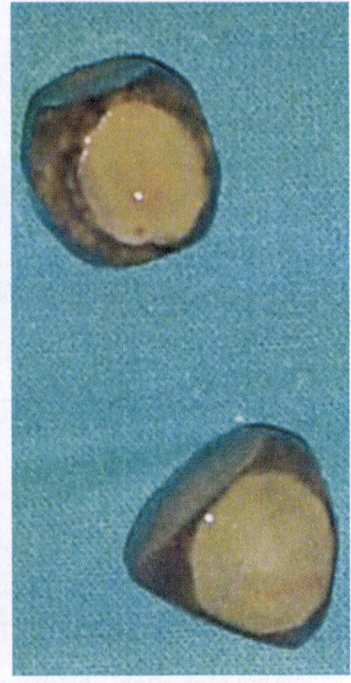

Fig. 25.6 Mixed stones - observe faceting

- It is single, solitary, occurs in aseptic bile. Sometimes they can be multiple. Precipitation of cholesterol gives rise to stone.
- Such stones can be silent for many years. They are radiolucent.
- Pigment can also get precipitated along with cholesterol.

2. Mixed stones (Fig. 25.6)

- They constitute about 80% of gall stones.
- They contain alternating layers of cholesterol and pigment with epithelial debris or vegetations, from infective organisms.
- They are multiple, small faceted by mutual pressure.

3. **Pigment stones** (Fig. 25.5)
- They are found in 5 to 10% of patients
- They are calcium bilirubinate stones
- Commonly occur due to haemolysis. Hence, they are black, multiple, small, irregular concretions or sludge particles.

CLINICAL FEATURES (COMPLICATIONS OF GALL STONES)

Key Box 25.3

IN THE GALL BLADDER

- Silent stones
- Flatulent dyspepsia
- Gall stone colic
- Acute cholecystitis
- Chronic cholecystitis
- Mucocoele
- Carcinoma of the gall bladder
- Mirizzi's syndrome

IN THE BILE DUCT

- Obstructive jaundice
- Cholangitis
- White bile (Page 427)
- Acute pancreatitis

IN THE INTESTINE

- Acute intestinal obstruction (gall stone ileus)

COMPLICATIONS IN THE GALL BLADDER

SILENT STONES

- This is usually a single, silent, cholesterol stone which is symptomless.
- They are accidentally discovered, may be by an ultrasound or plain X-ray abdomen (Since calcium contents are low in cholesterol stones, very rarely it is visible in a plain X-ray).
- This stone rarely causes obstructive jaundice.
- Hence, they are left alone without treatment.

FLATULENT DYSPEPSIA

- If an obese woman (Fatty, Fertile, Flatulent, Female in Forties) complains of gaseous distention, intolerance to fatty food and discomfort in the abdomen, heartburn, belching, she probably has gall stones. These patients benefit from cholecystectomy.

GALL STONE COLIC

- It usually occurs at night wherein a stone tends to block the cystic duct or neck of gall bladder in the supine position.
- It is a severe colicky upper abdominal pain felt in the right hypochondrium, may shoot to the back or between shoulder blades. The pain is continuous and lasts for a few hours.
- The pain is due to spasm of gall bladder
- It is associated with vomiting due to reflex pylorospasm, restlessness and sweating.
- There is tenderness in the right hypochondrium

ACUTE CHOLECYSTITIS

Definition: Acute bacterial inflammation of the gall bladder with or without stone.

Types

1. **Calculous-**Obstructive cholecystitis. It is the commonest variety.

2. **Acalculous-**Non-obstructive cholecystitis. It is not uncommon, seen in patients who are recovering from major illness (Key Box 25.4).

Key Box 25.4

ACALCULOUS CHOLECYSTITIS

- Mostly seen in ICU
- Usually associated with major illness such as polytrauma, burns, major surgery
- Distension of gall bladder, activation of factor VII, may be the causes
- Thrombosis of vessels, necrosis, oedema are features
- U/S and HIDA scan are useful investigations
- Percutaneous drainage of gall bladder or immediate cholecystectomy is necessary

---

3. Acute emphysematous cholecystitis

Key Box 25.5

EMPHYSEMATOUS CHOLECYSTITIS

- It means **'gas'** in the gall bladder
- Diabetes, renal failure, immunosuppression are precipitating factors
- Clostridium welchi is the causative factor
- It is a severe, fulminant form of acute cholecystitis, but rare
- Stones are absent in 30-50% of cases
- High incidence of gangrene and perforation
- Emergency cholecystectomy is indicated

Bacteriology of acute cholecystitis

1. Majority of the cases of calculous cholecystitis are due to organisms such as E. coli, Streptococci, Salmonella, Klebsiella, etc.
2. Typhoid fever can also cause **Typhoid Cholecystitis** around 2nd week of infection.
3. Clostridial infection of the gall bladder produces acute cholecystitis with toxaemia.
4. Bile stasis precipitates infection

Pathogenesis (Key Box 25.6)

- Acute calculous cholecystitis appears to be caused by obstruction to bile flow from gall bladder by stone or oedema formed as a result of local mucosal erosion and inflammation caused by stone. **Once mucosa is**

Key Box 25.6

STONE

Outlet obstruction   Mucosal erosion

Stasis   Destruction of cells by toxic bile salts

Bacterial proliferation   Bacterial proliferation

Necrosis and Perforation

---

eroded tissue planes are exposed to bile salts. Toxic bile salts destroy cells by their detergent action leading to necrosis and perforation of gall bladder.

- At the same time bacterial infection adds to the morbidity of acute cholecystitis. Positive bile cultures are found in 70% of cases of acute calculous cholecystitis.

Pathology

1. **Inflammation**: Entire gall bladder is inflamed, swollen and is friable. Inflammatory exudate surrounding the gall bladder when it collects under the diaphragm, results in pain radiating to the right shoulder (C3,4) due to phrenic nerve irritation. It may undergo complete resolution with antibiotic therapy but such recurrent attacks are common at a later date.

2. Extensive ulcerations of gall bladder may result in **perforation** of gall bladder with biliary peritonitis and carries a very high mortality rate.

3. If the obstruction is complete-gall bladder is converted into **mucocoele** or **pyocoele** (empyema). Empyema of the gall bladder can occur in diabetic patients with high grade fever and chills and rigors and can even cause septicaemia.

4. **Gangrene** of gall bladder can occur if the blood vessels get thrombosed. All these features are more in an obstructive variety.

   - If there is clostridial infection as in diabetics because of extensive gas production in biliary tree and associated toxicity, perfortion is likely even without a stone.

   - Perforation can occur when the stone is impacted in the Hartmann's pouch.

Clinical features

- A fatty, fertile, female is the typical victim who presents with severe upper abdominal pain. It is colicky in nature and more prolonged because of inflammation. Severe nausea and vomiting are present. In the initial phase, there is low grade fever, except in clostridial infection where there is high grade fever.

Signs

1. **Murphy's sign**
   - Keep the fingers in the right hypochondrium and ask the patient to take deep inspiration.

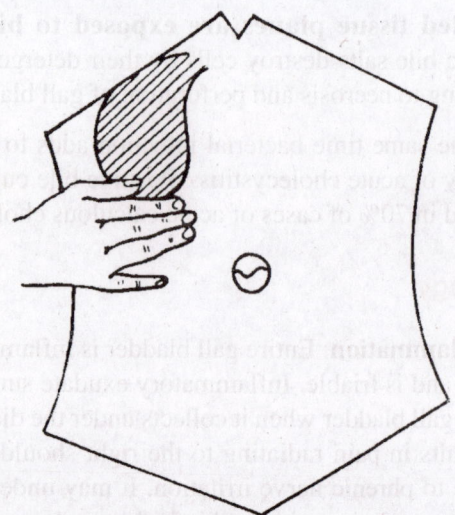

Fig. 25.7 Eliciting Murphy's sign

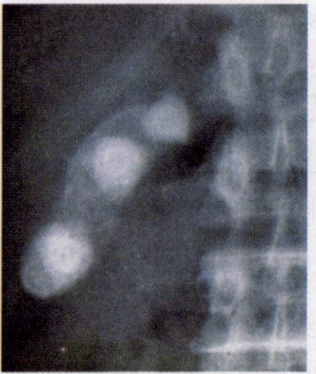 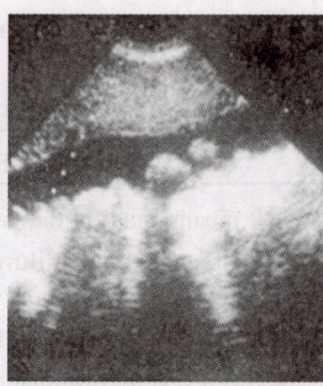

Fig. 25.8 Plain X-ray abdomen showing radioopaque shadows

Fig. 25.9 Ultrasonography showing posterior acoustic shadows

- At the height of inspiration there is a sudden catch in the inspiration.
- It is due to inflamed gall bladder coming in contact with fingers and producing pain. This is called **Murphy's sign positive**. It is a diagnostic sign of acute cholecystitis. (Fig 25.7)

2. **Boas' sign**
- An area of hyperaesthesia between 9th and 11th ribs posteriorly on the right side is a feature.

3. Upper abdominal **guarding, rigidity.**

4. **Vague mass** consisting of inflamed gall bladder, omentum, inflammatory exudate can be felt at times.

Investigations

1. **Total WBC** count is always raised.

2. **Blood and urine sugar** estimation to rule out diabetes mellitus

3. **Plain X-ray** abdomen erect position
- Gall stones can be demonstrated in 10% of the patients, as radio-opaque shadows in the right hypochondrium. In lateral view, the stone is seen in front of vertebral bodies (Fig. 25.8)
- To rule out other causes such as perforated peptic ulcer (air under diaphragm).
- Rarely, it may show calcified gall bladder (porcelain gall bladder).

4. **Emergency ultrasonography** (Fig. 25.9)
- To demonstrate stones, which cast **posterior acoustic shadow**

- It can demonstrate inflamed, thickened organ, in cases of acalculous cholecystitis.
- Demonstration of Murphy's sign, with the help of ultrasonography is possible which adds to the diagnosis.
- Ultrasound can also measure gall bladder function by using ultrasonic dimensions of the gall bladder.
- It can detect gall bladder polyps.

5. **HIDA scan / PIPIDA scan:**
- HIDA is **hepatic iminodiacetic acid**.
  ⁹⁹mTc labelled **HIDA** agent is excreted in the biliary tree, within one hour following I. V. administration.
- In acute cholecystitis, due to oedema of the cystic duct, even though the dye is excreted in the biliary tree, it does not enter the gall bladder. Hence, nonvisualisation of gall bladder is diagnostic of acute cholecystitis.
- Its importance lies in the **diagnosis of acalculous cholecystitis.**

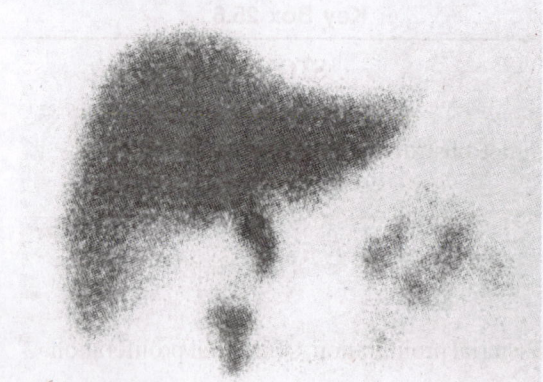

Fig. 25.10 HIDA scan showing nonvisualisation of gall bladder - a case of acute cholecystitis

Treatment

I. Conservative treatment is followed in majority of the cases

1. **Admission** in the hospital

2. **Aspiration** with Ryle's tube: Aspirating HCI decreases the stimulus to the secretion of bile. Spasm of gall bladder may come down.

3. **Antispasmodics:** Injection morphine 8-10 mg as analgesic, with injection atropine 1 ml to relieve spasm of sphincter of Oddi.

4. **Antibiotics:** Broad spectrum are given against gram +ve, gram -ve and anaerobic organisms. Patient is kept on nil orally for 2-3 days and during this time I.V. fluids are given. After 2-3 days pain comes down, signs (tenderness) disappear and abdomen becomes soft. Ryle's tube is removed, clear oral fluid is given for 2-3 days followed by soft diet. After 6 weeks patient is asked to come for elective cholecystectomy.

II. Early cholecystectomy

is done only in a few centres in the world. Due to acute cholecystitis extensive inflammatory oedema develops which masks the biliary tree. Hence, chances of injury to the cystic duct and CBD are high. Hence, it is not routinely done in many centers. However, it can be done provided:

- Set up is excellent, usually done within 48 hours (next available time).
- Experience of the surgeon should be good

CHRONIC CHOLECYSTITIS

- Recurrent attacks of cholecystitis will convert the gall bladder into a fibrosed, non-functioning, contracted, shrunken, small gall bladder. Gall bladder wall is grossly thickened. Stones are invariably present. Such patients present with classical fatty food intolerance. Murphy's sign is positive.

- They are diagnosed by ultrasound which reveals a small contracted gall bladder. Otherwise OCG (oral cholecystography) can be done to know the function of the gall bladder.

- **OCG-Graham Cole's test** (Fig.25.11). This test is done to know the function of the gall bladder.

Indication: Chronic cholecystitis.

Procedure: 2 days of fat free diet, previous night 6-8 tablets of telepaque (Iopanoic acid) is given orally. The dye reaches the liver through enterohepatic circulation and thus excreted into biliary tree.

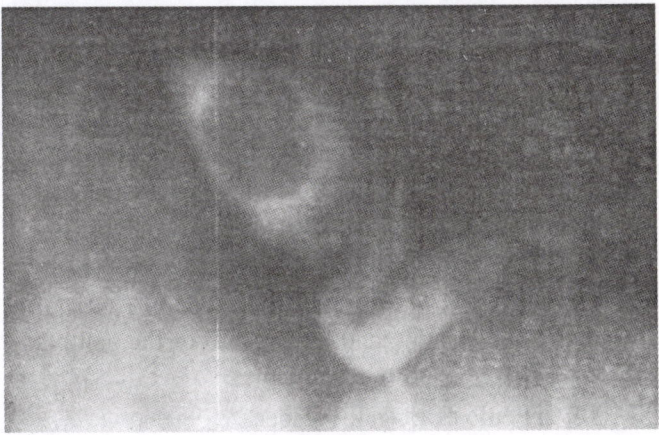

Fig. 25.11 OCG showing filling defect suggestive of stone

- On the day of OCG, one X-ray is taken in the morning, which shows dye filling the gall bladder. The patient is asked to take a fatty food and 1/2 an hour later another picture is taken. In chronic cholecystitis, the size of gall bladder is the same before and after fatty food and it is small. In the 2nd picture if the size is reduced by 50%, it is a functioning gall bladder.

OCG is a failure in cases of

1. Jaundice-hepatocytes cannot excrete the dye. Hence, gall bladder is not seen.

2. Acute cholecystitis-oedema of cystic duct prevents the dye entering the gall bladder.

3. Vomiting and diarrhoea

4. Iodine hypersensitivity

Usefullness of OCG:

In cases of acalculous cholecystitis, OCG can demonstrate non-functioning gall bladder or sometimes gall bladder is not visualised. That is an indication for cholecystectomy. With the increasing availability of ultrasound, OCG has become less popular.

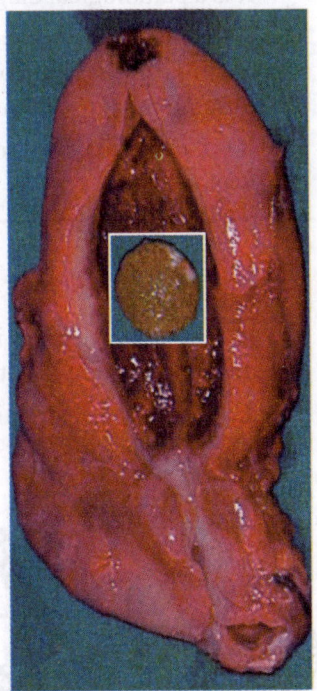

Fig. 25.12 Cholecystectomy specimen - observe thickened gall bladder wall

Treatment

- Cholecystectomy

CHOLECYSTOSES

Types :

I. Cholesterosis (Strawberry gall bladder): Aggregations of cholestrol crystals in the mucosa or submucosa.

II. Cholesterol polyposis (Gall bladder polyp): polypoidal projections of mucosa in the gall bladder.

III. Cholecystitis glandularis proliferans : Granulomatous thickening and hyperplasia of the gall bladder.

IV. Diverticulosis of gall bladder

V. Gall bladder wall with **fistula**

Clinical features

- Dyspepsia, upper abdominal discomfort, Murphy's sign is positive.

Management

- Ultrasound to confirm the diagnosis followed by cholecystectomy.

Key Box 25.7

XANTHOGRANULOMATOUS CHOLECYSTITIS

- It is a pathological diagnosis
- Gall bladder is chronically thickened, irregular with extension of yellow xanthogranulomatous inflammation to adjacent organs.
- It is thought to be due to bile penetrating gall bladder wall.

MUCOCOELE (Figs 25.13 , 25.14 and 25.15)

- It occurs when there is a stone blocking the cystic duct and the bile is not infected.
- As a result of obstruction, all the bile within the gall

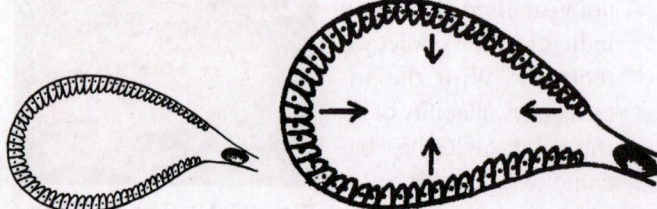

Fig. 25.13 Obstruction by stone

Fig. 25.14 Mucocoele

bladder is absorbed and is replaced by the mucus secreted from gall bladder epithelium.

- Clinically, it results in a soft, fluctuant, globular mass in the right hypochondrium which moves with respiration. It needs cholecystectomy.

EMPYEMA AND PERFORATION OF GALL BLADDER

- These are uncommon. Impacted stone, diabetes, virulent organisms precipitate pyocoele and perforation.
- Perforation can cause local abscess, if there are adhesions due to previous inflammation.
- Perforation into the general peritoneal cavity is rare but produces diffuse biliary peritonitis which has a high mortality rate.
- Urgent laparotomy, aggressive resuscitation, good antibiotic cover may help in reducing mortality. At laparotomy, removal of gall bladder is difficult. Hence, drainage of the pus and cholecystostomy with removal of gall stones can be done.

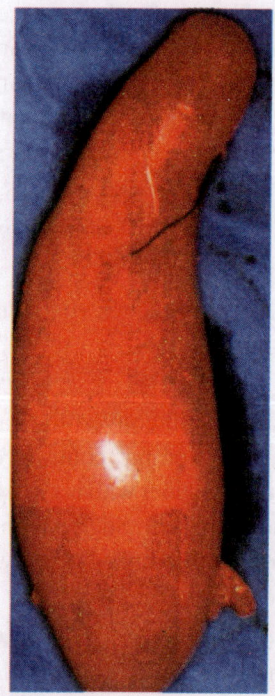
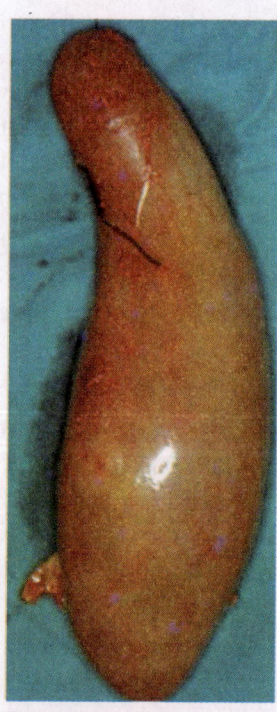

Fig. 25.15 Mucocoele of gall bladder

Fig. 25.16 Empyema of gall bladder

CARCINOMA OF GALL BLADDER

- Long-standing gall stones can bring about squamous metaplasia of gall bladder epithelium and can cause carcinoma of gall bladder. However, the incidence is very very rare. Hence, routine cholecystectomy is not advised for silent gall stones.

MIRIZZI SYNDROME

Type I : Compression of CBD without lumen narrowing.

Type II : Compression of CBD with lumen narrowing.

Type III : Compression causing CBD wall necrosis.

Type IV : Stone ulcerating into CBD resulting in cholecysto-choledochal fistula.

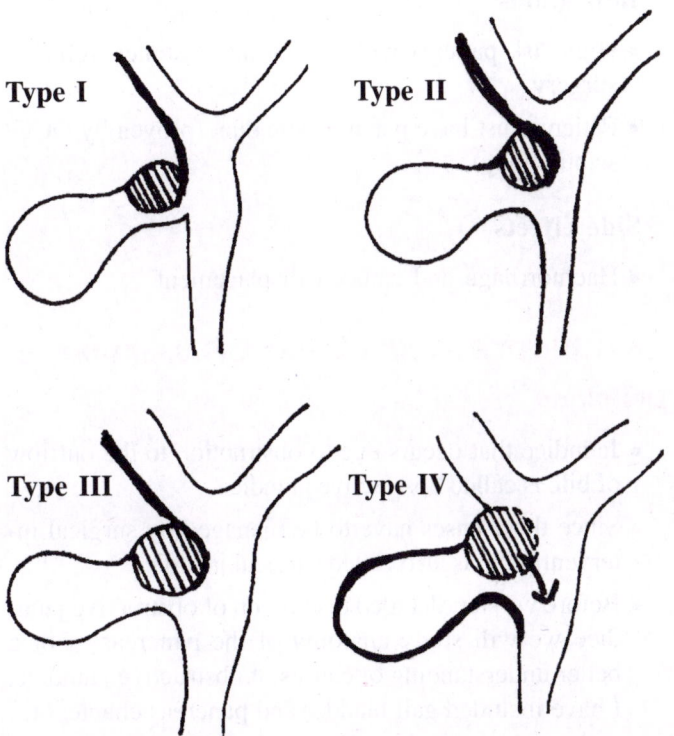

Fig. 25.17 Mirizzi's syndrome

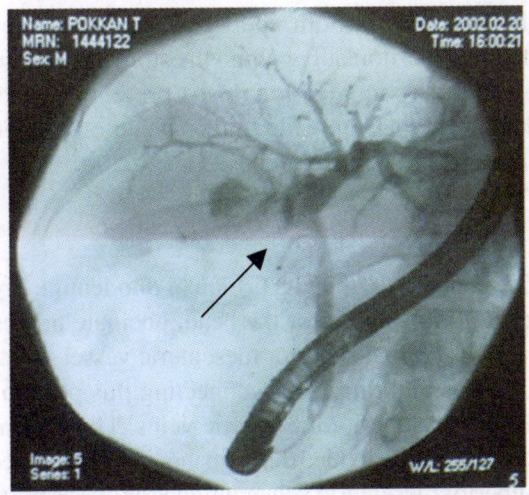

Fig. 25.18 ERCP showing Mirizzi's syndrome

Stone passing through the cystic duct into CBD is not Mirizzi Syndrome

TREATMENT OF GALL STONES IN GENERAL

1. **Emergency early cholecystectomy** is done only in a few centres.

2. **Open cholecystectomy** was the most popular method till recently.

3. **Laparoscopic cholecystectomy:** It has become the most popular method of choice today. More than 95% of gall bladders can be removed through a laparoscope. Some principles and procedure of laparoscopic cholecystectomy are discussed below.

Contraindications

1. Very badly contracted, fibrosed gall bladder

2. Very difficult gall bladder

Procedure (Fig 25.19, 25.20)

- 1cm long incision is made below the umbilicus, through which a pneumoperitoneum is maintained by CO_2 insufflation.

- Following this, a laparoscope is introduced and a camera is attached. 3 small 1cm incisions are made in epigastrium and in the right hypochondrium. These are used for suction, instrumentation, cauterisation, etc.

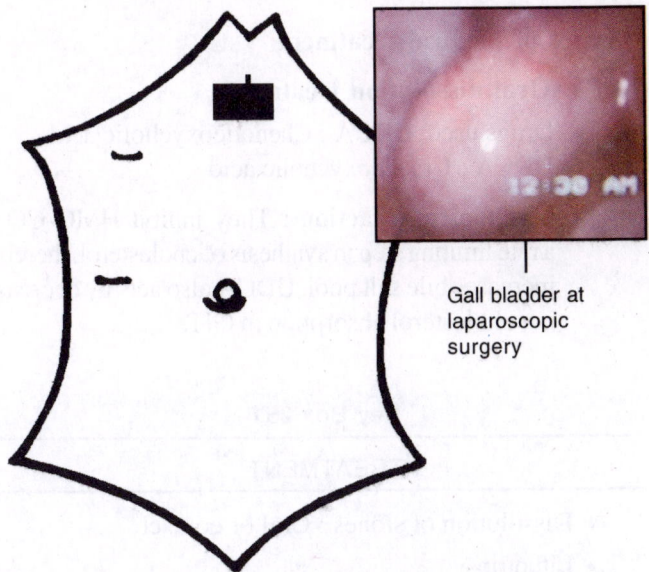

Gall bladder at laparoscopic surgery

Fig. 25.19 Incisions for laproscopic cholecystectomy

- Cystic duct and cystic artery are clipped and gall bladder is removed by gall bladder holding forceps and is brought outside through the epigastric port.
- Bleeding from liver is controlled by laser/cautery.
- Procedure is done under general anaesthesia. Procedure may take 1-3 hours depending upon the experience of the surgeon.

Advantages

1. Hospital stay is 1-2 days, recovery is very fast.
2. Pain is minimal. Hence, mobilization of the patient is much better and easy.
3. It gives an acceptable and better cosmetic result.
4. Complications like adhesions and incisional hernia are rare.

MEDICAL TREATMENT OF GALL STONES

- It is indicated for **pure cholesterol** stones only

Patient selection

- Patients with functioning gall bladder proven by OCG or scintigraphy
- Young thin, female patients
- Tiny < 5mm translucent, floating stones

Drawbacks

- Recurrence of stones once treatment is stopped
- Life long maintenance is needed

Types of medical treatment

1. Oral dissolution treatment

- Drugs used: CDCA : Chenodeoxycholic acid
  UDCA : Ursodeoxycholic acid
- **Mechanism of action :** They inhibit HMG-COA a rate limiting step in synthesis of cholesterol, thereby increases bile salt pool. UDCA also acts by decreasing cholesterol absorption in GIT.

Key Box 25.8
TREATMENT
• Dissolution of stones : Oral or contact
• Lithotripsy
• ESWL

2. Direct Contact Dissolution

- MTBE - Methyl Terbutyl Ether is the drug which is given through a catheter placed in gall bladder percutaneously.

Drawbacks

- Explosive and toxic if it enters bile duct or duodenum.

Indications

- High risk patients with symptomatic stones, refusing surgery
- Patient must have patent cystic duct (proven by OCG/scintigraphy)

Side effects

- Haemorrhage and catheter displacement

OBSTRUCTIVE JAUNDICE (SURGICAL JAUNDICE)

Definition

- Jaundice that occurs due to obstruction to the outflow of bile is called obstructive jaundice.
- Since these cases have to be managed by surgical intervention, it is also called surgical jaundice.
- Before we start detailed discussion of obstructive jaundice we will study anatomy of the pancreas. For a better understanding of causes of obstructive jaundice, I have included gall bladder and pancreas chapters together.

SURGICAL ANATOMY OF THE PANCREAS

The pancreas is both endocrine and exocrine organ situated retroperitoneally behind the stomach. It is soft and fleshy gland (pancreas-all flesh), extending from the duodenum on the right side to the spleen on the left side, the entire length being 6 inches.(Fig. 25.20)

PARTS

- The head lies within the C loop of duodenum. From the left inferior portion of the head, uncinate process presents, on which superior mesenteric vessel runs. There are 5-6 small thin veins connecting this portion of the head with superior mesenteric veins. These veins have to be carefully divided during pancreaticoduodenectomy. Superior mesenteric vein continues above as portal vein after joining the splenic vein. During

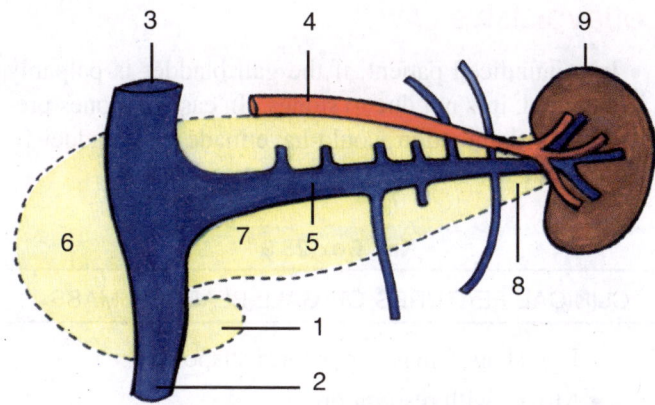

Fig. 25.20 Surgical anatomy of pancreas - 1. Uncinate process 2. Superior mesenteric vein 3. Portal vein 4. Splenic artery 5. Splenic vein 6. Head of pancreas 7. Body of pancreas 8. Tail of pancreas 9. Spleen

pancreaticoduodenectomy for periampullary carcinoma, before any major structure is divided, the infiltration into the portal vein should be ruled out. This is done by inserting a finger between the portal vein and head of pancreas-both from above and below.

- The neck is about 2 cm and is related posteriorly to superior mesenteric vessels.
- The body and tail: The head and neck continue as body which is placed transversely. It slopes upwards across the aorta and ends as tail of the pancreas, which is enclosed within lienorenal ligament along with splenic vessels. Large cystadenoma arising from the tail of the pancreas can move with respiration because of its contact with the spleen.

BLOOD SUPPLY OF THE PANCREAS

Arterial supply

- Splenic artery is the chief artery supplying the neck, body and the tail. Arteria pancreatica magna refers to one large branch of splenic artery.
- Superior and inferior pancreaticoduodenal arteries supply not only head of pancreas but also the adjacent duodenum. Thus, any surgery which involves excision of the head, the C loop of the duodenum also is removed. Thus, pancreaticoduodenectomy becomes a major surgery.

Venous drainage

- Body, neck and tail drain into splenic vein by means of multiple small veins.

- The head is drained by superior pancreaticoduodenal vein which drains into portal vein and inferior pancreaticoduodenal drains into superior mesenteric vein.

PANCREATIC DUCT

- The main pancreatic duct (duct of Wirsung), a tubular structure drains entire pancreas from tail to the head. It joins the common bile duct and forms ampulla of Vater. This ampulla opens on the duodenal papilla (a nipple-like elevation) in the 2nd part of the duodenum. Normal diameter of pancreatic duct is 2-3 mm. When it is dilated more than 6-8 mm, as in chronic pancreatitis, the longitudinal pancreaticojejunostomy can be done.
- Accessory pancreatic duct of Santorini drains the uncinate process and lower portion of the head and opens into the duodenum 2 cm above the opening of the main duct. The two ducts communicate with each other at many sites.

A CASE OF OBSTRUCTIVE JAUNDICE

AETIOLOGY (Fig 25.21)

I. Causes in the lumen

1. Stones in the common bile duct
2. Ova, cysts, worms of ascariasis
3. Hydatid cyst of biliary tree
4. Stone in the pancreatic duct

II. Causes in the wall

1. Periampullary carcinoma
2. Choledochal cyst
3. Stenosis of sphincter of Oddi (papillary stenosis)
4. Klatskin's tumour-Carcinoma of the bile duct where right and left ducts join.

III. Causes from outside (due to pressure)

1. Carcinoma head of pancreas
2. Chronic pancreatitis
3. Lymph nodes at the porta hepatis obstructing the biliary tree.

- Figures (25.21 and 25.22) highlight the importance of clinical examination of the abdomen. If gall bladder is palpable and hard with jaundice, it suggests carcinoma gall bladder.

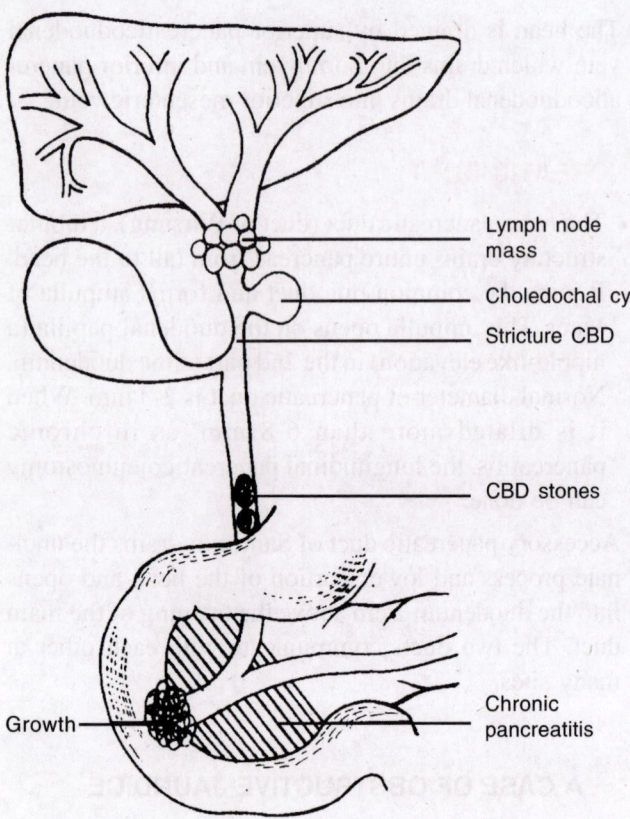

Fig. 25.21 Various causes of obstructive jaundice

Lymph node mass
Choledochal cyst
Stricture CBD
CBD stones
Growth
Chronic pancreatitis

COURVOISIER'S LAW

- In a jaundiced patient, if the gall bladder is palpably enlarged, it is not due to stones. In case of stones previous inflammation would have made gall bladder fibrotic, hence not palpable.

Key Box 25.9
CLINICAL FEATURES OF GALL BLADDER MASS
• Egg shaped mass / pyriform shape
• Moves with respiration
• Tensely cystic, sometimes tender
• Located in the right hypochondrium
• Superficially placed
• Intraabdominal, intraperitoneal

- From clinical point of view, 90% of cases of obstructive jaundice are due to stones and periampullary carcinoma or carcinoma of head of pancreas. Thus to get a better understanding in the clinics, these two topics have been discussed in Table 25.1 (Next page)

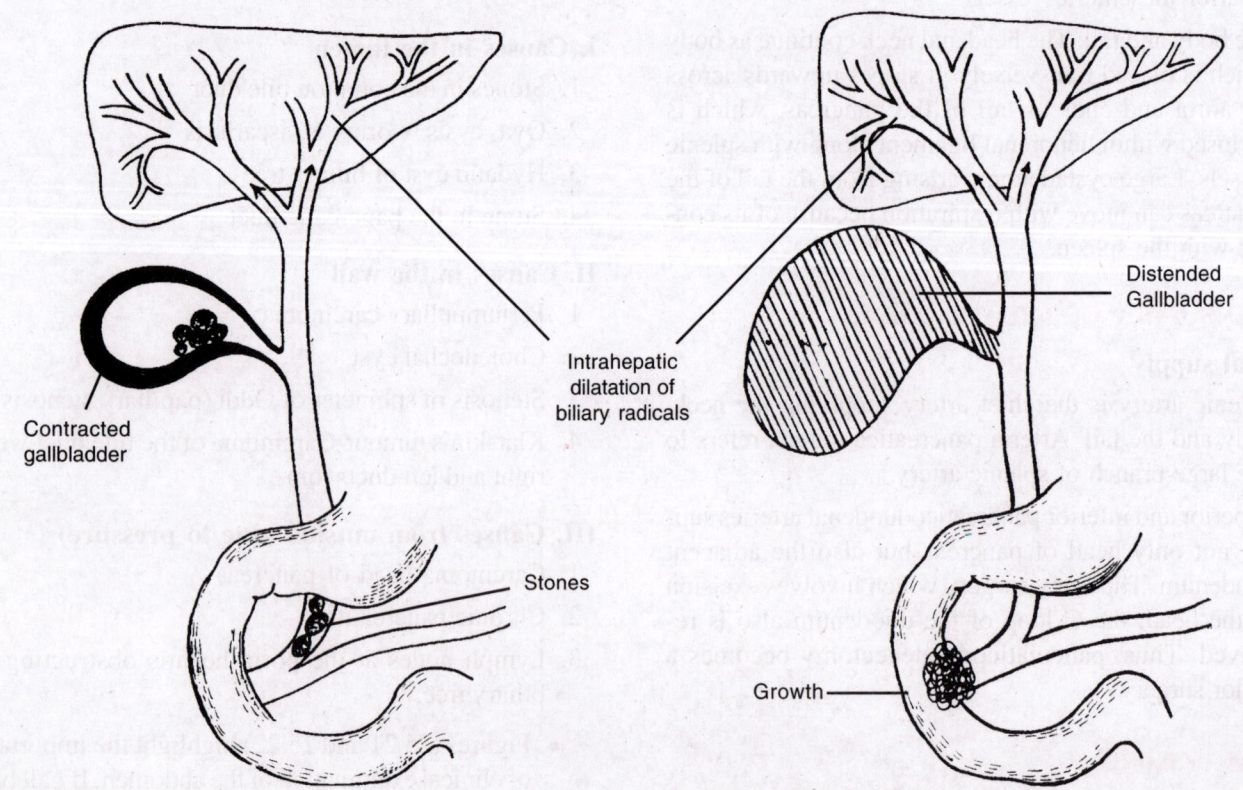

Contracted gallbladder

Intrahepatic dilatation of biliary radicals

Stones

Distended Gallbladder

Growth

Fig. 25.22 Contracted thick gall bladder due to stones hence not palpable

Fig. 25.23 Enlarged palpable gall bladder in cases of periampullary carcinoma

Table 25.1. Differences between stone in the CBD and periampullary carcinoma (Ca) / Ca head of pancreas

	STONE IN THE CBD	CA PERIAMPULLARY/HEAD OF PANCREAS
1. Age	30-50 years	50-70 years
2. Sex	More common in females	Common in both sexes equally
3. Duration of symptoms	Long duration	Short duration (1-3 months)
4. **Symptoms**		
Pain	It is due to a stone blocking the CBD resulting in spasm of CBD. It is severe colicky pain like gall stone colic.	There may be some discomfort in abdomen but colicky pain is not a feature. Pain is relatively rare in carcinoma head of the pancreas.
Fever	As a result of obstruction multiplication of organisms results in fever.	When obstruction becomes severe, there is bile stasis. Cholangitis, fever with chills and rigors can occur.
Jaundice	Occurs due to obstruction. Once inflammation subsides all these 3 symptoms are relieved partly but they occur after sometime. Hence, Intermittent pain, Intermittent fever, Intermittent jaundice are classical of a stone in CBD-**Charcot's Triad.**	As a result of slow developing obstruction at periampullary region, jaundice is **persistent, progressive, painless, pruritic.** In 5% of cases growth may ulcerate into the duodenum. It can cause melaena and jaundice may temporarily subside.
Stools	Since the obstruction is never complete, clay coloured stools are not commonly seen.	Clay coloured stools are common and when mixed with blood it is called **silvery stools** or aluminium paint stools.
Pruritus	May be present but mild	Severe-due to bile salts in the circulation.
Loss of appetite	No	Significant
Loss of weight	No	Significant
5. **Signs**		
Jaundice	Deep yellow	Sometimes greenish yellow
Anaemia	Absent	It is usually present.
6. **Per abdomen**	Liver can be enlarged due to the back pressure. It is smooth, with round border, firm in consistency.	Liver can be enlarged due to back pressure. If it is nodular, with sharp border, hard in consistency, it is due to secondaries in the liver.
7. **Gall bladder**	As a rule, gall bladder (GB) is not palpable	Gall bladder is palpable in 70-75% cases. (Key Box 25.9)
8. **Metastasis**	No	Left supraclavicular node, ascites etc.

Exceptions to Courvoisier's Law

1. Double impaction-One stone in CBD and one stone in cystic duct.
2. Periampullary carcinoma in a patient who has undergone cholecystectomy.
3. Primary oriental cholangiohepatitis causing stones in the CBD (gall bladder is normal in these cases).

Reynold's Pentad: (Key box 25.10)

Key Box 25.10
REYNOLD'S PENTAD OF ACUTE OBSTRUCTIVE CHOLANGITIS
1. Persistent pain 2. Fever 3. Persistent jaundice 4. Shock 5. Altered mental status

INVESTIGATIONS

1. **Hb %** is low in malignancy

2. **TC, DC** are increased in cases of infections

3. **BT, CT, PT** are altered in cases of obstructive jaundice

4. **Urine** for urobilinogen is negative in obstructive jaundice

5. **Serum alkaline phosphatase:** Normal value 60-300 units/litre. More than 500 units is suggestive of obstructive jaundice.

   • These are the enzymes which bring hydrolysis of phosphate esters in alkaline medium

   • Sources of alkaline phosphatase include liver, biliary tree, bone, intestine, kidney

   • Excretion mainly through biliary tree

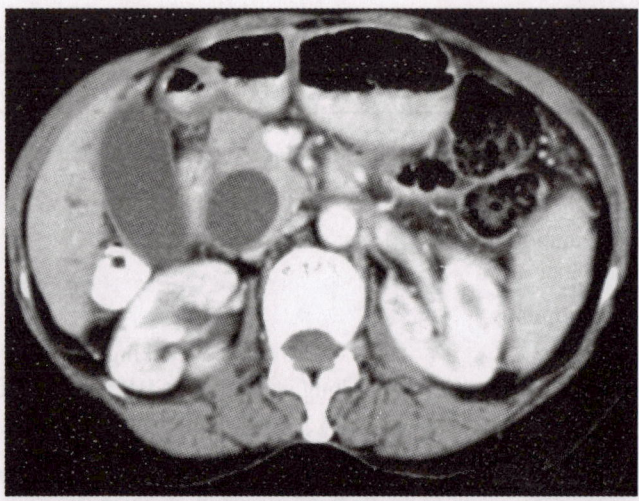

Fig. 25.24 CT scan showing hugely distended gall bladder and common bile duct - periampullary carcinoma

Key Box 25.11	
CAUSES OF INCREASEED LEVELS OF ALKALINE PHOSPHATASE	
GROSS ELEVATION	**MILD ELEVATION**
1. Obstructive jaundice	1. Metastasis in the liver
2. Biliary cirrhosis	2. Hepatic abscesses
3. Bone diseases	3. Hepatitis

6. **Abdominal Ultrasound:** It is the most useful, noninvasive, reliable and quick investigation for obstructive jaundice.

   • Dilated biliary radicles, both intrahepatic and extrahepatic can be demonstrated.

   • Stones can be diagnosed with their posterior acoustic shadow.

   • Mass lesion in the head region can be made out in cases of chronic pancreatitis or carcinoma head of the pancreas causing obstructive jaundice.

   • Ultrasound can detect multiple secondaries in the liver, thus, favouring the diagnosis of malignancy.

7. **CT scan:** The head mass of 2-3 cm in size, portal vein infiltration can be demonstrated by CT scan. Obliteration of fat plane between the mass and superior mesenteric vessels can be demonstrated by CT scan which decides the operability of periampullary carcinoma or carcinoma head of the pancreas.

   • CT scan can also detect coeliac nodes - presence of which is a contraindication for radical resections.

8. **Endoscopy** is useful to diagnose a periampullary carcinoma which may be seen as an ulcerative lesion in the second part of the duodenum. Biopsy can also be taken which shows adenocarcinoma.

   • In case of obstructive jaundice due to stones, smooth bulge can be seen in the second part of the duodenum. In carcinoma, ulcerated lesion can be seen.(Fig. 25.25)

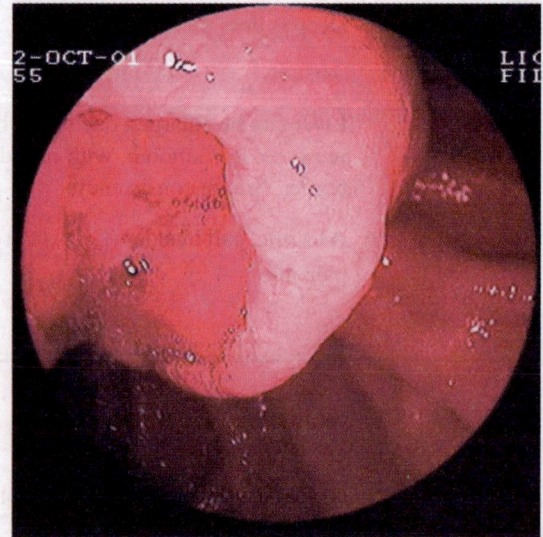

Fig. 25.25 Endoscopy showing growth in the periampullary region

---

1. With the availability of ultrasound and endoscopy this investigation has lost its importance.

9. **Barium meal**[1] follow through to see the C loop of duodenum (Fig. 25.26).

   - In periampullary carcinoma, there may be distortion of the medial border of the duodenum giving rise to **Inverted 3 sign.**

   In carcinoma head of the pancreas there may be widening of C loop of duodenum - **Pad sign**.

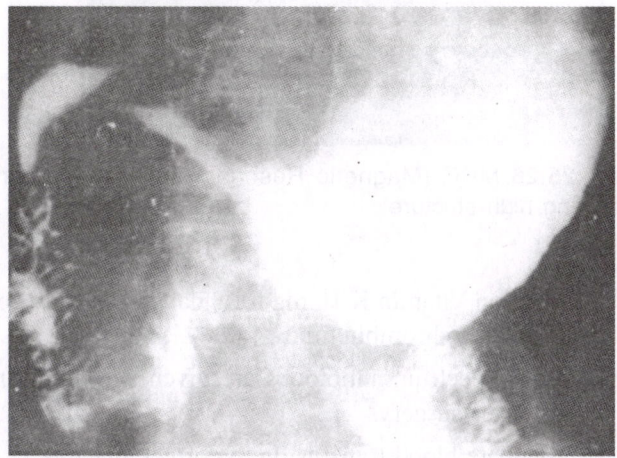

Fig. 25.26 Barium meal showing widening of C-loop of duodenum.

10. ERCP (Endoscopic Retrograde Cholangio-Pancreatography)

- With the help of a side viewing endoscope, ampulla of Vater is cannulated and a radio-opaque dye is injected.
- It fills up the biliary and pancreatic system.

Interpretation

1. Stones appear as filling defects in the CBD or in the common hepatic duct (CHD) (Fig. 25.27) which may be mobile (change position if patient is moved).

2. A periampullary carcinoma gives rise to an irregular filling defect or there may be total cut off in flow of dye.

3. Chronic pancreatitis may show the dilated duct and stones in the pancreatic duct, **chain of lakes appearance.**

Uses

1. If stones in the CBD are diagnosed, they can be treated in the following ways.

- Extraction by using a basket.
- Large stone can be crushed by using a lithotripter and can be extracted.
- Sphincterotomy (incise sphincter of Oddi) can be done to facilitate extrusion of small stones.

2. In patients with cholangitis with obstructive jaundice, stenting of common bile duct can be done to relieve

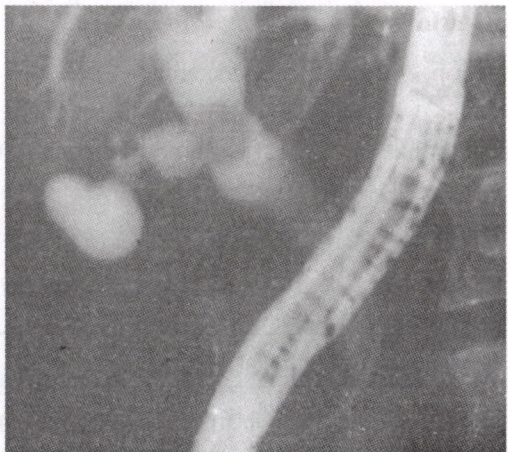

Fig. 25.27 ERCP showing stones in the CBD and contracted gall bladder.

obstruction. **Stent removal is necessary** at a later date.

3. In selected patients with **biliary strictures,** stent is placed after ERCP to relieve obstructive jaundice. (Sometimes permanent in malignancies).

4. In selected patients with **chronic pancreatitis**, pancreatic duct can be stented to relieve pain.

Complications

- Severe infection of biliary tree (cholangitis), acute pancreatitis can occur in 1-2% of the patients. Hence, prophylactic antibiotics are given before the procedure.

10. PTC (Percutaneous Transhepatic Cholangiography)

- Using an ultrasound image-intensifier, a dilated biliary radicle is identified within the liver and a fine needle (Chiba needle[1]) is introduced within, the stylet is removed and a radio-opaque dye is injected. Chiba needle is 15 cm long and 0.7 mm in diameter.

---

1. Chiba is the name of the university in Japan where this needle was developed.

Precautions

1. BT, CT, PT should be normal. Otherwise, Vitamin K injection 10 mg I.M. is given for 3 days.

2. If there is a bleeding tendency, this procedure should not be done.

3. Broad spectrum antibiotics are given before the procedure.

Complications

1. Infection, cholangitis, septicaemia

2. Biliary leak can be significant producing abdominal pain and guarding. Hence, P.T.C. should be done just prior to the surgery.

3. Haemorrhage

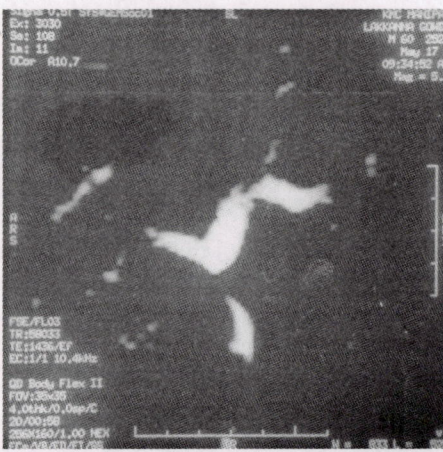

Fig. 25.28 MRC (Magnetic Resonance Cholangiogram) showing high stricture

---

Key Box 25.12

FACTS ABOUT PTC

1. In the diagnosis of high strictures, P.T.C is better than E.R.C.P.

2. It can also be used in ERCP failure cases.

3. In the diagnosis of Klatskin's tumour, P. T.C. is extremely useful. It can also delineate the dilated proximal duct, which helps in planning for a biliary-enteric anastomosis.

4. Catheter can be kept in the bile ducts to provide external drainage as in strictures or in inoperable malignancies with obstructive jaundice.

---

11. MRI scan (MRC) - Fig. 25.28

- It is the investigation of choice in a case of obstructive jaundice in cases of high strictures and cholangiocarcinomas.

- It is non invasive and delineates the bile ducts very well so that one can also plan for a biliary bypass.

TREATMENT OF OBSTRUCTIVE JAUNDICE

Pre-operative preparation

1. Adequate hydration before the surgery for 2-3 days.

2. I. V. mannitol 10% 200 ml, before, during and after surgery to prevent hepatorenal syndrome. Otherwise, injection dopamine 2 µg/kg/min is given to improve the urinary output.

3. Injection Vitamin K 10 mg for 3 days is given to correct the prothrombin time.

4. Broad spectrum antibiotics are given before, during and after surgery.

5. Adequate blood transfusion to correct anaemia.

TREATMENT OF CBD STONE

- Cholecystectomy is done first. This is followed by introduction of a cannula into the cystic duct and a radio-opaque dye is injected.

- This is called **OTC.**[1] (**O**n **T**able **C**holangiography). If the dye goes freely into the duodenum without filling defect, it is a normal OTC. If there are filling defects in the CBD, it is explored.

- **Precautions while doing OTC**

- There should not be any air bubble in the syringe.

  - 5-10 ml of dye has to be injected.

  - Leakage of the dye should not occur.

TYPES OF SURGERY FOR STONES IN THE CBD

There are three options available for treatment of stones in the CBD. Depending upon the merits of the cases and experience of the surgeon anyone of the methods can be selected.

1. **Supraduodenal CBD** is explored through an incision over the anterior wall and the stones are removed. It is called as supraduodenal choledocholithotomy. Operating choledochoscope is passed into the common

---

1. With availability of preoperative ERCP and basketting of the stones, OTC is less frequently done nowadays.

hepatic duct and its branches and the stones if present are removed. Closure of the CBD is done after inserting T tube. After 8-10 days, a T-tube cholangiography is done and if the dye goes freely into duodenum and no filling defect is seen in CBD, the T-tube is removed by gentle traction. By 10-12 days, a track is well formed. Hence, even if a minor leak occurs, the bile flows outside without causing peritonitis (Fig. 25.28).

Key Box 25.13

INDICATIONS FOR EXPLORATION OF CBD

1. History of Charcot's triad
2. Ultrasound proved stones in CBD
3. CBD dilated more than 1 cm in size
4. OTC shows filling defect
5. Palpable stones in the CBD

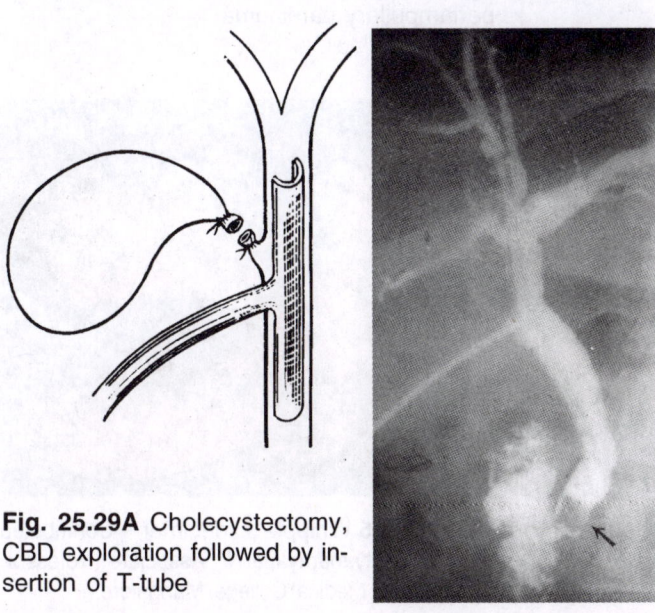

Fig. 25.29A Cholecystectomy, CBD exploration followed by insertion of T-tube

Fig. 25.29B T-tube cholangiogram showing residual stone in the lower CBD - It was removed through endoscopic papillotomy

II. Cholecystectomy + choledocholithotomy + choledochoduodenostomy: It can be done when CBD is dilated more than 1.5 cm in diameter and stoma should be at least 2-3 cm in size.

Advantages of choledochoduodenostomy

1. Biliary leak is negligible.
2. One need not worry even if there are retained stones in the CBD.

Key Box 25.14

INDICATIONS

- Recurrent stones in the CBD
- Multiple intrahepatic stones
- Stricture lower CBD

---

3. It is a permanent solution for a stenosis, stricture or multiple intrahepatic stones.

III. Pre-operative ERCP, sphincterotomy + extraction of stones followed by Laparoscopic cholecystectomy

- This method has become the choice today. Expertisation and sophisticated equipments are necessary for this.

TREATMENT OF PERIAMPULLARY CARCINOMA

SURGICAL TREATMENT

1. **Radical Pancreaticoduodenectomy- "Whipple's Operation"** (fig. 25.30).

   - In this operation growth along with 'C' loop of duodenum upto DJ flexure, removal of the head of pancreas upto the neck and partial gastrectomy is done followed by :
   - Pancreaticojejunal anastomosis (PJ), Gastrojejunostomy (GJ) and Choledochojejunostomy (CJ)
   - This is a major operation and carries 5-10% mortality due to pancreatic leakage, biliary leakage.
   - Whipple's operation is indicated in cases of mobile growth with no metastasis and general condition of the patients should be reasonably good.

2. **Pylorus preserving pancreaticoduodenectomy - PPPD**

   - In this operation, pylorus is preserved. Thus, gastric motility is not disturbed.

3. **Triple bypass : Cholecystojejunostomy + enteroenterostomy + gastrojejunostomy**

   - This is a palliative surgery in which distended gall bladder is anastomosed to a long loop of jejunum (40 cm) to relieve jaundice. To prevent food particles entering into the gall bladder, enteroenterostomy is done (Fig. 25.36).

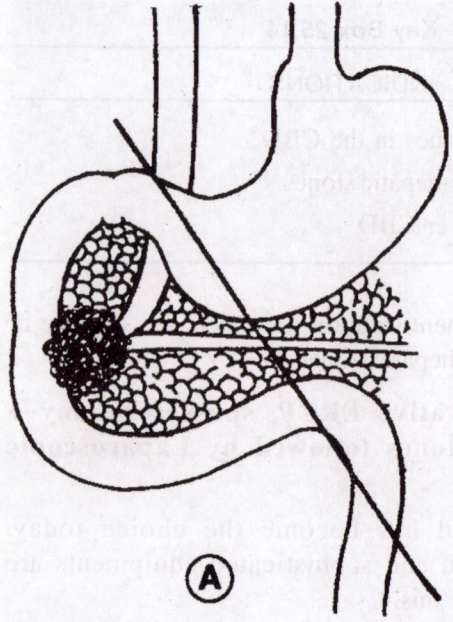

Fig. 25.30 Diagramatic representation of Whipple's resection.

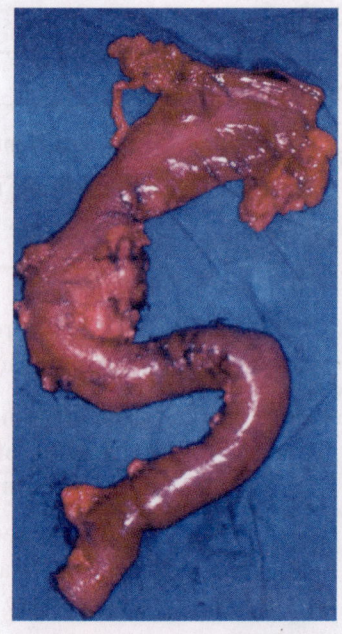

Fig. 25.31 Whipple's resection specimen

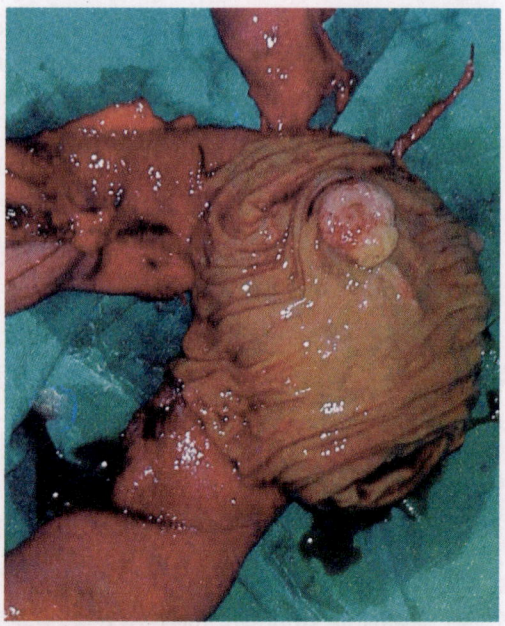

Fig. 25.32 See the ulcerative growth - periampullary carcinoma

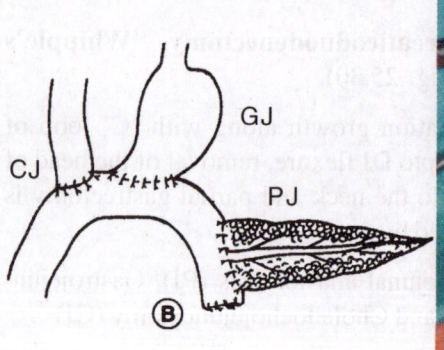

Fig. 25.33 Reconstruction following Whipple's operation

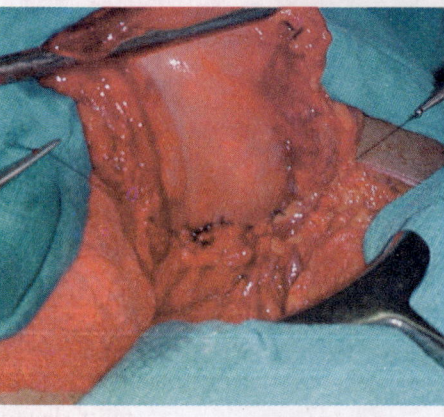

Fig. 25.34 Pancreatico gastrostomy (PG) is a better alternative to PJ

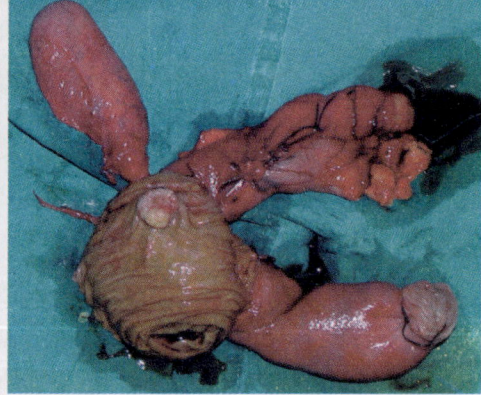

Fig. 25.35 Whipple's specimen - Contributed by Dr. Satyanarayana N., Associate Professor, Yenepoya Medical College, Mangalore

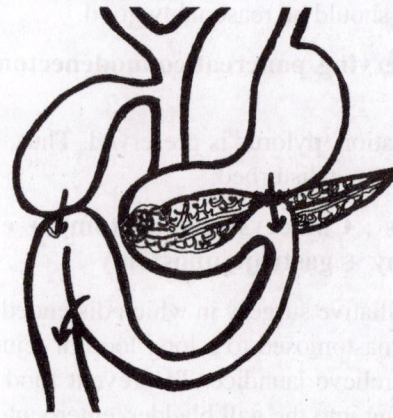

Fig. 25.36 Palliative tripple bypass

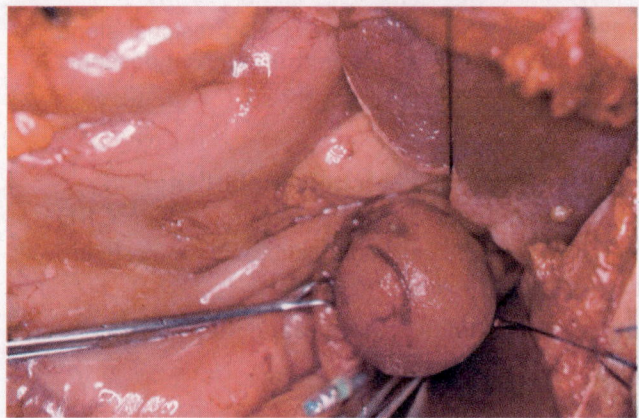

Fig. 25.37 Distended gall bladder ready for anastomosis

- Most of the patients in the postoperative period develop duodenal obstruction caused by the growth. Hence a palliative GJ is done at the same time.

NON SURGICAL TREATMENT

- Very elderly patients (age criteria not clear) who are not fit candidates for surgery and patients who have metastasis can be treated by palliative stenting. However, results of a surgical bypass is superior to stenting. Also, the stent needs to be changed frequently

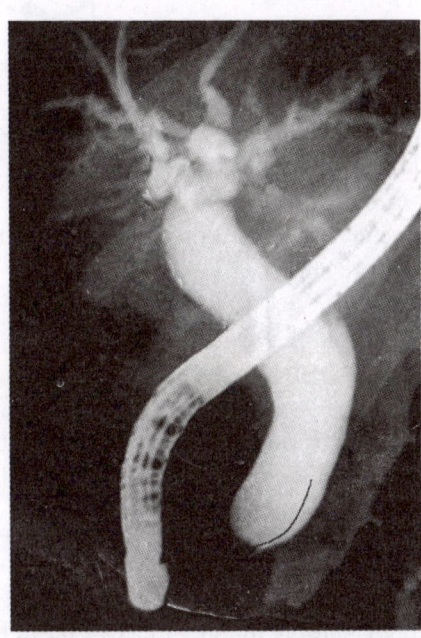

Fig. 25.38 Palliative stenting for carcinoma head of the pancreas

OTHER CAUSES OF OBSTRUCTIVE JAUNDICE

STRICTURE OF THE CBD

- 80% of strictures are following surgery on the biliary tree. They are called post-operative strictures. 20% are due to inflammatory pathology.
- It gives rise to slowly progressive, painless jaundice.
- Strictures account for 1-2% cases of obstructive jaundice.

Causes

1. Postoperative post-traumatic

- **Difficult cholecystectomy:** When the gall blad-

der is fibrosed, densely stuck to the right hepatic duct or to the common bile duct or as in early cholecystectomy due to oedema around Calot's triangle, injury can occur to the right hepatic duct or to the CBD or CHD resulting in stricture.(Fig 25.39)

Type I   Low common bile duct; stump > 2 cm

Type II   Middle common hepatic duct, stump < 2 cm

Type III   Hilar - confluence of right and left duct intact

Type IV   Right and left ducts separated

Type V   Involvement of the intrahepatic ducts

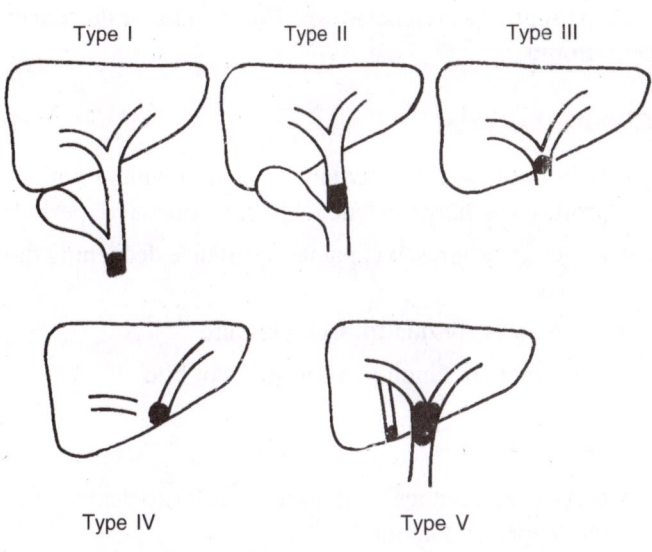

Fig. 25.39 Classification of benign billiary stricture - Bismuth classification

- **Dangerous** cholecystectomy: Sudden bleeding from cystic artery can occur due to traction on the gall bladder or due to lack of gentleness in ligating cystic artery. Sudden application of an artery forceps to control the bleeding may injure CBD. In such situations, packing the area, good suction and visualisation of the bleeding artery and ligation should be done. If the bleeding continues, the hepatic artery can be compressed between the finger and the thumb in the lesser omentum through the foramen of Winslow. This is called **Hogarth-Pringle manoeuvre**.

- **Dissection at fault**: Ignorance of anomalies like short cystic duct or too much traction of the gall bladder distorts CBD and predisposes to injury.

- It is the duty of the surgeon to show his assistants the Y junction which is formed by the cystic duct, common hepatic duct above and common bile duct below before dividing any structures in this area.

2. **Post-inflammatory** strictures follow recurrent attacks of cholangitis due to:

   - Stones in the CBD or CHD
   - Parasites like Ascaris lumbricoides in the biliary tree or **Asiatic cholangiohepatitis** produced by Chinese liver fluke infestation (Clonorchis sinensis).
   - Primary sclerosing cholangitis wherein the cause is not known.

3. **Malignant strictures are due to cholangio carcinoma**

Clinical features

- History of cholecystectomy in the past with or without profuse discharge of bile in the post-operative period
- A slowly progressive, painless jaundice deepening day by day
- Hepatomegaly due to back pressure
- Recurrent cholangitis due to stasis of bile

Investigations

- USG-to rule out residual stones in CBD, to demonstrate intrahepatic dilatation
- ERCP or PTC may demonstrate a stricture in the CBD or CHD with proximal dilatation
- T-tube cholangiography if T-tube is in place
- M.R.C. is noninvasive, better than PTC

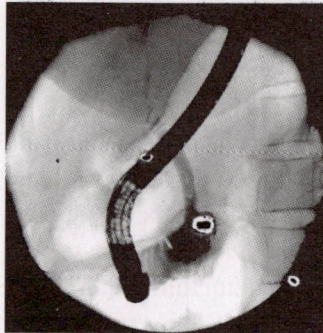

Fig. 25.40 ERCP showing partial clipping of CBD. Patient had developed jaundice in the immediate post-operative period

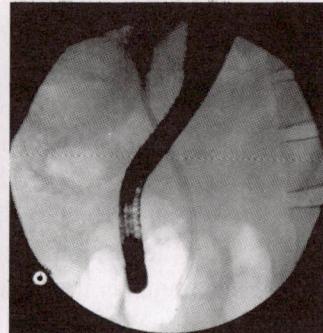

Fig. 25.41 Laparotomy, clip removal and stent insertion was done in the same patient. Stent was removed after one year

Treatment

- If it is due to laparoscopic clipping without transection of the CBD, it is better to re-explore and remove the clips and a T-tube or an endoscopic stent can be placed in the CBD.

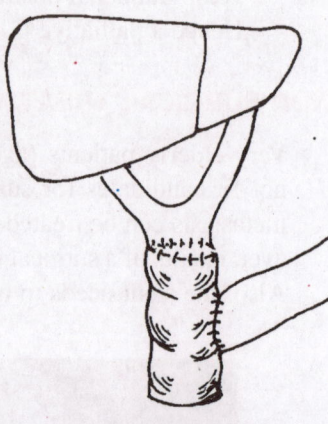

Fig. 25.42 Hepatico - jejunostomy

- Late cases can be managed by choledocho-jejunostomy or hepatico-jejunostomy by anastomosing a loop of jejunum to the dilated portion above the stricture.

However, the general condition of the patient should be improved before surgery.

SCLEROSING CHOLANGITIS

- It is characterised by development of multiple strictures and dilatation of CBD with features of fibrous thickening of CBD.

Types

- **Primary :** No cause is found. However it can be associated with following conditions

Key Box 25.15
ASSOCIATED CONDITIONS
• Ulcerative colitis • Crohn's disease • Grave's disease • Sjogren's syndrome

Secondary : It is due to stones or injuries.

Complications

- Due to long standing obstruction biliary cirrhosis and cholangiocarcinoma can develop.

Diagnosis

- **Ultrasound** can demonstrate intrahepatic dilatation.

- **MRCP** is a noninvasive investigation which can demonstrate multiple strictures and dilatation.
- **ERCP** is the investigation of choice which can demonstrate the strictures in the CBD and dilatation which is described as **beaded** appearance. However the risk of suppurative cholangitis is present.

Treatment: It is dificult

- Stenting is the choice, stents may have to be replaced or changed depending upon the blockage or if infection sets in.

CHOLEDOCHAL CYST

- It is a congenital cyst occurring in the CBD due to partial or complete weakness of the wall of the CBD.
- Majority of cases manifest by 1-2 years of age.

Classification : (Fig. 25.43 and Key Box 25.16)

Clinical features

1. Age: Majority of cases manifest in children within 1-2 years of age. It can also present in adults.
2. More common in **females** 4:1
3. **Abdominal distension** can be due to a large cyst and cyst can be palpated per abdomen in the right hypochondrium.
4. Slow progressive jaundice, recurrent attacks with abdominal pain and pyrexia

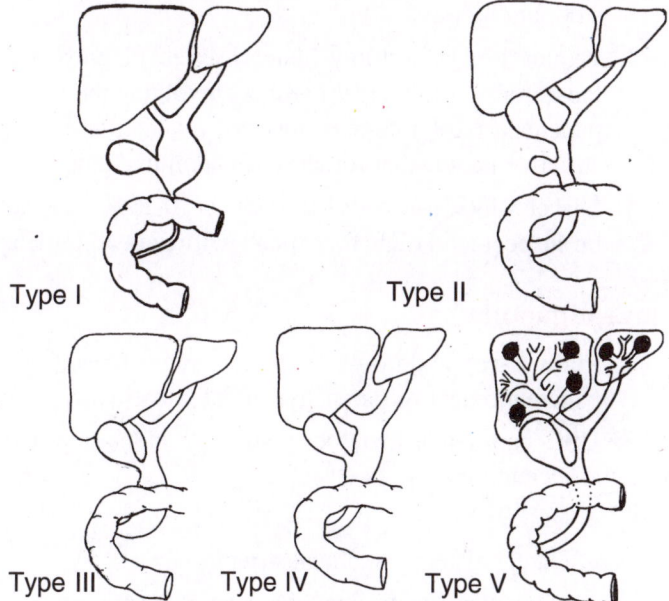

Fig. 25.43 Types of choledochal cyst

	Key Box 25.16	
Types	**TODANI CLASSIFICATION**	
Type I:	Fusiform dilatation of CBD - Commonest	
Type II:	Lateral saccular diverticulum of the CBD	
Type III:	Dilatation of intraduodenal segment of CBD (choledochocoele)	
Type IV :	Dilatation of CBD + intrahepatic biliary dilatation.	
Type V :	Multiple intrahepatic cysts.	

Investigations

1. **USG** will confirm presence of abnormal cyst. It is usually unilocular cyst.
2. **MRI:** It will reveal relation between lower end of the bile duct and pancreatic duct.
3. **ERCP** may be done but it will not give any extra information than MRI.

Treatment

- **This anomaly is premalignant.** Change to carcinoma is well recognised complication and it carries poor prognosis. **Hence excision of cyst and reconstruction is the treatment of choice.**

TypeI: Excision of the cyst followed by Roux-en-y-hepaticojejunostomy.

Type II: Excision of the diverticulum with suturing of CBD.

Type III: Endoscopic sphincterotomy is adequate (choledochocele)

Type IV: They are difficult to treat. Due to recurrent cholangitis, if total excision is not possible due to adhesions between the cyst and the portal vein, the **posterior wall of the cyst can be left**, after removal of mucosa. This is described as **Lilly's technique.**

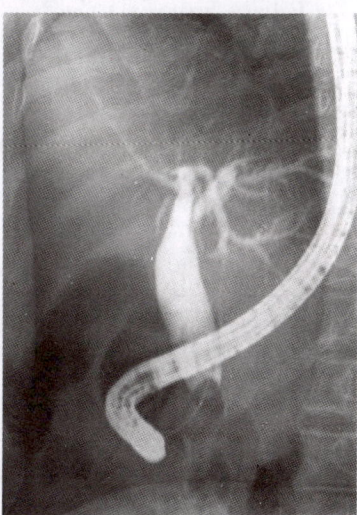

Fig. 25.44 ERCP showing choledochal cyst - type III treated by sphincterotomy

Complications

1. **Recurrent cholangitis** with high grade fever, resulting in biliary cirrhosis
2. **Rupture of the cyst** resulting in biliary peritonitis
3. **CBD stones**
4. **Carcinoma in the cyst** (25-30% of cases)

CAROLI'S DISEASE

- It is a congenital dilatation of intraheptic ducts with stenotic segments in between
- It is also an example for Type V choledochal cysts
- Diagnosed by ultrasound and CT scan. MRI and ERCP are other investigations.

Treatment

- Hepatectomy
- Liver transplantation

Complications

- Cholangitis: It occurs due to constant obstruction
- Stones: Obstruction and stasis precipitate stone formation.
- Biliary cirrhosis
- Cholangiocarcinoma

Key Box 25.17

ASSOCIATED LESIONS

- Congenital hepatic fibrosis
- Medullary sponge kidney

CHRONIC PANCREATITIS

DEFINITION

- Diffuse inflammatory process of pancreas involving head, body and the tail resulting in permanent structural and functional damage to the pancreas.

CAUSES

1. **Alcohol**: Alcohol stimulates the pancreatic secretion rich in protein. This forms plugs in the pancreatic duct and results in stasis of secretion and stone formation. Alcohol also causes spasm of sphincter of Oddi.
2. **Nutritional**: Common in Kerala and was thought to be due to **consumption of tapioca**. It is called Kerala pancreatitis or **tropical pancreatitis**. It is now thought to be due to malnutrition.

3. **Hereditary pancreatitis**: It is genetic disorder transmitted in Mendelian-dominant trait.
4. **Cystic fibrosis**: Generalised dysfunction of exocrine glands because of which secretions precipitate in the lumen.
5. **Hyperparathyroidism** favours precipitation of calcium intraductally. It can also activate pancreatic enzymes.

PATHOLOGY

- There is destruction of pancreas by ductal sclerosis, ductal strictures, glandular fibrosis and calcification, both intraductal and parenchymal.

CLINICAL FEATURES (M.O.P.E.D.)

1. **M**alabsorption occurs due to damage to exocrine glands resulting in steatorrhoea-10-15 stools per day, bulky, frothy, rich in fat, foul smelling. Malabsorption indicates late disease and results in weight loss. creatorrhoea refers to excessive loss of protein.
2. **O**bstructive jaundice can occur due to oedema of the head of pancreas. Later, fibrous constriction of CBD due to fibrotic indurated mass in the head region can cause jaundice by compressing the CBD.
3. **P**ain abdomen-upper abdominal pain radiating to the back in the region of L_1, L_2 due to retroperitoneal inflammation. Pain may be severe, sometimes radiating to both right and left sides. **Pain results due to multiple strictures in the pancreatic duct which increases intraductal pressure.** Pain is relieved on stooping forward.
4. **E**xploratory laparotomy-Many cases are diagnosed at laparotomy-irregularity, hardness involving the entire pancreas. Exploration is done for evaluation of obstructive jaundice or for chronic abdominal pain.
5. **D**iabetes-Incidence of diabetes is about 10-20%. It should be suspected in diabetic patients with pain abdomen.

Investigations

1. **Plain X-ray** abdomen can demonstrate stones in the pancreatic duct or parenchymal calcification.
2. **USG** can detect the stones, stricture, dilatation and associated cysts.
3. **ERCP**
   - Ductal distension, ductal stricture
   - Dilated pancreatic duct (diameter of the normal duct is 4-6 mm)

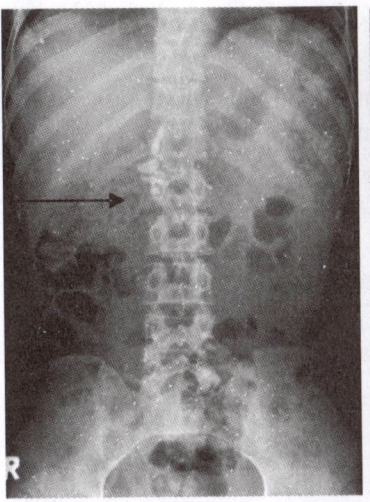
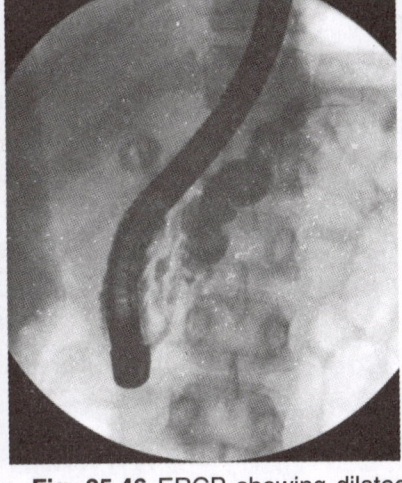
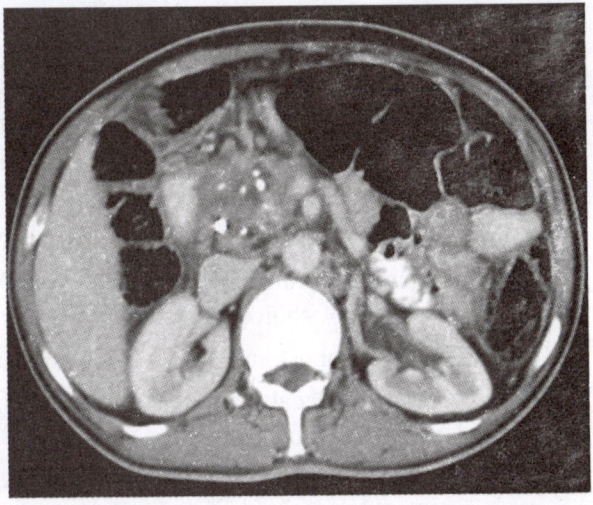

Fig. 25.45 Plain X-ray abdomen showing extensive calcification

Fig. 25.46 ERCP showing dilated pancreatic duct, chain of lakes

Fig. 25.47 CT scan showing chronic pancreatitis with head mass

- Demonstration of stones-appear as regular filling defect.
4. **CT scan**-can reveal ductal anatomy, head mass, size and configuration of pancreas.

Complications

1. Obstructive jaundice due to a mass lesion in the head region
2. Carcinoma of pancreas
3. Pseudocysts

Treatment

1. **Conservative**
   - Pain relief by analgesics, epidural analgesia, or splanchnic nerve block.
   - Supplement **pancreatic enzyme**, diet should be low in fat and **vitamin D** supplements should be given.
   - Control of diabetes, stop alcohol
2. **Surgery : Indications**
   - Persistent pain, obstructive jaundice and duodenal obstructions

Types of surgery (Figs. 25.48 and 25.49)

1. **Chronic pancreatitis involving tail of pancreas:** Distal pancreatectomy with removal of spleen.
2. **Diffuse chronic pancreatitis with dilated pancreatic duct:** Duct is laid open widely, strictures are cut open, stones are removed and it is anastomosed to a loop of jejunum-longitudinal pancreaticojejunostomy -

Puestow's operation (Roux-en-Y jejunal segment). The duct should be at least 8 mm in diameter. Sutures hold very nicely because of fibrosis of pancreas. Pain relief is obtained in about 80% of the cases. Pancreatic fistula is a complication of this surgery. Majority of the fistulae stop by themselves.

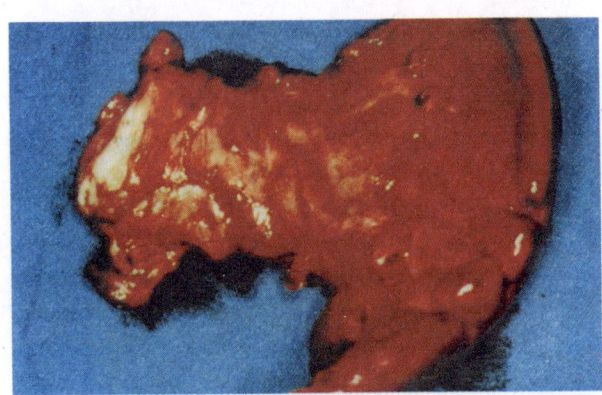

Fig. 25.48 Distal pancreatectomy

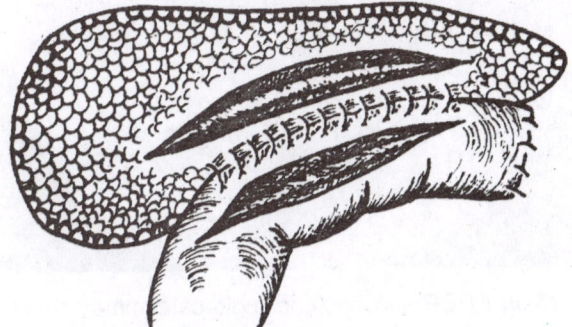

Fig. 25.49 Puestow's operation

3. **Chronic pancreatitis involving head mass:** In this situation doubt arises whether it is malignancy or not. Even trucut biopsy and frozen section are not full proof. Hence pancreaticoduodenectomy is advised, provided experience of the surgeon is good and the mortality rate is less than 5-10%.

4. **Chronic pancreatitis with bile duct obstruction**
   - If malignancy is ruled out, a bypass procedure is the treatment of choice.
   - Choledochojejunostomy is the ideal treatment
   - Pancreaticoduodenal resection (whipple) can also be done (as mentioned above).

5. **Chronic pancreatitis with duodenal obstruction**
   - Here also a resection of the head mass or gastrojejunostomy is the treatment of choice.

6. **Chronic pancreatitis with ascites:** Treatment of choice is Puestow's operation

CHOLANGIOCARCINOMA-BILE DUCT CARCINOMA

- It is an uncommon cause of obstructive jaundice
- Elderly males > 60 years are commonly affected
- Obstructive jaundice is the presenting feature
- Tender hepatomegaly is present due to congestion and may be due to cholangitis

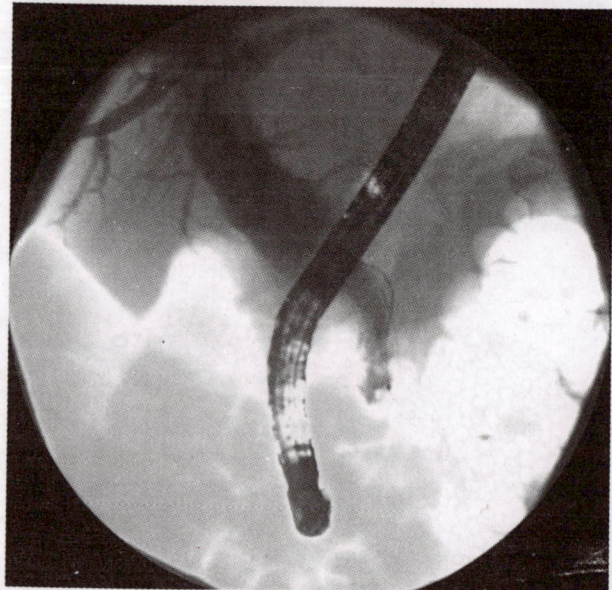

Fig. 25.50 ERCP showing cholangio carcinoma - there is a fear of introducing infection with ERCP. MRC would have been better

- Abdominal ultrasound, ERCP will help in localising the site of obstruction.
- Cholangiocarcinoma at the bifurcation of the hepatic duct is called **Klatskin's tumour.**
- Patients having following diseases have increased risk of developing cholongiocarcinoma.

Key Box 25.18

1. **C**holangitis - Primary sclerosing
2. **C**olitis - Ulcerative
3. **C**lonorchiasis
4. **C**holedochal cyst
5. **C**aroli's disease

- Treatment is difficult because most of the lesions are high up in the hilar region infiltrating the liver, portal vein etc. Resection and hepaticojejunostomy or endoscopic stent placement are the treatment modalities available.

CONGENITAL BILIARY ATRESIA

Aetiopathogenesis

- A disease of unknown aetiology, though rare, is fatal. Viral aetiology and defective embryogenesis have been blamed for the development of biliary atresia.

Types (Fig. 25.51)

- Type I : Common bile duct is involved
- Type II : Common hepatic duct is involved
- Type III : Atresia of right and left hepatic ducts

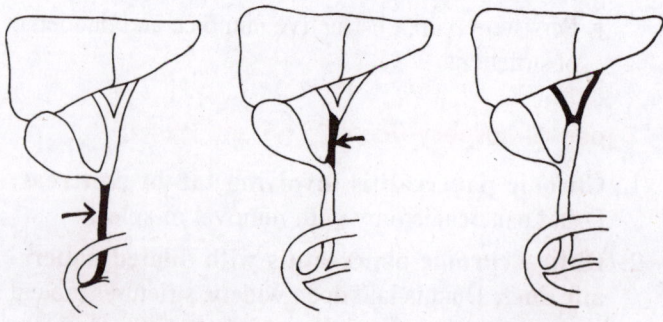

Fig. 25.51 Congenital biliary atresia - Type I, II and III

Clinical features

- It presents as jaundice at birth or in the neonatal period.
- Due to absence of bile in the gut, meconium is not bile stained. Hence, stools are pale.
- Gradually, due to the backpressure liver enlarges.
- Enlargement of the spleen may follow if there is development of portal hypertension.
- Steatorrhoea, pruritus and clubbing are the other features.

Treatment

- **Surgical drainage of bile** is the only available treatment provided patent bile duct or radical is seen. Anastomosis of Roux-en-Y loop of jejunum to the dilated bile duct or some times excision of bile duct tissue upto the liver capsule should be done followed by Roux-en-Y anastomosis. This is called **Kasai's portoentero stomy**.
- **Liver transplantation** is the choice when there is atresia of the intrahepatic duct.

Complications

1. Recurrent cholangitis giving rise to hepatic fibrosis
2. Bililary cirrhosis and portal hypertension

CARCINOMA OF THE GALL BLADDER

- **Incidence:** It is common in North eastern India.

AETIOLOGY

- **Gall stones:** 80-90% of gall bladder cancers are associated with gall stones.
- **Chemicals:** High incidence of gall bladder and biliary cancer is noted in people who work in rubber industries.
- **Gall bladder polyp**
- **Dietary :** Adulterated mustard oil for cooking is found to precipitate carcinoma gall bladder.

PATHOLOGY

- 85% of cases. It is adenocarcinoma, undifferentiated carcinoma, squamous carcinoma are also found.

CLINICAL FEATURES

- Significant weight loss, jaundice and mass in the right upper quadrant are common presentations.
- Few cases can present as chronic cholecystitis with a mass or acute cholecystitis.
- Obstructive jaundice, bleeding, ascites are late features.

INVESTIGATIONS

- Ultrasonography and endosonography are very useful investigations. Ultrasonographic guided FNAC can be done for histological diagnosis in suspected cases of gall bladder mass.
- CT scan is useful for staging
- ERCP if there is obstructive jaundice to localise the exact site and nature of obstruction.

TREATMENT

- If gall bladder cancer is found at cholecystectomy and if **mucosa only is involved**, then cholecystectomy is enough.
- If bladder wall is involved, then extended cholecystectomy is done. (Key Box 25.19)
- Radiation has very small benefits
- Chemotherapy also has been tried. 5FU, mitomycin C, doxorubicin are the drugs.

Key Box 25.19

EXTENDED CHOLECYSTECTOMY

Cholecystectomy

↓

Open the specimen

↓

Growth penetrating the wall

↓

Segmental wedge excision of liver

↓

Regional lymphadenectomy (lymph nodes in and around CBD, duodenum, pancreatico - duodenal regions)

Usual blunder committed is trying to do cholecystectomy for a diagnosis of stone but it is a case of carcinoma gall bladder - Inadequate surgery results in biliary fistula and speedens the death.

PROGNOSIS

- In general five year survival is very poor (refer Key Box 25.20).

Key Box 25.20

GALL BLADDER CANCER IS THE WORST - WHY

- Biologically very aggressive cancer (unlike basal cell cancer etc.)
- High incidence of lymphatic spread
- Easy spread into liver by direct infiltration
- Spreads by blood, neural, intra-peritoneal method
- Intraductal extension into CBD causing obstructive jaundice
- Infiltration into stomach, colon, duodenum, liver because of its location
- Radiation and chemotherapy is rarely of any benefit

Thus, we have discussed various causes of obstructive jaundice. Students should be able to differntiate between all these different causes and to offer an appropriate diagnosis in the examination.

CARCINOMA OF PANCREAS

- 70% of the cases occur in the head of the pancreas including periampullary region
- 30% occur in the body and the tail
- 70% of cases are adenocarcinoma of duct cell origin

AETIOLOGY

1. **Tropical pancreatitis** and hereditary pancreatitis are associated with pancreatic cancer-such malignancies can be multifocal.
2. **Haemochromatosis**-produces extensive calcification of pancreas. Also a precancerous condition.
3. **Diabetes-** Diabetic patients are 10 times more vulnerable for carcinoma of pancreas.
4. Other possible aetiological factors :
   - **Alcohol and smoking:** It is related to tobacco specific nitrosamines.

---
1. **Trousseau's sign** is also found in Buerger's disease.

- **Westernization of diet:** Fatty food, rich in animal proteins can cause pancreatic cancer.
- **Industrial carcinogens :** B11-naphthylamine, benzidine, gasoline are the possible agents.

PATHOLOGY

- Periampullary refers to carcinoma arising from ampulla of Vater, the duodenal mucosa or the lower end of the common bile duct.
- Microscopically, types are:
1. **Mucus** secreting carcinoma of ductal origin
2. **Non-mucus** secreting carcinoma of acinar origin.
3. **Anaplastic** carcinomas are poorly differentiated and tend to arise from the body of the pancreas.
4. **Cystadenocarcinomas** are rare, slow growing and tend to attain a large size.

CLINICAL FEATURES

- Periampullary and carcinoma head of pancreas present as obstructive jaundice (Page 399).

CARCINOMA BODY AND TAIL OF PANCREAS

SYMPTOMS

1. Severe pain radiating to the back in the region of L1 and L2. It is due to infiltration of retroperitoneal nerve plexuses or pancreatic duct obstruction
2. Gross weight loss in 3-6 months.
3. Anorexia, asthenia and generalised weakness.
4. Jaundice cannot occur in carcinoma body and tail of pancreas unless:
   - There are secondaries in liver.
   - There are lymph nodes at porta hepatis.
5. **Trousseau's sign**[1] (Thrombophlebitis migrans)
   - Migrating thrombophlebitis of the legs can occur in visceral malignancies particularly from carcinoma of pancreas, rarely carcinoma stomach, colon, etc.
   - It is supposed to be due to a sluggish blood flow resulting in thrombus formation.
   - It is superficial and affects the leg veins such as long saphenous vein.

SIGNS

1. **Anaemia** may be present as in any other malignancy.

Table 25.2 Differences between pancreatic mass and stomach mass

CARCINOMA BODY OF THE PANCREAS	CARCINOMA STOMACH
1. Pain radiating to the back is the presenting feature	Vomiting, dyspepsia is present. Pain is not a feature
2. Haematemesis is not a feature	Common feature
3. The mass will not move with respiration	Usually moves with respiration
4. Mobility is not a feature	Mobility is present
5. Knee elbow test-Mass does not fall forwards (retroperitoneal organ)	Stomach mass falls forward, (intraperitoneal) unless it is fixed
6. Percussion: Resonant note is obtained because of stomach/intestine anterior to it	Impaired note because of growth in the stomach

2. **Jaundice** is not a feature. Left supraclavicular node may be palpable.

3. **Per abdomen findings** (Table 25.2) : Majority of these cases are advanced fixed and are felt as a mass in the upper abdomen.

   I. Criteria of a pancreatic mass

   - It is situated on the left side involving left hypochondrium, umbilical region and epigastrium.
   - It does not move with respiration because it is retroperitoneal.
   - It does not fall forwards in knee elbow position of pancreas.
   - Can get above the swelling
   - On percussion it gives a resonant note because of anterior position of stomach

   II. Features of carcinoma are

   - Common in male, elderly patients
   - Hard, irregular, fixed lump

   III. Evidence of metastasis

   - Secondaries in the liver, ascites, rectovesical deposits, etc.

DIFFERENTIAL DIAGNOSIS

1. **Carcinoma stomach** infiltrating the pancreas
   - Such mass may not be mobile. It does not move with respiration because it is fixed to pancreas.
   - These patients will have vomiting first followed by backache at a later date.

2. **Carcinoma transverse colon**
   - Produces constipation and bleeding per rectum. Vertical mobility may be present.

   - Right to left peristalsis may be present
3. **Para-aortic lymph node mass** may be due to:
   - Intra-abdominal malignancies, lymphoma, testicular tumour, etc.

INVESTIGATIONS

I. Investigations for periampullary carcinoma and carcinoma of head of pancreas (discussed before).

II. **Investigations for carcinoma body and tail**

1. **USG**
   - Size of tumour: Can detect a mass as small as 2 cm.
   - **Extent of tumour:** Intraoperative ultrasound, to take a biopsy.
   - Infiltration of portal vein which makes it inoperable.

2. **CT scan**
   - Retroperitoneal invasion
   - Lymph node enlargement

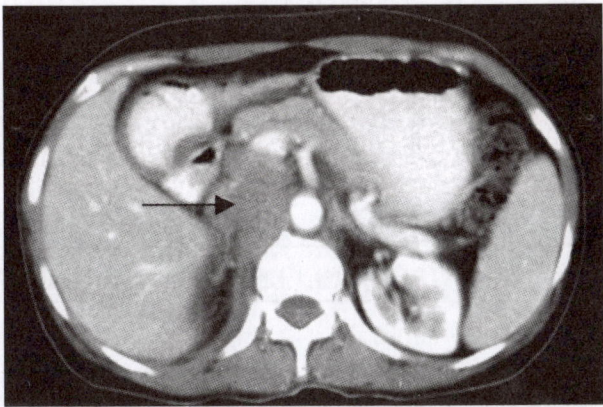

Fig. 25.52 Carcinoma body of the pancrease with para-aortic nodes

3. **Cancer antigen CA 19-9:** These are glycoproteins which are elaborated by malignancies. It is a tumour marker of pancreas to monitor carcinoma pancreas. Elevated in carcinoma of pancreas, colon, liver. It is also increased in pancreatitis.

TREATMENT

I. Periampullary carcinoma-Whipple's operation

II. Carcinoma of body and tail

A. If the tumour is very small, diagnosed very early, they are ideally treated by **Total pancreatectomy with removal of involved lymph nodes.**

B. Many cases are diagnosed late. They are inoperable either due to fixity to portal vein or due to metastasis. Hence, there is no role for curative surgery. For the confirmation of diagnosis, transabdominal USG guided fine needle aspiration cytology can be done. Surgery is not indicated in such cases; only palliative treatment can be offered. Prognosis is very poor.

- **Palliative radiotherapy**-4000-6000 cGy units can be given Response rate is 5-10%, It reduces size of the tumour and some pain relief is obtained.

- **Injection 5 - FU** 500 mg in 5% dextrose I.V. for 5 days per month for 6 cycles.

- **Coeliac plexus block** by using 50% alcohol 10-20 ml, on each side of coeliac ganglion.

- **Epidural analgesia**

ENDOCRINE TUMOURS OF THE PANCREAS

These tumours are members of APUDOMA arising from APUD cells (**A**mine **P**recursor **U**ptake **D**ecarboxylation). They are neuroectodermal in origin. Accordingly, following tumours can occur (Table 25.3).

These tumours can be :

- **Sporadic:** Usually occurs as a single tumour
- **Familial:** occur with other adenomas as in Multiple endocrine neoplasia syndrome-**MEN TYPE I** : Pituitary, parathyroid, pancreatic adenoma.

INSULINOMA (β-CELL TUMOUR)

- Majority of the insulinomas occur in the tail and body of pancreas and majority of them are benign, one third are malignant and one third are multiple.

- It can be a single adenoma or it can be due to diffuse hyperplasia or due to carcinoma.

- **Clinical features are that of hypoglycemia** (refer Key Box 25.21 for other causes of hypoglycemia)

Key Box 25.21
PERSISTENT HYPOGLYCAEMIA - CAUSES
• Insulinoma • Hepatoma • Hepatocellular damage • Hypopituitarism • Addison's disease • Large mesenchymal tumor

- In early stages, it can mimic a duodenal ulcer. Due to hypoglycaemia, hunger pain develops and tendency to ask for food is present.

- As it becomes severe, giddiness, dizziness, syncopal attacks, blurring of vision and diplopia can occur.

- Late stages-epilepsy, semiconsciousness and coma.

Whipple's triad of insulinoma

1. Attack of hypoglycaemia in morning hours, in the fasting state

2. Symptoms are relieved on taking glucose

3. Blood sugar in the fasting state is less than 45 mgs % during the attacks

Table 25.3 Endocrine tumours of the pancreas

ISLET CELLS	ACTIVE AGENT	SYNDROME	PRESENTATION
Alpha	Glucagon	Glucagonoma	Hyperglycaemia
Beta	Insulin	Insulinoma	Hypoglycaemia
Delta	Somatostatin	Somatostatinoma	
G	Gastrin	Gastrinoma	Hyperacidity

Investigations

1. **Serum insulin** levels done by immunoassay method are found to be very high
2. Persistent hypoglycaemia-blood sugar level of less than 50 mg/dl relieved by glucose is suggestive of insulinoma
3. **USG and CT scan** of abdomen can demonstrate the tumour if it is more than 2 cm.
4. Selective angiography will demonstrate tumour blush as majority of them are very vascular.

Treatment

- Enucleation is the treatment of choice.
- Resection of the tumour and if necessary distal pancreatectomy can also be done in selected patients.

CLINICAL NOTES

The author remembers a case of recurrent epilepsy getting admitted to the department of neurology. He was found to have hypoglycaemia and diagnosed as insulinoma only during the 4th admission. A 3 cm benign insulinoma was enucleated from the pancreas. Patient is asymptomatic till date.

GASTRINOMA (ZOLLINGER-ELLISON SYNDROME)

Two types are recognised

Type I (rare): These have antral G-cell hyperplasia, wherein gastrin is stored. Hypergastrinemia with chronic peptic ulceration is a feature. Pancreas is normal.

Type II: May be due to an ulcerogenic, non β-islet cell tumour or sometimes due to diffuse hyperplasia of the islet cells. Tumour secretes gastrin and is usually found in the tail of the pancreas. 50% of them are malignant.

- Intractable peptic ulceration, hypergastrinemia with massive acid hypersecretion of upto 500 ml/hour can occur.
- Diarrhoea, steatorrhoea and hypokalaemia results due to acid irritating the small bowel.

Gastrinoma should be suspected in following situations

1. **Unusual ulcer**: Ulcer not responding to intensive medical treatment
2. **Unusual recurrence:** Multiple recurrences inspite of the treatment
3. **Unusual number**: Multiple ulcers scattered in the GIT

4. **Unusual sites:** Ulcers present in the 2nd part of duodenum, an ulcer just **distal to the ligament of Treitz**, etc.
5. **Unusual age:** Sudden development of an ulcer in a young boy or in very elderly patients.

Site

- Commonly it occurs in the gastrinoma triangle also called as Psaros triangle. Following three points form **Psaros triangle.**
1. Junction of the cystic duct with the common bile duct.
2. Junction between head and neck of pancreas.
3. Junction between second and third parts of the duodenum.

Diagnosis

1. **Endoscopy** will reveal prominent mucosal folds and large amount of acid in the stomach.
2. **Serum gastri n** is increased above normal levels (normal value <150 ng/dl).
3. **CT scan and arteriography** may localise the tumour.

Treatment

1. **Type I:** Partial gastrectomy to remove G-cells bearing area.
2. **Type II:** If the tumour is small, removal of the tumour can be done (enucleation).
3. If the **tumour is large**, omeprazole 20 mg twice a day or somatostatin derivatives have been used to control the acidity. Total gastrectomy is the last resort, if gastrinoma is not found.

GLUCAGONOMA

- It arises from **alpha cells** producing glucagon. Around 90% are in the body and tail.
- Clinically, it presents with **extensive necrolytic migratory erythematous rashes.** Rashes occur due to low amino acid levels due to neoglucogenesis brought about by glucagon.
- **Mild diabetes**, weight loss, diarrhoea are the other features.
- Diagnosis is by elective arteriography and CT scan.
- **Treatment is enucleation.**

Thus, endocrine tumours of the pancreas are rare but when they occur they can present with varying clinical manifestations which confuses a clinician. A high index of suspicion is necessary. They may be benign but can be fatal if left untreated.

ACUTE PANCREATITIS

It is defined as an acute condition presenting with abdominal pain usually associated with increased pancreatic enzyme levels in the blood, as a result of inflammatory disease of pancreas. Clinically, it presents as vasomotor collapse, hypotension, shock. It carries 10-20% mortality rate.

- *Acute pancreatitis stings like a scorpion (produces severe pain).*
- *Acute pancreatitis drinks like a fish (produces dehydration).*
- *Acute pancreatitis eats like a wolf (pancreatic necrosis).*
- *Acute pancreatitis burrows like a rodent (produces fistula).*
- *Acute pancreatitis kills like a leopard (life-threatening).*

MARSEILLE'S CLASSIFICATION OF PANCREATITIS

1. Acute pancreatitis
2. Acute relapsing pancreatitis
   - In both these conditions, pancreas returns back to normal.
3. Chronic pancreatitis
4. Chronic relapsing pancreatitis
   - In both these conditions there is always permanent damage to the pancreas

AETIOLOGY

1. **Alcohol:** It is the major cause of acute pancreatitis in our country seen in about 50% of the cases. Alcohol stimulates pancreatic secretions rich in protein, forms protein plugs, results in obstruction to the pancreatic duct. Alcohol also stimulates trypsinogen. It causes spasm of sphincter of Oddi. All these factors result in inflammation.
2. **Biliary tract disease:** Stone in the biliary tree (gall stone pancreatitis) is the major cause of acute pancreatitis in the western world. In our country, it may be responsible for pancreatitis in about 20-30% of patients (Fig. 25.55).
3. **Collagen vascular disorders:** Autoimmune disease like polyarteritis nodosa can be a causative factor in acute pancreatitis.
4. **Drugs:** Corticosteroids, oestrogens, diuretics can cause pancreatitis.

5. **Endoscopic procedures:** Sphincterotomy, cannulation of CBD or pancreatic duct or basketing of stones from CBD can precipitate acute pancreatitis.
6. **Familial or Genetic** factors have been blamed for acute pancreatitis.
7. **Hyperparathyroidism** causing hypercalcaemia may stimulate pancreatic juices and can cause pancreatitis.
8. **Hyperlipidaemia** can also cause pancreatitis.
9. **Hypothermia** and **hypotension** can cause ischaemia to the pancreas resulting in acute pancreatitis.
10. **Injury to the pancreas** either postoperative or following blunt injury can result in pancreatitis.
11. **Infection:** Virus such as Mumps and Coxsackie can cause pancreatitis.

PATHOGENESIS (Fig. 25.53)

- It is an **autodigestion** following activation of trypsinogen. This is brought about by various agents mentioned above.
- It may be also due to reflux of bile into the pancreas.
- Trypsinogen is converted into trypsin. It acts and stimulates:

1. **Lipase:** Lipase splits the fat into fatty acids and glycerol. Fatty acids combine with calcium to form calcium soap. This is represented as fat necrosis seen in the omentum, subsynovial pockets of knee joint etc. This also explains hypocalcaemia and tetany seen in acute pancreatitis.
2. **Elastase:** It digests the elastic fibres of the blood vessels resulting in rupture and haemorrhage into the peritoneal cavity.
3. **Lysolecithinase:** This is derived from the bile. It produces extensive tissue necrosis resulting in destruction of pancreas.
4. **Prostaglandins, Bradykinins, Kallikrein, etc** : These are the inflammatory mediators. They produce profound hypotension, shock and collapse, due to loss of fluid in the retroperitoneum (III space loss).
5. **Extensive necrosis** of pancreas produces **MDF** (**M**yocardial **D**epressant **F**actor) which depresses ventricular contraction resulting in cardiac failure. Ultimate result is the development of **Multi Organ Failure**.

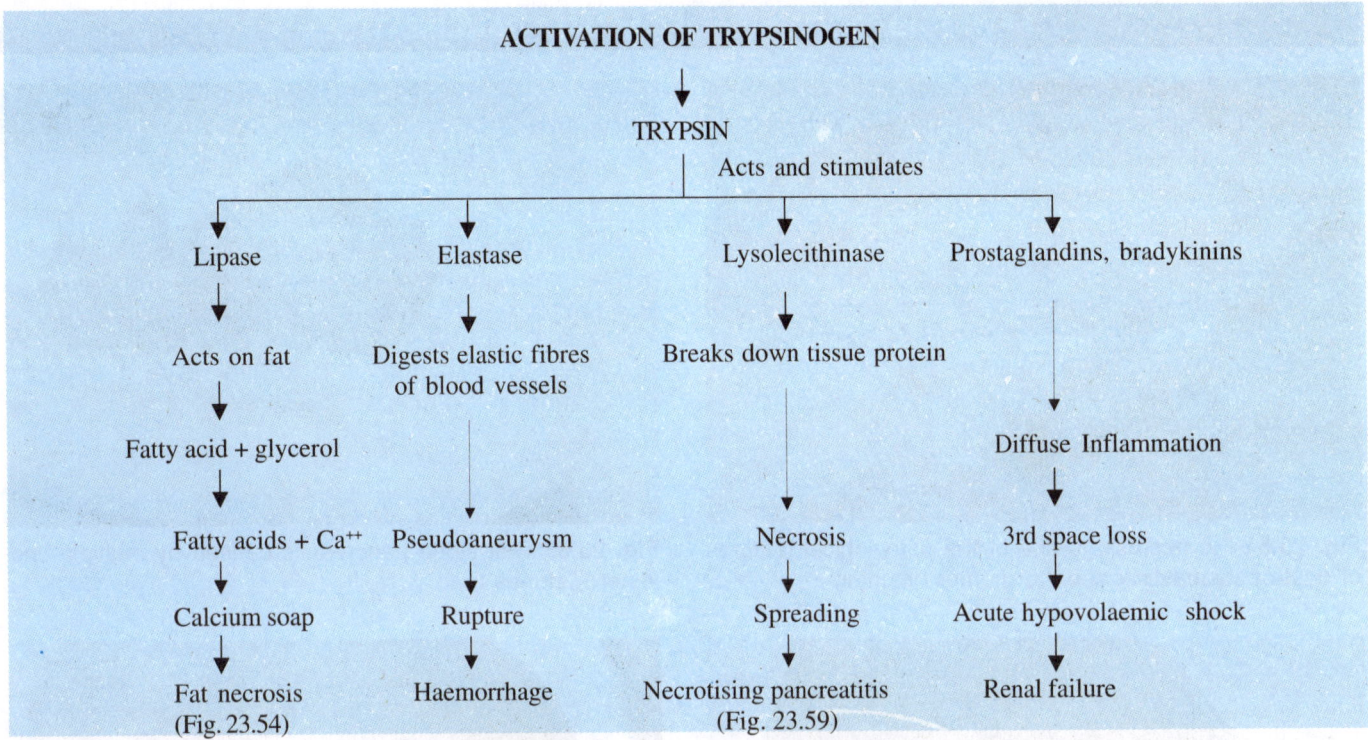

Fig. 25.53 Flowchart of pathogenesis of acute pancreatitis

CLINICAL FEATURES

Symptoms

1. Severe upper abdominal pain radiating to the back increases over a period of hours-illimitable agony is characteristic feature. It is partially relieved on stooping and bending forwards (Mohammedan Prayer sign).
2. Vomiting-Frequent and effortless due to reflex pylorospasm.
3. Fever-low grade
4. Haematemesis and melaena-poor prognosis-due to necrosis of duodenum.

Signs

1. **Febrile**, tachypnoeic patient in agony
2. **Cyanosis**-Improper perfusion of lungs
3. **Faint jaundice** due to oedema of the head of the pancreas.
4. **Features of shock**-feeble pulse, tachycardia, hypotension, cold extremities.
5. **Abdominal findings**
   - Tenderness in epigastrium
   - Upper abdominal guarding and rigidity
   - Abdominal distension due to either accumulation of blood or fluid in peritoneal cavity or due to paralytic ileus (Fig. 23.58).
6. **Cullen's sign** (Fig. 23.56)
   - Bluish ecchymotic discolouration seen around umbilicus.
7. **Grey Turner's sign** (Fig. 23.57)
   - Bluish discolouration in the flanks

Both these signs are due to peri-pancreatic and retroperitoneal haemorrhage and seepage of blood along fascial planes. Escape of pancreatic ferments (enzymes) into the anterior abdominal wall and spread through falciform ligament.

INVESTIGATIONS

1. **Haemogram (CBP)**: Hb % may be low due to haemorrhagic pancreatitis.
   - Total count is raised above 15,000 cells/cumm due to inflammation.
2. **Serum amylase** (widely used test)
   - Normal levels are 40-80 Somogyi units
   - Values around 400 are suggestive and values more than 1000 Somogyi units are diagnostic of acute pancreatitis.

FEW PHOTOGRAPHS OF ACUTE PANCREATITIS

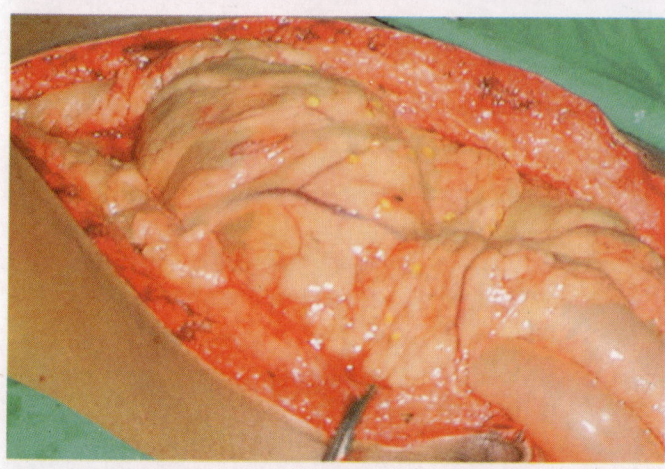

Fig. 25.54 Fat necrosis is one of the pathological features of acute pancreatitis - see the greater omentum

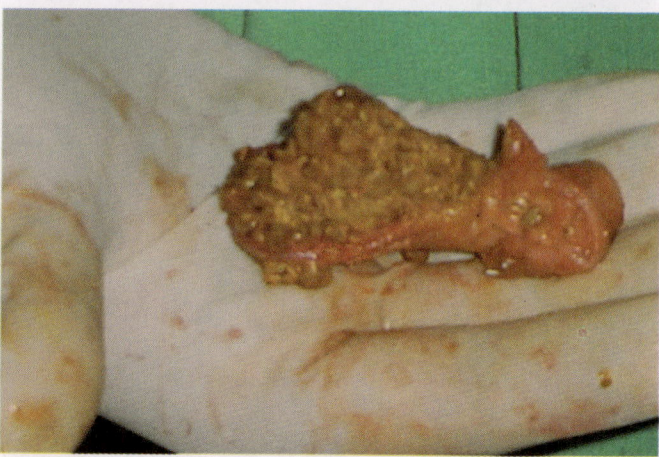

Fig. 25.55 Gall stone pancreatitis caused by multiple cholesterol stones

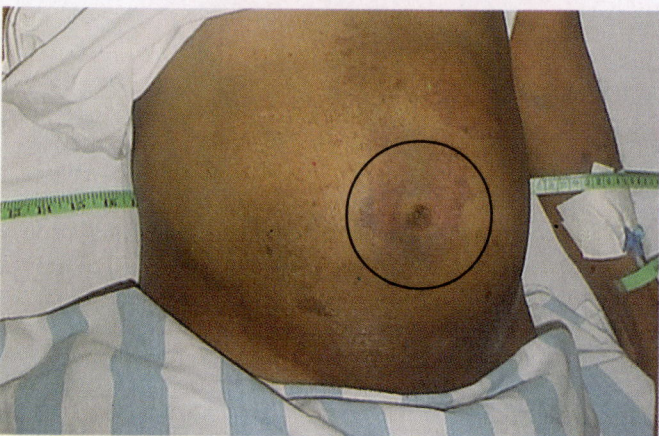

Fig. 25.56 Cullen's sign - discolouration arround the umbilicus

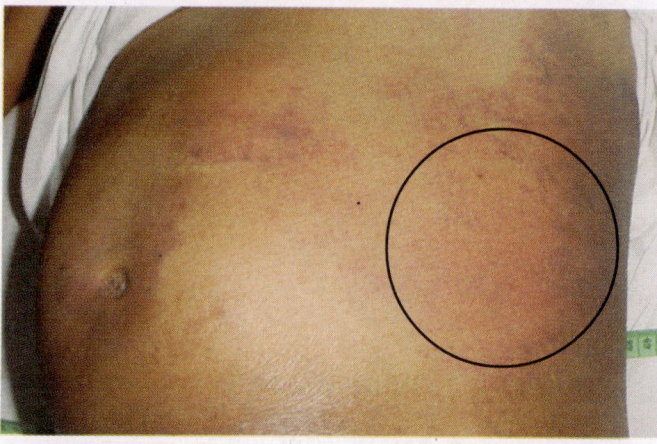

Fig. 25.57 Grey Turner's sign - discolouration in the flanks

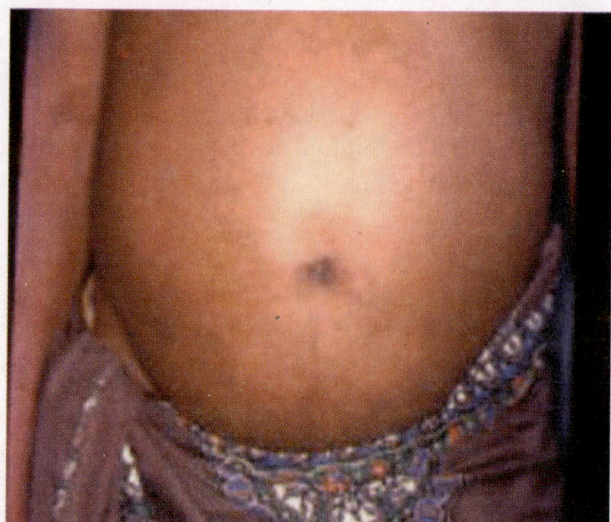

Fig. 25.58 Abdominal distension is due to paralytic ileus in the early stages. It can also be due to pancreatic ascites

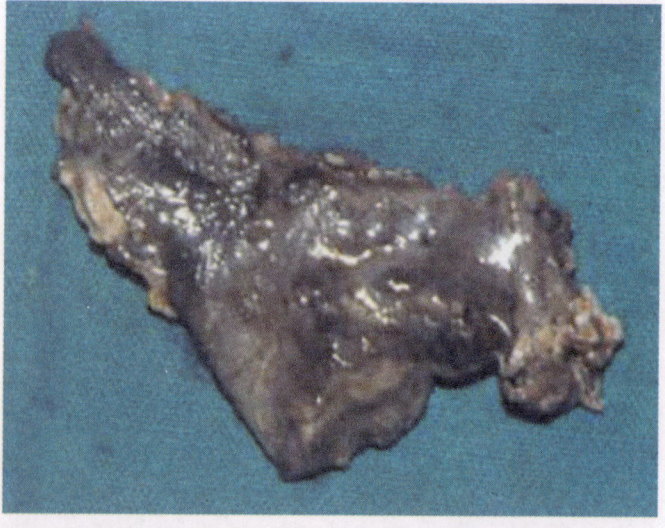

Fig. 25.59 Extensive pancreatic necrosis. Patient had multiorgan failure. After the necrosectomy he improved

---

Key Box 25.22

INCREASED AMYLASE LEVELS IS SEEN IN

- Acute pancreatitis
- Parotitis
- Afferent loop obstruction
- Spasm of sphincter of Oddi
- Biliary peritonitis - Duodenal injuries
- Mesenteric infarction
- Ruptured ectopic gestation

- It is increased in the first 24-48 hours and returns back to normal within 3-4 days.
- Persistent high level of amylase in acute pancreatitis indicates:
  - Unresolving inflammation
  - Recurrent attacks of pancreatitis
  - Complications-Pseudocyst, pancreatic abscess

3. **Blood for urea, creatinine**. to rule out renal failure

4. **Blood sugar estimation** - Glycosuria is present in almost 100% of patients.

5. **Serum calcium levels** - Hypocalcemia is seen, due to hypoalbuminaemia or fat necrosis.

6. **Total proteins are usually low, especially albumin**

7. **Plain X-ray abdomen (erect position)**

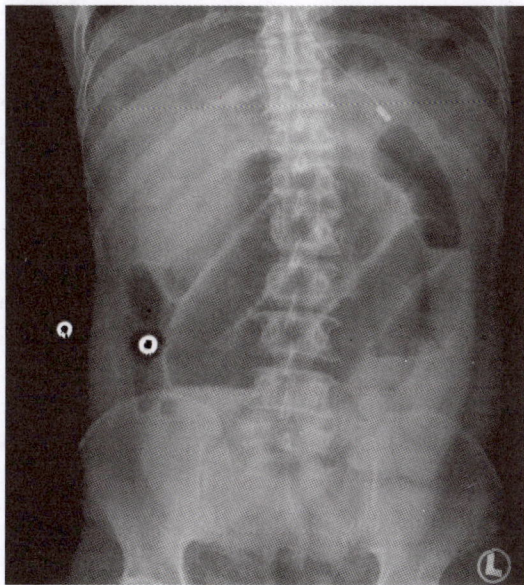

Fig. 25.60 Plain X-ray abdomen erect showing dilated jejunal loop due to paralytic ileus - Sentinel loop sign

- To rule out perforation of peptic ulcer.
- Sentinel loop sign - one dilated jejunal loop of intestine which is seen in the region of pancreas.
- Colon 'cut-off' sign refers to mild distension of transverse colon with collapsed descending colon.

8. **Abdominal ultrasound**-Can demonstrate oedematous pancreas, fluid in the abdomen or biliary tract disease.

9. **Serum lipase levels**-more specific but difficult to measure.

10. **Contrast enhanced CT scan** of abdomen is done after 3-5 days in patients who fail to respond to conservative treatment. **If CT scan demonstrates infected necrosis an urgent CT guided FNAC is done and gram stain is sent. If gram stain is positive, emergency necrosectomy should be done.**

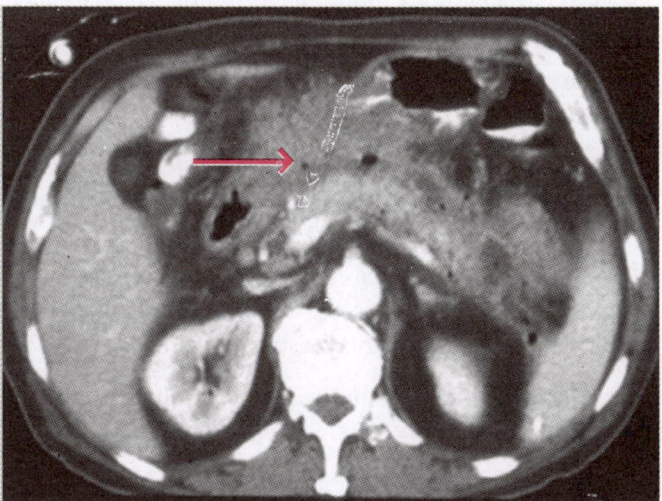

Fig. 25.61 CT scan showing extensive necrosis

MANAGEMENT: ALMOST ALWAYS CONSERVATIVE

Early aggressive fluid replacement is the key in the management of acute pancreatitis.

A. **A**spiration with Ryle's tube, to give rest to the pancreas.

B. **B**lood transfusion if Hb% is low, or fresh blood if proteins are low.

C. **C**harts-increasing pulse, increasing temperature indicates pancreatic abscess which needs laparotomy and drainage.

D. **D**rugs:

- Prophylactic antibiotics: doubtful value

- **Low molecular weight dextran** (Lomodex) 500 ml can be used to increase renal perfusion. Alternately, Dopamine 2 mg/kg body weight can be given I.V. which helps in renal perfusion.

- Injection **somatostatin** or injection octreotide is given to suppress the pancreatic juice. Octreotoide is given in the dose of 50 μg as a loading dose I.V. followed by 50 μg per one hour in 5% dextrose as maintenance dose. Injection hydrocortisone 100 mg I.V. as an anti-inflammatory agent can be given within 6 hours of acute pancreatitis. It can also be used to treat hypotension (doubtful value).

- Narcotics to reduce pain

E. **E**xploratory laparotomy, only when diagnosis is in doubt, when patient is not improving or when there is a complication of pancreatitis. such as pancreatic abscess, fistula or necrosis.

- At laparotomy, pancreas should not be handled. Peritoneal lavage is done followed with corrugated red rubber drain or tube drain. Lavage has shown some benefit.

- The wound can be left open as laparostomy or with mesh or with zip.

In cases of infected necrosis proved by CT guided FNAC and Gram stain, necrosectomy should be done.

F. Fluid should be given early. Rapid infusion of 3-4 litres of ringer lactate is used to treat hypovolaemic shock. Plasma or albumin may also be given.

Refer Table 25.4 for severity predictors in acute pancreatitis.

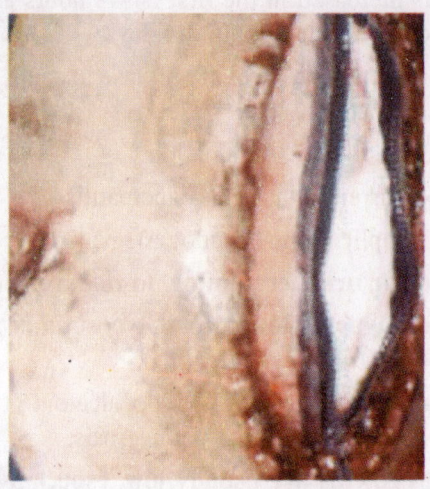

Fig. 25.62 After necrosectomy, it is better to perform zip laparostomy so that it can be opened any number of times for peritoneal toilet

Table 25.4 Severity predictors in acute pancreatitis

RANSON SCORE	GLASGOW SCALE
ON ADMISSION	
Age > 55 years	Age > 55 years
WBC count > 16 x 10^9 / Lit	WBC count > 15 x 10^9 / Lit
Blood glucose > 10 mmol / Lit	Blood glucose > 10 mmol / Lit
LDH > 700 units / Lit	Serum Urea > 16 m mol / Lit
AST > 250 Sigma Frankel unit	Arterial oxygen saturation (PaO$_2$) < 60 mm of Hg
WITHIN 48 HOURS	
Blood urea nitrogen levels > 5 mg%	Serum calcium < 2 mmol / Lit
Arterial oxygen saturation (PaO$_2$ < 60 mm Hg)	Serum albumin < 32 gm / Lit
Serum calcium < 2 mmol / Lit	LDH > 600 units / Lit
Base deficit > 4 mmol / Lit	AST/ALT > 600 units / Lit
Fluid sequestration > 6 Lit	

TREATMENT OF GALL STONE PANCREATITIS

- If gall stone is obstructing the ampulla of Vater and causing pancreatitis, endoscopic sphincterotomy can be done within 5-7 days of time. It has shown some benefit to the patients. After 2-3 weeks, once the jaundice subsides, cholecystectomy with removal of CBD stone is recommended.

COMPLICATIONS OF ACUTE PANCREATITIS

SYSTEMIC COMPLICATIONS

1. **Shock**

   - Hypovolaemia and hypoperfusion are the major factors responsible for renal failure. Due to collection of large amout of fluid in the **third space**-peritoneal cavity, pleural cavity and extravascular space, shock occurs. Fluid replacement with blood or albumin should be done at appropriate time to treat the shock.

   - Electrolyte abnormalities should be corrected.

2. **Respiratory insufficiency:** Factors responsible for this are: (Key Box 25.24)

   - Measurement of arterial blood gas values and administration of oxygen is enough in the initial stages. In late stages, pulmonary insufficiency needs to be treated with ventilatory support.

Key Box 25.24

RESPIRATORY FAILURE

- Abdominal distension and elevation of diaphragm
- Intravascular coagulation in the lung
- Lecithin present in the pulmonary surfactant is altered due to lecithinase resulting in defective capillary alveolar exchange.
- Defective ventilation caused due to pain
- Left-sided pleural effusion

---

3. **Hypocalcaemia** needs to be treated with calcium IV. It is due to hypoalbuminaemia and due to calcium soap.

4. **Pleural effusion** is treated by pleural tap (ultrasound guided), if it is symptomatic.

5. **Ards, mods**

LOCAL COMPLICATIONS

1. **Pancreatic abscess**

   - It develops after 3-4 weeks of pancreatitis. Secondary infection in a pseudocyst results in pancreatic abscess. It usually points out on the left flank.

   - It has to be drained by CT guided aspiration.

   - Laparascopy may be necessary not only for the diagnosis but also as a therapeutic means for removal of necrotic pancreas.

   - Otherwise open drainage of the abscess

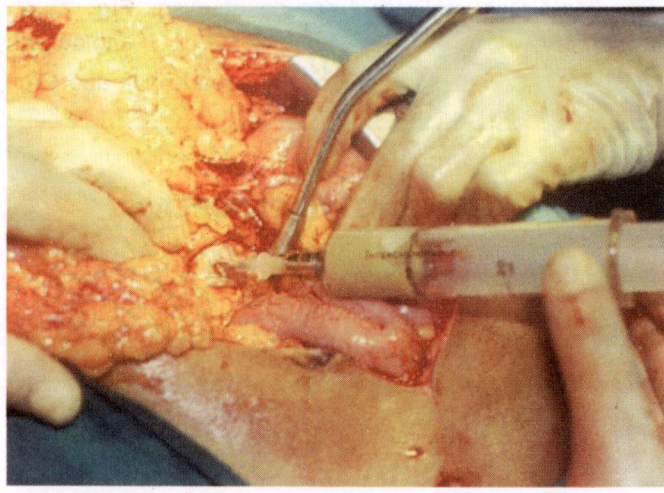

Fig. 25.63 Aspiration of pus from pancreatic abscess

2. **Pseudocyst of pancreas (vide infra)**

   - This complication is encountered after 2nd week following an attack of acute pancreatitis.

   - It is seen in about 20% of the patients

3. **Perforation** of colon or stomach

4. **Pseudoaneurysm** resulting in massive upper gastrointestinal or lower gastrointestinal bleeding. Bleeding into the pancreatic duct is called as **Haemosuccus pancreatitis** (Fig. 24.64, 25.65, 25.66)

   - This condition results due to enzymatic digestion of the blood vessles in the vicinity of pancreas. Thus splenic artery, gastroduodenal artery etc. are commonly involved.

   - It has very high mortality. Timely angiography followed by embolization is the treatment.

   - Otherwise, laparotomy, ligation of pseudoaneurysm with or without intracystic ligation of the bleeders is the treatment.

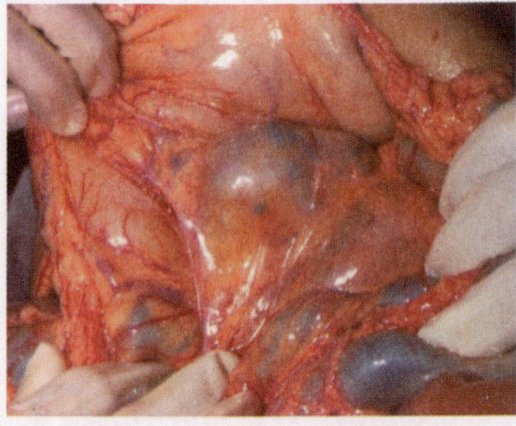

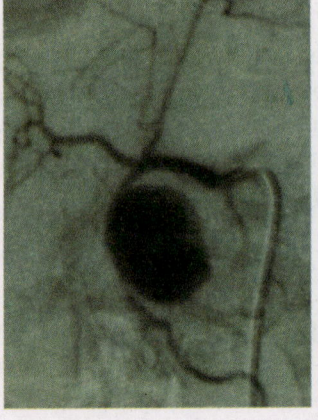

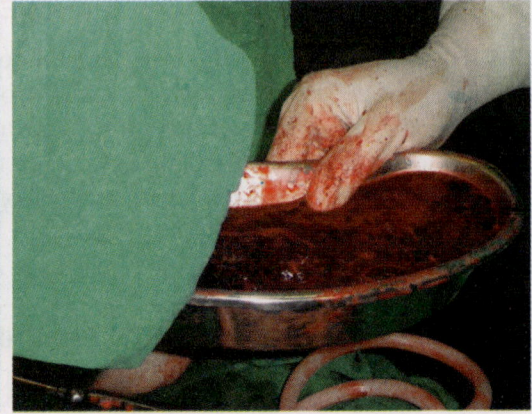

Fig. 25.64 Gastroduodenal pseudoaneurysm at surgery

Fig. 25.65 Diagnosis by angiography

Fig. 25.66 As a cause of massive upper gastrointestinal bleeding

Contributed by Prof. Annappa Kudva and Prof. B.H. Ananda Rao, Dept. of Surgery, KMC, Manipal

PSEUDOCYST OF PANCREAS

- **Definition:** Collection of free fluid in the lesser sac, due to pancreatic pathology.

It is called pseudocyst because it has NO EPITHE-LIAL LINING.

AETIOLOGY

1. Following an attack of **acute pancreatitis**, it usually appears after 2 weeks. The swelling appears in the upper abdomen.

2. **Blunt injury** of abdomen resulting in a ductal disruption wherein the pancreatic duct in the region of body is crushed against vertebral body.

3. Some cases of **chronic pancreatitis** may be associated with pseudocyst.

LOCATIONS OF PSEUDOCYST

1. Between stomach and transverse colon

2. Between stomach and liver (Fig. 25.67)

3. Behind or below the transverse colon

CLINICAL FEATURES

1. Tensely cystic mass in the epigastrium, umbilical region or in left hypochondrium. Tensely cystic mass feels firm on palpation. Classically upper border of the mass is not felt.

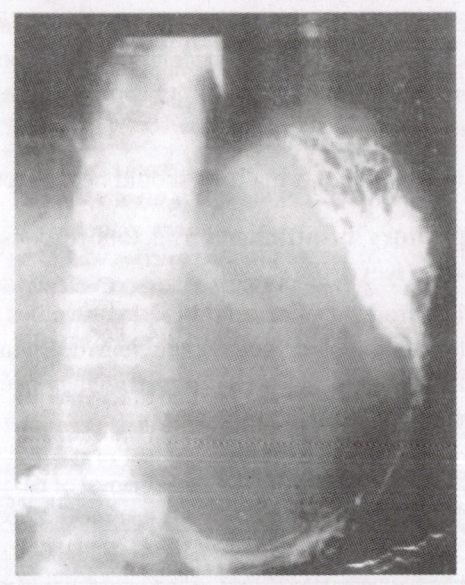

Fig. 25.67 Large pseudocyst behind the stomach demonstrated by barium meal

2. Does not move with respiration because it is retroperitoneal in location

3. It may have transverse mobility

4. It does not fall forwards

5. Percussion: It gives a **resonant note** because of stomach or intestine anterior to it

6. **Transmitted pulsation** from aorta can be felt.

7. If a Ryle's tube is passed, it can be felt over the swelling. It is called as **Baid sign**.

8. Depending upon the tension within the cyst it can be tender or non tender.

INVESTIGATIONS

1. USG - can detect size, location of cyst
2. Barium meal follow through. In a lateral picture, the stomach is pushed anteriorly and increased vertebro-gastric interval is seen (Not done nowadays)
3. ERCP may demonstrate communication of the cyst with the duct.

TREATMENT

I. Conservative line of treatment

- Majority of the pseudocysts following acute pancreatitis resolve by itself within 3-4 weeks.
- Hence, regular ultrasound examination is done to observe the pseudocyst.

II. Surgery

- Increase in size of cyst, severe pain, no response to conservative line of treatment are indications for surgery.

1. **Cystogastrostomy** (Figs. 25.68 to 25.71)

   Indications: Pseudocyst in relation to head and body of pancreas.

   - **Timing:** Surgery is done **after 6 weeks** because that is the time required for the wall to become fibrous.
   - **Size** of the cyst should be at least **6 cm.**
   - **Procedure:** Anterior gastrotomy is done and an incision in the posterior wall of stomach opens into the cyst cavity. Contents are drained. Opening is enlarged and cut end of stomach in posterior wall is sutured to cut edge of cyst wall. After one week cyst collapses. For reasons not known the food does not enter the cyst cavity. **Size of cystogastrostomy stoma is about 6 cm. This procedure can also be done by endoscopic method.**

2. Cyst confined to the tail of the pancreas-distal pancreatectomy with removal of tail and cyst.

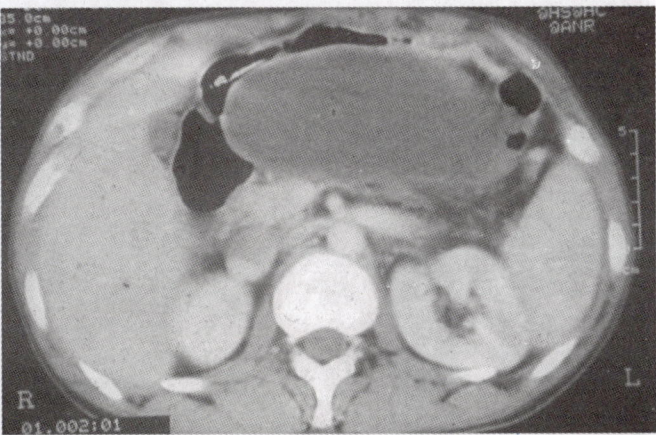

Fig. 25.68 CT scan - Classical pseudocyst pushing the stomach anteriorly - cystogastrostomy is ideal treatment

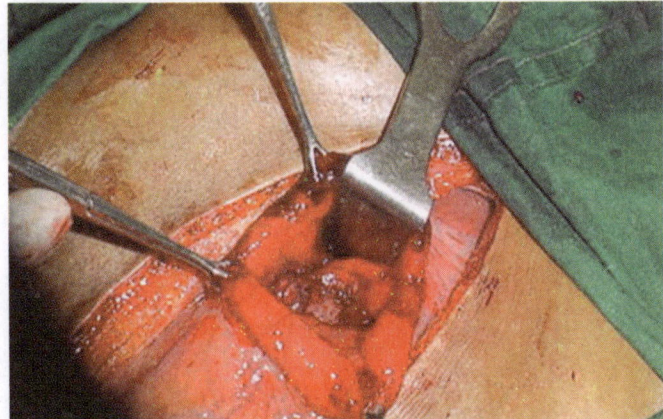

Fig. 25.70 Posterior gastric wall is sutured to anterior cyst wall after creating a stoma of 6 cm.

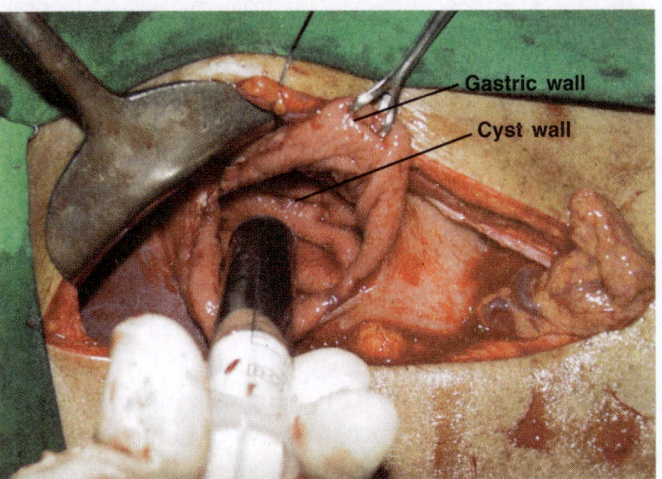

Gastric wall
Cyst wall

Fig. 25.69 Cystogastrostomy

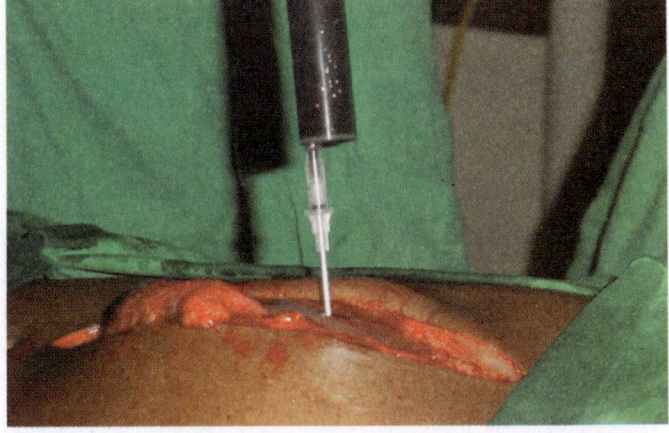

Fig. 25.71 Aspirated fluid has car engine oil appearance. Amylase contents of this cyst was very high

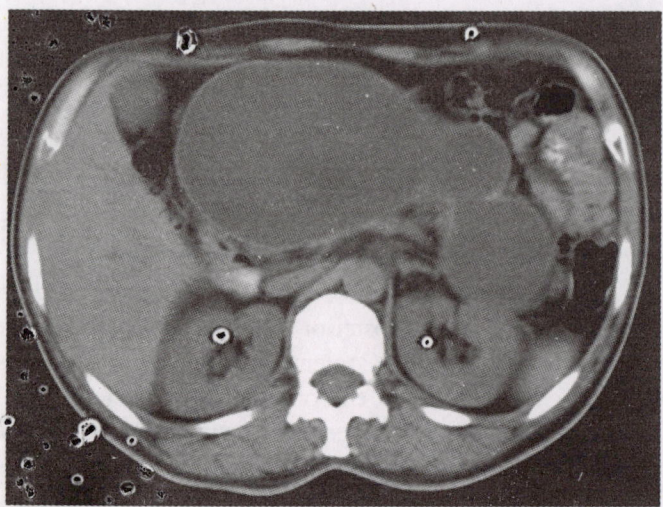

Fig. 25.72 CT scan showing large pseudocyst with multiple pockets. Cystojejunostomy is the ideal treatment

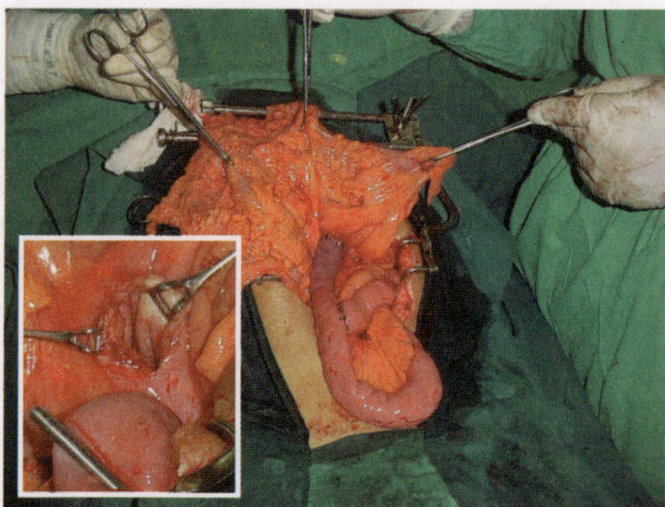

Fig. 25.73 Roux-en-Y Cystojejunostomy at surgery- inset shows the opened cyst wall which is thick

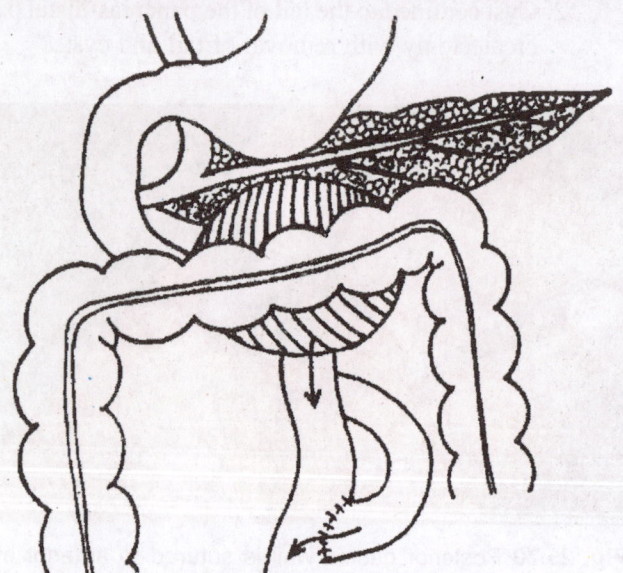

Fig. 25.74 Cystojejunostomy

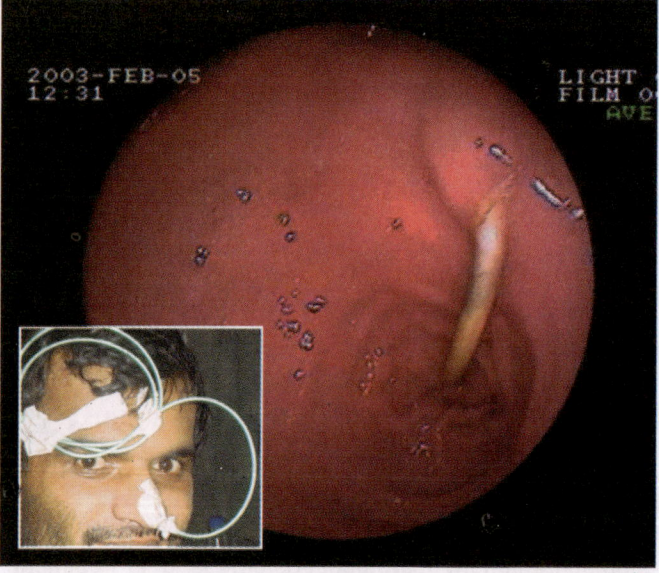

Fig. 25.75 Endoscopic cystogastrostomy - ideal to drain acute pseudocysts. Inset - After draining a nasobilliary catheter can be left in the cyst cavity. Contributed by Dr. Filippe Alvaris, KMC, Manipal

3. **Large cyst:** Cystojejunostomy by using Roux-en-Y loop can be done, by suturing jejunal loop, in the most dependent area (Fig. 25.74).

4. It can also be done by endoscopic method. This is easy, less invasive and ideal in draining acute psedocysts. This procedure can also be repeated. However, chances of introducing infection are present. Endoscopic method of draining the pseudocysts is also being done for chronic cysts (Fig. 25.75).

Young 18 year old engineering student got admitted with acute pancreatitis. At the end of 10 days, he developed an abscess in the left flank which was drained by a treating surgeon at a peripheral hospital and the case was then referred to our hospital. Patient was emaciated with swinging temperature. After 6 days of admission, faecal discharge started from left flank area indicating colonic necrosis. With difficulty, an emergency right transverse colostomy with necrosectomy was done. Fever persisted. One day, a call was attended by a duty doctor for breathlessness. The patient had a left pleural effusion. Aspiration of pleural cavity revealed bloodstained dirty fluid rich in amylase. He had developed pancreaticopleural fistula. He was managed conservatively in the sitting posture. Few days later, he developed severe convulsions and coma. Blood sugar was 20 mg% following administration of injection insulin because patient had developed diabetes. He was resuscitated. In the meanwhile injection somatostatin was airlifted from Switzerland (1987-1988 period). This boy stayed in the hospital for 90 days. He survived, went home with emaciation, malnutrition and permanent diabetes with plenty of cuts all over the body. He was a vegetarian and a teetotaler. This is a story of a patient who had developed complications such as abscess, transverse colon necrosis, left pleural effusion, respiratory failure, diabetes. What is the cause of pancreatitis? Nobody knows.

CONGENITAL ANOMALIES OF THE PANCREAS

ANNULAR PANCREAS (Key Box 25.25)

- It is a rare anomaly which occurs due to persistence of a portion of the ventral pancreatic anlage which fails to rotate. As a result of this, II part of the duodenum is surrounded by a thin rim of pancreatic tissue. Hence the name, annular pancreas.

Associated anomalies

- Intrinsic duodenal atresia or stenosis

Clinical features

- **Neonatal type:** It manifests early in life. It produces symptoms of acute intestinal obstruction with vomiting and inability to take food.
- **Adult type:** It manifests after the age of 20. Vomiting is bile stained. Due to stasis in the pyloric antrum, the features of duodenal ulcer may be present.

Investigations

1. **Plain X-ray abdomen:** Double bubble appearance occurs due to dilated stomach and dilated proximal duodenum.
2. **Barium meal** X-ray can demonstrate obstruction to II part of duodenum.

Key Box 25.25

ANNULAR PANCREAS

- Persistent ventral anlage
- Neonatal or adult age
- Plain X-ray - double bubble
- Barium meal - obstruction to II part of duodenum
- Duodenoduodenostomy is the treatment

Treatment

- **Duodenoduodenostomy** is the treatment of choice, Otherwise, duodenojejunostomy can be done.

It is tempting to divide the thin pancreatic rim. This should not be done as it will result in a pancreatic fistula.

Differential diagnosis

1. Pyloric stenosis
2. Wilkie's disease (chronic duodenal ileus)

ECTOPIC PANCREAS

- This condition is not uncommon. In some occasions, at laparotomy for some other conditions, a soft to firm irregular tissue or nodule, is found on the intestinal surface. Biopsy of this may come later as ectopic pancreas. Most of them are asymptomatic.
- It is found in the submucosa of the stomach, duodenum, small intestines, Meckel's diverticulum or in the hilum of the spleen.

Complications

1. In the stomach: It may undergo cystic degeneration.
2. In the intestine: It can cause intussusception.
3. In the intestine: Sometimes, it may be the source of gastrointestinal bleeding.
4. In the Meckel's diverticulum: any of the above complications, mentioned above.

CONGENITAL CYSTIC FIBROSIS

- It is inherited as an autosomal recessive disorder.
- It is a generalised dysfunction of exocrine glands resulting in defective mucus secretion.

- Malabsorption due to pancreatic insufficiency is a feature.
- Pulmonary disease due to bronchiolitis occurs later.

Pathology

- The viscid mucin which is produced results in obstruction of the ducts and ductules. Stasis of pancreatic secretions, alveolar rupture due to increased pressure takes place later. As a result of alveolar rupture, pancreatic enzymes leak outside resulting in pancreatitis.

Key Box 25.26

VISCID MUCUS

- Meconium ileus
- Cystic fibrosis of pancreas
- Respiratory tract infection
- Increased Na⁺ loss in the sweat

Clinical features

1. **At birth:** Meconium ileus or meconium peritonitis is an important manifestation of cystic fibrosis of pancreas.

2. **In infants**
   - Recurrent respiratory tract infection in the form of bronchiolitis and bronchiectasis results in cough with expectoration and dyspnoea.
   - Emaciation, steatorrhoea and stools are pale and sticky.

3. **Older children**
   - Steatorrhoea, gross emaciation and wasting are the features. Due to poor nutritional status, cirrhosis of the liver with portal hypertension can be a feature.

4. **In adults:**
   - Lucky survivors will suffer from gross wasting, diabetes, bronchiectasis, cirrhosis of the liver, sialadenitis and choroiditis.

Investigations

- Normal contents of the electrolytes in the sweat: Na - 70 mEq/litre, Chloride 60 mEq/litre, Potassium 20 mEq/litre.
- In these patients sodium excretion may be three to four times more than normal.

Treatment: Only symptomatic

I. **Nutritional support**
   - Fat intake should be low, protein should be increased.
   - Pancreatic enzyme preparations (5 to 10 gm) are given two to three times per day, to supplement pancreatic enzymes.

II. **Control infection**
   - Respiratory tract infection is treated with antibiotics, bronchodilators, mucolytic agents, etc.

III. **Role of surgery**
   - Indicated in meconium ileus to relieve intestinal obstruction.

PANCREATIC FISTULA

Causes

1. **External fistulae** result due to operative injury to the pancreas or due to a pancreatic anastomosis leak.
   - Injury to the tail of pancreas during splenectomy or adrenalectomy
   - Injury to the head and body during radical gastrectomy
   - Pancreaticojejunostomy for chronic pancreatitis or following Whipple's operation can also give rise to fistula in the post-operative period.
   - External drainage of an infected pseudocyst

2. **Internal fistulae:** It can occur following a blunt injury abdomen wherein the neck of the pancreas is crushed against lumbar spine resulting in injury. Internal fistulae can communicate with pleural space à pancreaticopleural fistula.

Clinical presentation

- In many cases, patients present with discharge of straw-coloured fluid from the drain site in the post-operative period.
- Internal fistula can manifest in a totally unexpected manner, some times as a case of pleural effusion.

Investigations

1. Amylase levels in the pleural fluid, peritoneal fluid and in the discharge will be high
2. Abdominal ultrasound is done to rule out a pseudocyst of the pancreas

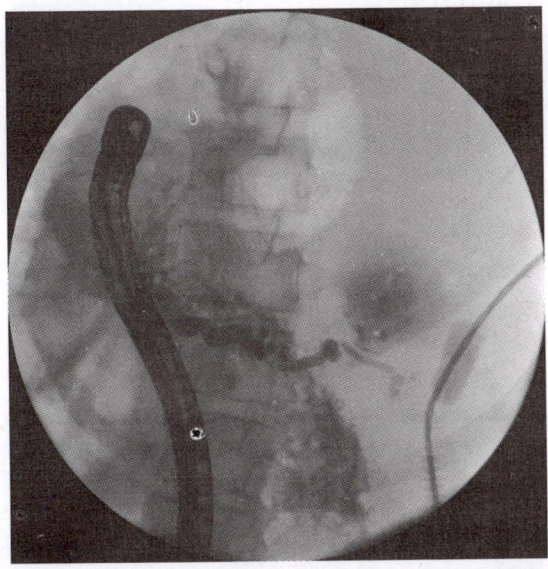

Fig. 25.76 Pancreatic fistula following acute pancreatitis

3. E.R.C.P.-It can demonstrate the leakage of the dye from the pancreatic duct into the surrounding area or along the fistulous tract and proximal obstruction if any.

Treatment

1. **Conservative treatment**
   - In majority of the cases following surgery, the fistulous discharge stops within one to three weeks of time. During this period, the skin is protected by application of zinc oxide cream. Electrolytes have to be checked frequently. Rarely, reexploration and ligation of the pancreatic duct may be necessary.

2. **Surgical treatment**
   - If the fistula persists in spite of conservative treatment fistulectomy with removal of involved part of the pancreas and body or tail has to be done.
   - In very difficult cases (plastured abdomen) fistulas on the anterior abdominal side, fistulo-gastrostomy can also be done.

Complications of pancreatic fistula

1. **Secondary infection**
2. **Massive bleeding:** It occurs due to digestion of elastin fibres of blood vessels resulting in pseudo-aneurysms. Morbidity is high.
3. **Ramification** which means branching pattern of the fistula which makes the surgery difficult.
4. **Bronchopancreatic fistula** - difficult to treat

CLINICAL NOTES

A patient was admitted to the hospital with acute breathlessness. He was found to have left sided pleural effusion (massive). He had blunt injury abdomen 2 months back during which time laparotomy and closure of a proximal jejunal perforation had been done. There was no obvious sign of pancreatic injury. Aspiration of pleural fluid revealed high amylase. It was a case of pancreaticopleural fistula.

MISCELLANEOUS CONDITIONS

WHITE BILE

- It is a misnomer.
- Long-standing cases of obstruction to the CBD; the bile in the CBD gets absorbed and is replaced by mucus secreted from the CBD.
- It is not white but straw coloured.
- It is not bile but is mucus

Significance

- It indicates a long standing obstruction.
- It has to be relieved as an urgent procedure.
- White bile is seen in :

1. Long standing stricture CBD, or
2. Due to the stones in CBD, and
3. Rarely, seen in periampullary carcinoma.

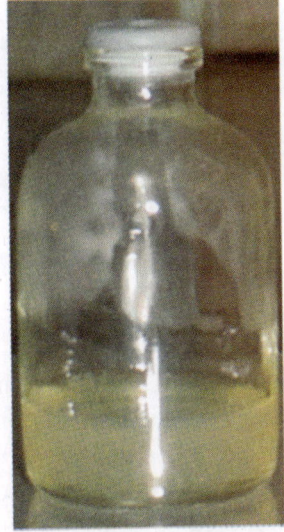

Fig. 25.77 White bile suggestive of severely impaired liver cell function

Spleen

26

- Surgical anatomy
- Functions of the spleen
- Congenital abnormalities
- Rupture
- Purpura
- Hereditary spherocytosis
- Thalassaemia
- Sickle cell anaemia
- Splenectomy
- Splenic artery aneurysm
- Hairy cell leukaemia
- OPSI

Diseases of the spleen and the causes of enlargement of the spleen is a great concern for physicians. Dozens of differential diagnosis of splenomegaly are being taught in medicine. However, a surgeon's role in the treatment of an enlarged spleen is minimal. But, he **does a 'magic' of removing** the spleen within minutes and saves the life of a patient for a ruptured spleen. A surgeon plays a major role by **treating hypersplenism with splenectomy**. In this chapter only topics related to surgeon's interest are dealt with. Other topics are mentioned briefly.

SURGICAL ANATOMY

The spleen is an anatomically small organ, hidden under the **9**th to **11**th rib, (dull note on percussion) measuring 1x 3 x 5 inches and weighing about 7 oz. It lies in intimate contact with the under surface of diaphragm. This explains why a splenic abscess can rupture through the diaphragm causing empyema. When blood collects due to splenic injury, it irritates the diaphragm causing referred pain to the shoulder tip. (**Kehr's sign**)

The **anterior border** is **notched** and is in contact with the stomach. It is enclosed by the **gastrocolic omentum**. The surgical importance of this is when traction is applied on the stomach during vagotomy, a splenic capsular tear can occur, resulting in bleeding. The **two leaves** of gastrocolic omentum pass backwards in front of the kidney forming the **lieno-renal ligament**. This ligament is responsible for some part of the posterior fixation of the spleen. When this ligament is divided the spleen can be brought to the surface of the wound during splenectomy.

The inferior part of the **hilum** of the spleen is (just) in contact with the **tail of the pancreas**. Often, during an emergency splenectomy, the tail of pancreas can get injured, resulting in a pancreatic fistula.

Blood supply

- **Arterial supply:** Splenic artery is a branch of coeliac artery. At the hilum of the spleen, it divides into four or five branches. Anatomical knowledge of these branches aids when performing partial splenectomy for ruptured spleen. [The blood flow rate through spleen is about 300 ml/min].
- **Venous drainage:** Four to five branches of the vein join and from the splenic vein. This forms the portal vein by joining with superior mesenteric vein behind the 2nd part of the duodenum.

Splenic parenchyma

- It is highly vascular

- Splenic pulp has red pulp and white pulp
- Red pulp is a honey combed vascular space which is made up of cords of reticular cells and sinuses.
- **White pulp consists of lymphatic tissue** and lymphoid follicles containing lymphocytes, plasma cells and macrophages.

Lymphatic drainage

- The lymph drains into hilar nodes → retropancreatic nodes → coeliac nodes. Because of its intimate contact with the fundus of the stomach and tail of the pancreas. spleen is removed along with the stomach (nowadays not done) and tail of the pancreas in cases of radical gastrectomy and distal pancreatectomy.

FUNCTIONS OF THE SPLEEN

- Destruction of aged, abnormal or damaged RBCS, platelets
- Immunological production of antibody
- Production of lymphocytes, monocytes and plasma cells
- Major site for synthesis of **tuftsin**, a peptide that stimulates phagocytic activity of leucocytes
- **Opsonins** are antibodies against bacteria and fungus produced by the spleen

Splenectomy and vaccination

- Splenectomy is avoided as far as possible in children below 5 years of age because incidence of **OPSI**

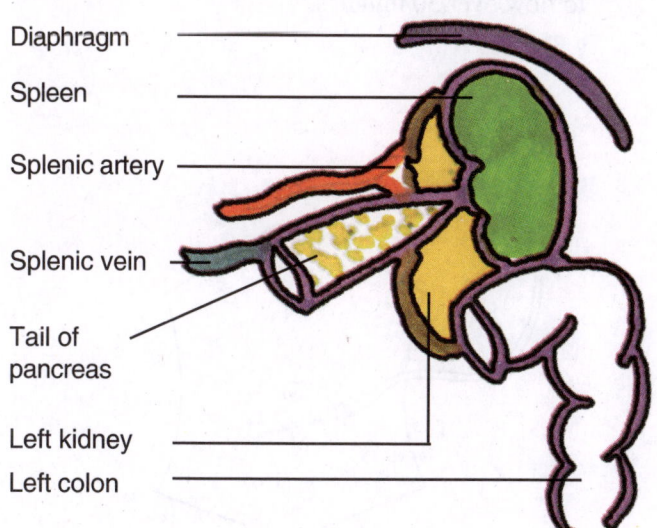

| Diaphragm |
| Spleen |
| Splenic artery |
| Splenic vein |
| Tail of pancreas |
| Left kidney |
| Left colon |

Fig. 26.1 Surgical anatomy of the spleen

(**O**pportunistic **P**ost **S**plenectomy **I**nfection) is higher in children following splenectomy.

- Anti pneumococcal vaccination and anti influenza are given 4-6 weeks prior to elective splenectomy.
- In emergency situations, vaccine should be given as soon as possible after splenectomy.

CONGENITAL ABNORMALITIES

1. **Accessory spleens: Splenunculi** : They are found in about 10-30% of population.
   - They can be found near the hilum of spleen, tail of pancreas, splenic ligaments or in the mesocolon.
   - In diseases of the spleen (Haemolytic, purpura) all these accessory spleens have to be removed along with spleen.
2. Splenic **agenesis** is rare.
3. **Polysplenia** is rare. It occurs due to failure of splenic fusion.
4. **Wandering spleen** is due to loose ligaments. It is more vulnerable for torsion.

RUPTURE OF THE SPLEEN

CAUSES

1. **Blunt injury abdomen**
   - Injury to the left side of chest, left lower rib fractures, due to fall from a tree, road traffic accidents can be associated with splenic rupture.
   - Retroperitoneal haemorrhage, fracture spine and renal injuries may be associated with splenic injury.
2. **Penetrating injuries** to the abdomen may cause **rupture of spleen**.
3. **Spontaneous** rupture of the spleen is seen in malaria and infectious mononucleosis, rarely in sarcoidosis, haemolytic anaemia, leukaemia.
4. **Iatrogenic**: Splenic capsule may be torn during surgical procedures like vagotomy, or gastrectomy due to traction on the stomach.

CLINICAL PRESENTATION

It can be divided into three groups
  I. **Tearing of splenic vessels**. Avulsion of splenic pedicle can result in severe haemorrhage and shock-

death can occur within a few minutes. Even in the best of the situations, death cannot be prevented often.

II. **A slow developing haemorrhagic** shock followed by recovery. Examination reveals evidence of intraperitoneal bleeding. This can occur due to a capsular tear or injury to the splenic parenchyma. Its clinical features are as follows:

- Anaemia-Pallor
- Pulse-Tachycardia, more than 100/min
- B.P. low/hypotension
- Cold, clammy extremities
- Abdominal distension
- Paralytic ileus develops slowly
- Guarding and rigidity
- **Kehr's sign** is positive. Irritation of under-surface of diaphragm by the blood causes irritation of phrenic nerve ($C_{3, 4}$). Thus, this pain is referred to shoulder region (supraclavicular nerve C_4).

Kehr's sign can be elicited by elevation of the foot end of bed for about 10 minutes.

- **Ballance's sign**: Blood in the vicinity of spleen is fresh blood which is coagulated and blood in the periphery is not coagulated. Hence, there will not be shifting dullness on the left side of the abdomen but can be present on the right side.
- **Saegesser's splenic point of tenderness**: An area of tenderness on the left side between sternomastoid and scalenus medius.

III. **Initial features of haemorrhagic shock, recovery and sudden haemorrhagic shock** after few hours to a few days. It is due to the following reasons.

- Greater omentum seals off a tear which gets re-opened after some time.
- A subcapsular haematoma which had developed, ruptures after some time.
- Associated injury to the tail of pancreas causes release of enzymes which digests the tissues at a later date. This variety is called as "delayed type of shock" or delayed rupture of spleen.

INVESTIGATIONS

1. **Hb%** estimation, PCV (packed cell volume) estimation (However in appropriate cases it should be re-

peated at frequent intervals to detect continuing haemorrhage).

2. **Four quadrant tap/aspiration** by using a fine needle (23 gauge) demonstrates blood either fresh or old. However, diagnostic peritoneal lavage (**DPL**) is more reliable (vide infra).

3. **Emergency USG** can reveal a splenic tear, a subcapsular haematoma and can rule out other injuries. It is the most important investigation in suspected cases of splenic injury. However, CT scan is more reliable but time consuming, hence it should be used only in cases of doubtful diagnosis and stable patients.

4. **Diagnostic peritoneal lavage (DPL)**
   - It is indicated in blunt injury abdomen where there are **equivocal signs** or **doubtful signs** of peritonitis.

Indications

- Unconscious patient with polytrauma with signs of abdominal injury.
- Unexplained shock.
- Associated spinal cord injury.

Procedure (Fig. 26.2)

- A 1 cm incision is made in the subumbilical region under local anaesthesia (L.A.) after emptying the bladder. Peritoneum is opened and a 12 or 14 Fr peritoneal dialysis catheter is introduced into the peritoneal cavity.
- Skin is closed and 1000 ml normal saline is allowed to flow over 30 minutes.

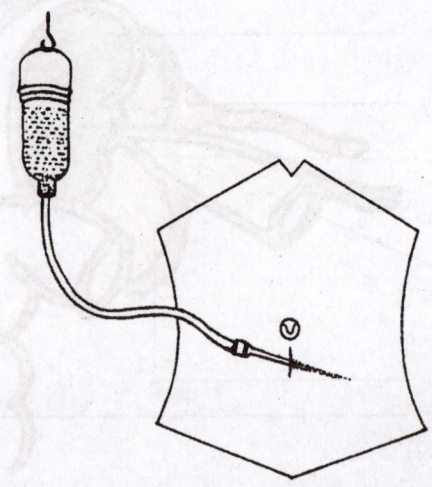

Fig. 26.2 Diagnostic peritoneal lavage

- Patient is turned to the right and left side and fluid is allowed to flow out.

- **DPL is positive when:**

1. Fresh blood of more than 20 ml is removed immediately after inserting dialysis catheter and it does not clot.

2. RBC count $1,00,000/mm^3$ or WBC $> 500/mm^3$.

3. Amylase level of over 175 units/dl.

4. Bile, food or any other fresh contents.

5. Gram stain is positive in the contents of lavage.

- Diagnostic accuracy is around 95% DPL is useful to rule out intestinal injury in addition to intra peritoneal bleeding.

5. **Plain X-ray abdomen**[1] erect (need not be done in an emergency situation).

  - Splenic outline may not be seen clearly
  - Fundic air bubble may be indented by the haematoma
  - Psoas shadow is obliterated (KUB X-ray)
  - Evidence of fracture of lower ribs
  - Evidence of fluid in the peritoneal cavity- **Ground glass appearance**

TREATMENT (Key Box 26.1)

Treatment can be discussed under 4 headings

Key Box 26.1
TREATMENT
• Emergency splenectomy
• Partial splenectomy
• Splenorrhaphy
• Nonoperative

1. In majority of cases the treatment of choice is **EMERGENCY SPLENECTOMY** because it is quick and easy to perform. The splenic artery is ligated first at upper border of pancreas followed by a splenic vein. In desperate situations the spleen is mobilised by incising the lieno-renal ligament, a large arterial clamp

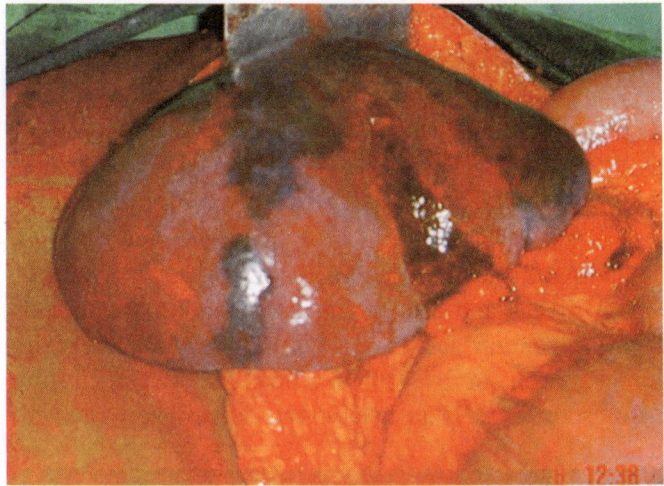

Fig. 26.3 Large laceration of the spleen

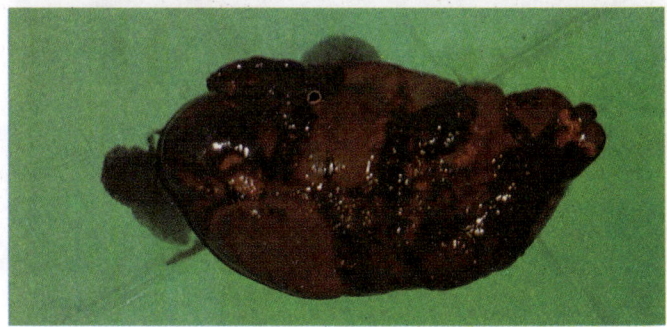

Fig 26.4 Splenectomy specimen

is applied at the splenic hilum and splenectomy is done (Fig. 26.3, 26.4).

2. **Splenorrhaphy (Fig. 26.5)**

  - It is a method of preservation of spleen when the general condition of the patient is reasonably good.

  - In this, a small tear is sutured by using chromic catgut and can be wrapped using greater omentum.

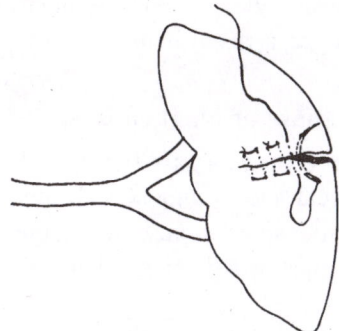

Fig 26.5 Splenorrhaphy

---

1. *Please do not make an unstable patient to stand for the sake of X-ray. He may collapse due to hypotension.*

3. **Partial splenectomy:**

- It can be done because the splenic artery gives an **upper polar branch and a lower polar branch** which divides into 2 branches. Hence, one of the branches of splenic artery is ligated, the bleeding stops and a partial splenectomy can be done comfortably.

- After splenectomy, the spleen can be cut into multiple pieces and can be implanted within the greater omentum and because of neovascularisation, the spleen survives and functions like a spleen in the production of antibodies. This can be done in children.

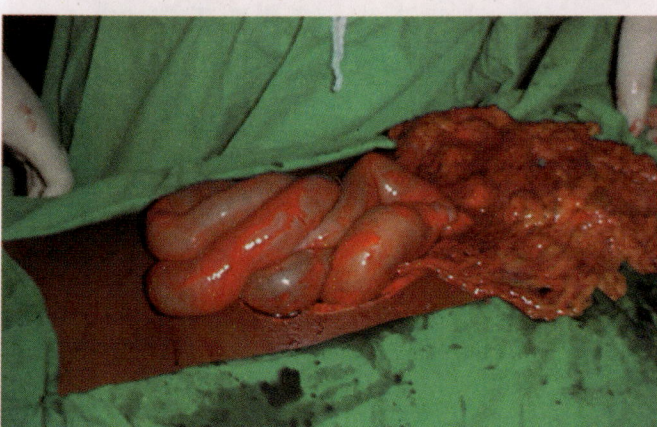

Fig 26.6 Haemoperitoneum

4. **Nonoperative or conservative treatment :**

- It is safe in selected adult and paediatric patients with isolated splenic injuries.

- Small risk of delayed rupture should be explained to the patient. (Key box 26.2)

COMPLICATIONS OF SPLENECTOMY

1. **Haematemesis** can occur due to congestion of stomach mucosa, as a result of ligation of short gastric vessels.

2. **Left basal (base of lung) collapse**

3. **Post-splenectomy sepsis (OPSI):** Incidence of meningococcal and pneumococcal infection is more in children after splenectomy. Hence, the pneumococcal vaccine must be administered in the postoperative period.

4. **Splenosis :** This refers to multiple small implants of splenic tissue on the peritoneal surface following traumatic rupture of spleen. They can give rise to adhesions.

Key Box 26.2

PATIENT SELECTION

1. Haemodynamically stable patients

2. No other associated organ injuries which require laparotomy

3. No extraabdominal injuries which may preclude assessment of abdomen

4. Facilities for emergency resuscitation, ultrasonography, CT scan should be available

5. Patient must be willing for hospitalisation and close observation

6. Regular monitoring by duty doctors, expert nursing staff who maintain hourly vital charts

---

HAEMATOLOGICAL INDICATIONS FOR SPLENECTOMY

IDIOPATHIC THROMBOCYTOPAENIC PURPURA (I.T.P.)

- This condition occurs due to development of autoantibodies against patient's own platelets (Key Box 26.3)

Key Box 26.3

OTHER CAUSES OF PURPURA

- ↓ Production: Cytotoxic drugs, aplastic anaemia
- ↑ Consumption of platelets : DIC as in septicaemia
- ↑ Destruction: S.L.E., infectious mononucleosis.
- ↑ Capillary fragility: Steriod induced or Henoch-Schonlein pupura

---

- The normal levels of platelets are between 1,50,000-4,00,000 cells per mm^3.

- Spleen is probably responsible for sequestration of platelets and for production of antibodies.

CLINICAL FEATURES

- Condition is common in females. F : M = 3 : 1.

- Purpuric patches (ecchymosis refers to skin discolouration due to extravasation of blood) are found on buttocks and petechial (a spot) haemorrhages commonly occur in the limbs. These are dependent areas having high intravascular pressure.

- All types of haemorrhages are common and can be mild or moderate (See the Key Box 26.4)

Key Box 26.4
COMMON TYPES OF HAEMORRHAGES
• Epistaxis • Menorrhagia • Haemetemesis • Bleeding gums • Haemarthrosis • Haematuria

- Intracranial haemorrhage is found in 1-2% of patients but it may be the cause of death.
- In 25% of cases, the spleen is just palpable (small size).
- **Hess's tourniquet test** : More than 20 petechiae in a circle of 3 cm diameter in cubital fossa suggests purpura.

INVESTIGATIONS

- Bleeding time is prolonged in purpura-clotting and pro-thrombin times are normal.
- Platelet count is reduced
- Bone marrow biopsy: Precursor of platelets (mega karyocytes) are increased

TREATMENT

In children

- Spontaneous regression occurs in majority of cases.
- Short course of corticosteroids are beneficial. Tablet prednisolone in the dose of 10 mg/ day over a period of 6 weeks is given.

In adults

- **Splenectomy** is indicated when **ITP has presented for more than 6-9 months.** When ITP has **relapsed** in spite of steroids, the patient is given a trial of prednisolone, 1 mg/kg/day. **Platelet count rises within 7 days of starting steroids.**

RESULTS

- 70-80% of patients respond permanently and do not require any further treatment. Counts rise above 1,00,000/mm^3 in 7 days. Even if counts are not raised, recurrent bleeding rarely takes place.

SURGERY FOR ITP

- Can be done even when platelets are as low as 10,000 cells/mm3.
- **Diathermy** is used to open layers of the abdomen.
- **Splenectomy is not difficult**. **Accessory spleens** (15-30%) if present should be **removed**.
- Platelet transfusion may be required post-operatively, if there is bleeding.

HAEMOLYTIC ANAEMIA

- This type of anaemia results from an increased red cell destruction which occurs in the spleen. The life span of red blood cells is also shortened. Hence, irrespective of the cause of haemolytic anaemia, these cases can benefit from splenectomy. **Anaemia, jaundice and splenomegaly** are the triad of haemolytic anaemia.

Types of haemolytic anaemia

1. Hereditary spherocytosis
2. Acquired autoimmune haemolytic anaemia
3. Thalassaemia

HEREDITARY SPHEROCYTOSIS

- This hereditary disorder is transmitted by either parent as Mendelian autosomal dominant. The disease is characterised by a **defect in cell wall protein of the red cell, namely spectrin,** which increases reflux of sodium into the cell. This causes the biconcave red cell to swell and become spherical. Hence, the name spherocytosis.

CONSEQUENCES OF SPHEROCYTES IN CIRCULATION

1. The spherocyte is already weak. Adding on to this, there is greater loss of membrane phospholipid which results in a delicate fragile spherocyte.
2. Because of the altered shape, **oxygen and energy requirements of RBCs increase which cannot be met by the spleen**. In the spleen, they are destroyed and release excessive haemoglobin which is converted into bilirubin.

- The amount of bilirubin produced is increased and most of it is unconjugated. It gets attached to albumin as it is **lipid soluble** and therefore cannot be excreted in the urine. Hence, this type of jaundice is also known as acholuric jaundice.

Most of this bilirubin is excreted in the biliary tree resulting in pigment stones in the biliary tree.

CLINICAL FEATURES

- Seen equally in both sexes
- History of recurrent attacks of jaundice can be elicited from childhood
- Jaundice is mild, never deep, not associated with itching or bradycardia
- **Pallor** is an important feature due to destruction of the red cells
- **Acute haemolytic crisis**: It is precipitated by an acute infection or stress. Abdominal pain, nausea, vomiting, pyrexia, pallor are the features. The condition can be confused for an abdominal emergency. In severe cases, anaemia, thrombocytopenia, leukopenia can occur.
- Spleen is **moderately enlarged**. The liver is also palpable in a few cases
- In adults, **gall stone colic** and obstructive jaundice due to **CBD** stone can also complicate the disease process. Incidence of gall stone disease is around 50%. **It is common after the age of 10 years**.
- Leg ulcers may occur as a result of anaemia

INVESTIGATIONS

1. Peripheral smear-Spherocytes are present
2. Reticulocyte count is increased (15-25%). These are immature red cells which are discharged by the bone marrow due to the loss of red cells.
3. Coombs' test is negative
   - Serum bilirubin is mildly elevated and most of it is unconjugated
4. **Fragility test**
   - Normal red cell haemolysis occur in **0.47%** saline solution. Here, it occurs at **0.6%** or even in weaker solution.
5. Ultrasound is done to rule out gall stones

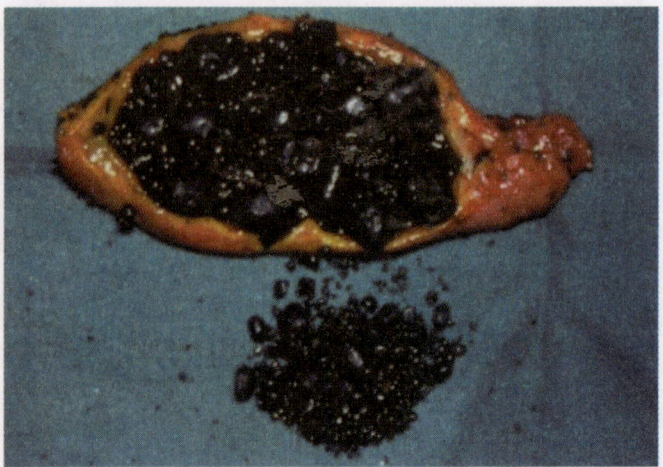

Fig 26.7 Pigment stones

TREATMENT

- **Splenectomy is the treatment** including removal of accessory spleen. Ideally, it should be done between the age of 6 to 10 years. It helps in following ways:
  1. By decreasing erythrocyte destruction, anaemia improves, thus avoiding blood transfusions.
  2. Erythrocytes acheive normal life span. Hence, jaundice also disappears.
  3. Leg ulcers heal quickly.

Hereditary elliptocytosis is also a genetic disorder wherein RBCs are oval in shape. It also responds to splenectomy.

ACQUIRED AUTOIMMUNE HAEMOLYTIC ANAEMIA

Due to an autoimmune reaction, the red cell surface is damaged and it gets destroyed in the splenic red pulp. Antibodies develop against red cell antigens. In 50% of cases, the cause is not known. The following are the probable causes.

- SLE, lymphoma, chronic lymphocytic leukaemia
- Drugs: Methyldopa, mefenamic acid

CLINICAL FEATURES

- More common in females after 50 years of age
- Splenomegaly, moderate in size
- Gall stones are found in around 25% of cases

INVESTIGATIONS

- Anaemia is present
- Spherocytes may be present because of the red cell surface damage
- Coombs' test is positive

TREATMENT

- It is a self-limiting disorder. Reassurance plays an important role.
- **Corticosteroids**, short course prednisolone 60 mg/day is given.
- Splenectomy is done when steroid response is not satisfactory.

THALASSAEMIA

- It is also called as Cooley's anaemia, Mediterranean anaemia, Heinz body haemolytic anaemia.

AETIOPATHOGENESIS

- It is a hereditary disorder transmitted as a **dominant trait.** It is characterized by a defect in haemoglobin peptide chain synthesis. Depending on type of peptide chain involvement, it is classified into α, β and γ. However, b-thalassaemia is more common. There is a decrease in haemoglobin and red cells will be destroyed prematurely due to intracellular precipitates (**Heinz bodies**).
- When it is a heterozygous disorder, it is called as beta-thalassaemia minor and homozygous disorder is called as beta-thalassaemia major (Cooley's anaemia). **The abnormal gene is inherited from both the parents.**

CLINICAL FEATURES

- Severe anaemia resulting in weakness, lethargy, leg ulcers etc.
- Splenomegaly mild to moderate in size. Sometimes, it is massive resulting in abdominal discomfort or may cause abdominal distension.
- Jaundice due to haemolysis. Liver can also be enlarged.
- To compensate for anaemia, bone marrow hyperplasia occurs resulting in bossing of skull and prominent malar bones. Thalassaemia major usually manifests in the first year of life.

COMPLICATIONS

1. **Haemosiderosis** (deposition of iron in tissues) of pancreas results in chronic pancreatitis and diabetes.
2. **Hepatic cirrhosis** due to liver haemosiderosis
3. **Aplastic crisis** with severe life threatening infections
4. **Gall stones** occur in about 20% of cases

INVESTIGATIONS

- Peripheral smear demonstrates microcytic hypochromic anaemia.
- Haemoglobin electrophoresis reveals reduction or absent levels of haemoglobin A (Hb-A). There is a compensatory increase in foetal haemoglobin (Hb-F).

TREATMENT

- Blood transfusion-multiple repeated transfusions may be necessary.
- Surgical-Splenectomy is indicated in a very few cases who require multiple transfusions and patients with gross splenomegaly.

SICKLE CELL ANAEMIA OR SICKLE CELL DISEASE

- This is a hereditary haemolytic disorder in which haemoglobin A is replaced by haemoglobin S (HbS). This results in crescent shaped erythrocytes. This HbS molecule crystallises if there is hypoxia, strenuous work or due to dehydration. As a result of this, red cells are distorted and elongated. Therefore, blood viscosity is increased, causing obstruction in the splenic circulation.(Key Box 26.5)

Key Box 26.5

FUNCTIONAL ABNORMALITIES IN SICKLE CELL ANAEMIA

- Spleen sometimes acts as a large reservoir for red cells and the sickle cells are destroyed
- Antibody production is decreased
- Spleen's ability to filter Streptococcus pneumoniae is reduced

EFFECT OF HbS BLOCKAGE

- Splenic microinfarcts
- Splenomegaly or **autosplenectomy** due to repeated infarcts (Fig. 26.8).

CLINICAL FEATURES

- The disease is very common in Africans. Most of the patients in India have high Hb-F levels which protect Hb-S. Hence, symptoms are not seen in the first few weeks.
- Abdominal pain is due to recurrent infarcts or due to gall stones in a few patients.
- Skin ulcers occur due to anaemia or hypoxia.

Microinfarction of carpal and tarsal bones resulting in bony pains which is described as Hand-Foot syndrome

INVESTIGATIONS

- Peripheral smear demonstrates sickle cell
- Haemoglobin electrophoresis to identify the type of haemoglobin

TREATMENT

- Folic acid supplements
- Splenectomy has a doubtful value. It is indicated only when excessive numbers of RBCs are sequestrated causing anaemia

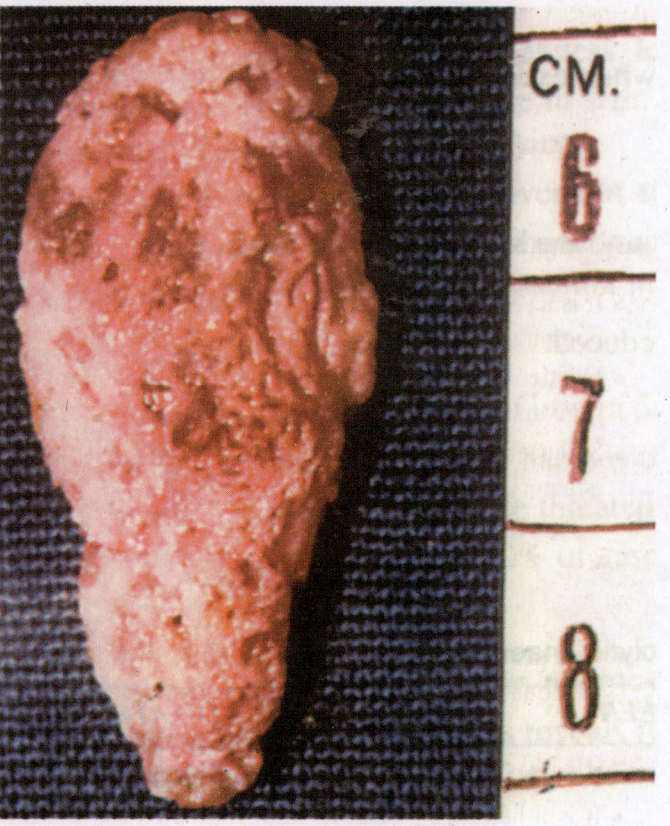

Fig 26.8 Sickle cell anaemia - nugget spleen (3 cms size). An example for autosplenectomy

COMPLICATIONS

- Infarct of cerebrum resulting in hemiplegia
- Mesenteric infarction resulting in gangrene of the bowel
- Pulmonary infarction resulting in chest pain

    Refer Table 26.1 for comparison

	AETIOLOGY	SHAPE OF RBC	SPLEEN	INVESTIGATION	TREATMENT
1. Hereditary sphrerocytosis	Increase in red cell permeability to sodium	Spherocyte	Large	Reticulocyte count	Splenectomy very beneficial
2. Autoimmune haemolytic anaemia	SLE, Drugs	Spherocyte	Medium size	Coomb's test is positive	Steroids: splenectomy in steroid failure cases
3. Thalassaemia (Cooley's anaemia)	Reduction of β-chain of haemoglobin	Small thin and no shape	Moderate size	Resistance to osmotic lysis Electrophoresis Hb-A	Splenectomy for bulky spleen and for frequent transfusion cases
4. Sickel cell	Hb-A is replaced by Hb-S	Sickle shape	Mild and later Not palpable	Electrophoresis Hb-S	If hypersplenism splenectomy

Table 26.1 Summary of haemolytic anaemias

SPLENECTOMY FOR OTHER CONDITIONS

1. **Hypersplenism**: It is defined as pancytopenia in the presence of normal or hypercellular bone marrow. Following are the causes of hypersplenism:

   - Portal hypertension

   - **Tropical splenomegaly** due to malaria, kala-azar or schistosomiasis, etc. Since these diseases are endemic in tropical countries, it is called as tropical splenomegaly. Gross enlargement of the spleen and hypersplenism are indications for splenectomy in such cases.

   - Myeloproliferative disorders

   - Tuberculosis

   - Primary hypersplenism wherein the cause is not found

2. **Cysts of the spleen** (Fig. 26.9)

   - Parasitic cyst is rare. Typically, it is caused by echinococcal disease (hydatid disease).

   - Traumatic cysts are due to a haematoma giving rise to liquefaction. These are false cysts of the spleen.

   - Congenital cysts can be due to a dermoid cyst, haemangioma or lymphangioma.

3. **Tumours of the spleen**

   - **Lymphoma** is the commonest cause of enlargement of spleen. Spleen used to be removed as a part of a staging laparotomy. Now, it is very rare.

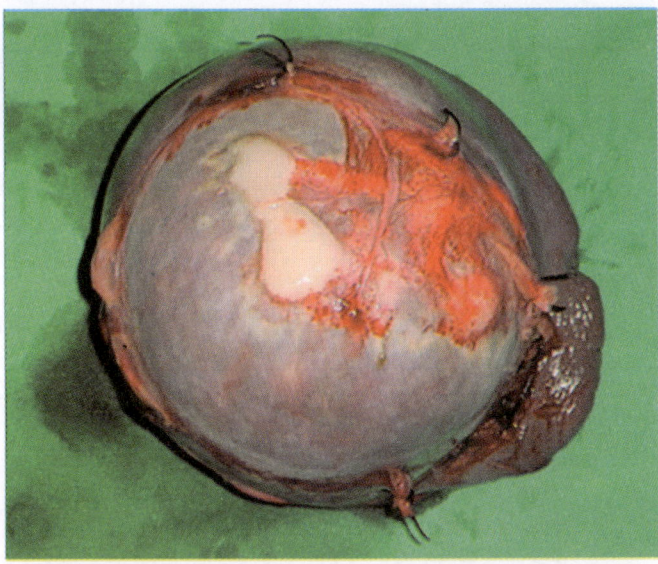

Fig 26.9 Simple cyst of the spleen resulting in compression of the spleen - appearance like that of a *globe*

   - **Fibrosarcoma or angiosarcoma** are rare malignant tumours.

4. **Miscellaneous indications**

   - **Splenic abscess** can occur due to infected septic emboli from otitis, typhoid fever or due to thrombosis of splenic vein causing infarction followed later by infection.(Key Box 26.6)

   - Tubercular abscess of the spleen is rare. It is usually affected secondary to abdominal or pulmonary tuberculosis (Fig. 26.10, 26.11 and 26.12).

   - **Felty's syndrome** refers to splenomegaly, neutropaenia with rheumatoid arthritis. After

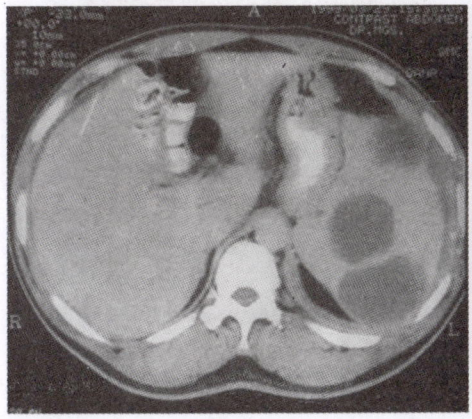

Fig 26.10 CT scan showing multiple spleenic abscesses

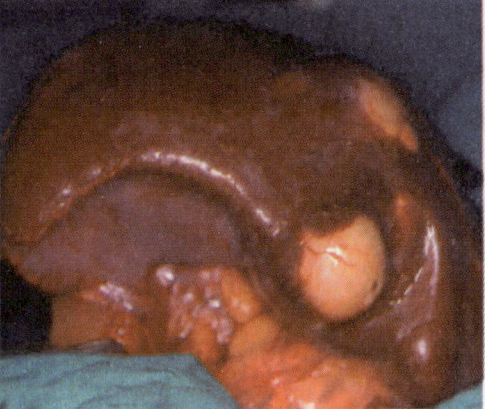

Fig 26.11 Same patient as in Fig. 26.10 with multiple abscesses in the spleen

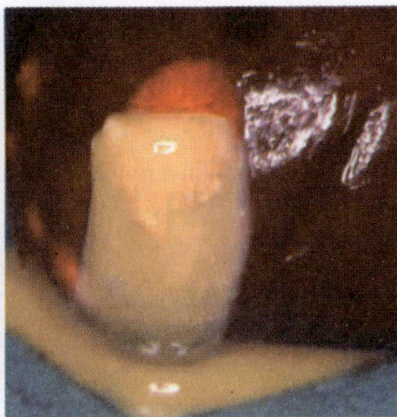

Fig 26.12 Incision of the abscess after splenectomy

Key Box 26.6

CAUSES OF SPLENIC ABSCESS

- Typhoid, paratyphoid fever
- Osteomyelitis
- Otitis media
- Puerperal sepsis
- May be associated with pancreatic necrosis

splenectomy, leg ulcers will heal quickly and neutropaenia also improves. Steroids may act better now and incidence of recurrent infection become less.

- Patients with **large spleen** of chronic myeloid leukaemia, Gaucher's disease and hairy cell leukaemia also will benefit after splenectomy.

- **Splenic artery aneurysm :** It is an uncommon condition. More common in women.

SPLENIC ARTERY ANEURYSM

Causes

- **Atherosclerosis :** Commonly seen in elderly patients
- **Congenital :** Young patients : These patients may present first time during pregnancy with enlargement or rupture.
- **Acute pancreatitis :** Inflammatory process may give rise to pseudoaneurysm formation.

Clinical features

- Pain and vomiting
- Thrill or Bruit
- Calcification in a routine X-ray

Investigations

- Ultrasound / CT scan
- Angiography

Treatment

- **Nonoperative:** Embolisation of splenic artery

- **Operative:** Ligation of splenic artery at the upper border of pancreas after opening lesser sac followed by splenectomy.

HAIRY CELL LEUKAEMIA (HCL)

- The cells on a blood smear have an irregular outline due to the presence of filament like cytoplasmic projection hence the name hairy cells.
- HCL is a clonal proliferation of abnormal B cells. (very rarely T cells).

Clinical features

- Anaemia
- Recurrent infection
- Massive enlargement of spleen

Investigations

- Blood counts are low. White cell count may be raised with circulating hairy cells.
- Bone marrow has increased cellularity with characteristic infiltration by **hairy cells**

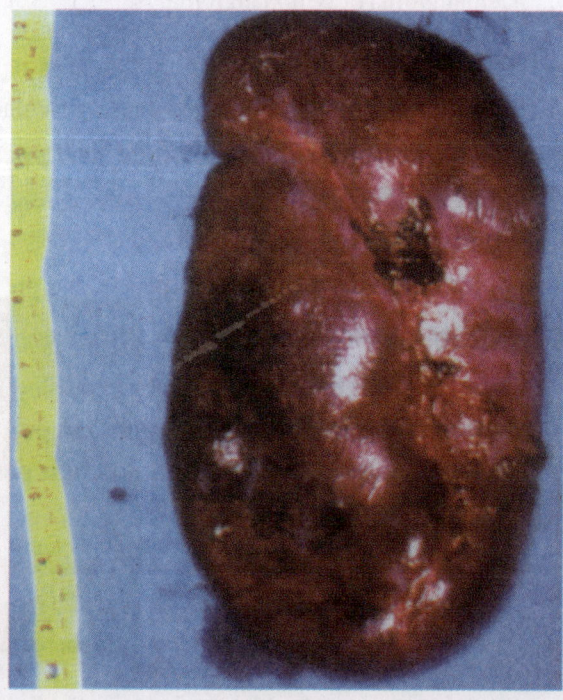

Fig 26.13 Splenectomy was done for large spleen causing discomfort - reported as Hairy cell leukaemia

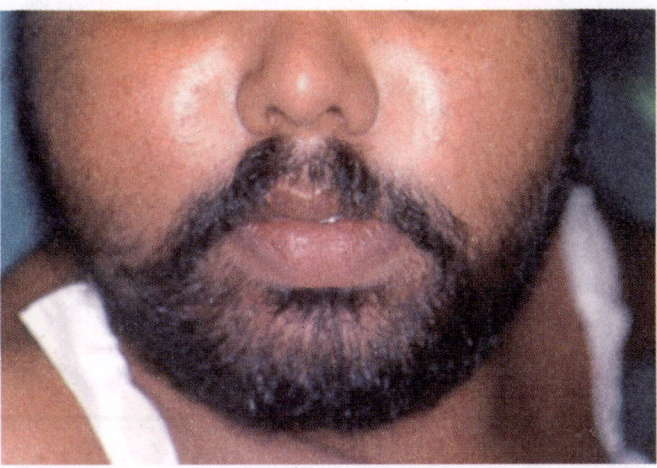

Fig 26.14 Same patient (as in Fig. 26.13) had received steroids for one year without a proper diagnosis - Observe Cushingoid face

Treatment

- Drug : 2 - chloradenosine acetate (2-CDA) has been beneficial. It can induce remission.
- Splenectomy is indicated in cases of diagnostic difficulties and very large spleens.

OPSI (OPPORTUNISTIC POST SPLENECTOMY INFECTION)

- Following splenectomy, specially children are vulnerable for opportunist infection such as pneumococcus, H. influenza and Meningococcus.

Recommendations for

I. Elective splenectomy

- All children aged over 2 years, should receive pneumococcal vaccination.
- Haemophilus influenza type b vaccination for all irrespective of age.
- Meningococcal protection for only those who travel to high risk areas.

II. After Emergency splenectomy

- Vaccines should be given as early as possible, however protection is **not always** guaranteed.
- Daily dose of oral prophylaxis with penicillin, erythromycin or amoxycillin to all children till 10 years who undergo splenectomy before the age of 5.

Classification of the indications of splenectomy

1. Rupture of the spleen
2. Haematological indications
3. Hypersplenism
4. Cysts of the spleen
5. Tumours of the spleen
6. Miscellaneous conditions

Benefits of splenectomy (Table 26.2)

Table 26.2

SPLENECTOMY BENEFITS		
MAXIMUM	**MODERATE**	**MILD**
1. Rupture of the spleen	1. Tropical splenomegaly	1. Chronic myeloid leukaemia
2. Hereditary spherocytosis	2. Autoimmune haemolytic anaemia	2. Thalassaemia
3. Idiopathic thrombocytopaenic purpura (ITP)	3. Felty's syndrome	3. Sickle cell disease
4. Cysts of the spleen		4. Gaucher's disease
5. Tumours of the spleen		5. Hodgkin's lymphoma
6. Hypersplenism		6. Hairy cell leukaemia
7. Left sided portal hypertension		

Peritoneum and Peritoneal Cavity

27

- Peritoneal cavity
- Acute peritonitis
- Pelvic Abscess
- Subphrenic abscess
- Laparostomy
- Post-operative peritonitis
- Biliary peritonitis
- Pneumococcal peritonitis
- Pseudomyxoma peritonei
- Abdominal compartment syndrome

THE PERITONEAL CAVITY

- It is the largest cavity in the body accommodating various viscera. The peritoneum lining the inner side of parietes is called as parietal peritoneum which is very sensitive, innervated by both somatic and visceral afferent nerves. This explains the sharp localised cutting pain of peritonitis. Diaphragm and central part of the peritoneum is supplied by phrenic nerve (C4) and partly by intercostal nerve. Rest of the peritoneum is supplied by intercostal nerves and lumbar nerves.

Visceral peritoneum

- It covers viscera and is supplied by autonomic nervous system. Hence, it is not sensitive. Thus, gastrojejunostomy can be done without anaesthesia but distension and traction to the bowel causes pain. During herniorrhaphy under spinal anaesthesia, handling of bowel or traction on the bowel produces uncomfortable upper abdominal pain.

Peritoneal cavity

- It is divided into greater and lesser sac (omental bursa) which communicate by the foramen of Winslow or epiploic foramen.

Fluid

- It normally contains 100 ml fluid. When it is insulted by infection, large amount of fluid can collect in this space giving rise to severe fluid and electrolyte imbalance. This is described as III space loss, e.g. peritonitis, pancreatitis.

Peritoneum

- Peritoneum is lined by flattened single layer of cells and thin layer of fibroelastic tissue. A large peritoneal defect heals within a few hours because of these mesenchymal cells. Applying this principle, some surgeons do not close the peritoneal layer after laparotomy.

Absorption and exudation

- This takes place through capillaries and lymphatics present in between two layers of peritoneum.

ACUTE PERITONITIS

DEFINITION

- Inflammation of the peritoneum is called peritonitis.

CAUSES

- They can be classified into primary or secondary.

I. Primary peritonitis

1. Spontaneous peritonitis of childhood
2. Spontaneous peritonitis of adults
3. Tuberculous peritonitis
4. Peritonitis associated with dialysis

II. Secondary peritonitis

- This term refers to peritonitis due to intraabdominal source and it is the most common form of peritonitis. Following are causes for secondary peritonitis.

1. **Perforation of the hollow viscus** (Fig. 27.1)
   - Perforated duodenal ulcer, gastric ulcer
   - Perforated enteric ulcer, tubercular ulcer
   - Perforated Meckel's diverticulum
   - Perforated colonic ulcer

2. **Direct spread-post-inflammatory**
   - Acute cholecystitis
   - Acute appendicitis
   - Gangrene of the intestine

3. **Penetrating injuries to the abdomen, where the organisms are carried from outside.**

4. **Postoperative peritonitis** is due to the introduction of infection during surgery which might be due to
   - Improper sterilization technique
   - Improper fumigation
   - Unsterile technique of surgery
   - Foreign body (mop) in the abdomen (Fig. 27.2)

5. **Parturition peritonitis:** It refers to peritonitis after pregnancy and delivery.

PATHOGENESIS

Due to anyone of the reasons mentioned above, infection sets in and causative organisms multiply in the peritoneal cavity.

- **Gram-negative organisms:** Escherichia coli (E. coli), Proteus, Klebsiella. They are present in the small and large bowel.

- **Enterococci :** Streptococci faecalis needs bile to grow. It is present in the urinary tract, genital tract and also in the intestines. However, both aerobic and anaerobic streptococci are the common organisms second only to gram negative organisms They are the chief organisms in puerperal sepsis.

- **Bacteroids :** They are anaerobic organisms, present mainly in the lower intestine.

- **Bacteria from outside alimentary canal:** Gonococci. pneumococci, tubercular organisms, etc.

- These organisms proliferate in the peritoneal cavity resulting in peritonitis. As a result of this, there is secretion of a large amount of fluid in the peritoneal cavity resulting in 3rd space loss which leads to severe **hypovolaemic shock.** This fluid is rich in proteins, bacteria and toxins. Due to powerful endotoxins released by gram negative bacteria, endotoxic shock or septic shock (refer shock), ensues.

- The fluid is rich in fibrinogen which forms fibrin and helps in localisation of infection.

- Peritoneum loses its shiny surface, becomes reddish and oedematous covered with thick fibrinous exudate.

CLINICAL FEATURES

It depends upon whether it is localised peritonitis or generalised. In cases of retrocaecal appendicitis, the abdominal signs may be minimal but guarding and rigidity of the back muscles is characteristic. Features of generalised peritonitis are as follows:

- **Severe abdominal pain** which is cutting in nature, becomes worse on movement of the abdominal wall. Hence, the patient lies still on the bed.

- **Persistent vomiting** is due to irritation of parietal peritoneum.

- **The pulse rate is increased.** An increase in the pulse rate may be an early indication of peritonitis, in cases of gangrene of the bowel or peritonitis following blunt injury abdomen.

- **High grade fever with chills and rigors** indicates a septicaemic process.

- **Cough tenderness** indicates parietal peritoneal inflammation. Abdominal tenderness is elicited in all quadrants of the abdomen.

- **Rebound tenderness** (Blumberg's sign): Abdomen is pressed, for a few seconds. The patient experiences pain. Sudden release of pressure causes severe pain. It is due to sudden movement of the sensitive parietal peritoneum (Fig. 27.3).

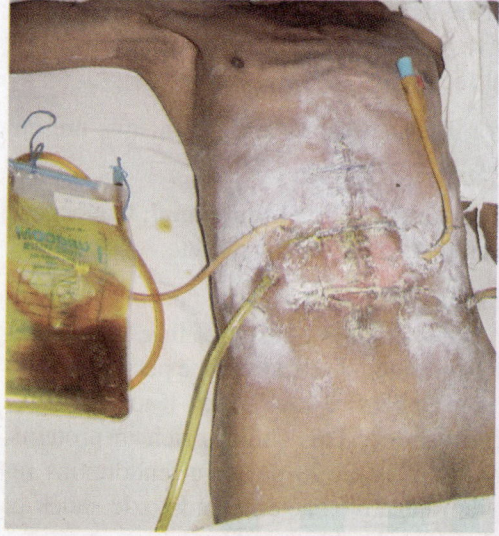
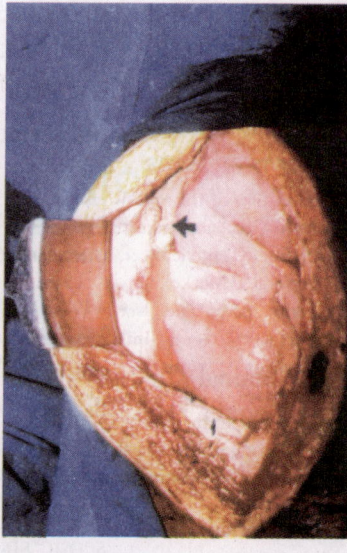
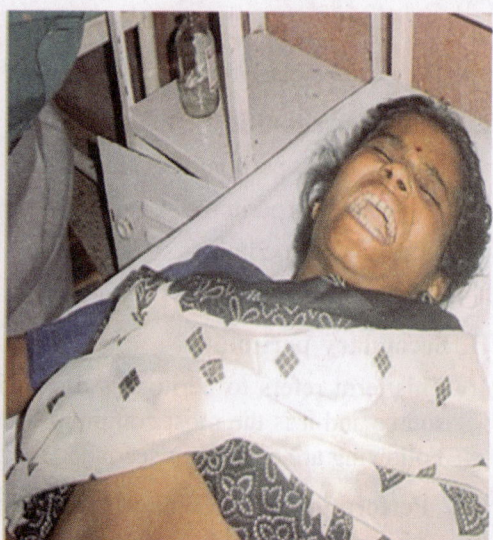

Fig. 27.1 Peritonitis due to perforation of duodenal ucler - post operative billiary fistula

Fig. 27.2 Mop in the peritoneal cavity. This patient had postoperative peritonitis

Fig. 27.3 Rebound tenderness is the diagnostic sign of peritonitis

- **Guarding and rigidity** of abdominal wall
- Bowel sounds are absent. Distension of the abdomen occurs within few hours due to accumulation of fluid and due to paralytic ileus (Also refer Key Box 27.2).
- **End stage disease :** Hippocratic facies

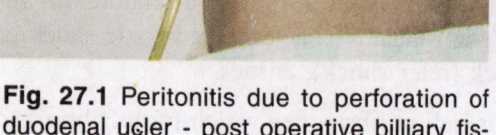

Key Box 27.1
FACTORS AFFECTING DIFFUSE PERITONITIS

- Speed of peritoneal contamination. Eg: perforation of Meckel's diverticulum
- Stimulation by purgatives
- Virulence of organisms
- Perforation in a closed loop obstruction
- Immuno compromised status
- Young children - omentum is thin and small

Key Box 27.2
HIPPOCRATIC FACIES

- Hollow, bright eyes
- Pale and pinched face
- Cold perspiration in the head and brows
- Blue lips
- Dry, cracked tongue

INVESTIGATIONS

1. Complete blood picture shows **high total count** with predominant neutrophil count.

2. Urine and blood examination for **sugar** is done to rule out diabetes mellitus.

3. Plain X-ray abdomen erect (Fig. 27.4)
   - **Gas under the diaphragm** - Perforation
   - **Ground glass appearance-** a smooth homogenous appearance due to accumulation of fluid.
   - Obliteration of psoas shadow and pre peritoneal fat planes.

4. Abdominal USG to detect **fluid in abdomen**

5. **Four quadrant abdominal tap** (Fig. 27.5)
   - Aspiration of blood indicates haemoperitoneum or gangrene of the bowel.
   - Aspiration of bile indicates biliary peritonitis due to perforated duodenal ulcer, gall bladder perforation or intestinal perforation.
   - **Aspiration of frank pus** indicates peritonitis due to gram negative bacteria. Foul smelling pus is due to anaerobic bacteria producing free fatty acids and their esters.
   - Amylase estimation should be done to rule out pancreatitis.

6. Diagnostic laparoscopy can be used in suspected cases of peritonitis. (Key Box 27.3)

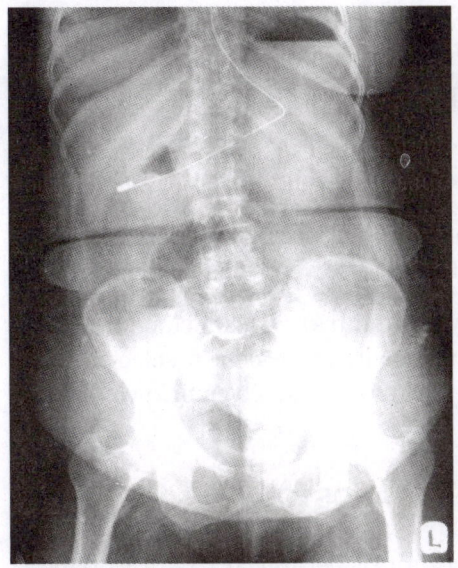

Fig. 27.4 Plain X-ray abdomen showing ground glass appearance

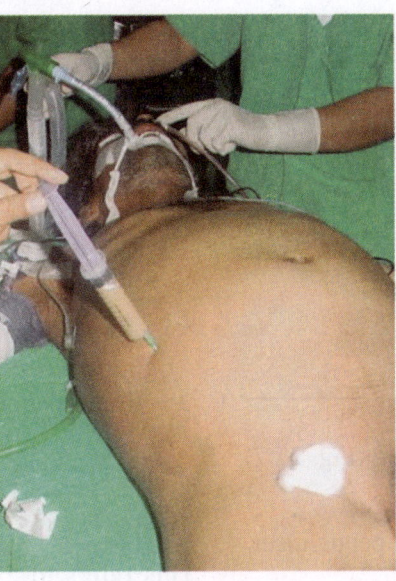

Fig. 27.5 Diagnostic tap showing pus

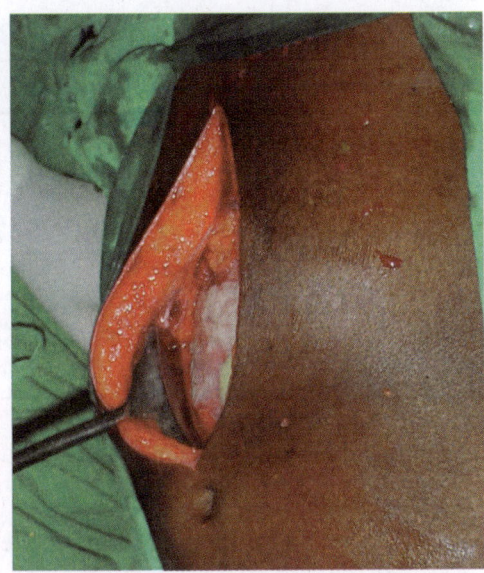

Fig. 27.6 Peritonitis due to perforated carcinoma of the stomach

Key Box 27.3
DIAGNOSTIC LAPAROSCOPY
<ul><li>It can be used to reconfirm peritonitis</li><li>It can diagnose pancreatitis (laparotomy may be avoided).</li><li>It can also treat primary cause. Eg: Laparoscopic closure of duodenal ulcer perforation</li><li>Also peritoneal toilet can be given</li></ul>

Key Box 27.4
SELECTION OF ANTIBIOTICS
<ul><li>2nd or 3rd generation cephalosporins should be started as early as possible</li><li>Once culture reports are available (after surgery), antibiotics can be changed</li><li>Antibiotics should also cover aerobes and anaerobes</li><li>Should not have serious toxicity</li></ul>

MANAGEMENT

1. **Aspiration:** Nasogastric aspiration with Ryle's tube helps in decreasing gastrointestinal secretion. Thus it reduces abdominal distension. It also prevents vomiting and gives rest to the gut.

2. **Bowel care and blood:** Purgatives should not be given as it may result in perforation. Blood is arranged for surgery.

3. **Charts:** Temperature, pulse rate, respiratory rate, intake-output charts are maintained.

4. **Drugs** are given against gram-positive, gram-negative and anaerobic organisms.(Key box 27.4)

5. **Exploratory laparotomy** and appropriate surgery is done followed by thorough peritoneal toilet/wash with normal saline (Key Box 27.5)

6. **Fluids**-Intravenous fluids are given before, during and after surgery.
   - In all such cases, an **emergency cut down** (venesection) - cephalic or basilic vein is done followed by fluid infusion. Pre-operatively the aim is to maintain at least 30 ml/hour of urine. Venesection also has the advantage of measuring **CVP**.

PRINCIPLES OF SURGERY FOR PERITONITIS

1. Generous **midline** or **paramedian** incision is used.

2. As soon as the peritoneal cavity is opened purulent fluid comes out. The fluid is collected and sent for **culture and sensitivity**. Greenish fluid indicates a hollow viscus perforation. All the fluid is drained, the source of peritonitis is identified and appropriate

Key Box 27.5

PRINCIPLES OF SURGERY

- Appropriate antibiotics
- Generous incision
- Good Surgery
- Peritoneal wash
- Drain
- Tension sutures

surgical procedure is done. Examples are (Fig. 27.7)

- Appendicectomy for appendicitis.
- Closure of perforation for perforated peptic ulcer.
- Closure or resection for ileal perforation.
- Resection of the bowel for gangrene.

3. It is better to use **nonabsorbable suture** material like silk to do an intestinal anastomosis or for closure of perforation. In the presence of infection, absorbable sutures like catgut gets digested very fast.

4. A thorough **peritoneal wash/toilet** is given by using warm saline (upto 10 litres) to avoid intraperitoneal abscesses. Antiseptic agent like betadine solution is also used as a cleaning agent.

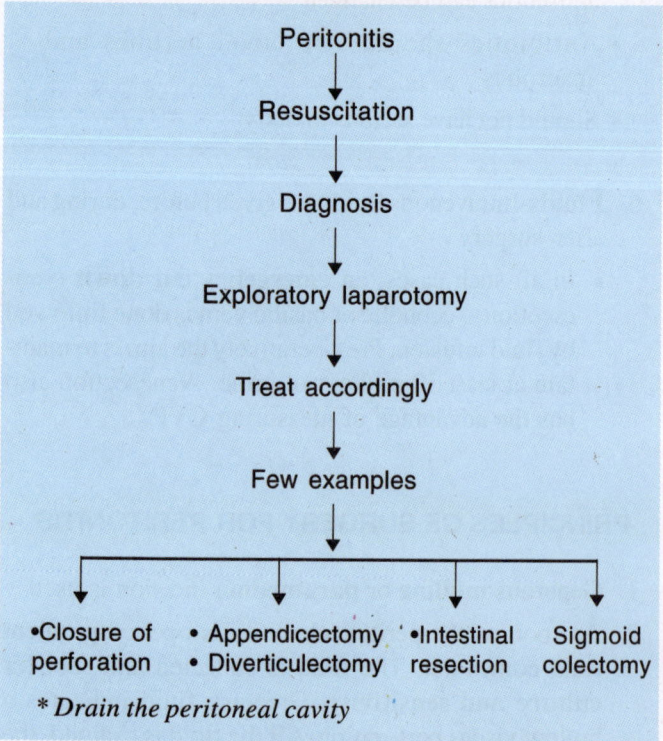

Peritonitis

↓

Resuscitation

↓

Diagnosis

↓

Exploratory laparotomy

↓

Treat accordingly

↓

Few examples

- Closure of perforation
- Appendicectomy
- Diverticulectomy
- Intestinal resection
- Sigmoid colectomy

Drain the peritoneal cavity

Fig. 27.7 Management of peritonitis

5. Peritoneal cavity is drained to the exterior by using **corrugated rubber drain** or by using **tube drains**. These are kept in the sub-hepatic space and in the pelvic cavity.

6. The wound is irrigated with **antiseptic agents**.

7. **Tension sutures** are put depending upon the severity of the peritonitis to prevent burst abdomen.

8. **Laparostomy (vide infra) :** This method of exposing the peritoneal cavity can be done in selected cases. Details about laparostomy are given below.

LAPAROSTOMY

This refers to exposure of peritoneal cavity to outside without approximation of anterior abdominal wall.

Types

1. **Open laparostomy:** Abdominal fascia and peritoneum is not sutured.

   Advantages: Abdominal compartment syndrome can be prevented (Page 453)

   Disadvantages: Significant fluid loss and secondary infection.

2. **Closed laparostomy or Mesh laparostomy:** Here the fascial layer is closed by using marlex mesh or prolene mesh or even a zip to protect exposed viscera.

   Advantages: One can minimize infection.

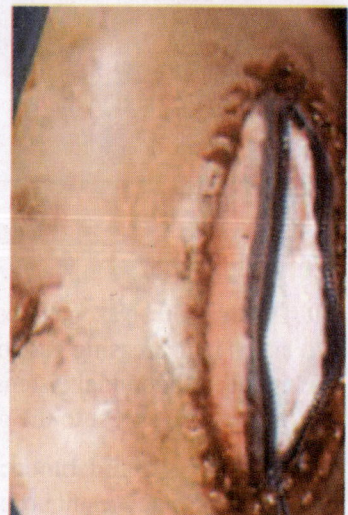

Fig. 27.8 Zip closure of peritoneum

   Disadvantages: Abdominal compartment syndrome and perforation of bowel can occur.

Indications of laparostomy: When a second look procedure is contemplated. Examples: Acute pancreatitis, Mesenteric ischaemia.

COMPLICATIONS OF PERITONITIS

1. **Severe hypovolaemic shock** giving rise to renal failure. It can be prevented by adequate hydration of the patients and careful usage of antibiotics like gentamycin.

2. **Septic shock, multi-organ failure** and death occurs in late cases of peritonitis.

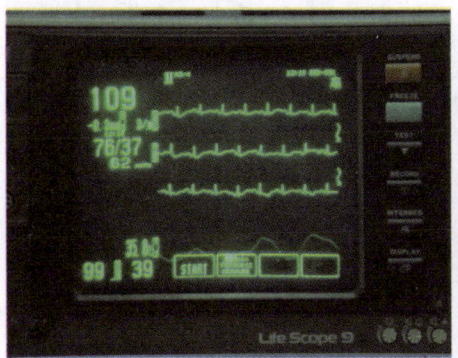
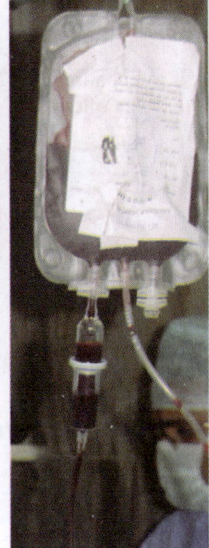

Fig. 27.9 Close monitoring of patient with vital signs and blood transfusion in addition to antibiotics play a major role in the management of septic shock

No doubt, drainage of the septic focus is the most important step

3. **Subacute intestinal obstruction** due to post-operative adhesions
4. **Pelvic abscess**
5. **Subphrenic abscess**

PELVIC ABSCESS

This refers to accumulation of pus in the rectovesical pouch or pouch of Douglas (Rectouterine pouch).

Causes

- **Any peritonitis,** commonly after acute appendicitis following perforation or following salphingo-oophoritis. The rectovesical pouch is the most dependent part in the body. Hence, the septic emboli accumulated in peritoneal space give rise to pelvic abscess.
- Anastomotic leakage is also an important cause.

Clinical features

- History of surgery/peritonitis

- Post-operative high grade fever
- History of discharge of mucus per rectum first time in a patient who is recovering from peritonitis suggests pelvic abscess. It occurs due to irritation of the rectum. Increased frequency of micturition occurs due to irritation of bladder.
- Deep tenderness in the suprapubic region

Diagnosis

- Confirmed by per rectal examination. A tender boggy swelling is felt in the anterior wall of rectum. Ultrasound can define an abscess and can detect the size of the abscess.
- CT scan is very useful in defining pelvic abscess, its extent and to detect foreign body.

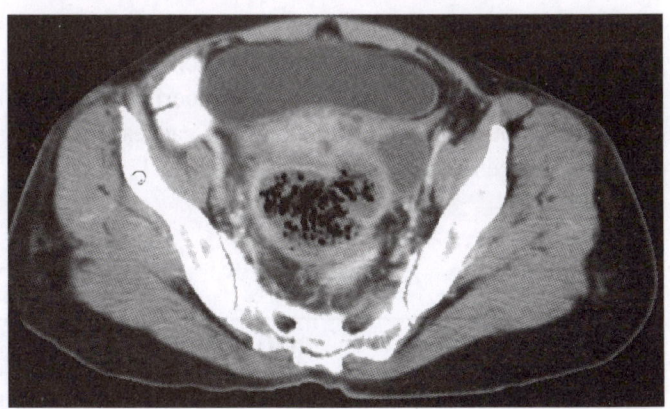

Fig. 27.10 CT scan showing gauze pieces

Treatment (Fig. 27.11)

- Under general anaesthesia, a proctoscope is introduced and a nick is made in the anterior wall of the rectum which opens into the abscess cavity. Pus is drained with a sinus forceps through the rectum. There is no peritoneal contamination. The cavity collapses after a few days. Postoperatively, the patient is given broad spectrum antibiotics.

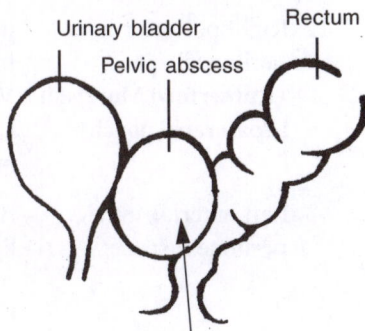

Fig. 27.11 Drainage of pelvic abscess through the rectum

- In females pus can be drained through posterior fornix.

CLINICAL NOTES

30 year old lady had persistent discharge of pus through vagina following vaginal hysterectomy. CT scan of the pelvis showed foreign body - gauze pieces. A re-exploration was done through posterior fornix and 12 gauze pieces were removed.

SUBPHRENIC ABSCESS

As a result of peritonitis, residual abscess can collect in the intraperitoneal cavity. Pus that collects under the diaphragm is described as subphrenic abscess. Subphrenic abscess is the commonest intraabdominal abscess.

SURGICAL ANATOMY

• There are 5 subphrenic spaces between the diaphragm and the liver bounded by various peritoneal folds. Four are intraperitoneal and one is extraperitoneal. The spaces, boundaries and the common causes of pus in these spaces is described in Table 27.1 and Fig. 27.12.

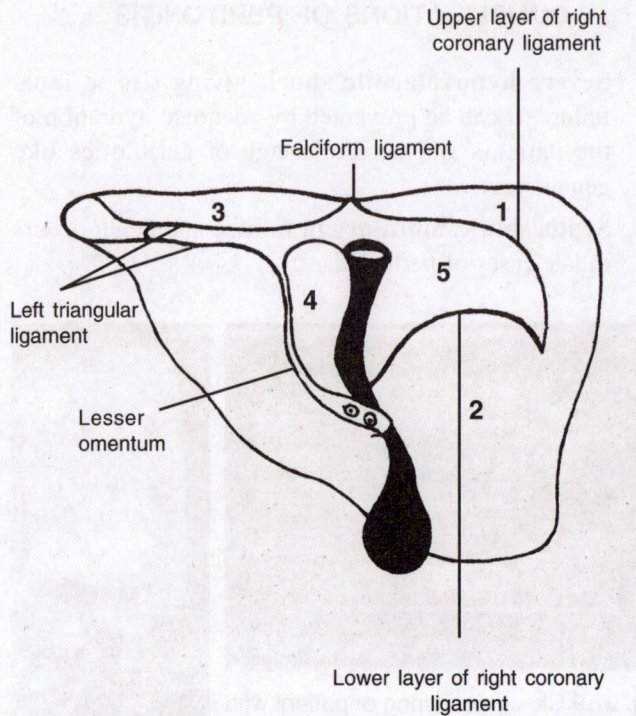

Fig. 27.12 Subphrenic spaces - refer Table 27.1 for numbers

Table 27.1		
SPACES	**BOUNDARIES**	**COMMON CAUSES**
1. Right anterior intra-peritoneal space	It lies between right lobe of the liver and diaphragm Posteriorly-anterior layer of the coronory ligament and right triangular ligament. On the left side is the falciform ligament	Perforated duodenal ulcer gastric ulcer, cholecystitis
2. Right posterior intra-peritoneal space (**Rutherford Morrison's hepatorenal pouch**)	It lies below the right lobe of the liver. Inferiorly-hepatic flexure and transverse colon. Medially-second part of the duodenum. Laterally-abdominal wall. This is the biggest intraperitoneal space	Appendicitis, Cholecystitis Perforated duodenal ulcer Upper abdominal surgery
3. Left anterior intra-peritoneal space	Above-diaphragm. Posteriorly-left triangular ligament, left lobe of the liver, lesser omentum, anterior surface of the stomach. Right side-falciform ligament Left side-spleen	Surgery on stomach-gastrectomy. Distal pancreatectomy. Left hemicolectomy
4. Left posterior intra-peritoneal space (lesser sac)	In front-by lesser omentum and posterior surface of the stomach. Behind-pancreas, suprarenal, left kidney. On the right side-foramen of Winslow through which it is communicating with the greater sac.	Pseudopancreatic Cyst Perforated gastric ulcer
5. Midline extraperitoneal space (bare area of the liver)	Above-upper layer of coronary ligament Below-lower layer of coronary ligament Left-inferior vena cava	Amoebic hepatitis Pyogenic liver abscess

AETIOPATHOGENESIS (Fig. 27.13)

- The causative organisms of peritonitis are Escherichia coli, enterococci, Klebsiella, Enterobacter, Proteus, Bacteroids, etc.

- The high incidence of subdiaphragmatic abscess is due to constant circulation of fluid from below upwards because of following reasons:

  1. Upward movement of diaphragm during expiration.
  2. Decreased intra-abdominal pressure
  3. Capillary action

Subphrenic abscess is common on the right side because of the following reasons

1. Left paracolic gutter is narrow and colophrenic ligament is present on the left side.

2. Right paracolic gutter is wide and deep and colophrenic ligament is absent.

3. Majority of diseases affect right side (perforation, liver abscess, appendicitis, gall bladder disorders etc).

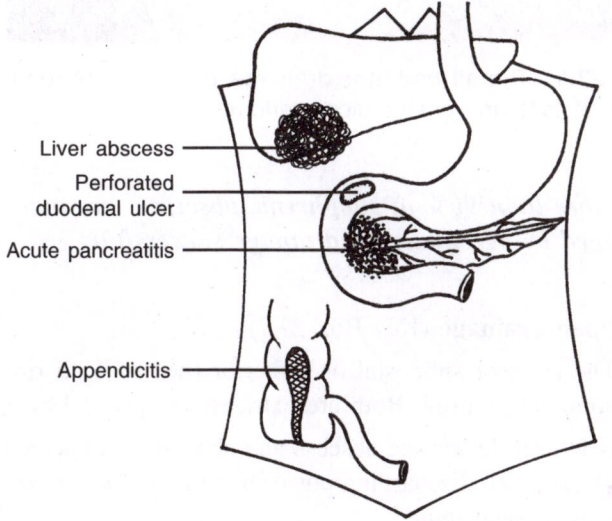

Fig. 27.13 Common causes of subphrenic abcess

Clinical features

- A patient who is recovering from peritonitis complains of fever with sweating. Initially, fever is low grade, continuous. Later, there is high grade fever with chills and rigors.

- Deterioration of health occurs very fast with wasting and anorexia.

- Shoulder pain is due to irritation of under surface of the

diaphragm by the pus (sensory fibers of the phrenic nerve are irritated-$C_{3,4}$)

- Tenderness is present in the epigastrium on deep palpation.

- Common causes of post-operative fever are absent, e.g. thrombophlebitis, urinary tract infection, etc.

Hence, it is said:

> *Pus nowhere, Pus somewhere, Pus under the diaphragm -Harold Barnard*

INVESTIGATIONS

1. Total count with neutrophil count

2. Plain X-ray abdomen (erect)-may show gas and fluid level under the diaphragm (Fig. 27.14)

3. Fluorescent radiography may reveal absence of movement of right side of diaphragm on inspiration.

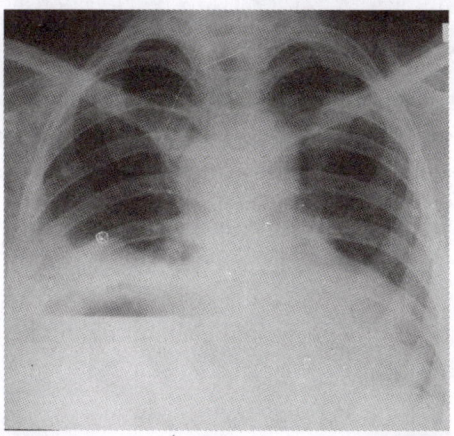

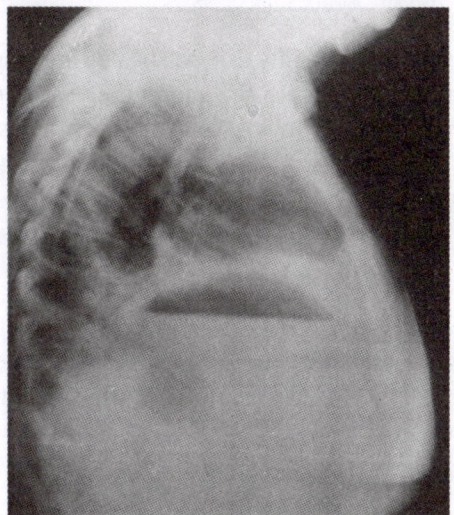

Fig. 27.14 Plain X-ray - gas and fluid level under diaphragm - PA view and lateral view

4. **Ultrasonography** confirms the site of abscess, number of abscesses, loculations, etc.
   - Abscess is characterised by hypoechogenic cavity surrounded by sharp distinct echogenic wall.
5. **CT scan** demonstrates well defined, low density mass, the rim is enhanced after intravenous injection of contrast medium. The mass tends to be round because of centripetal expansion.

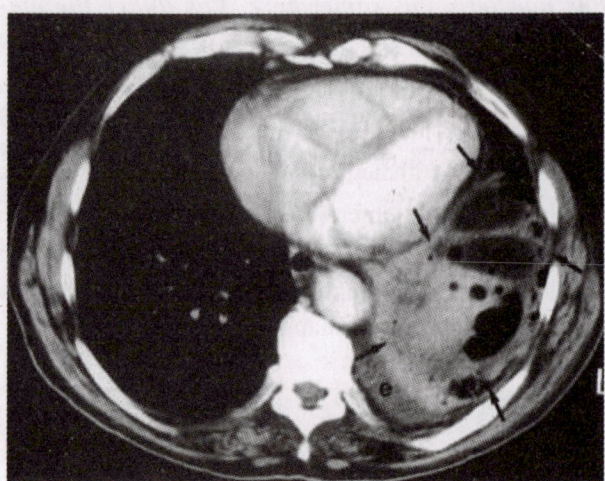

Fig. 27.15 CT scan showing left subphrenic collection following acute pancreatitis - a pigtail catheter is inserted (also refer Fig. 27.16)

6. **Isotope imaging** using Gallium 67 citrate or Iridium 111.

TREATMENT

Today with the availability of sophisticated imaging facilities, percutaneous drainage has become the choice of therapy rather than surgery. Both have been given below.

I. Percutaneous drainage can be done with the help of ultrasound or CT scan, provided the abscess cavity is unilocular, and the track should be safe.

Types

1. **Pigtail catheter** (using Seldinger's technique) : It is a small tube used to drain bile, urine, pancreatic fluid or abscess
2. **Trocar catheter:** 12- 16 French trocar is used.
3. **Sump catheter:** It has a double lumen which permits irrigation as well as drainage and allows a good suction.

Key Box 27.6
INDICATIONS FOR REMOVAL OF CATHETER

- Drainage less than 10 ml/day
- No fever, no pain
- WBC counts return to normal.

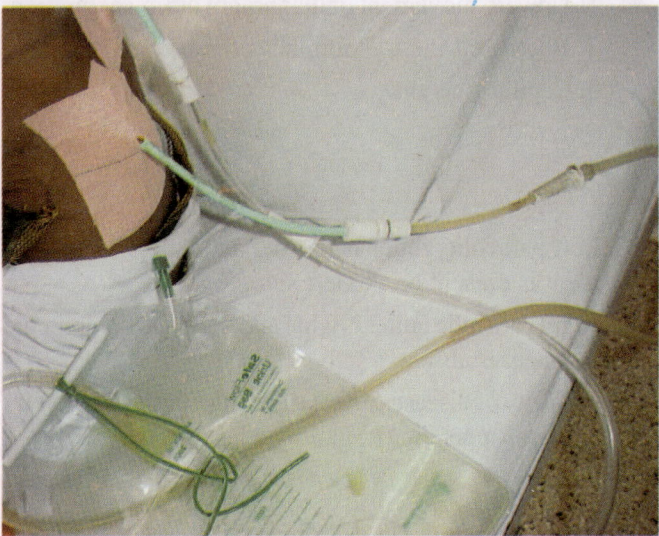

Fig. 27.16 Pigtail catheter drainage of left subphrenic abscess following gastric ulcer perforation.

- *More than 90% of subphrenic abscesses are managed by percutaneous drainage successfully.*

II. Open drainage (Key Box 27.7)
- The anterior subcostal or posterior (bed of 12th rib) approach is used. Both are extraserous approaches.
- However, lesser sac abscess and abscesses connected with bowel, discharging pus or bile are drained by intraperitoneal route.
- Open drainage is ideal in cases of multiloculated abscess.
- Surgery is always done undercover of broad sprectrum antibiotics.

Key Box 27.7
INDICATIONS FOR OPEN DRAINAGE

1. Multiloculated abscess
2. Persistent fistula discharging pus
3. Thick viscid content

SPECIAL TYPES OF PERITONITIS

POST-OPERATIVE PERITONITIS

- It should be suspected following surgery on intestines or biliary tract, when a patient who is recovering from paralytic ileus starts deteriorating.

Causes of delay in the diagnosis

- Presence of fever is attributed to other sources of infection like urinary tract infection, thrombophlebitis etc.
- Presence of pain and tenderness is attributed to recent laparotomy scar.
- Tachypnoea, hypotension are attributed to pre-existing medical conditions like COPD, cardiac failure.
- Steroid therapy masks the local signs and symptoms.
- Administration of antibiotics would have reduced the severity of peritonitis (masking effect) only to manifest as septicaemia some time later.

How to suspect post-operative peritonitis

- Deterioration after 3-5 days of operation (the time when anastomotic dehiscence takes place)
- Delay in recovery from paralytic ileus
- Evidence of toxaemia
- Free drainage of bile and faecal matter or pus from the drain site or from the main wound (Fig. 27.17).
- Oliguria may be an early indicator of post-operative peritonitis.

Treatment (Key Box 27.8)

Key Box 27.8
TREATMENT
• Danger lies in delay, not in re-operation
• Leak or abscess cavity is confirmed by abdominal ultrasound
• Exploration (preparation like a routine laparotomy)
• Resection or resuturing
• Drainage of abscess cavity
• Refashioning of colostomy, if it is retracted
• Once abscess is drained or leakage is prevented, recovery is wonderful

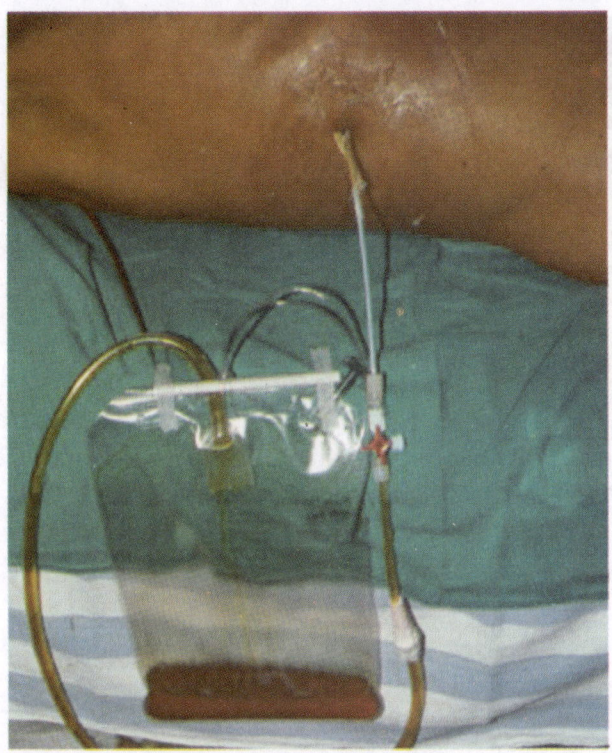

Fig. 27.17 Post cholecystectomy bile leak due to injury to the common bile duct

CLINICAL NOTES

In 1973, when ultrasound facilities were not available, a 35 year old male who had undergone appendicectomy for a gangrenous appendix was found to have high spiking fever on the 3rd post-operative day. All possible causes of post-operative fever including malaria were ruled out. On the 10th post-operative day, the patient developed a purulent discharge of 1000 ml through the lower part of the main wound following which he had a dramatic recovery.

BILIARY PERITONITIS

- Leakage of bile into the peritoneal cavity results in biliary peritonitis, especially when the drainage tube is not provided.

CAUSES

1. **Surgery on the gall bladder**
   - Leakage from the cystic duct
   - Injury to the right hepatic duct
   - Leak from accessory cholecysto-hepatic duct

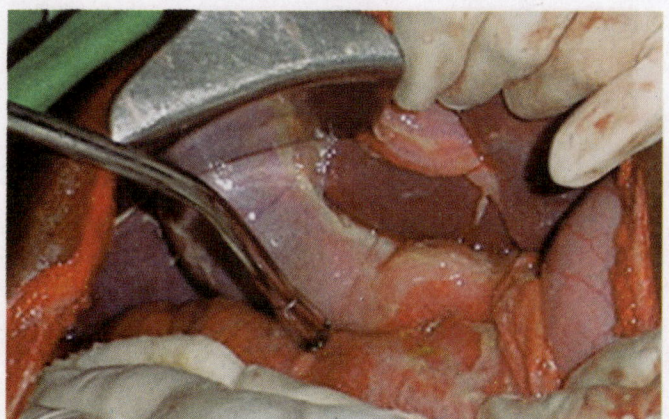

Fig. 27.18 Biliary peritonitis following duodenal ulcer perforation.

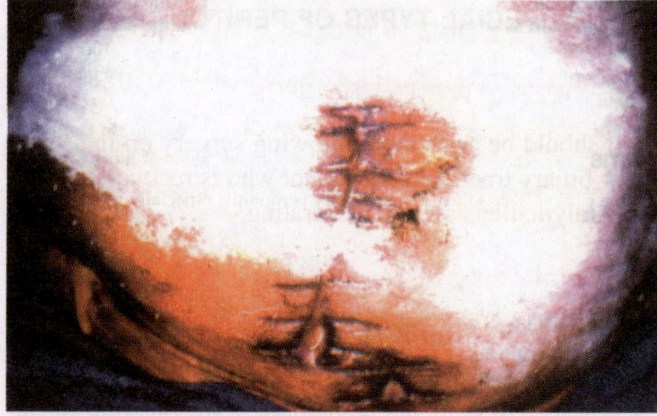

Fig. 27.19 Injury to the terminal ileum during tubectomy-with faecal fistula

2. Surgery on the CBD

- Retained stones in the lower CBD
- Loose sutures over CBD
- T-tube not anchored properly

3. Surgery on the duodenum

- Sphincteroplasty
- Partial gastrectomy
- Re-perforation of sutured duodenal ulcer

4. Injury to the duodenum

- During nephrectomy, hemicolectomy
- Blunt injury

5. Instrumentation

- ERCP, stenting or following duodenal polypectomy

6. Diseases of the gall bladder

- Perforation or gangrene of the gall bladder

CLINICAL FEATURES

- In majority of the cases the local signs are confined to one quadrant of the abdomen in the form of guarding and rigidity. There may be excoriation of the skin due to drainage of bile to the exterior. However, when the anastomosis gives way, generalised peritonitis can occur and in untreated cases septicaemic shock can develop.

TREATMENT

1. Most of the biliary fistulae will heal within 2-3 weeks with conservative line of treatment.
2. If it does not heal, re-exploration and resuturing or resection has to be done.

3. Feeding jejunostomy is a very useful procedure in all cases of reperforation of sutured duodenal ulcers or difficult duodenal ulcer closures.

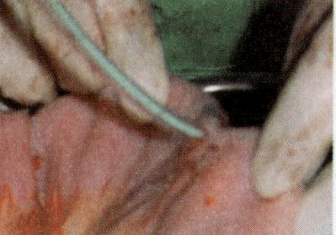

Fig. 27.20 Feeding jejunostomy

PNEUMOCOCCAL PERITONITIS

- Primary variety is more common. Girls of 3-6 years of age are usually affected. Infection spreads from female genital tract through vagina
- Malnourishment precipitates pneumococcal peritonitis
- In boys, blood spread can occur following upper respiratory tract infection

Clinical features

- High grade fever with features of toxaemia
- Bloody diarrhoea and frequency of micturition indicative of pelvic peritoneal inflammation.
- Other features of peritonitis are present

Diagnosis

- Aspiration of peritoneal fluid demonstrates high WBC count-30,000/mm^3. More than 90% are polymorphs.

Treatment

- Laparotomy and drainage of pus (odourless and sticky initially and creamy or purulent in the later stages), to be followed by appropriate antibiotics.

PRIMARY STREPTOCOCCAL PERITONITIS

- Infants and children less than 4 years are commonly affected.
- Peritoneal exudate is cloudy and contains flakes of fibrin.
- Symptoms of gastroenteritis-greenish watery stools are present.
- Source of infection is tonsillitis, pharyngitis, etc.
- Treated with injection crystalline penicillin.

PARTURITION PERITONITIS OR ABORTION PERITONITIS

This occurs after a delivery if proper aseptic precautions are not taken. The incidence has come down in the recent years. Attempted abortions by using instruments which are not sterile results in peritonitis. Most of the time, peritonitis is confined to pelvis with paralytic ileus, mucous diarrhoea and offensive lochia. Late cases develop generalised peritonitis, intra-abdominal abscess, intestinal obstruction and infertility. Refer Table 27.2 for summary of various types of peritonitis.

Key Box 27.9
ABORTION PERITONITIS
<ul><li>Instrumentation</li><li>Puerperal sepsis</li><li>Offensive lochia</li><li>Pelvic peritonitis</li><li>Infertility</li></ul>

SPONTANEOUS (PRIMARY) BACTERIAL PERITONITIS (SBP)

- As the name suggests, in this condition, there is no de-

Key Box 27.10	
RISK FACTORS	
CHILDREN	**ADULTS**
<ul><li>Malnutrition</li><li>Malignancy</li><li>Chemotherapy</li><li>Splenectomy</li></ul>	<ul><li>Cirrhosis</li><li>Nephrotic syndrome</li><li>Chronic renal failure</li></ul>

monstrable intra-abdominal disease responsible for peritonitis.

TYPES (Key Box 27.10)

1. **In infants:** It is more common in female children. Spread is by haematogenous route. The causative organisms are streptococcus pneumoniae. It may follow respiratory tract or urinary tract infection. (See the box)

2. **In adults:** Male alcoholic patients are commonly affected followed by patients with chronic liver disease. Causative organisms are E. coli, S. faecalis, etc.

- Portal hypertension increases permeability of gut wall. thus increasing bacterial migration. These bacteria which colonise in the small bowel reach systemic circulation because of shunting of blood around liver sinusoids to systemic circulation. Portal lymph also gets contaminated, giving rise to increased ascitic fluid.

CLINICAL FEATURES

- Dull aching pain in the abdomen with low grade fever
- Rebound tenderness is present, bowel sounds are absent or sluggish
- Cirrhotic patients may develop coma with onset of primary bacterial peritonitis
- Septic shock is a late feature with high mortality rate

Table 27.2. Summary of various types of peritonitis

TYPE	AGE	ROUTE	EXUDATE
Pneumococcal	3-6 years	Vagina	Odourless, sticky, turbid pus with high grade fever
β-haemolytic streptococci	Children	Vagina	Cloudy and fibrin flakes +
Parturition	20-40 years	Vagina	Thick pus +
Tuberculous	20-40 years	Pulmonary tuberculosis	Straw coloured fluid + Tubercles +
Perforation peritonitis	20-40 years	Hollow viscus	Foul smelling exudate +

DIAGNOSIS

- **Peritoneal tap and gram staining** of the fluid
- **Laparoscopy** may help to rule out intrabdominal emergencies such as perforations, etc.
- **Ultrasound** can detect nature of the liver and amount of fluid in the abdomen.

TREATMENT

- Conservative treatment is followed, provided secondary bacterial peritonitis is ruled out.
- Broad spectrum antibiotics like aminoglycosides with cephalosporins is the ideal choice. Metronidazole is always added.
- Instillation of antibiotic solution into ascitic fluid to achieve a quick and high concentration.
- If laparotomy is done, peritoneal wash or toilet is given.

MISCELLANEOUS

PSEUDOMYXOMA PERITONEI

- In this condition, peritoneal cavity is filled with mucoid substance (jelly-like) brownish or yellowish.
- Well differentiated pseudomucinous cystadenoma or carcinoma of ovary gives rise to this condition or rupture of mucocoele of the appendix. Some authors believe primary lesion arises from appendix and later spreads to ovaries (Fig. 27.21)
- Primary tumour is **very slow growing** and metastasis is exceptional.

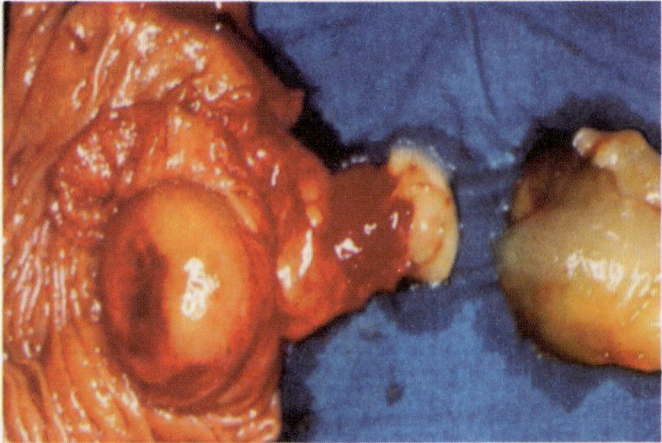

Fig. 27.21 Rupture of mucocoele of the appendix. Contributed by Dr. Stanley Mathew, FRCS, Associate Prof., Dept. of Surgery, KMC, Manipal

---

Key Box 27.11

SITES

- Ovary, most common
- Appendix
- Uterus
- Bowel
- Urachus

CLINICAL FEATURES

- Patients can present with slow painless and progressive abdominal distension. No shifting dullness.
- More common in females.
- It can also present with features of intestinal obstruction.

TREATMENT

- Aggressive surgery is the main mode of treatment. Masses of tumour tissue (jelly) should be resected or scooped out. Thus debulking, bilateral oophorectomy, appendicectomy, omentectomy is done.
- Combination chemotherapy by using cisplatin and/or intraperitoneal alkylating agents have been used.
- Recurrence can occur, because the tumor is locally malignant.

CARCINOMA PERITONEI

- This name is applied to an advanced stage of intra-abdominal malignancy involving the entire peritoneal cavity.

Features at laparotomy

- Multiple firm to hard nodules on the visceral and parietal peritoneum.
- Dense adhesions between the intestinal loops and other viscera
- Plaques on the intestinal surface
- Widespread secondaries in the liver
- Ascites-straw coloured or haemorrhagic
- Greater omentum being the **police-man** and a great drain pipe of the abdomen with rich lymphatics, is studded with nodules.
- Low protein ascites is more vulnerable for risk of

Key Box 27.12

COMMON CAUSES

Carcinoma of the:
- Stomach, colon, pancreas
- Breast, ovary

---

developing peritonitis. **Incidence of peritonitis in malignant ascites cases is low because of increased immunoglobulin levels in malignant ascites and increased opsonic activity.**

Differential diagnosis

- The most common differential diagnosis is tuberculosis (peritoneal). These nodules are firm and greyish.

Other causes include

- Acute pancreatitis with fat necrosis
- Ruptured hydatid cyst
- Lymphomatous nodules

TREATMENT

1. Radioactive gold (^{198}Au) instillation into peritoneal cavity
2. Tamoxifen is useful for ascites due to carcinoma of the breast

GRANULOMATOUS PERITONITIS

- Talc, gauze, starch, etc. are causative factors.
- It occurs many weeks after surgery.
- Low grade fever, weight loss, distension, crampy abdominal pain are the features.
- Laparoscopy is the key investigation - can visualize granuloma and biopsy can be taken. Also, fluid can be aspirated and sent for histopathology. High concentrations of lymphocytes are present in both.
- Symptomatic treatment - sinus, fistula needs to be treated.

PERIODIC PERITONITIS

- It is of unknown aetiology
- It affects children, young adults and females

- Presents as abdominal pain, tenderness, pyrexia and increased total WBC count.
- When in doubt, laparotomy should be done.

ABDOMINAL COMPARTMENT SYNDROME (ACS)

- Tense, distended abdomen with pressure of > 85cm of H_2O resulting in failure to ventilate is defined as ACS.

Aetiology

Thus any factors which increase intra abdominal pressure can give rise to ACS. Some important examples are:
- Peritonitis with or without abscess.
- Massive bleeding
- Acute gastric dilatation
- Laparoscopic procedures
- Reduction of massive hernia
- Intestinal obstruction / ileus.

Consequences

- Decreased venous return inspite of normal arterial pressure results in decreased cardiac output. As a result of this, renal, mesenteric and coeliac blood flow decreases resulting in renal and bowel ischaemia, etc.

Grading of intra abdominal hypertension

Key Box 27.13

BURCH GRADING

Grade I	:	10-15 cms of water
Grade II	:	15-25 cms of water
Grade III	:	25-35 cms of water
Grade IV	:	> 35 cms of water

Treatment

- Resuscitation with IV fluids and inotropic agents.
- Decompression - nasogastric tube will help in cases of Grade I and II ACS.
- Otherwise, laparostomy and release of pressure followed by simple closure is required.

- Anatomy
- Physiology
- Abdominal tuberculosis
- Tuberculous peritonitis
- Glandular tuberculosis
- Intestinal tuberculosis
- Inflammatory bowel diseases
  Ulcerative colitis, Crohn's disease
- Surgical complications of enteric fever
- Intestinal amoebiasis
- Peutz - Jegher's syndrome
- Carcinoid tumour
- GIST
- Short gut syndrome

ANATOMY

Small intestines consists of proximal $^2/_5$ jejunum and distal $^3/_5$ ileum. Thus it is about 6 metres in length.

Small intestine starts at duodenojejunal flexure just to the left of the inferior mesenteric vein.

Surgical importance: To identify the first (short) loop of jejunum for gastrojejunostomy.

Small intestine ends at ileocaecal junction

Blood supply (Fig. 28.1)

Superior mesenteric artery is the **artery of the midgut** which supplies the entire midgut (entire small intestine). Jejunal arteries are end arteries.

Venous drainage is through superior mesenteric vein.

Key Box 28.1

DIFFERENCES BETWEEN JEJUNUM AND ILEUM

	JEJUNUM	ILEUM
• **Length**	$^2/_5$	$^3/_5$
• **Diameter**	Wider	Less
• **Wall**	Thick and double (mucous membrane can be felt)	Thin
• **Colour**	More red	Red
• **Peyer's patches**	Very very less	More
• **Blood supply**	Long and few vasa rectae (1or 2)	Short and numerous (5 or 6)
• **Mesentery**	Transparent	More fat

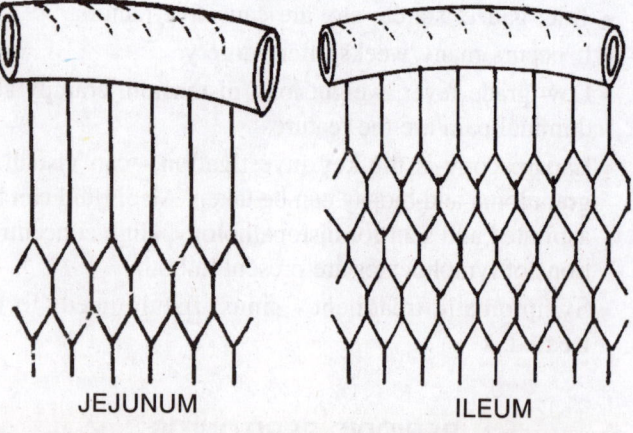

JEJUNUM   ILEUM

Fig. 28.1 Blood supply - jejunum and Ileum

MICROSCOPIC ANATOMY AND FUNCTIONS
(Key Box 28.2)

- The basic unit of small bowel mucosa is villus, which is a finger – like projection. Each villi is covered with tall columnar epithelium.
- Goblet cells, Paneth cells and endocrine cells are seen in the crypts.

Key Box 28.2
FUNCTIONS OF THE SMALL INTESTINE

- Digestion and absorption
- Synthesis of lipoproteins
- Secretion of regulatory peptides
    - Secretin
    - Cholecystokinin
    - Somatostatin
    - VIP
- Immune function : Production of immunoglobulins (IgA). The **B** cells and **T** cells help in phagocytosis and secretion of cytokines.

ABDOMINAL TUBERCULOSIS (TB)

Definition

The term abdominal tuberculosis includes tuberculous infection of gastrointestinal tract, mesenteric lymph nodes, peritoneum, omentum and solid organs related to gastrointestinal tract. Examples - Liver, Spleen.

Classification (Key Box 28.3)

The commonly encountered four forms of tuberculosis are given below:

1. Tuberculous peritonitis
2. Tuberculous mesenteric lymphadenitis-Glandular tuberculosis
3. Intestinal tuberculosis
4. Tuberculosis of solid viscera, like liver and spleen

Routes of spread of infection and pathogenesis

1. Intestinal tuberculosis is caused by mycobacterium due to swallowed sputum (pulmonary tuberculosis) or milk

Key Box 28.3
VARIOUS FORMS OF ABDOMINAL TB

I. Peritoneal tuberculosis : Acute, chronic
A. Chronic forms
  1. Ascitic type (wet)
    • Generalised
    • Localised
  2. Fibrous type (dry)
    • Adhesive
    • Plastic
    • Miliary nodule type
B. Tuberculosis of peritoneal folds
  1. Mesenteric adenitis
  2. Mesenteric cysts / abscess
  3. Bowel adhesion
II. Gastrointestinal
  1. Ulcerative
  2. Hyperplastic
  3. Sclerotic / plastic
III. TB of solid viscera
  1. Liver
  2. Spleen

    borne infection (Mycobac. bovis). From intestinal tuberculosis, mesenteric nodes get involved and later in continuity, the peritoneum can get involved.
2. **Blood spread** infection from pulmonary tuberculosis, during bacteraemic phase.
3. **Lymphatic spread** from tuberculosis of intestines.
4. **Genitourinary tuberculosis:** From here upward spread occurs, thus peritoneum gets affected.
5. **From bile:** Granuloma in liver, excrete bacilli in bile.

TUBERCULOUS PERITONITIS

It can be of two types: acute and chronic. Basically, it produces the following pathological changes:

1. Intense exudation which causes ascitic form
2. Exudation with minimal fibroblastic reaction-loculated form
3. Extensive fibroblastic reaction-plastic form
4. Fibroblastic with secondary infection-purulent form

• In most of the cases, tuberculous peritonitis results from reactivation of latent primary peritoneal focus.

Types

1. ASCITIC FORM (Fig. 28.2) (Generalised variety)

• It is common in children and young adults. The child is brought to the hospital with abdominal distension.

• Omentum can be felt as a rolled up transverse mass, which is nodular due to extensive fibrosis. Abdomen has a doughy feel with fluid giving rise to shifting dullness.

• Aspiration of peritoneal fluid reveals exudate, which is rich in lymphocytes.

• Peritoneal cavity contains pale-straw coloured fluid and the peritoneal surface is studded with tubercles.

• Umbilical hernia or congenital hydrocoele appears in children due to increased intra-abdominal pressure.

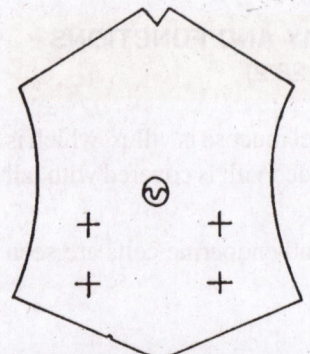

Fig. 28.2 Ascitic form

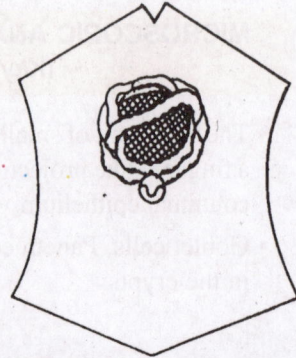

Fig. 28.3 Encysted ascites

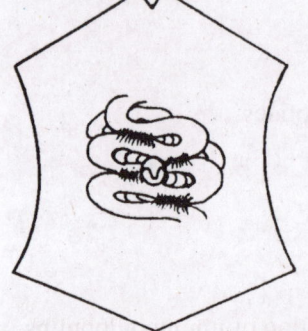

Fig. 28.4 Fibrous peritonitis

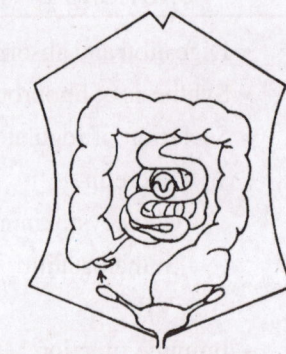

Fig. 28.5 Purulent type

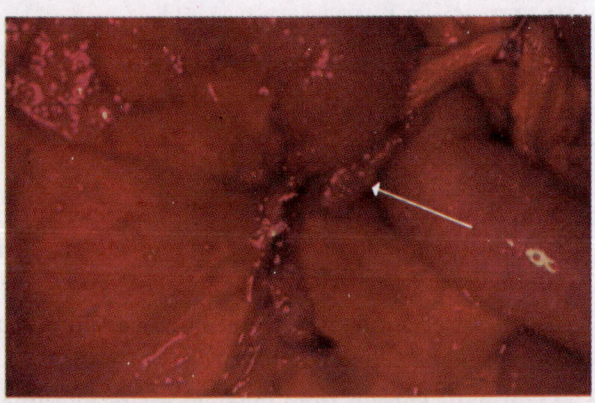

Fig. 28.6 Fibrous bands

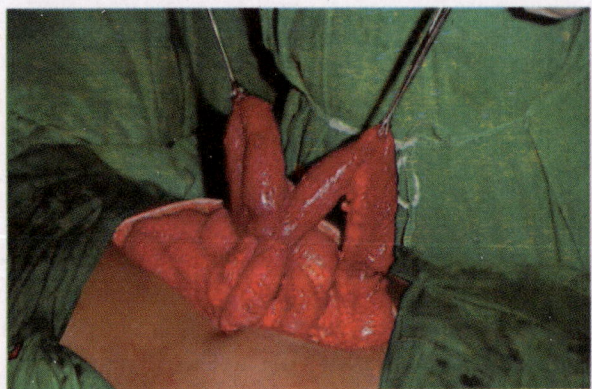

Fig. 28.7 Adhesive form

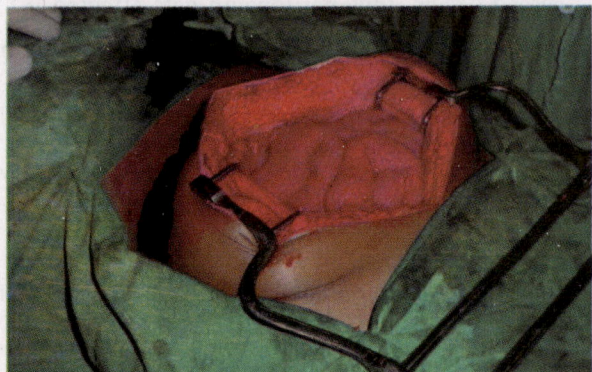

Fig. 28.8 Tubercle on the peritoneal surface

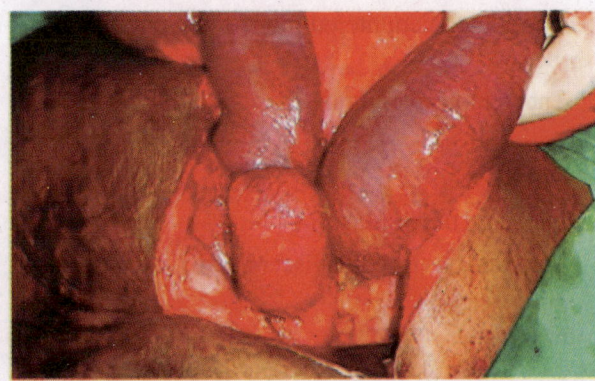

Fig. 28.9 Tuberculous peritonitis

2. LOCULATED OR ENCYSTED FORM (Fig. 28.3)

- In this variety, ascitic fluid is present in one quadrant of the abdomen which is sealed off by matted intestinal coils surrounded by omentum. It gives rise to localised swelling. These patients have no shifting dullness.

- It commonly presents in adults.

- Other cystic swellings in the abdomen such as pseudocyst of the pancreas, mesenteric cyst, retroperitoneal cyst are the differential diagnosis.

3. FIBROUS PERITONITIS (PLASTIC) (Fig. 28.4)

- In this variety, there is no ascites but there is extensive fibrosis which results in dense adhesions between the coils of intestines. Intestines are matted, distended, not able to empty properly due to adhesions and bands. It is associated with strictures.

- This gives rise to blind loop with steatorrhoea and emaciation.

- Usually, presents with intestinal obstruction at a later date due to fibrous band which needs to be divided to relieve obstruction. On some occasions, it is not possible to enter into the peritoneal cavity, due to dense adhesions.

4. PURULENT VARIETY (Fig. 28.5)

- Seen in females as a complication of genitourinary tuberculosis (tuberculous salpingitis).

- The spread occurs through the female genital tract and there is always secondary infection.

- It presents with acute peritonitis and on opening, the peritoneal cavity is studded with tubercles, cold abscesses and pus.

- Laparotomy, drainage of pus, followed by antituberculous treatment is the choice of therapy.

- It carries poor prognosis because of complications like toxaemia and faecal fistula formation.

- Tuberculous peritonitis can be associated with infections of pleural space and pericardial space (effusion) **POLYSEROSITIS** syndrome.

TUBERCULOUS MESENTERIC LYMPHADENITIS

Clinical presentation

1. **As a calcified lesion** (Fig.28.10) along the line of mesentery, which extends from L_2, at the left of vertebral column to the right sacroiliac joint. In 50% of cases, there is no active infection, but in the remaining, there is infection. If the symptoms are that of tuberculosis, anti-tuberculous treatment should be given. The shadow caused by lymph nodes are round to oval, mottled and may or may not be regular.

2. **Acute mesenteric lymphadenitis** (Fig. 28.11)
   - Common in children, clinically mimics acute appendicitis.
   - Pain in right iliac fossa, vomiting, fever, rigidity can be present.
   - On palpation, tender mass of swollen lymph nodes can be felt in the right iliac fossa.
   - Laparotomy, appendicectomy and biopsy of the lymph node is the procedure of choice.

3. **Chronic lymphadenitis** (Fig. 28.12) in children presents as **failure to thrive**. Fever, loss of weight, loss of appetite, emaciation, pallor are present. The child's abdomen is protuberant. On deep palpation, nodes can be felt in the right iliac fossa. These nodes have to be differentiated from nodes that enlarge due to lymphoma.

4. **As pseudomesenteric cyst** (Fig. 28.13)
   - This is due to caseation of mesenteric lymph nodes confined within two leaves of mesentery.

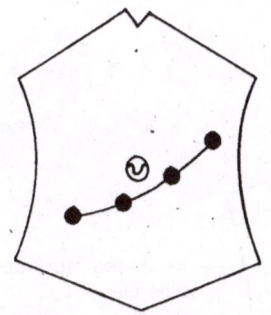

Fig. 28.10 Mesenteric lymph node.

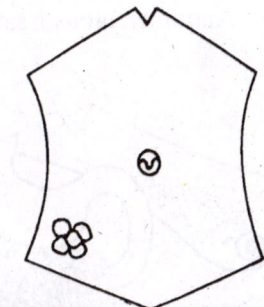

Fig. 28.11 Acute lymphadenitis.

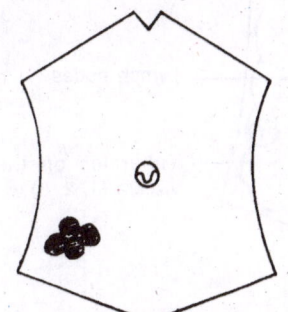

Fig. 28.12 Chronic lymphadenitis

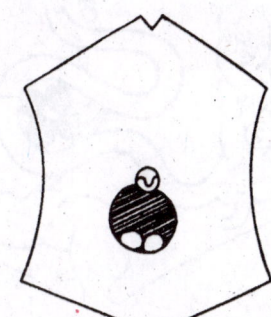

Fig. 28.13 Pseudo-mesenteric cyst

- Due to the adhesions, intestines can get kinked or twisted causing intestinal obstruction.

General investigations in tuberculous peritonitis and tuberculous mesenteric lymphadenitis

- Diagnosis is generally by indirect methods. It is difficult to demonstrate tubercular bacilli.

1. ESR may be raised in about 50% of patients
2. Chest X-ray may reveal pulmonary tuberculosis
3. Abdominal X-ray may reveal calcified mesenteric nodes or dilated bowel loops, air fluid levels.
4. **Ascitic fluid aspiration** (Key Box 28.4)
5. **Laparoscopy and peritoneal biopsy** can give a tissue diagnosis. Biopsy can be taken from omental nodule, peritoneal surface or from a thickened band.

> *One can avoid a laparotomy with the advent of laparoscopy and biopsy - Fig. 28.14, 28.15*

6. **CT guided lymph node biopsy** in selected cases.
7. **Ultrasound** not only can detect ascites, but also dilated loops and peritoneal tubercles (**echo-poor**), isolated/matted nodes with evidence of central caseation may also be seen.

Treatment:

- Antituberculous treatment

Key Box 28.4
ASCITIC FLUID ANALYSIS (STRAW COLOURED FLUID)

- Increased white cell count (>500/cc), predominantly lymphocytic.
- Increased total protein (>2.5 gm/dl)
- SAAG < 1.1 (Serum Albumin - Ascitic fluid albumin)
- LDH > 90 units/L.
- Decreased pH
- Increased adenosine deaminase
- Bacterial isolation and culture is possible in 20-45% of patients.

* SAAG= Serum - Ascitic Albumin Gradient

CLINICAL NOTES

An 18 year old girl presented with colicky abdominal pain, low grade fever, gross emaciation etc. Barium meal follow through demonstrated strictures of the small bowel. Laparotomy was done. There were dense adhesions. Minimal dissection resulted in two openings in the terminal ileum. Peritoneum was studded with tubercles from which biopsy was taken. Abdomen was closed with a drainage tube. Postoperatively patient was given antituberculous treatment. After three months, patient came to the outpatient department and had put on 14 kg weight. She was asymptomatic. This case history illustrates the presence of tuberculosis as a major cause of illness in India. It also highlights the importance of anti-tuberculous treatment and recovery.

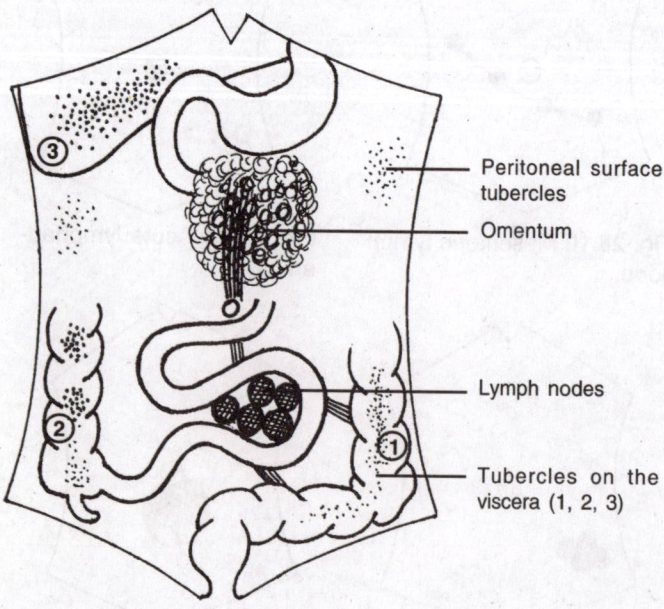

Peritoneal surface tubercles

Omentum

Lymph nodes

Tubercles on the viscera (1, 2, 3)

Fig. 28.14 Various sites from where laparoscopic biopsy can be taken in suspected case of abdominal tuberculosis

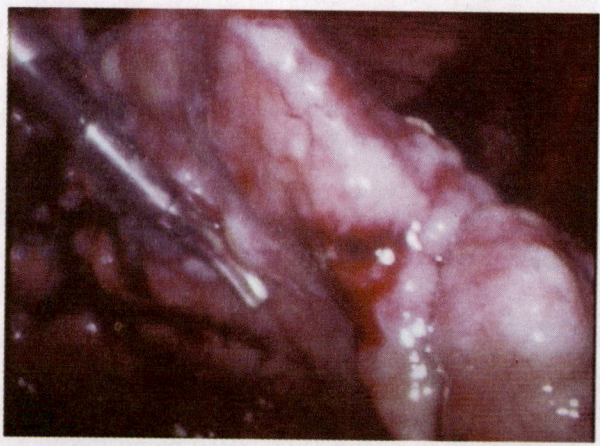

Fig. 28.15 Extensive abdominal tuberculosis - laparoscopic biopsy being done

INTESTINAL TUBERCULOSIS

Ileocaecal region is commonly involved in tuberculosis because of the following reasons:

1. Rich lymphatics in Peyer's patches
2. Presence of alkaline media favours the growth of the organisms.
3. Presence of iliocaecal valve precipitates stasis
4. Terminal ileum is the area of maximum absorption

TYPES (Table 28.1 for comparison)

1. Ulcerative variety
2. Hyperplastic variety
3. Mixed (Sometimes)

CLINICAL FEATURES

In general, abdominal tuberculosis presents with following symptoms:

- **Abdominal pain** which can be dull vague pain or colicky pain (stricture) which increase after taking food or relieved by vomiting.
- **Diarrhoea :** Watery, small quantity, abnormally foul smelling. It may alternate with constipation.
- **Nonspecific symptoms** such as flatulence, noisy sounds in the abdomen (borborygmi) are not uncommon.
- **Abdmonial distension :** It is due to ascites and subacute intestinal obstruction.

SIGNS

- Typically patients are **malnourished and pale.**

- **Visible intestinal peristalsis** may be seen.
- **Distended bowel loops** can be palpated.
- **Doughy abdomen** in case of peritoneal invovement.
- **Rolled up omentum,** mass in the right iliac fossa or lumbar region, loculated ascites, etc are other features.

INVESTIGATIONS

- The investigations such as ESR, Chest X-ray, sputum AFB, abdominal ultrasound are routinely done.
- Barium studies (Fig. 28.18, 28.19) can be done provided there is no acute obstruction.
- Colonoscopy and visualisation of the terminal ileum provides better information than barium enema.

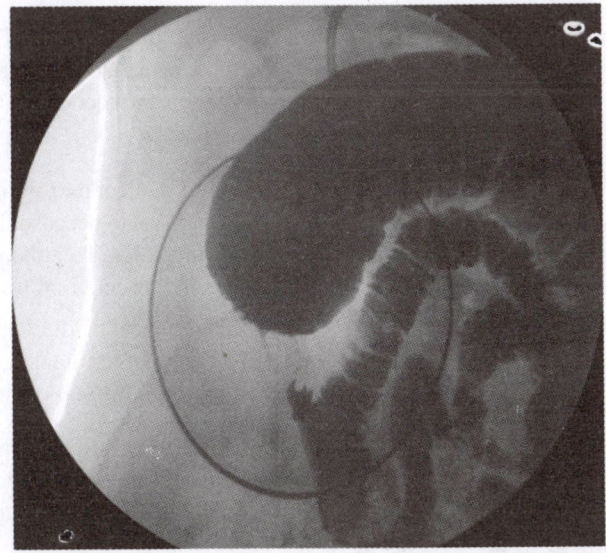

Fig. 28.18 Enteroclysis showing stricture of the jejunum with proximal dilatation

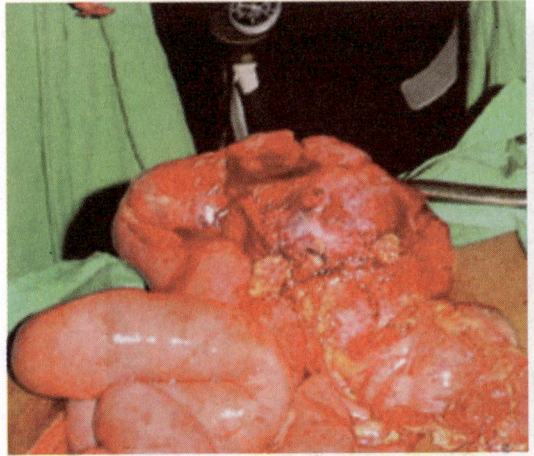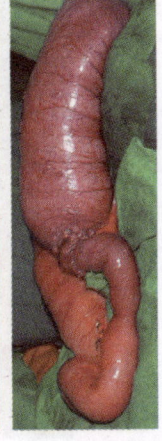

Fig. 28.16 Mass in the right iliac fossa - hyperplastic variety

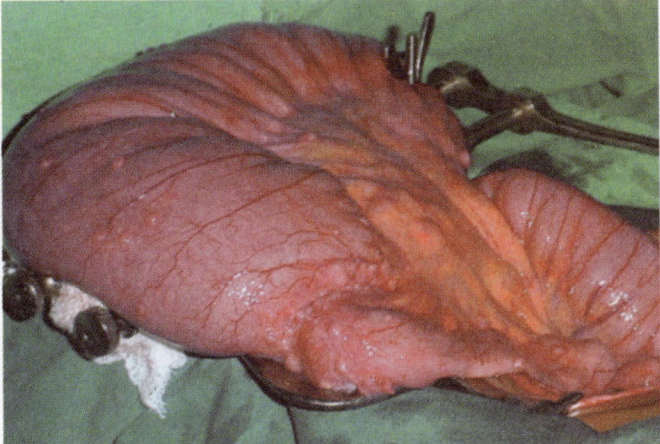

Fig. 28.17 Tuberculous stricture with intestinal obstruction - observe the stricture, tubercles and massive proximal dilatation

Table 28.1 Comparison of two forms of intestinal tuberculosis (TB)

	ULCERATIVE VARIETY	HYPERPLASTIC VARIETY
1. Aetiology	Secondary to pulmonary TB. Occurs due to swallowing of TB bacilli - (Mycobacterium TB)	It is a primary intestinal TB, due to M. bovis. Milk-borne infection or due to Mycobacterium TB -low grade infection
2. Site	Terminal ileum	Ileocaecal region
3. Virulence of the organism	Very virulent	Less virulent
4. Resistance of body	Very poor	Good
5. Pathology	Multiple ulcerations in the terminal ileum with/without involvement of lymph nodes. Ulcers are transverse. Serosa is reddened and oedematous.	It is low grade, chronic continuous inflammation involving ileo-caecal region resulting in cicatrising granuloma in right iliac fossa (mass in right iliac fossa)
6. Clinical features	Symptoms of pulmonary TB and blood and mucous in stool resulting in gross emaciation and cachexia. Diarrhoea is also a feature	Abdominal pain and diarrhoea may be the initial symptoms for a long time and later fever, weight loss and subacute intestinal obstruction occur
7. Complications	• **Acute** TB, ulcer perforation-ulcers are transverse because they follow the lymphatics. Treatment is laparotomy and resection of bowel. • **Chronic:** healing of ulcer resulting in stricture of terminal ileum --> subacute intestinal obstruction.	Nodular, fixed, firm mass in the right iliac fossa which later produces subacute intestinal obstruction
8. Barium meal follow through	Demonstrates a stricture, or multiple strictures. In the initial stages, ileum is not seen due to hypermotility.	**Barium enema** can demonstrate (i) contracted caecum, (ii) Pulled up caecum (subhepatic), (iii) Luminal obstruction, (iv) obtuse ileo-caecal angle
9. Chest X-ray and sputum AFB	Positive	Negative
10. **Colonoscopy and biopsy**	To confirm the diagnosis	To rule out carcinoma caecum

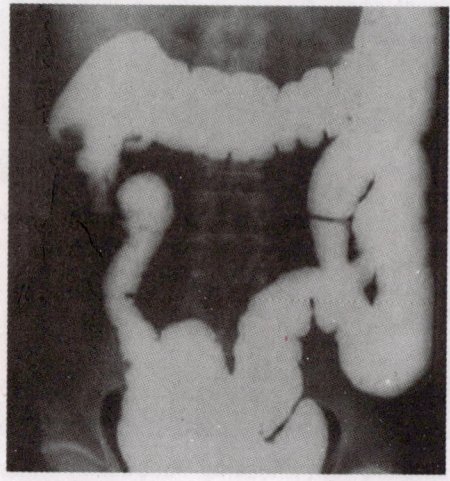

Fig. 28.19 Barium enema - pulled up caecum

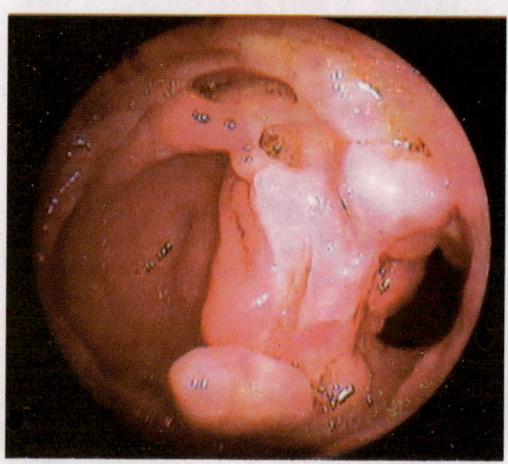

Fig. 28.20 Colonoscopy showing nodular leison in the ascending colon biopsy proved tuberculosis

TREATMENT OF INTESTINAL TUBERCULOSIS

1. No evidence of intestinal obstruction: Antituberculous treatment

2. With obstruction (stricture) (Fig. 28.21)

A. **Solitary stricture:** it is best treated by stricturoplasty by incising the stricture longitudinally and suturing it transversely.

B. **Multiple strictures** at long intervals: Stricturoplasty is the ideal treatment.

C. **Multiple strictures within a short segment.** Resection is the ideal treatment.

Stricture within 10 cm from the ileocaecal junction is best resected (Fig. 28.22)

3. **Surgical treatment of hyperplastic tuberculosis:** Limited resection is the treatment of choice. It includes removal of terminal 8-10 cm of the diseased ileum, caecum with appendix, diseased portion of the ascending colon, followed by ileocolic anastomosis (Fig. 28.20). All these cases have to be given antituberculous treatment for a period of 9-12 months. The nutritional requirements such as albumin levels and improving the haemoglobin by blood transfusion before surgery and after surgery helps in smooth recovery in the postoperative period.

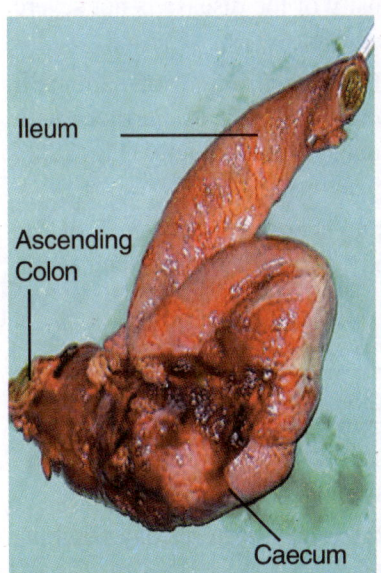

Fig. 28.21 Limited resection

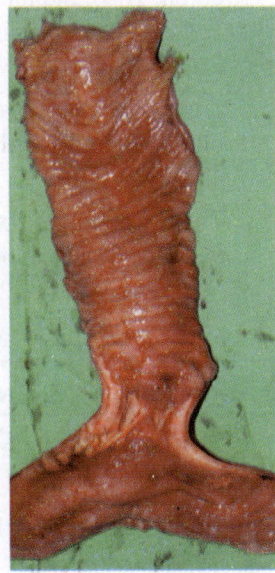

Fig. 28.22 Resection of the stricturous segment

INFLAMMATORY BOWEL DISEASES

Definition

These are the diseases involving small and large bowel, of unknown aetiology, characterised by multiple ulcerations in the bowel, clinically manifest as blood and mucous in stools. Ulcerative colitis and Crohn's disease (regional enteritis) are included under this heading. However, both these diseases are uncommon in India. Hence, amoebic dysentery, intestinal TB, enteric fever with intestinal manifestations can also be included in this.

ULCERATIVE COLITIS

AETIOLOGY

1. **Autoimmune factor:** Even though exact mechanism of ulcerative colitis is not clear, there are some factors which may point out at autoimmune reaction. They are :
   - **Cytotoxic T lymphocytes** against colonic epithelial cells in the lamina propria of the bowel.
   - Presence of **anticolon antibodies**.

2. **Dysfunctional immunoregulation** in the intestinal wall results in inappropriate production of **cytokines**. This creates an imbalance between various interleukins resulting in inflammatory changes.

3. **Psychosomatic and personality factors:** Ulcerative colitis is more common in western women. Emotional stress, family stress, stress from divorce are the contributing factors.

Western, white, worrying women's disease is ulcerative colitis.

4. **Dietary factors**
   - Westernization of the diet which is rich in red meat has been blamed. Vegetarian diet is supposed to protect the colon's mucosa.
   - **Allergy to milk protein** is responsible for ulcerative colitis in a few patients.

5. **Defective mucin production** and a defective mucosal immunological reaction is considered as a chief factor responsible for ulcerative colitis.

Appendicectomy and smoking has been protective factors for development of ulcerative colitis.

PATHOLOGY (Key Box 28.5)

- Disease always starts in the rectum and spreads in a backward manner, thus involving the entire colon in majority of cases. 5% of cases, terminal ileum can also be involved-**back wash ileitis**.

- Disease manifests as multiple, small superficial ulcers – **Pinpoint ulcers**.

- As the disease progresses, inflammation spreads into the submucosa of the colon. Attempt at healing may produce **Pseudopolyp**.

- There is epithelial hypertrophy in between the ulcers, resembling polyp. Healing with fibrosis results in a narrow, contracted colon, called **Pipe Stem Colon.**

- Microscopy: Pus (abscess) in the crypts and pus cells (inflammatory cells) in the lamina propria are typical of ulcerative colitis.

Key Box 28.5

PATHOLOGY

1. **P**inpoint ulcers
2. **P**seudopolyposis
3. **P**ipe stem colon
4. **P**us cells

CLINICAL FEATURES

1. More common in female. Female: male ratio is 2 :1.

2. Age: The common ages of presentation is 3rd decade followed by 4th decade and 2nd decade,

3. Disease is characterised by passage of 15-20 stools per day and contains blood and mucous. Sometimes, watery diarrhoea. (Key Box 28.6) As the rectum looses elasticity and lumen collapses, tenesmus occurs.

4. Relapses and remission are common and are related to emotional distrurbances.

5. Severe dehydration, malnutrition, anaemia, hypoproteinaemia are late features.

6. Acute fulminating attack is associated with high grade fever, bloody dysentery, distension of the abdomen and tenderness all over the abdomen with profound weakness. Hypokalaemia, acidosis, anaemia, shock are other features.

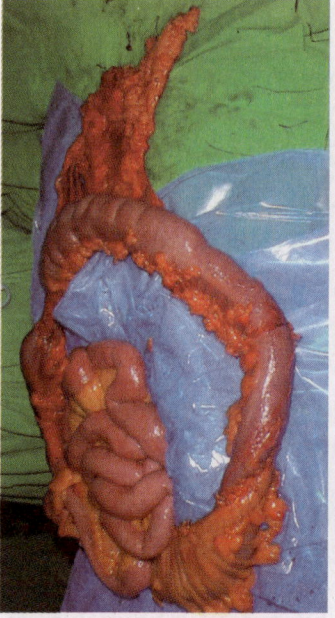 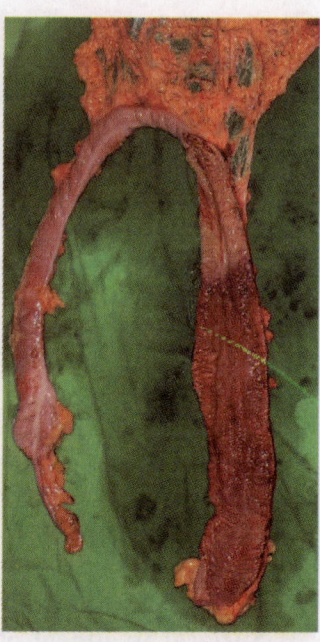

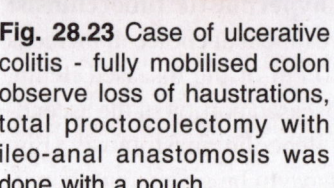

Fig. 28.23 Case of ulcerative colitis - fully mobilised colon observe loss of haustrations, total proctocolectomy with ileo-anal anastomosis was done with a pouch

Fig. 28.24 Sharp demarcation at the splenic flexure may be due to an incomplete marginal artery ending at point of demarcation. Case of left sided colitis

TYPES OF ULCERATIVE COLITIS (depending upon the extent of the colon involved)

1. **Proctitis:** In about 20-25% of the patients, the disease involves only rectum. In such patients stools are semisolid because of absorption of water by normal colon. Also, the intensity of the disease is not severe and risk of cancer is 2-5%.

2. **Left sided colitis:** Is found in 15 % of patients.It presents as severe recurrent attacks of diarrhoea with blood in stools, without systemic toxicity (Fig. 28.23 and 28.24).

3. **Total proctocolitis:** Is seen in about 25 % of the patients. Severe bloody diarrhoea, hypoproteinaemia

---

Key Box 28.6

TYPES - DEPENDING UPON SEVERITY

- **Mild colitis:** Refers to < 4 stools per day without systemic signs and symptoms
- **Moderate colitis:** Refers to < 6 stools/day without systemic toxicity
- **Severe colitis:** Refers to > 6 stools/day with systemic toxicity

are its features. Chances of cancer and complications are high in this group.

COMPLICATIONS

1. **Toxic megacolon:** It is an abdominal emergency encountered with fulminating colitis. Severe abdominal pain and tenderness, toxaemia , high fever, tachycardia, leucocytosis, toxaemia are the features. **Plain X-ray** abdomen **which shows colon** with **diameter more than 6 cm** gives **the diagnosis**. It requires emergency treatment by laparotomy and colectomy. Supportive treatment and intravenous corticosteroids are necessary.

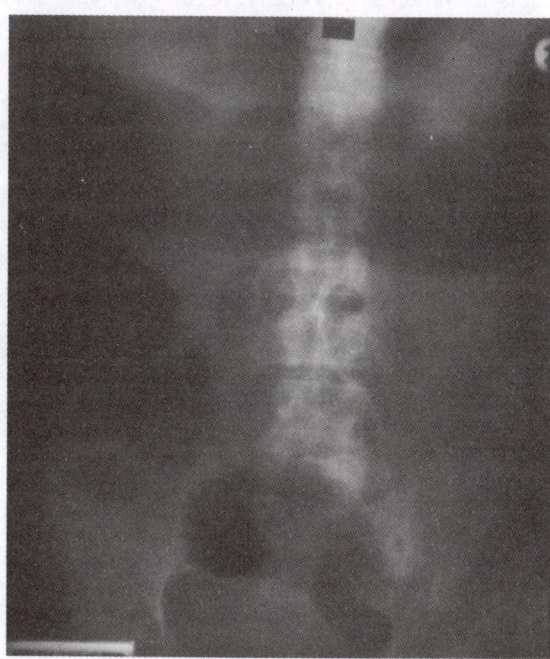

Fig. 28.25 Plain X-ray abdomen showing dilated transverse colon more than 6 cm - Toxic megacolon.

Key Box 28.7

FACTORS PRECIPITATING TOXIC MEGACOLON

- Barium enema
- Opiates, antidiarrhoeal drugs, anticholinergic agents
- Not known

Key Box 28.8

TOXIC MEGACOLON -CAUSES

- Ulcerative colitis, salmonella colitis
- Pseudomembranous colitis, amoebic colitis

---

2. **Massive haemorrhage** per rectum is uncommon. It is treated by blood transfusion.

3. **Perforation** is to be treated as peritonitis with resection of colon. Mortality rate is around 25-50%. Steroids may mask the symptoms.

4. **Carcinoma of the colon** (Key Box 28.9)
   - Overall incidence is 3% when the disease is present for 15 years.
   - At the end of 25 years, the incidence may be around 20%.
   - Hence, routine sigmoidoscopy and biopsy have to be done when the disease is present for more than 10 years and if it shows epithelial dysplasia, it should be considered as premalignant.
   - Incidence is more in total proctocolitis and when the disease has started in the early age group.

Key Box 28.9

ULCERATIVE COLITIS AND COLORECTAL CANCER (CRC)

- CRC is more aggressive
- Multicentric and synchronous
- UC patients with PSC (Primary sclerosing cholangitis) have increased risk of CRC
- More advanced stage at the time of presentation
- Risk increases with duration of the disease
- Malignancy develops on a background of dysplasia (dysplasia associated lesion or Mass (**DAL-M**))

---

5. Recurrent perianal abscess resulting in perianal fistula, in about 15-20% of patients.

6. **General complications (Extraintestinal)**
   - **Protein malnutrition** resulting in cirrhosis. Primary sclerosing cholangitis is also found in many cases. Fatty acid infiltration is seen in 40% of cases. It is reversible after control of disease.
   - **Skin ulcerations**, pyoderma, erythema nodosum, etc reflects protein malnutrition.
   - Conjunctivitis, iritis, arthritis involving large joints are also the other features.
   - Incidence of **bile duct cancer** is high in these patients.

Peripheral arthritis and ankylosing spondylitis are the two most common extraintestinal manifestations.

INVESTIGATIONS

1. Sigmoidoscopy: (Key Box 28.10)

- Can demonstrate inflammatory changes in the mucosa
- Mucous, pus and blood are visible
- Multiple ulcers are visible with bleeding

Key Box 28.10	
SIGMOIDOSCOPY-FINDINGS	
AMOEBIC ULCER	*ULCERATIVE COLITIS*
• Large	• Small - pinpoint
• Deep-flask shape	• Superficial
• Mucosa in between ulcer is healthy	• Unhealthy mucosa in between

2. Barium enema findings in ulcerative colitis: (Should not be done in acute cases) (Fig. 28.26)

- Contracted colon/Pipe stem colon
- Absence of haustrations, and mucosal irregularity
- Pseudopolyposis appears as stippled appearance

3. Colonoscopy (Fig. 28.27. 28.28)

- To confirm the diagnosis by biopsy
- To find out the extent of involvement of colon
- To follow up patients who are on treatment
- To rule out carcinomatous changes

4. Plain X-ray abdomen: To rule out megacolon and perforation.

5. C-reactive protein: Its level is very high in case of acute fulminating attack or toxic megacolon.

TREATMENT OF ULCERATIVE COLITIS

I. Conservative line of management

- Hospitalization and bed rest
- Correction of fluid and electrolyte imbalance
- Blood transfusions to correct anaemia and TPN hypoproteinaemia (Fig. 28.29).
- **Salazopyrines** are given in the dose of 2 gm/day. Mode of action: When given orally, it gets split into 5-aminosalicylic acid and sulphapyridine in the colon. This

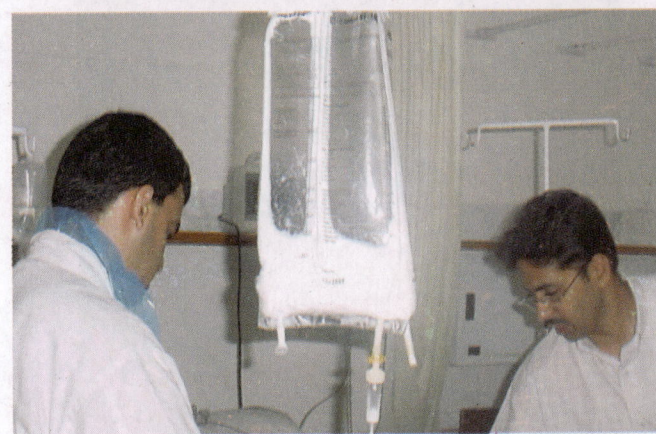

Fig. 28.29 Total parenteral nutrition (TPN) before and after surgery for ulcerative colitis plays an important role in the recovery of the patient, as these patients are grossly emaciated and hypoproteinaemic

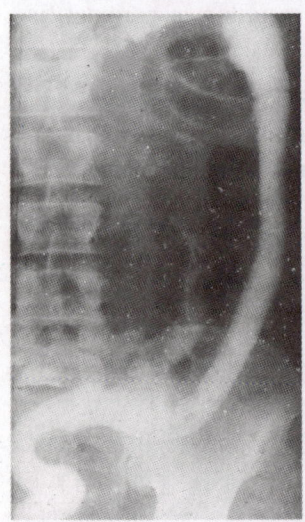

Fig. 28.26 Barium enema showing pipe stem colon

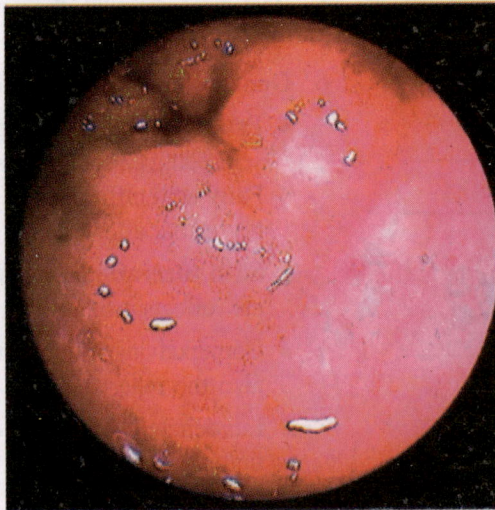
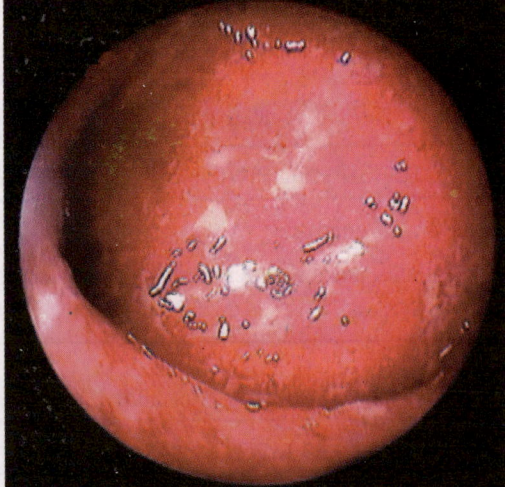

Fig. 28.27, 28.28 Colonoscopy - pin point ulcers with bleeding - Contributed by Dr. Filipe Alvaris, Medical gastroenterologist, KMC, Manipal

suppresses activity of prostaglandins E1 and E2 and thus reduces inflammation. They are used mainly to induce remission.

Role of corticosteroids

- Less severe cases not responding to salazopyrines are given a trial of oral prednisolone 60 mg/day. They decrease the frequency of stools. The dose is tapered off over 3-4 weeks.
- In acute attacks, IV hydrocortisone 100 mg is given.
- Prednisolone retention enema : 20 mg in 200 ml saline in intractable diarrhoea. It avoids systemic toxicity. Prednisolone 20-40 mg/day can also be given orally for 3-4 weeks.
- **Role of cyclosporin :** Those patients who do not respond to corticosteroids, can be given IV cyclosporin 4 mg/kg/day. It can induce remission.

II. Surgery

Indications for surgery

- Complications like dysplasia, toxic megacolon
- Active disease in spite of medical line of management
- Steroid dependence
- Haemorrhage

1. **Total proctocolectomy** followed by permanent ileostomy (ileoanal anastomosis should not be done because of incontinence). Ileostomy is connected to ileostomy bag. Adhesive obstruction and chronic perineal sinus are late complications. This is the procedure with least complications (Fig. 28.30, 28.31).

2. **Restorative proctocolectomy** with ileal pouch:

- This can be done as one or two stage procedures.
- Total proctocolectomy is done first.
- A mucosectomy of the upper anal canal is done.
- A pouch is created by anastomosing the loops of ileum. J shaped pouch is the most popular followed by W pouch (Figs. 28.32, 28.33 and 38.34).

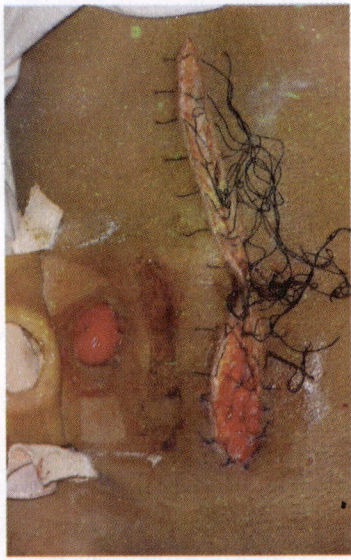

Fig.28.34 Total proctocolectomy with the pouch with protective ileostomy

- Pouch is anastomosed to the dentate line (junction of upper and lower anal canal) by using stapler or by hand sutures.

Protective ileostomy is done and it can be closed after two months.

Advantages of a pouch

1. Avoids ileostomy
2. Continence is preserved and patient is able to pass the stools via naturalis.
3. At the same time, all the diseased **mucosa** has been removed. Thus, the risk of cancer is negligible.

- Pouchitis is a complication

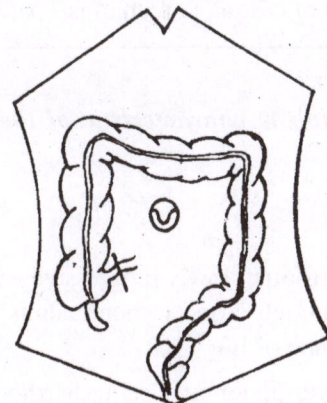

Fig. 28.30 Total colectomy

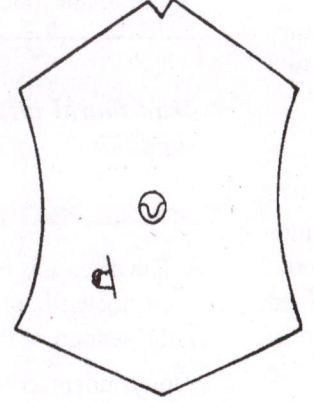

Fig 28.31 Ileostomy

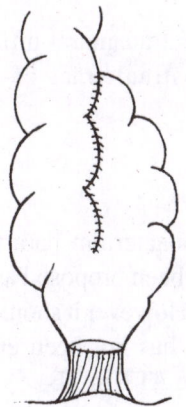

Fig. 28.32 J pouch

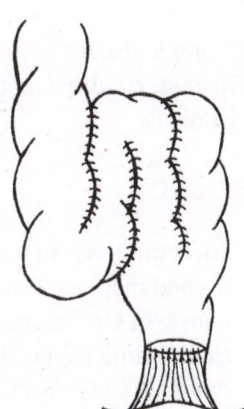

Fig. 28.33 W pouch

ILEOSTOMY

- End ileostomy is done following total procto-colectomy. It is a permanent ileostomy. Ileum is brought out through the lateral edge of rectus abdominis. It should project at least 4 cm outside.

- Loop ileostomy is to divert gastrointestinal contents to protect ileo pouch anastomosis. It is a temporary ileostomy which is closed after 6-8 weeks of time.

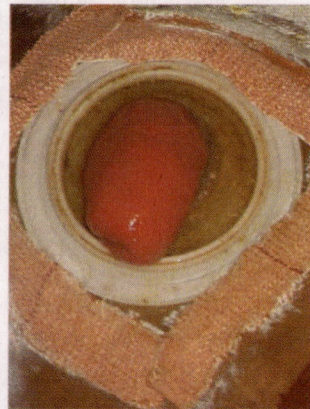

Fig. 28.35 Ileostomy - It should project out for atleast 5 cms.

- Ileostomy care is done by fluid and electrolyte care, disposable ileostomy bag, skin protection.

- Complications of an ileostomy are like that of colostomy-retraction, prolapse, bleeding, stenosis.

- Permanent ileostomy is also required following total colectomy for carcinoma colon. (Fig. 28.35)

CROHN'S DISEASE

It was called regional ileitis because the disease was first reported in the terminal ileum. However today it is called **regional enteritis** because the disease can occur in jejunum, ileum, colon, oesophagus etc. Involvement of ileum is more common, followed by colon.

DEFINITION

- Crohn's disease is a chronic transmural inflammatory disease of the Gastrointestinal tract of unknown aetiology.

AETIOLOGY

1. **Infectious agents :** Mycobacterium para-tuberculosis and measles virus have been proposed as potential causes of Crohn's disease. However it should be noted that antimicrobial therapy has not been effective in eradicating Crohn's (unlike ATT in TB).

2. **Immunologic factors:** Similar to UC. Focal ischaemia due to autoimmune reaction also has been considered.

3. **Genetic factors:** Single strongest risk factor for development of Crohn's is a relative with Crohn's disease.

PATHOLOGY (KEY BOX 28.11)

- Disease **starts in terminal ileum** as ulcerations of intestine in about 60% of cases.

- There is extensive inflammatory oedema and mucosal ulcers are present. Fibrotic thickening of the intestines results in **Hose Pipe Rigidity** of the intestine.

- There are **skip areas** which are characteristic of Crohn's disease (one segment of intestine is normal in between).

- **Mesenteric nodes are enlarged.** They can cified but do not show any caseation.

- **Intense infiltration of mononuclear cells** and lymphoid hyperplasia is common.

- As the disease progresses, there is cicatrising granuloma of bowel wall, resulting in narrowing of lumen resulting in intestinal obstruction. **Caseation is characteristically absent.**

- Once inflammation spreads to the serosa, adhesions develop between bowel loops or other structures. Abscesses occur in the mesentery, which rupture resulting in internal fistula.

Key Box 28.11
CROHN'S - PATHOLOGY
• Linear ulcers
• Transmural inflammation
• Skip areas
• Small intestine affected in 35% of cases
• Large intestine in 15% of cases and rectum is spared

Transmural inflammation is characteristic of the condition.

CLINICAL FEATURES

- The disease is often **insidious**, slowly progressive with protracted course, commonly affects young adults in the second or third decade of life.

Intermittent colicky lower abdominal pain, diarrhoea, weight loss is common. Depending upon symptoms it can be classified as follows.

Key Box 28.12

CLINICAL FEATURES AND COMPLICATIONS

- **C**olitis - Ileocolitis
- **R**ectal - Anorectal disease
- **O**bstruction due to stricture
- **H**ollow viscus fistulae
- **N**utritional deficiencies

  You can remember it as **CROHN**

1. **Stage of ileocolitis:** Clinically, presents as pain abdomen and mucous in stools, in younger patients. It may be associated with fever. Presence of pain and tenderness in the right iliac fossa mimics appendicitis. If there is a mass, it may be confused for an appendicular mass.

2. **Stage of subacute intestinal obstruction** due to stricture of the terminal ileum. Strictures can be multiple.

3. **Stage of fistula formation :** It can be Entero-enteric or Entero-cutaneous. Following are the examples of fistulae encountered in Crohn's disease-Ileovesical, Ileocolic, Ileoileal, Ileovaginal etc.

4. **Perianal disease** in the form of multiple ulcers in the anorectal region, perianal abscesses, multiple fistulae in ano are much more common than in ulcerative colitis.

> *Anal fissure is the most common anal problem in Crohn's Disease*

- Extraintestinal complications are similar to ulcerative colitis.

INVESTIGATIONS

1. **Small bowel enema:** Enteroclysis:

   - **Cobble stone** reticulation because of multiple ulcers and islands of normal mucosa in between.
   - Absence of peristalsis in terminal ileum
   - **String sign of Kantor** is demonstrated in terminal ileum due to narrowing of the lumen.
   - Multiple strictures and dilated segments in between can be demonstrated.

2. Sigmoidoscopy and colonoscopy may demonstrate inflamed mucosa, which is granular with **aphthoid ulcers**, which are **discrete**.

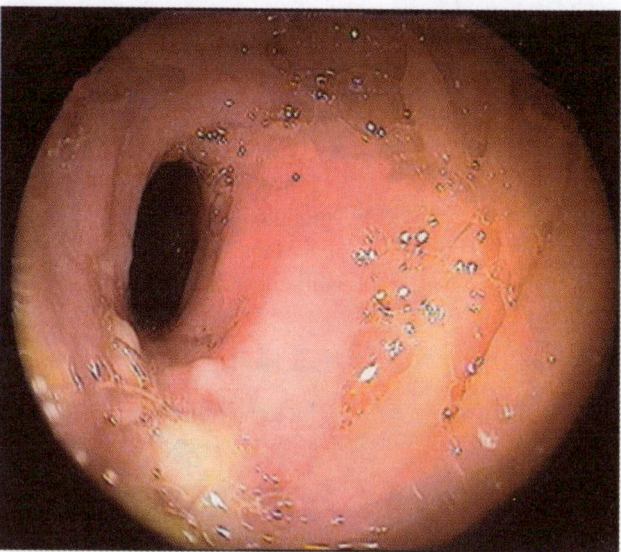

Fig. 28.36 Colonoscopic view of Crohn's disease

3. Fistulography to localise the internal fistula

4. **CT:** It is done to detect thickening of bowel and extraintestinal disease.

TREATMENT

I. Conservative (medical) treatment is similar to ulcerative colitis.

- Even though salazopyrines and corticosteroids have been beneficial in Crohn's disease, salazopyrines do not induce remissions. They are used in acute ileocolitis.

- Immunosuppressive therapy using azathioprine and 6-mercaptopurine are also effective.

- Most recent and promising drug is **Infliximab** - a monoclonal antibody to Tumour Necrosis Factor (TNFα) - it mainly helps in **closure of fistula.**

- Metronidazole has shown some benefit.

II. Surgical treatment: Resection **is not the aim** of surgery but it may have to be done in cases of obstruction, perforation, intraabdominal abscesses, internal fistulae, bleeding and malignancies. Depending upon the involvement of the bowel, various resections are possible. Examples:

1. Stricture-stricturoplasty or resection

2. Ileocaecal resection

3. Colectomy and ileorectal anastomosis

Table 28.2 Summary of tubercular ileocolitis, ulcerative colitis and Crohn's colitis

	TUBERCULOSIS	CROHN'S	ULCERATIVE COLITIS
1. Bacteria	Mycobacterium	No	No
2. Pathology	Continuous spread. Caseating granuloma, lymph node caseation. Transmural inflammation present	Skip areas. Cobblestone granuloma present No caseation. Deep longitudinal ulcers Transmural inflammation	Continuous, pseudopolyposis. Pinpoint ulcers. Crypt abscesses. Superficial ulcers Mucosa and submucosa involved
3. Site	Ileocaecal	Terminal ileum and colon	Rectum and colon
4. Bowel wall	Thick and fibrotic	Thick fibrotic	Thin
5. **Clinical**			
Bleeding	Uncommon	Uncommon	Very common
Diarrhoea	Uncommon	Very common	Very common
Fever	Common	Common	Rare
Mass	Very common	Common	Rare
Anal disease	Rare	Very common	Rare
Toxic megacolon	Never	Rare	More common
Fistulae	Uncommon	Very common	Uncommon
Stricture	Common	Common	Rare

4. If the fistulae are present, they are disconnected from the bowel and are excised.

   * Comparison of intestinal tuberculosis, ulcerative colitis and Crohn's disease is given in table 28.2.

SURGICAL COMPLICATIONS OF ENTERIC FEVER

During the third week of enteric fever, Salmonella typhi, paratyphi, (enteric bacilli) multiply in Peyer's patches and can give rise to following problems:

1. **Haemorrhage** is seen in about 5-10% of cases due to ulceration of Peyer's patches. It can be occult, obvious or rarely massive bleeding. It is managed conservatively in majority of cases.

2. **Perforation of terminal ileum**: An oval, vertical perforation resulting in peritonitis. Enteric perforation need not give rise to all signs of peritonitis-guarding, rigidity can be minimal because of poor, immunocompromised nature of the diseases and due to **Zenker's degeneration**. It is a single perforation in about 85% of the cases. It is situated in the anti-mesenteric border of the terminal ileum. Typically, it occurs on the third week of enteric fever. Bradycardia, dehydration, toxicity are the other features.

- Hyperplasia of reticuloendothelial system including lymph nodes, liver and spleen is characteristic of typhoid fever.

- Diagnosis of perforation is based clinically on the acute abdominal pain, bleeding per rectum with / without guarding and rigidity. (Guarding is minimal in enteric fever because of degeneration of the muscles - Zenker's degeneration)

- **Plain X-ray abdomen** may not reveal gas because of small sealed off perforation.

- The most useful investigation is **CT scan** which not only can reveal pneumoperitoneum but also pericolic collection, which can be missed by ultrasound (See next page case report).

Treatment

- Emergency laparotomy, resection of bowel and end to end anastomosis or closure of the perforation by using nonabsorbable sutures. Abdomen is closed with a tube drain kept in right iliac fossa. Wound infection is common in such cases.

- **Small bowel exteriorisation:** This can be considered in cases after resection when both ends of the intestine are friable. This is a very safe option. After 2-4 weeks relaparotomy and closure of the perforation is done.

3. **Paralytic ileus** due to toxic dilatation of intestine, results in distension of abdomen - it is the most common complication

4. **Typhoid cholecystitis** is not uncommon. Chances of gall bladder perforation are present.

5. **Typhoid pyelonephritis**, cystitis, epididymo-orchitis.

6. **Typhoid osteomyelitis**

7. **Typhoid conjunctivitis**

8. **Thrombosis** of the common iliac vein occurs probably due to sluggish blood flow.

9. **Perforation** of large intestine can occur in paratyphoid 'B' infections.

- Most of these complications occur due to bacteraemia produced in the early septicaemic phase of enteric fever. Liver, spleen, bone, bowel are commonly affected.

CLINICAL NOTES

Patient with enteric fever partially treated presented on the 10th day with acute abdominal pain and fever. Lower abdominal guarding and rigidity was present. Plain X-ray abdomen could not reveal gas under the diaphragm. Ultrasonography did not reveal pericolic collection. A CT scan of the abdomen was done. It revealed pneumoperitoneum and pericolic collection. Immediate laparotomy and closure of the perforation was done and peritoneal cavity was drained. Patient recovered dramatically.

INTESTINAL AMOEBIASIS

- Disease is caused by Entamoeba histolytica and transmitted mainly by contaminated drinking water.

- After the cysts are swallowed, they are broken down in the intestine by trypsin into trophozoites which produce inflammation of the colon. Trophozoites swallow red blood cells and multiply by mitosis. They enter into crypts of Lieberkuhn. They produce multiple submucous loculi which later result in multiple ulcers which are flask-shaped (bottle neck) ulcers with healthy intervening mucosa.

- Some trophozoites are transformed into cysts and excreted outside.(Fig. 28.37)

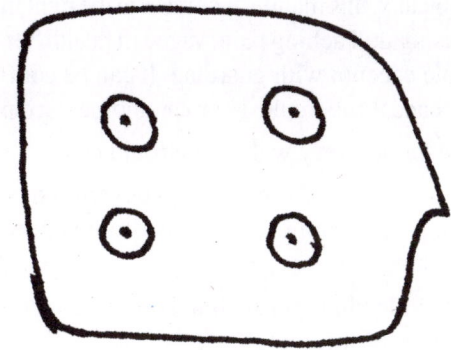

Fig. 28.37 Quadrinucleate cyst of Entamoeba

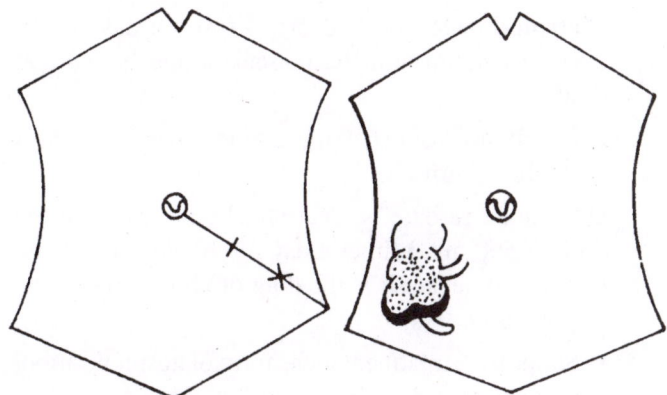

Fig. 28.38 Sir Philip Manson Bahr's amoebic point

Fig. 28.39 Amoeboma, tender mass

Clinical features

1. **Amoebic typhilitis**: Inflammation of the caecum by amoeba is described as amoebic typhilitis. It produces pain in the right iliac fossa and it can be confused for appendicitis. However, in this condition there is also tenderness in the left iliac fossa. The corresponding McBurney point on the left side is called Sir Philip Manson Bahr's amoebic point of tenderness (Fig. 28.38).

2. **Amoebic dysentery**: It can be acute or chronic. An acute attack is associated with gripping pain abdomen with blood and mucous in stool, an urgency to pass stools. High grade fever with tenesmus are the other features. Chronic dysentery is more common, 2-4 foul smelling stools per day with mild to moderate colicky abdominal pain, etc.

3. **Amoeboma**: Chronic, low grade, persistent inflammation of the caecum produces granulomatous hyperplasia of the caecum, with thickening of the pericaecal tissue (producing mass in the right iliac fossa) (Fig. 28.39).

- Clinically, this manifests as mass in the right iliac fossa causing dull aching pain, vague ill health, tender palpable caecum with guarding. It can be confused for ileocaecal tuberculosis or carcinoma caecum.
- It responds very well to metronidazole.

4. Amoebic perforation of caecum or sigmoid can occur resulting in pericolic abscess. Peritonitis needs emergency surgery.

5. Massive bleeding per rectum is rare. It occurs due to separation of the slough.

Treatment

1. **Metronidazole** 400-600 mg, 3 times a day for 10 days. It acts on amoeba present on the lumen and tissue.

2. Diiodohydroxyquin 650 mg, 3 times a day for 20 days is another alternative.

3. Diloxanide furoate is ideal for chronic cases in the dose of 500 mg 3 times a day for 10 days. It acts on luminal amoebae. It is the drug of choice in chronic cyst passers.

- Supportive treatment in the form of hospitalisation, correction of dehydration, antispasmodics and bed rest also to be advised. The stool culture must be done before and after treatment with anti amoebic drugs.

PEUTZ-JEGHER'S SYNDROME (FAMILIAL HAMARTOMATOUS POLYPOSIS)

This syndrome is characterised by:

1. **Familial** tendency
2. **Melanosis** of mucosa of lip, cheek, interdigital space and even, perianal skin (Fig. 28.40).
3. **Multiple polyps** in the small bowel, mainly in the jejunum. They are hamartomatous polyps.

Clinical presentation

1. Runs in families
2. As a cause of bleeding per rectum, results in chronic anaemia.
3. Can cause adult intussusception
4. Rarely, it can turn into malignancy

Treatment

- Blood transfusion to correct anaemia

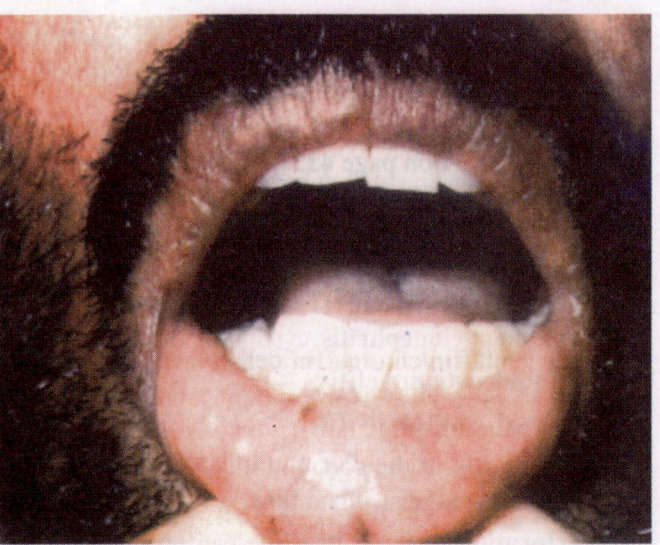

Fig. 28.40 Melanosis of lips, cheek

- Resection of that portion of bowel containing polyp, in cases of bleeding or intussusception.

CLINICAL NOTES

We had 3 interesting cases of Peutz-Jegher's syndrome. **First case** was of a boy of 14 years, who presented with acute intestinal obstruction. At laparotomy, there were 3 intussusceptions in the jejunum due to polyps. About 15 large polyps were removed after doing an enterotomy.

Second case was of a 50 year old lady, who presented with duodenal carcinoma. Endoscopy revealed polyps in the stomach and duodenum. Specimen of pancreaticoduodenectomy revealed it as a case of Peutz-Jegher's syndrome. This lady did not have pigmentation of the oral mucosa.

The third case was of a 35 years old male who has been coming to our hospital with intermittent bleeding with anaemia. Endoscopy revealed multiple polyps in the stomach and duodenum. Small bowel enema demonstrated multiple polyps in the small bowel. Even proctoscopy showed multiple polyps in the rectum. He is being managed conservatively.

SMALL BOWEL TUMOURS

- Benign tumours such as lipoma, hamartoma, polyps can occur.
- Malignant tumours such as adenocarcinoma, gastrointestinal stromal tumours (**GIST**), carcinoid and lymphoma can occur in the small intestine.

ADENOCARCINOMA

- Duodenum is the commonest site. They present with pain, bleeding, intestinal obstruction. Diagnosis is by enteroclysis and CT scan. Resection is the best treatment. However, these tumours are rare (Key Box 28.13).

Key Box 28.13
MALIGNANCY IN SMALL INTESTINE IS RARE - WHY?
<ul><li>No stasis, rapid transit of food</li><li>Secretion of immunoglobulins - IgA</li><li>Various carcinogens are diluted by secretions</li><li>Comparatively low and inactive bacteria in the small bowel</li></ul>

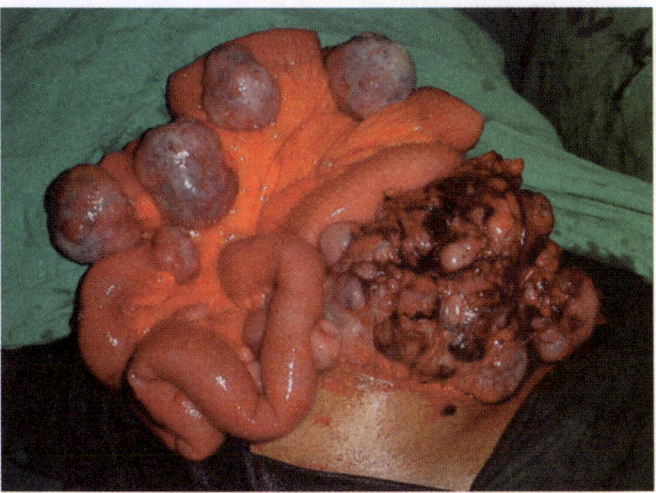

Fig. 28.42 GIST involving terminal ileum, caecum and ascending colon. Contributed by Dr. Stanley Mathew, FRCS, Associate Professor, KMC, Manipal

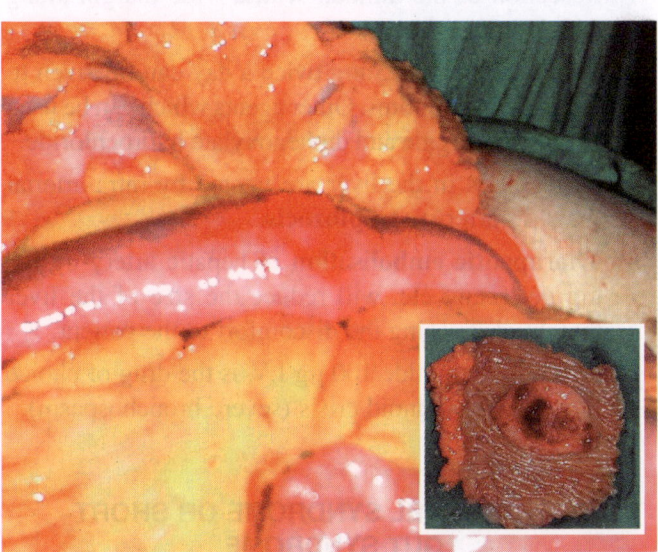

Fig. 28.41 This patient presented with abdominal pain, melena and loss of weight. CT scan of the abdomen revealed mass in the jejunum. It was resected. (Inset) Mucosal surface showed ulceration. Histopathology report was adenocarcinoma

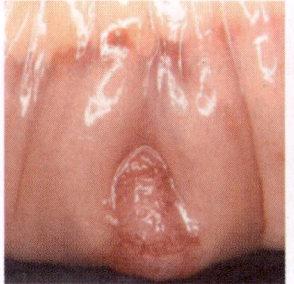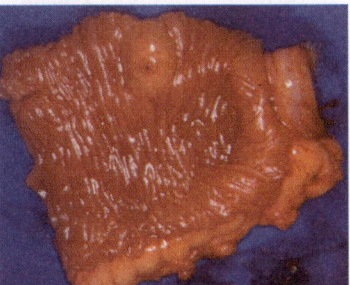

Fig. 28.43 GIST involving jejunum - resected specimen showing mucosal ulceration - Contributed by Dr. Padmanabha Bhat, Dept. of Surgery, KMC, Manipal and Prof. H.D. Shenoy, Father Muller's Hospital, Mangalore

CARCINOID TUMOUR (ARGENTAFFINOMA)

It arises from argentaffin/chromaffin cells which are present in the crypts of the villi of intestine. These cells are called as Kulschitsky cells. These cells stain for ammoniacal silver salt solution to black colour. Hence, they are called as argentaffinoma, chromaffinoma. They secrete **5 HT** (Serotonin or **5** Hydroxytryptamine). They can be single or multiple and can be associated with adenocarcinoma.

Site

- Appendix: 65%. **It is the most common site.** It more commonly occurs in females.
- **Terminal ileum:** 30%. Most of them are **malignant**.
- Bronchial carcinoid produces bronchial obstruction and produces carcinoid syndrome without secondaries in liver (refer Table 28.3).

GIST: GASTROINTESTINAL STROMAL TUMOUR

- Earlier called as leiomyoma and leiomyosarcoma, they occur in jejunum or ileum
- They present as bleeding / mass / perforation
- Very often massive bleeding may be the only presentation
- Diagnosis is by endoscopies and CT scan
- Treatment is similar to above in the form of resection
- Diagnosis of malignancy is by mitotic figures

Table 28.3 Comparison of carcinoid tumours at various sites

	FOREGUT	MIDGUT	HINDGUT
Site	Duodenum, stomach, bronchus, pancreas, etc.	Jejunum, ileum, right colon	Rectum
Incidence	Rare	Common	Uncommon
Hormones	5 HT, histamine	5 HT, prostaglandins, insulin, ACTH, etc.	DO NOT secrete

- When the tumour occurs in the appendix it is usually benign, hard and occurs in distal one-third of appendix.
- When the tumour occurs in the ileum it is usually malignant, and produces multiple bulky secondaries in the liver, even when primary is very small.
- The hormones produced by the tumour **5 HT** (serotonin) are not metabolised because of the secondaries. So, they are absorbed into the circulation and produce various symptoms. This is called as carcinoid syndrome (Fig. 28.44, Table 28.3).
- **Carcinoid syndrome** consists of following features:
  1. Carcinoid tumour which is malignant
  2. Secondary in the liver
  3. Symptoms are red, blue cyanosis of skin flushing attack and asthmatic attacks, intestinal hyperperistalsis causing diarrhoea and pulmonary and tricuspid stenosis with CCF.

Diagnosis

- 24 hours urine for 5 Hydroxyindole acetic acid. Normal levels 2-9 mg/24 hours. Very high values are found in this condition.

Treatment

1. Resection of the tumour, with a wide margin along with lymph nodes.
2. **Bromocryptine** 2.5 mg twice a day can be given to reduce the symptoms. Other agents which can be used are methylsergide and diphenoxylate hydrochloride.
3. Secondaries in the liver are treated by intra-arterial (hepatic artery) **streptozocin**.
4. **Therapeutic embolisation** of hepatic artery by using gel foam, etc. will reduce the size of the liver thereby decreasing the discomfort to the patient.
5. Injection octreotide 100 μg I.V. is the drug of choice in cases of carcinoid crisis (severe bronchospasm)

SHORT BOWEL SYNDROME OR SHORT GUT SYNDROME

This is the result of massive resection of bowel (mainly small bowel), which results in severe nutritional deficiencies which eventually is fatal. This most unfortunate event is caused by a benign lesion.

Causes of short gut syndrome (Key Box 28.14)

- Short gut syndrome results due to **massive resection** of the bowel resulting in loss of length of the bowel, loss of absorptive area of the bowel and loss of valves. Superior mesenteric artery being an end artery, thrombosis at the origin is invariably fatal.
- **Midgut volvulus** of neonates is congenital due to arrested rotation resulting in floating caecum and mobile intestine. We had an interesting case of midgut volvulus in an 18 year old boy consequent to a laparotomy done for perforated duodenal ulcer. While replacing the

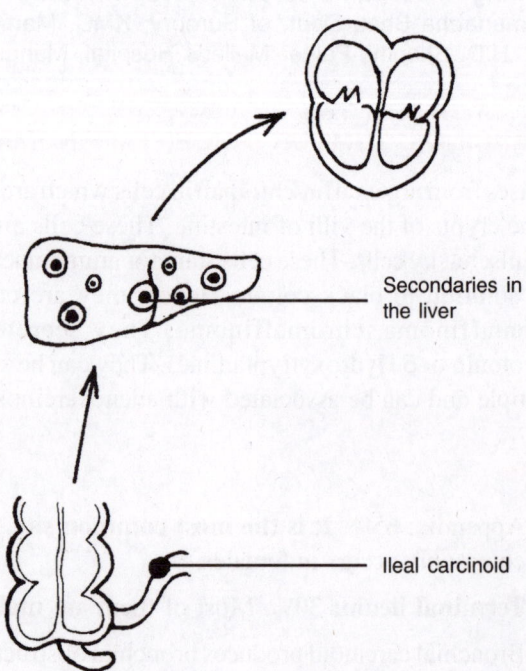

Secondaries in the liver

Ileal carcinoid

Fig. 28.44 Carcinoid syndrome

coils of bowel within the abdomen, probably the mesentery was twisted resulting in massive gangrene. This boy has about 100 cms of the small bowel with valve surviving on "Baby food" for the last 5 years.

- **Necrotising enteritis** (enteritis necroticans) is a complication of infection of small bowel by clostridium perfringens. It usually occurs after a heavy feast wherein pork is consumed. There is extensive suppuration of mucosal and submucosal layer of jejunum (also ileum). Serosa may show multiple dark bluish patches. Massive resection is done for a necrotic, perforated, unhealthy bowel which results in short gut syndrome.

- **Radiation enteritis** or radiation enteropathy results in

patients who also receive radiotherapy to the abdominal and pelvic regions (e.g. carcinoma cervix). Arrest of all division resulting in mucosal thinning, ulceration followed by oedema and later fibrosis are characteristic of this condition. Endarteritis and vasculitis also adds to these changes resulting in stricture, perforations, abscess, mal-absorption and multiple resection, etc.

Pathophysiological effects (Fig. 28.45), (Key Box 28.15)

It depends upon

- Extent of resection
- Site of resection
- Presence/absence of ileocaecal valve
- Age of the patients
- Infants tolerate extensive resections better than adults. Patients with less than 100 cm of the small bowel will develop severe nutritional deficiencies and may require parenteral nutrition.

1. **Malabsorption of fat and fat soluble vitamins** after ileal resections occur due to interruption of enterohepatic circulation of bile salts. These bile salts enter the colon and are converted into secondary bile salts. These bile salts block absorption of water and electrolytes.

2. **Gastric hypersecretion**

- Due to delayed clearance of gastrin, as in proximal

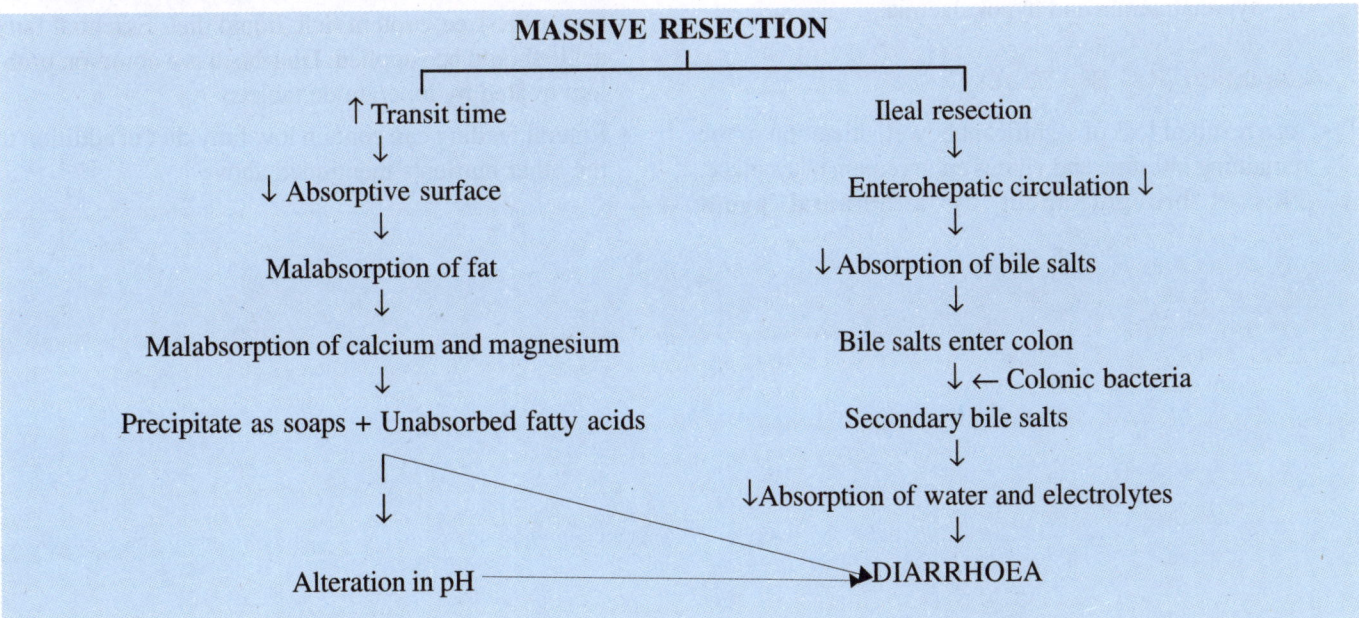

Fig. 28.45 Flowchart of nutritional deficiency in short gut syndrome

Key Box 28.15
EFFECTS OF SHORT GUT
<ul><li>Severe malabsorption</li><li>Gall stones</li><li>Fatty infiltration of liver</li><li>Urinary stones</li><li>Gastric hyperacidity</li></ul>

Key Box 28.16
ADAPTATION
<ul><li>Villous size↑</li><li>Length of bowel ↑</li><li>Transit time ↑</li><li>Absorption from colon↑</li></ul>

jejunal resections, there is increased gastric secretion of acids resulting in hyperacidity.

3. **Liver disease**
   - Fatty infiltration of the liver and mild hyperbilirubinaemia is a feature in massive resections and jejunoileal bypass. Acute fulminant hepatic failure can also occur.

4. **Gall stone formation**
   - There is increased incidence of cholesterol stones as a result of reduced bile salt pool, after ileal resection and jejunoileal bypass.

5. **Urinary stones**
   - All types of urinary stones are common due to low levels of calcium excretion in the urine and high levels of oxalate.
   - Water and salt depletion and loss of K^+ causes hyponatraemia and hypokalaemia.

Adaptation (Key Box 28.16)

- As a result of loss of significant bowel, dilatation of the remaining intestine and villous enlargement takes place. This is brought about by a humoral agent enteroglucagon. In children, length of the bowel is increased. Also, the number of cells in the villi is increased (work hypertrophy). There is also evidence to suggest gradual slowing of the transit time.

Treatment

- Treatment of short-gut patients is difficult. It needs a special set up of dieticians who plan a "proper food" for these patients in consultation with treating surgeons. It is a gradual process of feeding the patient starting from parenteral nutrition to normal low fat diet after few months.

- In the initial 2-3 months following massive resection, total parenteral nutrition including supplementation of fluid and electrolytes is the ideal treatment. Sips of plain water or oral hypotonic solutions can be used.

- After 2-3 months, when adaptation of bowel takes place, enteral feeding is started gradually with baby food, fat-free, fibre-free, protein rich, liquid diet. Essential fatty acids should be supplied. Diarrhoea is a common problem treated by loperamide tablets.

- Enteral feeding can contain low fatty diet in addition to the other nutrients mentioned above.

Large Intestine

29

- Surgical anatomy
- Function
- Blood supply
- Tumours
- Carcinoma
- Diverticular disease

SURGICAL ANATOMY

- Large intestine extends from ileocaecal valve to anus. It has five segments: right colon, left colon, transverse colon, sigmoid colon, rectum and anal canal. (Fig. 29.1)

- Average length is about 135 - 150 cms.

- Interestingly, alternating portions of the colon is mobile and fixed. Ascending colon and descending colon are fixed but caecum, transverse colon and sigmoid colon are mobile. Mobile structures can undergo twisting (volvulus).

- **Right colon** is big and hepatic flexure is broad.

- **Left colon** is small and splenic flexure is acute, hence ischaemic colitis commonly affects splenic flexure. Splenic flexure is deeply situated, therefore the malignancy in this area can easily be missed.

- **Muscle coat:** Outer longitudinal muscle is arranged in the form of three strips called as taenia coli. All three join at the rectosigmoid junction and form a complete longitudinal layer of the rectum. These three taenia coli converge at the base of the appendix. This is an important method to localise appendix.

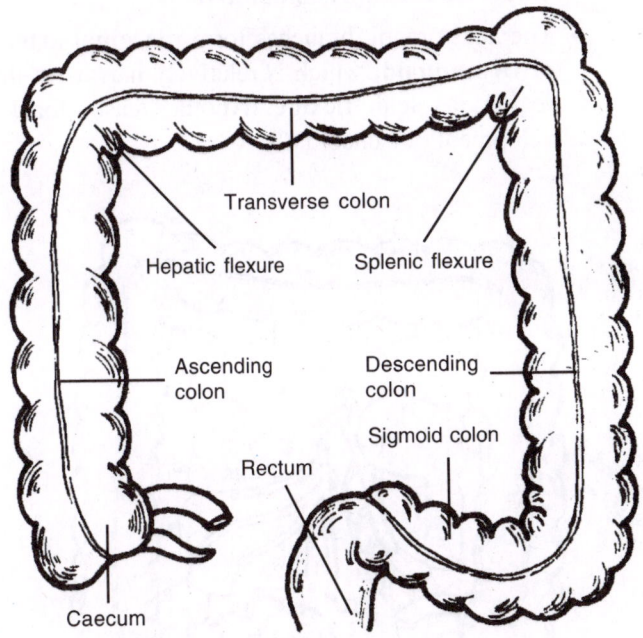

Fig. 29.1 Parts of the large intestine

BLOOD SUPPLY OF COLON

Arterial supply

1. **Superior mesenteric artery**, a branch of abdominal aorta is given at the level of first lumbar vertebra (L_1). It supplies the entire small bowel and the right colon up to 1/3rd of transverse colon. **Branches** of superior mesenteric artery (SMA) are

   A. **Middle colic artery** supplies the transverse colon mainly. It divides into right and left branches.

B. **Right colic artery** which supplies right colon.

C. **Ileocolic artery** supplies the terminal ileum and ascending colon. It divides into anterior and posterior caecal branches and supplies caecum and appendix through appendicular artery.

2. **Inferior mesenteric artery (IMA),** a branch of abdominal aorta given at the level of L_3 supplies the left colon, up to mucocutaneous junction at the lower end of anal canal (Hilton's line). Its branches are :

A. **Left colic artery** which anastomoses with branches of middle colic artery. It divides into upper and lower branches supplying the descending colon.

B. **3 sigmoidal branches.**

C. **Superior haemorrhoidal artery.**

• The anastomotic branches form **marginal artery of Drummond,** which is relatively narrow in the region of splenic flexure. (Another reason for development of ischaemia)

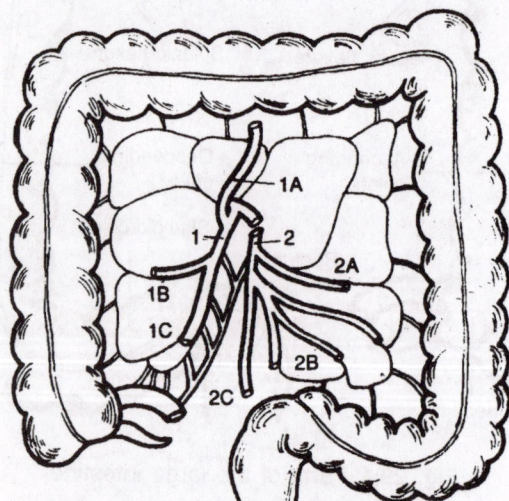

Fig. 29.2 Blood supply of the colon

Venous supply

• Follows the corresponding artery and empty into superior and inferior mesenteric veins, ultimately draining into the portal vein.

COLONIC FUNCTION

1. Absorption

• Water content is reduced from 1000 to 1500 ml, per day. Thus stools become solid. Similarly, sodium, potassium and bile salts are also absorbed.

Significance: In cases of diarrhoea there would be loss of water, sodium, potassium and other electrolytes.

2. Secretion

• Colon also secretes K^+ and cl^-. It is increased in colitis. Chloride secretion is increased in cystic fibrosis.

3. Motility

• Colon has 4 types of motility. Propulsive, retropulsive, mass peristalsis and gastrocolic reflux. Thus contents travel aborally.

4. Recycling

• Recycling of various nutrients takes place in the colon. Few examples; fermentation of carbohydrates, short chain fatty acids, urea cycling etc.

• Butyrate is the main product of bacterial fermentation. It is required mainly for fuel for colonic epithelium.

> *More distal the colon- more protein metabolism and putrefaction resulting in carcinogens and greater exposure to colonic mucosa. Hence, two thirds of colonic cancer occur in the left colon.*

TUMOURS OF THE LARGE INTESTINE

Benign tumours are usually referred to polyp, which means **elevated from the surface.** They are as follows:

1. ADENOMATOUS POLYP

• It may be a villous adenoma which is a flat lesion or a tubular adenoma having a pedicle. Tubular is more common.

• They give rise to bleeding, diarrhoea and hypokalaemia.

• They can be single or multiple

• They are premalignant and the risk of malignancy is greater with increase in the size of the adenoma.

• Today, they can be removed with the colonoscope-polypectomy.

• Malignant potential of villous adenoma is more than tubular adenoma.

• Adenoma less than 1 cm-risk of malignancy is 1%; 1-2 cm is 10%; > 2 cm is 30%.

2. HAMARTOMATOUS POLYP

- This can occur in the colon as in Peutz-Jegher's syndrome. Risk of malignancy is very limited. Symptomatic polyps need to be treated.

- **Juvenile polyps** are usually single and occur in children. They give rise to bleeding and are easily resected. They do not have malignant potential.

3. FAMILIAL POLYPOSIS COLI (FPC) OR FAMILIAL ADENOMATOUS POLYPOSIS

- It is a genetic disorder inherited as a Mendelian dominant. The gene is APC (Adenomatous Polyposis Coli) and is located in the short arm of chromosome 5. Prevalence : 1 in 10,000.

- It is transmitted from both sexes. The incidence is same in either sex.

- When it is associated with desmoid tumour, craniofascial osteoma, epidermoid cysts, congenital hypertrophy of retinal pigment epithelium, it is described as **Gardner's syndrome**.

- When familial polyposis coli is associated with central nervous system tumour and glioblastoma it is called as **Turcot's syndrome**.

- 50% of them have benign gastric polyps and 90% of them have duodenal polyps.

Clinical features

- Runs in families; other members of the family are affected

- Manifests at the age of 20 years in the form of blood and mucous in the stool, loose stools, etc. It produces crampy lower abdominal pain.

- Anaemia and protein malnutrition occur slowly

- Mean age of development of carcinoma is 39 years

Diagnosis

- Confirmed by sigmoidoscopy or colonoscopy which reveal multiple polyps varying from few millimetres to centimetres and are sessile. Biopsy has to be taken. Polyps are visible after 15 years, certainly by the age of 30 years.

Complication

- Incidence of malignancy is **100%**

Treatment

- **NSAID: Sulindac** 300 mg. twice a day and **aspirin** 325 mg. once a day have been found to decrease the size of polyps.

- Patients, who are above the age of 30 years have high chances of having a carcinoma in the colon. Hence even when there is no malignancy, surgery is advisable.

Types of Surgery

- Many patients do not like ileostomy. Hence, a subtotal colectomy with ileorectal anastomosis can be done. This is done provided that rectum is examined frequently and endoscopic snaring of the polyps is done regularly, especially in a young patient.

- **Restorative proctocolectomy** with ileoanal anastamosis by using a pouch is another alternative. (Refer Page 465 for details)

  However, it is a major surgical procedures and should be undertaken only by an experienced surgeon.

Screening

- Starts from the age of 10 years by sigmoidoscopy

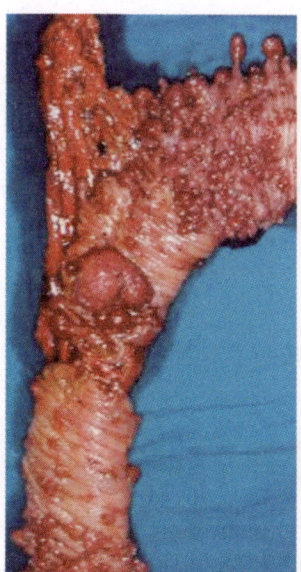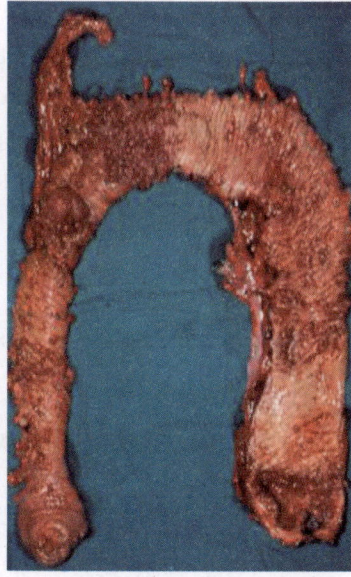

Fig. 29.3 and Fig. 29.4 Familial polyposis coli with two malignancies - lower rectum and hepatic flexure. This patient was being treated for chronic diarrhoea for 7-8 years with various medications. Colonoscopy was done first time in our hospital. Total proctocolectomy specimen - Contributed by Dr. Challa Srinivas Rao, Associate Professor, Dept. of Surgery, G.S.L. Medical College, Rajamundri, Andhra Pradesh

Table 29.1 Summary of colonic polyps.

TYPE	CAUSE	MALIGNANT POTENTIAL	FEATURES/SYNDROME
1. Adenomatous polyp	Benign tumour	1-10%	Hypokalaemia, diarrhoea
2. Hamartomatous polyp	"Misfire"	Negligible	Peutz-Jeghers syndrome
3. Familial polyposis coli	Genetic disorder	100%	Gardner's and Turcot's syndrome
4. Metaplastic polyps	Hyperplasia	Nil	Asymptomatic

4. METAPLASTIC POLYP

- Also called as hyperplastic nodules. They are of viral aetiology. They do not have malignant potential. (Refer Table 29.1 for comparison)

HNPCC (HEREDITARY NONPOLYPOSIS COLORECTAL CANCER)

- Autosomal dominant, **No POLYPS**
- **Lynch Syndrome I :** Site specific colorectal cancer
- **Lynch II:** Cancer family syndrome - They have extracolonic cancers such as endometrial cancer, ovarian cancer, Transitional cell cancer etc.

Diagnostic criteria

1. Atleast 3 members in a family should have colorectal cancer - two of whom are first degree relatives.
2. At least two consecutive generations
3. At least one relative should have colorectal cancer by less than 50 years of age

Screening

- Increased incidence of proximal colonic cancer

CARCINOMA COLON

Carcinoma colon is the most common malignancy in the Western world after the age of 50. If the diagnosis is made early it is still a curable cancer. Over a period of years the understanding of development of carcinoma has changed and more and more molecular biology of colonic cancer is being discussed. (Key Box 29.1)

PRECANCEROUS CONDITIONS (Key Box 29.2)

1. Polyps: Environmental and genetic factors favour the

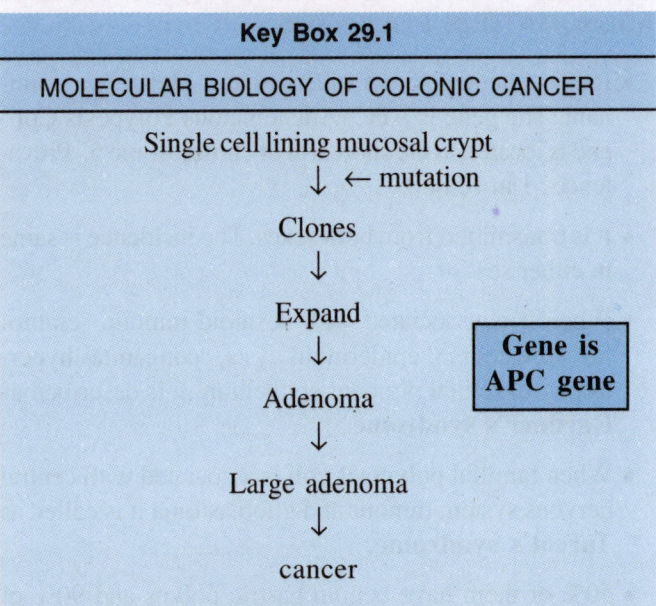

Key Box 29.1

MOLECULAR BIOLOGY OF COLONIC CANCER

Single cell lining mucosal crypt
↓ ← mutation
Clones
↓
Expand
↓
Adenoma
↓
Large adenoma
↓
cancer

Gene is APC gene

development of colonic polyps and their transformations into malignancy. The incidence of malignancy is increased when the polyp is more than 1 cm, polyps are multiple or flat (refer Table 29.1).

Familial polyposis coli has 100% chance of carcinoma.

2. Inflammatory bowel disease

   A. **Ulcerative colitis** is a definite precancerous con-

Key Box 29.2

PREMALIGNANT CONDITIONS CARCINOMA COLON

- Familial polyposis coli
- Ulcerative colitis
- Adenomatous polyp
- Crohn's colitis
- Hamartomatous polyp - very very rare

dition. Presence of dysplasia diagnosed by colonoscopic biopsy is an indication for colectomy.

   B.Crohn's involving colon also has a mildly increased risk of developing carcinoma when compared to ulcerative colitis.

Aetiological factors

1. **SAD factors:** *It is sad to know that* **SAD** *factors are responsible for carcinoma colon.* They are: S-Smoking, **A**-Alcohol, **D**-Dietary factors. Diet rich in red meat has high animal fat, this alters intestinal bacteria, which converts primary bile acids into secondary bile acids. This is the beginning of formation of carcinogenic polycyclic aromatic compounds. After cholecystectomy, there is increase in free bile acid concentration, thus increasing the risk of colonic cancer.

2. **Genetic factors** have been found in carcinoma of the colon. Colorectal families have been identified.

Calcium salts are protective. They form insoluble bile salt complexes, thus reduce the concentration of bile acids in the colon.

Pathological types (Fig. 29.5)

Rectum (40%) and sigmoid (20%) take a major share in colorectal carcinoma followed by caecum (12 to 15%). Multiple synchronous cancers are also common in the colon.

   A. **Annular stricture**-Common in left colon (splenic flexure, pelvic colon).

   B. **Tubular stricture**-Common in left colon and at the rectosigmoid junction.

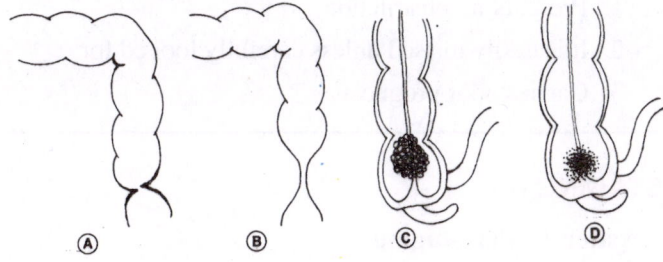

Fig. 29.5 Types of carcinoma colon.

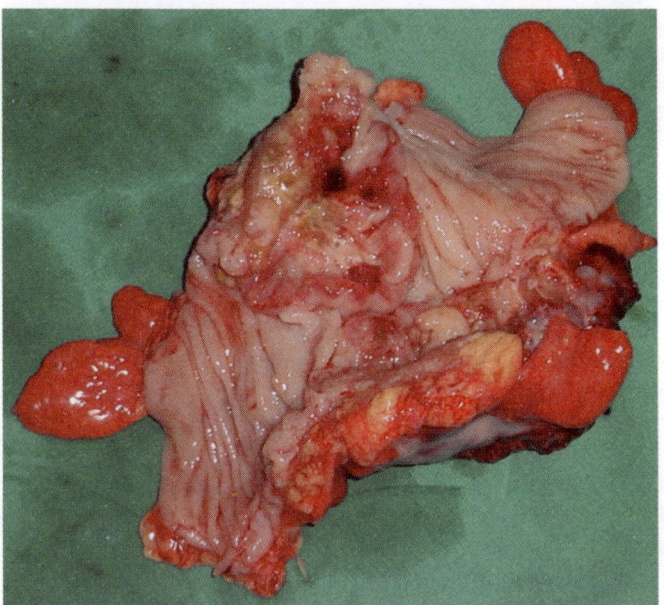

Fig. 29.6 Ulceroproliferative growth in the descending colon

   C. **Ulcerative lesion** - Ascending colon or caecum

   D. **Proliferative growth** - More in right colon, the least malignant, fleshy and bulky polypoid lesion

   • It is a columnar cell adenocarcinoma. In about 5% of cases, it undergoes mucoid degeneration. Such tumours carry poor prognosis. They spread to the liver very fast and secondaries produce mucoid material.

CLINICAL FEATURES OF CARCINOMA COLON (MNEMONIC = T.M.A. PAI)[1]

1. **Tumour**: The mass produced by carcinoma caecum and even hepatic flexure is palpable. It is firm to hard, irregular and with or without fixity (Fig. 29.6).

   • Occasionally, growth at pelvirectal junction can be felt on rectal examination.

   • However, on left sided constrictive lesions, growth is not often felt. It is the hard faecal matter and lymph nodes which are felt as a mass.

2. **Metastasis:** 5-10% patients present with metastasis to liver (mucoid adenocarcinoma), ascites, etc. Distant metastasis is not common (Fig. 29.7).

3. **Anaemia** is an important feature of carcinoma caecum. It may be due to blood loss or a proliferative growth secreting toxins causing suppression of bone

---

1. *Late* **Dr. T. M. A. Pai** *is the founder of Kasturba Medical College and Hospital, which is a part of Manipal Academy of Higher Education, (M.A.H.E. University) Manipal 576 104, Karnataka, South India.*

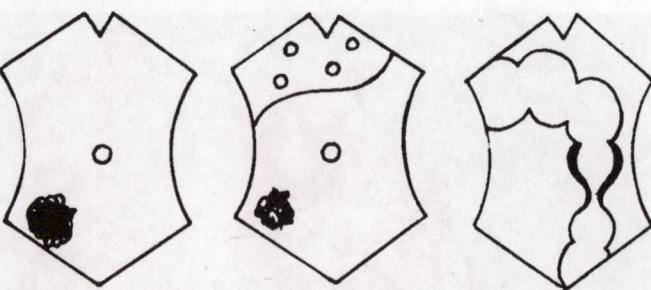

Fig. 29.7 Carcinoma caecum **29.8** Carcinoma caecum with secondaries in the liver **29.9** Carcinoma left colon with intestinal obstruction

marrow. Asthaenia and anorexia are the other features.

4. **Pain** abdomen: Dull aching pain may be present. Colicky pain is due to chronic obstruction as in left sided growths (napkin ring stricture).

5. **Alteration** in the bowel habits: A recent constipation, increase in the dose of laxatives followed by attacks of diarrhoea can be due to carcinoma colon. Diarrhoea is due to hard faecal balls, irritating the colonic mucosa resulting in increasing secretion of mucous produced by proximal colon.

6. **Intestinal obstruction** is caused by constricted left sided lesions (Fig. 29.9). On the left side, diameter of colon is narrow, contents are solid and growth is constrictive. Lower abdominal distension, right to left peristalsis are the late features. Carcinoma sigmoid can cause colovesical fistula.

Key Box 29.3

PECULIARITIES OF CARCINOMA SIGMOID

- Commonly presents as obstructive lesion - constipation / intestinal obstruction
- Colovesical fistula: Carcinoma sigmoid is the 2nd commonest cause
- It can cause colovaginal fistula
- It can also infiltrate ureter, uterus and ovary
- It can present as abscess in the lateral abdominal wall

Obstructed and perforated carcinoma colon have poor prognosis.

Key Box 29.4

PECULIARITES OF CARCINOMA OF CAECUM

1. Incidence is more in females
2. Presents with anaemia and a mass
3. Can present as acute appendicitis when the lumen of appendix is obstructed (in elderly patients)
4. It is a cause of intussusception (secondary) (Fig. 29.10)

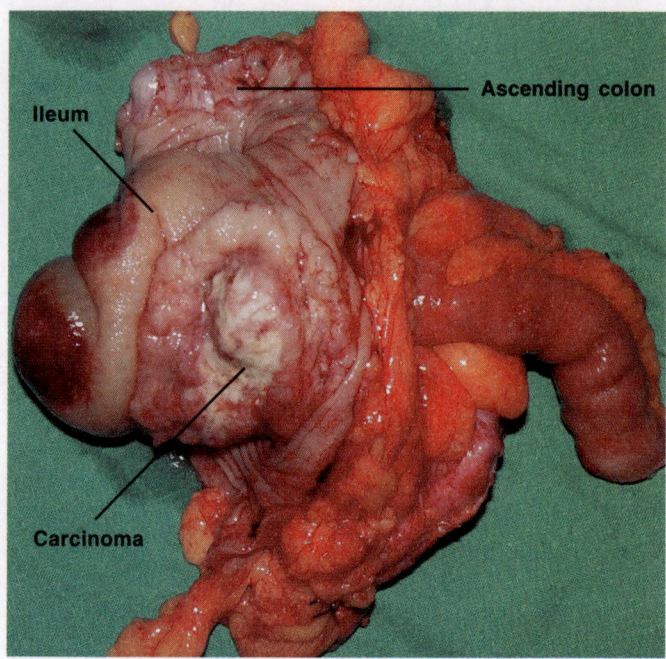

Fig. 29.10 Intussusception due to carcinoma caecum

Key Box 29.5

PECULIARITES OF CARCINOMA SPLENIC FLEXURE

1. Presents as obstruction
2. It is easily missed unless carefully looked for
3. Carries poor prognosis

STAGING

Astler Coller staging

A : Limited to mucosa

B_1: Extend into muscularis propria

B_2 : Extend into entire bowel wall

B_3: Extend into adjacent organs

C_1: B_1+ Lymph nodes

C_2: B_2 + Lymph nodes

C_3: B_3 + Lymph nodes

SPREAD

1. **Local**: For a long time, the lesion is confined to mucosa and submucosa. They grow in annular fashion and later longitudinally. Once serosa is involved, spread occurs rapidly into neighbouring structures like ureter, bladder, uterus etc. The involvement of these structures is **not a contraindication** for surgery.

2. **Lymphatic spread**
   - **N1 :** Epicolic, paracolic nodes are the first to get involved.
   - **N2 :** Nodes at the origin of ileocolic and middle colic artery.
   - **N3 :** Nodes at the origin of superior and inferior mesenteric artery are involved in approximately 50% of the patients at presentation to the hospital.

3. **Blood spread:** It occurs late, resulting in secondaries in the liver, etc.

Because of the drainage into the portal system, colonic cancers spread to the liver first. On the other hand, rectal cancers spread to the lungs because of drainage into inferior vena cava

COMPLICATIONS

1. **Intestinal obstruction.** (Fig. 29.11)

2. **Pericolic abscess :** Pain is present in the tumour site and may radiate to back or to the leg or hip as in caecal perforations. It is due to irritation to the psoas muscles or due to irritation of femoral nerve.

- Diagnosis is confirmed by ultrasound / CT scan.

- Percutaneous aspiration, followed later by elective resection is the best treatment.

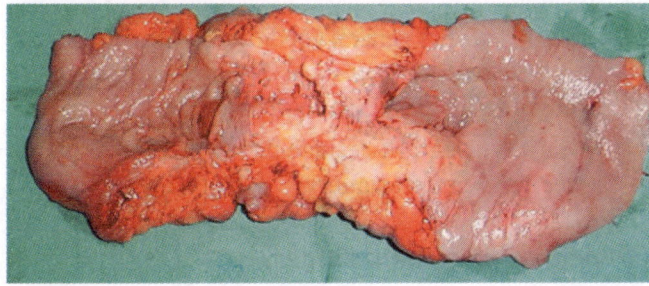

Fig.29.11 Intestinal obstruction due to recto-sigmoid stricture

3. **Faecal fistula** (Fig. 29.12)
   - Pericolic abscess when it is incised or drained to the exterior may result in faecal fistula if there is malignancy.
   - Carcinoma caecum may result in appendicitis and appendicectomy may invariably result in faecal fistula.

4. **Internal fistula:** Colovesical, colocolic, coloenteric are not uncommon complications by malignancies. They are managed by resection. However, preoperative assessment of fistulae by investigations should be done.

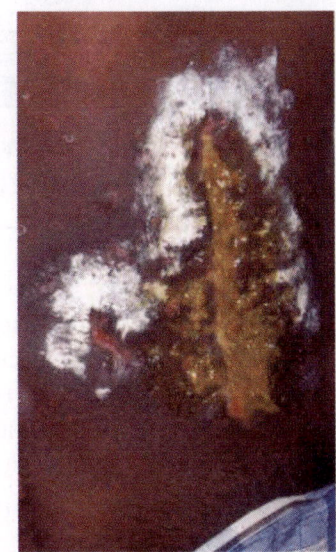

Fig. 29.12 Carcinoma colon perforated - pericolic abscess - which on draining resulted in faecal fistula

Involvement of local structures is not a contraindication for radical resection

INVESTIGATIONS

1. Complete blood picture demonstrates low Hb%

2. **Double contrast barium enema** may show irregular filling defect-intrinsic, persistent. It may also show an apple core deformity (Fig. 29.13, 29.14).

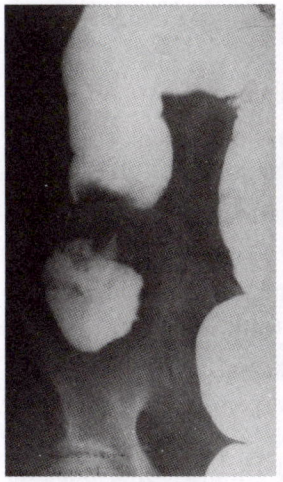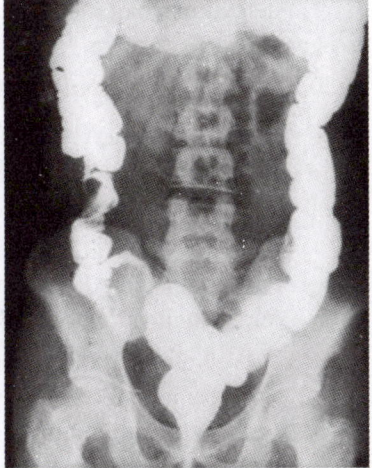

Fig. 29.13 Barium enema showing apple core deformity
29.14 Intrinsic irregular persistent filling defect

Key Box 29.10

BARIUM ENEMA

- Gives good anatomic and topographic information
- Can detect diverticular disease (associated)
- Small ulcerative lesions can also be diagnosed

3. **Colonoscopy** is done to take a biopsy from growth and also to rule out synchronous malignancy as in 5% of the cases (more than one malignancy at the time of diagnosis). If biopsy cannot be taken, as in obstruction, brush cytology can be taken.

- Small risk of perforation is present and it is an invasive procedure. (Fig. 29.15)

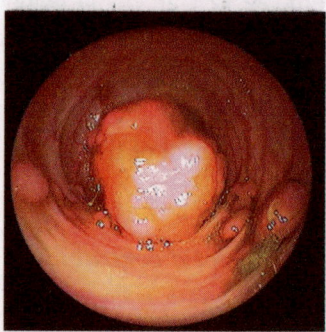 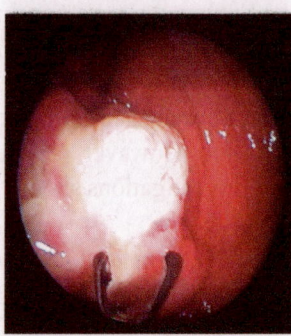

Fig. 29.15 Colonoscopy showing growth and biopsy is being taken. Contributed by Dr. Filipe Alvaris

4. **Ultrasound and CT** are baseline investigations today mainly to detect the spread of the disease - locally and distally (secondaries in liver, paraaortic nodes etc). Contrast enhanced CT is better than ultrasound in detecting small metastasis in liver. Guided biopsy can also be taken.

5. **Carcino Embryonic Antigen (CEA)**
   - It is a fetal glycoprotein, not present in normal human beings (minute quantities).
   - Present in last trimester in foetus.
   - If it appears in adults, the following diseases have to be considered: Carcinoma colon, pancreas and embryonal carcinoma of testis
   - Levels above 1000 international units are diagnostic of carcinoma colon. However, it has a prognostic rather than a diagnostic value. After treatment of the primary, CEA level should come back to normal. If it is increased, it suggests either recurrent tumour or secondaries in the liver.

Also in node negative colonic cancer, if preoperative CEA are increased, chemotherapy is recommended.

PROGNOSTIC FACTORS OF CARCINOMA COLON

1. **Spread**: Limited to mucosa, no nodes. 5 years survival is 90-100%.
2. **Histologic grade**: Well differentiated carcinoma is better than poorly differentiated variety.
3. **Anatomic location**: Splenic flexure growth has the worst prognosis. Ascending colon and rectosigmoid growths have better prognosis.
4. **Clinical presentation**: Patients who present with obstruction and perforation do worse than other patients.

MANAGEMENT

Key Box 29.11

GOALS

1. Remove primary tumour with adequate margin
2. Regional lymphadenectomy
3. Restoration of GI tract

Preoperative preparation

1. **Mechanical bowel preparation** by regular enemas, two to three days before surgery is necessary to reduce the bacterial load in the colon. This reduces incidence of anastomotic leakage.
   - **Whole gut irrigation by oral polyethylene glycol** is found to be superior than enemas. It is the method of choice today.
2. **Antibiotics :** Oral antibiotics neomycin/metronidazole or neomycin/erythromycin afternoon and evening before surgery are given mainly to decrease wound infection.
3. Improvement of general condition by correcting albumin levels and if necessary, TPN will definetely decrease the incidence of anastomotic leakage.
4. A fat free diet, low residue diet is prescribed two to three days before surgery.

Principles of colonic surgery

1. **No touch technique** of Turnbull by dividing the vas-

cular pedicle at the beginning of surgery will reduce the incidence of tumour embolism.

2. **Curative surgery** includes wide local excision, margin clearance, regional lymphadenectomy, removal of fat, fascia, etc.

3. Cut ends should have **good bleeding**

4. **Right sided** obstructive lesions are treated by **resection**.

5. **Left sided** obstructive lesions are better managed by a **temporary colostomy** followed two weeks later by elective colectomy.

SURGERY (Key Box 29.11)

- Over a period of years, the radical resections for carcinoma of colon have become less radical to the extent of bowel resection. For example: One need not remove terminal 30 cm of ileum for carcinoma caecum today. Only 6-8 cm of removal of ileum is more than enough in a right hemicolectomy.

Different types of surgery

1. **Carcinoma right colon including caecum**: If it is operable, the treatment is right radical hemicolectomy. Structures removed in this operation are (Fig.29.14, 29.15 and Key Box 29.12):

- **Terminal 6-8 cm of ileum**[1]
- Caecum, appendix and ascending colon
- 1/3 of transverse colon

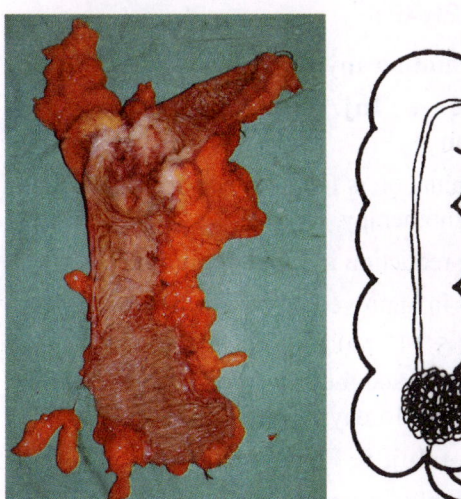
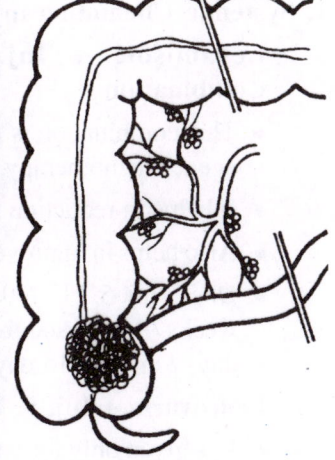

Fig. 29.16, 29.17 Right radical hemicolectomy

---

1. *One need not remove two feet of terminal ileum.*

- Fat, fascia, lymphatics and lymph nodes like ileocolic nodes, pericolic nodes, etc.

- If the growth is fixed to posterior abdominal wall, common iliac vessels, palliative ileotransverse anastomosis is done (ileotransverse colostomy)

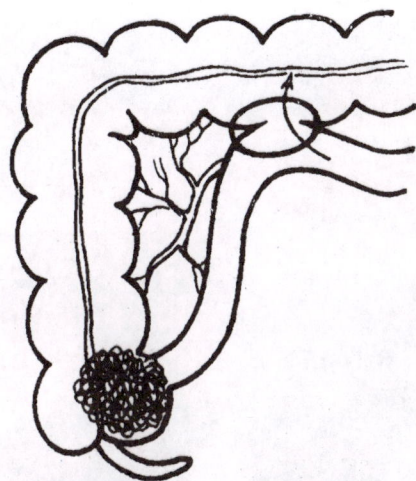

Fig. 29.18 Ileotransverse bypass.

2. **Carcinoma transverse colon**-'V' resection. The area supplied by middle colic artery is removed followed by end to end anastomosis. One may land up removing entire transverse colon (Fig. 29.18).

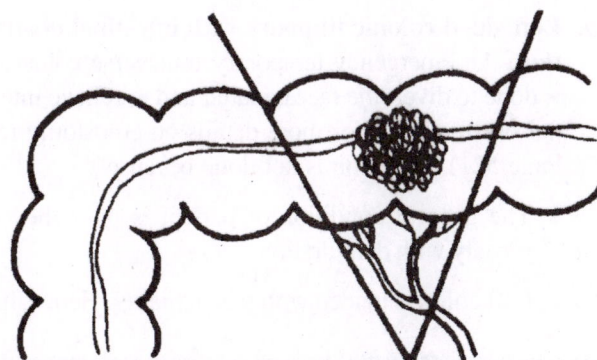

Fig. 29.19 Wide V-resection for carcinoma transverse colon.

Key Box 29.12
RIGHT HEMICOLECTOMY STRUCTURES WHICH CAN GET INJURED
• Duodenum • Ureter • Gonadal vessels

3. **Carcinoma left colon** - Left radical hemicolectomy.

   • Left half of the transverse colon and descending colon are removed followed by anastomosis of transverse colon to sigmoid colon-this is the area supplied by left colic artery (Fig. 29.20).

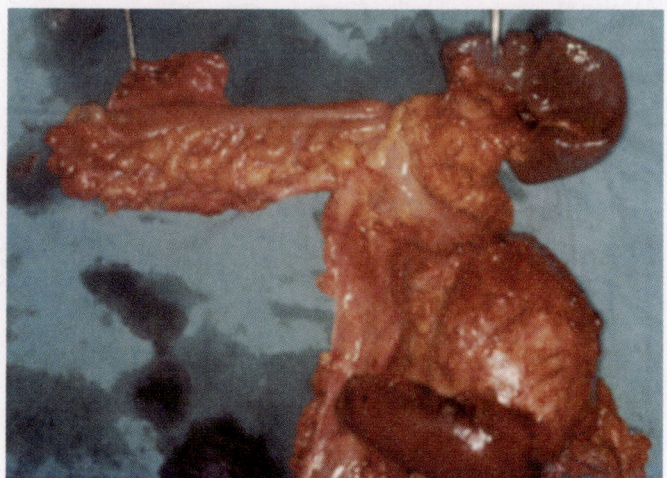

Fig. 29.20 Left radical hemicolectomy including removal of the spleen as the growth was infiltrating the spleen

4. **Carcinoma sigmoid colon**-Radical sigmoid colectomy followed by anastomosis of descending colon to the rectum (colorectal anastomosis) (Fig. 29.21).

5. **Left sided colonic tumours with intestinal obstruction.** An emergency temporary transverse colostomy is done to divert the faecal matter and to relieve intestinal obstruction. (For more details on colostomy refer Page 521) Resection is not done because

   • The general condition of patient is poor they are grossly with dehydration.

   • Left colon is loaded with faecal matter. Hence, high chances of anastomotic leakage and faecal peritonitis are present.

   • After 2 weeks, laparotomy is done once again. The primary tumour is resected and end to end anastomosis done. This is followed by closure of the colostomy 8 weeks later-**3 Stage operation**.

Single stage resection

• Obstructive lesions can also be managed by single stage resection provided, thorough colonic irrigation through appendicular stump (after appendicectomy), is successful in cleaning the entire colon.

• General condition of the patient should allow another **2 hours of extra time** for irrigation, resection and anastomosis.

• It avoids another 2 surgical procedures

• One stage resection and end to end anatomoses with protective colostomy is an another alternative procedure. Colostomy is closed after 6 weeks.

Wangensteen's second look operation

Since carcinoma of the colon has a good prognosis, regular follow-up of the patient is essential. For the first year, ultrasound examination of abdomen can be done once in 3 months, colonoscopy and CEA levels once in 6 months. If there is any suspicion of recurrence, a second look operation is advised, so that an early recurrent tumour can be resected. A solitary metastasis in the liver can be removed.

ADJUVANT THERAPY

I. Systemic Chemotherapy :Types

1. **Levamisole + Inj. 5 Flurouracil (5.FU) Combination**

   • This combination is found to be superior to single agent chemotherapy.

   • It helps in reduction in further recurrence

   • Also helps in improved survival

   • Dose : Inj. 5. FU 400 mg/m^2/day, I.V. x 5 day per 4 weeks / 1 year and Levamisole : 150 mg/day for 3 days / once in 15 days/ 1 year.

2. **Leucovarin + Inj. 5. Flurouracil**

   • It is given only for 6 months

   • Dose: Inj. 5. FU 400 mg/m^2/day, I.V. x 5 day per 4 weeks and Leucovarin: 20mg/m^2 /day x 5 days per 4 weeks per 6 months.

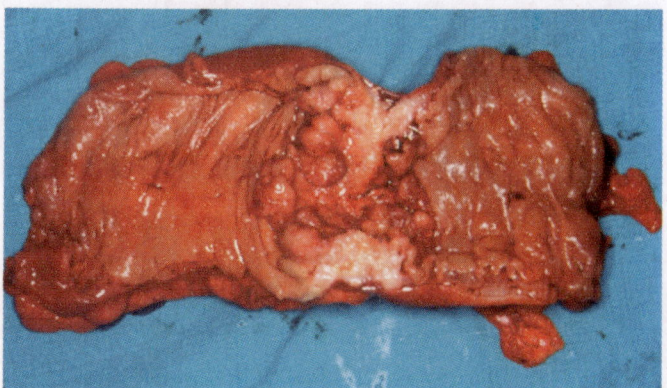

Fig. 29.21 Sigmoid colectomy

3. Adjuvant chemotherapy using injection 5-FU infusion and leucovorin with oxali platin is also being tried. The results are better with this regimen.

Key Box 29.13

INDICATIONS FOR CHEMOTHERAPY

1. All node positive patients
2. In node negative patients if:
   - T_4 lesions involving free mesothelial surface
   - Major microscopic vein involvement
   - Signet cell carcinoma
   - High pre-operative CEA
   - Aneuploidy on flow cytometry

II. Immunotherapy

- Autologous tumour vaccines and monoclonal antibodies have been tried as nonspecific stimulation of immune system.

III. Radiotherapy (Key Box 29.14)

- Adenocarcinoma colon does not respond well to radiotherapy unlike carcinoma rectum.

Key Box 29.14

INDICATIONS FOR RADIOTHERAPY

- Soft tissue infiltration into psoas or abdominal wall
- Inoperable or recurrent tumours

Follow up (Key Box 29.15)

- Most of the colonic cases are curable if diagnosed and treated early. Also metachronous lesion can occur in the rest of colon. Hence certain tests are necessary during follow up.

Treatment of recurrent or metastatic cancer

- Recurrence or metastasis is suspected during follow up by abnormal values of investigation.
- Recurrent tumour should be resected enblock - it may amount to a more radical procedure - it may amount to resection of duodenum, liver, kidney etc.
- Metastasis in the liver (Key Box 29.16)

Key Box 29.15

FOLLOW UP OF COLORECTAL CANCER

Tests	Duration	In yrs.
1. Haemoccult	Once in 3-6 months	3
2. Colonoscopy	6 months after surgery, later once in a year	3
3. Alkaline phosphatase	Once in 3-6 months for 3 years	3
4. CEA	Once in 6 months	3
5. Chest Xray	Yearly	

Key Box 29.16

INDICATIONS FOR RESECTION

- Solitary metastasis or metastasis confined to one lobe
- < 3 metastasis in both lobes
- Absence of extrahepatic disease

DIVERTICULAR DISEASE OF COLON

- It is an acquired condition, in which colonic mucosa herniates through the circular muscle fibres at weak points, where blood vessels penetrate the colonic wall. Since it is acquired it lacks the muscle coat. Hence, they are thin, more prone for infections and perforation. Hence they are pseudodiverticuli.

AETIOPATHOGENESIS

- The disease is common in western population wherein diet is very **poor in fibres** because of refining of sugar and flour. **NSP (nonstarch polysaccharides)** or low dietary fibres are the chief factor for **diverticulosis of colon.** As a result of this, the contents of the bowel are hard. Very high pressure can develop within colon which causes increased **segmentation** and circular muscle thickening resulting in diverticular disease. In Africans and Indians, the disease is rare because of high fibre content of the diet.

- The disease starts after the age of 40. Any stress, emotional disorders may add to the constipation already caused by dietary factors and result in diverticular formation.

- **90% of them affect sigmoid colon.** Rectum is spared in majority. Rarely it affects right colon.

Key Box 29.17

NSP AND DISEASES

- Diverticular disease
- Obesity and diabetes
- Constipation, piles
- Breast cancer and colonic cancer

- Diverticula project between antimesenteric and mesenteric borders with taenia, but they never penetrate taenia.

- There is **muscle hypertrophy,** which project into the lumen as obstructive folds. The mucosa is essentially normal. Slowly luminal diameter is narrowed.

- **Inflammation** occurs in the pericolonic tissue with or without abscess formation.

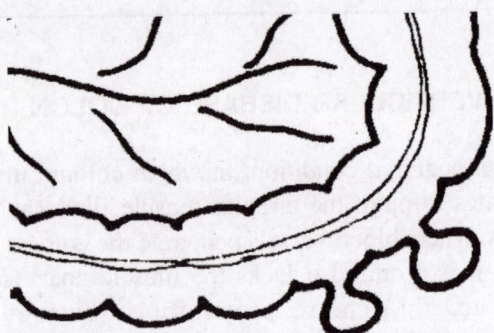

Fig. 29.22 Diverticula in the sigmoid colon

CLINICAL FEATURES

1. **Diverticulosis:** It refers to presence of divelticulosis without much symptoms. But on careful questioning, patients do have lower abdominal distention, heaviness, flatulence, etc. Vague abdominal pain is also felt in the left iliac fossa.

2. **Diverticulitis:** Left-sided lower abdominal pain, moderate to severe, associated with passage of loose stools. Pain is partially relieved on passing flatus.

   - Bleeding per rectum can be the presenting feature, sometimes it can be massive.

   - Low grade fever, tenderness, rigidity and even mass may be present in the left iliac fossa (like left-sided appendicitis). Mass is thickened, inflamed, tender, sigmoid. Such attacks result in abscess which rupture into hollow organs and give rise to fistulae.

3. **Internal fistulae:** Colovescical fistula gives rise to pneumaturia (flatus in the urine) and rarely faeces in the urine

The most common fistula in acute diverticulitis is colovescical followed by colovaginal

INVESTIGATIONS

1. **Sigmoidoscopy:** Mucosa may be normal or may show erythematous and oedematous changes. Ulcers are absent. Opening of diverticulae can be seen.

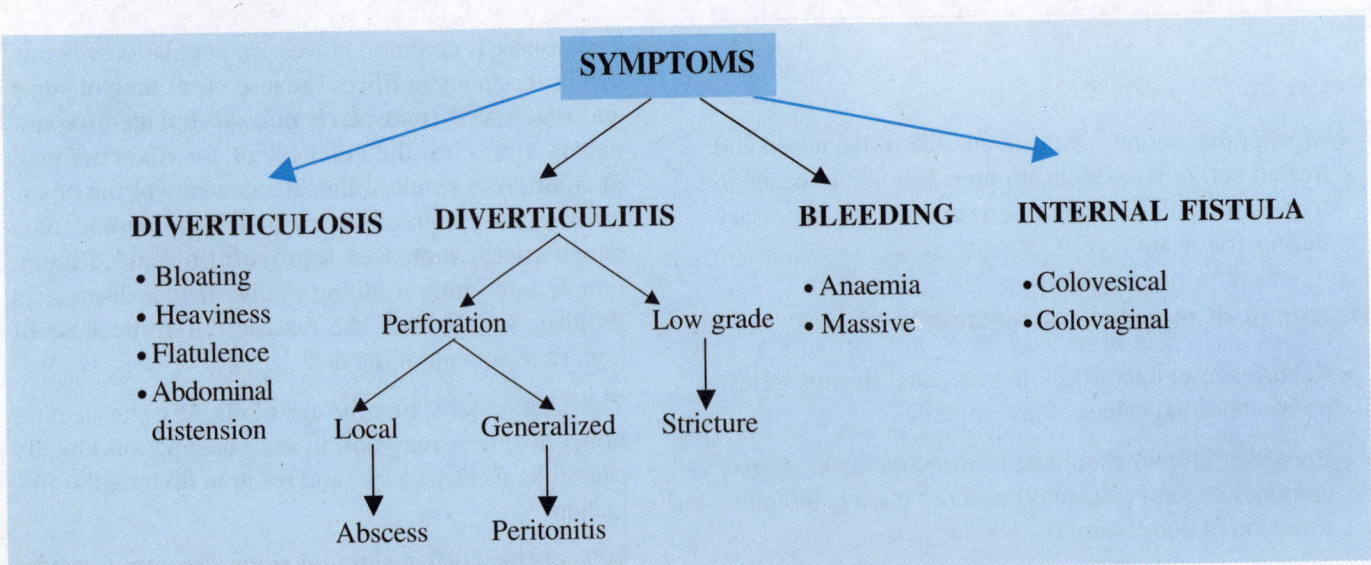

Fig. 29.23 Summary of the symptoms of diverticular disease

2. **Barium enema: Contraindicated in acute cases.**
   - It may show **"saw tooth"** appearance due to muscle hypertrophy.
   - It may show a long stricture
3. **Colonoscopy** to confirm the findings and to rule out **carcinoma colon**. (Fig. 29.24)

Sigmoidoscopy, colonoscopy and barium enema are contraindicated in acute diverticulitis.

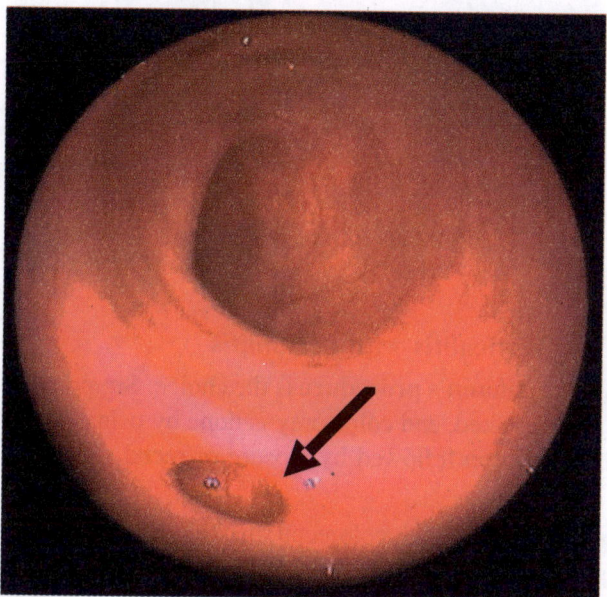

Fig. 29.24 Colonoscopy showing opening of diverticula

4. Ultrasound and CT scan is the investigation of choice in acute diverticulitis. (Fig. 29.25)

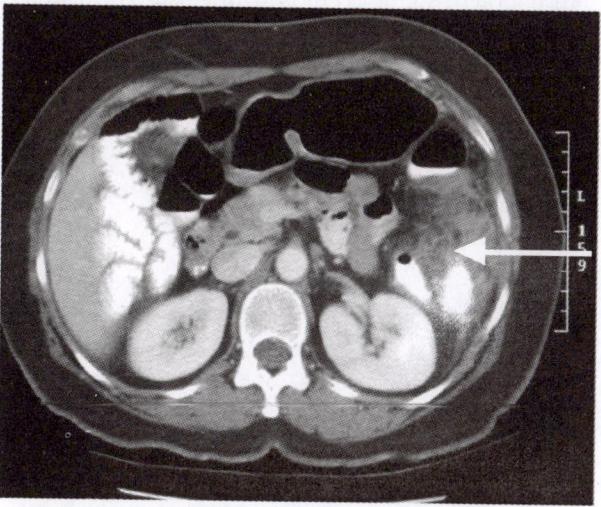

Fig. 29.25 CT Scan showing pericolic abscess

Key Box 29.18

CT SCAN ACUTE DIVERTICULITIS

- Can detect thick muscular folds - thus confirm the diagnosis
- Detect an abscess - thus confirm complication
- Detect extraluminal air or contrast - thus confirm perforation
- Can rule out other causes - acute pancreatitis with pericolic collection etc.
- It is the investigation of choice in acute diverticulitis

COMPLICATIONS

1. **Massive haemorrhage** per rectum: Haemorrhage is due to vessels in the base of diverticula, more so in atherosclerotic or hypertensive patients.
2. **Stricture** of sigmoid colon can develop due to recurrent attacks resulting in intestinal obstruction.
3. **Perforation** may result in peritonitis, pericolic abscess or pelvic abscess (Fig. 29.26).

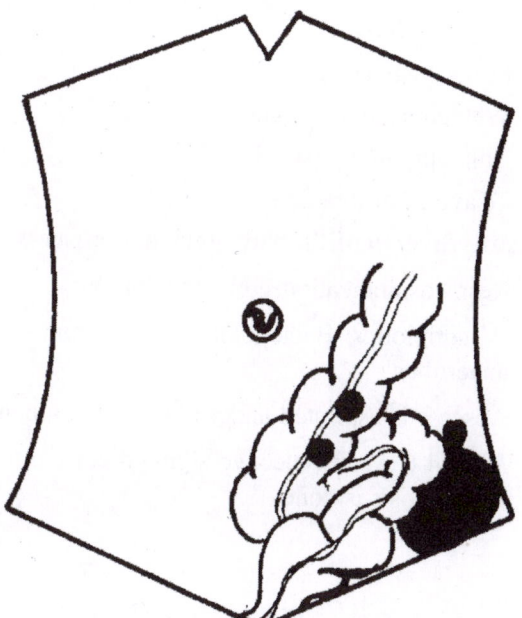

Fig. 29.26 Pericolic abscess

4. **Fistula formation:** Internal fistulae occur due to inflammatory adhesions and abscess formation which ruptures resulting in fistula. Thus, colovesical, colovaginal, colointestinal fistula can occur (Fig. 29.27).

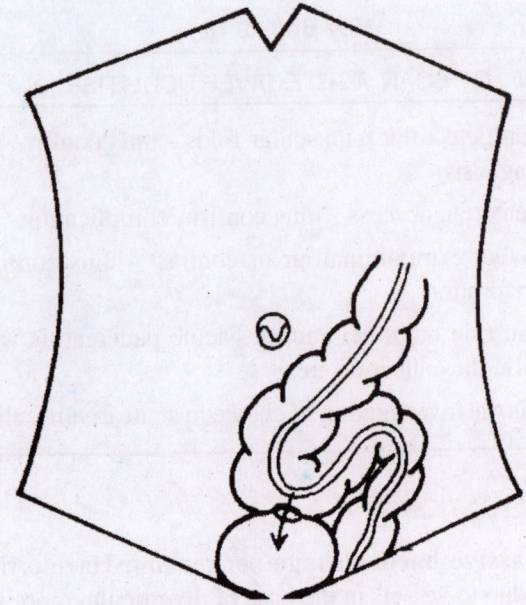

Fig. 29.27 Colovesical fistula

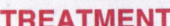

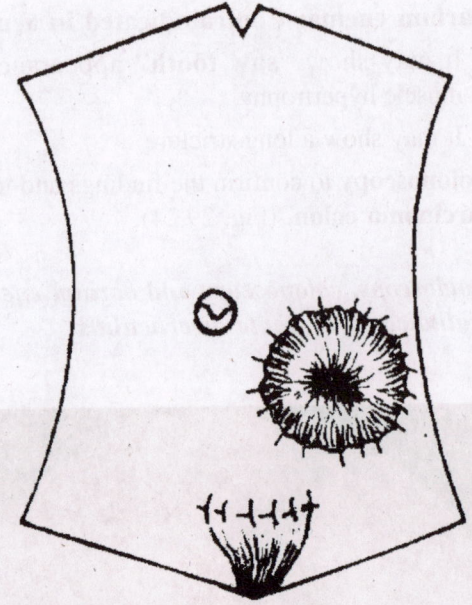

Fig.29.28 Hartmann's procedure

TREATMENT

1. **Stage of diverticulosis** or in those patients who have recovered from one attack of diverticulitis.

   • High residue diet

   • Fruits, vegetables

   • Wholemeal bread, flour

   • Bulk purgative - Isogel

   • To avoid constipation

2. **Acute diverticulitis with pericolic abscess**

   • Rest, hospitalization, correct hydration

   • IV antibiotics: Bactericidal against gram -ve and anaerobes

   • Abscess is aspirated under ultrasound guidance.

   • After 4-6 weeks, elective sigmoid colectomy and anastomosis is done.

3. **Diverticulitis with peritonitis**

A. **Hartmann's procedure** is the choice: Sigmoid colon is resected, end colostomy is done by using descending colon followed by closure of rectal stump. (Fig. 29.28)

   • After 4-6 weeks, colorectal anastomosis is done.

B. However if a **perforation is small**, general condition is good, after the resection, colon is irrigated with 8-10 litres of saline till the contents are clear, followed by colorectal anastomosis in the same sitting.

4. **Treatment of fistulae:** As an elective procedure, with good preparation, after confirming the site of fistula, resection of sigmoid colon with closure of fistula can be done.

Intestinal Obstruction

30

- Intestinal obstruction
- Sigmoid volvulus
- Meckel's diverticulum
- Adhesions and bands
- Gall stone ileus
- Intussusception
- Food bolus obstruction
- Mesenteric ischaemia
- Hirschsprung's disease
- Atresia and stenosis
- Volvulus neonatorum
- Imperforate anus
- Paralytic ileus
- Pseudointestinal obstruction

INTESTINAL OBSTRUCTION

- When the intestinal contents are prevented from travelling distally, it is called intestinal obstruction.

CLASSIFICATION

I. Depending upon the nature of obstruction

A. **Dynamic** obstruction/mechanical obstruction

B. **Adynamic** obstruction-paralytic ileus or neurogenic ileus

II. Depending upon the cause of obstruction

A. **In the lumen of the gut:**
- Gall stones ileus
- Food bolus obstruction
- Roundworm mass
- Foreign body (rare)
- Meconium ileus

B. **In the wall of the gut**
- Stricture eg. tuberculosis
- Crohn's disease
- Carcinoma
- Atresia
- Adhesions

C. **Outside the wall of the gut**
- Volvulus, intussusception
- Congenital bands
- Meckel's diverticulum with band
- Obstructed hernia

III. Depending upon severity of obstruction

A. **Acute obstruction:** Signs and symptoms appear very early. Usually, it affects small bowel, e.g. volvulus, obstructed hernia.

B. **Chronic obstruction** (eg. carcinoma colon) affects large bowel (colic comes first, distension later) diverticular disease can also produce chronic obstructions.

C. **Acute on chronic obstruction** develops in carcinoma colon, wherein an acute obstruction suddenly results due to the accumulation of faecal matter in the proximal bowel.

IV. Depending on the blood supply

A. **Simple obstructions:** Blood supply is not seriously impaired.

B. **Strangulated obstruction:** Blood supply is seriously impaired.

C. **Closed loop obstructions:** This occurs in carcinoma of the right colon with constrictive lesions. If the ileocaecal valve is competent and if the obstruction is total, the intraluminal pressure within the colon increases. As a result of which, the caecum may perforate. Thus, closed loop obstruction can be dangerous (Fig. 30.1).

PATHOPHYSIOLOGY (Figs. 30.2 and 30.3)

- As a result of obstruction, the proximal bowel undergoes hyperperistalsis which is responsible for colicky pain abdomen. The peristalsis may continue for a few days and later the intestine may be paralysed and flaccid. After 3-4 hours, distal to the obstruction, all physiological activities of the bowel are stopped. Intestine becomes contracted, pale and does not exhibit peristalsis. After a few hours, the proximal bowel gets dilated secondary to obstruction.

- The causes of distension of intestinal loop are:

A. Gaseous distension

- Swallowed air (70%). Because of colic and anxiety, the swallowed air is increased. Oxygen is absorbed and nitrogen is released which cannot be absorbed. This results in distension.

- Diffusion of air from the blood into bowel lumen produces carbon dioxide which diffuses very rapidly.

- Gas due to bacterial activity releases H_2S, NH_3 etc.

B. Distension due to fluids:

- 1500 ml of saliva
- 2 litres of gastric juice
- 3 litres of intestinal secretions
- 1 litre of bile and pancreatic juice

Normally, all this fluid is absorbed in the bowel. In cases of intestinal obstruction, this fluid absorption is delayed. It accumulates in the intestinal loop. Excretion of water and electrolytes into the lumen is also increased.

Strangulation (Key Box 30.1)

- **Interference with blood supply**: As the tension within the loops become more and more, venous congestion takes place resulting in oedema of the bowel wall.

- If the obstruction is not relieved, capillary rupture and haemorrhage into bowel may ensue. In cases of volvulus and intussusception, the arterial compromise takes place rapidly causing gangrene of bowel wall very early. Bacterial proliferation takes place and endotoxins released.

- Transmigration of gram-negative organisms, anaerobes and gram-positive organisms through the gangrenous bowel results in peritonitis.

- The organisms release powerful endotoxins which are absorbed from the peritoneal surface and cause gram-negative shock or septic shock. It carries very high mortality rate.

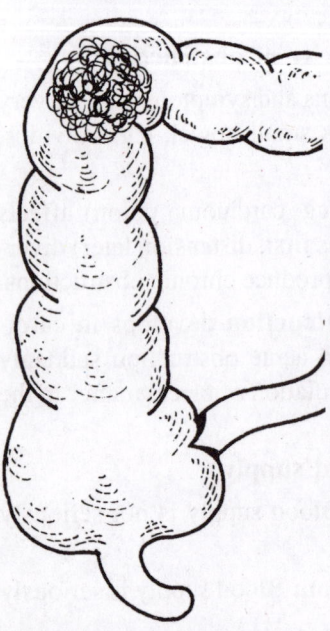

Fig. 30.1 Closed loop obstruction

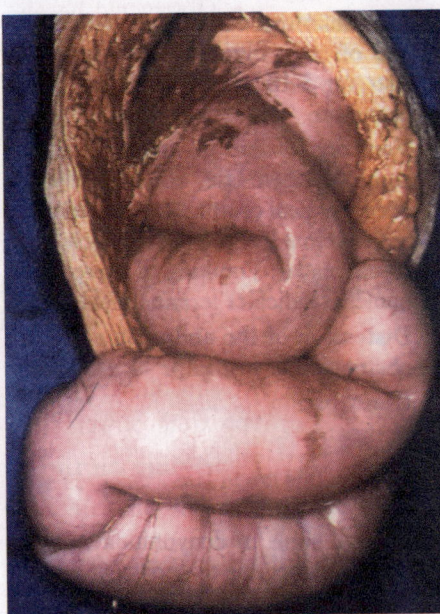

Fig. 30.2 Dilated small intestinal loops in a case of ileal obstruction

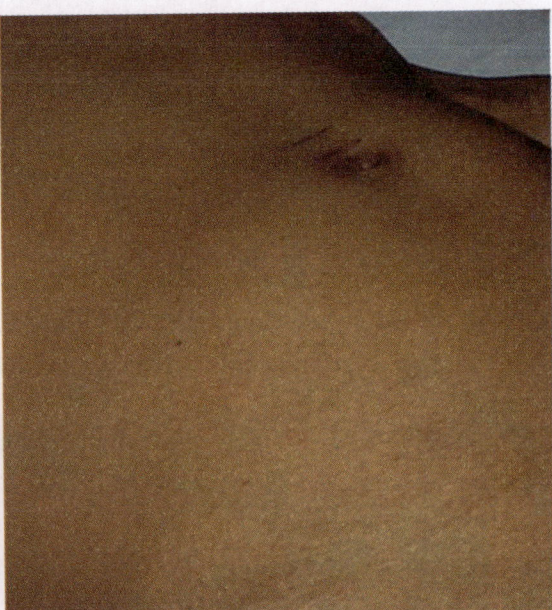

Fig. 30.3 Distension of the abdomen - watch step ladder peristalsis

Key Box 30.1

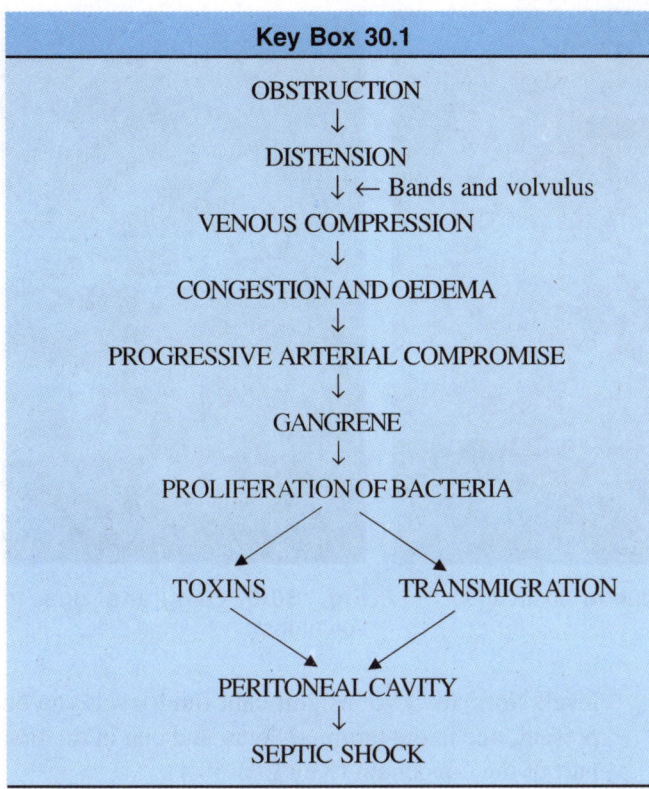

OBSTRUCTION

↓

DISTENSION

↓ ← Bands and volvulus

VENOUS COMPRESSION

↓

CONGESTION AND OEDEMA

↓

PROGRESSIVE ARTERIAL COMPROMISE

↓

GANGRENE

↓

PROLIFERATION OF BACTERIA

↓   ↓

TOXINS   TRANSMIGRATION

↓   ↓

PERITONEAL CAVITY

↓

SEPTIC SHOCK

- Early gangrene without obstruction is a feature of mesenteric thrombosis or embolism.
- Loss of blood volume is an important feature of massive gangrene.

CLINICAL FEATURES

1. **Pain abdomen:** Central abdominal pain is a feature of small intestinal obstruction and peripheral pain is a feature of large intestinal obstruction. It is a colicky pain, that lasts for 5-10 mins, intermittent. On pressure, it decreases.

2. **Vomiting** is due to reverse peristalsis, first stomach contents, then bile, followed by faeculent vomiting. Faeculent is not faecal matter but terminal ileal contents which undergo bacterial degradation and fermention resulting in the smell of faecal matter. Vomiting of altered blood indicates haemorrhage and gangrene.

Vomiting of faeculent contents indicates terminal ileal obstruction.

3. **Distension of the abdomen**: Central abdominal distention in ileal obstruction and peripheral in large bowel obstruction, or it may be localised to one or two quadrants as in sigmoid volvulus.

4. **Constipation** because the distal bowel does not act.

Constipation to faeces and flatus is called obstipation. Exceptions are given below.

Key Box 30.2

INTESTINAL OBSTRUCTION WITH DIARRHOEA

- Faecal impaction
- Richter's hernia
- Gall stone ileus
- Mesenteric vascular occlusion

Signs

1. **General signs of dehydration:** Dry skin, dry tongue, sunken eyes, feeble pulse, with low urinary output results due to persistent vomiting and sequestration of fluid and electrolytes.

2. **Abdominal findings**
   - Distension, **tympanitic note** on percussion
   - **Step ladder peristalsis** in terminal ileal obstruction. Right to left colonic peristalsis in left sided colonic obstruction-large bowel obstruction.
   - On auscultation-loud, noisy intestinal sounds are heard. They are called borborygmi.
   - Hernial orifices have to be looked for, especially a small femoral hernia in females.

Sings of strangulation

- It should be suspected when features of obstruction are present along with features of shock. (Also refer Key Box 30.3)
- Features of septic shock - fever, hypothermia, renal failure, respiratory failure
- **Rebound tenderness:** It is called Blumberg's sign. It is a classical sign of peritonitis.
- **Guarding and rigidity** of the abdominal wall.
- **Absent bowel sounds** because rest of the bowel loops undergo paralytic ileus.
- Sudden symptoms - spasmodic pain and continuous pain suggest strangulation.
- Features of strangulation and perforation occurs quickly in cases of closed loop obstruction (Key Box 30.3).

Rectal examination

- In small bowel obstruction, rectum is empty and is often ballooned out.

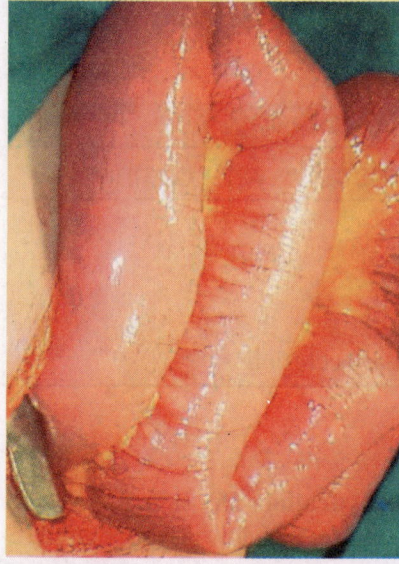

Fig. 30.4 Dilated intestinal loops

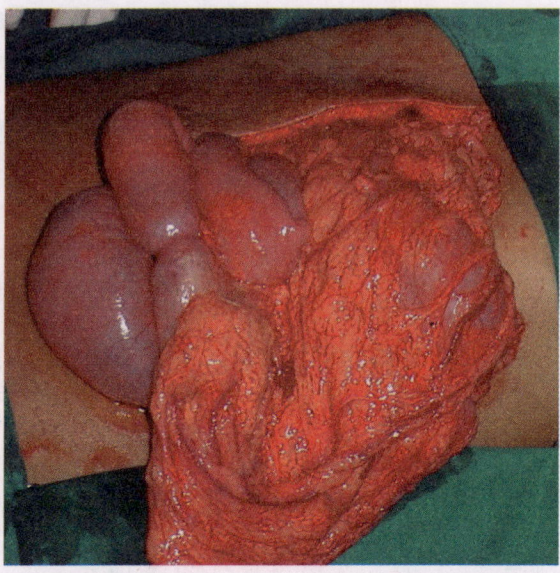

Fig. 30.5 Perforation due to obstruction.

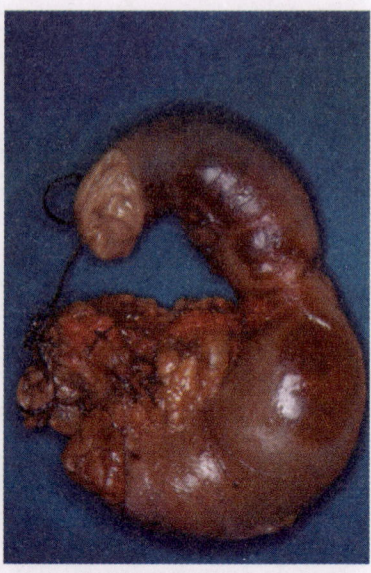

Fig. 30.6 Gangrene due to volvulous

Key Box 30.3

CLOSED LOOP OBSTRUCTION

- This occurs when the bowel is obstructed at both proximal and distal points (Fig. 30.4)
- Proximal bowel is not distended as much in this condition
- Gangrene and perforation can occur fast (Fig. 30.5)
- Retrograde thrombosis of mesenteric vein, can result in distension of the bowel
- Few examples of closed loop obstruction include sigmoid volvulus, strangulated hernia, carcinoma right colon (Fig. 30.6)

- Carcinomatous growth with or without stools can be felt. Finger may be stained with blood.

INVESTIGATIONS

1. **Complete blood picture:** Low Hb % indicates underlying malignancy. Increased total WBC count indicates infection and sepsis.
2. **Electrolytes:** Most of the electrolytes are low in cases of intestinal obstruction.
3. **Plain X-ray abdomen** in the erect position is an important investigation in cases of intestinal obstruction. Multiple gas fluid levels are pathognomonic of intestinal obstruction. Gas levels appear earlier than fluid

level. Normally two insignificant fluid levels can be present, one in the terminal ileum and one in the first part of the duodenum (Key Box 30.4).

- Supine films indicate the distal limit of obstruction.

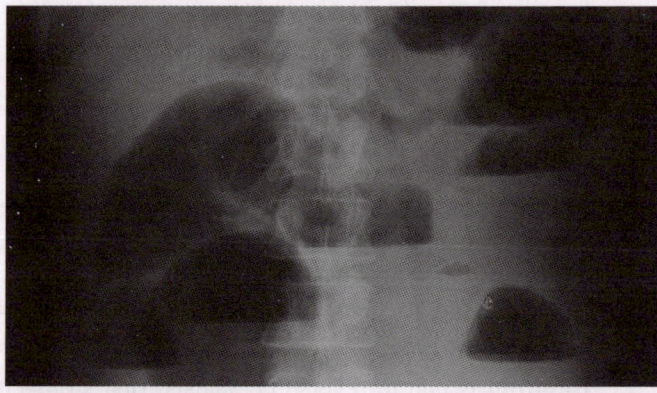

Fig. 30.7 Multiple gas fluid levels- plain X-ray erect abdomen

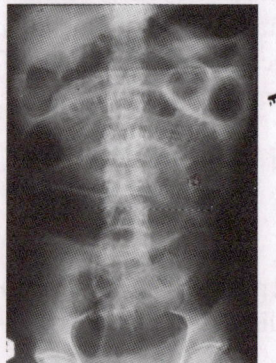

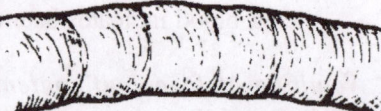

Fig. 30.9 Volvulae conniventes

Fig. 30.8 Plain X-ray supine - distended intestines

Key Box 30.4

PLAIN X-RAY FINDINGS

- Plain X-ray may demonstrate gall stone ileus or foreign body
- Gas is absent in the small bowel as in mesenteric vascular ischaemia
- Sigmoid volvulus appears as a large dilated loop
- Jejunum is characterised by regularly placed mucosal folds called **Volvulae Conniventes** (Fig. 30.9) placed opposite to each other (Herring bone pattern). They are produced by valves of Kirckring.
- Large bowel is characterised by **haustrations** (Fig. 30.10) - Incomplete, large mucosal folds, not placed opposite to each other
- **Caecum has no haustrations.** It appears as a round gas shadow in the right iliac fossa
- Ileum has no characters - **Characterless loop of Wangensteen**

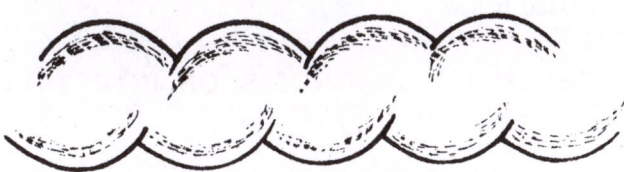

Fig. 30.10 Haustrations

MANAGEMENT

- Preoperative preparation includes correction of dehydration, electrolytes and broad spectrum antibiotics. Principles in the management of intestinal obstruction are as follows:

A. **Aspiration** with Ryle's tube - this is the most important step in the management of intestinal obstruction. It helps in decreasing the distension and also prevents vomiting. This will, help in preventing respiratory complications, such as aspiration following general anaesthesia.

B. **Bowel care:** No purgatives[1], nothing is given by mouth because purgation can cause perforation.

C. **Charts:** Temperature, pulse, respiration and intake output chart. In cases of conservative management such as obstruction due to adhesions, change in temperature, increasing pulse rate suggests perforation or gangrene. These cases have to be explored immediately.

D. **Drugs** to cover gram-positive, gram-negative and anaerobic organisms.

E. **Exploratory laparotomy** is done and depending upon the findings obstruction is treated. Few examples are given below in the Key Box 30.5.

F. **Fluids** should be given before, during and after surgery. It forms the most important treatment of intestinal obstruction.

Key Box 30.5

EXPLORATORY LAPAROTOMY - PRINCIPLES

- Long midline incision
- Resection of gangrene and anastomosis
- Adhesion - Release
- Bands - Divide
- Gall stone ileus - Remove the stone
- Volvulus - Untwist or resection
- Obstructed hernia - Reduce. Gangrene-Resect
- Stricture - Resection or Stricturoplasty

PRINCIPLES OF MANAGEMENT OF INTESTINAL OBSTRUCTION

Ask the following questions to yourself and proceed.

1. What is the probable cause of obstruction?
2. Is it small bowel obstruction at laparotomy?
3. Is it large bowel obstruction at laparotomy?
4. Is it simple obstruction?
5. Is It strangulation?
6. Is it some kind of a surprise or a difficult case?

1. Probable cause of obstruction

- A previous laparotomy scar may indicate it could be an adhesive obstruction (most common).
- An obvious obstructed hernia (inguinal or femoral) can be managed without a laparotomy.

---

1. *An innocent patient comes to a doctor and says since last two days I have not passed stools nor flatus. I have got colicky abdominal pain. Kindly give me purgatives.*

- An elderly man, hypertensive and atherosclerotic, with features of blood in the stools with acute abdominal pain may be having superior mesenteric ischaemia.
- Constipated elderly man in poor health, with acute or chronic obstruction may be having carcinoma of the colon.

2. Diagnosis of small bowel obstruction at laparotomy

- Caecum is collapsed
- Dilated loops of small intestine are present
- A stricture or a mass lesion may be obvious at laparotomy

3. Diagnosis of simple obstruction

- It is done when bowel is not gangrenous
- In doubtful cases, because of long-standing ischaemia, wrapping the bowel with warm and moist pack and administration of pure oxygen may help the bowel to recover from ischaemia (Key Box 30.6).

Key Box 30.6

VIABLE BOWEL - FEATURES

- Normal peristalsis
- Normal peritoneal sheen is present
- Normal pulsations are visible or felt at the mesentery
- Normal pink colour is present

---

4. Diagnosis of large bowel obstruction at laparotomy

- Caecum is distended. (Key Box 30.7)
- A growth may be palpable and obvious in the transverse colon or in the hidden colon i.e. splenic flexure.
- It is very important to examine the entire colon (synchronous carcinoma is more common).

5. Diagnosis of strangulation

- Black, dark, foul smelling bowel is seen as soon as laparotomy is done.
- Peritoneal fluid contains blood stained fluid
- Precautions are being taken not to contaminate peritoneal cavity when gangrenous segment is removed.

Don't hesitate to take the help of senior experienced surgeons in treating uncommon situations such as massive ischaemia and gangrene of small bowel and colon (due to mesenteric vascular occlusion), synchronous carcinoma and ileosigmoid knotting, etc.

Key Box 30.7

LARGE BOWEL OBSTRUCTION

- Carcinoma and impacted faecal matter are the two most common causes
- Generally occur in elderly patients
- Pseudoobstruction to be kept in mind (conservative treatment)
- Right sided obstructive lesions are managed by resection (one stage)
- Left sided tumours are managed by single stage or two stage procedures

---

6. It is a surprise

- Surprises are well known in intestinal obstruction. Congenital bands, foreign bodies, internal herniation, lymphomatous strictures are a few examples.
- The detailed management of individual cases are discussed below.

DIFFERENTIAL DIAGNOSIS OF INTESTINAL OBSTRUCTION (Fig. 30.11)

VOLVULUS OF THE SIGMOID COLON

- Common in North India (Punjab), Eastern Europe, Uganda.
- In certain parts of India as mentioned above, it is one of the common surgical emergencies in elderly population (Refer Key Box 30.8).

Key Box 30.8

CERTAIN FACTS ABOUT SIGMOID VOLVULUS

- More common in males
- 2/3 cases sigmoid volvulus and 1/3 being caecal volvulus
- Common in middle age and above > 60
- It consists about 10 to 15% of cases of intestinal obstruction in India
- More common in rural population
- It is not an uncommon event during pregnancy

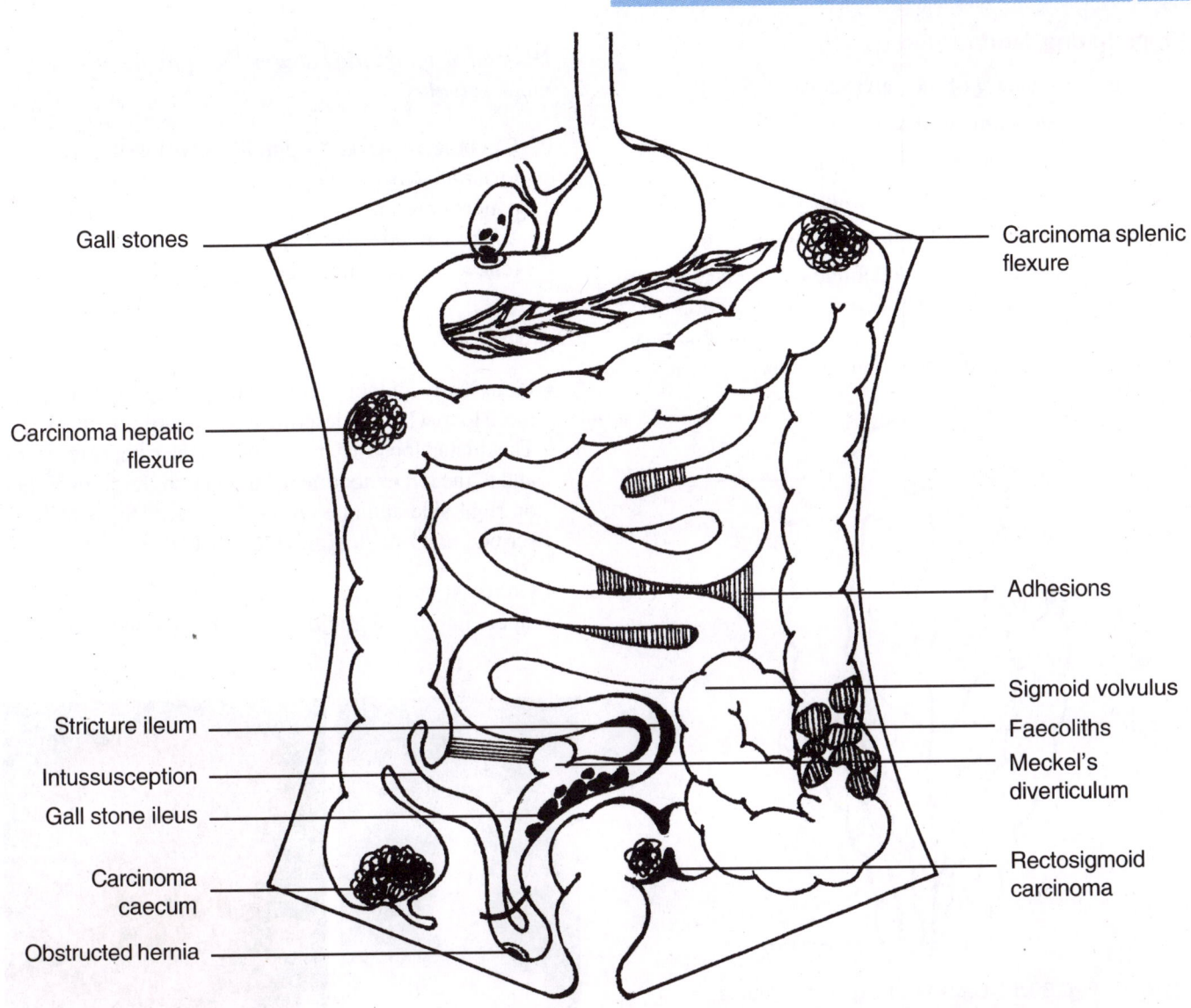

Gall stones

Carcinoma hepatic flexure

Stricture ileum

Intussusception

Gall stone ileus

Carcinoma caecum

Obstructed hernia

Carcinoma splenic flexure

Adhesions

Sigmoid volvulus

Faecoliths

Meckel's diverticulum

Rectosigmoid carcinoma

COMMON CAUSES OF ILEAL OBSTRUCTION

- Obstructed hernia
- Stricture
- Intussusception
- Ileocaecal tuberculosis
- Adhesions
- Bands
- Worm ball
- Ileal atresia

COMMON CAUSES OF GANGRENE

- Volvulus
- Intussusception
- Obstructed hernia
- Mesenteric vascular occlusion
- Twisting around a band

COMMON CAUSES OF COLONIC OBSTRUCTION

- Carcinoma colon
- Sigmoid volvolus
- Faecal impaction
- Mesenteric ischemia
- Stricture colon
- Sliding hernia
- Hirschsprung's disease
- Anorectal malformations

Fig. 30.11 Differential diagnosis of intestinal obstruction - diagramatic representation

Precipitating factors (Fig. 30.12)

1. Long mesentery of the pelvic colon
2. Narrow attachment at the base
3. Long redundant, pendulous sigmoid
4. Loaded colon due to high residue diet
5. Diverticulitis with a band, or adhesions
   - Sigmoid volvulus is a definite occurrence in mentally disturbed patients, hypothyroidism, Parkinson's disease, multiple sclerosis etc probably due to severe constipation due to medications.

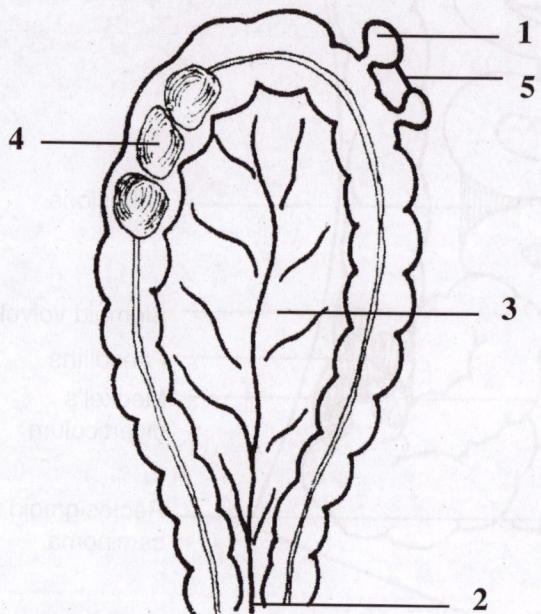

Fig. 30.12 Causes of sigmoid volvulus

> *Ogilivie's syndrome precipitates volvulus*

CLINICAL FEATURES

1. **Acute sigmoid volvulus** presents as intestinal obstruction. It starts usually after straining at passing stools. Volvulus is usually in anticlockwise direction and after $1^1/_2$ turns, the entire loop becomes gangrenous.

   - Enormous distension of the abdomen takes place, which gives a tympanitic note all over the abdomen. It is due to diffusion of CO_2. Due to gross distension, results in severe hypovolaemic shock develops within 6-8 hours of volvulus. Gangrene sets in, which gives rise to features of strangulation. A dilated loop can be seen and felt. Features of peritonitis are seen within 1-2 days. PR : Rectum is empty.

> *Distended tympanitic drum like abdomen - Sigmoid volvulus*

2. **Chronic recurrent sigmoid volvulus-**It occurs due to partial twisting and untwisting of the bowel. Elderly patients present with recurrent lower abdominal pain on the left side, distension of the abdomen, which is relieved on passing large amount of flatus.

DIAGNOSIS

- Plain X-ray abdomen erect shows a hugely dilated sigmoid loop which is described as **'bent inner tube sign'**. The dilated loop may be visible on the right side, centre and to the left of abdomen, having two fluids levels one on right side and one on the left side. This is also described as **Omega sign** (Fig. 30.13).

- **Contrast enema :** As the barium enters the rectum, it tapers into the sigmoid colon - **Bird's beak sign.**

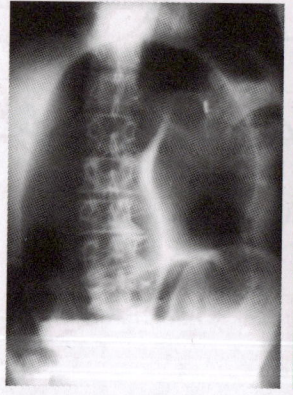 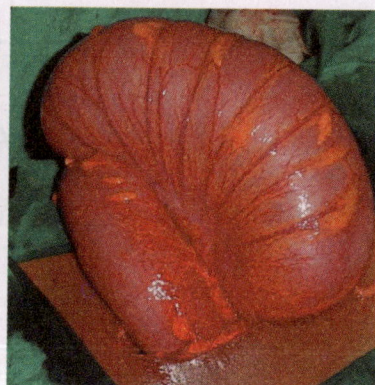

Fig. 30.13 Plain X-ray abdomen showing distended sigmoid loop

Fig. 30.14 Sigmoid colon at surgery - huge distension results in severe hypovolaemic shock

TREATMENT

Non-operative

- A successful passage of flatus tube or sigmoidoscope upto 25-30 cms results in release of large amount of flatus and fluid and obstruction is relieved. If obstruction is completely relieved or if there is no gangrene and the general condition of the patient improves an elective resection is done after 7 days. If resistance is found while passing flatus tube, instill barium for guidance.

Operative treatment (Fig. 30.14)

1. **Single stage resection:** This can be done provided general condition of the patient is good. If the loop is gangrenous, resection followed by end to end anastomosis is done, after giving on table lavage using saline washes till the contents of the colon are clear.

2. **Hartmann's procedure:** If the loop is gangrenous and proximal bowel is loaded with faecal matter, resection of the sigmoid colon is done. Proximal descending colon is brought out as an end colostomy and rectum is closed (**Hartmann's procedure**). After 6 weeks, colorectal anastomosis is done.

3. **Sigmoidopexy:** If the loop is not gangrenous, untwist the sigmoid loop and fix the sigmoid to the posterior abdominal wall (sigmoidopexy). If the mesentery is long, it can be made short by plication.

4. **Exteriorisation:** Paul Mickulicz procedure is done when general condition of the patient is poor in elderly patients, in severely dehydrated with impending septicaemia. In such cases, the gangrenous loop is brought outside and resected, with a proximal colostomy and a distal mucous fistula (Fig. 30.15).

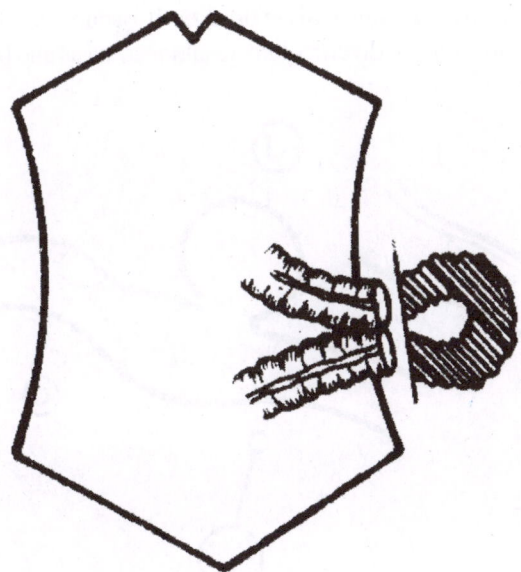

Fig. 30.15 Paul-Mickulicz procedure

CAECAL VOLVULUS

- It is a rare cause of intestinal obstruction.(Fig. 30.16) Also refer Key Box 30.9)

Key Box 30.9
COMPARISON OF CAECAL VOLVULUS AND SIGMOID VOLVULUS

CAECAL VOLVULUS	SIGMOID VOLVULUS
• Rare	• Common
• Clockwise twist	• Anticlockwise
• Mobile caecum is the cause	• Long mesentery
• Middle aged	• Elderly debilitated
• Kidney shaped gas shadow with single fluid level on the left side.	• Omega sign Coffee bean shaped
• Treated only by surgery	• Nonoperative treatment should be attempted in all cases (provided no ischaemia)

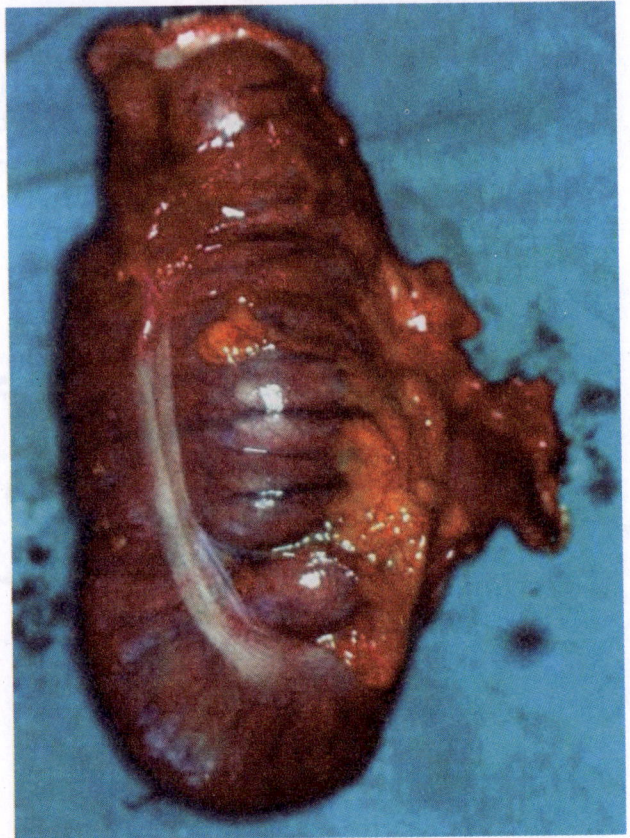

Fig. 30.16 Caecal volvulus with gangrene.

- In a plain X-ray abdomen, caecum produces round shadow in the centre of the abdomen.
- Resection is the ideal treatment

MECKEL'S DIVERTICULUM WITH A BAND

It is a congenital diverticulum which occurs due to persistent intestinal end of Vitello Intestinal Duct. **Being congenital, it has all layers of the bowel.**

ANOMALIES OF VITELLOINTESTINAL DUCT (Fig. 30.17)

A. Entire duct is obliterated & resulting in **fibrous band.** Bowel can twist around the band, resulting in volvulus.

B. Persistent **intestinal end**-Meckel's diverticulum.

C. **Meckel's diverticulum with the band** attached to the umbilicus can give rise to intestinal obstruction.

D. **Umbilical fistula** results when entire duct is patent. Even though it is connected to the terminal ileum, the opening is very small. The discharge is rarely faecal. Many a time, it is the mucous secreted from the lining of the duct (Omphaloenteric fistula).

E. **Umbilical sinus** results due to persistent umbilical end discharging mucous. Slowly umbilical adenoma results when epithelial lining of the sinus gets everted.

F. **Intra-abdominal cyst** results when both ends are obliterated. The central portion of the duct persists and secretes mucous. This is very, very rare.

MECKEL'S DIVERTICULUM

• It is present in 2% of the cases, 2 inches long, 2 feet away from ileocaecal region in the **antimesenteric border**. (Ileal duplication can occur in the mesenteric border)

Key Box 30.10
MECKEL'S[1] DIVERTICULUM AND OTHER ASSOCIATED ANOMALIES
• Angiodysplasia of the caecum
• Anorectal atresia, atresia of the oesophagus
1. The most common congenital anomaly of small intestine

• In 12% of the patients, heterotrophic gastric tissue is found which can produce peptic ulceration. In a few other patients, it can contain pancreatic and colonic tissue (Key Box 30.10).

CLINICAL PRESENTATION

1. Massive bleeding per rectum-in the form of melaena is not uncommon. In many other patients, mild chronic bleeding can result in anaemia (Key Box 30.11)

2. **Acute Meckel's diverticulitis**-It occurs due to food blocking the diverticulum, resulting in stasis and bacterial

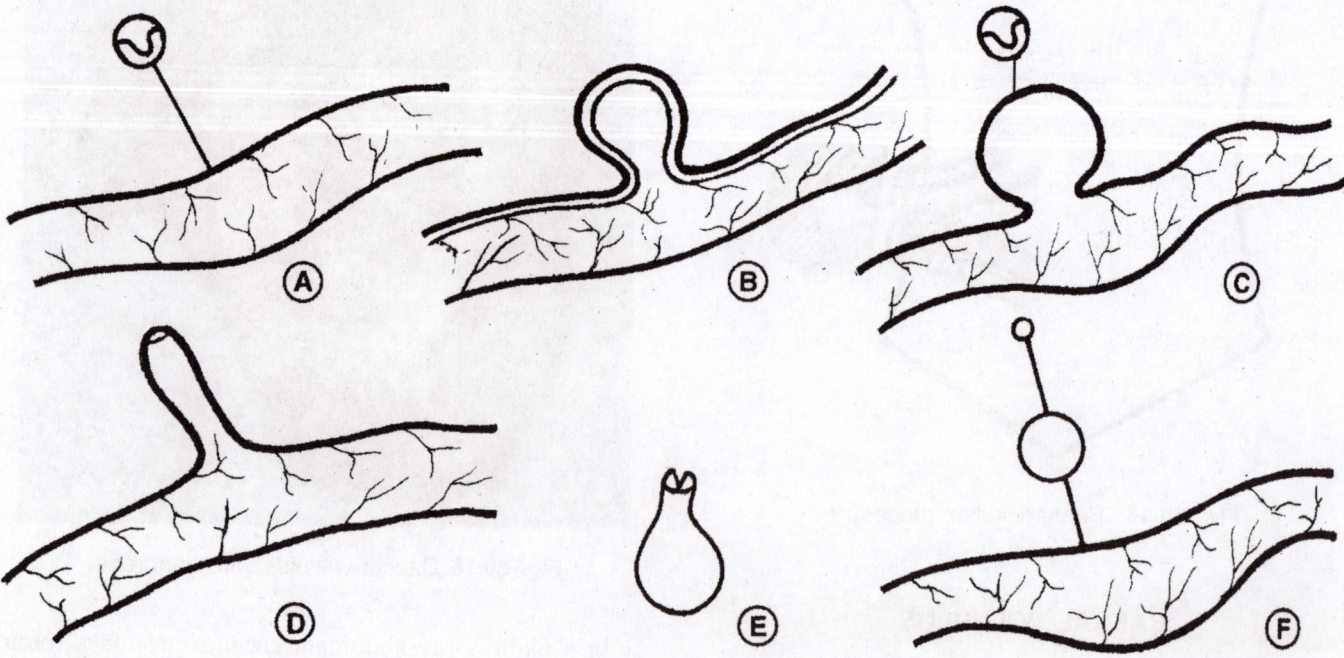

Fig. 30.17 Anomalies of vitellointestinal duct (A-F)

proliferation. Such cases can perforate very often. It is impossible to differentiate it from ruptured appendix. This is treated by laparotomy and resection of diverticulum with intestine. In majority of appendicular perforations, local abscess will occur because of retrocaecal position of the appendix (70%), However, perforation of Meckel's diverticulum, even though a rare cause of peritonitis, has a high mortality rate. This is because infection spreads very fast as diverticulum is intraperitoneal and contents are faeculent.

3. As a cause of **intestinal obstruction,** when it is associated with a band or due to volvulus.

4. **As a cause of intussusception:** Here also, inflamed heterotrophic tissue can be found in the diverticulum.(2% cases)

5. **Pain** can occur due to chronic peptic ulceration.

6. **Neoplasm :** Carcinoids and GIST are common than small intestine in Meckel's diverticulum.

Hernia of Littre is a hernial sac containing Meckel's diverticulum (Key Box 30.12).

Key Box 30.11

MECKEL'S DIVERTICULUM AND BLEEDING

- It is due to peptic ulceration in an ectopic gastric mucosa

- Painless, major, brick red sometimes massive lower GI bleeding in healthy infant

- Intermittent or chronic bleeding results in anaemia

- Technitium 99m scan is usually diagnostic

- It is one of the very very rare causes of upper GI bleeding

Key Box 30.12

MECKEL'S DIVERTICULUM AND INTESTINAL OBSTRUCTION

- Intussusception
- Band
- Volvulus due to band
- Internal herniation beneath mesodiverticular band
- Diverticulitis with band
- Littre's hernia

INVESTIGATIONS

1. No investigation can prove diagnosis of Meckel's diverticulum. Small bowel enema may demonstrate the diverticulum if opening is wide. (fluoroscopy is more ideal).

2. ^{99m}Tc-labelled **pertechnetate** given I.V., may localise the heterotrophic gastric mucosa in the Meckel's diverticulum, in about 90% of patients. This radionuclide is taken up by mucin secreting cells and parietal cells and immediately it is secreted. Thus, if ^{99m}Tc appears in the stomach as well as in other part of bowel, it indicates functioning hetertrophic tissue. Even when bleeding is at a rate of 0.1 ml/minute, it can detect Meckel's diverticulum. Hence, it is superior to angiography. **Very useful in children with bleeding.**

The pertechnitate anion $99Tc^m$ is selectively taken up by gastric mucosal cells, thyroid, salivary glands and choroid plexus.

TREATMENT (Fig. 30.18)

1. Incidentally found Meckel's during laparotomy for some other cause can be left alone provided it has wide mouth. However, a note of it must be made in the operation register (Key Box 30.13).

2. Meckel's diverticulum with bleeding, band, perforation and narrow mouth is treated by removal of diverticulum with adjacent intestine because the gastric tissue may often line the intestine also.

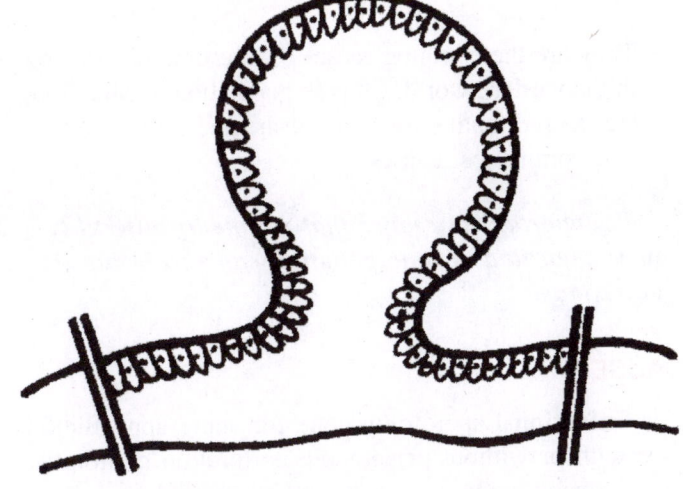

Fig. 30.18 Meckel's diverticulectomy should include normal intestine also

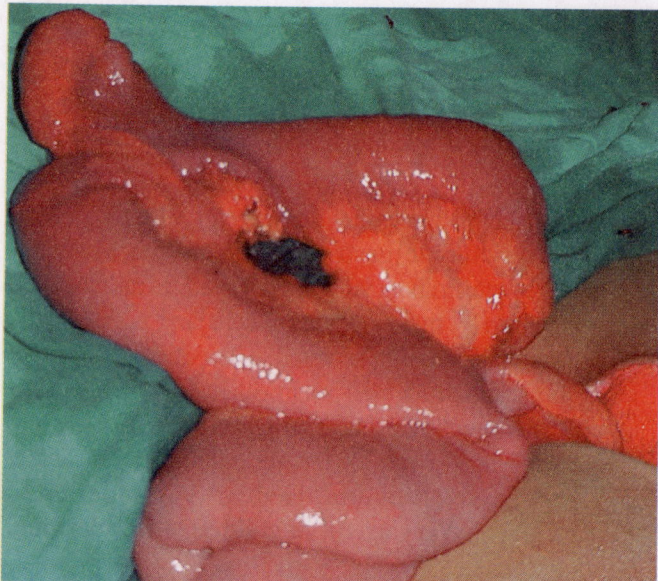

Fig. 30.19 Inflammed Meckel's diverticulum

Key Box 30.13

INDICATIONS FOR REMOVAL OF INCIDENTALLY FOUND MECKEL'S DIVERTICULUM (MD)

- Children under 2 year of age
- Meckel's with a band
- Meckel's with adhesions
- Meckel's with narrow base
- Long Meckel's diverticulum

ADHESIONS AND BANDS

- They are the common causes of intestinal obstruction in the western world, Chinese population of Malaysia, etc. In India adhesions and obstructed hernia are the two commonest causes.

It is important to realise that secondary infertility in women and ectopic gestation can result due to adhesions.

CAUSES

1. **Infection**-Laparotomy done for acute appendicitis with or without perforation, perforation peritonitis, intraabdominal abscess have higher incidence of adhesions. Surgery is the commonest causes of peritoneal adhesions.

2. **Iatrogenic** refers to talc, silk thread, foreign body (mop), etc. used for surgery which can induce extensive adhesions due to foreign body reaction.

3. **Ischaemia**-Lack of blood supply, particularly venous occlusion can cause adhesions, e.g. mesenteric vascular occlusion.

4. **Injury** to the bowel can result in adhesions.

5. **Irradiation** enteritis is becoming common due to irradiation of carcinoma of the cervix cases.

PATHOGENESIS

- Ischaemia and irritation of the intestines are the chief factors responsible for adhesions.(Key Box 30.14)

Key Box 30.14

PATHOGENESIS OF ADHESIONS

- Peritoneal injury / ischaemia / irritation
  ↓
  Inflammation
  ↓
  Fibrinous exudate
  ↓
  Fibrous Adhesions

  Complete resolution   Dense fibrous adhesions

- Peritoneal plasminogen activators release results in lysis of adhesion.

TYPES

1. **Fibrinous adhesions** (bread and butter adhesions): They are the causes of early postoperative obstruction, which settles down within 3-5 days. Majority of them will disappear in due course of time.

2. **Fibrous adhesions:** If the infection is continuing or if foreign body is present, the fibrinous material is converted to fibrous band. They also occur at the site of ischaemia. They will cause late intestinal obstruction.

3. **Tuberculous adhesions** are dense adhesions to develop which results in matting of intestinal coils. Separating them at laparotomy is extremely difficult.

INVESTIGATIONS

1. **Plain X-ray abdomen:** Small bowel enema are very useful investigations to prove the obstruction.

2. **Computed Tomogrphy (CT)** enhanced with oral contrast

- Detect air fluid level : complete obstruction
- The absence of mass lesion.
- Dilated and collapsed loop junction.
- CT has a sensitivity of 100% and specificity of 88%.
- Thus CT and and MRI are very helpful in patients with small bowel obstruction.

TREATMENT

I. Conservative treatment in the form of nasogastric aspiration, replacement with intravenous fluid to correct dehydration and electrolytes may be successful in early post-operative obstruction. If it is not successful, reoperation is required. Generally 48-72 hours is the waiting period in patients who present to the hospital as late adhesive obstruction. Further delay may result in perforation or gangrene of the bowel.

II. Surgical methods (Key Box 30.15)

- In other cases where fibrous bands are the cause, they need to be divided to relieve obstruction.
- Laparoscopic adhesiolysis is more often being used and it is indicated in pelvic adhesion, selected cases of abdominal adhesion, single band adhesion, obstruction with mild distention.
- Recently absorbable and nonabsorbable membrane barriers such as expanded polytetra- fluoroethylene (PTFE) and membrane composed of Hyaluronic acid and carboxymethyl cellulose has been used.

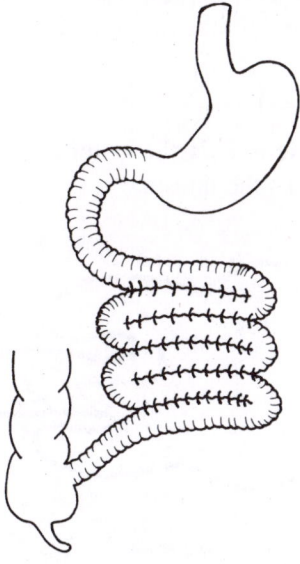

Fig. 30.20 Surgery for adhesions - Noble's plication

Key Box 30.15

PRECAUTIONS

- Handle the bowel carefully. Good suturing without tension. Avoid anastomotic leak
- Raw peritoneal areas should not be sutured
- Thorough peritoneal toilet in cases of peritonitis with saline or dextran to drain pus, bile, blood clots
- Avoid spillage of contents - Bile, faecal matter
- Prefer a Pfannensteil incision than midline incision
- Noble's plication (Fig. 30.20)
- Laparoscopic method produce decreased adhesions than laparotomy

---

BANDS

The most common bands are due to peritonitis either bacterial or due to tuberculosis.

Key Box 30.16

TYPES OF BAND

- Congenital : Transduodenal band of Ladd
  : Vitello Intestinal duct associated band
- Acquired : Following peritonitis
  : Diverticulum
  : Greater omentum as a band

GALL STONE ILEUS - GALL STONE OBTURATION

- It should be suspected in a patient who has gall stones who presents with intestinal obstruction.
- Elderly females above the age of 60 are usually affected.
- Gall stone reaches the terminal ileum by forming 'cholecystoduodenal fistula' due to recurrent attacks of cholecystitis (Fig. 30.21, 30.22 and 30.23). Terminal ileum is the narrowest portion of gut wherein gall stone gets impacted. Sometimes, the stone may ulcerate from gall bladder into jejunum, colon, etc.

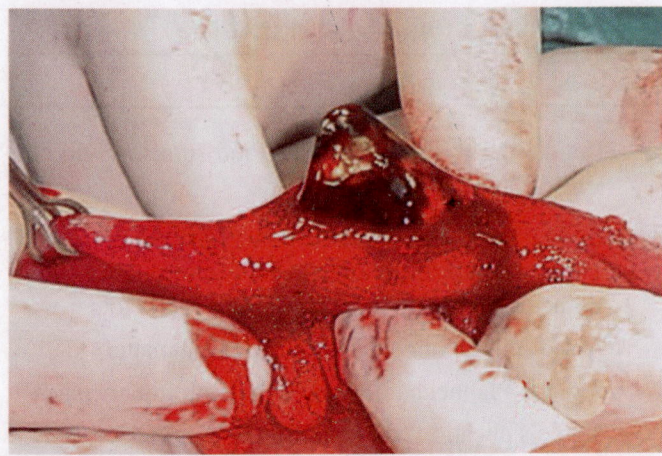

Fig. 30.21 Gall stone ileus. Contributed by Prof. M.G.Shenoy and Dr. G.N. Prasad, KMC, Manipal

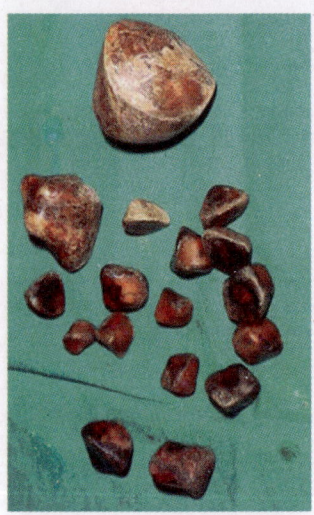

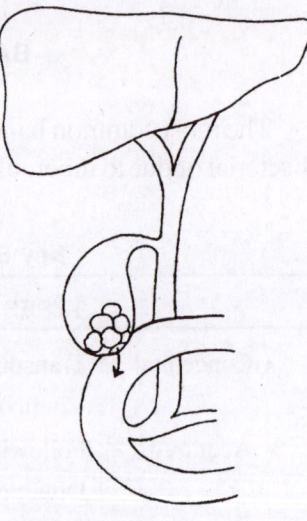

Fig. 30.22 17 gall stones were removed in this case

Fig. 30.23 Cholecysto-duodenal fistula

Investigations

1. **Plain X-ray** abdomen (erect position) may demonstrate multiple gas and fluid levels and stone in the gall bladder and also in the lower abdomen suggesting gall stone ileus
2. **Presence of air** in the biliary system (Key Box 30.17)
3. **Small bowel enema** may demonstrate partial obstruction.

Treatment

1. **Laparotomy**, locate stone and if possible, **crush with finger.** If it is successful, no further treatment is necessary. After 6 weeks, cholecystectomy is advised. If

---

> **Key Box 30.17**
>
> ### AIR IN THE BILIARY TREE
>
> - Cholecystoduodenal fistula
> - Choledochoduodenostomy, sphincteroplasty
> - Emphysematous cholecystitis

a large stone is felt in the gall bladder, stone is removed with an incision on the gall bladder.

2. Otherwise enterotomy, removal of the stone and closure of intestine is done. Search the entire length of the intestine for possibility of other stones.

INTUSSUSCEPTION

DEFINITION

Invagination of one segment of intestine within the other (usually the proximal into distal) is called as intussusception.

It is the most common cause of intestinal obstruction in infants aged 6 to 18 months.

TYPES

1. Simple ileocolic is the most common type, followed by ileoileal or colocolic
2. Compound-ileoileocolic
3. Retrograde jejunogastric intussusception, a complication of gastrojejunostomy (GJ) is a rare but it is an interesting type of intussusception (Page 351).

PARTS (Fig. 30.24)

1. **Intussuscipiens**-It is the outer tube (distal bowel which receives the intestine).

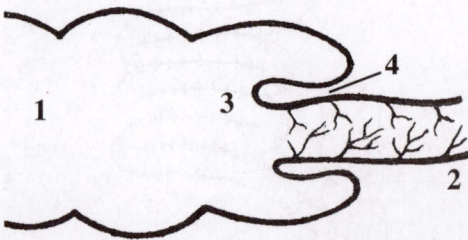

Fig. 30.24 Parts of intussusception - See the text for numbers

2. **Intussusceptum**-proximal bowel (inner tube) which enters inside.

3. **Apex** is the part which advances further into the distal bowel.

4. **Neck**, the narrowest portion of intussusception, is the junction of entering layer with the mass.

- The whole mass that develops is called intussusception.

AETIOPATHOGENESIS

1. Idiopathic intussusception: Actual cause is not known. It is seen in infants. Possible factors:

- **Dietary factor:** Around the age of 6-9 months, weaning of breast milk is done. Weaning causes alteration in the bacterial flora in the GIT, causing swelling of the Peyer's patches. These protrude into the terminal ileum and may precipitate intussusception.

- **Infective factor:** It usually follows upper respiratory tract infection with virus (adenorotaviruses) which produce inflammation of Peyer's patches.

2. **Adult secondary intussusception**: In adults there is always a cause for intussusception.

Key Box 30.18
CAUSES - ADULT INTUSSUSCEPTION
• Meckel's diverticulum
• Polyps: Peutz-Jegher's syndrome (hamartomatous polyps)
• Carcinoma-a proliferative growth in the caecum or in the transverse colon
• Submucous lipoma or lipomatosis bowel
• Purpura with submucosal haemorrhages causing swelling of the intestine

PATHOPHYSIOLOGY

- As the apex advances, it drags the mesentery containing blood vessels which get obstructed at the neck resulting in mucosal ulcers and haemorrhages. Marked lymphadenopathy and hypertrophy of Peyer's patches is found at operation.

- If the neck is too tight, gangrene sets in very early, as in ileocolic intussusception (Fig. 30.25).

---

1. *Hindi speaking mother says Baccha Rota Hai Aur Sota Hai*

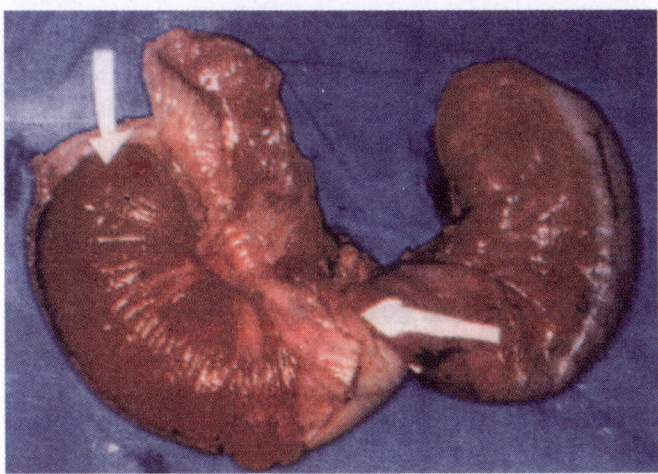
Fig. 30.25 Intussusception

- All other features of strangulation, dehydration, distension and septicaemic shock develop later.

CLINICAL FEATURES

- **First born male infants** between 6-9 months are commonly affected.

- Child screams with abdominal pain[1] (intestinal colic) which is associated with facial pallor.

- One attack of **red currant jelly stools** is characteristic. Bleeding is due to mucosal ulcer, mucous is due to irritation of intestines. This is followed by absolute constipation. **Red currant jelly stools are not found in adult intussusception.**

- Vomiting 3-4 times, initially due to pylorospasm. Later, due to obstruction.

- In between the spasm, the child sleeps but gets up suddenly with the pain.

Signs

- The mother is asked to feed the baby in sitting position and the examination should be done with left hand, standing in front of the mother.

- A contracting, hardening mass in and around the umbilical region can be felt (Sausage shaped).

- Emptiness in the right iliac fossa **Signe De Dance**.

- There may be a visible step ladder peristalsis.

- Rarely, intussusception can be seen outside the anus due to long mesentery.

- Rectal examination reveals blood-stained mucous on the examining finger.

- Features of peritonitis occur in untreated cases.

INVESTIGATIONS (Fig. 30.26)

- **Barium enema:** Claw (pincer) ending is diagnostic of intussusception. This is also called as meniscus sign. If there is any suspicion of gangrene, this test should not be done. In many cases, the diagnosis is established on clinical grounds.

- **Ultrasound** has been used increasingly nowadays. It can detect **target sign** and detect **mass (Doughnut sign)**

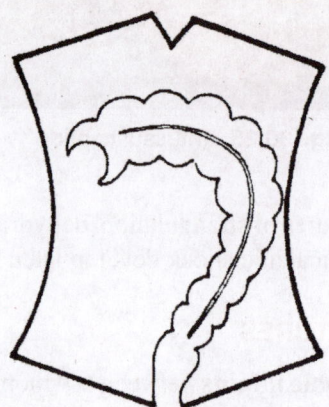

Fig. 30.26 Claw ending

TREATMENT

I. Conservative treatment (Key Box 30.19)

- **Hydrostatic reduction** can be attempted when gangrene is ruled out as in early intussusception. A lubricated catheter is introduced into the rectum and 1-2 litres of saline from a height of 1-2 metres is allowed to run. Catheter is removed and buttocks are pressed together. 50-70% of cases are reduced by this method. 1 : 3 barium sulfate in warm isotonic saline can also be used.

Key Box 30.19
HYDROSTATIC REDUCTION IS SUCCESSFUL WHEN
1. Passage of flatus and faeces with barium.
2. Symptom-free, comfortable child.
3. Small bowel loops are filled with contrast.
ADVANTAGES
• Easy, non-operative method.
COMPLICATION
• Rarely, colonic perforation.

Contraindications

- Peritonitis with shock
- Total intestinal obstruction

II. Surgical treatment

Laparotomy and reduction of intussusception.

- Intussusception is reduced by milking (squeezing) the colon in opposite direction, which is facilitated by breaking the adhesions at the neck using the little finger. Appendicectomy is also done, as it avoids any future confusion as to the reason for the abdominal scar. Fixing the caecum is not necessary, because idiopathic intussusception rarely recurs. If the loop is gangrenous, resection and ileocolic anastomosis is done

- **Recurrent intussusception is rare**. If it occurs, terminal ileum is sutured to the side of the ascending colon.

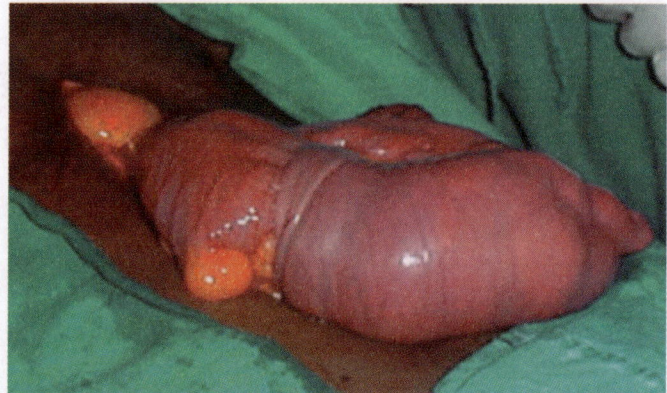

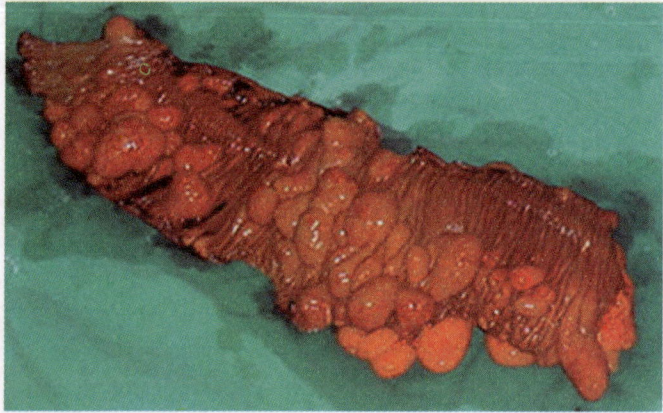

Fig. 30.27, 30.28 Adult intussusception due to jejunal lipomatosis. This patient was a 24 years old male who presented with intestinal obstruction. A mass was palpable in the umbilical region, at laparotomy this mass was resected. Opened specimen shows extensive segmental lipomatosis - Contributed by Dr. Gabriel Rodrigues, Dr. Mahesh Gopa Setty, Dr. Lavanya K., KMC, Manipal

FOOD BOLUS OBSTRUCTION

This complication can occur, particularly when a GJ or partial gastrectomy is done.

Factors precipitating this condition are

- Unmasticated, undigested particles
- Coconut pieces, jackfruit seeds and gulped coins, etc.
- They get impacted in the terminal ileum which is the narrowest portion of the gut.

Treatment

- Squeeze the bolus into the caecum. Otherwise, enterotomy and removal may be necessary.

OBSTRUCTION DUE TO INTERNAL HERNIA

1. These are the rare causes of intestinal obstruction. Due to some congenital defects in the mesentery, the floating, mobile intestines can herniate.
   - A defect in the mesentery.
   - A defect in the transverse mesocolon.
   - A defect in the broad ligament.
   - Hence, whenever a surgical procedure is done for resection of the bowel or GJ, etc., once the anastomosis is compeleted, the **rent in the mesocolon** as in GJ or **rent** in the small bowel mesentery should be closed.
2. Herniation can also occur through one of the potential spaces (fossae) in and around the viscus.

Duodenal fossa

1. Left paraduodenal fossa-Inferior mesenteric vein lies very close to the free border here.
2. Right duodenojejunal fossa-Superior mesenteric artery runs in its free border.

Colonic fossa

1. Superior ileocaecal fossa
2. Inferior ileocaecal fossa
3. Sigmoid fossa

They are the rare causes of intestinal obstruction to be kept in mind.

MESENTERIC VASCULAR OCCLUSION

- It is common in elderly patients who are **hypertensive** and usually obese. It is due to **atherosclerosis** causing thrombosis of the superior mesenteric artery or due to emboli which originate from atheromatous plaques or from the infarcted heart.
- **Superior mesenteric vein** can also get thrombosed due to injury during pancreatectomy or thrombosis as a result of oral contraceptive pills.

Key Box 30.20
CAUSES OF EMBOLI

- Atheroma
- Mural thrombus due to valvular diseases of the heart
- Myocardial infarction
- Subacute bacterial endocarditis
- Septic emboli

EFFECTS

- The pathological effects of arterial occlusion and venous occlusion are the same. Superior mesenteric artery supplies the entire midgut starting from the duodenojejunal flexure to right one third of the transverse colon, it is an end artery. As a result of thrombosis, the entire small bowel and portion of the large bowel becomes gangrenous (if there is a thrombus at the origin of superior mesenteric artery).

CLINICAL FEATURES

- Clinically, the patient presents with severe abdominal pain, vomiting, distension and bloody diarrhoea instead of constipation. Abdominal examination may reveal a tender, distended loop of the bowel. Localised rebound tenderness indicates underlying gangrene. Most of the patients present with advanced gangrene with septic shock. High index of suspicion is necessary to make a clinical diagnosis of this condition when the patients come early.

INVESTIGATIONS

1. **Total counts** are raised, if there is gangrene
2. **Plain X-ray abdomen** (erect) reveal absence of gas within the bowel loops

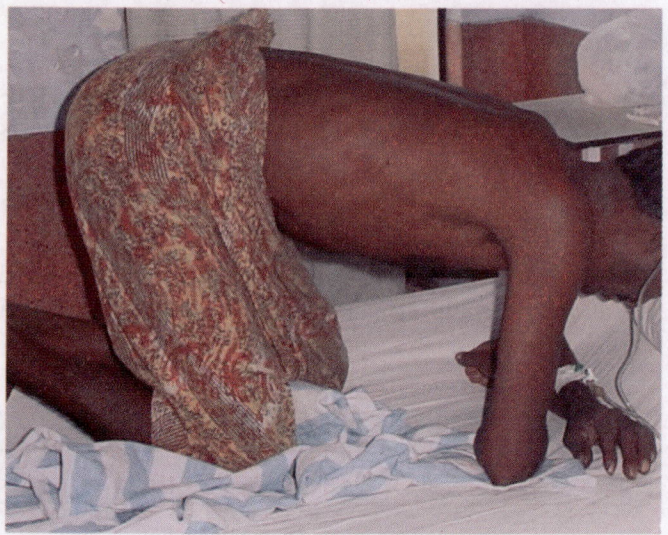

Fig. 30. 29 Attitude of a patient with severe ischaemia due to superior mesenteric vascular occlusion. In these cases pain is disproportionate to the abdominal signs

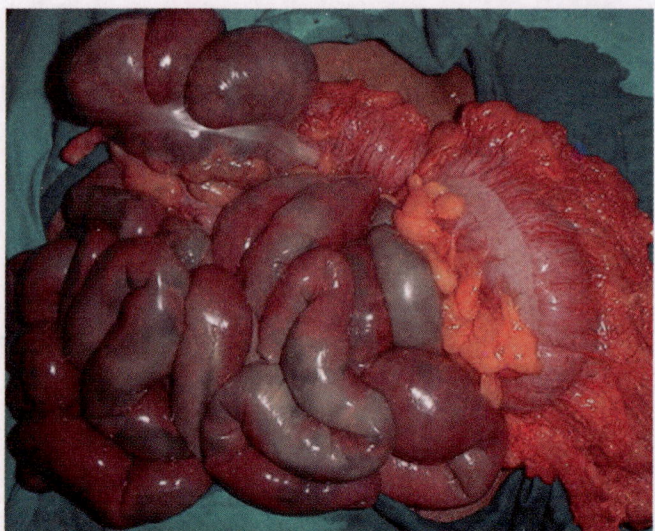

Fig. 30. 30 Massive gangrene of small intestines and right side of the colon due to thrombosis at the origin of superior mesenteric artery

3. **Serum phosphate** levels are raised within 3-4 hours following ischaemia as small bowel is rich in phosphates.

4. **Emergency angiography** can be done within 6 hours of ischaemia. It can demonstrate arterial thrombosis at the origin or distally in one of the branches.(It can be therapeutic also, see below)

TREATMENT

1. Majority of the patients present late with massive gangrene. **Massive resection** of the gangrenous bowel followed by end to end anastomosis is done. These patients suffer from short bowel syndrome (vide infra).

2. If patients come within 4-6 hours of ischaemia, emergency angiography followed by **papaverine infusion** into the superior mesenteric artery can be tried. Otherwise emergency laparotomy is done and the superior mesenteric artery is explored. A Fogarty catheter is introduced and embolectomy is done. These patients may require a second look operation within 24-48 hours to rule out gangrene developing later due to rethrombosis of the artery.

PROGNOSIS

- Majority of the cases present with the massive gangrene. Even after a massive resection, they succumb to the sepsis and multiorgan failure.

- Common causes are Tubercular stricture of the ileum or jejunum in India and Crohn's disease in the Western World.
- Radiation stricture, ischaemic strictures and nonspecific strictures are the other causes.
- Small bowel enema or enteroscopy is very useful investigations. (Refer Page 459)

NEONATAL INTESTINAL OBSTRUCTION

CAUSES

1. **Hirschsprung's disease** — congenital megacolon
2. Atresia and stenosis
3. Arrested rotation with bands
4. Volvulus neonatorum
5. Meconium ileus
6. Imperforate anus (Page 510)

HIRSCHSPRUNG'S DISEASE

It is also called as congenital megacolon, **aganglionic megacolon** or primary megacolon. It is one of the common causes of neonatal intestinal obstruction.

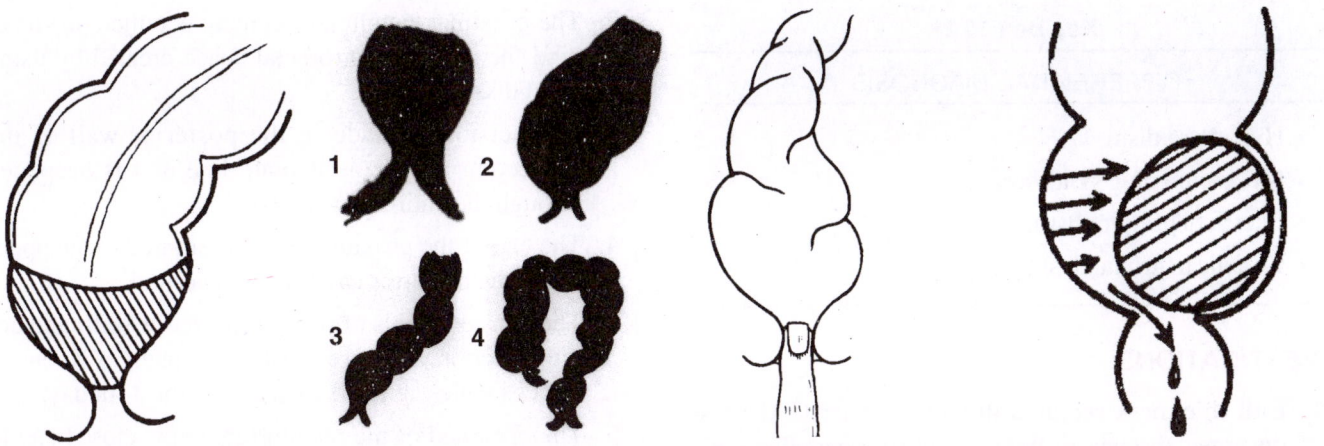

Fig. 30.31 Pathophysiology **Fig. 30.32** Types **Fig. 30.33** Rectal examination **Fig. 30.34** Acquired megacolon

PATHOPHYSIOLOGY (Fig. 30.31)

- The disease always involves the anus and rectum wherein parasympathetic ganglion cells are absent in the neural plexus of the intestinal wall. The defect involves internal sphincter.

- As a result of this, there is a **terminally constricted, non-relaxing segment**, in the rectum and sigmoid (lower part), above which the pelvic colon (sigmoid) is enormously dilated. Rectosigmoid area is involved in 80% of cases.

- There is **circular muscle hypertrophy,** mucosal hyperaemia, ulcers, etc., present in the dilated segments.

- In between, there may be a **transition zone,** which contains a few parasympathetic ganglion cells (cone).

- Rarely, Hirschsprung's can also involve the entire sigmoid colon, entire colon, etc.

- Hirschsprung's rarely occurs in adults also.

TYPES OF HIRSCHSPRUNG'S DISEASE (Fig. 30.32)

1. **Ultrashort segment :** Anal canal and terminal rectum is aganglionic.
2. **Short segment :** Anal canal and rectum is completely involved.
3. **Long segment :** Anal canal, rectum and part of colon involved.
4. **Total colonic :** Anal canal, rectum and whole length of colon is involved.

CLINICAL FEATURES

- Male children are commonly affected, when compared to females.

- Incidence: 1 in 4000 to 5000 live births.

> ***The most common associated anomaly is Down's syndrome (5 to 10%)***

- The child presents with acute neonatal intestinal obstruction manifesting failure to pass meconium or delay in passing meconium with abdominal distension.

- Within 12-24 hours, all features of intestinal obstruction can be found. If it is complicated by **enterocolitis,** it may result in **perforation** and septicaemia. A severe diarrhoea with blood and mucous, abdominal distension and vomiting can occur within a few hours, followed by hypovolaemic shock.

- Rectal examination reveals that the rectum is empty, finger is gripped by anal sphincter and there is **no perianal soiling** (Fig. 30.33). On the other hand, in acquired megacolon, rectum is loaded with faecal matter, perianal soiling is present and there is no sphincter activity (Fig. 30.34).

- **Chronic variety:** Chronic constipation manifesting in the first few weeks of life-child may be brought with abdominal distension. Stools are goat pellet like.

DIFFERENTIAL DIAGNOSIS (Key Box 30.21)

- Acquired megacolon: Usually manifests by one to two years of age. Rectum is loaded with faecal matter.

COMPLICATIONS

- Intestinal obstruction, perforation, peritonitis
- Enterocolitis
- Growth retardation

Key Box 30.21

DIFFERENTIAL DIAGNOSIS

- Hypothyroidism
- Meconium plug syndrome
- Intestinal pseudoobstruction
- Colonic neuronal dysplasia

INVESTIGATIONS

1. **Full thickness rectal wall** biopsy under G.A. demonstrates absence of parasympathetic ganglion cells and hypertrophic nerve fibres in the nerve plexus. It should be taken above the anorectal junction.

Today submucosal suction biopsy is more popular than biopsy since it avoids haemorrhage, infection and scarring.

2. **Barium enema**
- 3.6% solution is used, the intermediate zone appears as a cone with proximal dilatation and distal narrow zone which is characteristic of Hirschsprung disease.

TREATMENT

I. Emergency cases

- Right transverse loop colostomy: In most of the cases, aganglionic segment is limited to rectosigmoid region.
- A full thickness biopsy of the colostomy is sent for histopathological examination.

II. Definitive surgery

- Can be done usually between the age of 3-6 months (8 to 10 Kg of weight)
- Resection of aganglionic bowel (anorectum) followed by a pull through procedure. **Maintaining continence is the main aim.**
- Few points of comparison between Duhamel's and Swenson's pull through is mentioned below.

Duhamel's	**Swenson's**
1. Retrorectal pull through.	1. Endorectal pull through.
2. Technically easy.	2. Difficult.

Steps of Duhamel pull through surgery

1. The rectum is transected above the pectineal fold and is closed.

2. The proximal ganglionic segment is pulled down behind the rectum (Retrorectal space created by using blunt dissector.)

3. An incision is made in the posterior wall of the anorectum above the dentate line and is deepened through the entire bowel wall.

4. The end of the proximal colon is sutured to the opening in the posterior anal canal all around.

5. The adjacent walls of rectum (posterior wall) and colon (anterior wall) are crushed by using a Kocher's forceps which falls off by itself by the 14th day.

6. The open end of the rectum (above) is closed end to side, to the colon.

Other types of Surgery : Soave's mucosectomy and pull through operation.

ATRESIA AND STENOSIS

- Commonly, it affects the duodenum, followed by ileum and jejunum (Fig. 30.35).
- There may be single/multiple atresia

It is the most common cause of intestinal obstruction in neonates.

- Clinical features of obstruction manifest within 48-72 hours in the form of obstruction.
- Atresia means imperforation; stenosis means narrowing.
- Duodenal atresia presents as vomiting with or without bile, minimal distension and visible gastric peristalsis.

Key Box 30.22

TYPES OF DUODENAL ATRESIA

Type I : Membranous web (commonest)

Type II : Fibrous cord

Type III : Complete atresia

Key Box 30.23

DUODENAL ATRESIA - ASSOCIATED LESIONS

- Annular pancreas
- Down's syndrome
- Maternal hydramnios

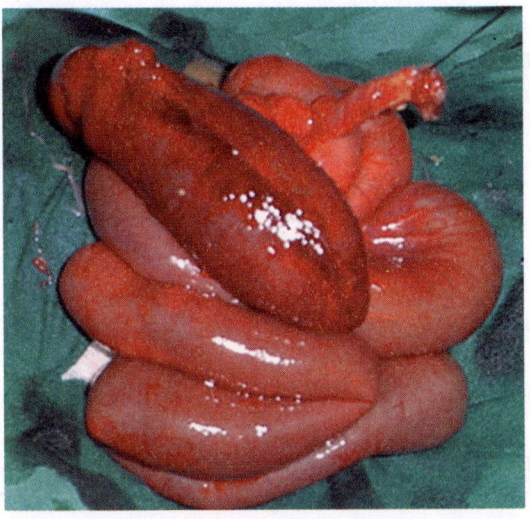

Fig. 30.35 Ileal atresia

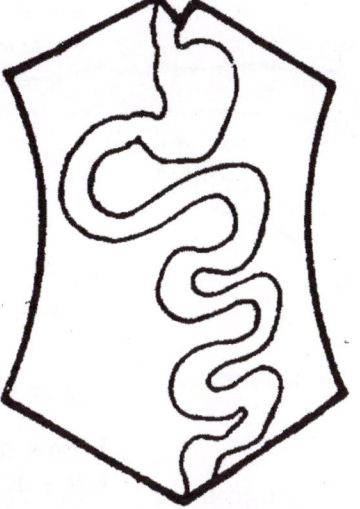

Fig. 30.36 Arrested rotation with band

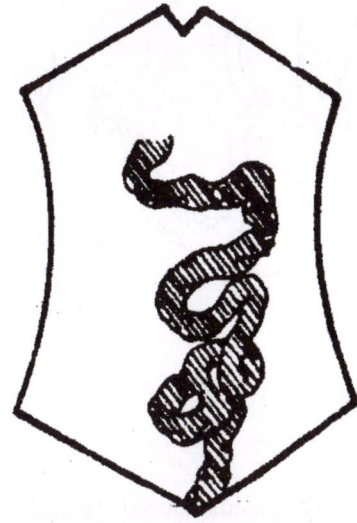

Fig. 30.37 Volvulus neonatorum

- Ileal atresia presents with central abdominal distension and vomiting.
- **X-ray abdomen erect: Double-bubble** in duodenal atresia and multiple fluid and gas levels in ileal atresia.

Treatment

- **Duodenal atresia**: Duodenojejunostomy by anastomosing dilated duodenum above the atresia to the jejunal loop.
- **Intestinal atresia** : Resection and anastomosis is the treatment.

ARRESTED ROTATION WITH BANDS

- It is a congenital anomaly wherein the caecum and right colon are found on the left side (Fig. 30.36).
- As a result of this there are peritoneal bands which run across from left to right, and cause intestinal obstruction (duodenal obstruction).
- One such band is called as **Transduodenal Band of Ladd** which compresses the second part of duodenum and gives rise to obstruction (features like duodenal atresia).
- Differential diagnosis is duodenal atresia.

Treatment

- Laparotomy, division of band and fixation of the caecum in the right iliac fossa.

VOLVULUS NEONATORUM

It is a complication of arrested rotation with bands which predispose to midgut volvulus (small bowel). These unfortunate infants undergo massive resection of the bowel if it is gangrenous (Fig. 30.37). Such massive resections give rise to short gut syndrome. Thus, the patient becomes a digestive cripple. If the loop is not gangrenous, it is treated by laparotomy, untwisting of bowel and division of bands.

MECONIUM ILEUS

- It is a neonatal manifestation of mucoviscidosis of the pancreas wherein the mucous is thick and viscid. This, along with meconium produces obstruction. There may be an ileal atresia, which might have precipitated meconium ileus. Majority of meconium ileus is coupled by complications like gangrene, perforation and peritonitis. As a sequelae to peritonitis, calcification and adhesive meconium obstruction develops.
- Infants present with abdominal distension, bilious vomiting and failure to pass meconium.
- Plane X-ray shows distended bowel and mottling due to calcification.
- **Soap bubble sign** or Neuhauser sign : Ground glass appearance in the right lower quadrant due to viscid meconium mixed with air.
- **Ultrasonography :** Dilated loops of bowel filled with

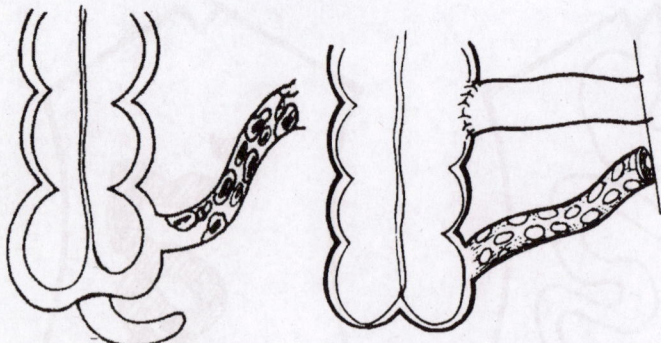

Fig. 30.38 Meconium ileus

Fig. 30.39 Bishop-Koop operation

echogenic material are highly suggestive of meconium ileus rather than ileal atresia.

- If perforation is ruled out, barium enema can be done which shows microcolon.

Treatment

I. Conservative treatment

- It is indicated if there is no peritonitis, general condition of the child is reasonably good or if there is partial obstruction. Dilute gastrograffin is introduced into the colon as enema. It fills up terminal ileum. It absorbs fluid from the interstitial space into the lumen because it is hyperosmolar. Consequently, the meconium becomes soft and it is passed naturally. Hypervolaemia is to be corrected during this period.

II. Surgical treatment - Bishop-Koop operation (Fig.30.38, 30.39)

- Ileum is divided in the proximal healthy part. This proximal ileum is anastomosed to the ascending colon to relieve obstruction—end to side anastomosis.

- Distal ileum containing thick meconium pellets is brought outside as a fistula and regular saline washes are given to dilute the meconium. Mucous fistula needs to be closed after a few weeks.

ANORECTAL ANOMALIES

Developmental anatomy

- To start with, there is a common chamber called as Cloaca, which is later divided into 2 chambers, anteriorly allantois gives rise to urinary bladder and posteriorly post-allantoic gut gives rise to rectum and upper 2 cm of anal canal.

- Post-allantoic gut fuses with proctodeum, thus giving rise to anal canal. If there is a defective fusion of this, it results in imperforate anus.

IMPERFORATE ANUS

Incidence

- 1:4500 live births. Common in female children

Types of imperforate anus

I. Low Anomaly : It refers to termination of the bowel below the anorectal bundle.

1. **Covered anus** (Fig. 30.40A)
   - The anal orifice is covered by a tag of skin

2. **Membranous anus** (Fig. 30.40B)
   - Covered with a thin membrane

3. **Anterior ectopic anus** (Fig. 30.40C)
   - Anus is situated anteriorly

4. **Stenosed anus** (Fig. 30.40D)
   - Anal orifice is microscopic

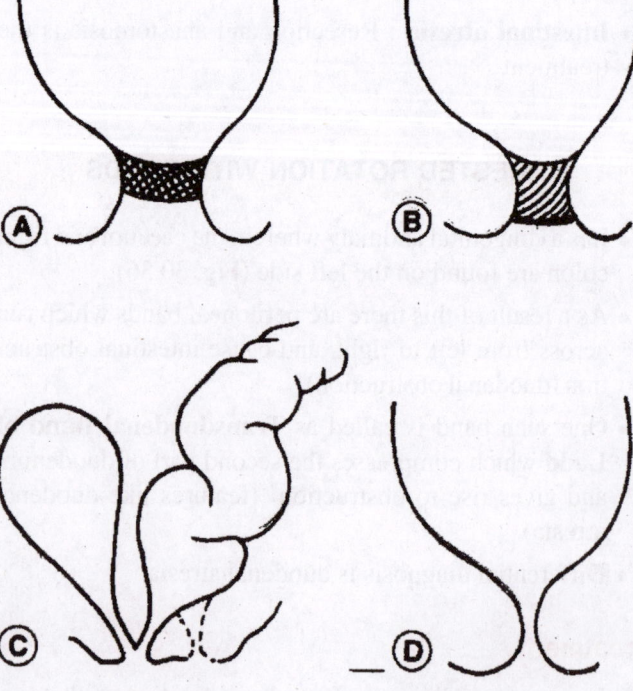

Fig. 30.40 Low anorectal anomalies

II. High anomalies : They are supralevator - The bowel terminates above the anorectal bundle.

1. Anorectal agenesis, with fistula : Rectovesical, rectovaginal, rectourethral fistulae (Fig. 30.41A).

2. Rectal atresia : Colon ends as a blind pouch below (Fig. 30.41B).

3. Cloaca : In this variety, bowel, urinary and genital tracts open into a common chamber. This occurs in females only.

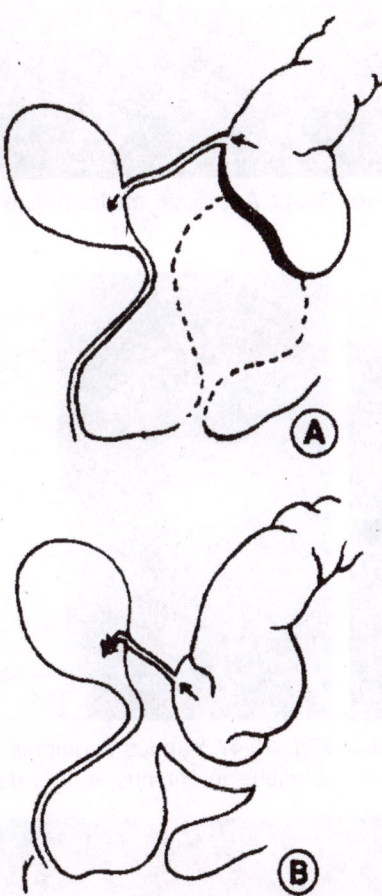

Fig. 30.41 High anorectal anomalies

Diagnosis -Wangenstein's Invertogram

- 12 hours after birth, the child is held upside down (12 hours is the time for the gas shadow to reach the distal portion of the gut). A metal coin is strapped to the site of anus and X-ray is taken. If the gas shadow is above the pubo-coccygeal line, it is high anomaly. If the distance between the coin and gas shadow is more than 2.5 cm, it is a high anomaly. If the gas shadow is below the pubococcygeal line, it is a low anomaly.

Treatment

I. Low anomaly

- Easy to treat, division of membrane or skin followed by dilatation is all that is required with some amount of plastic reconstruction. (Anoplasty is necessary).

II. High anomaly : Repaired by 3 stage procedure :

- 1st stage : Preliminary transverse colostomy to relieve intestinal obstruction.

- 2nd stage : When the child is 8-10 kg of weight, a "Pull through" operation is done with division of fistula.

- 3rd Stage : After 2 months, colostomy is closed.

CAUSES OF INTESTINAL OBSTRUCTION DEPENDING UPON THE AGE GROUP

NEONATE- 0 TO 7 DAYS (Fig. 30.42 to 30.49 Next page)

1. Atresia and stenosis
2. Hirschsprung's disease
3. Arrested rotation with bands
4. Volvulus neonatorum
5. Meconium ileus
6. Imperforate anus

YOUNG PATIENTS UPTO 30 YEARS

1. Obstructed hernia
2. Adhesions
3. Tuberculous stricture ileum
4. Crohn's disease of ileum
5. Tuberculous peritonitis with adhesions
6. Meckel's diverticulum with band
7. Adult intussusception

MIDDLE AGE PATIENTS 30-60 YEARS

1. Adhesions
2. Obstructed hernia
3. Carcinoma left colon
4. Diverticulosis with stricture left colon
5. Gall stone ileus
6. Sigmoid volvulus
7. Mesenteric vascular occlusion
8. Adult intussusception

VARIOUS CAUSES OF INTESTINAL OBSTRUCTION IN CHILDREN

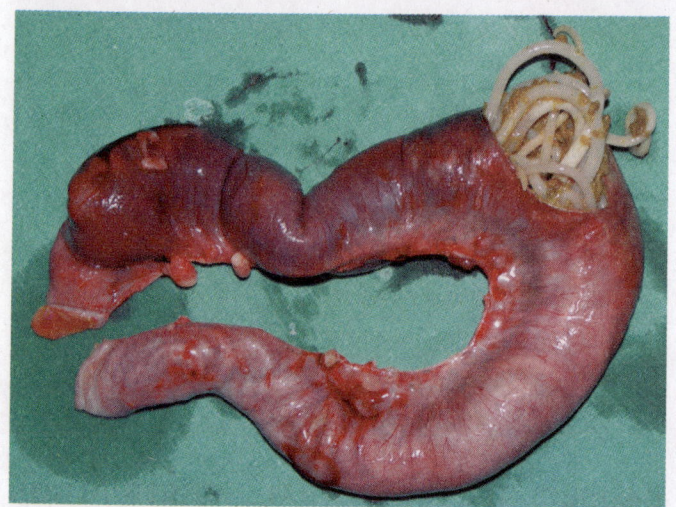

Fig. 30.42 Worm ball obstruction

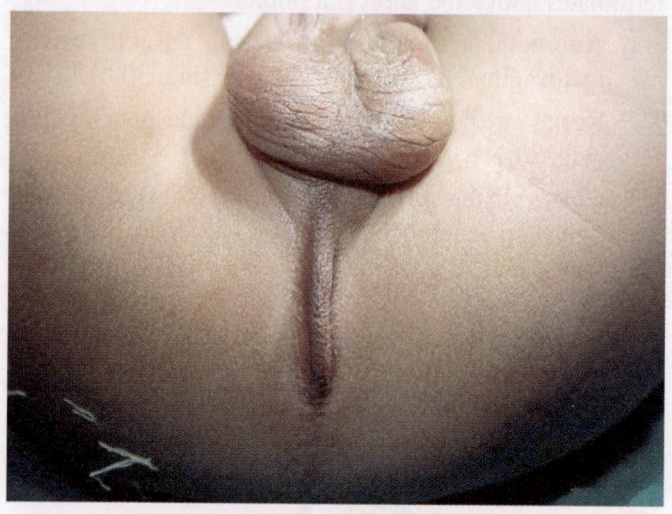

Fig. 30.43 Anorectal malformation

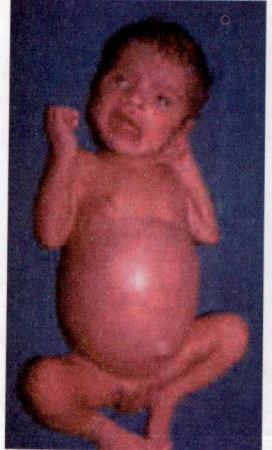

Fig. 30.44 Ileal obstruction

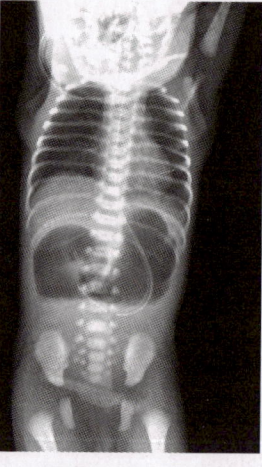

Fig. 30.45 Double bubble appearance

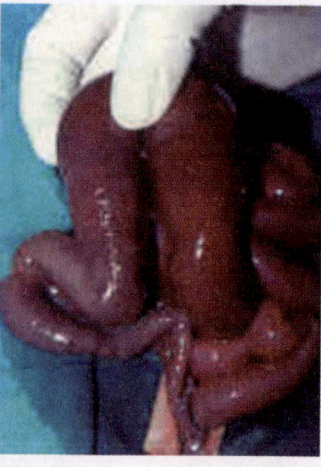

Fig. 30.46 Hirschsprung's disease

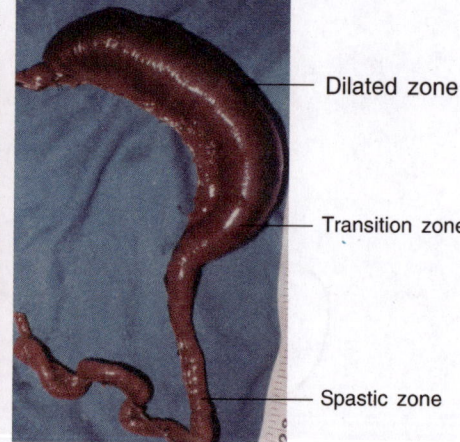

Fig. 30.47 Various segments of the large intestine in Hirschsprung's disease

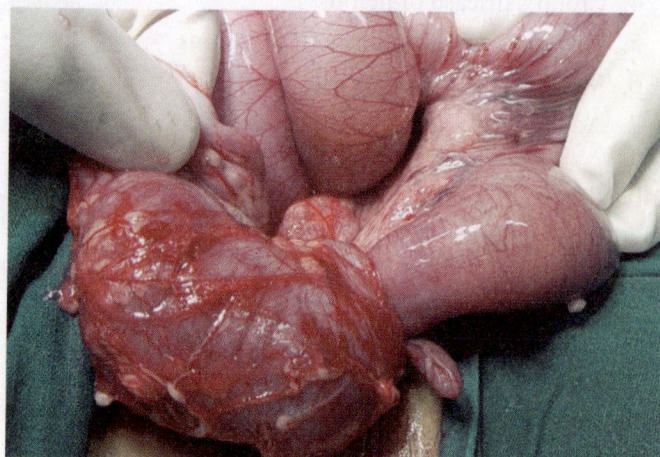

Fig. 30.48 Ileo-caecal intussusception

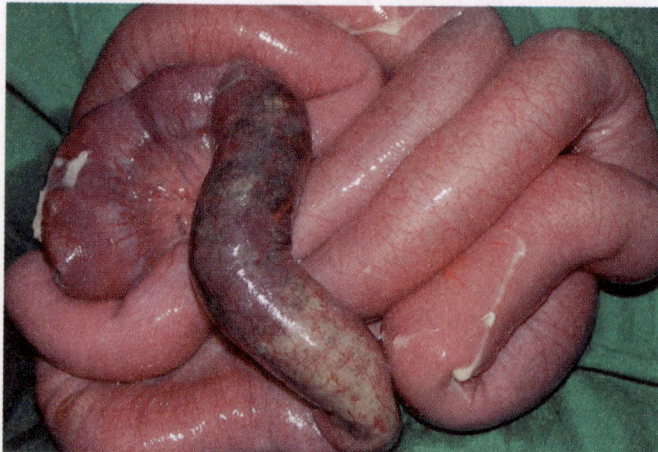

Fig. 30.49 Necrotising enterocolitis with patchy gangrene

Contributed by Prof. Vijaykumar, Head of the Dept. of Paediatric surgery, KMC, Manipal

PARALYTIC ILEUS (NEUROGENIC ILEUS)

- In this condition, there is a failure of transmission of parasympathetic impulses from one segment to the other. That means, there is a failure of parasympathetic mechanism, which results in paralysis of bowel. It gives rise to large collection of fluid and gas within the bowel resulting in distension.

Causes

1. **Post-operative**
   - Exposure of the intestines, handling of the intestines, contamination with blood, foreign body, etc., causes temporary suppression of parasympathetic activity and results in paralytic ileus. This gets aggravated by allowing oral fluids too early.
2. **Following peritonitis**
   - The pus is the chief cause. Bile, blood, etc. are other causes. Bacterial toxins also prevent movement of the bowel.
3. **Reflex :** Following fracture spine, retroperitoneal haemorrhage, etc.
4. **Hypokalaemia:** K⁺ is the chief ion of muscles. Hypokalaemia causes generalised muscle weakness including muscles of the bowel.

Clinical features

1. **Abdominal distension** is gross. Tympanitic note all over is a feature. Respiratory and cardiac functions are impaired.
2. **No colicky pain** abdomen (in dynamic obstruction, colicky pain is a feature). Dull pain occurs due to distension of the abdomen.
3. **Failure to pass flatus,** effortless vomiting is also characteristic of paralytic ileus.
4. On auscultation, **tinkling sounds** are heard due to shift of fluid from one coil of bowel to the other.
5. Severe fluid, electrolyte and protein depletion occurs.

Key Box 30.24

THREE TYPES OF BOWEL SOUNDS

- Normal: Once in 20 seconds, low pitch
- Borborygmi: Loud, noisy which occurs once in 5-10 seconds
- Tinkling sounds: Mild metallic sounds as in paralytic ileus

---

Investigations

1. Plain X-ray abdomen erect demonstrates distended loops of bowel
2. Electrolyte study and correction of any abnormality.

Treatment

- Basic principle in treating paralytic ileus is **DRIP AND SUCTION.**
- The cause of paralytic ileus has to be treated first, e.g. if there is hypokalaemia supplement potassium. If there is pus in the peritoneal cavity then drain it.
- Ryle's tube aspiration, to give rest to the gut.
- Intravenous fluids, supplementation of ions, correction of dehydration, oliguria, etc. Such treatment is continued for 3-4 days.
- Ryle's tube is removed when abdomen is soft, bowel sounds are heard and patient has present flatus. Clear oral fluids are started for 2-3 days followed by soft diet. Small bowel activity returns within 12-18 hours, followed by colon which starts functioning within 36-48 hours. However, gastric functions may return ranging from 18 hours to 4 days.

PSEUDOINTESTINAL OBSTRUCTION

- Acute colonic pseudoobstruction (ACPO) is also called as **Ogilvie's Syndrome.**

Pathogenesis

- It occurs mainly due to malfunctioning of sacral parasympathetic nerves. (S2-S4) It results in atony of the descending colon resulting in functional obstruction. **It is interesting to note that the junction of the dilated and collapsed bowel is near the splenic flexure.** This is the place wherein parasympathetic supply by vagus ends and sacral autonomic nervous system starts. An increased sympathetic tone result in colonic dilatation due to inhibition of contraction (Key Box 30.25).

Clinical features

- Elderly and old patients with abdominal distension are the victims.
- Failure to pass faeces and flatus for several days.
- Tachypnoea due to elevation of the diaphragm due to distended colon is common.

Key Box 30.25

CAUSES

1. Retroperitoneal irritation
   - Blood
   - Urine
   - Fracture spine and pelvis
2. Drugs
   - Levodopa
   - Tricyclic antidepressants
3. Metabolic
   - Uraemia
   - Diabetes
   - Myxoedema
   - Hypokalaemia
4. Viral infections

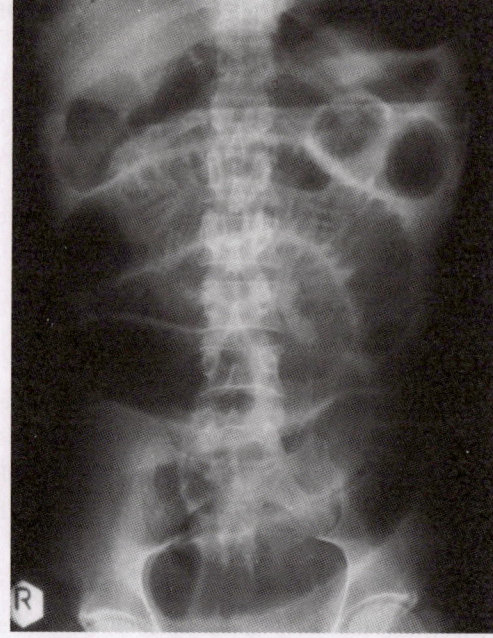

Fig. 30.50 Plain X-ray abdomen showing dilated bowel loops

- Rectal examination reveals some faeces (in cases of mechanical obstruction, rectum is empty).
- Plain X-ray abdomen erect may not show or may show one or two air fluid levels. Distension is mainly colonic.
- Carcinoma colon is to be differentiated by barium enema.

Treatment

- It is conservative, provided acute abdomen is ruled out.

- Prokinetic drugs such as Cisapride or Mosapride have been tried in selected cases.
- Rarely even after colonoscopic decompression if distension continues, caecal tenderness persists laparotomy followed by tube caecostomy may have to be done.

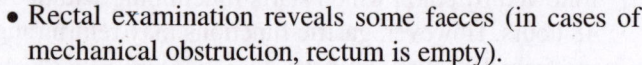

- Intestinal obstruction is a challenging surgical emergency encountered by general surgeons. This can affect any age group starting from neonate to an old man. It can affect a school going boy, working woman or a man during their peak of life. Sometimes it can be fatal either due to delay in the diagnosis, delay in the treatment or complications related to surgery. Abdomen is a pandora's box. Sometimes, it is difficult to pinpoint the cause of obstruction. However, students should be able to diagnose intestinal obstruction, resuscitate the patients and refer the patient for further surgical treatment. With the availability of sophisticated investigations like CT scan, diagnosis can be established in majority of cases before surgery. However in other cases - **'Exploratory Laparotomy'** will give the diagnosis.

Rectum and Anal Canal

31

- Surgical anatomy
- Carcinoma rectum
- Solitary rectal ulcer syndrome
- Prolapse rectum
- Surgical anatomy of anal canal
- Haemorrhoids
- Anorectal abscess
- Fistula in ano
- Fissure in ano
- Pilonidal sinus
- Sacrococcygeal teratoma
- Malignant tumours of the anal canal
- Stricture of the anal canal and rectum
- Anal incontinence

SURGICAL ANATOMY OF THE RECTUM (Fig. 31.1)

The rectum starts at the rectosigmoid junction, opposite the **third piece of sacrum**. It descends in the sacral hollow, passes through the pelvic floor, and ends in the anorectal junction, which is about 4 cm away from the anal verge. Anorectal junction is enclosed by puborectalis muscle posteriorly and in the lateral aspects. The rectum is 15-18 cm in length.

Peritoneal covering

- Upper one third is completely covered by peritoneum. (>11cms from anal verge)

- Middle one third is covered in front and lateral aspects. (6-11 cms)

- Lower one third (0-6 cms) has no peritoneal covering, but has two fascial condensation layers. Posteriorly, the strong **Waldeyer's** layer separates the rectum from lower sacral pieces and coccyx. At surgery stripping of this fascia results in uncontrollable bleeding from sacral plexus of veins, which is underneath the Waldeyer's fascia.

- Anteriorly, weak **Denonvillier's** fascia separates the rectum from prostate and bladder. Stripping of this fascia results in troublesome bleeding from prostatic venous plexuses.

- **Valves of Houston:** Rectum is never straight in adults. It has one convexity on the left and two convexities on

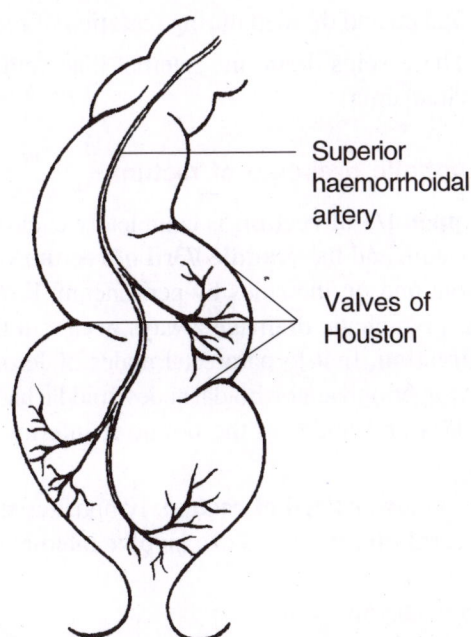

Superior haemorrhoidal artery

Valves of Houston

Fig. 31.1 Surgical anatomy of the rectum

515

the right side. There are 3 **valves of Houston**. (Prominent mucosal folds) two on the left and one on the right.

- That portion of the rectum resting on the pelvic floor is called **ampulla** - dilated portion of the mid rectum.

Arterial supply

1. **Superior haemorrhoidal artery,** branch of the superior rectal artery is the continuation of the inferior mesenteric artery, which divides into right and left branches. Right branch divides into anterior and posterior branches which supply the rectum.

2. **Middle haemorrhoidal artery,** branch of internal iliac artery, runs in the lateral ligament of the rectum.

3. **Inferior rectal artery,** a branch of internal pudendal artery supplies the lower rectum.

Venous return

The rich submucous plexus of veins surrounding the ampulla form external rectal plexus. The venous drainage from here flows in two directions.

1. **Upwards** to drain into superior rectal veins, which joins inferior mesenteric veins, which in turn drain into the portal system.

2. **Across** to drain into middle rectal veins, which run in the lateral ligament of the rectum along with middle rectal artery. Hence, the lateral ligaments have to be ligated and divided during resection of rectum.

   These veins drain into internal iliac veins (Systemic circulation).

Lymphatic drainage of rectum

- **Upper 1/3 of rectum** is completely enclosed by peritoneum and the **middle l/3rd of rectum** is covered in front and on the sides by peritoneum. From these areas, lymphatic drainage always occurs in the **upward direction,** first to pararectal nodes of Jerota followed by superior haemorrhoidal nodes, middle haemorrhoidal nodes and nodes at the origin of inferior mesenteric artery.

- From **lower l/3rd of rectum**, lymphatics spread in the **lateral direction** and can involve internal iliac nodes.

Nerve supply

- **Sympathetic:** The fibres come from hypogastric plexus, which is located at the aortic bifurcation at the level of L_5. Injury to this can cause absence of emis-

sion or dry orgasm. Fibres also come along with inferior mesenteric artery and superior rectal artery

- **Parasympathetic:** (S_2, S_3, S_4) by means of nervi erigentes from the hypogastric plexus and supply motor fibres to detrusor. Pain and ability to distinguish flatus and faeces is because of these fibres. Loss of mucosa of the rectum results in the loss of these sensations. During division of lateral ligaments or during anterior dissection of the bladder base, injury to nervi erigentes can occur.

CARCINOMA RECTUM

AETIOPATHOGENESIS

Similar to carcinoma colon. However, precancerous conditions and risk factors are mentioned below.

Precancerous conditions

- Polyps in FAP, Villous adenoma (Page 476, 477)
- Ulcerative colitis (Page 461)
- Crohn's disease (Page 466)

Risk factors

- **S**moking, **A**lcohol, **D**iet (Page 479)
- Genetic
- Colorectal family

PATHOLOGICAL TYPES

1. **Annular** variety is common at the **rectosigmoid** junction. It presents with constipation and intestinal obstruction. It takes about 12 months for the growth to completely encircle the lumen of the gut (napkin ring deformity).

2. **Polypoidal** lesions are common in the **ampulla** of the rectum.

3. **Ulcerative** lesions can occur anywhere in the rectum with **raised edges** and the growth occurs in the transverse direction.

4. **Diffuse** variety is similar to linitis plastica. It develops from ulcerative colitis. It has a poor prognosis.

5. **Colloid** variety is rare. The tumour contents are **gelatinous** due to increased mucous production. This variety is seen in young patients.

CLINICAL FEATURES OF CARCINOMA RECTUM

1. **Constipation** requiring increasing doses of purgatives due to annular growth at rectosigmoid junction.

2. **Bleeding per rectum,** frank blood or mixed with stools is common. It is never massive, painless and is the earliest symptom of carcinoma rectum. Very often, it is confused for haemorrhoids.

3. **Early morning spurious diarrhoea** is due to accumulation of mucous overnight in the ampulla of rectum (dilated middle portion of rectum), which causes an urgency to pass stools but results in only mucous with minimal stools. There is always a sense of incomplete defaecation.

4. **Tenesmus**
   - Painful, incomplete defaecation associated with bleeding is called as tenesmus.
   - This symptom is common with stricturous growths.

5. **Bloody slime** (Key Box 31.1)
   - An attempt at defaecation results in mucous mixed with blood.

6. Loss of appetite, loss of weight due to **liver secondaries**, abdominal distension due to obstruction are late features.

7. **Rectal examination** should be done, in every case of bleeding per rectum.

An indurated, cauliflower-like growth or infiltrative ulcer can be felt in more than 90% of the cases of carcinoma rectum. After removal of the finger, very often it is stained with blood. Hence, in every case of bleeding per rectum, rectal examination with the gloved finger followed by proctoscopy should be done.

> *Rectal cancer presenting as a fistula in ano is the equivalent to a perforated colonic cancer, it is a bad prognostic sign.*

Key Box 31.1
CLINICAL FEATURES
• Bleeding per rectum • Constipation • Early morning spurious diarrhoea • Bloody slime • Tenesmus

CLINICAL NOTES

A 22-year-old girl was treated with iron tablets for anaemia due to occasional bleeding per rectum. She was treated with metronidazole, because she was passing mucous along with the stools. She developed intestinal obstruction after 6 months during which time a surgeon was consulted. Rectal examination revealed a large growth, fixed all around. She died after 6 months because of advanced disease. The case illustrates the importance of rectal examination and that carcinoma of the rectum very often occurs in young patients.

DIFFERENTIAL DIAGNOSIS: (Key Box 31.2)

1. **Proctitis:** It could be due to inflammatory bowel diseases, tuberculosis, radiation or could be an amoeboma (rare).

Key Box 31.2
RECTAL ULCERS
1. Carcinoma rectum 2. Amoebic ulcers 3. Ulcerative colitis 4. HIV infections 5. Solitary rectal ulcers 6. Radiation proctitis

2 Solitary Rectal Ulcer Syndrome (SRUS)

- **Site:** Commonly occurs in the anterior wall of lower rectum, an area of muscosal change.

- **Mucosa:** It is erythematous, heaped up and bleeds on touch.

- It is a single, depressed ulcer.

- The cause, eventhough not clear - probably due to trauma.

- **Clinical features are:** Passage of blood and mucous in stools and mucosal prolapse may be a feature.

- Biopsy is a must to rule out carcinoma rectum.

- **Treatment is conservative:** to avoid constipation/straining.

SPREAD OF CARCINOMA RECTUM

1. Local spread

- It takes 18 months for a growth to encircle the lumen of rectum, as in annular strictures at the rectosigmoid junction.
- Then, it involves muscle coat and spreads into extra-rectal tissues.
- Anteriorly, it involves prostate, seminal vesicles and bladder base in males and vagina and uterus in females.
- Posteriorly, sacral plexus gets involved in late cases and causes sciatica-like pain.

2. Lymphatic spread

3. Blood spread

- It results in secondaries in the liver, lungs, etc. They are common in young patients with anaplastic variety and in colloid carcinoma.

4. Peritoneal spread

- It results in ascites, carcinomatous nodules over the peritoneum, etc.

DUKES STAGING OF CARCINOMA RECTUM

Stages

A Growth confined to the rectal wall

B Growth involving perirectal pad of fat and tissues. No nodes

C Nodes are involved

C_1 Local lymph nodes—pararectal

C_2 Distal Lymph nodes—in the course of the blood vessels

ASTLER-COLLER MODIFICATION OF DUKES SYSTEM

Stages

A Limied to mucosa — No nodes

B_1 Extention into muscularis propria — No nodes

B_2 Extension into entire bowel wall — No nodes

B_3 Extension into adjacent organs — No nodes

C_1 Extension into muscularis propria — Positive nodes

C_2 B_2+Lymph nodes

C_3 B_3+Lymph nodes

D Distant metastasis

PROGNOSIS AS PER DUKES STAGING

- Duke's A: 5 year survival is 90 to 100%
- Duke's B: 5 year survival is 50 to 80%
- Duke's C: 5 year survival is less than 50%

INVESTIGATIONS

1. **Proctoscopy:** It should be done in all cases of bleeding per rectum. It is done as an out-patient procedure. The left lateral position with buttocks elevated on a small pillow is the ideal position for protoscopy. However, knee-elbow position can also be used. The growth appears as an ulcer with everted edges. A biopsy is taken to prove the diagnosis. The histological grading of the tumour is as follows:

   A. **Well-differentiated carcinoma—Low grade variety**

   B. **Moderately differentiated carcinoma—The most common variety**

   C. **Anaplastic carcinoma—The most aggressive variety**

2. **Sigmoidoscopy:** To take a biopsy from rectosigmoid growths, sigmoidoscopy is essential.

3. **Barium enema:** It is indicated when proctoscopy and sigmoidoscopy fail to give a diagnosis due to spasm of the colon. When carcinoma arises in multiple polyposis coli or ulcerative colitis, barium enema is done to rule out synchronous malignancies.

4. **Colonoscopy:** If synchronous carcinoma exists (8 to 10%) biopsy can be taken to prove the diagnosis.

5. **C.E.A.:** The increased levels of carcinoembryonic antigen indicates metastasis.

6. **Ultrasound:** Some cases of carcinoma rectum present with metastasis like secondaries in the liver, ascites with paraaortic nodes, etc. (colloid carcinoma).

7. **Endorectal ultrasonography: EUS**

Key Box 31.3
EUS

- It is also called as **T**rans **R**ectal **U**ltra **S**onography - TRUS
- To know the level of penetration
- Detect perirectal lymph node enlargement
- Invasion of adjacent structures - Levator ani, bony plevis etc.

8. Computed Tomography (CT) Scan

- It helps to detect the lesion
- To know the extension of the tumour
- To know the fixation to adjacent structures (ureter, uterus, bladder base etc.)

TREATMENT OF CARCINOMA RECTUM

Principles

1. Aim is to have a **curative resection**
2. **Palliative resection** is worth doing even in presence of metastasis.
3. Eventhough surgical treatment is the main modality, **radiotherapy and chemotherapy** are beneficial.
4. At surgery, **ligation of vascular pedicle** is done first to prevent tumour embolisation.
5. **Ligation of bowel,** proximal and distal to the tumour helps to prevent transluminal dissemination.
6. 40% ethanol is used as tumouricidal agent to prevent suture line recurrence.
7. Distal surgical margin should be about 2.5 cms to 3 cms.
8. An attempt should be made to perform a **Total Mesorectal Excision (TME)** - (Key Box 31.4).

DIFFERENT TYPES OF SURGERIES FOR CARCINOMA RECTUM

Carcinoma upper 1/3 of rectum (Figs. 31.2 & 31.3)

- High anterior resection, which includes removal of growth along with the nodes, followed by colorectal

---

Key Box 31.4

TOTAL MESORECTAL EXCISION

- Mesorectum is the perirectal fat surrounding the rectum
- This fat is rich with lymphatics and pararectal nodes
- By sharp dissection, growth should be removed along with mesorectum. This is called as Total Mesorectal Excision

anastomosis is the treatment of choice. This is the operation of choice when the growth is situated between **11-15 cm** from the anal verge. The lymphatic spread from upper 1/3 is always in the upward direction. Hence, the sphincter is saved. If the bowel is well prepared, protective colostomy is not necessary (Sphincter saving surgery).

Carcinoma lower 1/3 of rectum (Figs. 31.4 & 31.5,6,7)

A. This refers to growth within **7 cm** from the anal verge. To achieve a radical cure, the sphincter has to be sacrificed. Radical surgery is called as Abdomino Perineal Resection or abdomino perineal excision (APR). Patient is put in Lloyd Davis position (supine with lithotomy). Two surgeons operate simultaneously, one from the abdomen and one from the perineum. Abdomen is opened first and the growth is mobilised from the sacrum and from the urinary bladder. At this stage, anus is closed by a perineal surgeon. Rectum and anal canal is mobilized. The entire specimen of rectum and anal canal and the nodes are removed followed by *'Permanent End Colostomy'* by bringing the sigmoid colon outside in the left iliac fossa (Sphincter sacrificing surgery).

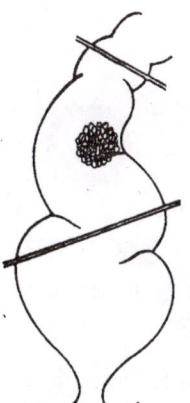
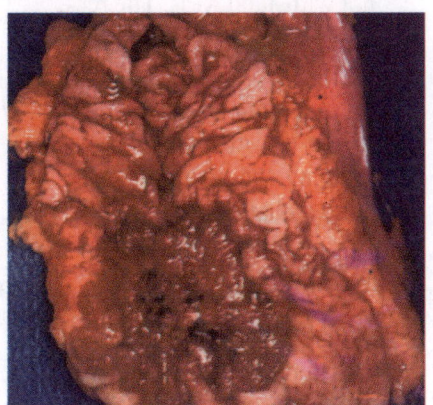

Fig 31.2 Carcinoma upper rectum

Fig 31.3 High anterior resection

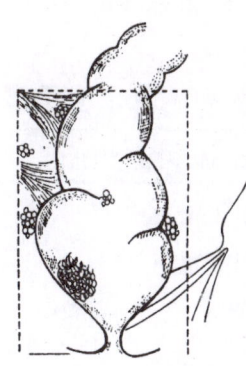
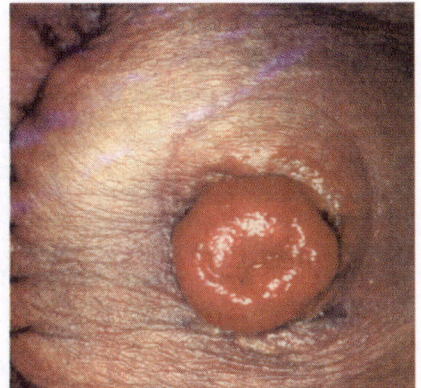

Fig 31.4, 31.5 The field of clearance in APR followed by permanent end colostomy

Key Box 31.5

STRUCTURES REMOVED IN APR

- Growth with entire rectum and anal canal
- Fascia propria with pararectal nodes
- Two thirds of the sigmoid colon and mesocolon with lymphatics and lymph nodes
- Muscles and peritoneum of pelvic floor
- Wide area of perianal skin, with part of ischiorectal fossa

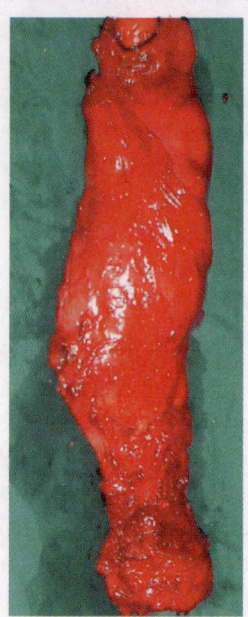 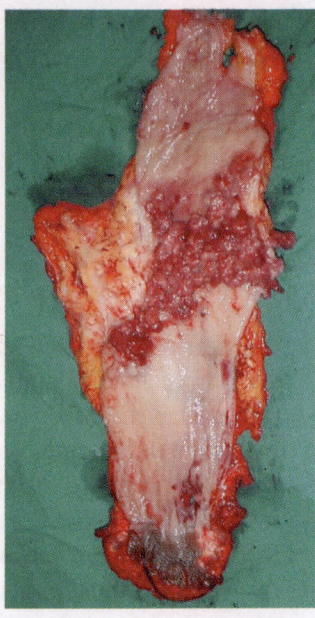

Fig 31.6 APR specimen. Observe the entire mesorectum has been removed **Fig. 31.7** Nodular lesion 3 cms away from the anal verge

B. Local excision: In our country 95% of low rectal cancers are treated and offered by abdominal perineal resection. Very small percentage of patients may be considered for local treatement - **local excision** (Key Box 31.6).

Key Box 31.6

LOCAL EXCISION OF CARCINOMA RECTUM

- Mobile tumours less than 4 cms in diameter
- Less than 40% of rectal wall involvement
- Located within 6 cms of anal verge
- Lesion should be T1 or T2
- No vascular or lymphatic invasion
- No nodal involvement - pre-operative MRI or EUS

Carcinoma middle 1/3 of rectum

- This refers to growth between 7-11 cm from the anal verge. The decision to save the sphincter can be taken at laparotomy. In cases of well-differentiated carcinoma, 2 cm margin is adequate. **In anaplastic carcinoma, 5 cm clearance is necessary.** In female patients with broad pelvis after mobilisation of the rectum, the 7 cm growth may appear around 10 cm from the anal verge. Thus, sphincter can be saved. If the sphincter can be preserved, low anterior resection (LAR) is done—sutures can be applied by hand or with staples. If sphincter cannot be preserved, APR is done (APR is also done if the tumour is bulky and high grade).

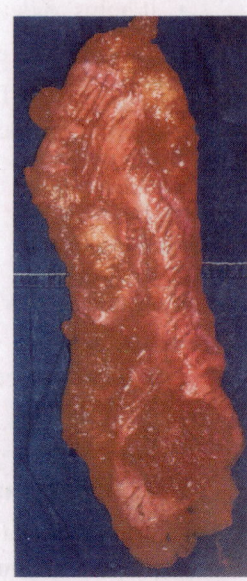

Fig 31.8 Low anterior resection

Inoperable cases

- Locally advanced growths present with severe pain, bleeding and with subacute intestinal obstruction. Temporary loop colostomy is done in the left iliac fossa by bringing the sigmoid colon outside. Postoperatively, radiation and chemotherapy is given.

Hartmann's operation (Fig. 31.9)

- This is indicated in old and debilitated patients who may not withstand APR. The rectum is excised, the lower end of the rectum is closed and a colostomy is performed. When the growth is slow-growing, this operation gives good palliation.

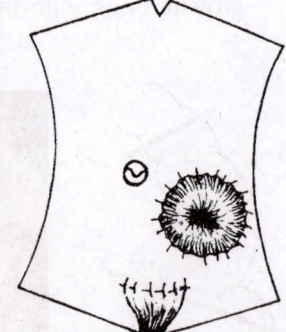

Fig 31.9 Hartmann's operation

- It involves wide retraction followed by good visualisation of lesion followed by complete thickness excision followed by direct suturing. It can be done by trans-anal, trans-sacral or trans-sphincteric approach.

ROLE OF RADIOTHERAPY IN CARCINOMA RECTUM

- Response rate of adenocarcinoma rectum is much better than rest of the gastrointestinal adenocarcinomas. Rectal cancers are more radiosensitive and colonic cancers are more chemosensitive. Neutron beam irradiation is used in the dose of 4000-5000 cGy units.

- **Preoperative radiotherapy** is indicated when the tumour is extended through the bowel wall. It reduces the size of the tumour and thus the tumour may be operable. The dose given is 45 cGy units (down staging of tumour).

Key Box 31.7

ADVANTAGES OF PREOPERATIVE RADIOTHERAPHY

- ↓ Tumour seeding at surgery
- ↑ Radiosensitivity due to more oxygenated cells
- Conversion of APR to LAR

- **Post-operative radiotherapy** is given to reduce the local recurrence.

- **Papillon's intracavity radiation** is indicated for a small, localised, well-differentiated and exophytic carcinoma as curative radiotherapy. Dose is 4000-5000 cGy units in 3 minutes.

ROLE OF CHEMOTHERAPY

1. Injection **5 fluorouracil** (5FU) in the dose of 475 mg/m^2/day/I.V. into 5 days with Injection **Leucovorin** 30 mg/day for 5 days.
   - 3 such courses are given at 4 weekly intervals.
   - Leucovorin or folinic acid is added to Injection 5FU as an immunomodulator.

2. Injection 5 FU in the same dose mentioned above can be used along with **Levamisole** in the dose of 150 mg twice a day for 3 days once in 15 days for one year.
   - However, the first combination using Leucovorin is more popular than levamisole.

Rectal cancers are more radiosensitive and colonic cancers are more chemosensitive.

COLOSTOMY

- Opening of the colon to the exterior, either temporary or permanent, for the drainage of faecal matter is called as colostomy.

TYPES

1. Temporary colostomy

A. In cases of acute left-sided colonic obstructions, proximal half of right transverse colon is brought out through the upper part of the right rectus abdominus muscle. Later, radical resection of the left colon is done followed by closure of the colostomy.

B. In cases of traumatic or congenital fistula affecting the left colon temporary colostomy is indicated (Fig. 29.24). The loop of the colon which is brought outside and held by glass rod which is passed through the transverse mesocolon and held by rubber tubing. This rod is removed after 5 days.

2. Permanent colostomy

It is indicated after abdomino-perineal resection, wherein the end of the sigmoid colon is brought outside in the left iliac fossa as permanent colostomy. The colostomy site should be 3 cm away from anterior superior iliac spine so that colostomy bag can be fitted properly. (Fig. 31.5)

3. Double barrelled colostomy

In this the adjoining walls of intestine are crushed. Both ends of the loop are defunctioned. This type of colostomy is not frequently done now. It was done earlier for sigmoid volvulus, resection of colonic stricture, etc.

INDICATIONS FOR COLOSTOMY

- **Congenital:** In Hirschsprung's disease and anorectal anomalies, temporary colostomy is done first.
- **Carcinoma:** Following APR, permanent endsigmoid colostomy is done.
- **Colonic fistulae:** Fistulae due to diverticulitis, Crohn's disease or due to tuberculosis.
- **Colonic injuries:** Trauma due to stab injuries or due to operative injuries following nephrectomy, pelvic operations PCNL (percutaneous nephrolithotomy).

ADVANTAGES OF COLOSTOMY

• Distal bowel takes complete rest, regains normal size and bacterial colonisation is reduced. It becomes empty and sterile so that chances of leakage at a later operation is reduced.

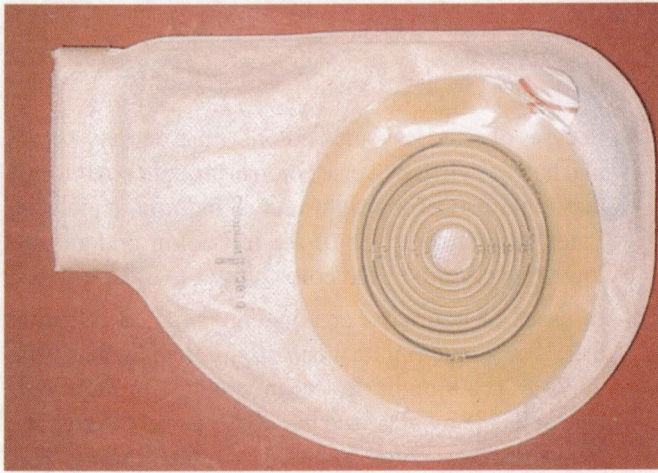

Fig 31.10 Disposable colostomy bags are available with or without flange. Depending upon the size of the stoma, it can be cut open so as to fit into the colostomy

COMPLICATIONS OF COLOSTOMY

• Bleeding, necrosis, retraction, prolapse and colostomy diarrhoea are some complications.

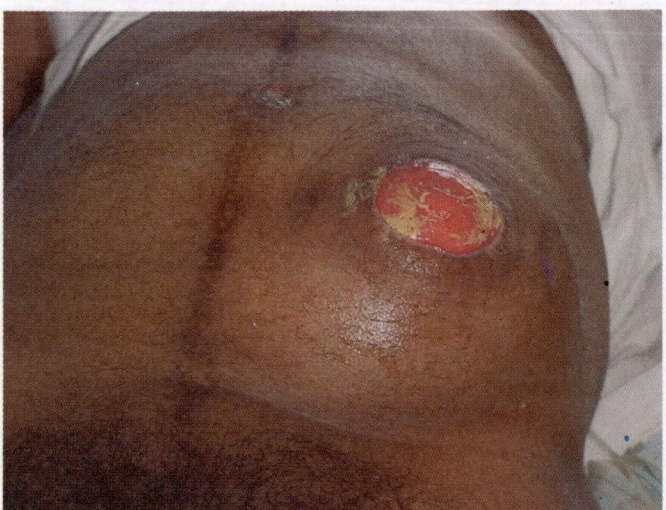

Fig 31.11 Paracolostomy hernia

Colostomy should be done by experienced surgeon as patient has to live with the colostomy life long.

PROLAPSE OF RECTUM

• Protrusion of the mucous membrane or the entire rectum outside the anal verge. This condition is common in children and elderly patients.

TYPES

• Prolapse can be of two types: Partial prolapse and complete prolapse.

Partial prolapse

• In this variety, the protrusion is between 1.25-3.75 cm outside the anal verge (Fig. 31.12)
• It is usually a mucosal prolapse.

Causes

1. In infants, it is due to **undeveloped sacral curve** and in children it can be secondary to **habitual constipation.**
2. It can follow after an attack of **whooping cough or excessive straining.**
3. It can follow an attack of diarrhoea resulting in **loss of fat** in the ischiorectal fossae, which supports the rectum.
4. In adults it is common in females probably due to **"Torn Perineum".**

Treatment

1. **Digital reposition :** In infants, partial prolapse is temporary. Mother is advised to push the prolapse inside after lubricating with lignocaine jelly.
2. **Injection of ethanolamine oleate** into the submucosa of the rectum. It causes aseptic fibrosis. Thus, mucosa gets tethered to the other layers.
3. Partial prolapse can be **excised**, after applying **Goodsall's ligature.**

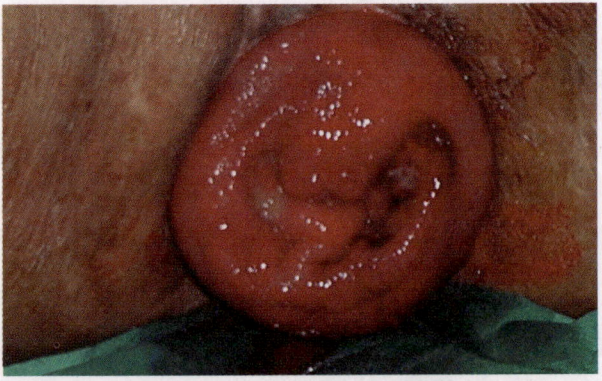

Fig 31.12 Partial prolapse

COMPLETE/TOTAL PROLAPSE

- It is also called as procidentia
- It is defined as protrusion of the rectum for more than 3.75 cm outside the anal verge. Very often, it is the entire rectum which protrudes out on straining, sometimes with the peritoneal sac.
- Very often, it is associated with prolapse uterus

Causes

1. **Common in elderly women who are multipara.** Probably, it is due to repeated **birth injuries** to the perineum causing damage to the nerve fibres. As age advances, muscles become weak, added by fatty degeneration of the muscle, resulting in a prolapse rectum.

2. **Excessive straining** causing weakness of the supports of the rectum.

3. **Defective collagen maturation** resulting in failure of rectal support by levators and pelvic fascia.

4. Presence of **deep rectovescical pouch** and excessive mobility of the rectum (mesorectum) predisposes to prolapse of the rectum.

5. Many people believe that prolapse of the rectum starts as an **intussusception** in the first stage, initiated by certain factors such as diarrhoea, constipation and disorder of the pelvic floor.

Clinical features

- Constipation is an important feature of rectal prolapse.
- Excessive mucous discharge causing irritation to the perianal skin.
- On asking the patient to strain at stool[1], the rectum descends down, which clinches the diagnosis.
- Some degree of incontience of faeces and flatus is always present. It will give rise to urgency and perianal soiling.
- Rectal examination—lax anal sphincter and wide gaping on straining.

Palpation of prolapse between finger and thumb reveals double thickness of tissue, especially anteriorly because of deep pouch of Douglas.

Differential diagnosis

- Large third degree haemorrhoids
- Large polypoid tumour
- Prolapse of sigmold colon

Complications

- Proctitis, ulceration and rarely bleeding
- Gangrene of the rectum

Treatment: Surgical procedures - Aim

1. Safe procedure to correct with minimal morbidity without mortality. They are classified as perineal procedures and abdominal procedures.
2. To cure or to improve **incontinence**

Perineal procedures

1. **Delorme's procedure:** In this, the prolapse is completely everted, mucosa is stripped and muscle coat is plicated. Mucosal continuity is maintained by suturing anal canal mucosa below to the rectal mucosa above. This is an easy operation to do in elderly patients. However, relapse rates are high and it does not correct the defect.

2. **Altmeir's procedure:** In this operation, full thickness of the prolapsed rectum with part of sigmoid is excised followed by anastomosis of part of the sigmoid to the anal canal from below. To improve continence, plication of levator ani and puborectalis muscle is done. Urgency and incontinence are the features because of removal of rectum.

3. **Thiersch wiring:** In this operation, a steel wire or a thick silk suture is applied all around the anus after reducing the prolapse. The knot is tightened around a finger. Patients with poor surgical compliance benefit from this operation. However, breakdown of the wire, perianal sepsis and anal stenosis are the complications.

Abdominal procedures

1. **Wells' operation :** A laparotomy is done, rectum is pulled upwards and is sutured to the sacrum posteriorly with the help of a polyvinyl alcohol sponge kept behind the rectum. The sponge is sutured posteriorly and

---

1. In fact surgeon should see the prolapse of the rectum outside when patient strains to make the clinical diagnosis.

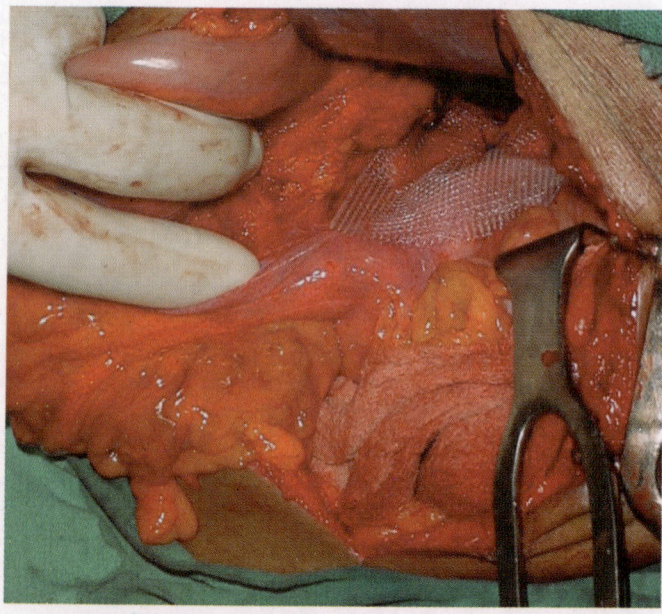

Fig 31.13 Mesh fixation for total prolapse of the rectum

laterally to the walls of the rectum. Dense fibrotic reaction occurs resulting in fixation of the rectum to the sponge.

2. **Ripstein's sling operation:** After a laparotomy, the rectosigmoid junction is sutured to the sacrum by using **Teflon Sling**, below the sacral promontory. One complication of this operation is constipation due to rectosigmoid angulation. Hence, sigmoidectomy has been suggested along with this operation.

3. **Mesh rectopexy:** Instead of polyvinyl sponge, a marlex mesh can be kept behind the rectum. This is sutured behind, to the sacrum and then to the posterior and lateral surfaces of rectum. Today laparoscopic method of fixing the mesh has become poplular.

4. **Lahaut's operation :** Anchoring rectosigmoid to rectus sheath (extraperitonisation).

SURGICAL ANATOMY OF ANAL CANAL

It is 3 cm long, starts as the continuation of rectum, passes through pelvic diaphragm and ends at the anal verge (skin).

INTERNAL SPHINCTER

• It is the continuation of circular muscle fibres of rectum and ends 0.5 cm below pectinate line.

• It is involuntary and 2.5 cm long.

• Internal sphincter with fibres of external sphincter and puborectalis which maintains the anorectal angle, form the **anorectal bundle, and maintains continence.**

• Its fibres are transversely placed. Motor fibres come from presacral plexus.

EXTERNAL SPHINCTER

• It is formed by **striated muscle fibres** intermingled with longitudinal muscle fibres of the rectum which get attached to the skin of perianal region. It has superficial, deep and cutaneous portions.

• Levator and puborectalis have an attachment with internal sphincter.

• Nerve supply (motor) comes from inferior haemorrhoidal branch of internal pudendal nerve and perianal branch of the 4th sacral nerve (motor to levator ani also).

• It is voluntary and gives temporary continence.

DEVELOPMENT

• Anal canal is developed from fusion of **post-allantoic gut** with **proctodeum.**

• The junction of these is the dentate line or pectinate line. **Anal valves of Ball** are remnants of proctodeal membrane.

• At the level of dentate line, the mucosa is folded in the form of longitudinal columns - *columns of Morgagni.*

• In between the columns of Morgagni, 4-8 anal glands open into the small anal sinuses.

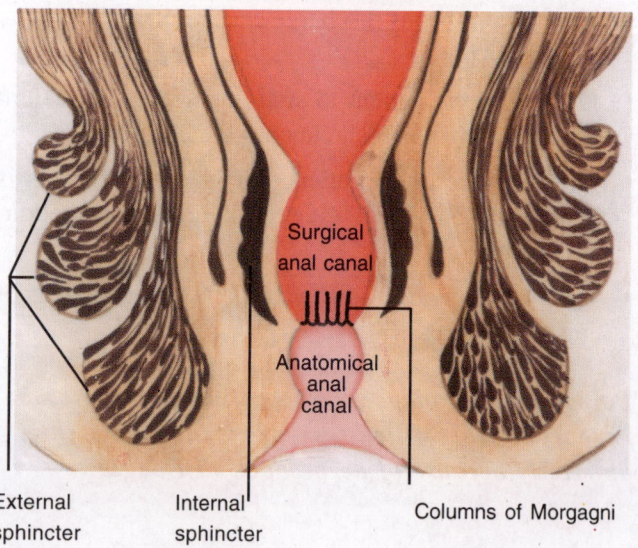

Fig 31.14 Anatomy of the anal canal

Table 31.1 Comparison of anal canal above and below the dentate line

	ABOVE THE DENTATE LINE	BELOW THE DENTATE LINE
1. Nomenclature	Surgical anal canal	Anatomical anal canal
2. Epithelium	Cuboidal epithelium	Skin - squamous epithelium, without hair and sweat glands
3. Nerve supply	Parasympathetic, hence painless	Spinal nerves, inferior haemorrhoidal nerve, very painful
4. Venous drianage	Portal system	Systemic veins (external iliac vein)
5. Colour	Pink	Skin colour
6. Development	Post-allantoic gut	Proctodeum
7. Lympatic drainage	Para-aortic nodes	Superficial and deep inguinal nodes

Comparison of anal canal above and below the dentate line is given in Table 31.1.

HAEMORRHOIDS (PILES)

DEFINITION

Dilated plexus of superior haemorrhoidal veins, in relation to anal canal.

CLASSIFICATION

I. Primary/Idiopathic haemorrhoids

Causes

1. **Standing position** of the human being is partly responsible for piles because blood has to flow against gravity.
2. **Anatomical factor**—the veins passing through the submucosa of the rectum, get constricted during the act of defaecation.
3. **Familial or genetic**—absence of valves or congenital weakness of vein wall.
4. **Constipation** causes excessive straining.
   - Thus gravity, straining and irregular bowel habits are important factors in the development of **Piles**.

II. Secondary haemorrhoids

Causes

1. Carcinoma of rectum, by blocking the veins, can produce back pressure and can manifest as piles.
2. **Portal hypertension** is an uncommon cause of piles (rectal varices).

3. **Pregnancy**, due to compression on superior rectal veins or due to progesterone which relaxes smooth muscle in the wall of the veins, can cause haemorrhoids.

III. Depending upon the location of haemorrhoids

1. **Internal haemorrhoids**—above the dentate line, covered with mucous membrane.
2. **External haemorrhoids**—at anal verge, covered with skin.
3. **Interno-external** — both varieties together.

LOCATION

Classically situated in the 3, 7, 11 o'clock positions (Fig. 31.14) (Left lateral, right posterior and right anterior respectively).

- Superior haemorrhoidal artery (vein) gives 2 branches on right side and 1 branch on left side. Hence, piles are two on right side and one on left side.

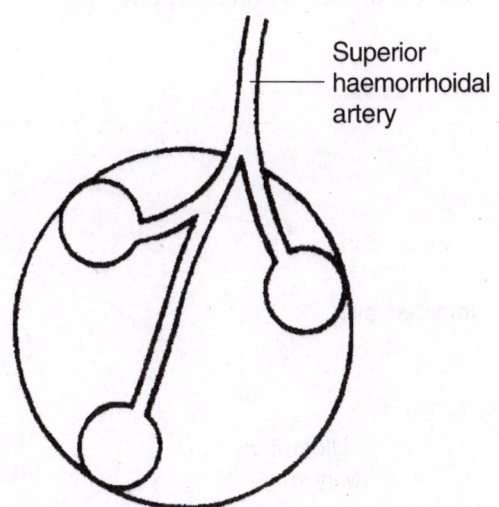

Superior haemorrhoidal artery

Fig 31.15 Classical location of pile masses

CLINICAL FEATURES

- Painless bleeding — fresh bleeding occurs after defaecation — **Splash in the Pan.** This causes chronic anaemia. Haemorrhoids which bleed are called Grade I haemorrhoids.

- The capillaries of the lamina propria are only protected by a single layer of epithelial cells, hence minor trauma precipitates bleeding.

- As the straining increases, the haemorrhoids partly prolapse outside. After defaecation, it returns back (Grade II) or can be digitally replaced (Grade III haemorrhoids).

- Permanently prolapsed pile outside (Grade IV) haemorrhoids. Patient complains of pain or discomfort.

- Most of the patients complain of constipation.

- Discharge of mucous and irritation of perianal skin— pruritus is a common feature.

INVESTIGATIONS

- Per rectal examination is done mainly to rule out carcinoma rectum or other causes of bleeding per recum. Haemorrhoids cannot be felt by rectal examination unless they are thrombosed or fibrosed.

- Proctoscopy—As the obturator is removed, piles prolapse into the lumen of proctoscope as cherry red masses.

- Sigmoidoscopy and proctoscopy are done to rule out proximal cancer.

COMPLICATIONS OF PILES (FIG. 31.16)

1. It can cause chronic anaemia. Rarely massive bleeding can occur due to portal hypertension.

2. A prolapse outside presents with pain (severe) in the perianal region -piles gripped by internal sphincter results in venous congestion and oedema followed by strangulation. Such patients are treated by:

- Elevation of foot end of bed
- Metronidazole 400 mg, 3 times a day for 5 days.
- Saline dressings to reduce oedema
- Local lignocaine jelly application

3. Ulceration and secondary infection

4. Thrombosis and fibrosis

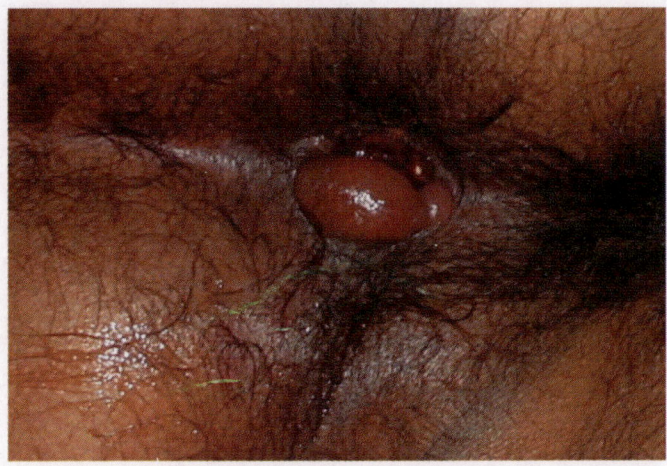

Fig 31.17 Prolapsed piles

TREATMENT OF PILES

1. **Lord's dilatation:** Under G.A., the internal sphincter it widely stretched which is supposed to relieve the venous congestion, and improve the piles. This is indicated in grade I varices. It is supposed to rupture pecten

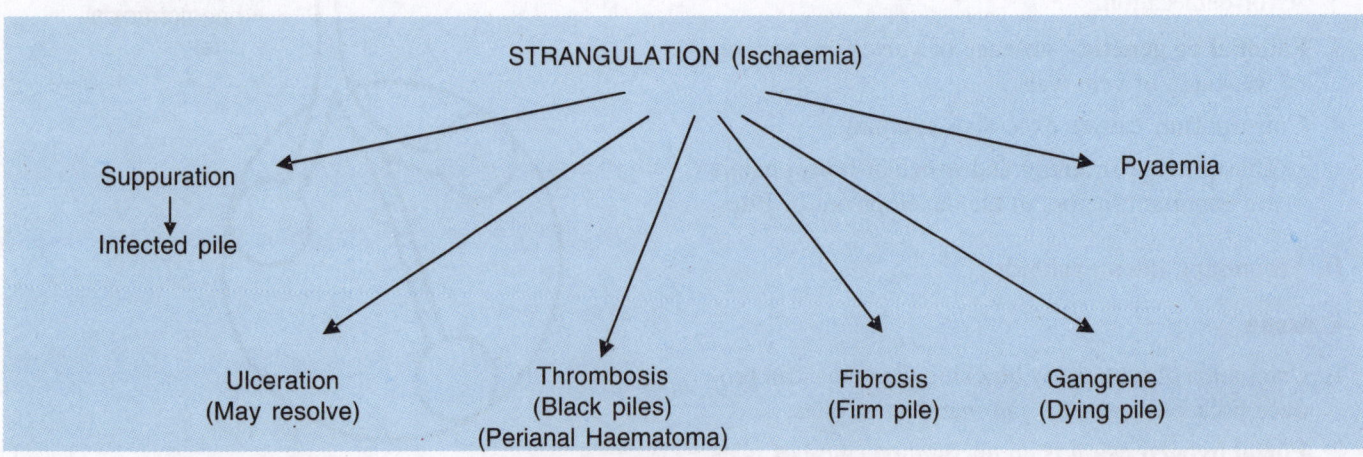

Fig 31.16 Complications of piles

bands. It also results in dilatation and disruption of the few fibres of internal sphincter.

2. **Injection of sclerosant:** 5% phenol in almond oil is injectcd into **submucosa** above the dentate line.Hence, it is painless. It produces **aseptic thrombosis** of pile mass and is indicated in grade I. The injection is **perivascular.**

3. **Barron's band application :** It is indicated for grade II and grade III haemorrhoids, wherein bands are applied at the neck of the haemorrhoids. It causes necrosis and thus, piles get fibrosed. One or two can be banded at a time.

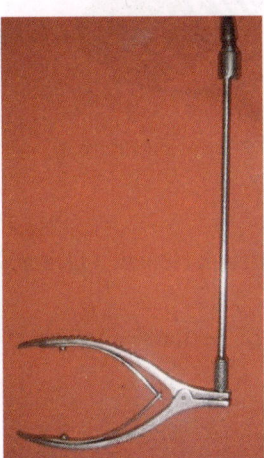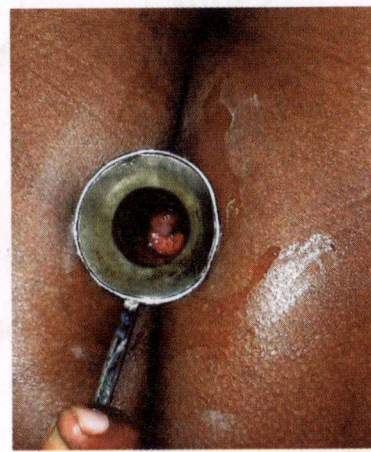

Fig 31.18 & 31.19 Barron's band ligator and band has been applied to one of the pile masses

4. **Haemorrhoidectomy:** Excision of the pile masses up to base is indicated in grade II and grade III haemorrhoids. It can be done by two methods: Open and closed method. (Vide infra)

5. **Cryosurgery:** Liquid nitrogen at -196°C is applied to pile masses which coagulates the tissues. The procedure is painless and there will be continuous mucous discharge for 3-4 weeks.

Key Box 31.8	
TREATMENT OF PILES	
• Neglect	Conservative
• Inject	Grade I and II
• Ligate	Band ligation - Grade II or Grade III
• Dilate	Lord's dilatation
• Dissect	Surgery

HAEMORRHOIDECTOMY

1. Open method — Miligan Morgan ligature and excision.

- Stretch the sphincter
- Identify the positions of pile masses
- Dissection upto the base (pedicle)
- Transfixation ligature with **nonabsorbable silk**
- Excision of the piles
- Trimming the wound
- Haemostasis obtained
- Wound packed with roller gauze
- A tube drainage is provided so that the blood (oozing) can escape outside

2. Closed method (Hill-Ferguson):

- Basic steps are the same as above
- Cut mucosa and skin edges are sutured with absorbable catgut sutures

Postoperative management

1. Strong analgesics, in the form of injection pethidine or morphine, are given to reduce the pain.

2. Antibiotics along with metronidazole are given to prevent secondary infection.

3. Bulk purgatives are given to avoid constipation.

4. **Sitz bath** twice/day is given by using warm saline or $KMnO_4$ solution.

Postoperative complications

1. **Retention of urine** is common in men due to severe pain. It can be managed by treating the pain and hot water fomentation in the suprapubic region. Catheterisation is done as a last resort.

2. **Secondary haemorrhage** can occur due to infection. It manifests 6 to 8 days later. If the bleeding is significant, exploration in the operation theatre may be necessary. It should be done under anaesthesia. With good illumination it is possible to identify the bleeding points and ligate them.

3. **Anal stenosis** can occur if too much skin is excised during haemorrhoidectomy. It needs regular dilatation.

4. **Wound infection:** Minor degree of wound infection does occur which can be managed by sitz bath, antibiotics and regular dressings.

ANORECTAL ABSCESS

- It is due to **pyogenic infection of an anal gland**. It starts at the base of anal crypt in between sphincters and then it spreads.
- Culture usually shows E. coli in about 70-80% of cases.
- Staphylococcus aureus, Streptococcus, Bacteroides are the other organisms.
- Blood-borne infection can occur in diabetic patients.

Key Box 31.9
CAUSES OF ANORECTAL ABSCESS
• Infection
• Irritation (Crohn's, Ulcerative colitis)
• Immunity low (Diabetes, AIDS)

TYPES (Fig. 31.20)

1. Perianal abscess

- It occurs due to infection of anal glands in the perianal region.
- It may be due to a boil or due to anal gland infection or due to thrombosed external pile.
- It produces severe pain, throbbing in nature and on examination a soft, tender, warm swelling is found.
- Rectal examination reveals a tender, boggy, swelling under the anal mucosa.

Treatment

- Antibiotics, incision and drainage and excision of part of skin (roof).

2. Submucous abscess

- Collection of pus under the mucous membrane of rectum or anal canal.
- It can also be due to infection of injected haemorrhoids. It can be opened by using proctoscope.

3. Ischiorectal abscess

- Collection of pus in the ischiorectal fossa, which is lateral to rectum and medial to pelvic wall.
- Bounded above by levator ani and inferiorly by pad of fat in the ischiorectal fossa.

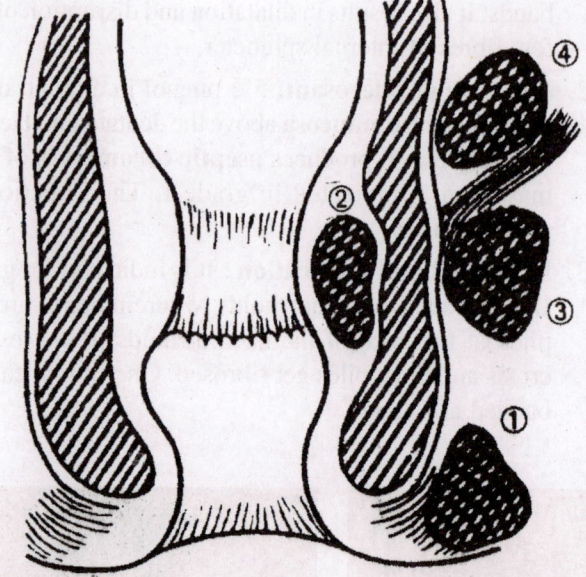

Fig 31.20 Types of anorectal abscess (Refer text)

- Ischiorectal fat is poorly vascularised. Hence, it is more vulnerable for infection.
- Abscess occurs due to spread of perianal abscess or due to blood-borne infection.

Clinical features

- Severe throbbing pain is characteristic of ischiorectal abscess.
- Induration in the ischiorectal fossa.
- Frank evidence of abscess like fluctuation need not be seen (Key Box 31.10) and is a late sign.
- High grade fever with chills and rigors.
- Common in diabetic men.
- Per rectal examination is painful and bogginess can be appreciated on the side of the lesion.

Key Box 31.10
DEEP ABSCESS WITH NO FLUCTUATION
1. Ischiorectal abscess
2. Breast abscess
3. Parotid abscess
4. Prostatic abscess
5. Midpalmar abscess

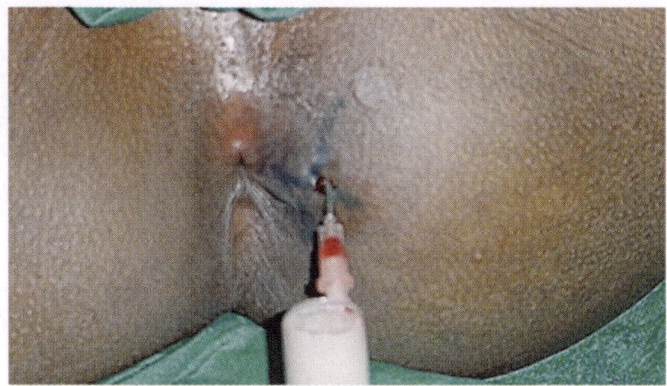

Fig 31.21 Aspiration of ischiorectal abscess

Treatment

- Under anaesthesia, a cruciate incision (+) (Fig. 31.22) is made and the 4 flaps are raised. All the pus is evacuated and the wound is packed with iodine roller gauze

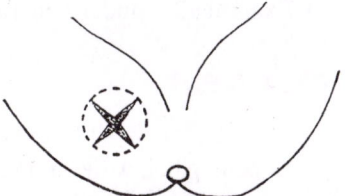

Fig 31.22 Cruciate incision - drainage

and left open. Edges of the skin are trimmed to leave an opening so that drainage of pus occurs freely. It heals with granulation tissue within 10-15 days. Appropriate antibiotics are given for a period of 10 to 15 days.

4. Pelvirectal abscess

- It is a pelvic abscess, which is drained through the rectum. The common causes are pelvic peritonitis, appendicitis, septic abortions, etc. The details of the causes, clinical features and the management are discussed in page 445.

FISTULA IN ANO

Abnormal communication between anal canal and rectum with exterior (perianal skin). Eventhough multiple openings are seen in the perianal skin, **the internal opening is always single.**

AETIOPATHOGENESIS

1. They occur due to persistent anal gland infection, which results in anorectal abscesses which rupture inside as well as outside resulting in a fistula. Once a fistula occurs, it persists because of infection and absence of rest to the part.

2. Patients with pulmonary tuberculosis have got 1-2% chances of developing multiple fistulae in ano. Such fistulae are **not indurated and there is watery discharge without pus.**

3. In Western countries, ulcerative colitis, Crohn's disease are responsible for multiple fistulae in ano.

4. Colloid carcinoma of rectum can present as multiple fistulae in ano. Hence, PR should be done in every case of fistula in ano.

Other causes of fistula (Key Box 31.11)

Key Box 31.11
SPECIAL TYPES OF FISTULA IN ANO
• **F**istula carcinoma
• **I**leitis - Crohn's
• **S**chistosomiasis
• **T**uberculosis
• **U**lcerative colitis
• **L**ymphogranuloma venereum
• **A**nal fissure abscess
* *Students can remember as* ***FISTULA***.

CLASSIFICATION

1. Standard classification (Fig. 31.23)

1. Subcutaneous
2. Submucous
3. Low anal
4. High anal
5. Pelvirectal

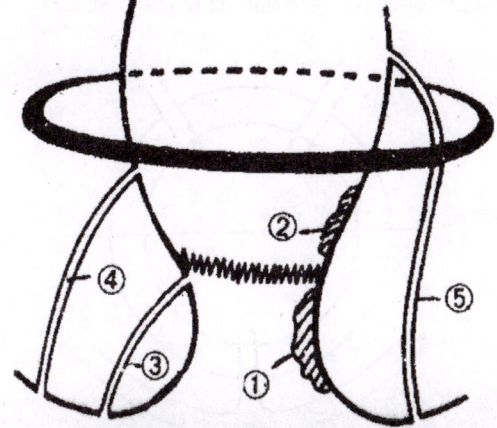

Fig 31.23 Standard classification

II. Parks' classification (Fig. 31.24)

1. Intersphincteric
2. Transsphincteric
3. Supralevator (internal opening is situated above the anorectal bundle)

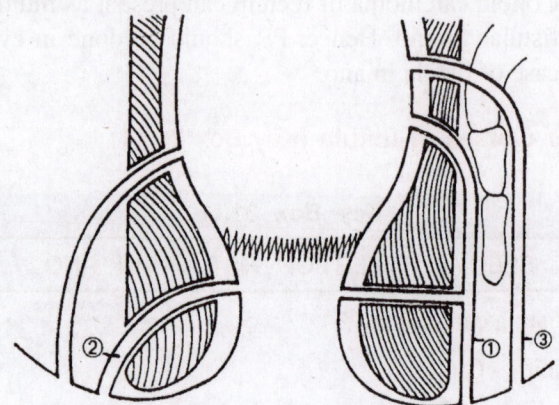

Fig 31.24 Parks' classification

CLINICAL FEATURES

- Persistent seropurulent discharge, keeps the part always wet.
- Previous history of anal gland infection, with recurrent abscess.
- External opening can be single/multiple, with pouting granulation tissue, may discharge blood.
- Internal opening in carcinoma felt as a 'buttonhole' defect inside the rectum.
- **Goodsall's Rule:** A fistula, with an external opening in the anterior half of anus within 3.75 cm tends to be direct type and in the posterior half indirect type or curved and sometimes horse-shoe type. It may communicate with the opposite side (Fig. 31.25).

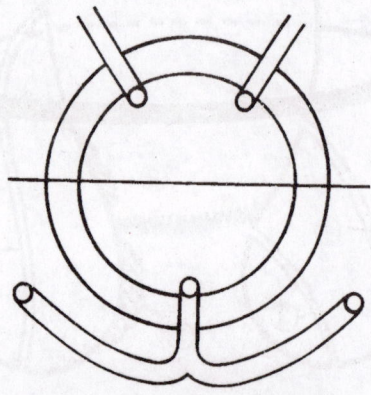

Fig 31.25 Goodsall's rule

DIAGNOSIS

- External opening is found at the bottom of a depressed area or with granulation tissue or it is seen with discharging pus.
- Internal opening may be felt on digital examination as **indurated** area or sometimes can be seen with proctoscopy or after sigmoidoscopy.
- The entire track may be palpable as indurated cord like structure.
- **Endorectal ultrasonography** and **MRI** seems to identify internal openings and fistula. However they can be selectively used in deserving cases.
- Examination under general or regional anaesthesia

TREATMENT

I. Fistulotomy: It is indicated in low fistula (internal opening below the anorectal bundle). A probe is passed through the external opening into the rectum and along the length of this tract the fistula is laid open. It is done under anaesthesia. The wound is left open and allowed to heal by granulation tissue developing from the floor of the fistula (marsupialisation).

Intersphincteric and low trans-sphincteric fistulas of recent origin are treated by fistulotomy and marsupialization.

Advantages:

- Least chances of recurrence
- Relatively easy procedure
- Minor degree of incontinence

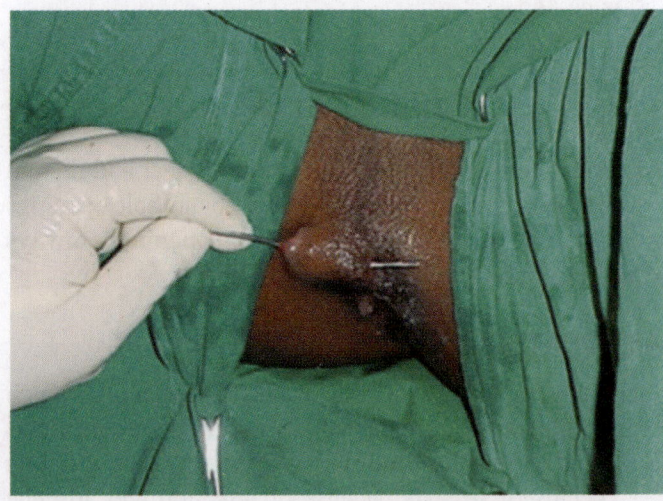

Fig 31.26 Fistulotomy by passing a fistula probe

II. Fistulectomy: All **chronic fistula (low) are treated by fistulectomy** by excising the entire fibrous tissues and track. Here also wound is kept open. This can also be done for **posterior semihorseshoe and horseshoe** fistula. Some incontinence can occur.

III. Fistulectomy with or without colostomy: It is indicated in high fistula in ano. The internal opening is situated above the anorectal bundle. Hence, during fistulectomy, there is a chance of injury to the anorectal bundle and may cause incontinence. Temporary or permanent colostomy may be necessary. If there is a cause, treat the cause. Surgery of intersphincteric fistula and trans-sphincteric fistula may result in incontinence.

IV. Use of Seton or medicated thread (Ksharsutra): It is passed through the entire tract and both ends are tied and tightened once a week so that by 6 weeks it cuts through.

FISSURE IN ANO

Longitudinal tear in the lower end of anal canal results in fissure in ano. It is the **most painful condition** affecting the anal region. Commonly seen in young patients.

AETIOPATHOGENESIS (KEY BOX 31.12)

- 90% of fissure-in-ano occur in the posterior part of anal canal and 10% anteriorly. It is initiated by hard stool causing a crack. As a result of this, defaecation results in pain. Fissure-in-ano are more common midline posteriorly, this is because of relative ischaemia.
- **Due to pain, internal sphincter spasm** takes place which makes constipation worse resulting in a chronic fissure (Fig. 31.27).
- **Anterior fissures** occur in elderly women secondary to repeated pregnancies. This is due to damaged pelvic floor and lack of support to anal mucous membrane.

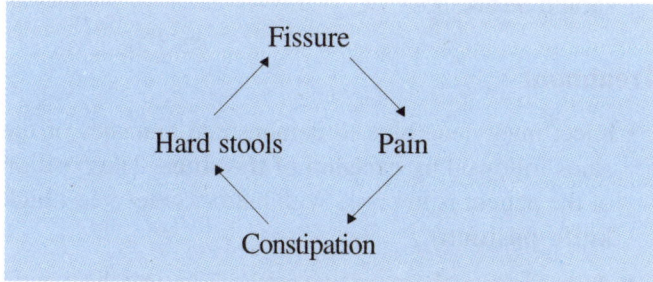

Fig 31.27 Aetiopathogenise of anal fissure

Key Box 31.12

VARIOUS FACTORS WHICH PRECIPITATE FISSURE IN ANO

- Faeces - Hard
- Ischaemia
- Surgical procedures - Haemorrhoidectomy
- Sphincter hypertonia
- Underlying diseases - Crohn's, STDs etc.
- Repeated child birth
- Enthusiastic usage of ointments and abuse of laxatives

Fissure away from midline should raise the possibility of Crohn's disease, STDs etc.

CLINICAL FEATURES

- Severe pain during and after defaecation, burning in nature, lasting for about 1/2 hour to 1 hour because of which defaecation is postponed.
- Severe constipation is present.
- Stools are hard, pellet like and there is a drop of blood or streak of fresh blood.

Drop of blood is due to Fissure in Ano.
Splash of blood is due to Haemorrhoids.

- Sentinel pile refers to tag of skin at the outer end of the fissure
- In some cases, fissure may be associated with a small perianal abscess resulting in worsening of pain.

DIAGNOSIS

1. When the buttocks are spread apart, a longitudinal tear and a hypertrophied, thickened skin is seen near the lower end of fissure - **sentinel pile**.
2. Per rectal examination can be done (with lignocaine jelly application) and **sphincter spasm** can be appreciated.
3. Proctoscopy is contraindicated because the condition is very **painful**.

TREATMENT

1. Conservative

- Avoid constipation - encourage fibre diet, mild laxatives, not to postpone defaecation.

- Surface anaesthetic creams : lignocaine jelly
- Metronidazole and antibiotics
- Sitz bath

II. Agents which decreases sphincter pressure

- **Glyceryl trinitrate** topical application : significant headache and 50% recurrence are drawbacks.
- **Purified botulinum toxin** injection into internal spincter: It inhibits presynaptic release of acetylcholine from cholinergic nerve endings and cause temporary paresis of striated muscle. Cost, perianal thrombosis are drawbacks.

Key Box 31.13

ROLE OF BOTULINUM TOXIN INJECTION

- Achalasia cardia and other oesophageal motility disorders
- Anal fissures
- Sphincter of Oddi dysfunction
- Frey's syndrome

- **Calcium channel blockers** - Nifedipine, diltiazem oral as well as topical application also have been used.

III. Surgical Treatment:

1. **Lateral sphincterotomy** (or dorsal) is another alternative procedure. Here internal sphincter is divided away from fissure either in right or left lateral positions. The procedure can be easily done by using a bivalved speculum in the anal canal. This is the procedure of choice.
2. **Lord's dilatation** It is also called as **blunt sphincterotomy** - few fibres of internal sphincter are divided. It relieves the spasm and the fissure heals. Rarely, in female patients it may result in incontinence.
3. **Fissurectomy and local advancement flap** This is indicated in presistent, chronic, non-healing fissure. After excision of the fissure, the resulting defect in the anal canal is closed by a small (**rhombold**) advancement flap.

Lateral sphincterotomy is very popular and gives good results.

PILONIDAL SINUS (JEEP BOTTOM)

Means **nest of hairs** in Greek. Also called as **Jeep-Bottom** because it was very common in jeep drivers.

It is an acquired condition, commonly found in hairy males. More common in dark people than fair people. **It is acquired due to the following reasons:**

- Appears between the age of 20-30 years
- Hairy men are more affected
- The **hair follicle is never demonstrated in the wall of the pilonidal sinus** but hair is the content of pilonidal sinus.
- Hair accumulates due to vibration and friction causing shedding of the hair. Thus, it accumulates in the gluteal cleft and enters the opening of the sweat glands.

Key Box 31.14

SITES OF PILONIDAL SINUS

- Midline over the coccyx
- Umbilicus
- Interdigital

Clinical features

- External opening of the sinus seen just above the anal verge in the midline over the coccyx
- History of discharge of pus
- History of recurrent abscesses which rupture, discharging pus
- Can be asymptomatic

Diagnosis

- Osteomyelitis of the coccyx is the only differential diagnosis for pilonidal sinus. Hence, X-ray of the coccyx should be taken.

Treatment

- Inject methylene blue to demonstrate branches of the sinus followed by **excision of the sinus**. The position of the patient is in prone with buttocks elevated (**Jack knife position**).
- After excision there are two methods to treat the wound - Open and closed methods.

- **Open method:** The wound is left open after excision followed by regular packing with iodine or Eusol gauze pieces.
  - It may take 3-4 weeks for the healing of pilonidal sinus. Regular 'sitz bath' is also given.
  - This method carries the least recurrence.
- **Closed method:** The wound is closed by 'z' plasty. This method carries 10-20% chances of recurrence.

Very very rarely carcinoma can arise in a chronic pilonidal sinus.

SACROCOCCYGEAL TERATOMA

- It is a congenital condition affecting the sacrococcygeal region.
- In this region, totipotential cells persist for a longer period compared to rest of the area. Hence, it is the site of teratomas.

Clinical features

- 20% of the cases are stillborn babies. It is common in a female child.
- Presents as swelling in the sacrococcygeal region pushing the rectum anteriorly.
- The surface of the swelling ulcerates. Many cystic areas are present in the swelling.
- The swelling is fixed to the sacrum and coccyx from which it is impossible to separate/isolate.

Complications

- Ulceration
- Secondary infection
- Haemorrhage
- Teratocarcinomatous change occurs by one year of age

Treatment

- Excision of the teratoma with part of sacrum and coccyx.

MALIGNANT TUMOURS OF ANAL CANAL

- They are not uncommon tumours which present with bleeding per rectum, burning and itching in the anal region.

- The diagnosis is obvious in many cases once buttocks are separated or by digital examination.
- Tissue diagnosis is a must before radical treatment.

TYPES

1. **Squamous cell carcinoma:** Papillomas are the chief predisposing factors. Local excision or APR is the treatment with external RT in appropriate cases.

2. **Basaloid carcinoma:** It is a highly malignant non-keratinising squamous cell carcinoma. Treatment is similar to squamous cell carcinoma.

Basal cell carcinoma is very rare in the anal canal.

3. **Melanoma:** Beware of a patient who comes with bilateral groin nodes which are bulky. Patient may be having malignant melanoma of anal canal - Bluish/blackish ulcer in the anal canal. APR is potentially curable and local excision if metastases are present.

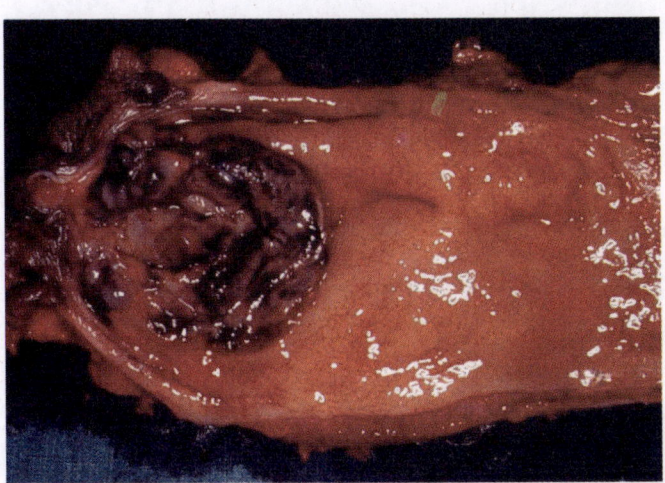

Fig 31.28 Malignant melanoma of the anal canal - APR specimen

4. **Adenocarcinoma** is rare, it can occur from the anal glands in preexisting fistula in Ano. APR with 5, FU and radiation therapy is indicated.

Please note Bowen's disease, Paget's disease or verrucous carcinoma, squamous and Basal cell carcinoma can also occur in the skin of anal margin.

STRICTURE OF ANAL CANAL AND RECTUM

CAUSES

1. **Post-operative:** Haemorrhoidectomy, pull through operations, repeated diathermy fulguration of polyps.

2. **Irradiation:** It occurs one to two years after irradiation.

3. **Senile strictures**

4. **Lymphogranuloma inguinale**: A sexually transmitted disease affecting both male and female patients. Initially pararectal lymph nodes are enlarged followed by development of rectal strictures.

5. **Inflammatory bowel diseases :** Both ulcerative colitis and Crohn's disease results in rectal strictures (5-10%).

6. **Rare :** Congenital, amoeboma, carcinoid, endometriosis, tuberculosis, CMV colitis.

Clinical features

• Increasing constipation is the characteristic feature of stricture of the rectum. It may be associated with hard stools, bleeding and pain in some cases. Per abdominal examination may reveal loaded colon with scybalous masses. Rectal examination can detect a stricture.

However, it is mandatory to rule out carcinoma rectum which is the most common cause of stricture.

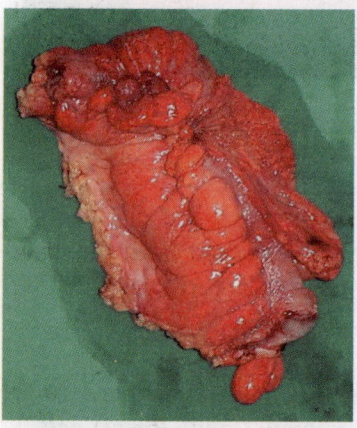 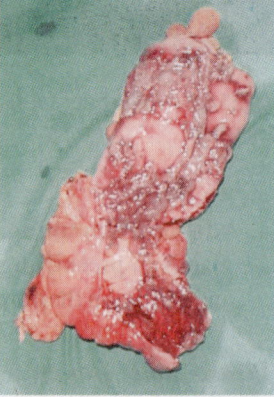

Fig 31.29 Rectal stricture due to CMV colitis - Contributed by Dr. Satyanarayana N., Dr. Srinivas Pai, Dr. Madhu, KMC, Manipal

Treatment

1. Conservative treatment includes bulk purgatives, a vegetable diet, etc.
2. Regular dilatation may be necessary for the strictures situated low in the rectum and anal canal.
3. Intractable strictures need to be resected.
4. Treatment of the primary disease.

ANAL INCONTINENCE

Mechanism of anal continence

• Distension of rectum causes tonic contraction of external sphincter. This is controlled by cerebrum and the centre is in the lumbosacral region of the spinal cord.
• Faeces in contact with anal canal stimulates the specialised nerve endings.
• Nerve endings are also present in the puborectalis.
• High pressure in the anal canal (25-120 mm of Hg) and angle between rectum and anal canal (80°) are the important factors which maintain anal continence.

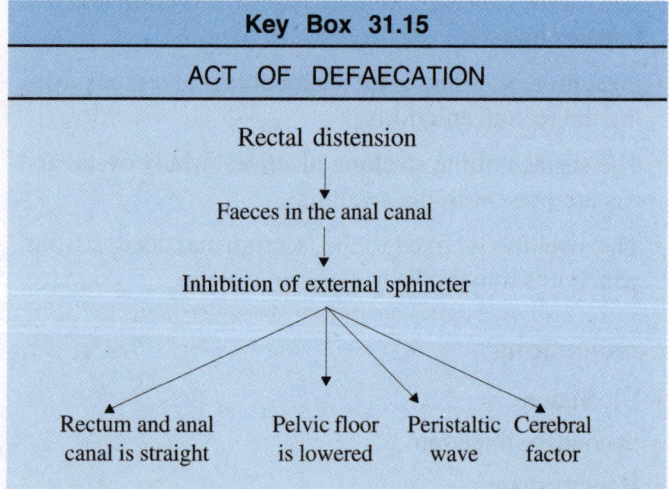

Key Box 31.15

ACT OF DEFAECATION

Rectal distension
↓
Faeces in the anal canal
↓
Inhibition of external sphincter
↓

| Rectum and anal canal is straight | Pelvic floor is lowered | Peristaltic wave | Cerebral factor |

Anorectal ring

• It marks the junction between the rectum and anal canal. It is formed by puborectalis, highest part of internal sphincter, longitudinal muscle and external part of sphincter.

Causes of anal incontinence

1. **Traumatic:** Injury to the anorectum due to sharp penetrating objects, occurs due to accidents.

2. **Surgical procedures:** Damage to the internal and external sphincter can occur due to Lord's dilatation, a procedure done for fissure-in-ano. However, most of it is temporary.
   - Division of high fistula-in-ano may result in incontinence.
   - Following pull-through procedures done for anorectal anomalies, Hirschsprung's disease.

3. **Mass in the anorectum:** Prolapse piles, prolapse rectum and carcinoma rectum may produce temporary incontinence which subsides after surgical procedures.

4. **Neurological causes:** In females, pudendal nerve neuropathy which results due to chronic straining may result in incontinence. Spinal injuries, spina bifida, meningo-myelocoele are associated with anal incontinence.

5. **Miscellaneous:** Old age (senility), general debility and faecal impaction are the other causes.

TREATMENT

I. **Temporary incontinence:** Reassurance. Perineal exercises to improve the tone of internal and external sphincter.

II. **Permanent incontinence:**

1. Divided sphincter can be reunited, followed by overlapping the remaining muscles.

2. Inter-sphincteric repair of puborectalis sling and plication of the external sphincter.

3. Gracilis muscle can be used to create a new anal sphincter by transposing it followed by electrical stimulation using a pacemaker.

PROCTALGIA FUGAX

- This condition is characterised by attacks of severe cramp-like pain arising in the rectum
- Anxiety status, straining at stools or ejaculation are the few precipitating factors
- The pain may be unbearable, may recurr at irregular intervals. It is possibly due to segmental cramp in the pubococcygeus muscle. Pain usually lasts for a few minutes and subsides (**Fleeting perineal pain**)
- Symptomatic treatment in the form of analgesics are given

PRURITUS ANI

Definition

- This is intractable itching around the anus

Causes

1. **Perianal and anal discharge:** Anal fissure, fistula in ano, prolapsed piles, polyps, genital warts are a few conditions which renders the anus moist.

Mucous discharge is an intense pruritic agent

2. **Poor hygiene,** lack of cleanliness, excessive sweating and wearing tight and rough underclothing are common causes

3. **Parasitic** causes - **Threadworms**

4. **Psychoneurosis**

5. **Allergy, diabetes,** are the other causes

Sexually transmitted diseases such as herpes, anal warts and HIV infection must be excluded.

Treatment

- Hygienic measures
- Prednisolone topical cream 1% with antifungal agent (miconazole nitrate 2%)
- Moisturising cream/lotion
- Antihistamine - promithazine hydrochloride 10-25mg at night times

Key Box 31.16
PRURITIS ANI - **TO AVOID**

- Toilet paper
- Soap
- Too tight underclothing
- Too many ointments
- Local anaesthetic cream

The Appendix

32

- Surgical anatomy
- Congenital anomalies
- Acute appendicitis
- Differential diagnosis
- Appendicular mass
- Complications
- Faecal fistula

SURGICAL ANATOMY OF THE APPENDIX

- It is 8-10 cm long, may vary from 3-30 cm in length.
- It is situated 2 cm posteromedial to ileocaecal junction, at the point of convergence of the three taeniae coli.

Positions of the appendix (Fig. 32.1)

1. Retrocaecal in about 70% of patients (12 O'clock)
2. Pelvic in 20% of cases (4 O'clock)
3. Preileal and postileal (2 O'clock)
4. Subcaecal (6 O'clock)
5. Paracaecal
6. **Subhepatic appendix** is associated with subhepatic caecum. It occurs due to **malrotation of the gut.**

Layers of the appendix

- Mesoappendix is the continuation of mesentery of the ileum above. It comes down carrying blood vessels in the mesoappendix.
- It has got serosa, mucosa lined by columnar epithelium

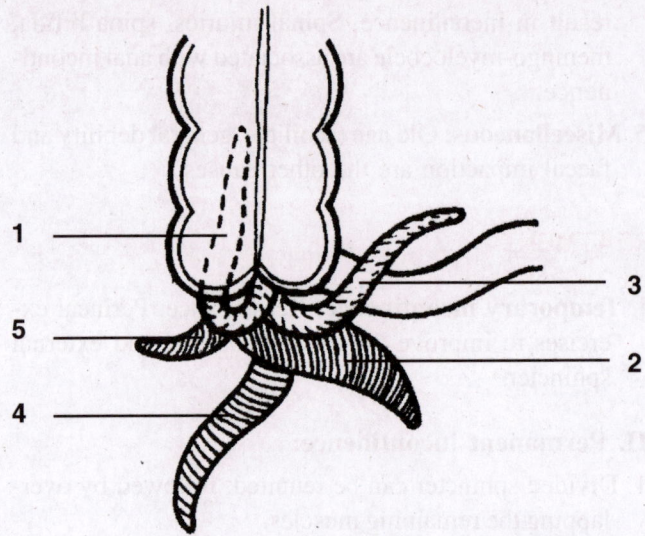

Fig. 32.1. Postitions of the appendix

(similar to intestinal mucosa). It has circular muscle fibres and longitudinal muscle fibres

- Submucosa has rich lymphoid follicles. The lymphatic tissue decreases as age advances. Hence, incidence of **appendicitis is less after the age of 30 years**.
- Appendicular orifice is occasionally guarded by an indistinct semilunar fold of mucous membrane, known as Valve of Gerlock.

Blood supply of the appendix

- Appendicular artery is a branch of ileocolic artery. Accessory appendicular artery of Sheshachalam (a branch of posterior caecal artery) is a branch of ileocolic artery, which runs in the mesoappendix.

- Veins follow the artery and end in the superior mesenteric vein. Thus draining into portal vein.

Locating the appendix (Fig. 32.2)

Trace the taenia coli or trace ileal loops at laparotomy. Taenia coli point at the base to the appendix. However, surface marking of the appendix is done as follows: Draw a line from anterior superior iliac spine to the umbilicus. The junction of lateral 1/3 and medial 2/3 of this line indicates the location of appendix. This is the point of maximum tenderness in appendicitis. This is called as **McBurney's point.**

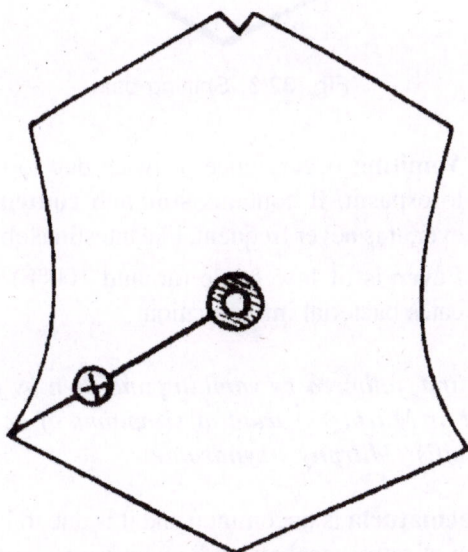

Fig. 32.2. McBurney's point

Lymphatics

The lymphatic channels which are 4 to 6 in number drain into ileocolic nodes, ileocaecal nodes and appendicular nodes in mesoappendix.

CONGENITAL ANOMALIES

1. **Subhepatic appendix :** This occurs due to malrotation of the gut. Appendicitis in a subhepatic appendix causes confusion about the diagnosis and management.

2. **Congenital absence** and duplication of the appendix are very very rare conditions.

3. In **situs inversus viscerum** the appendix may be found in the left lower abdomen.

ACUTE APPENDICITIS

It is one of most common surgical emergencies encountered by general surgeons.

AETIOLOGY

1. **Racial and dietary factors**
   - It is common in white races more often than dark coloured persons. Young males are affected more often.
   - It may be related to westernization of food - a diet rich in meat precipitates appendicitis and a diet rich in fibre (cellulose) protects the person from appendicitis.

2. **Familial susceptibility**
   - It is related to having a long retrocaecal appendix in which case the blood supply is diminished to the distal portion, which may precipitate appendicitis.

3. **Socio-economic status**
   - Appendicitis is common in middle class and rich people. The exact reasons are not known.

4. **Obstructive theory**
   - Obstruction to the lumen of the appendix due to faecoliths, worms, ova, cysts of entamoeba causes obstructive appendicitis.

5. **Non-obstructive theory**
   - It is due to bacteria like E. coli, Enterococci, Proteus, Pseudomonas, Klebsiella and anaerobes which produce diffuse inflammation of appendix and cause appendicitis.

PATHOLOGY

I. In non-obstructive cases (catarrhal appendicitis)

Process of inflammation is slow and gradual.

- A mild attack may completely resolve or mucosal and submucosal oedema can occur.
- Ulceration of the appendix results in slow bacterial invasion of lymphoid tissue.
- Gangrene and perforation are rare.

II. In obstructive cases symptoms are abrupt, vomiting is more, pain is more and tenderness is more.

- It is a more dangerous variety. Due to obstruction, the contents get infected fast and the tension increases. The appendix becomes a closed loop, which results in septic thrombosis of vessels. Gangrene of appendix, perforation, peritonitis, followed by a local abscess, can occur (Key Box 22.1).

- In children greater omentum is very thin. Hence, it cannot localize the infection. In adults, omentum is like a fatty apron which localizes the infection.

- In **aged patients,** because of atherosclerosis, **gangrene** occurs **very fast** resulting in peritonitis. Obstruction is caused by faecoliths, worms and bands which cause tenting. Obstructed appendicitis is one of the examples for closed loop obstruction. Other causes are volvulus, carcinoma hepatic flexture, etc.

- Common bacteria encountered in acute appendicitis are Bacteroides fragilis, Escherichia coli, Clostridium perfringens, Streptococcus faecalis, Pseudomonas aeruginosa etc.

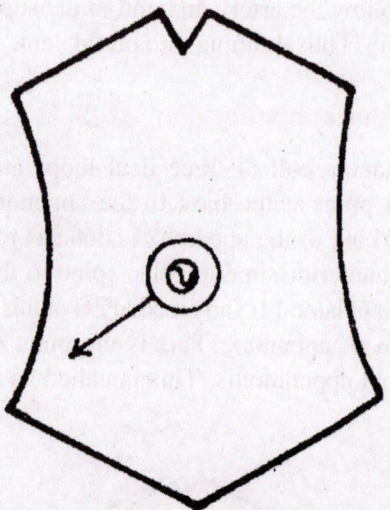

Fig. 32.3. Shifting pain

Key Box 32.1
WHY APPENDICITIS IS DANGEROUS ?

- The appendix is a cul-de-sac (closed at one end) and can be easily blocked
- The appendicular artery is an end artery (gangrene can occur fast)
- Inflammatory oedema causes easy and early thrombosis of appendicular artery
- The appendix has no muscular coat, hence perforates easily
- The lumen of the appendix is very very narrow - 1-3 mm in diameter

CLINICAL FEATURES

- Peak incidence is in the second and third decades. Very uncommon before the age of 2 years.

Symptoms

- **Pain** is severe colicky type, initially felt in the umbilical region and it is due to distension of appendix. This is a visceral pain. After a few hours, the pain localizes to the right iliac fossa. It is a somatic pain which is due to inflammation of parietal peritoneum. This is called as shifting pain of acute appendicitis (Fig. 32.3).

- **Vomiting** occurs once or twice due to reflex pylorospasm. It contains **stomach contents.** However, it is never frequent, like intestinal obstruction.

- **Fever** is of low grade (around 100°F) and indicates bacterial inflammation.

Pain first, followed by vomiting and then by fever is called as Murphy's[1] triad of symptoms of acute appendicitis (Murphy's syndrome).

- **Haematuria** is uncommon and it is due to inflammation of retrocaecal appendix which irritates the ureter in the retroperitoneum.

- **Constipation** is the usual feature, except in pre- and postileal appendicitis, where they produce diarrhoea due to irritation of ileum.

Signs

1. *Cough tenderness* (Fig. 32.4) indicates inflammation of parietal peritoneum. This is an important physical sign which differentiates acute appendicitis from right sided ureteric colic.

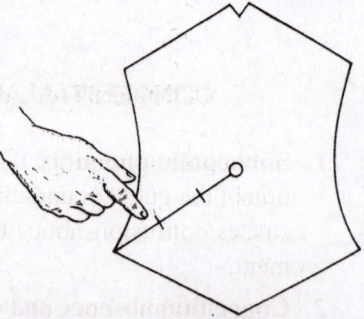

Fig. 32.4. Cough tenderness

---

1. *Can you find out what is Murphy's sign and Murphy's punch test?*

2. *Tenderness and rebound tenderness* are present at Mc Burney's point. Rebound tenderness is called as Blumberg sign. It is due to inflammation of the parietal peritoneum. This physical sign can be elicited in all cases of peritonitis.

3. *Guarding and rigidity* in the right iliac fossa: However, guarding and rigidity of back muscles (erector spinae) indicates retrocaecal appendicitis (Also refer Key Box 32.2).

4. *Rovsing sign:* Palpation of left iliac region of abdomen producing pain on the right iliac region. It is because of displacement of colonic gas and small bowel coils impinging upon the inflamed appendix.

5. *Hyperaesthesia* in the Sherren triangle (Fig. 32.5): It is formed by anterior superior iliac spine, umbilicus and pubic symphysis. It is due to irritation of lower abdominal nerves.

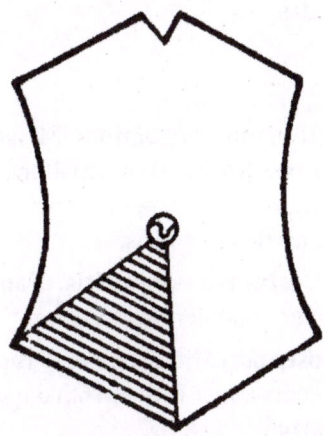

Fig. 32.5. Hyperaesthesia in the Sherren triangle

6. *Cope's psoas test:* Seen in retrocaecal appendicitis. There will be irritation of psoas major which produces flexion at the hip. If any attempt is made to extend it, it produces pain.

7. *Cope's obturator test:* Seen in pelvic appendicitis due to irritation of the obturator muscle. Flexion and medial rotation produces pain.

8. *Features of generalised peritonitis* are seen only when there is a rupture. Gangrene and perforation is more common in elderly patients because of atherosclerosis. In infants, omentum is very thin without much of fat. Hence, diffuse peritonitis occurs very fast.

9. *Rectal examination:* There is tenderness in the right rectal wall—**differential tenderness**.

Key Box 32.2
VARIATIONS IN ACUTE APPENDICTIS

1. **Retrocaecal** : Silent (no rigidity in the right iliac fossa)

2. **Pelvic** : Causes diarrhoea

3. **Post-ileal:** Causes diarrhoea—called as missed appendix

4. **Subhepatic :** Manifests as pain in the right iliac fossa, very difficult to remove from grid-iron incision

5. **In pregnancy :** The location of the pain is shifted higher up and laterally

SCORING SYSTEM

To avoid negative appendicectomies, many scoring systems have been developed considering signs, symptoms and investigations. Most commonly used Alvarado scoring system is given below.

Table 32.1 Alvarado Scoring System

FEATURES	SCORE
Symptoms :	
Migrating RIF pain	1
Anorexia	1
Nausea, vomiting	1
Signs :	
Tenderness RIF	2
Rebound tenderness	1
Elevated temperature	1
Laboratory :	
Leucocytosis	2
Shift to left	1
Total	10

Score less than 5	:	Not Sure
Score 5-6	:	Compatible
Score 6-9	:	Probable
Score more than 9	:	Confirmed

• Eventhough Alvarado scoring is highly suggestive of appendicitis it is only a simple and cost effective scoring system. This can be applied when sophisticated investigations such as ultrasonography and CT scan are not available.

INVESTIGATIONS

1. Total WBC count is almost always increased above 10,000 cells/cumm.

2. Plain X-ray abdomen erect is taken to rule out perforation. It may show dilated small bowel loops in the right iliac fossa.

Presence of faecolith is highly suggestive of acute appendicitis in plain x-ray.

3. Abdominal ultrasound to rule out other causes including gynaecological causes. Ultrasound can demonstrate a non-compressible, aperistaltic tubular organ with a thick wall. It can be used to elicit probe tenderness.

4. However **CT Scan is the investigation of choice.** Please remember cost of the CT scan has to be weighed upon the economic status of the patient, in our country.

5. C-reactive protein is elevated in any inflammatory conditions like appendicitis.

DIFFERENTIAL DIAGNOSIS OF ACUTE APPENDICITIS

Innumerable conditions may mimic some signs of appendicitis. A few important conditions have been considered here.

IN CHILDREN

1. **Enterocolitis** is common in children. It presents with severe diarrhoea with blood and mucous in the stools.

2. **Meckel's diverticulitis** can present with abdominal pain, vomiting, fever—signs and symptoms are similar to acute appendicitis (difficult to differentiate clinically).

3. **Worm ball** is common in children in the developing countries. However, features of intestinal obstruction will be present.

4. **Acute iliac lymphadenitis** - nonshifting pain, rebound tenderness is absent.

IN YOUNG ADULTS

1. **Right-sided ureteric colic:** Haematuria, severe pain from loin to groin, absence of cough tenderness help in excluding acute appendicitis.

2. **Amoebic typhilitis** is associated with diarrhoea, blood in the stools and tenderness in left iliac fossa (Manson Barr's amoebic point of tenderness).

3. **Torsion of undescended testis:** Absence of testis in the scrotum clinches the diagnosis.

4. **Meckel's diverticulitis**

IN MIDDLE AGE

1. **Acute pancreatitis :** Inflammatory exudate collects and gravitates in the right iliac fossa resulting in pain, guarding and rigidity in the right iliac fossa. History of alcohol intake, severe backache and tenderness in the epigastrium helps in diagnosing acute pancreatitis.

2. **Perforated duodenal ulcer** can present with pain in the right side of the abdomen due to similar causes mentioned above.

3. **Acute cholecystitis** can also present with features of acute appendicitis. However, it is common in elderly females.

IN FEMALES

1. **Ruptured ectopic gestation:** Missed periods, features of haemorrhagic shock (pallor), extreme tenderness on cervical movement on per vaginal examination clinches the diagnosis.

2. **Bilateral salpingo-oophoritis:** Pain on both sides of the lower abdomen is a feature.

3. **Mid menstrual** (Mittelschmerz) rupture of ovarian follicle occurs about 14th to 16th day and can produce abdominal pain.

4. **Torsion of ovarian cyst** produces very severe abdominal pain with a mass.

Any female patient with right-sided lower abdominal pain should undergo gynaecological examination to rule out the causes mentioned above, before subjecting for appendicectomy.

SYSTEMIC DISEASES

1. **Pleurisy** and **pneumonia.**

2. **Porphyria:** Violent intestinal colic occurs due to spasm. It is precipitated by barbiturates. Urine is orange coloured and when it is exposed to sunlight, the colour changes to amber.

3. **Potts spine** causes compression of nerve roots—radicular pain.

4. **Preherpetic pain** of 10th and 11th dorsal nerve is located over the same area, marked hyperaesthesia is present.

5. **Purpura** and bleeding disorders

CLINICAL NOTES

• A 30 year old lady was diagnosed to have acute appendicitis with classical features—pain, fever, vomiting and tenderness in the Mc Burney's point. Gynaecological examination revealed pelvic infection. An infected copper T was removed which was the cause of abdominal pain.

• A 22 year old man underwent appendicectomy for right sided abdominal pain. At laparotomy, appendix was normal. However, it was removed. He continued to have abdominal pain. An ultrasound of the abdomen revealed torsion of undescended testis. **Nobody had examined his external genitalia!!**

• 36 year old male who had previous history of abdominal pain underwent appendicectomy for tenderness and rebound tenderness in right iliac fossa. Operative surgery notes say the appendix was slightly inflamed and seropurulent fluid was in right iliac fossa. After 2-3 days, greenish fluid (bile) started draining out through the tube. Condition of the patient deteriorated and reexploration this time, by midline incision revealed perforated chronic duodenal ulcer!!

TREATMENT

• **Emergency appendicectomy:** Emergency appendicectomy is offered when patient comes within 24 to 48 hours of abdominal pain. It is very important to rule out or detect a mass, especially if a decision is made to operate around 2nd or 3rd day. If a mass is palpable, it is better not to operate now. (Please refer to operative surgery, Appendicectomy) A few important steps are given here (Fig. 32.6, 32.7).

  • Appendix is identified by tracing taenia coli which converges onto the base of the appendix. Mesoappendix is divided in between ligatures. Purse-string suture is applied all around the appendix in the caecum. The appendix is divided in between ligatures, the stump is invaginated and the purse-string is tightened. Abdomen is closed in layers.

  • Laparoscopic appendicectomy has become more popular nowadays.

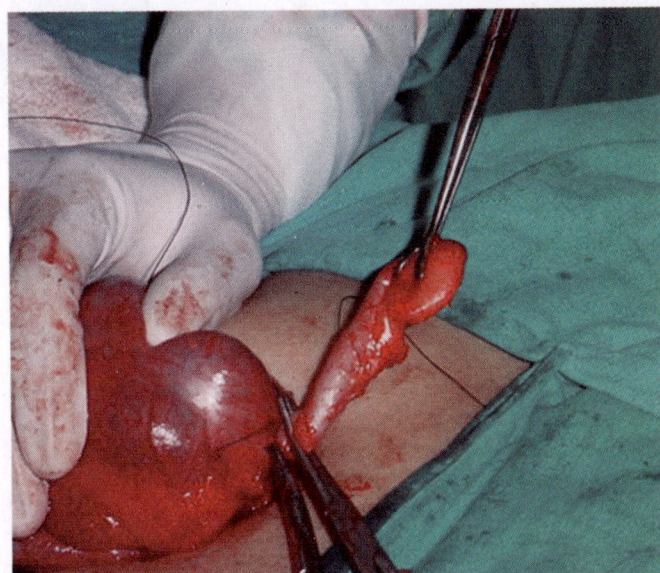

Fig. 32.6 Emergency appendicectomy - base is crushed

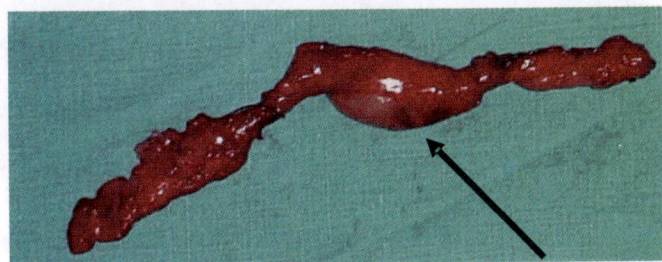

Fig. 32.7 Large faecolith resulting in acute appendicitis

COMPLICATIONS OF ACUTE APPENDICITIS

1. **Rupture** of appendix causes generalised peritonitis with 10-20% mortality rate. Emergency laparotomy, appendicectomy, peritoneal wash followed by drainage of peritoneal cavity is the treatment to be done.

2. **Appendicular mass** (Fig. 32.8):

• Following an attack of acute appendicitis, infection is sealed off by greater omentum, caecum, terminal ileum, etc., which results in a tender, soft to firm mass in right iliac fossa.

• Presence of a mass is a contraindication for appendicectomy because it is very difficult to remove appendix from such a mass and attempt to remove may result in a faecal fistula.

• It is treated by **Oschner and Sherren's regime.**

  - **A**spiration with Ryle's tube to give rest to the gut.

  - **B**owel care—purgatives should not be used (may cause perforation).

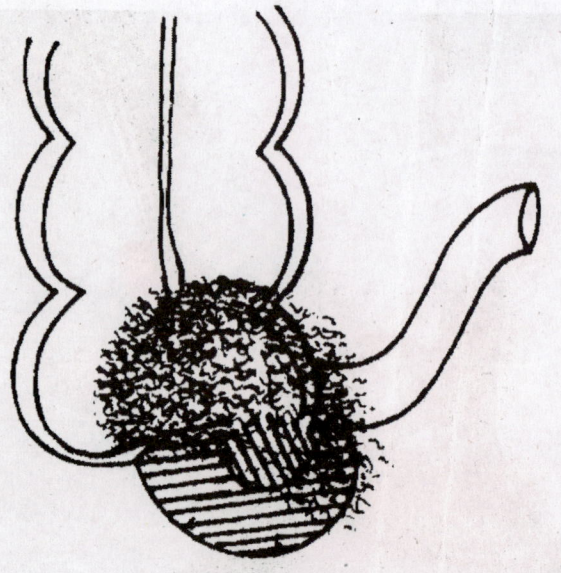

Fig. 32.8. Appendicular mass

- **C**harts—temperature, pulse, respiration, diameter of the mass. Swinging temperature, and increase in size of mass indicates an appendicular abscess.

- **D**rugs to cover all the organisms—gram-positive, gram-negative, anaerobic organisms.

- **E**xploratory laparotomy should not be done; However, when, the condition of the patient is not improving, there is a suspicion of an abscess and when doubtful of the diagnosis, exploration is indicated.

- **F**luid

Patient is kept nil orally for a few days. During this time. intravenous fluids are given to correct dehydration.

- After 3-4 days, the abdomen becomes soft, tenderness decreases and once stools are passed, Ryle's tube is removed. Clear oral fluids followed by soft diet is given. By one week, the patient is back to normal. **After 6-8 weeks,** patient is advised **elective appendicectomy.**

- 60 year old lady was diagnosed to have appendicular mass and was undergoing conservative management. On the fourth day she developed features of early septic shock. As the patient was not improving, laparatomy was done. It was a case of **volvulus of the caecum.**

3. Appendicular abscess (Fig. 32.9)

- Following an attack of appendicitis, if the infection is not controlled properly, an abscess can occur in rela-

tion to appendix. They are retrocaecal (a), subcaecal (b), preileal, postileal (c), pelvic (d) and lumbar abscesses. Clinically, it presents with high grade fever with chills and rigors and a tender boggy swelling in the right iliac fossa or in the right lumbar region. Pelvic abscess presents with diarrhoea.

TREATMENT

1. **Retrocaecal abscess** is drained by extraperitoneal approach. An incision of 5 to 6 cm is made in the right iliac fossa and all muscles are divided. However, peritoneum is not opened. It is swept medially and pus is drained outside. Appendicectomy is done at a later date (Fig. 32.10)

2. **Preileal and postileal** abscesses are drained by a laparotomy.

3. **Pelvic abscess** is drained via the rectum (Page 445)

4. **Lumbar abscess** (perinephric abscess) is drained by a loin incision.

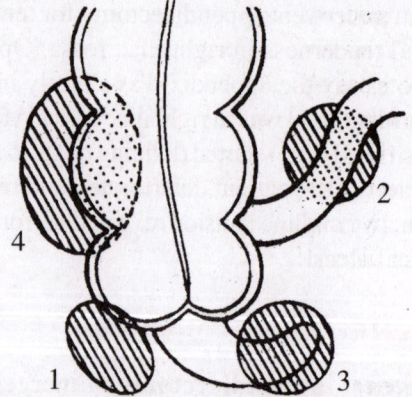

Fig. 32.9 Appendicular abscess (Refer text)

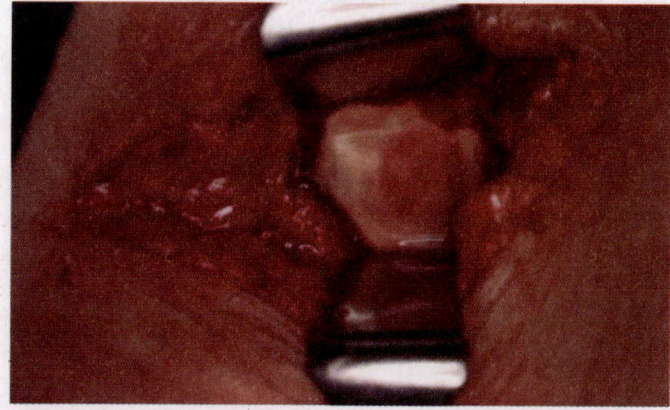

Fig. 32.10 Appendicular abscess drained by extraperitoneal route

FAECAL FISTULA

- It can occur after appendicectomy especially when gangrene of the appendix extends to base of the caecum. It can also occur if purse-string suture is not properly applied or else injury to the terminal ileum or caecum etc.

- Discharge of faeculent contents or faecal matter after appendicectomy suggests faecal fistula.

- Usually discharge stops after a few days provided there is no distal obstruction.

- Cases which do not respond to conservative treatment are managed by resection of the diseased portion of the caecum or ascending colon.

Carcinoma caecum and ileocaecal tuberculosis are important diseases for faecal fistula in India and Crohn's disease in the west.

CLINICAL NOTES

- A female medical student underwent laparoscopic appendicectomy for recurrent appendicitis. On the seventh day of post-operative period faecal fistula developed from the port site. Treating surgeon assured her that the discharge will stop. The discharge persisted for two months during which time, she lost 7 Kg. weight and she used to get intermittent pain, swelling, fever followed by discharge. She was explored to find the clip which was applied to the appendicular stump had given way.

Key Box 32.3
FAECAL FISTULA - CAN OCCUR

- After drainage of appendicular abscess
- After appendicectomy - if purse-string sutures are not properly applied
- If the caecum is also involved by inflammation
- If the cause of appendicitis is carcinoma
- If chronic diseases develop or present -Tuberculosis, Crohn's or Actionomycosis
- It appendicitis is associated with carcinoma caecum

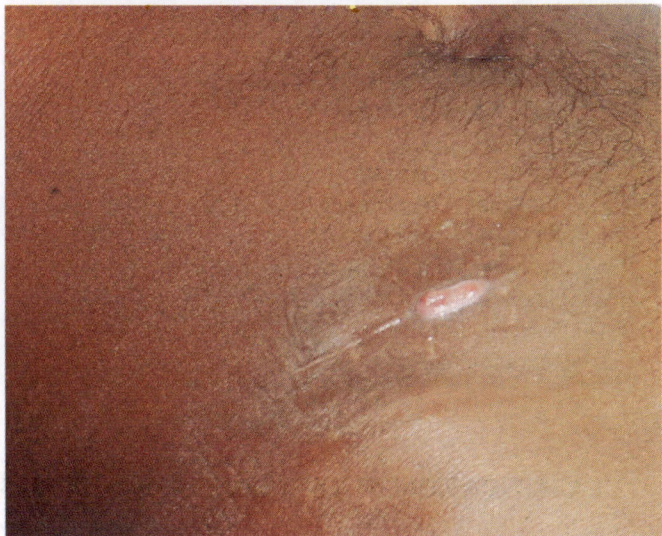

Fig. 32.11 This patient had faecal fistula which healed after two weeks of conservative management

Umbilicus and Abdominal Wall

33

- Classification of umbilical diseases
- Umbilical infections
- Umbilical fistulae
- Umbilical neoplasms
- Abdominal dehiscence
- Divarication of recti
- Rectus sheath haematoma
- Meleney's gangrene
- Desmoid tumour
- Endometriosis

Key Box 33.1
UMBILICAL CORD STRUCTURES

IN FOETAL LIFE

I. Umbilical vein
2. Right and left umbilical arteries
3. Urachus

IN EMBRYONIC LIFE

• Vitellointestinal duct and structures mentioned above.

CLASSIFICATION OF DISEASES OF UMBILICUS

I. Inflammtation

A. Omphalitis
B. Granuloma
C. Dermatitis
D. Pilonidal sinus

II. Fistulae

A. Faecal

1. Patent vitellointestinal duct (Key Box 33.1)
2. Carcinoma transverse colon
3. Tuberculous peritonitis

B. Urinary: Patent urachus

C. Biliary

III. Neoplasms

A. Benign

1. Adenoma: Raspberry tumour
2. Endometrioma

B. Malignant

1. Primary carcinoma
2. Secondary carcinoma from:
   • Stomach, colon
   • Ovary, breast

IV. Umbilical hernia

V. Umbilical calculus (umbolith)

INFLAMMATION

A. OMPHALITIS

- Inflammation of the umbilical cord due to Staphylococcus aureus and Streptococci occurs in the neonatal period 3-4 days after birth. The incidence is increased in hospital births.

- Rarely, gram-negative organisms and Clostridium tetani can cause omphalitis[1], if strict aseptic precautions are not taken. If infection is not controlled, it can result in further complications.

1. **Abscess of the abdominal wall:** Pus can be seen coming out of umbilicus. It may need drainage with antibiotic cover. Gentle squeezing will help, followed by antiseptic dressings and systemic antibiotics.

2. **Extensive ulceration of the abdominal wall** similar to Meleney's ulcer, is a rare complication (Subcutaneous synergistic gangrene) of omphalitis.

3. **Septicaemia** can occur due to organisms entering into umbilical vein and then into portal vein. This results in pyelephlebitis with jaundice, fever, chills and rigors.

4. **Neonatal jaundice** due to intrahepatic cholangitis.

5. **Portal vein thrombosis** resulting in extrahepatic portal hypertension (pre-hepatic).

6. **Umbilical hernia** results due to sepsis producing a weak scar.

B. GRANULOMA

- Granuloma indicates persisting inflammation underneath. It is a cause of great concern and worry to the patients. This can be destroyed by **application of copper sulfate or silver nitrate solution.**

C. DERMATITIS

- Dermatitis more often occur in adults wherein chronic infection of the umbilicus sets in with foul smelling discharge.

D. PILONIDAL SINUS

- Umbilicus is a low area compared to the surface of abdominal wall. Hence, hairy men may shed their hair which accumulates in the umbilicus and may result in pilonidal sinus. It may need removal of sinus with tuft of hair or rarely umbilicus.

UMBILICAL FISTULAE

A. FAECAL

1. **Persistent vitello-intestinal duct** is an uncommon congenital anomaly. Many a time the intestinal opening is so small that only mucoid contents come out of umbilicus. Rarely, if the opening is big, omphaloenteric faecal fistula results. (Also refer page 498)

2. **Internal hollow viscus malignancies,** especially carcinoma of the transverse colon can erode through umbilicus resulting in a faecal fistula.

3. **Tuberculous peritonitis** induces dense adhesions, strictures and perforations. A perforation which is sealed off by coils of matted bowel and omentum results in local abscess which may perforate through a weak point i.e. umbilicus resulting in a faeco-biliary fistula. If a diagnosis can be proved by wall biopsy of the sinus/fistula antituberculous treatment can cure the disease. Laparotomy is extremely difficult in such cases. One may end up with creating more holes in the bowel—better avoided.

> *One innocent disease (V. I. DUCT), one prevalent disease (TB), one malignant disease (Carcinoma bowel) are the causes of umbilical faecal fistula.*

B. PATENT URACHUS (FIG. 33.1)

- The ventral urogenital sinus which forms the urinary bladder is continued cranially as urachus which extends into the umbilical cord—allantoic stalk. If this portion persists, patent urachus forms which connects umbilicus with urinary bladder. If it is fibrosed, as it occurs normally, it is called **median umbilical ligament.**

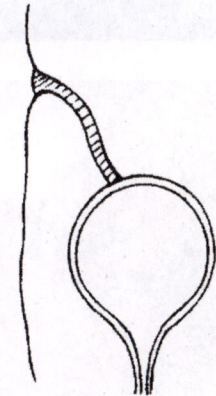

Fig. 33.1 Patent Urachus

- A patent urachus may manifest as urinary discharge

Key Box 33.2
ABNORMALITIES OF URACHUS
1. Patent urachus
2. Urachal sinus
3. Urachal cyst
4. Urachal diverticulum

---

1. *Application of cowdung to the umblical cord is still prevalent in a few places in our country. In addition to causing omphalitis, it will also cause neonatal tetanus.*

from umbilicus. It manifests usually in childhood and early adult life. In most cases, there will be some kind of obstruction to the normal passage of urine. Entire urachus is excised after correcting distal obstruction.

C. BILIARY FISTULA

• Rarely perforation of gall bladder due to severe form of cholecystitis may result in local abscess which may rupture through umbilicus resulting in biliary fistula. Instances are recorded wherein stones have come out of umbilicus.

NEOPLASMS

1. **UMBILICAL ADENOMA** is a pedunculated swelling having **raspberry colour.** Hence, the name **raspberry tumour.**

   • It is due to unobliterated vitello-intestinal duct.

• Mucosa of the persistent duct prolapses through umbilicus and gives rise to this adenoma.

• It is moist with mucous and tends to bleed (columnar epithelium rich in goblet cells).

Treatment

• If the tumour is pedunculated, a ligature is tied around it and by a few days, the adenoma drops off.

• If tumour reappears, excision of umbilicus is advised.

2. **ENDOMETRIOMA** of umbilicus is rare but patients have typical history to tell i.e. it bleeds during menstruation.

3. **MALIGNANT:** Secondary carcinomatous nodule in and around umbilicus reflects advanced malignancy commonly from stomach and colon carcinoma, ovary, uterus, breast are other causes. The nodule is tender, fixed and reddish in colour (Fig. 33.2).

* See also figures 33.2 to 33.7

SOME INTERESTING DISEASES OF UMBILICUS

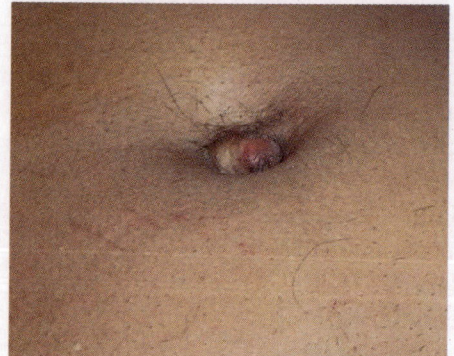
Fig. 33.2. Sister Mary Joseph's nodule

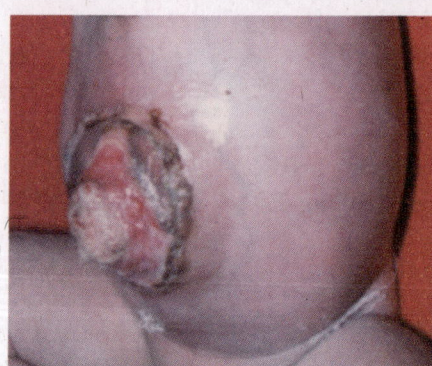
Fig. 33.3 Exomphalous major

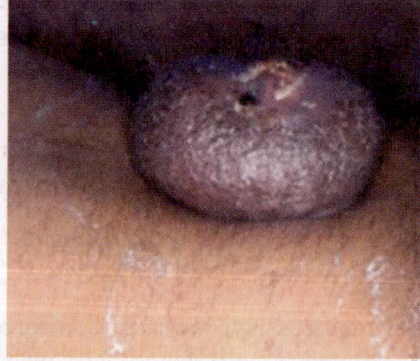
Fig. 33.4. Irreducible umbilical hernia in a cirrhotic patient

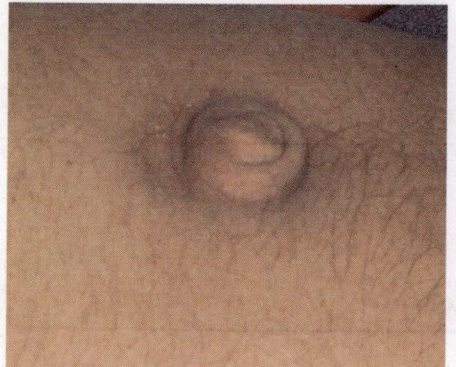
Fig. 33.5. Umbilical hernia

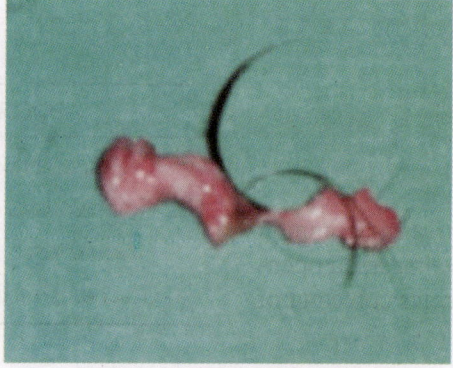
Fig. 33.6. Pilonidal sinus

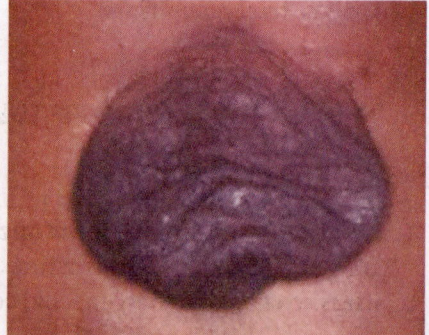
Fig. 33.7. Observe skin of umbilical hernia in cirrhosis of liver, resembling scrotal skin

UMBILICAL HERNIA

- Umbilicus is one of the weak points in the body. Hence, it is one of the sites of hernia. All the details of umbilical hernia has been discussed in page 566.

UMBOLITH

It is composed of desquamated epithelium which becomes inspissated and gets collected in the umbilicus. With secondary infection, there will be blood stained discharge. It is treated by controlling infection, debridement and if necessary removal of umbilicus.

- This umbolith or umbilical calculus is black in colour.

ABDOMINAL WALL

PYOGENIC ABSCESS (Fig. 33.8)

- Abdominal wall is one of the sites of pyogenic abscess specially in diabetic patients. It is a part of pyaemia. Localised tenderness suggests an abscess. Diagnosis can be confirmed by ultrasound and it is treated by incision and drainage.

ABDOMINAL WALL VEINS (Fig. 33.9)

- Veins are seen in portal hypertension. In relation to umibilicus, they are called as caput medusae. Direction of the veins are important which can be demonstrated by emptying the vein observing the direction of re-filling.

BURST ABDOMEN-ABDOMINAL DEHISCENCE

A soundly healed abdominal scar can withstand any amount of intraabdominal pressure. However, 1-2% of the abdominal wounds (incisions) give way resulting in prolapse of intraabdominal contents outside. This causes great concern, or anxiety to the patient, and more so for relatives. It is said that the anxiety and worry caused by the intestines prolapsing out is much more than that is caused by emergency re-explorations for open cardiac surgery. It is not possible to prevent wound dehiscence totally because causative agents are multifactorial.

Factors responsible for wound dehiscence

1. **Surgery :** It depends upon the type of surgery done. Surgery done for grossly contaminated cases like peritonitis,biliary fistula, or faecal fistula have a high incidence of wound dehiscence (Fig. 33.10).

2. **Sepsis :** Uncontrolled infection (sepsis) can digest the suture material used and will result in burst abdomen.

3. **Suture material used :** The absorbable sutures like catgut gives rise to increased incidence of wound dehiscence than nonabsorbable sutures.

4. **Surgeon related factors :** Meticulous dissection, haemostasis, gentle handling of tissues, a good tensionless tight closure, carefully judged incisions will have reduced incidence of burst abdomen.Midline vertical incisions have decreased chance of wound dehiscence than paramedian incision.

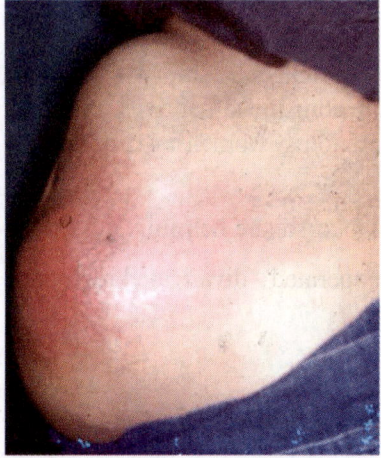

Fig 33.8 Abdominal wall abscess in a diabetic patient

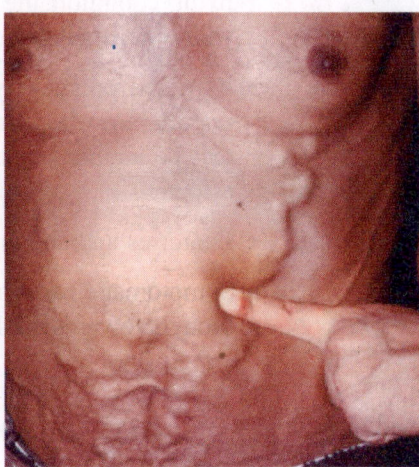

Fig 33.9 Dilated tortuous veins due to portal hypertension

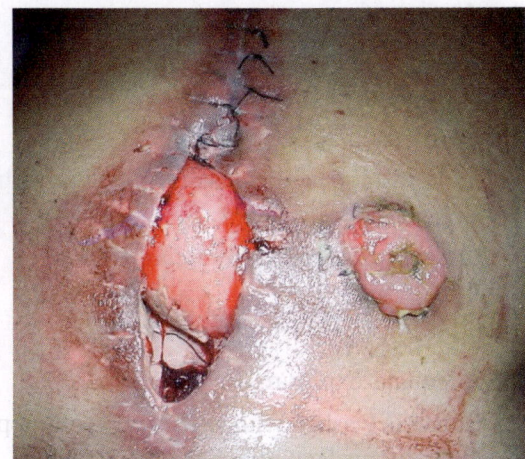

Fig 33.10 Wound dehiscence in a case of APR - probably due to placement of colostomy nearer to the suture line

Key Box 33.3

BURST ABDOMEN - FACTORS

- **Surgery** → Peritonitis
- **Sepsis** → Uncontrolled infection
- **Sutures** → Absorbable—catgut
- **Surgeon** → Poor quality
- **Sick patient** → Malignancy, diabetes, uraemia, jaundice
- **Straining** → Coughing, vomiting

Students can remember the causes of burst abdomen as 6S.

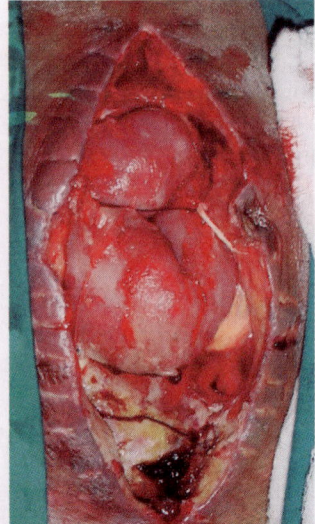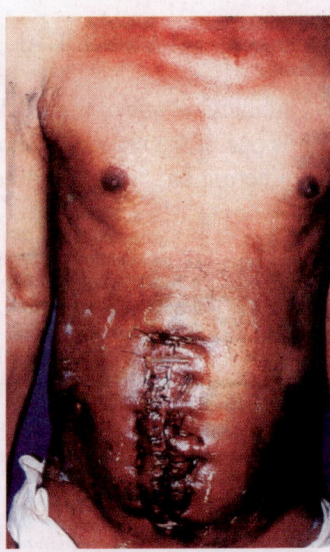

Fig 33.11 & 33.12 Wound dehiscence due to gangrene of the intestine - laparotomy was done, resection followed by closure of the abdomen with tension sutures

5. **Sick patient:** Patients with malignancy, jaundice, obesity, anaemia, hypoproteinaemia, uraemia have poor wound healing.

6. **Straining :** In the postoperative period, violent cough, persistent vomiting, abdominal distension due to paralytic ileus predisposes to burst abdomen.

Clinical features

- Patients who are recovering reasonably well in the postoperative period suddenly complain of pink or brownish coloured serosanguinous discharge. It is the pathognomonic sign of burst abdomen.
- It usually occurs on the 6th to 8th postoperative day.
- If skin sutures are removed, omentum or small bowel coils will be seen outside.

Interestingly, it is a painless, shockless disruption (with) full of apprehension.

Treatment

- Reassurance.
- The bowel or the contents are covered with pads and bandage.
- Emergency surgery and closure is done.

Principles of surgery

1. Adequate exposure.
2. Bowel is washed with saline and gently replaced into the peritoneal cavity.
3. Edges of the wound/incision are trimmed.
4. A single layer closure of the abdominal layer, by taking

suture bites through whole thickness of the abdominal wall is done.

- A few tension sutures are placed which are tied over a rubber or a plastic tube and they are removed after 2 weeks.
- It should be remembered that **secondary wound healing is better than primary wound healing** and rarely infection occurs.

DIVARICATION OF RECTI

- In this condition, the two rectus abdominal muscles are widely separated (not in the midline).
- Repeated pregnancy in quick succession is the most important cause. Chronic constipation or overstraining may be another factor. Obviously women are commonly affected.
- Exercises and abdominal corset are helpful.
- Symptomatic cases are operated - divaricated recti are brought towards midline.

RECTUS SHEATH HAEMATOMA

Collection of blood in relation to rectus sheath and muscles occur due to tearing of one of the branches of inferior epigastric artery. A parietal haematoma occurs usually at the level of the arcuate line. It is an uncommon condition. However, the causes can be as follows :

1. **Trauma :** A sudden blow to the abdominal wall.
2. **Straining :** Sudden straining such as violent cough or vigorous exercise in a muscular man can cause haematoma.
3. **Pregnancy:** Rarely, the cause of haematoma can be pregnancy, in later trimester. The exact cause is not known.

Clinical features

- History of sudden straining or coughing, etc.
- A tender lump develops just below and to the side of umbilicus at the level of arcuate line where posterior rectus sheath is absent.
- Nausea, vomiting, pyrexia are the other features.

Differential diagnosis

- Spigelian hernia. (It is very, very rare.)

Treatment

- The condition is self-limiting. With antibiotics and analgesics, a haematoma subsides within 5-7 days.
- If it persists or progresses or if there is a doubt about the diagnosis, exploration and evacuation of haematoma should be done and the bleeding vessels are ligated. The results and recovery are excellent.

CLINICAL NOTES

- A 60 year old diabetic, male patient had a large pyaemic abscess on the abdominal wall below and to the right of umbilicus. An incision and drainage of the abscess was done. Within 2 hours of surgery, the surgeon was called to see this patient who had hypotension and blood was pouring out of the incision. Exploration of the wound revealed large 'clots' and bleeding from inferior epigastic artery, which was ligated. Probably, while breaking all the loculi of the abscess cavity, the vessel would have been injured.

MELENEY'S PROGRESSIVE POSTOPERATIVE SYNERGISTIC GANGRENE

This dangerous complication is rare nowadays, thanks to the good pre- and postoperative antibiotics.

Aetipathogenesis

- It is caused by synergistic action of microaerophilic non-haemolytic streptococcus and staphylococcus aureus.
- Surgical operations which have increased risk of Meleney include perforated appendicitis, biliary tract surgery, colectomy, etc.
- Atherosclerosis, diabetes are the other precipitating factors.
- Starts as cellulitis with reddish skin and post-operative fever.
- The spread may occur within 3-5 days, with extensive gangrene and sloughing of the skin of the adominal wall with purulent discharge.

Clinical features

- Postoperative patient with cellulitis of abdominal wall
- Fever of moderate degree, an extremely tender abdominal wall, with purulent discharge
- Toxicity and deterioration of general health may follow soon

Treatment

1. **At the stage of cellulitis:** Broad spectrum antibiotics to cover not only the organisms mentioned above but to cover anaerobic organisms. Thus benzyl penicillin, gentamicin and metronidazole combination is used.
2. **At the stage of gangrene:** Emergency aggressive debridement is the treatment. Dead skin and subcutaneous tissue is excised, pus is drained, slough is removed.
3. **Hyperbaric oxygen** may be very useful.
4. The skin grafting is done, once the wound is healed with granulation tissue.

DESMOID TUMOUR

- It is an uncapsulated fibroma which occurs in the abdominal wall.
- It arises from muscles and aponeurotic layer of the abdominal wall.
- Childbirth, trauma or operative scars are the possible aetiological factors.
- Desmiod tumour is one of the components of Gardner's syndrome (Page 477).

- It is bengin but it has a tendency to infiltrate the muscles and some fibromas do exhibit dysplastic changes. The cut surface is compared to an onion - whorled fibroma with spindle-shaped cells.

- Sarcomatous changes and metastasis does not occur.

- However, simple excision results in recurrence. Hence, **wide excision with 2-3 cm** of normal **healthy margins** is necessary with reconstruction of the abdominal wall.

- In spite of adequate surgery, 10-20% chances of recurrence occurs (Key Box 33.4)

Drugs like sulindac and tamoxifen have also been used here, with some success.

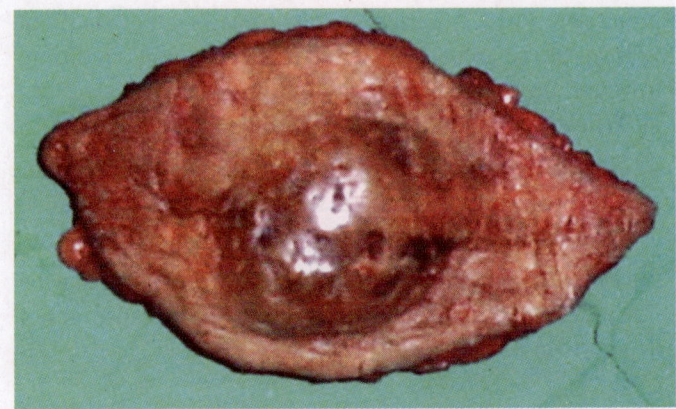

Fig 33.13 Wide excision of desmoid tumour

Key Box 33.4

PECULIARITIES OF DESMOID TUMOUR

- Uncapsulated fibroma
- Infiltrates muscles, even though benign
- Does not change into sarcoma
- It may be a part of Gardner's syndrome
- Simple excision results in recurrence
- Wide excision is recommended

ENDOMETRIOSIS OF THE ABDOMINAL WALL

- It occurs due to mechanical implantation of endometrial cells during surgery (Sites - Key Box 33.5)

- Painful, palpable swelling more symptomatic at the time of menstruation is characteristic feature

- Cyclical bleeding peri-menstrually can occur

- Oral contraceptive pills may control the symptoms

- Otherwise excision of the nodule has to be done

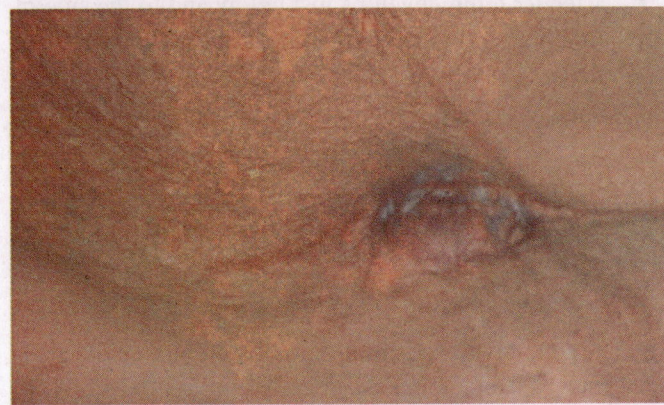

Fig 33.14 Scar endometriosis

Key Box 33.5

SITES OF ENDOMETRIOSIS

- Laparoscopic port — Umbilicus
- Gynecological surgery — Abdominal incision
- Episiotomy — Perineum

Hernia

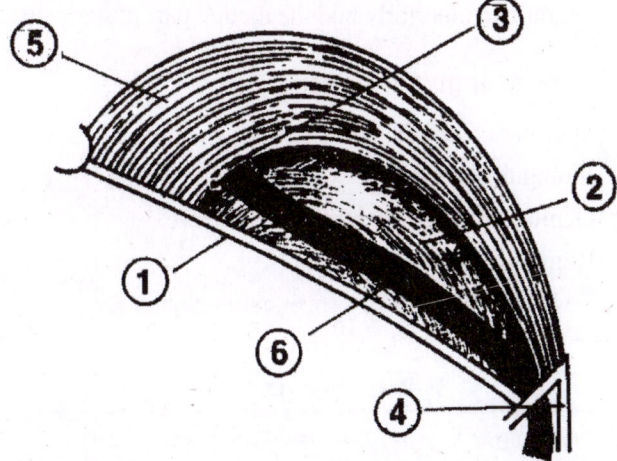

Fig. 34.1 Anatomy of the inguinal region (Refer text for details)

Abnormal protrusion of a viscus or a part of it through a weak point in the body is known as a hernia. Inguinal hernia occurs either through the deep inguinal ring (indirect hernia) or through the posterior wall of the inguinal canal (direct hernia).

ANATOMY OF THE INGUINAL REGION (Fig.34.1)

Inguinal ligament (Poupart's ligament) (1)

- It is the ligamentous portion of the external oblique aponeurosis which folds inwards and extends from anterior superior iliac spine to the pubic tubercle.
- The midpoint between these 2 structures is called midpoint of the inguinal ligament.

- The midpoint between the anterior superior iliac spine and pubic symphysis is called midinguinal point.

Inguinal canal (2)

- It is 4 cm in length extending from the deep inguinal ring to the superficial inguinal ring.

Deep ring (internal ring) (3)

- It is a 'U' shaped defect in the fascia transversalis which forms the posterior wall of the inguinal canal. It lies 1.25 cm above the mid point of the inguinal ligament.

External ring (superficial ring) (4)

- Superficial ring is a triangular defect in external oblique

551

aponeurosis. It is in bounded by the lateral and medial crura formed by the external oblique aponeurosis and the base of the triangle is formed by the pubic crest.

Boundaries of inguinal canal

- **Anterior:** External oblique aponeurosis and a few fibres of the **conjoined muscle** (especially of internal oblique) laterally.

- **Superior :** Arched fibres of the **conjoined muscle.** (5)

- **Inferior :** Inguinal ligament and the lacunar ligament on the medial side (Gimbernat's ligament).

- **Posterior :** Fascia transversalis and the conjoined tendon medially. Thus, the inguinal canal is strong in the lateral part anteriorly and the medial part posteriorly.

Contents of inguinal canal

1. Spermatic cord (Key Box 34.1)
2. Ilioinguinal nerve
3. Genital branch of genitofemoral nerve
4. Round ligament in females
5. Vestigeal remnant of processus vaginalis sac

Key Box 34.1
CONTENTS OF THE SPERMATIC CORD
1. Vas deferens
2. Testicular artery
3. Artery to the vas
4. Cremasteric artery
5. Pampiniform plexus of veins
6. Lymphatics
7. Sympathetic nerves
8. Genital branch of genitofemoral nerve
9. Processus vaginalis

INGUINAL DEFENCE MECHANISM

1. Obliquity of inguinal canal (in children it is straight).
2. During straining or coughing, the conjoined tendon contracts, and since it forms the anterior, superior and posterior boundaries, it closes the inguinal canal - **shutter or sphincter-like effect.**
3. Increased intra-abdominal pressure produces plugging effect at the external ring. The deep ring is pulled up-

wards and laterally because it is adherent to the posterior surface of **transversalis muscle.** This occludes the ring and prevents herniation - **Ball valve** effect.

CLASSIFICATION OF HERNIA

I. Anatomical classification

1. Indirect hernia
2. Direct hernia

II. Nyhus classification

This classification is based **primarily on defect,** which helps in planning an appropriate repair.

Type I. Indirect hernia with normal deep ring

Type II. Indirect hernia with dilated deep ring

Type III. Based on posterior wall defect

 a. Direct

 b. Pantaloon

 c. Femoral

Type IV. Recurrent hernia

INDIRECT HERNIA

It is a herniation of abdominal contents through the deep ring into the inguinal canal. **Indirect hernia occurs due to persistent processus vaginalis sac.** It is the most common type of hernia in the body. The preformed sac passes through the deep ring, traverses the inguinal canal and may extend into the scrotum through the external ring. As it comes into the inguinal canal, it is invested by the following coverings:

1. External spermatic fascia derived from external oblique aponeurosis
2. Cremasteric fascia derived from internal oblique
3. Internal spermatic fascia from fascia transversalis

TYPES OF INDIRECT HERNIA

1. **Complete hernia** (scrotal) (Fig. 34.2A): When the sac is patent up to the bottom of the scrotum, it is a **Complete scrotal hernia.**
2. **Funicular** (Fig. 34.2B)

 The processus vaginalis sac is patent upto the root of scrotum **Incomplete indirect hernia.**

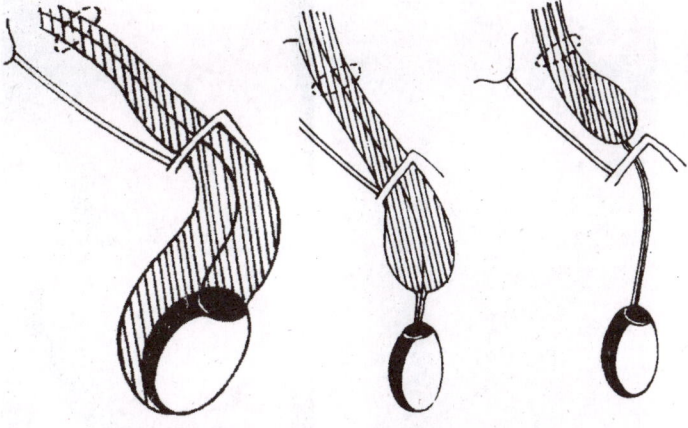

Fig. 34.2A, B & C Types of indirect herina

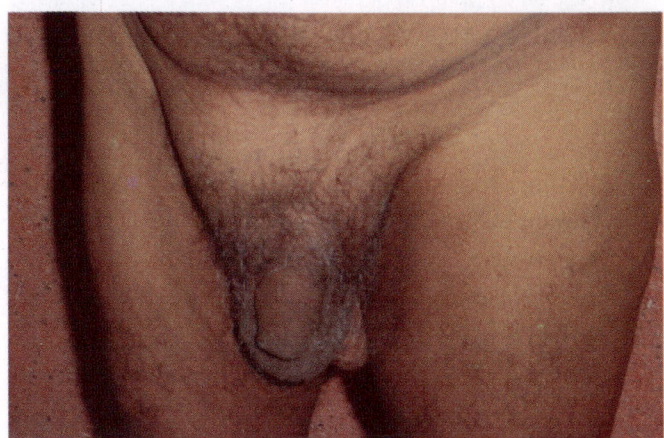

Fig. 34.3 Direct hernia

3. Bubonocoele (Fig. 34.2C): Processus vaginalis sac is confined to the inguinal region or the inguinal canal only. Such hernias are seen in young patients.

PARTS OF THE HERNIA

Hernia sac is the part of peritoneum which is dragged into the inguinal canal. The mouth of the sac is in the peritoneal cavity. The neck is the narrowest portion (deep ring). The actual hernial sac has a body and a fundus. Depending upon the contents it can be named as follows: Omentum—Omentocoele, Intestine—Enterocoele, Littre's hernia—Hernia containing Meckel's diverticulum. It may also contain ovary or appendix. **When part of the wall of the gut is involved it is know as Richter's hernia.**

The coverings of indirect inguinal hernia from outside to inside:

1. Skin
2. Two layers of superficial fascia - fatty and membranous
3. External spermatic fascia, a continuation of the external oblique aponeurosis
4. Cremaster muscle and fascia, a continuation of the internal oblique
5. Internal spermatic fascia - derived from the fascia transversalis
6. Extraperitoneal fat
7. Peritoneum

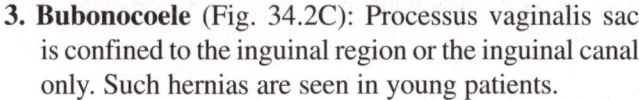

DIRECT HERNIA

- It is always acquired. It occurs through Hesselbach's triangle, a weakness in the posterior wall of the inguinal canal (transversalis fascia). Its boundaries are:

medially by lateral border of the rectus abdominis; laterally by inferior epigastric artery; and below by the inguinal ligament.

Coverings of the direct inguinal hernia from outside in are:

1. Skin
2. Two layers of superficial fascia
3. External oblique aponeurosis
4. Conjoined tendon
5. Fascia transversalis
6. Peritoneum

Precipitating factors

1. Weakness of fibres of transversus abdominis or congenital absence of a few fibres is a major factor responsible for direct hernia.

2. **In elderly patients it is precipitated by:**
   - Chronic cough giving rise to chronic bronchitis
   - Difficulty in passing urine due to BPH (Benign Prostatic Hypertrophy)
   - Chronic constipation due to habitual constipation or malignancy of left colon

> *As the direct hernia pushes through the posterior wall, it is very unusual for it to descend into the scrotum.*

Ogilvie hernia

This is a type of direct hernia where in hernial sac appears through a circular defect (congenital) in the conjoined tendon.

CLINICAL EXAMINATION OF A CASE OF HERNIA

HISTORY

- Swelling in the inguinal region which is gradually increasing in size.
- To start with, the swelling disappears on lying down and increases on straining, walking, etc. Later it cannot be reduced (due to adhesions).
- History of (H/o) dragging pain indicates omentocoele.
- Since the omentum is attached to the stomach above and supplied by T_{10}, pain is referred to the umbilical region.
- Sudden, severe pain in the hernia, vomiting and irreducibility indicates "obstructed hernia."
- H/o chronic cough, constipation, difficulty in passing urine should be asked. If present, it may suggest the cause of hernia.
- Division of ilio-inguinal nerve during appendicectomy may cause denervation of fibres of the right transversus abdominis, which forms 'U' shaped ring, resulting in weakness of the abdominal wall.

INSPECTION (For example, a model case of incomplete hernia)

It should be done in the standing position. Both sides should be checked.

- There is a swelling in the inguinal region extending to the root of scrotum measuring about 6 x 3 cm, **surface is smooth, borders are round and skin over the swelling is normal.**
- Ask the patient to cough - **expansile impulse on cough is present**. If peristalsis is present, it indicates an enterocoele. Expansile impulse on cough is diagnostic of hernia.
- Presence of scar indicates a recurrent hernia. Ragged scar indicates infection.
- Direct hernia pops out as soon as the patient stands.

PALPATION

- Inspectory findings should be confirmed.
- Swelling is soft, and gurgles if it is an entercocle.
- It may be firm or granular if it is an omentoceole.

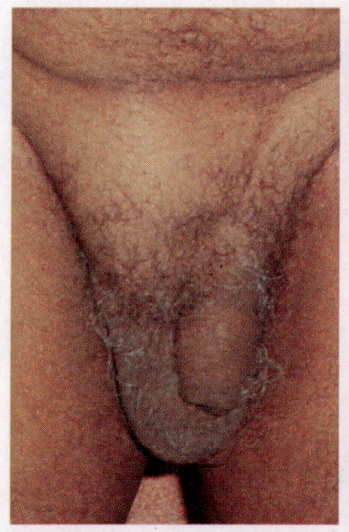 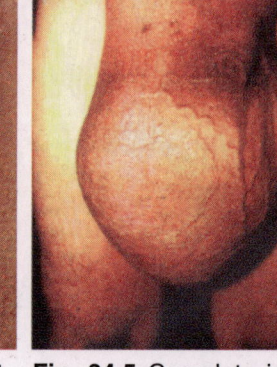

Fig. 34.4 Incomplete indirect hernia

Fig. 34.5 Complete indirect hernia

1. **Ask the patient to cough**—expansile impulse is felt at the root of scrotum.

Key Box 34.2
EXPANSILE IMPULSE ON COUGH
• Hernia • Meningocoele • Dermoid cyst with intracranial communication • Laryngocoele • Lymphatic cyst in children • Empyema necessitans

2. **Getting above[1] the swelling** should be done in the standing position. (Not possible in Fig. 34.5)

- At the root of scrotum, the spermatic cord is palpated between the finger and the thumb. In cases of incomplete indirect hernia, spermatic cord cannot be felt as a naked structure, because it is covered anterolaterally by the sac. This is called as **getting above the swelling not possible** (negative).

This is a test to differentiate scrotal swellings from inguinoscrotal swellings

---

1. *This test has no meaning or usefulness in bubonocoele. It is a test to differentiate scrotal swelling from inguino-scrotal swelling.*

3. **Reducibility**—ask the patient to lie down.

- If the swelling becomes smaller or disappears, it is a hernia (hydrocoele is not reducible).
- If it is difficult to reduce, ask the patient to reduce it. Otherwise, flex and medially rotate the hip and try to reduce it.
- If in spite of this, the swelling is not reduced, it is called as an irreducible hernia.

4. **Finger invagination test**

- At the root of the scrotum, skin is gathered and lifted up with the little finger. It is then invaginated into the external ring. As the external ring is stretched in indirect hernia, the finger goes obliquely and laterally. In a direct hernia, the finger goes backwards, and the superior ramus of the pubic bone can be felt as a bare bone. On asking the patient to cough, the impulse touches the pulp of the finger in direct hernia and the tip in indirect hernia.

This test results in discomfort to the patient. It cannot be done in female patients because the labial skin is thick and not lax. Hence, it is not a relevant test. However, in very early doubtful cases of indirect hernia an impulse on cough may be appreciated at the deep ring in this test.

5. **Internal ring occlusion test** (Deep ring occlusion test). Reduce the swelling first.

- Locate the deep ring $1/2$" above the midpoint of inguinal ligament and occlude it with the thumb and ask the patient to cough.
- a. If impulse and the swelling is seen, it is a direct hernia—because it occurs in the Hesselbach's triangle (medial to deep ring).

b. If the swelling is not seen, it is an indirect hernia.

Problems of deep ring occlusion test

- a. If occlusion is not done properly, results may vary.
- b. Pantaloon hernia (Romberg hernia, saddle bag hernia, dual hernia). It is a direct hernia having indirect component.

6. **Leg raising test** or (Head raising test)

- Weakness of oblique muscles is manifested by Malgaigne's bulgings above the iliac crest and inguinal ligament. *It is an absolute indication for hernioplasty.*

7. **Zieman's method:** Three finger method

- Keep index finger at deep ring, middle finger at the posterior wall above and lateral to the external ring and ring finger at femoral ring. Now ask the patient to cough. Depending upon the type of hernia, impulse is felt. It is not necessary to perform this test in incomplete or complete indirect hernias.

8. **Evidence of stricture urethra**—young patients with urinary complaints with hernia may be suffering from stricture urethra. Lift the scrotum and feel for any strictures in the bulbar urethra.

9. **Examination of respiratory system** is done to rule out chronic bronchitis, tuberculosis, etc.

10. **Per rectal examination** should be done in elderly patients to rule out prostatic enlargement.

Examine the opposite side also.

Diagnosis

- Right side, indirect, incomplete, uncomplicated, reducible omentocoele. (See Table 34.1 for comparison)

		Table 34.1. Differences between direct and indirect hernia	
		DIRECT HERNIA	**INDIRECT HERNIA**
1.	Aetiology	Weakness of posterior wall of inguinal canal	Preformed sac
2.	Precipitating factors	Chronic bronchitis, enlarged prostate	—
3.	On standing	Pops out	Does not pop out
4.	Side	usually bilateral	Unilateral (30% bilateral)
5.	Internal ring occlusion test	The swelling is seen	Swelling is not seen
6.	Malgaigne's bulgings	May be present	Absent
7.	Complications	Not common because neck is wide	Common, neck is narrow
8.	Relationship of sac to the cord	Sac is posterior to the cord	Sac is anterolateral to the cord
9.	Direction of the sac	It comes out of Hesselbach's triangle	Sac comes through the deep ring

DIFFERENTIAL DIAGNOSIS OF A GROIN SWELLING

Groin refers to the junction of lower abdomen with the thigh. Hence, swellings in the inguinal region and upper thigh close to the inguinal ligament are included under groin swellings.

1. **Inguinal hernia**

2. **Femoral hernia:** The main sac is below and lateral to pubic tubercle.

3. **Vaginal hydrocoele:** Fluctuation and transillumination tests are usually positive and getting above swelling is possible.

   (Please note in infantile hydrocoele and hydrocoele en-bisac getting above swelling is not possible)

4. **Retractile testis :** It can present as a firm swelling in the inguinal region. Scrotum is empty.

5. **Saphena varix :** Patient can present with a swelling in the thigh. Swelling is usually about 2.5 cms below the inguinal ligament. A swelling that disappears on elevation of the leg is characteristic of any swelling of **venous origin.**

6. **Funiculitis :** A funiculitis can occur with or without acute epididymo-orchitis. Severe pain in inguinal re-gion, tender swelling, high grade fever with chills and rigors are characteristic. Spermatic cord is thickened and swelling is not reducible.

7. **Inguinal lymphadenitis:** Pain and nodular swelling below inguinal ligament is a feature. It is not reducible and some sources of infection in the lower limb are usually present.

8. **Lipoma of the cord :** It presents as a soft, lobulated but not irreducible swelling in the inguinal region.

INVESTIGATIONS

- Routine investigations like complete blood picture (CBP) and urine examination is done. In elderly patients, chest X-ray, electrocardiography or even pulmonary function tests may be necessary. Patients with urinary complaints are evaluated for prostatic enlargement and for stricture urethra.

PRE-OPERATIVE PREPARATION

- A patient with chronic bronchitis and bronchial asthma should be properly treated with bronchodilators, antibiotics, mucolytic agents, etc. Cigarette smoking should be stopped.

- Elderly patients with bilateral hernia mostly suffer from

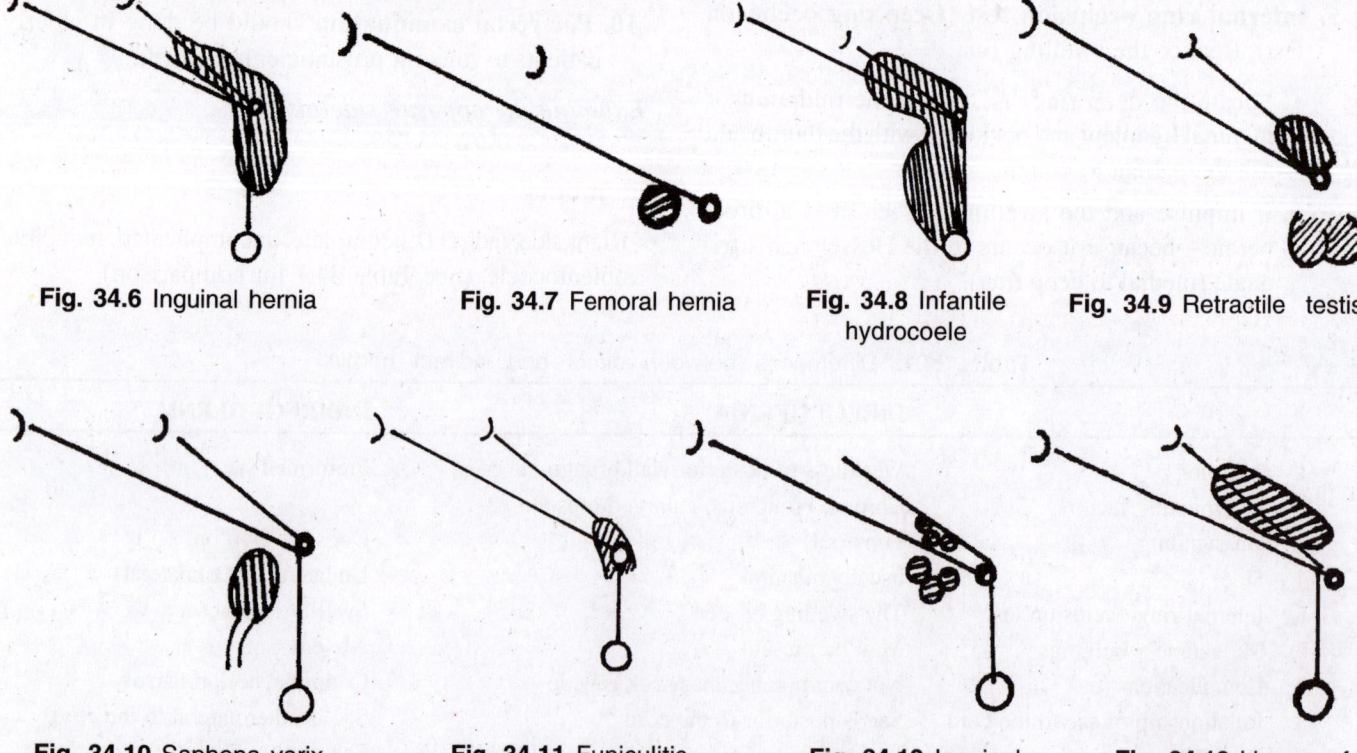

Fig. 34.6 Inguinal hernia   **Fig. 34.7** Femoral hernia   **Fig. 34.8** Infantile hydrocoele   **Fig. 34.9** Retractile testis

Fig. 34.10 Saphena varix   **Fig. 34.11** Funiculitis   **Fig. 34.12** Inguinal lymphadenitis   **Fig. 34.13** Lipoma of the cord

benign prostatic hypertrophy. Prostatectomy should be considered first followed by repair of hernia, in such cases.

- Young adults with difficulty in passing urine may have a stricture urethra. They should undergo proper treatment for the stricture.

TREATMENT

> *Herniotomy, herniorrhaphy and hernioplasty are the three "key" operations for inguinal hernia.*

1. Herniotomy

- Excision of the sac alone is done in patients upto 14 -16 years of age (children). Hernia occurs due to preformed sac. Hence, **no repair is necessary.**

2. Herniorrhaphy (Fig. 34.14)

- It can be of two types - Bassini's and Shouldice.
- **A. Bassini's herniorrhaphy:** Herniotomy with approximation of posterior wall of the inguinal canal by suturing the conjoined tendon (above) to the inguinal ligament below, by using interrupted, nonabsorbable suture material like nylon, thick silk or polypropylene. This is the most popular method. Repair of stretched deep ring by narrowing and laterally displacing the spermatic cord is done (**Lytle's repair**) in selected cases at the end of the procedure.

  If there is tension, an incision over the anterior rectus sheath will help in doing the repair (**Tanner's slide**).

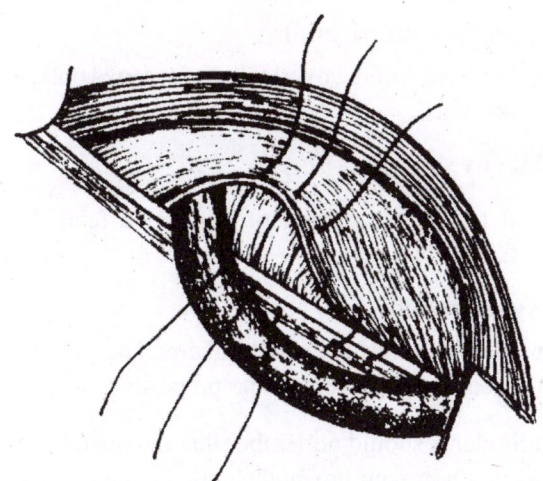

Fig. 34.14 Bassini's herniorrhaphy

Indications for Bassini's herniorrhaphy

1. Indirect hernia with good muscle tone.
2. Direct hernia with good muscle tone.

Criticism for Bassini's herniorrhaphy

1. It is a repair with tension
2. Conjoined tendon and inguinal ligament approximation is **not physiological.**

> *Hence irrespective of the type of hernia, Mesh repair (Lichtenstein) is recommended today as first line of repair.*

B. Shouldice repair

- It is the most popular tensionless method wherein only local tissues are used.
- After opening the inguinal canal herniotomy is done.
- Transversalis fascia which forms the posterior wall, is incised from the internal ring till pubic tubercles.
- Thus, upper and lower flaps of transversalis fascia are sutured in a double-breasting manner by using non-absorbable sutures like 34 gauge stainless steel wire, polyamide or polypropylene. This is the **first layer** of Shouldice repair.
- The **second layer** is like Bassini's, wherein conjoined tendon is sutured to the inguinal ligament by using nonabsorbable sutures.
- The **third layer** is completed by suturing upper flap of external oblique aponeurosis to the inguinal ligament.
- The results have been good in Shouldice's hands. The operation needs **expertise.**

3. Hernioplasty: It refers to strengthening the posterior wall of inguinal canal. There are 2 types of hernioplasties which are commonly practised.

Key Box 34.3
SHOULDICE REPAIR
• First layer : Double breasting of the transversalis fascia
• Second layer : Conjoined tendon is sutured to inguinal ligament
• Third layer : Upper half of external oblique aponeurosis is sutured to inguinal ligament

A. Strengthening the posterior wall of inguinal canal by a Prolene mesh or Marlex mesh. The fibroblasts and capillaries grow over the mesh, thus converting it into a thick fibrous sheath (Fig. 34.15). **(Lichtenstein repair).** Mesh is to be sutured to the transversalis fascia, lacunar ligament and inguinal ligament. Lacunar ligament is that portion of the inguinal ligament which extends backwards and upwards to the pectineal line and forms the medial margin of the femoral ring.

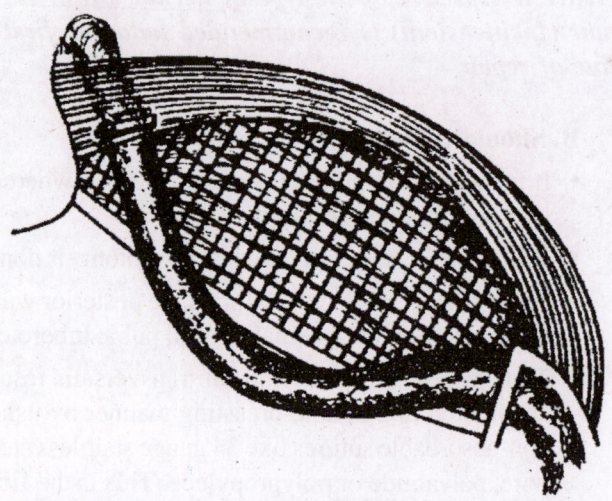

Fig. 34.15 Prolene mesh repair - Lichtenstein repair

B. Prolene darning: Suturing the conjoined tendon to the inguinal ligament without tension in a criss cross manner by using prolene suture material (handmade mesh). This is preferred in direct and indirect hernias (Fig. 34.16).

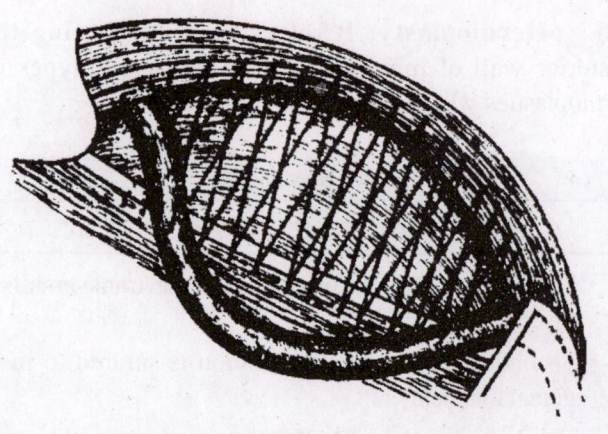

Fig. 34.16 Prolene darning

Indications for hernioplasty

1. Indirect or direct hernia with a good muscle tone. In such cases, darning can be done.
2. Indirect or direct hernia with weak muscle tone—meshplasty is preferred
3. Recurrent hernia

OTHER SURGERIES FOR INGUINAL HERNIA

1. Kuntz operation (Fig. 34.17)

- In this operation the spermatic cord is divided at the deep ring and it is removed along with the testis, so that the deep ring can be permanently closed, and hernia never recurs. It is indicated in elderly patients with recurrent hernia and poor abdominal muscle tone.

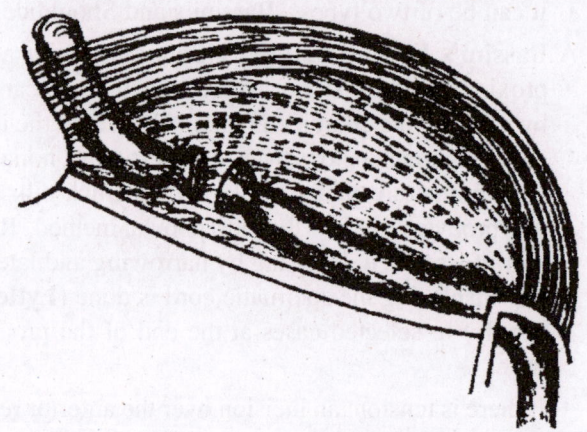

Fig. 34.17 Kuntz operation

2. Andrew's imbrication

- In this operation, overlaping of external oblique aponeurosis

3. Mcvay

- It refers to suturing of conjoined tendon to the Cooper's ligament.

4. Nyhus repair

- Ideally indicated in bilateral direct hernia wherein a broad mesh is kept in the preperitoneal space.

Note : Students should remember that the operation which you have seen in your hospital should be mentioned in the clinical examination.

COMPLICATIONS OF HERNIA

1. **IRREDUCIBILITY:** Occurs due to adhesions formed between omentum, sac and the contents. Irreducibility produces dull aching pain.

2. **OBSTRUCTED HERNIA:** Irreducible hernia + obstruction to the lumen of the gut give rise to obstructed hernia. Clinically, it produces severe colicky abdominal pain, abdominal distension, vomiting and step ladder peristalsis.

Key Box 34.5

FACTORS RESPONSIBLE FOR OBSTRUCTED HERNIA

- Narrow neck
- Irreducibility
- Sudden straining
- Too many contents
- Long duration of hernia

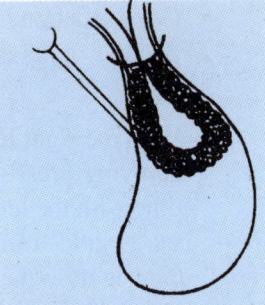

Fig. 34.18 Strangulated hernia

Key Box 34.4

DIAGNOSIS OF IRREDUCIBLE HERNIA

- Hernia is tense
- Tender
- Irreducible
- No impulse on cough
- Recent increase in size of swelling

Treatment

- Urgent division of the neck of the sac followed by herniorrhaphy or hernioplasty.

3. STRANGULATED HERNIA

- Irreducibility + obstruction + impairment of blood supply to intestine (Key Box 34.5, Fig. 34.18).

Pathology

- Strangulation commonly occurs in femoral hernia, obturator hernia and in indirect hernia.
- Initially the venous return is occluded, the part gets congested, mucosal ulceration and haemorrhage occurs into the gut wall. It also results in oedema due to capillary exudation.
- If the obstruction is not relieved, constriction of the artery takes place resulting in gangrene of bowel. If this happens, there is a proliferation of bacteria (Fig. 34.20).
- Such a gangrenous segment contains decomposed blood in which gram-negative organisms multiply. They produce endotoxins resulting in endotoxic shock. If the gangrene extends into the intra-abdominal segment of the bowel, peritonitis can occur.
- The deep ring and the external ring are the common constricting agents.

Clinical features

- Sudden, severe, prolonged pain with some features of shock are indicative of strangulation.
- Clinical examination of such hernia reveals:
1. Tense
2. Tender
3. No impulse on cough
4. Irreducible
5. Recent increase in the size of swelling
6. General condition of patient is poor :
   - Feeble pulse
   - Hypotension
   - Rebound tenderness
   - Guarding and Rigidity if infection has spread
   - Absent bowel sounds
   - Toxic look

Treatment

I. General measures

1. The patient is hospitalised. The foot end of the bed is raised so that an irreducible hernia may reduce by gravity. However, if there is a suspicion of gangrene, this step is not recommended.
2. A Ryle's tube is introduced to decompress the stomach, thus preventing vomiting and reducing abdominal distension.
3. Intravenous fluids are given to correct dehydration and to prevent renal failure.
4. Narcotic analgesics are required to reduce the pain.
5. An attempt should be made to reduce the swelling when there is no gangrene by the following measures.

- Good sedation
- Patient's thigh is flexed, adducted and medially rotated.
- With the right hand, the sac is gently squeezed by applying pressure over the scrotum. At the same time with the left hand, the proximal portion of the sac is guided into the inguinal canal. This procedure is described as taxis. **TAXIS is contraindicated if there is gangrene.**
- **Complications of forced reduction** include, contusion of intestinal wall, the rupture of the sac at the neck and reduction-en-mass i.e. the entire sac with the contents are reduced into the abdominal cavity. But, intestine still remains strangulated.

6. The patient is prepared for surgery and blood is arranged for it.

II. Surgery (Key Box 34.6)

- With broad-spectrum antibiotic coverage, the hernia is explored by an inguinoscrotal incision and hernial sac is defined. At this stage, *don't divide the constricting ring.* First aspirate all the toxic fluid from the sac. Now the constriction is divided by using a grooved director or hernia bistoury. **While dividing the constricting ring, the inferior epigastric vessels may be damaged.** Therefore, care has to be taken to protect these vessels.
- If the bowel is gangrenous, resection of gangrenous segment and anastomosis is done. Closure of incision includes placement of corrugated red rubber drain or tube drain, which is brought out through a separate incision.
- If viability of the bowel is doubtful, the intestinal loops are covered with hot wet mops for a period of 5-10 minutes and 100% of oxygen is given to the patient (request the anaesthetist). Return to pink

colour, peristalsis of bowel and pulsations in the mesentery indicate viability.

- If the general condition of the patient permits, repair of the hernia can also be done.
- If evidence of peritonitis is present or if gangrene is spreading within, laparotomy should be done.

4. INCARCERATED HERNIA

- It is an obstructed hernia due to obstruction caused by faecal matter. It generally occurs in a sliding hernia.

5. INFLAMMED HERNIA

- It occurs when the contents of hernia get inflamed, e.g. appendicitis in a hernial sac, Meckel's diverticulitis in hernial sac.

Thus, complications of hernia can be dangerous. It may range from a simple obstruction to a life-threatening strangulation. Hence, early diagnosis and early treatment is necessary in all cases of indirect hernia. In few selected cases of direct hernia, where in the defect is big, the chances of strangulation are less. However, if there are no medical contraindications, surgery has to be advised (Key Box 34.7).

Following are few examples of strangulations without obstruction. They have diarrhoea and bleeding per rectum rather than constipation (Key Box 34.8).

Key Box 34.6

SURGERY FOR STRANGULATION

- Generous inguinal incision, identify the sac
- First aspirate toxic fluid
- Divide constricting agent
- Check for viability
- Resection of gangrene
- Repair of hernia
- Broad spectrum antibiotics

Key Box 34.7

SUMMARY OF COMPLICATIONS OF HERNIA

- Irreducibility
- Obstructed hernia
- Strangulation
- Incarcerated hernia
- Inflammed hernia

Key Box 34.8

STRANGULATIONS WITHOUT OBSTRUCTION

- Omentocoele
- Richter's hernia
- Littre's hernia

TYPES	CLASSIFICATION	REPAIR
I	• Snug internal ring • Preperitoneal indirect sac • Does not admit 1 finger	• Herniorrhaphy or hernioplasty
II	• Moderately enlarged internal ring • Bubonocoele • Admits 1 finger	• Herniorrhaphy or hernioplasty
III	• Large defect - 2 or 3 finger breadth internal ring. May be sliding hernia	• Preperitoneal mesh by slitting transversalis fascia
IV	• Large direct hernia with full defect • Internal ring is normal	• Mesh repair
V	• Direct hernia with punched out hole/defect in the transversalis fascia • The internal ring is intact	• Plug the defect or purse-string closure of the defect followed by mesh repair
VI	• Pantaloon hernia	• Mesh repair
VII	• Femoral hernia	• Femoral hernia repair

Table 34.2 Gilbert's classification and suggested repair

GILBERT'S CLASSIFICATION (Table 34.2)

- It is based on the defect in the posterior wall (direct hernia) or defect in the internal ring (indirect).
- Depending upon the defect the suggested repair is given above. However, basic principles are the same.
- The last two types - Type VI and Type VII are modifications by Robbin.

RECURRENT HERNIA

CAUSES

Pre-operative

1. Chronic cough
2. Weak muscle tone
3. Straining while passing urine
4. Obesity, ascites, etc.

Intraoperative

1. **Improper excision of the sac :** The sac should be ligated at the level of deep ring (neck). This is called as **high ligation of the sac**. Very often, as soon as the inguinal canal is opened the sac is seen. If it is ligated at the fundus or body (low ligation), it invariably results in recurrence.

2. **Absorbable sutures** like catgut have life span of 2-3 weeks. If they are used for reconstruction, they invariably result in recurrence.

3. **Bleeding :** At the end of the surgery, small bleeding points should be coagulated by using diathermy or ligatures. Haematoma formation predisposes to infection, which can be the cause of recurrences.

4. **Tension** between suture lines can cause strangulation and fibrosis of muscle fibres. Hence, care and gentleness is important while suturing conjoined tendon to the inguinal ligament.

Post-operative

1. **Persistent post-operative cough** weakens the suture line.

2. **Haematoma** can get secondarily infected resulting in pus formation. The sutures give way leading to recurrence. Hence, if there is a significant haematoma, it should be drained.

3. **Infection:** Eventhough hernia is a clean surgery, if hernioplasty is done in the form of meshplasty or the prolene darning, antibiotics are necessary.

4. **Exertion:** Too much exertion in the postoperative period, in the form of lifting heavy weights or carrying heavy weights on the shoulder, may weaken the suture line, resulting in hernia.

Most of the recurrences occur within one year. Incidence of recurrent hernia may vary from 2-8% even in experienced hands. In a case of recurrent hernia, it is difficult to say whether it is a direct hernia or indirect hernia. From the management point of view it does not matter.

Treatment

• If the sac is present due to incomplete excision at the previous surgery, it should be completely excised up to the level of deep ring, followed by hernioplasty.

• Meshplasty is the surgical treatment for a recurrent hernia. However, if mesh cannot be placed either due to infection or due to non-availability, prolene darning can be done.

• In all these cases, precipitating factors if present should be treated first.

• The only way to totally prevent recurrences is by closure of the deep ring. This can be done only after dividing the spermatic cord (Kuntz procedure). It is indicated in elderly patients who have multiple recurrences.

SPECIAL HERNIAS

DUAL HERNIA

• It has two sacs, one direct and another indirect connected by an isthmus which is behind the inferior epigastric artery. It is also known as saddle bag hernia or **pantaloon hernia.**

Significance

• **Deep ring occlusion test**: The inference of the test may not be correct.

• It is the **cause of recurrence** if one sac is not treated properly.

PREVESICAL HERNIA

• It is also called as **funicular direct hernia**. It is a hernia containing a portion of the bladder with pre-vesical fat through the defect in the conjoined tendon on the medial side. History of the swelling becoming less prominent after micturition may be present.

LITTRE'S HERNIA (Fig. 34.20)

• It is referred to a hernia containing Meckel's diverticulum. When the diverticulum gets infected, such hernias are called inflammed hernias. The cause of infection may be precipitated by partial obstruction to the diverticulum by constricting agents.

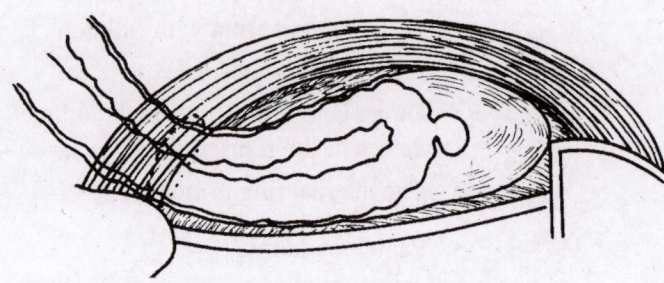

Fig. 34.19 Littre's hernia

MAYDL'S HERNIA (HERNIA- EN-W) (Fig.34.20)

• It is a **W** hernia wherein the intra-abdominal bowel loop segment becomes gangrenous very early, but in the scrotum there are no signs of gangrene.

• The patient presents with obstructed hernia and at operation the inguinoscrotal segment has no gangrene. The intra-abdominal segment has to be examined and the gangrenous portion should be excised. It can also be called retrograde strangulation. Clinically, there is tenderness above the inguinal ligament.

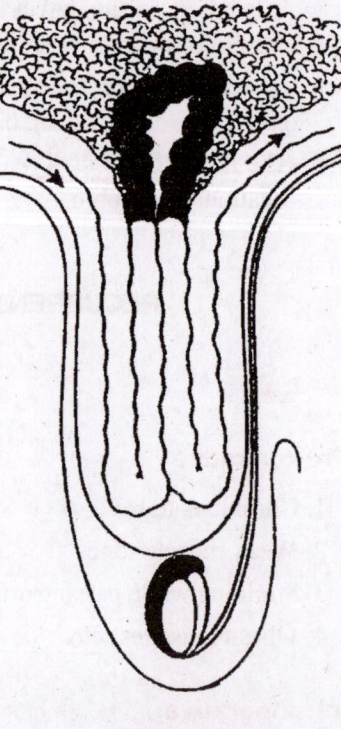

Fig. 34.20 Maydl's hernia

SLIDING HERNIA (Hernia-en-glissade)

- Incidence : 1-2%
- It occurs as a result of the slipping of posterior peritoneum along with the retroperitoneal viscus under the cellular tissue. As a result of which, the caecum, on the right side and the sigmoid colon on the left side, form the posterior wall of the sac. **If the caecum and appendix are the contents of the hernia sac, it is not a sliding hernia.** However, a true hernial sac containing omentum or intestines exists.
- Urinary bladder can also be the content of the hernia sac (Fig. 34.21).

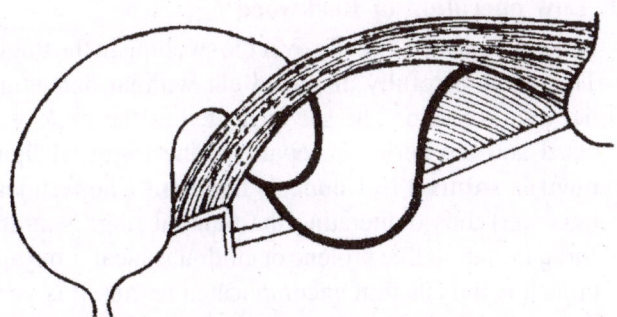

Fig. 34.21 Sliding hernia

Clinical features

- It almost always occurs in males.
- It can be suspected when there is a large hernia descending down into the scrotum. Left sided is more common than right sided hernia.
- It practically always occurs in long standing cases of inguinal hernia.
- They are not completely reducible.

Complications

- These hernias can easily strangulate and since its wall contents include the large intestine, the mortality and morbidity increases.

Treatment

1. Truss is absolutely contraindicated.
2. Once the hernial sac is opened, the sac should not be twisted a purse string suture is applied within to avoid injury to caecum/sigmoid colon. The sac is removed and the repair of the hernia done.
3. In elderly patients, orchidectomy is advised to give a permanent cure for hernia.

FEMORAL HERNIA

Herniation of intra-abdominal contents through the femoral canal is described as femoral hernia. Women are more often involved, as compared to men with the ratio being 2:1, which is doubled in parous women. However, it should be remembered that **in women, inguinal hernias are the most common type of hernia, followed by incisional hernia.** Femoral hernia is the third most common type of hernia.

Commonly the hernia is unilateral, the right side being affected more than the left side. It is bilateral in about 15-20% of the patients.

ANATOMY OF FEMORAL CANAL AND FEMORAL RING (Fig. 34.22)

- The femoral canal extends from the femoral ring to the saphenous ring. It is $1\frac{1}{2}$ inches below and lateral to the pubic tubercle. It is the innermost compartment of femoral sheath.
- It is similar to a truncated cone **which is narrow at the femoral ring.**
- **Contents of femoral canal are :**
    - Fat
    - Fascia
    - Lymphatics-lymph node of Cloquet
- Femoral vein is in the middle compartment of the femoral sheath and femoral artery is in the lateral compartment.
- Femoral nerve is outside the femoral sheath.
- Femoral sheath : Fascia transversalis is continued downwards behind the inguinal liagament as the anterior layer of the femoral sheath. Fascia iliaca continues behind the femoral vessels as the posterior layer of the femoral sheath.

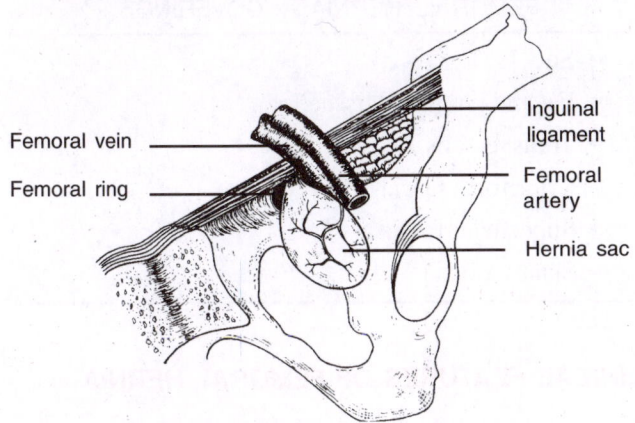

Fig. 34.22 Anatomy of femoral ring and canal

BOUNDARIES OF FEMORAL RING

- *Anterior :* Inguinal ligament.
- *Posterior :* Ligament of Cooper, ileopectineal ligament.
- *Medial :* Lacunar ligament (Gimbernat's ligament).
- *Lateral :* Thin septum which separates the femoral canal from femoral vein (silver fascia).

CAUSES FOR FEMORAL HERNIA

> *Femoral hernia is never congenital*

1. **Pregnancy:** Nature has provided all human beings with an empty femoral sheath on the medial side so that as gravid uterus compresses the external iliac vein, the femoral vein can also expand within femoral sheath. Thus, increased abdominal pressure due to repeated pregnancies is one of the chief factors responsible for femoral hernias. The maximum incidence is around 30-40 years of age.
2. **Wide femoral canal:** This is due to the narrow insertion of iliopubic tract into the pectineal line of the pubis and may be responsible for a few cases of femoral hernia.

COURSE OF THE HERNIAL SAC

- As the hernia comes into the femoral canal, it is an oblong swelling due to the rigid femoral canal. When it comes out through the saphenous opening, it expands and becomes retort shaped because Scarpa's fascia is attached to the deep fascia of thigh below the saphenous opening.

Key Box 34.9

FEMORAL HERNIA - COVERINGS

- Sac
- Fat and lymphoid tissue
- Transversalis fascia
- Cribriform fascia
- Superficial fascia
- Skin

CLINICAL FEATURES OF FEMORAL HERNIA

- Females between the age of 20 to 40 years are commonly affected.

- Right side is more commonly affected because of the dominant nature of right side of the body.
- To start with, there is a small swelling below the inguinal ligament, which goes unnoticed very often.
- Expansile impulse is often not present due to the narrow canal.
- Reducibility may be present.
- Typically, the swelling is below and lateral to the pubic tubercle (inguinal hernia is above and medial to pubic tubercle).

TREATMENT

1. Low operation of Lockwood

- Incision is placed directly over the swelling in the thigh. The sac is carefully dissected out without damaging the femoral vein. The sac is ligated at the neck, excised and the hernia is repaired—the **inguinal ligament is sutured to Cooper's ligament** (iliopectineal ligament) thus obliterating the femoral ring. Non-absorbable suture like prolene or ethilon is ideal. Low approach is indicated in uncomplicated hernia. It is very difficult to manage a gangrenous loop of bowel with this approach.

2. Inguinal operation

- Through an **inguinal incision,** the inguinal canal is opened. The transversalis fascia is incised. Hernial sac is visualised. This is followed by excision of the sac. The high approach is preferred when there is a strangulated femoral hernia. This offers a very good view of the abnormal obturator artery from above, if it is present.
- Repair is done by suturing the conjoined tendon to iliopectineal line.

3. Combined approach - high operation of McEvedy

- Inguino-femoral approach: A vertical incision is made over the swelling and extended above the inguinal ligament, and the sac can be dissected from both above and below. This approach has the advantages of both operations mentioned above.

COMPLICATIONS OF FEMORAL HERNIA

1. As the femoral ring is narrow and so is the neck of the sac, obstruction and strangulation are very common.
2. Richter's hernia

- Commonly seen in femoral hernias and obturator hernias, which have narrow necks.

- This occurs when a **portion of the circumference of the bowel** is caught within the hernial sac and is constricted by the narrow ring. Signs and symptoms of intestinal obstruction are absent, even though it is an obstructed hernia, because the lumen is not obstructed.

- The hernia is tense, tender, irreducible and has no cough impulse.

- As the lumen is patent, there may be bloody diarrhoea rather than constipation. Gangrene can soon occur.

Treatment

- Combined or inguinal approach to deal with gangrene.

Summary of femoral hernia (Key Box 34.10)

Key Box 34.10
FEMORAL HERNIA
• Rarely occurs in males (5-10%) • Commonly associated with Richter's hernia • Fatty female with small swelling under a big belly usually goes undetected • Dangerous because of early strangulation • Cannot be controlled by a truss • Surgical repair is a must

RARE TYPES OF FEMORAL HERNIA

1. Lacunar hernia (Laugier's hernia)

In this case, the hernia passes through a small defect in the lacunar ligament.

2. Prevascular hernia

In this case, the hernial sac is located in behind the femoral vessels and behind the inguinal ligament. It may be associated with congenital dislocation of the hip (Narath hernia).

3. Pectineal hernia

In this case, the hernia passes between the pectineus muscle and its fascia, behind the femoral vessels. It is also called Cloquet's hernia.

4. External femoral hernia

It is a hernia lateral to the femoral artery (Hesselbach's hernia).

DIFFERENTIAL DIAGNOSIS OF FEMORAL HERNIA

1. **Inguinal hernia :** An inguinal hernia is above and medial to pubic tubercle. The femoral hernia is below and lateral to pubic tubercle (Fig. 34.23).

2. **Saphena varix :** It is the dilated, saccular, upper end of long saphenous vein with varicosity. It disappears on lying down because of gravity. Thrill may be felt on coughing.

3. **Lipoma :** Soft and lobular, slips under palpating fingers.

4. **Psoas abscess :** It is an iliopsoas abscess due to tuberculosis of spine. There are two swellings, one above and one below the inguinal ligament. Cross fluctuation can be elicited between these two swellings. The tenderness over the spine and X-ray of the spine help in making a diagnosis.

5. **Enlarged femoral lymph nodes** are firm and round. They can be enlarged in lower limb infections, abrasions, wounds in the perineum and also in carcinoma penis.

6. **Femoral artery aneurysm** is rare. It presents as a pulsatile swelling in the groin with a continuous murmur. Peripheral pulses are often weak.

7. **Psoas bursa:** Osteoarthritis of the hip can produce distension of psoas bursa, which disappears on flexing the hip.

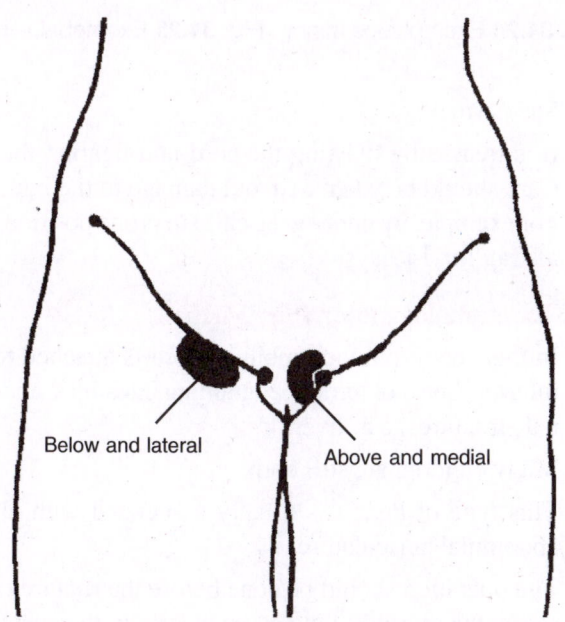

Below and lateral   Above and medial

Fig. 34.23 Femoral hernia (Rt) and indirect hernia (Lt).

UMBILICAL HERNIA

- It can be discussed under three headings
1. Umbilical hernia of newborn
II. Umbilical hernia of infants and children
III. Umbilical hernia of adults

UMBILICAL HERNIA OF NEWBORN

- It is called as *Omphalocoele—Exomphalos.*
- It is found 1 in 6000 live births.
- Failure of midgut as a **whole or part** to enter coelomic cavity during embryonic life, resulting in exomphalos.
- It is also associated with weakness of abdominal musculature (few fibres may be absent). Two types have been recognised.

1. Exomphalos minor (Fig. 34.24)

- In this condition, the umbilical cord is attached to the summit of the sac.

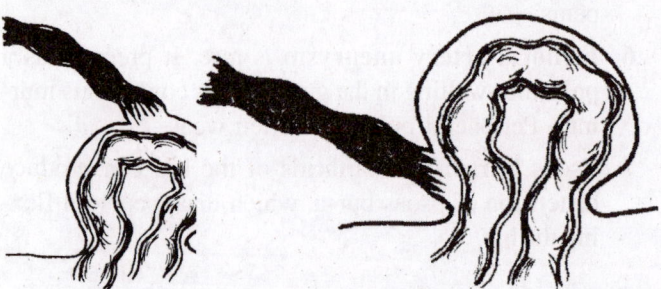

Fig. 34.24 Exomphalos minor   **Fig. 34.25** Exomphalos major

- Sac is small.
- It is treated by twisting the cord and ligating the sac. Care should be taken to avoid damage to the intestine. For example, by nursing the child in prone position with a strap for 14 days.

2. Exomphalos major (Fig. 34.25)

- In this condition, the umbilical cord is attached to the inferior aspect of the sac, containing intestines, abdominal structures, e.g. liver.
- Many children are still born.
- This type of hernia is usually associated with absent abdominal musculature.
- The operation should be done before the rupture of the sac as the morbidity increases greatly in the event of a rupture of the sac.

- During the operation, skin flaps are raised on both sides to cover the defect. A true repair is necessary which is done at a later date.

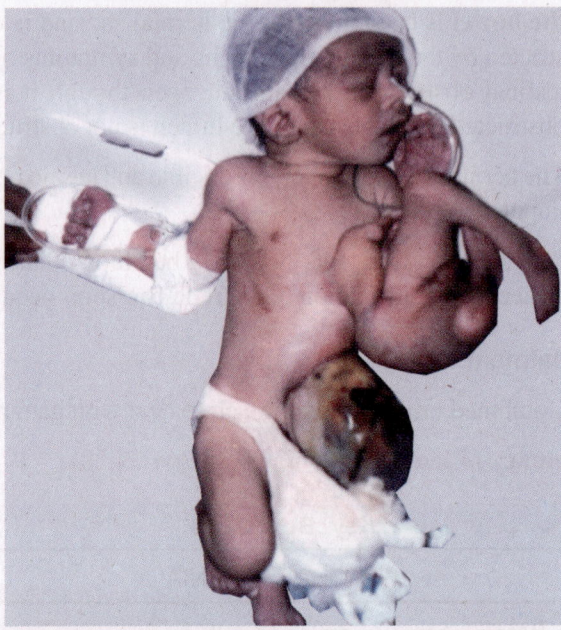

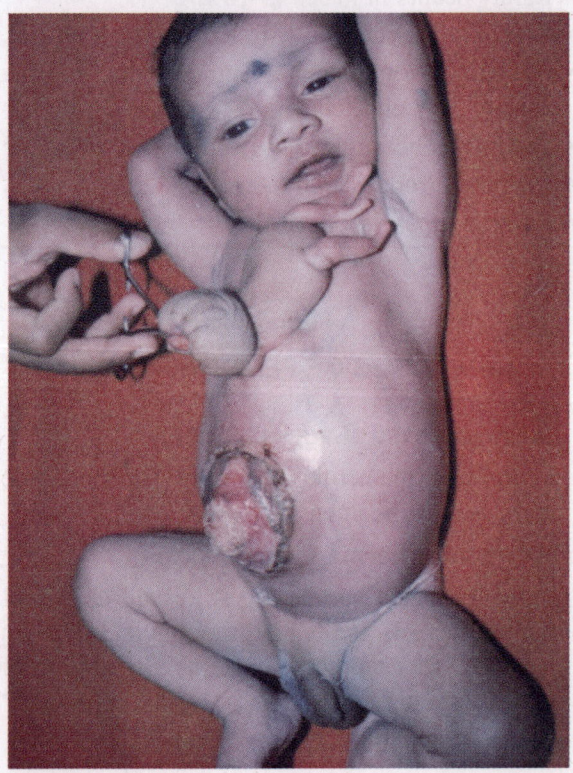

Fig. 34.26 Epigastric heteropagus with exomphalos major
Fig. 34.27 Same child on the 21st post-operative day. The repair is done by rotating flaps from gluteal region of the parasitic baby. Contributed by Prof. Vidyadhar Kinnal, Prof. R.S. Channagiri, Dr. Channanna, Dept. of Surgery, Vijayanagar Institute of Medical Sciences, Bellary, Karnataka

UMBILICAL HERNIA OF INFANTS AND CHILDREN

- It occurs as a complication of umbilical sepsis, which weakens the umbilical scar.
- It is a true umbilical hernia containing either omentum/intestines.

Clinical features

- Common in male children
- Child is brought with the complaint of swelling in the umbilical region whenever the child cries.
- Most of the cases are symptomless. Parents are anxious about the swelling.
- Strangulation is rare

Treatment

- **Reassurance** is the most important advice given to the parents.
- **No treatment is required** other than **strapping** the abdominal wall by keeping a pad in front of umbilicus.
- Majority of the hernias get corrected by 2 years of age (90%).
- If the hernia does not correct itself, repair is necessary to close the defect in the linea alba.

UMBILICAL HERNIA OF ADULTS

- It is not a true umbilical hernia but it is a para-umbilical hernia in which the hernia occurs either above, below or to the side of the umbilicus, through the linea alba.
- The contents are the greater omentum, transverse colon or small bowel. Due to adhesion, it is often irreducible.

Aetiology

- Females in the 5th decade are commonly affected. Male: female ratio is 1 : 5.
- **Obesity** with flabby abdominal muscle predisposes to paraumbilical hernia.
- Repeated **pregnancies** also weakens the abdominal wall.

Clinical features (Refer also Table 34.3)

- Patients present with a swelling in the umbilical region, which increases on straining or coughing,
- On asking the patient to cough, **expansile impulse** is present.
- **Reducibility can be present.**
- **Dragging pain** is usually due to omentum which is felt as a firm or granular mass. If gurgling is present, it is indicative of small intestines in the hernial sac.
- After reducing the swelling, the **defect** can be made out in the linea alba.

Complications

1. **Irreducibility** is common due to adhesions between the omentum and the sac.
2. **Obstruction** presents with colicky abdominal pain and vomiting. Distension follows soon. Untreated cases develop strangulation. Very often, these patients present with **incarcerated** hernia due to the presence of transverse colon in the sac.
3. As the sac enlarges, due to its weight and gravity, it sags down resulting in friction of skin and this causes **intertrigo.**

Table 34.3. Comparison of umbilical hernia of infants and paraumbilical hernia of adults		
FEATURES	**INFANTS**	**ADULTS**
Age in years	0 - 3	50 - 60
Sex	Common in male child	Common in females
Causes	Neonatal sepsis	Obesity, weak muscles, pregnancy
Defect	A small defect in the umbilical scar	Above or below the umbilicus
Symptoms	Symptomless	Symptoms are present
Strangulation	Rare	Very common
Treatment	Conservative (strapping), surgery (rare)	Mayo's repair

Treatment (Fig. 34.28)

1. Reduction of weight

2. *Mayo's repair* (surgical treatment)

- A curvilinear incision is made below the umbilicus or a double semilunar incision can be used. Umbilical cicatrix is then removed (in small hernias it can be preserved).

- Skin flaps are raised (upper and lower)

- The sac is dissected all around and the defect in the linea alba is defined.

- Contents of the sac can be reduced with or without opening of the sac

- Extra **redundant** sac is excised

- Peritoneum is closed

- Defect or cut in the linea alba is extended on both sides **(laterally)** and then upper and lower aponeurotic flaps are sutured together by using double breasting technique.

- Suture material used is prolene or nylon

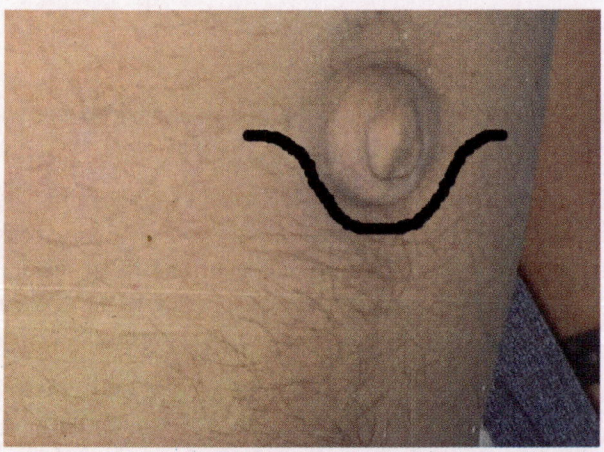

Fig. 34.28 Curvilinear incision

Key Box 34.11
MAYO'S UMBILICAL HERNIORRHAPHY
• Excision of umbilicus • Reduction of contents and excision of the sac • Double breasting of the fibrous aponeurotic layer • Haemostasis, suction and obliteration of dead space • Additional lipectomy and umbilicoplasty

INCISIONAL HERNIA

- It is also called as **ventral hernia** or post-operative hernia. It is a hernia that occurs through a weak scar. Very common in females.

FACTORS WHICH PRECIPITATE INCISIONAL HERNIA (Key Box 34.12)

1. **Infection:** Cases operated for peritonitis such as perforated duodenal ulcer, gangrene of the intestines etc. usually develop incisional hernia. The drainage tubes which are placed inside the peritoneal cavity help in reducing the post-operative incisional hernias, by draining peritoneal contents outside.

2. **Anatomical site:** The midline[1] is especially weak in the lower abdomen because of absence of posterior rectus sheath below the arcuate line or semilunar line.

3. **Obesity with weak muscle tone** predisposes to incisional hernia.

4. **Faulty technique** of closure of the abdomen or **faulty sutures** are also responsible for incisional hernia.

5. **Ascites, distension and persistent postoperative** cough further weakens the incision.

6. **Wrongly placed incisions** wherein nerves of the abdominal muscles are cut, precipitate incisional hernia. Lumbar incisions, lower midline incisions and large transverse incisions often give rise to incisional hernias.

Key Box 34.12
CAUSES OF INCISIONAL HERNIA
• Infection uncontrolled • Incision wrongly placed • Improper suture material • Increased intra-abdominal pressure

CLINICAL FEATURES

- Serosanguinous discharge on the 4th post-operative day through the main suture line is a signal of the development of wound dehiscence, partial or total. Such cases later develop an incisional hernia.

---

1. *Is that the reason why we see many cases of incisional hernia after gynecological operations*

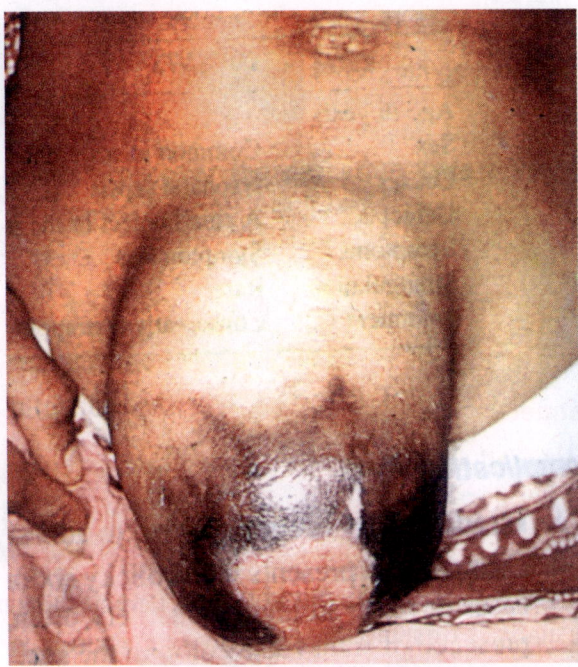

Fig. 34.29 Incisional hernia

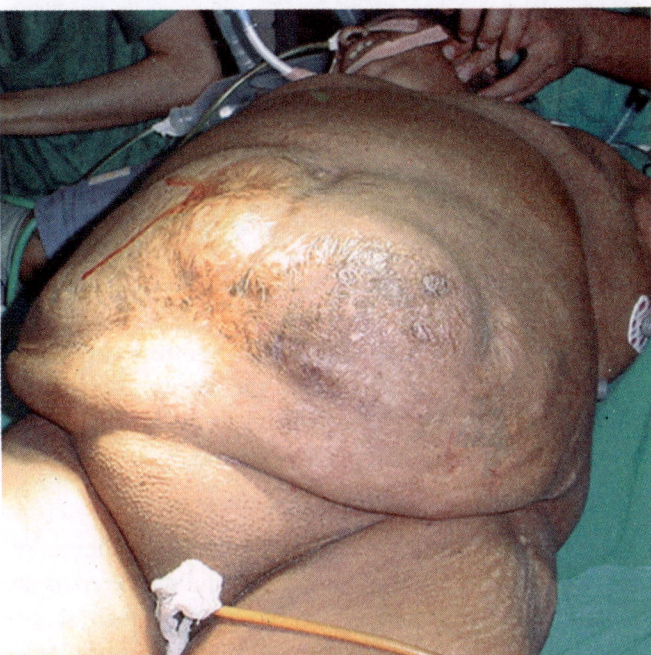

Fig. 34.30 Three times operated case of incisional hernia - huge recurrence

- History of infection during the first surgery, post-operative cough is usually present.
- There is a bulge/swelling in relation to the scar.
- Scar is thin and evidence of secondary healing in the form of irregular scar may be present.
- Expansile impulse on cough and reducibility may be present.
- After reduction of the contents, a defect can be palpated through the scar. Defect depends upon number of stitches that have given way.

TREATMENT

- Surgical treatment is necessary if the **defect is narrow,** if there is **discomfort** to the patient or if there is a **danger** in the form of obstruction.
- Pre-operative preparation includes reduction of weight, control of cough, etc.
- There are various operations for the treatment of incisional hernia depending upon the size of the defect, anatomical location of the incision and presence of precipitating factors.

1. Anatomical repair

- In this operation, all the anatomical layers such as peritoneum, posterior rectus sheath, linea alba and the sub-cutaneous tissue are identified. Closure is done layer by layer by using non-absorbable suture material.

2. Mesh repair

- As most of the incisional hernias are due to a large defect in the main incision and the majority of it occurs in obese women, repair using mesh has become the most popular method.
- In this operation, the sac is opened, greater omentum is excised, the contents are reduced followed by closure of the peritoneum. A mesh is kept in place which is sutured all around to the locally available tissues, without tension. Prolene mesh or marlex mesh is commonly used. **In all these repairs, tensionless, nonabsorbable suture repairs are done.** The mesh is placed in the peritoneal space covered by rectus muscles.

3. The Keel operation

- It is also known as the Keel operation of Rodney-Maingot. It can be recommended for small hernias with good locally available tissues.
- In this operation, the scar is excised; the sac is dissected and is pushed back into the abdomen *without opening the peritoneum.*Inverting sutures are applied, bites taken through the peritoneum with the aponeurotic layer which is available by using non-absorbable suture

material. **This repair on cross section** *resembles the keel of the ship.* Since the *peritoneum is not opened, recovery is smooth* and paralytic ileus is not a feature in the post-operative period.

- This operation is considered obsolete now.
- There are dozens of operations for incisional hernia repair. However, anatomical repair and mesh repair are frequently being done. In any type of repair there should be a tension-free repair. Hence, mesh repair is considered as the best repair, especially in obese multipara female patients with poor muscle tone.

EPIGASTRIC HERNIA

- It is also called as **fatty** hernia of the linea alba.
- This type of hernia occurs in the epigastrium through the linea alba which extends between the xiphoid process and umbilicus.

Precipitating factors

- Sudden straining or heavy exercise results in the tearing of a few fibres of linea alba and is responsible for precipitating an epigastric hernia. Initially there is a small protrusion of extra peritoneal pad of fat. Rarely, if it enlarges, it is due to the dragging of the peritoneal sac. The opening is very narrow. Hence, the hollow viscus cannot enter the sac. Diastasis of rectus muscles which results in a wide linea alba can also precipitate an epigastric hernia.

Clinical features

- Common in muscular men, manual labourers.
- Typically the swelling is situated in the upper abdomen midway between xiphoid process and umbilicus. Many a time, it contains only an extraperitoneal protrusion of the fat.
- An expansile impulse on cough is rare.

- Dull aching pain is due to the fatty contents which are partially strangulated. However, tenderness is an important feature of epigastric hernia.
- Many cases are associated with peptic ulcer disease.

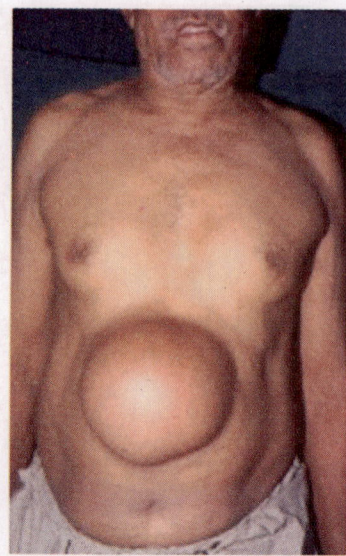

Fig. 34.31 Large epigastric hernia

Treatment

- A small incision is made over the swelling, the fatty tissue is isolated. It is ligated and excised because usually a tiny blood vessel enters the pad of fat. If a hernial sac is present, it is opened and contents are reduced followed by closure of the defect by using nonabsorbable sutures.

RARE EXTERNAL HERNIAS

INTERPARIETAL HERNIA

- It is also known as interstitial hernia.
- Basically, they are inguinal hernias. However, the processus vaginalis sac instead of following the normal route into the scrotum, traverses between various layers of the abdominal wall (parietes) resulting in interstitial hernias.
- Patients with Down's syndrome and Prune belly syndrome are commonly affected.

Types

1. **Preperitoneal:** In this variety the hernial sac lies between the transversalis fascia and peritoneum. It is seen in about 20% of patients. The sac is like a small diverticulum.

2. **Interparietal:** It is also called as intermuscular type. It is the commonest variety wherein the sac passes between the external oblique and internal oblique muscles. The swelling caused by the hernial sac causes discomfort to the patient. Sometimes, this can be a bilocular sac.

3. **Extraparietal:** It is also known as inguino-superficial variety. In this variety the hernial sac passes exterior (superficial) to the external oblique aponeurosis beneath superficial fascia of the abdominal wall. It is commonly associated with undescended testis or ectopic testis.

   - Majority of such cases present with features of intestinal obstruction.

- They are treated by identifying the sac, excision followed by closure of the defect or repair by using nonabsorbable sutures.

SPIGELIAN HERNIA[1]

- It is an interstitial hernia which occurs through the Spigelian fascia. This is a thin strip of fascia which runs parallel to the outer border of rectus sheath from the tip of the 9th costal cartilage to the pubic tubercle.

- Since it is very wide in the region of umbilicus/arcuate line, spigelian hernias occur commonly at this level.

- Spigelian fascia contributes a few fibres to form rectus sheath.

Precipitating factors

- Repeated pregnancies, advancing age, obesity, muscular degeneration, sudden strain due to coughing, weight lifting, etc. give rise to spigelian hernias.

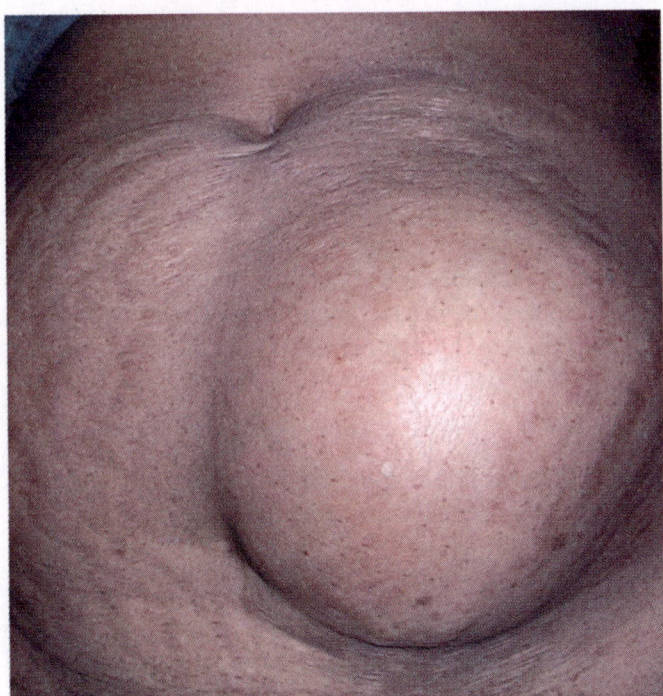

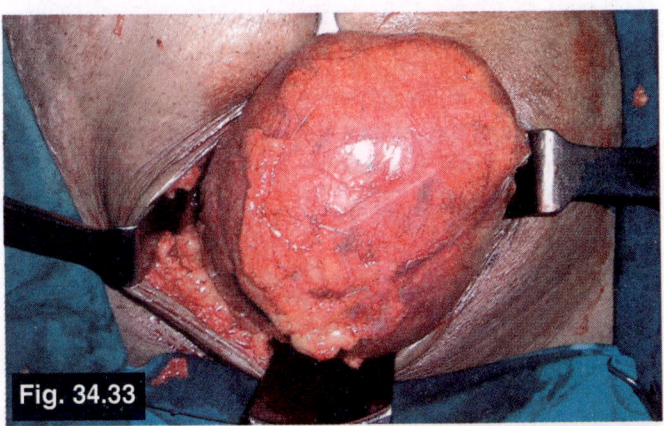

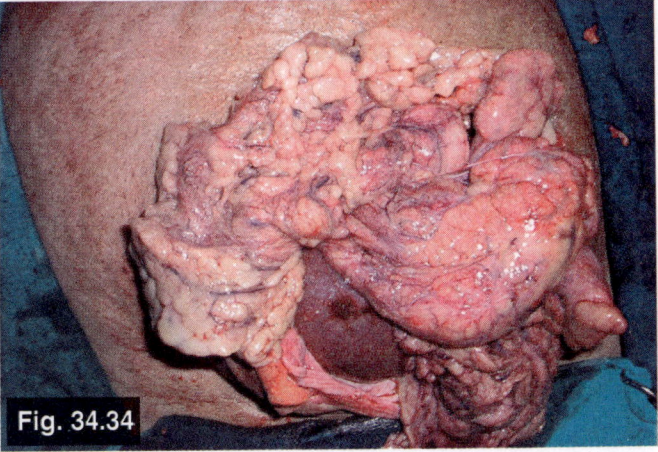

Fig. 34.32 Obstructed Spigelian hernia in a 70 year lady - first presentation to the hospital
Fig. 34.33 Delivary of the sac **Fig. 34.34** Contents of the sac. Contributed by Prof. M.G. Shenoy and Dr. G.N. Prasad, KMC, Manipal

---

1. *Prof. Spieghel, Anatomy and Surgery Professor not only described spigelian fascia but also the caudate lobe of the liver.*

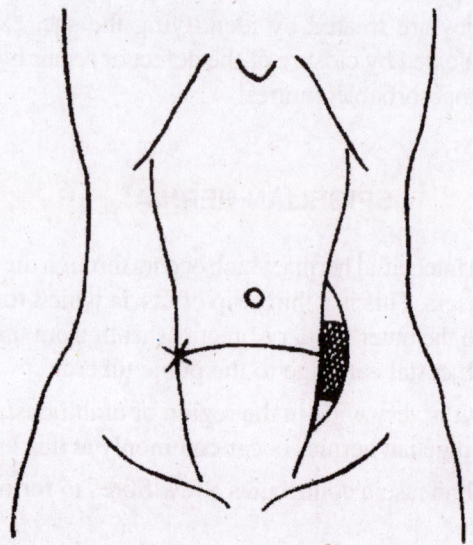

Fig. 34.35 Spigelian fascia and the site of hernia

Clinical features

1. Seen in both sexes equally around 50 years of age.

2. A round, soft, reducible swelling situated just below and lateral to the umbilicus—located typically at the junction of the arcuate line and lateral border of rectus abdominis. Sometimes, it is tender.

3. The swelling gives rise to an expansile impulse on cough.

4. As the hernia enlarges, it insinuates between external and internal oblique muscle. Hence, it is an example for interparietal hernia.

Investigations

1. An ultrasound can define the defect in the semilunar line.

2. X-ray abdomen, lateral view shows coils of bowel outside the peritoneal cavity.

Differential diagnosis

- Haematoma within the rectus sheath. However it will not give rise to impulse on cough.

Complication

- Strangulation is common due to the rigid fascial ring surrounding the hernial sac. Richter's hernia also can occur here.

Treatment

- An incision of about 5 to 6 cm is made over the swelling and abdominal wall muscles are split or cut. The sac is excised after reducing the contents followed by repair of the defect. Recurrence occurs in about 5% of the patients.

LUMBAR HERNIA

Two types of lumbar hernia are well recognised. They are as follows :

1. **Primary** which occurs through an anatomical defect :

   - **Through the inferior lumbar triangle of Petit.** Its boundaries are :

     - Inferiorly : Iliac crest
     - Laterally : External oblique
     - Medially : Latissimus dorsi

   - **Through the superior lumbar triangle.** Its boundaries are :

     - Above : 12th rib
     - Medially : Sacrospinalis
     - Laterally : Internal oblique

2. **Secondary** to a renal operation done through a loin incision. It is an example of a *lumbar incisional hernia*, which occurs due to either infection or weakness of loin muscles. The operation done for tuberculosis of spine through a loin incision, very often gives rise to a secondary lumbar hernia (it is an incisional hernia).

Differential diagnosis

1. **Lipoma** is common in the lumbar region (loin). It is soft, lobular, and slips under the palpating fingers.

2. **Cold abscess** secondary to tuberculosis of the spine gives rise to a nontender swelling in the para-vertebral space. Tenderness is present over the spine which gives a clue to the diagnosis. Patients may have deformity of the spine in the form of gibbus.

Treatment

- Small defects can be closed with simple sutures. Large defects need to be closed with or without mesh.

Primary lumbar hernias are very very rare.

OBTURATOR HERNIA

- This hernia occurs through the obturator canal which is bounded above by the superior ramus of pubis and below by the sharp edge of the obturator membrane.
- As the hernia is covered by the pectineus muscle, it is often overlooked.

Precipitating factors

- In females, the obturator foramen is wider in the transverse direction (it is triangular in shape in females and oval in males).
- Repeated pregnancies
- Loss of body weight
- Chronic lung diseases

Clinical features

- The most common presentation is acute intestinal obstruction with strangulation (80%). Recurrent attacks of intestinal obstruction which get resolved spontaneously is also common.
- This hernia causes more pain than any other type of hernia. Pain often radiates along the obturator nerve and may even be referred to the knee via its geniculate branch—*called as Howship Romberg sign.* The leg is usually kept in the *semiflexed position* and movement of the limb gives rise to pain. If the limb is flexed, abducted and rotated outwards the hernia becomes prominent. Patients are usually over 60 years of age and women are more frequently affected than men.

Key Box 34.15

OBTURATOR HERNIA

- The most common presentation is not a swelling but acute intestinal obstruction
- Can present as only pain in the knee - **(Howship Romberg sign)**
- Vaginal examination: Tender mass can be felt on the lateral side
- Very high chance of strangulation

- A few patients (20%) complain of palpable **hernial mass** in the groin.
- Per vaginal examination can reveal a tender lump on the lateral side of the vault.

Treatment

- Constricting agent in case of obstruction is the obturator fascia, which needs to be divided. Nerves and vessels are posterolateral to the hernial sac. Since majority of the cases present with intestinal obstruction and strangulation, a lower laparotomy is done. A grooved director is used to divide the obturator fascia.
- Contents are reduced or if there is gangrene, the affected bowel is resected.
- Closure of the obturator opening is done by stitching the broad ligament over the opening or by using monofilament nylon.

Bleeding Per Rectum

35

Lower gastrointestinal (GI) bleeding refers to bleeding which occurs below the ligament of Treitz. Bleeding per rectum may be a manifestation of upper GI bleeding, the causes of which have been discussed under haematemesis. In this chapter, bleeding per rectum due to lower GI causes will be discussed.

Investigating a case of lower GI bleeding is like investigating a 'crime' by C.B.I. officer. One should not jump to conclusions as soon as one cause of bleeding is found. **There are innumerable examples of piles being treated for bleeding, totally missing a growth above in the rectum.**

CAUSES

DEPENDING ON AETIOLOGY

I. Congenital
- Polyps: Congenital polyp, Peutz-Jeghers' syndrome, familial polyposis coli
- Meckel's diverticulum
- Hereditary Haemorrhagic Telangiectasia (HHT)

HHT is the most important inherited anomaly which produces bleeding.

II. Inflammatory
- Tubercular ulcers in the small intestine
- Enteric ulcers
- Crohn's ileocolitis
- Ulcerative colitis
- Necrotising enterocolitis
- **Dysentery**; Amoebic, bacillary strongyloides infestation

III. Neoplastic
- Papilloma of rectum
- Carcinoma colon and rectum
- Leiomyoma of the intestines
- Lymphoma
- Carcinoma small bowel
- Diverticular disease

IV. Vascular
- Angiodysplasia
- Ischaemic colitis
- Vasculitis-polyarteritis nodosa
- Haemangioma

V. Clotting disorders
- Haemophilia
- Thrombocytopenia
- Leukaemia
- Warfarin therapy
- Disseminated intravascular coagulopathy

VI. Miscellaneous
- Piles
- Prolapse
- Fissure in ano
- Injury to the rectum

DEPENDING ON SITE OF BLEEDING

I. Small intestine
- Peutz-Jeghers' polyps
- Meckel's diverticulum
- Tubercular ulcers
- Crohn's ulcers
- Leiomyoma

II. Large bowel
- Angiodysplasia right colon
- Carcinoma colon
- Ulcerative colitis
- Dysentery
- Diverticular disease

III. Anorectal conditions
- Piles
- Prolapse rectum
- Fissure in ano
- Fistula in ano (rare)
- Injuries to the rectum

Most of the causes have been discussed in the respective chapters. Angiodysplasia and Haemobilia are discussed here (Key Box 35.1 and 35.2).

Key Box 35.1
ANGIODYSPLASIA

- They are acquired lesions
- Caecum and right colon are common sites
- Small bowel (proximal) is second common site
- Small red mucosal lesions between 2-10 mm, flat or raised lesions
- Recurrent painless and self limiting bleeding
- They can be treated endoscopically-coagulation with heat probe, bipolar electrode or laser etc. But recurrence or failure can occur
- Surgery by resecting the segment is a definitive procedure

Key Box 35.2
HAEMOBILIA

- Rare cause of UGI or LGI bleeding
- **Triad of Sandblom**- maelena, biliary pain, jaundice
- External trauma
- Iatrogenic   - Transhepatic puncture (PTC, Stenting)
  - Surgery on biliary tree or pancreas
  - After dilatation of biliary strictures etc.
- Endoscopy   - Blood emerging from ampulla of Vater

CLINICAL EXAMINATION

1. **Age of the patient**
   - Children and young boys: Polyps, Meckel's diverticulum, necrotising enterocolitis (Fig. 35.1)
   - Young age group: Piles, tuberculosis, Crohn's, dysentery
   - Middle and old age: Carcinoma (Fig. 35.2), piles, prolapse, diverticular disease.

2. **Colour of blood**
   - Bright red : Piles, fissure, polyp
   - Altered blood : Carcinoma, tubercular ulcer, Crohn's colitis, dysentery
   - Maroon colour : Meckel's diverticulum

3. **Blood with mucous**
   - Intussusception
   - Dysentery
   - Inflammatory bowel diseases (Fig. 35.3)
   - Carcinoma

4. **Other special features**
   - Severe pain with bleeding: Fissure in ano
   - Splash in the pan: Piles
   - Red currant jelly stools: Intussusception
   - Streak of blood : Fissure in ano
   - Bloody slime: Carcinoma rectum
   - Blood with cherry-red mass coming out (piles, polyps)

5. **Palpable mass abdomen**
   - Hard mass in the colon : Carcinoma colon
   - Firm to hard mass in the right iliac fossa: Ileocaecal tuberculosis (Fig. 35.5)
   - Contracting mass : Intussusception

6. **Rectal examination**
   - Very, very painful : Fissure in ano
   - Pedunculated mass : Rectal polyp (Juvenile polyps)
   - Ulcerations in the rectum : Solitary rectal ulcer
   - Indurated ulcer or cauliflower like growth: Carcinoma rectum

7. **Evidence of bleeding tendencies**
   - Purpuric spots
   - Haematoma

DIFFERENTIAL DIAGNOSIS OF LOWER GI BLEEDING

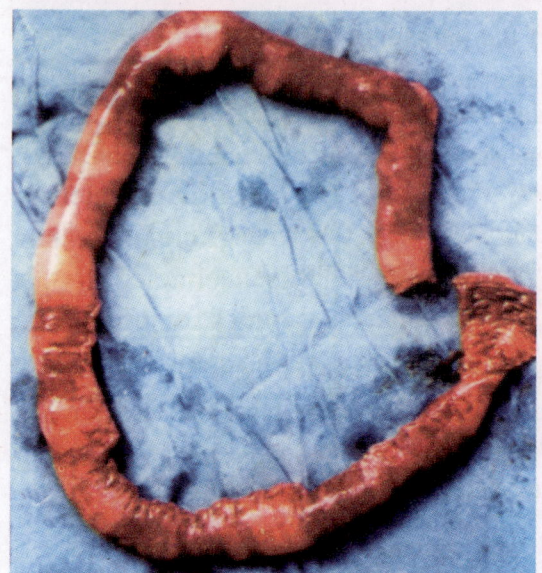

Fig. 35.1 Necrotising enterocolitis

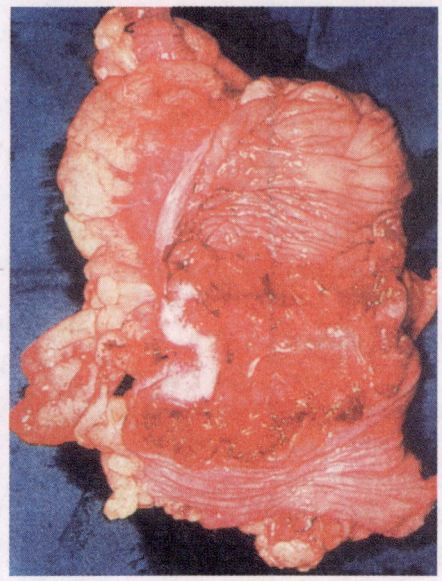

Fig. 35.2 Carcinoma colon

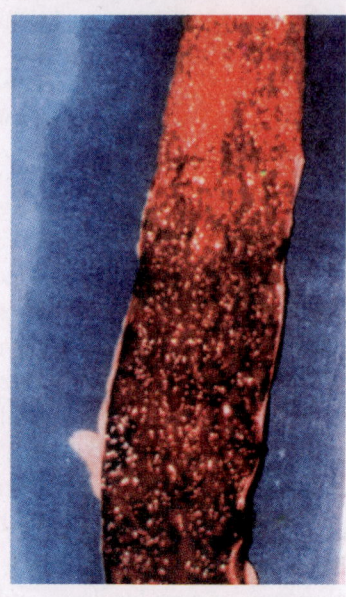

Fig. 35.3 Ulcerative colitis

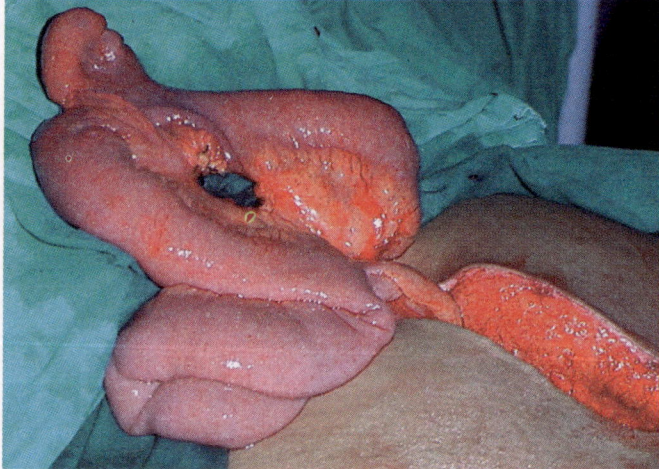

Fig. 35.4 Meckel's diverticulum

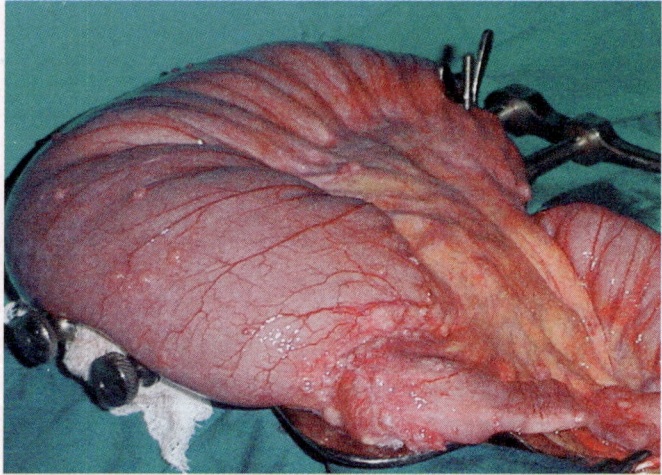

Fig. 35.5 Intestinal tuberculosis

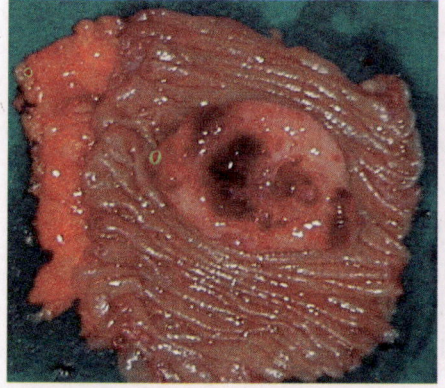

Fig. 35.6 Adenocarcinoma jejunum

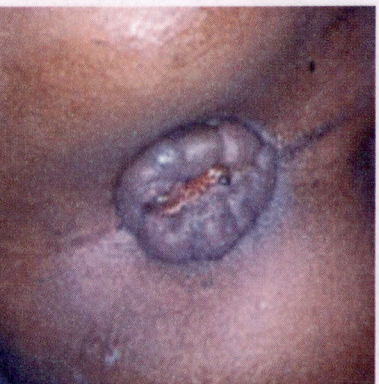

Fig. 35.7 Haemorroids

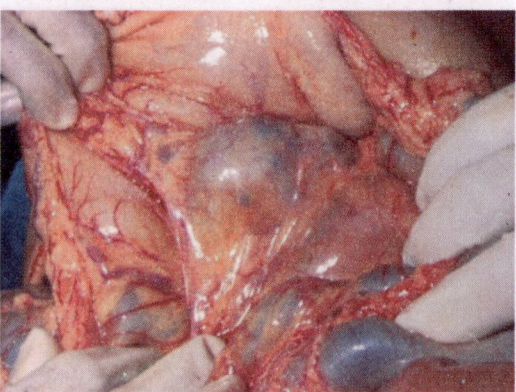

Fig. 35.8 Pancreatic pseudoaneurysm

Key Box 35.3

COMMON CAUSES OF LOWER GI BLEEDING

- Carcinoma colon
- Ulcerative colitis
- Haemorrhoids
- Intestinal tuberculosis
- Amoebic dysentery

Key Box 35.4

BLEEDING PER RECTUM WITH ACUTE ABDOMEN

- Mesenteric ischaemia
- Intussusception
- Ischaemic colitis
- Necrotising enterocolitis

INVESTIGATIONS (Fig. 35.9 to 35.19)

1. Proctoscopy
- Cherry red to pink mucosal bulges: Haemorrhoids
- Bleeding ulcer or a growth: Cancer of rectum
- Single anterior ulcer: Solitary ulcer rectum

2. Sigmoidoscopy
- Multiple small pinpoint ulcers : Ulcerative colitis
- Large deep flask-shaped ulcer : Amoebic ulcers
- Multiple small polyps: Hereditary polyposis coli

3. Colonoscopy
- Today colonoscopy is the number one investigation in lower GI bleeding. It can detect 3 important diseases such as carcinoma, inflammatory bowel diseases (IBD) and diverticular diseases. It can also detect ischaemic colitis, polyps and angiodysplasia. It needs to be repeated.

4. Stool examination
- Amoebiasis, bacillary dysentery
- Hookworm infestations

5. Barium enema
- Irregular filling defect in the colon: Cancer colon
- Contracted pipe-stem colon: Ulcerative colitis
- Pincer ending: Intussusception
- Saw-tooth appearance : Diverticular disease

6. Small bowel enema (Enteroclysis)
- Diverticulum in the terminal ileum is Meckel's diverticulum, multiple ulcers and stricture terminal ileum can be due to tuberculous ulcer.
- Barium studies have little value in the presence of acute haemorrhage. They can be used in intermit tent bleeding where in endoscopy has failed to detect the cause.

7. Special investigations:
They are indicated when the diagnosis of lower GI bleeding cannot be made out. They are more useful where there is active bleeding.

A. Visceral angiography
- All three vessels - coeliac, superior mesenteric and inferior mesenteric are used.
- Extravasation of contrast into the bowel lumen is suggestive of a 'lesion'.
- Bleeding rate should be at least 0.5 ml/mt.
- Thus meckel's diverticulum, angiodysplasia, small bowel tumours, vasculitis etc. can be diagnosed.

B. Radionuclear scanning
- ^{99m}Tc-labelled sulphur colloid or autologous red cells with ^{99m}Tc may be given which can detect the bleeding site.
- Less precise but less invasive with least complications.

FEW IMPORTANT TIPS AT EXPLORATORY LAPAROTOMY

- Midline incision is **preferred**
- Careful inspection and palpation of entire small and large bowel.
- Empty small bowel then palpate for hidden lesions.
- Intraoperative enteroscopy if no obvious lesion is found.
- Endoscopic evaluation of transilluminated gut wall.
- On table colonoscopy via appendiceal opening after appendicectomy.
- Rarely, blind right hemicolectomy or blind resection of proximal jejunum may be necessary in obscure bleeding (keeping in mind angiodysplasia).

ROLE OF ENDOSCOPY IN LOWER GI BLEEDING

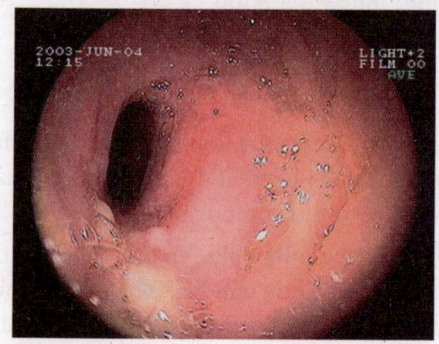

Fig. 35.9 Crohn's disease

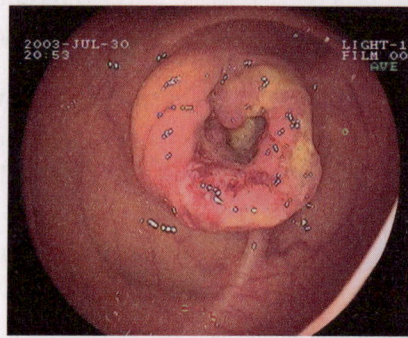

Fig. 35.10 Carcinoma caecum

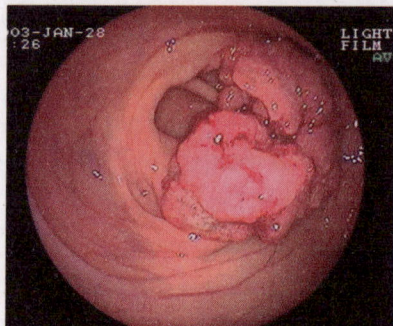

Fig. 35.11 Carcinoma sigmoid colon

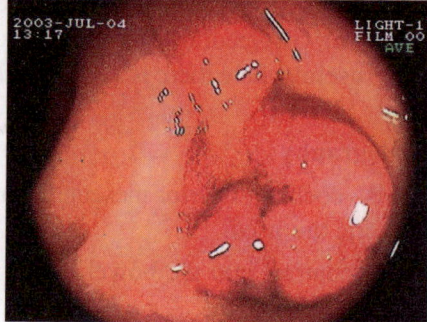

Fig. 35.12 Colonic polyps

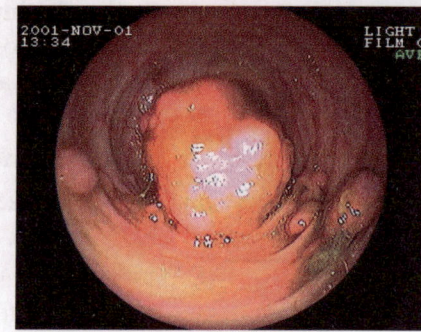

Fig. 35.13 Colonic polyposis

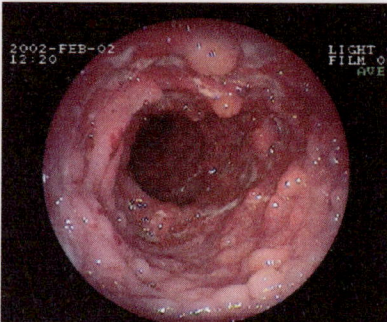

Fig. 35.14 Intestinal tuberculosis

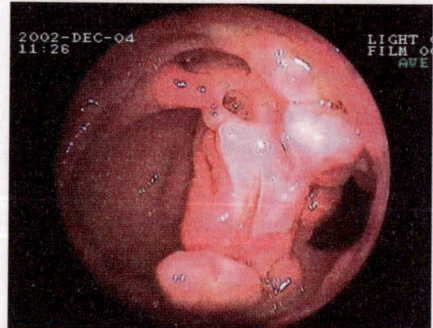

Fig. 35.15 Tuberculosis of the colon

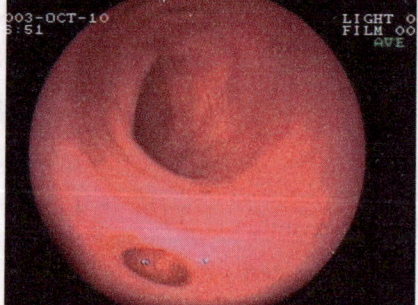

Fig. 35.16 Colonic diverticula

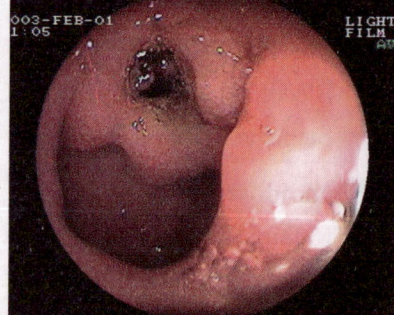

Fig. 35.17 Duodenal ulcer

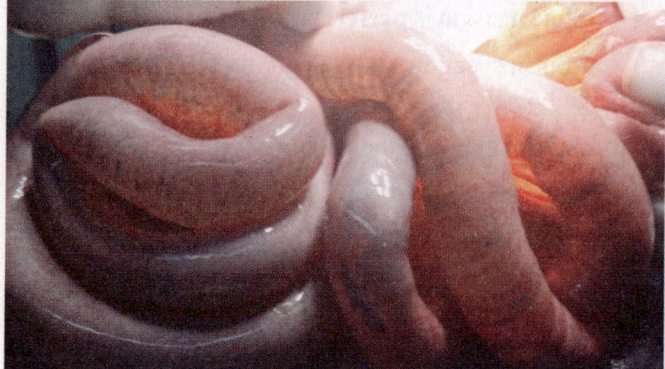
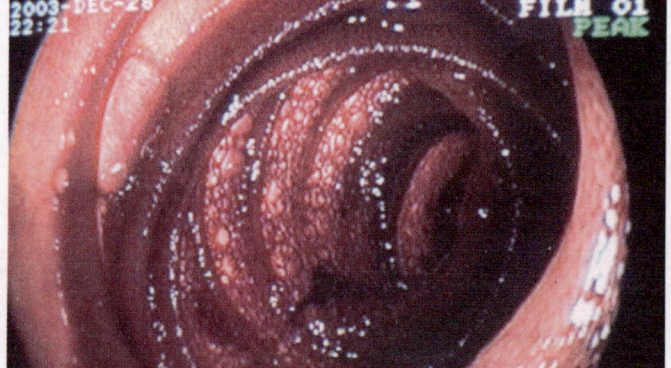

Fig. 35.18, 35.19 Enteroscopy done at laparotomy for suspected case of angiodysplasia of the jejunum - resected successfully. All these endoscopic pictures are contributed by Dr. Filipe Alvaris, Gastroenterologist, KMC, Manipal

FEW IMPORTANT TESTS IN LOWER GI BLEEDING

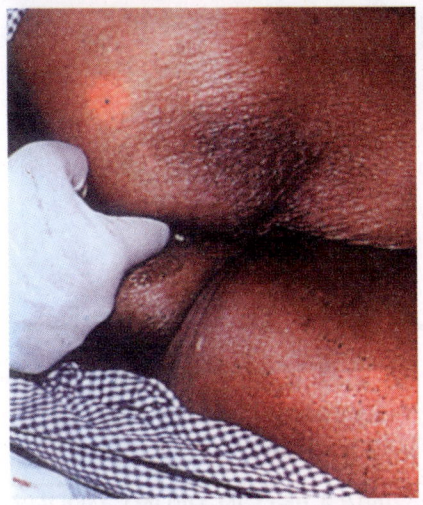

Fig. 35.20 Rectal examination

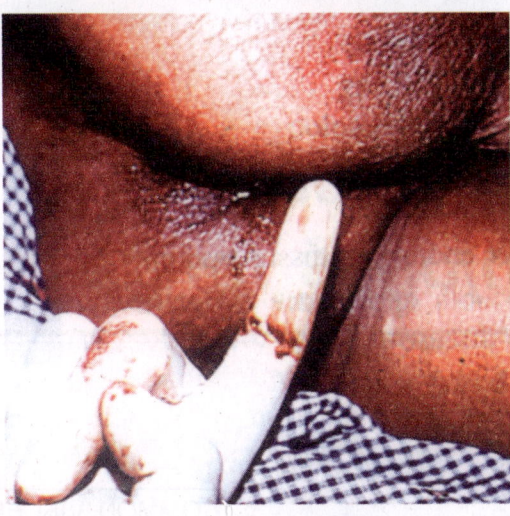

Fig. 35.21 Glove streaked with blood-Ca rectum

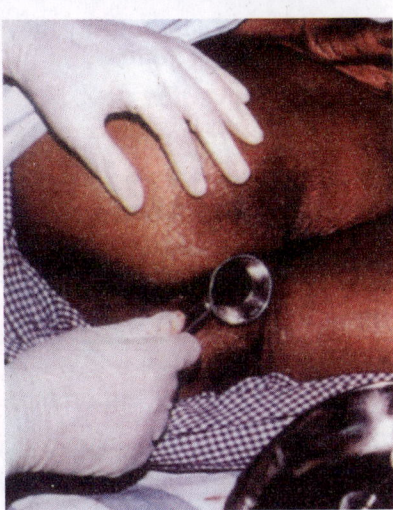

Fig. 35.22 Proctoscopy

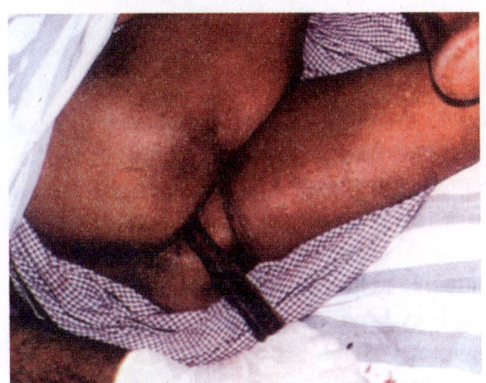

Fig. 35.23 Sigmoidoscopy

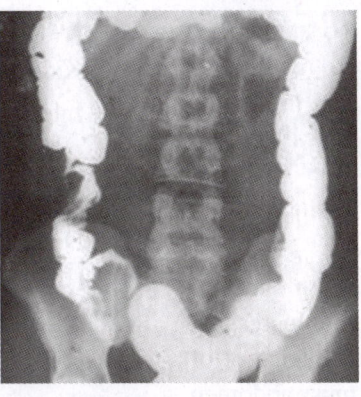

Fig. 35.24 Barium enema - Carcinoma ascending colon

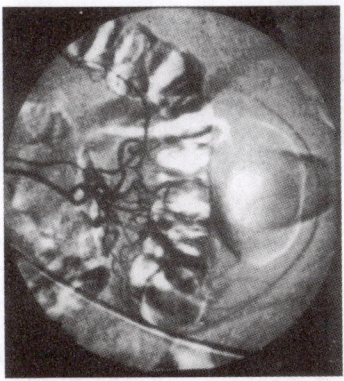

Fig. 35.25 Inferior mesenteric angiography showing leakage of dye into the lumen of sigmoid colon - Sigmoid angiodysplasia

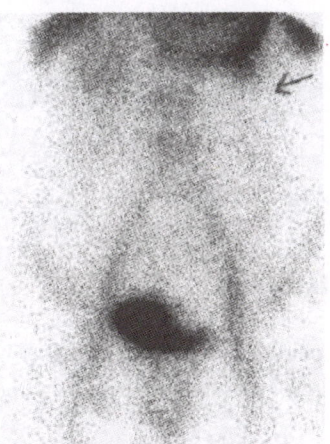

Fig. 35.26 Angiodysplasia of proximal jejunum diagnosed by 99mTc red blood cells scan (Page 768)

CLINICAL NOTES

28 years old male patient had an urgency to pass stools early morning. He collapsed while passing stools, with a massive bleeding. He was brought to the hospital in a state of shock. He was resuscitated, blood transfusions were given. All investigations were normal. He had another bout of massive bleeding the next day, during which time, even an angiography could not detect the cause. Urgent laparotomy was done. A 4 cm small bowel tumour (haemorrhagic) was excised from jejunum and histology confirmed it as leiomyoma. **Leiomyoma is called as bleeding tumour of the small bowel.** The case history highlights the importance of **exploratory laparotomy. Leiomyomas are included under GIST.**

Abdominal Trauma, War And Blast Injuries Triage

36

- Liver injuries
- Small bowel injuries
- Duodenal injuries
- Pancreatic injuries
- Renal injuries
- Blast injuries
- Warfare injuries
- Missile wounds of abdomen
- Triage

Blunt injury abdomen is one of the common surgical emergencies encountered by general surgeons. Increasing number of vehicles, high speed and poor maintenance of the roads are the contributing factors. Blunt injury abdomen with polytrauma is one of the commonest causes of death in the younger population. Thus, it is important for a house officer to recognise a polytrauma patient, to diagnose and to suspect intraabdominal injury, so that urgent resuscitation and treatment can be offered to the patient at proper time, at the proper hospital and by a proper surgeon. Major systems involved are given in the box.

Craniospinal and chest injuries are discussed in their respective chapters. Pelvic and skeletal injury is beyond the limits of this book. In this chapter, blunt injury of the abdomen is discussed.

CAUSES OF BLUNT INJURY ABDOMEN

1. Rail and road traffic accidents (most common)
2. Fall from a height and dashing against an object
3. Seat belt syndrome
4. Assault

Key Box 36.1

COMMON VISCERA INVOLVED IN BLUNT INJURY

1.	Spleen	Significant bleeding
2.	Liver	Significant bleeding
3.	Kidney	Significant bleeding.
4.	Intestines	Perforation- Peritonitis
5.	Pancreatico-duodenal injuries	Usually missed
6.	Diaphragm	Missed- Tachypnoea
7.	Urinary bladder	Urinary peritonitis

Key Box 36.2

MAJOR SYSTEMS INVOLVED

- Craniospinal
- Chest
- Abdomen
- Pelvis
- Skeletal

LIVER INJURIES

Liver injury should be suspected when a patient with suspected blunt injury abdomen is brought with the following features :

- Right lower ribs fracture
- Injury marks on the lower chest or upper abdomen

- *Almost 70-75% of cases are due to involvement of first four organs. Splenic injury is responsible in about 25% of cases (Page 429).*

- Patient with persistent hypotension or patient who had shock following blunt injury abdomen.
- Child can have liver injury without fracture of ribs because of elastic nature of the rib cage.

CLINICAL PRESENTATION

- The most common presentation is features of intraperitoneal haemorrhage, which includes hypotension, thready pulse, abdominal distension, etc. (refer splenic injury, Page 429). Peritoneal signs are minimal as early bleeding does not produce much peritoneal irritation.
- However, massive lacerations of the liver including stellate fractures present with rapidly developing hypotension and shock, which are life threatening.

INVESTIGATIONS

- Ultrasonography and more precisely CT scan should be done in all patients who are hemodynamically stable with or without support.

TREATMENT

1. **Simple lacerations which are not bleeding at lap-**

Key Box 36.3

CT SCAN WITH IV CONTRAST

- It can grade the liver injury
- It can guide a conservative or operative treatment.
- It also rules out other injuries
- Grade I and Grade III injuries can be managed by non-operative treatment
- Free contrast in and around the liver is indicative of active bleeding

---

arotomy : A drain is kept in the liver bed, blood and clots are sucked out and peritoneal wash is given,

2. **Simple laceration with bleeding :** It is sutured by interlocking horizontal mattress sutures by using special liver suturing needle. If too much tension is applied while suturing, cutting through can occur. Omentum can be used as a 'Plug' in between the laceration (Fig. 36.1). Absorbable sutures are used.

3. **Subcapsular haematoma :** If present, should be evacuated.

4. **Deep laceration with bleeding :** In such situations, wound should be opened. Dead liver parenchyma is removed, bleeding vessel at depth and biliary radical is ligated. It is described as tractotomy.

Table 36.1. Liver injury scale

GRADE	INJURY	DESCRIPTION
I	Haematoma	Subcapsular Haematoma; <10% surface area
	Laceration	Capsular tear , <1 cm parenchymal depth
II	Haematoma	Subcapsular, 10-50% surface area;
		intraparenchymal extension < 10 cm diameter
	Laceration	<10 cm long; 1-3 cm parenchymal depth
III	Haematoma	Subcapsular, > 50% surface area; expanding
		intraparenchymal haematoma of >10cm or expanding
	Laceration	>3 cm, intra parenchymal depth
IV	Laceration	Parenchymal disruption of 1-3 Couinaud's
		segments within a single lobe
V	Laceration	Parenchymal disruption. >3 Couinaud's
		segments within a single lobe
	Vascular	Retro hepatic vena cava / central major hepatic veins
VI	Vascular	Hepatic avulsion

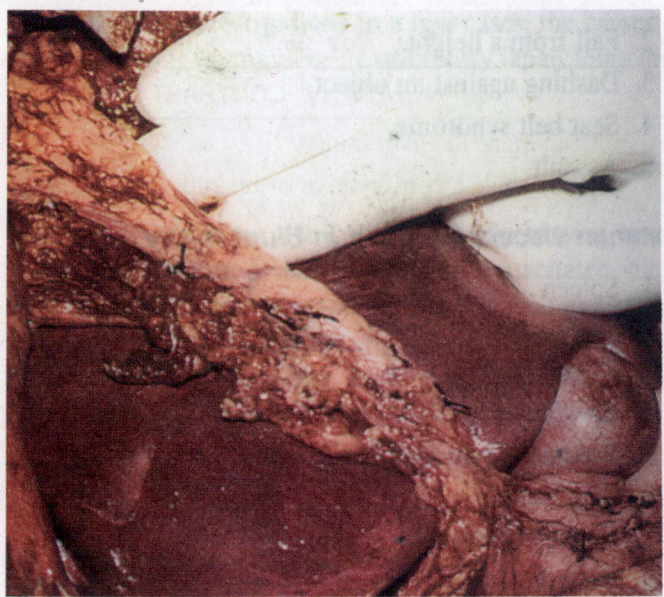

Fig. 36.1 Liver injury - use of omentum

3. Haematoma can rupture into the peritoneal cavity resulting in leakage of bile—biliary peritonitis.

4. Haemobilia refers to rupture of the haematoma into the bile duct—it may result in massive haemetemesis or melena.

5. **Severe lacerations:** These injuries present with massive bleeding. Temporary control is done by compression of portal vein and hepatic artery in gastrohepatic omentum in front of foramen of Winslow (Pringle manoeuvre). If bleeding stops, portal veins or branches of hepatic artery are damaged. If bleeding continues, hepatic veins are the source of bleeding. Visualisation of source of bleeding with debridement of avascular liver tissue is done by finger fracture method (Fig. 36.2). **Perihepatic packing** can be used to compress the liver as a temporary measure to buy time for resuscitation or to explore rest of the abdomen or as a definitive treatment when other measures fail. Pack is usually removed after 24-48 hours.

- Non anatomical resection may have to be done, in few cases.

6. **Complex liver injuries:** These injuries involve hepatic veins, retrohepatic vena cava or branches of portal vein resulting in massive haemorrhage. This type of massive injury can be managed by large thoracoabdominal incision or abdomino-sternal incision by doing sternotomy. Division of the right triangular ligament helps in visualizing bleeding from hepatic veins.

COMPLICATIONS OF LIVER INJURIES

1. Massive bleeding, hypovolaemia and cardiac arrest.
2. Haematoma can get infected resulting in an abscess.

SMALL BOWEL INJURY

- The shearing injuries produce either disruption or laceration of the bowel between fixed and mobile points, i.e. at the **duodenojejunal flexure or at ileocaecal junction.** These are the most common sites of small bowel injuries.

- Injury to the small bowel can also occur due to crush injury between spine and a steering wheel or handle bars, etc.

- Mesentery and its vessels also get damaged and

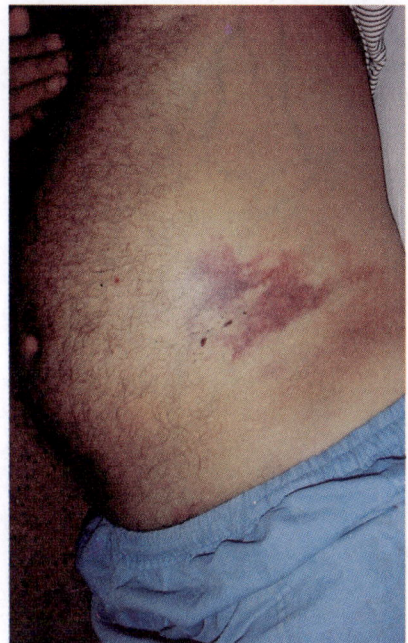

Fig. 36.2 Observe London's Sign: Bruising over the abdominal wall signifying hollow viscous perforation

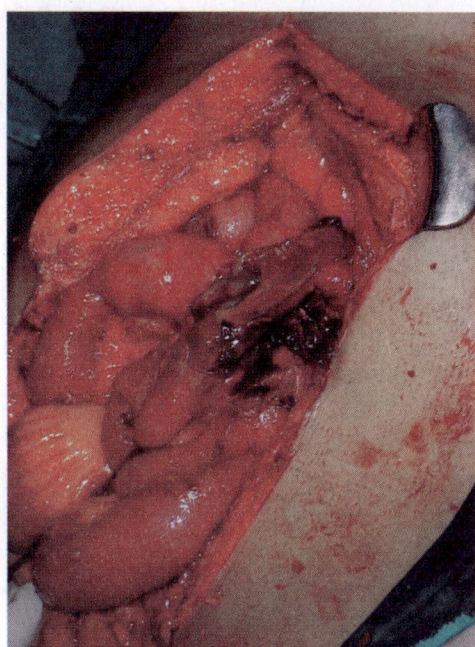

Fig. 36.3 Gangrene of the jejunal loop due to injury to the mesenteric blood vessels in the same patient (Fig. 36.2)

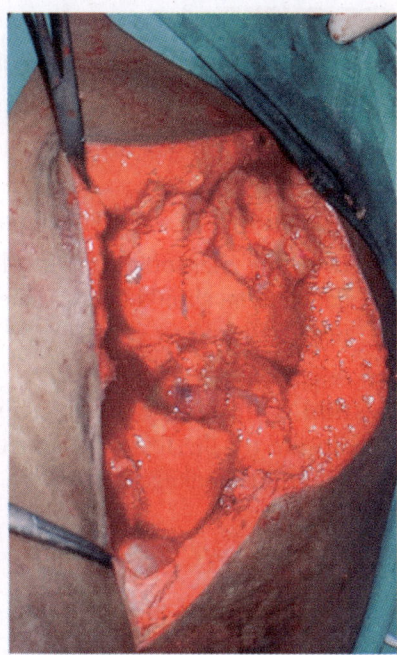

Fig. 36.4 Peritonitis following ileal perforation

bleeding can be sufficient to produce hypovolaemia and shock.

CLINICAL PRESENTATION

1. **Acute abdominal pain:** Features are like that of any perforation peritonitis with guarding and rigidity and erect abdominal X-ray shows gas under diaphragm.

2. **Features of peritonitis** with haemoperitoneum is the result of bowel injury with bleeding from the mesentery.

3. **Occult or hidden perforation:** A small perforation gets sealed off by coils of bowel and omentum. Most of these patients present with abdominal pain. But very often, peritonitis features are missed as a result of other associated injuries like fracture pelvis or retroperitoneal haematoma. After 3-4 days, a localised abscess may form and rupture into the peritoneal cavity, resulting in peritonitis. This is aggravated by intake of oral fluids which stimulate peristalsis. **Repeated examination is the most honoured, most fruitful investigation in blunt injuries of the abdomen.** (See clinical notes Page 684)

X-ray abdomen erect demonstrates free gas under the right dome of the diaphragm in majority of cases. Four quadrant tap or diagnostic peritoneal lavage is also useful.

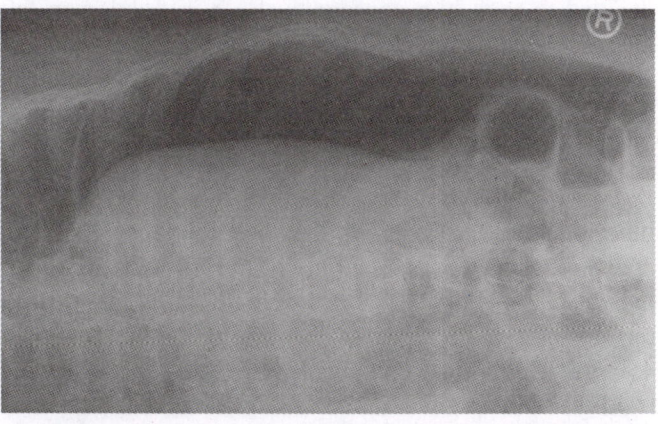

Fig. 36.5 Lateral decubitus picture is extremely useful in polytrauma cases wherein patient is unable to stand due to fractured limbs. However, CT scan is the best investigation in blunt injury abdomen

Key Box 36.6
SMALL BOWEL INJURY
• Acute abdominal pain
• Guarding and rigidity
• Rebound tenderness
• Gas under diaphragm in plain X-ray abdomen erect
• Laparotomy and closure of perforation

TREATMENT

Golden time to operate is within 6 hours.

- **Perforation :** Single or multiple, have to be closed, after trimming the edges by using non-absorbable sutures like silk.

- A **lacerated** or a macerated bowel has to be resected.

- Bleeding mesenteric vessels have to be ligated and haematoma should be evacuated and bowel should be inspected for any ischaemia.

- A perforation of ileum **close to the ileocaecal junction** is treated by **ileocolectomy** rather than simple closure for the fear of enterocutaneous fistula, due to suture line leakage.

CLINICAL NOTES

23 year old male with fracture femur and pelvic fracture was admitted to the hospital after 12 hours of injury. A general surgeon was consulted to rule out an intraabdominal injury. Pulse rate was 100/min and on deep palpation, there was tenderness in the right iliac fossa. Keeping in mind associated pelvic injury, it was decided to treat him conservatively. X-ray abdomen left lateral decubitus (erect film could not be taken as patient could not stand) film did not show free intraperitoneal air (gas). Ultrasound revealed a retroperitoneal haematoma of 8 cm x 3 cm.

The patient was treated conservatively with Ryle's tube for 3 days. On the 4th day, oral fluids were started, as patient passed stools once. On 7th day morning, patient had tachypnoea. Pulse was 120/min, BP was 90/60 mm of Hg. Previous 24 hours urine output was only 450 ml. Abdominal examination revealed guarding and rigidity in the right iliac fossa. It was decided to do a laparotomy. At laparotomy, there was a small 2 cm perforation in the ileum with bilioma surrounded by intestinal loops and gross contamination of peritoneal cavity. Perforation was closed and the peritoneal cavity was drained. Patient made a good recovery from septicaemia thanks to antibiotics and surgery.

DUODENAL INJURIES

- Retroperitoneal duodenum is commonly injured.

- Streering wheel or belt or a blow in the epigastrium may injure the duodenum as it is crushed against the spine.

CLINICAL FEATURES

- Peritonitis features are not common as it is the retroperitoneal duodenum (II & III part) that is injured.

- Tenderness is present on deep palpation.

- Being retroperitoneal, these injuries manifest late as abscess formation or fluid in lesser sac, etc

INVESTIGATION (Fig 36.6)

- X-ray abdomen

  - Obliteration of psoas shadow

  - Air outlining the kidney

  - Absence of air in the duodenum

- Raised serum amylase, is one of the biochemical parameters that should arouse a suspicion of pancreatic injuries (or both).

TREATMENT

- Golden time to operate is within 6 hours.

- When in doubt, about narrowing of lumen, duodenojejunostomy may be indicated.

- When in doubt regarding duodenal fistula, tube duodenostomy is done.

- Duodenal haematoma is managed conservatively.

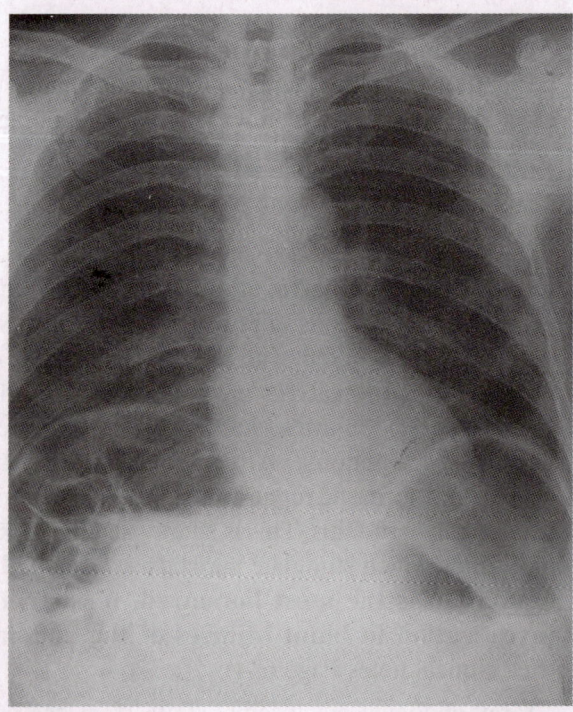

Fig. 36.6 Air outlining small portion of the kidney and air pockets under the diaphragm - cheladiti sign

PANCREATIC INJURIES

Because of anatomical close approximation of pancreas with vertebral column, blunt injury abdomen in the epigastrium, kicks or **seat belt injuries** crush the pancreas against **the vertebral column (Key Box 36.7, 36.8).**

DIAGNOSIS

- Pancreatic injury alone is diagnosed when patient presents with a pseudocyst of the pancreas 2-3 weeks following an injury.
- Very often, laparotomy is done for haemorrhage or perforation. In such situations, retroperitoneal bleeding or collection of bile or collection of fluid in the lesser sac arouses suspicion of pancreatic injuries.

Key Box 36.7
PANCREATIC INJURIES
• Anatomically hidden • Very often, injuries missed • Peritonitis features are not seen • Dangerous because of enzymatic activation • Can manifest as pleural effusion

Key Box 36.8
PANCREATICODUODENAL INJURIES
• Diagnosed late • Peritonitis features are minimal • Shock is very rare • At laparotomy, they are missed • Surgical treatment needs more skill and experience • Feeding jejunostony is very useful • Mortality and morbidity around 50%

TREATMENT

1. **Pseudocyst** following blunt injury abdomen invariably requires **surgical drainage e.g. cystogastrostomy** because of injury to pancreatic duct.
2. Injury to body and tail require **subtotal pancreatectomy** with splenectomy.

3. Rarely, **pancreaticoduodenectomy** may be required for significant injury to the head of pancreas with injury to the duodenum.

COMPLICATIONS

- Pancreatic fistula
- Pancreatic pseudocyst
- Pleural effusion

RENAL INJURIES

TYPES (Fig. 36.7)

I. **Minor:** Subcapsular haematoma, minor laceration and renal contusions.

II. **Major injuries:** Bleeding into renal pelvis from laceration of medulla, corticomedullary rupture, hilar injury.

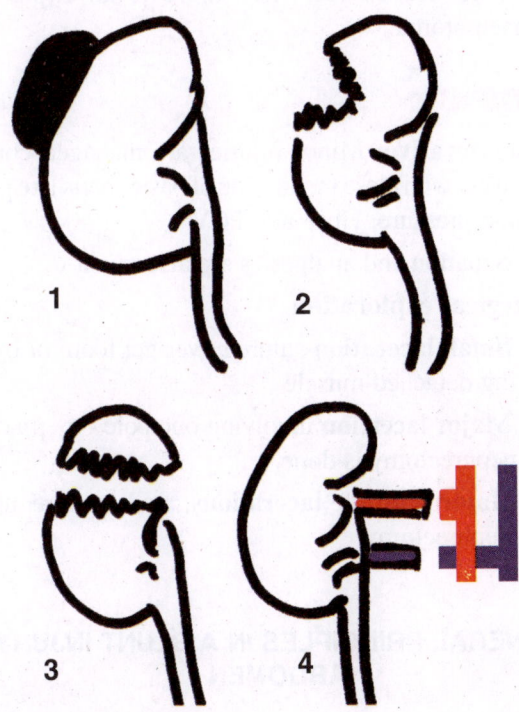

Fig. 36.7 Closed renal trauma.1. Subcapsular haematoma, 2. Laceration 3. Avulsion of on of the poles 4. Avulsion of renal pedicle

CLINICAL FEATURES

- **Haematuria** is the most important (80-90%) sign of renal injury. It may be mild, or sometimes can be massive depending upon the extent of injury. It may be absent in renal pedicle avulsion.

- **Loin bulge** due to perinephric haematoma
- **Bruising** of soft tissue in the loin
- Retroperitoneal haematoma compressing on splanchnic nerves (meteorism) results in paralytic ileus, which causes **abdominal distension**
- Associated injuries like fractures of the transverse process of lumbar spine

INVESTIGATIONS

1. Intravenous pyelography can demonstrate:
   - Intrarenal extravasation
   - Extrarenal extravasation (pararenal pseudohydrone -phrosis due to extravasated blood and urine slowly occluding pelviureteric junction)
   - Function of injured kidney
   - Function of opposite kidney
2. Ultrasound and C.T. scan are other investigations which are useful when there is an expanding haematoma.

TREATMENT

1. **Conservative:** Minor injuries are managed conservatively with close monitoring of basic charts like pulse, blood pressure, Hb% and PCV.
   - Sedation and analgesics are also given
2. **Surgical exploration**
   - **Small laceration** sutured over gel foam or by using detached muscle
   - **Major lacertion** involving one pole - a partial nephrectomy is done
   - **Major multiple lacerations**, avulsions, require nephrectomy

GENERAL PRINCIPLES IN A BLUNT INJURY ABDOMEN

- A patient should be admitted, to the hospital and carefully monitored if there is a slight doubt regarding blunt injury abdomen.
- **Repeated examination,** careful monitoring of pulse rate, temperature and blood pressure, chest X-ray, es-

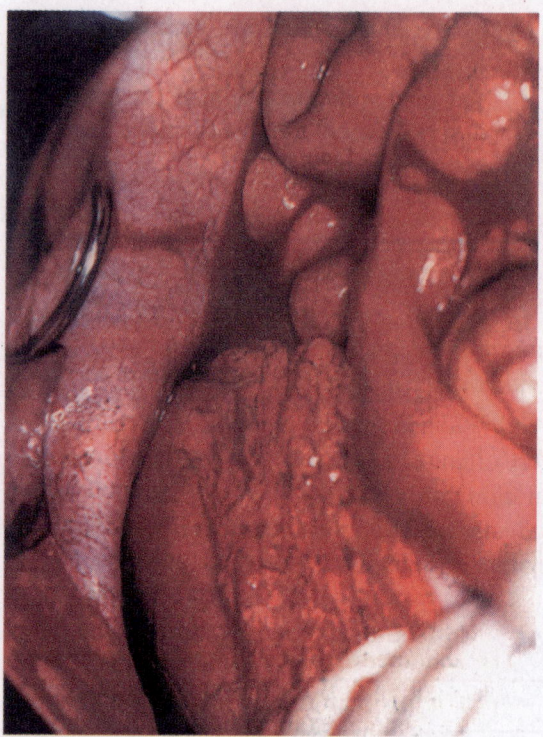

Fig. 36.8 A case of missed liver injury with haemoperitoneum. Repreated examination reveled deteriorating general condition. CT scan proved the diagnosis

timation of Hb%, frequently helps in many cases of silent blunt injuries.

- Most of the cases today are **polytrauma** cases, Hence, all systems should be examined. Among all these, priority should be given to life-threatening, salvageable injuries like **extradural haematoma, haemothorax, splenic injuries, liver injuries, etc.**
- It is easier to make a diagnosis of fracture[1] (revealed injuries) which can be treated later. FRACTURE CAN WAIT BUT NOT RUPTURE. Concealed injuries should be carefully looked for.
- Undoubtedly, diagnostic peritoneal lavage, plain X-ray abdomen erect and ultrasound (the immediate noninvasive investigations) help in diagnosis of more than 90% of cases of blunt injury abdomen (Fig. 34.6).
- Adequate blood, appropriate antibiotics, aggressive resuscitation before surgery to treat hypovolaemia and shock are the major factors which decide the outcome of surgery.

---

1. *Even a grandmother can diagnose fractures. However, it needs lot of experience and skills in diagnosing blunt injury abdomen.*

- In a major accident involving many patients, quick decision should be taken regarding **triage**—who can be saved, who cannot be saved.

BLAST INJURIES

- Bursting of bombs or shells rupture their casing and impart high velocity to resulting fragments. These fragments cause more devastating injuries than bullets. All explosives are accompanied by a complex blast wave.

- **The two main components are: Blast pressure wave** (dynamic over pressure) with positive and negative phase and mass **movement of air (blast wind)**

- Positive phase of blast wave lasts few milliseconds (close to the explosion it may be over 7000 k N/M^2) (Tympanic membrane ruptures at 150 K/m^2)

- Like sound waves blast pressure waves flow over and around an obstruction and affect persons sheltering behind a wall. The pressure affecting such a person is known as incident pressure (pressure at 90^0 to direction of travel of blast shock front).

- Person standing in front of a wall facing an explosion is subject to added effect of reflected pressure. Mass movement of air displaces air at supersonic speed. This disrupts environment, hurting debris and people. Blast wave under the water travels at great speed and to greater distance. Injuries tend to be complex and severe.

- **Structures injured by primary blast wave are ear, lungs, heart, gastrointestinal system.**

- Most will have combination of blunt, blast and thermal injuries. Deafness, lung contusion, capillary leakage and haemorrhage into alveoli, ARDS precipitated by over transfusion are the features. Perforation of the intestines and penetration injuries to the eye are the other features.

- Management consists of resuscitation in a well equipped trauma unit, blood transfusions, intensive care monitoring, antibiotics and appropriate surgical procedures.

WARFARE INJURIES

- Penetrating missile wounds, injuries from blast phenomena and burns are typical features of modern conventional war. The most common wounding agent in surviving casualties is a fragment wound and not a bullet wound as many erroneously believe. The aim in modern war is to incapacitate and **not to kill**. Hence large number of surviving casualties are a major financial and logistic burden on a nation engaged in war.

WOUND BALLISTICS AND MECHANISMS OF INJURY

- Bullets fired from hand guns are propelled at low velocity, have low available energy and result in low velocity transfer wounds (100-500 J), whereas those from assault rifle have high velocity and have high available energy (2000-3000 J) and they cause high energy transfer wounds. **Low energy** transfer wounds leave injury confined to wound tract. **High energy** transfer wounds causes local laceration, crush injury and also cause remote injury from wound tract due to temporary cavitation phenomena.

MANAGEMENT

- Entrance and exit wounds do not indicate considerable damage that may have occurred to deeper structures.
- Resuscitate as per ATLS guidelines
- Record the wounds in case sheets, take photographs if necessary
- Under anaesthesia excise skin around entry and exit wounds, give liberal longitudinal incision through skin and deep fascia, which allows proper visualization of underlying structures.
- Debride (cut till healthy tissues are seen) all dead tissues - dead muscle does not bleed or contract, it looks dusky.
- Identify neurovascular bundles and examine them
- Dissect and mark injured nerves for possible future repair
- Repair arteries and veins if injured
- Give thorough wash and let out all the dirt
- Injured tendons are trimmed and tied for easy identification at future surgery
- Fix bones by appropriate methods
- Cover the wound with absorbable dressing
- Appropriate antibiotics and injection tetanus toxoid are given
- Amputation may be necessary if limb is grossly mutilated
- Delayed primary closure is done (4-6 days later) once the wound starts healing

MISSILE WOUNDS OF ABDOMEN

- Every penetrating and perforating missile wound of the abdomen should be explored by laparotomy. A full midline incision from xiphisternum to pubis is recommended and it may be extended to thorax if necessary.

- The rest of the treatment depends on the nature of injury. Bleeding mesenteric vessels are ligated, injured small bowel is repaired by suturing or by resection and anastomosis. In colonic injuries, simple closure or closure with protective colostomy is necessary depending upon the nature of the colon and contamination.

- Liver, splenic, pancreatic and renal injuries have been discussed in respective chapters.

PENETRATING TRAUMA OF THE ABDOMEN

- Today all penetrating injuries of the abdomen need not be explored by laparotomy. A good physical examination of the patient, entry point and exit point, and haemodynamic status of the patient followed by investigations such as ultrasonogram and CT scan will guide the decision for laparotomy.

Key Box 36.9

INDICATIONS FOR LAPAROTOMY

- Tenderness, guarding, rigidity
- Unexplained shock
- Evisceration of contents
- Positive investigations
  - Positive DPL
  - Gas under diaphragm
  - IVP, cystoscopy, cystogram
  - Ultrasonogram or CT scan

TRIAGE

- The term **triage** is derived from the French word **tries**, meaning **to sort out**. This is a method of sorting out injured patients, during mass casualties depending on the severity of injury. If you are the first on the scene, first priority is to get expert help, (call up fire services, regional trauma centre etc).

- Triage is a skilled activity where in there is a leader (usually senior most doctor / Surgeon) and there are many assistants. The leader sorts out patients (people) depending upon their severity of injury.

- Each of the patients can be color coded. (a colored flag is attached to them), Examples:

1. **Immediate help is necessary -** Red Otherwise will die in a few minutes if no treatment is offered. Eg. Obstructed airway, tension pneumothrorax

2. **Urgent help is necessary -** Yellow These patients may die in 1-2 hrs if no treatment is given. Examples are cases of massive bleeding and hypovolaemia.

3. **Delayed -** Green These patients can wait. Examples are minor fractures.

4. **Expectant -** Blue An attempt to treat them, may delay those patients who are salvageable

5. **Dead people are flagged -** white or black

The leader assesses the patient - flags and moves forward and it is his assistant who carries out the further necessary resuscitation. Leader should not resuscitate a single patient. There are others waiting for his expert help.

A COMMON SCHEME

1. **Can the patient walk?**

   Yes - Delayed (Green)

   No - Check for breathing

2. **Is the patient breathing?**

   No - Open the airway

   Are they breathing him?

   Yes - immediate (Red)

   No - DEAD (white)

   Yes - Count or estimate respiratory rate (over 15sec).

   <10 to >30 per minutes - immediate (Red)

   10 -30 per minute - check the circulation

3. **Check the circulation**

   Pulse >120 (capillary refill >2sec) - immediate (Red)

   Pulse < 120 (capillary refill < 2sec) - urgent (yellow).

- If any regional trauma centre is well equipped and nearby, one has to transport all the injured patients to hospital (scoop and run), where expert help is available.

Meanwhile trauma centre can be alerted about the arrival of casualties. If expert help is far away, then one may have to treat the patients at the accident site (stay and play). Resuscitation is done as per ATLS guidelines.

- During these exercises do not forget to take care of your own safety, in burning vehicles, burning or falling buildings etc.

MANAGEMENT

An initial quick evaluation of the patient for anaemia, level of consciousness, if necessary volume replacement , application of C collar to the neck etc. are done.

Key Box 36.10

FUNDAMENTAL STEPS

- Airway management
- Breathing
- Circulation
- Disability and assessment of level of consciousness by Glasgow coma scale
- Exposure of the patient fully for thorough examination
- Finger evaluation and tubes

- These six initial steps are included under primary survey and resuscitation in ATLS (Advanced Trauma Life Support)

Airway with cervical spine protection

- Rapid assessment of signs of obstruction - foreign body, laryngeal and faciomaxillary fracture, fallen back tongue.
- Lift the jaw, introduce airway, good suction of throat, intubation or even tracheostomy if necessary.
- In polytrauma, assume cervical spine fracture and C - Collar is applied immediately (Fig. 36.9).

Breathing and O$_2$ administration

- Rule out tension pneumothorax, multiple fractures of ribs and haemothorax, surgical emphysema etc.

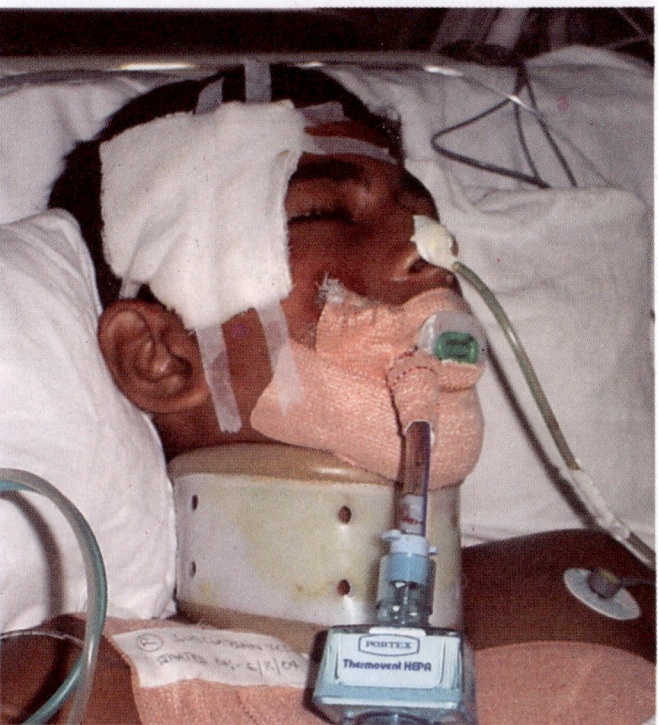

Fig. 36.9 Management of a polytrauma patient in an intensive care unit - C collar has been applied and patient is being ventilated

Tension pneumothorax is a clinical diagnosis don't delay the treatment waiting for chest x-ray.

- All trauma patients should receive high-flow oxygen.

Circulation and control of bleeding

- Immediate and quick assessment of circulation status, evidence of shock and evidence of internal or external bleeding should be looked for.
- Feeble thready pulse, hypotension indicates volume or blood loss. Splenic, liver or mesenteric injuries can be diagnosed by ultrasound. Bleeding into the pleural space or pericardium needs further tests - CT scan or Echo cardiography etc.

The immediate goal is to arrest the bleeding rather than replacing the blood.

Disability

- Glasgow coma score and assessment of pupils can help immediately to assess the status of the patient.

Exposure with control of environment

Key Box 36.11

- Clothing removal
- Examine anterior and posterior surface of the patient
- Covering with blankets
- Warm the patient

Fingers and tubes

- Quick examination of all orifices. Examples : Bleeding from the ear, nose or oral cavity, rectal and vaginal examination, bleeding from urethra etc.
- Nasogastric tube, endotracheal tube, catheter, intravenous line or central line are the immediate requirements of a polytrauma patient.

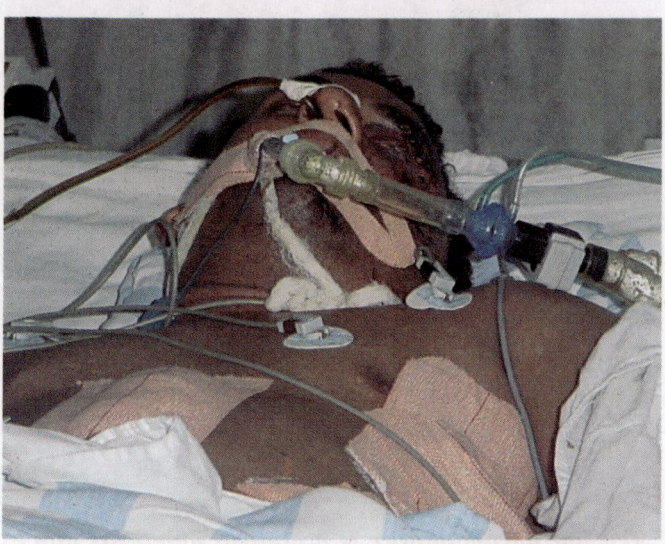 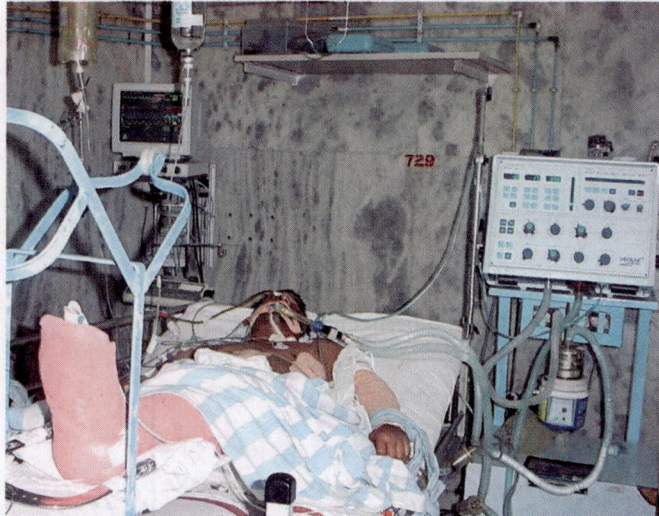

Fig. 36.10 Polytrauma patient with tubes
- Nasogastric tube bleeding suggests contusion of the stomach
- Endotracheal tube is life saving - bleeding indicates contusion of the lungs
- Intercostal tube bleeding indicates haemothorax
- Urinary catheter bleeding indicates renal and bladder injuries
- Intravenous lines and central venous pressure catheters are important to monitor the volume load

Abdominal Mass

37

CLINICAL EXAMINATION OF ABDOMINAL MASS (CLINICS)

The abdomen is like Pandora's box. However, a student who is examining a case of abdomen is like an investigating C.B.I, officer. He has to collect information at every level of examination i.e, history, past history, general examination and abdominal examination. An attempt has been done here to highlight the importance of history and clinical examination. **Ten Points** in the history, if taken properly and analysed properly may give a definite **clue** in majority of cases. After getting this **clue**, clinical examination of the mass may become easy.

REGIONS IN THE ABDOMEN

- Abdomen is divided into nine regions (quadrants) by two horizontal lines and two vertical lines.

- Upper horizontal line or transpyloric line is midway between xiphisternum and umbilicus.

- Transtubercular line is at the level of the two tubercles on the iliac crest about 5 cm behind anterior superior iliac spine.

- The vertical lines are drawn on either side through midpoint between anterior superior iliac spine and symphysis pubis. Following are the nine quadrants of the abdomen:

1. Right hypochondrium
2. Epigastrium
3. Left hypochondrium
4. Right lumbar region
5. Umbilical region
6. Left lumbar region
7. Right iliac fossa
8. Hypogastrium
9. Left iliac fossa

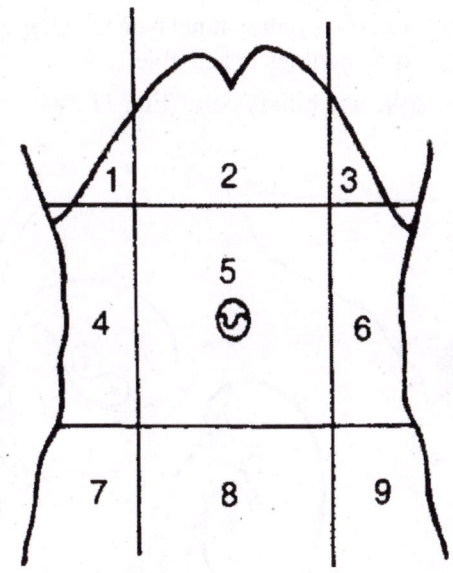

Fig. 37.1 Regions of the abdomen (Refer text)

591

HISTORY

1. **Abdominal pain** is present in most of the cases of abdominal mass. Abdominal pain can be of the following types:

A. Dull aching pain: It suggests a solid organ enlargement. It is a continuous pain felt in the anatomical location of the swelling. Many a time, patients describe it as a discomfort rather than pain.

Examples

- Liver enlargement: Pain in the right hypochondrium. It occurs due to stretching of parietal capsule (Fig. 37.2A)
- Splenic enlargement: Pain in the left hypochondrium
- Renal enlargement: Pain in the back and costal region or costovertebral pain (37.2C)
- Enlarged lymph nodes (para-aortic), pancreatic tumours: Backache

B. Colicky pain suggests hollow viscus obstruction. This pain is due to hyperperistalsis. It is severe, intermittent (comes and goes). Each attack may last for 5-10 minutes. Patient bends himself, holds the abdomen and puts pressure on the abdomen which gives some kind of relief. Being visceral type of pain, it is not very well localised. Following are few examples :

- Mass in the right iliac fossa (carcinoma caecum or ileocaecal tuberculosis). Initially there may be vague discomfort. However, when partial obstruction occurs, it results in a colicky abdominal pain which is centrally located and sometimes unbearable
- Ureteric colic and biliary colic (Fig. 37.2B)

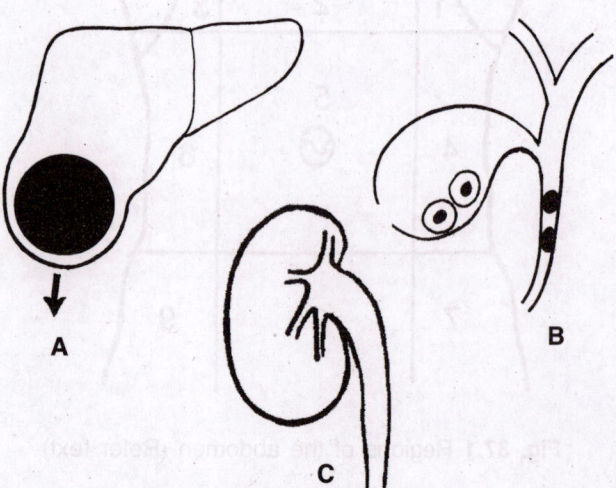

Fig. 37.2 Source of the pain

- Carcinoma pyloric antrum or pyloric stenosis produces colicky upper abdominal pain with gastric peristalsis. However, this type of pain is not an unbearable one.

C. Referred pain : Tuberculosis of spine is a common problem in India. Often patients present with iliopsoas abscess. Patients can complain of referred pain in the lower abdomen.

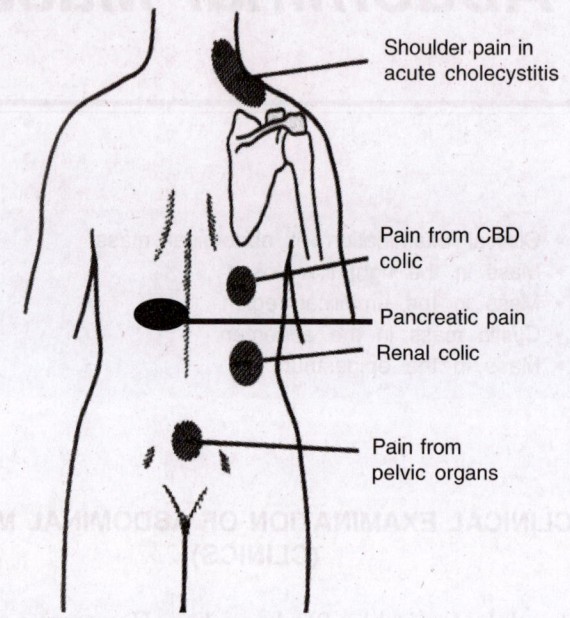

Shoulder pain in acute cholecystitis

Pain from CBD colic

Pancreatic pain

Renal colic

Pain from pelvic organs

Fig. 37.3 Referred pain

2. Sensation of fullness

- Carcinoma of the stomach and pyloric obstruction. Also hepatoma or large pancreatic tumours can cause extraluminal compression on the stomach resulting in sensation of fullness in the abdomen.

3. Vomiting

- Persistent, profuse, projectile and non-bilious vomiting suggests pyloric stenosis. Chronic duodenal ulcer and carcinoma stomach are the common causes of pyloric obstruction.
- Persistent, profuse, projectile, bilious vomiting—Intestinal obstruction. For example, ileocaecal tuberculosis, stricture of the small bowel, adhesions, etc.

4. Haemetemesis

- Epigastric mass suggests carcinoma stomach
- Splenomegaly may be an indication of portal hypertension.

5. Bleeding per rectum

- Fresh blood with or without melaena—Carcinoma colon
- Melaena—Carcinoma stomach, Portal hypertension

6. Loss of appetite and loss of weight

- Carcinoma pancreas, carcinoma stomach, etc. Please note that these two symptoms are seen not only in intra-abdominal malignancies, but also in many diseases like tuberculosis. However, it should be noted that one of the earliest signs of carcinoma stomach is loss of appetite and severe weight loss is an early important feature of carcinoma body of the pancreas.

7. Bowel habits

- Fresh bleeding per rectum: Carcinoma colon
- Blood and mucus (Bloody slime): Carcinoma rectum
- Alternate constipation and diarrhoea: Carcinoma colon

8. Jaundice

- Progressive persistent, pruritic jaundice: Periampullary carcinoma or carcinoma head of pancreas. However in periampullary carcinoma, fluctuation can occur if growth ulcerates.
- Mild recurrent jaundice: Haemolytic anaemias.
- Intermittent jaundice, pain, fever - Charcot's triad—stone in the common bile duct.

9. Haematuria

- Fresh bleeding/clots: Renal cell carcinoma.

10. Fever

- High grade fever, with chills and rigors: Stone in common bile duct
- Low grade fever: Hepatoma, renal cell carcinoma, lymphoma. Fever is due to some pyrogens released into circulation or due to tumour necrosis.

ON EXAMINATION

INSPECTION

- The patient is asked to breathe well with mouth open.
- Students should spend a few minutes watching the abdomen carefully.

1. Shape of the abdomen

- Scaphoid in normal cases
- Generalised distension with fullness in the flanks is usually due to ascites.
- Localised distension can be due to a mass
- Presence of step ladder peristalsis indicates small bowel obstruction, visible gastric peristalsis indicates pyloric stenosis and right to left peristalsis indicates colonic obstruction.

2. Restricted movement of any one region of the abdomen indicates an inflammatory pathology. However, this is diffcult to appreciate.

3. Umbilical nodule (Sister Joseph's) indicates intraabdominal malignancy.

4. If the mass is prominent or visible, details about the mass such as size, shape, surface, borders, movement with respiration has to be mentioned.

   - If the details about the mass cannot be appreciated or if mass is not clear on inspection, it is better to say "there is fullness" rather than trying to manipulate the details about the mass.

5. Inspection of male genitalia - if scrotum is empty it could be a case of undescended testis[1].

PALPATION

Methods of palpation

Following are the methods of palpation available for the clinician depending upon the merits of the case :

1. **Superficial palpation:** Gentle superficial palpation of the abdomen gains confidence of the patient. It can detect superficial lesion of the abdominal wall such as lipomatosis, neurofibromas or fibromas etc. It can also detect an area of tenderness, so that clinician is careful while doing deeper palpation. Superficial palpation is done with the flat of the hand or finger.

2. **Deep palpation:** These are important requirements for deeper palpation:

   - Patient should be well relaxed, with flexion of the knee for about 45 degrees.
   - The face should be turned to opposite side and the patient is asked to breathe comfortably with open mouth.

---

1. *A case of mass abdomen diagnosed to be soft tissue sarcoma or lymphoma of the para-aortic node region by ultrasound proved to be a seminoma in an undescended testis. Patient says 6 months back his right testis was removed by a 'groin' incision.*

- Deep palpation should be started from the quadrant situated diagonally opposite the site of pain.
- Palpation should cover not only 9 quadrants of the abdomen, it should include 2 more quadrants i.e the 2 renal angles and 12th quadrant—external genitalia in males[1]
- The deep palpation is carried out with the palmar surface of the fingers and some degree of angulation depending upon on the depth of palpation.

TESTS

1. **Movement with respiration:** This test is done by placing the fingers (hand) over the lower border of the swelling and the patient is asked to take a deep breath. Movement with respiration is positive when there is "up and down" movement or anteroposterior movement. Any structure in contact with diahragm moves with respiration. Examples :

- Liver, stomach, spleen, gall bladder move very well with respiration.
- Splenic flexure growths, due to contact with the lower pole of the spleen may move with respiration and hepatic flexure growths due to contact with liver have very limited movement.
- Renal swelling moves with respiration because kidney is enclosed by fascia of Gerota, which is attached above to the diaphragm.

2. **Finger insinuation test:** This test has relevance in an upper abdominal mass.

- Liver and spleen are under right and left costal margins respectively. Hence, it is not possible to get the upper margin or upper border of these organs. An attempt to invaginate between the costal margin and these masses is NOT POSSIBLE. On the other hand, finger invagination under the costal margin is possible in a stomach mass.

3. Size, shape and surface

- An egg-shaped mass or globular mass suggests gall bladder lesion (Fig. 37.4A)
- A horse-shoe shape may indicate a horse-shoe kidney (Fig. 37.4B)
- Reniform shape suggests a renal swelling (Fig. 37.4C)

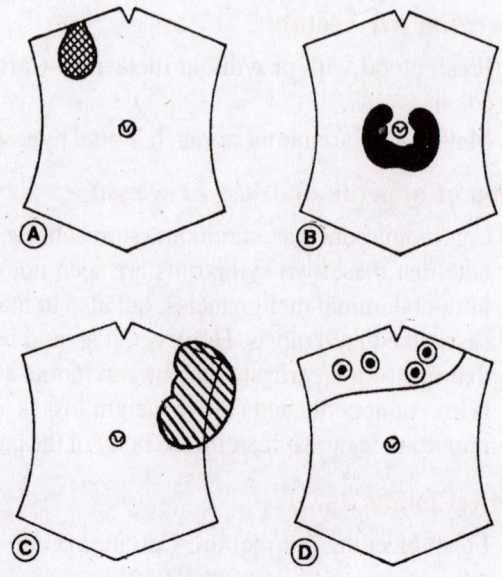

Fig. 37.4 A-D

- **Large nodular surface** is seen in following conditions (Fig, 37.4D):
  - Polycystic kidney
  - Secondaries liver
  - Group of lymph nodes
- **Smooth surface** usually indicates a benign lesion.
  - Splenomegaly, hydronephrosis, ovarian cyst, gall bladder swelling, etc.
- **Irregular surface** is an important feature of malignancy like carcinoma of the stomach, carcinoma liver, etc.

4. Consistency

- **Hardness** is a feature of malignant lump. Thus, hepatoma, carcinoma stomach, pancreatic carcinoma presents as hard lump. However, it should be remembered that often the malignant lump is firm and not hard.
- **Firm** consistency is found in ileocaecal tuberculosis, nodes of lymphoma, etc,
- A peculiar **doughy** feel is described of tuberculous abdomen.
- It is difficult to elicit fluctuation test for intraabdominal swellings, and often tensely cystic swellings feel firm on palpation, e.g. pseudocyst of pancreas, hydronephrosis, etc.

---

1. *Dont forget the 12th man in a cricket match. He is also an important player.*

- Indentation or pitting on pressure can be found in a colon loaded with faeces.
- Temporary contraction of a stomach (visible gastric peristalsis) should not be confused as a **mass.**

5. Margins or borders

- Upper border cannot be made out in liver, splenic and renal swellings.
- Lower border is not appreciated in pelvic masses, e.g. uterine fibroid, ovarian cyst (pelvic).
- A characteristic notch is felt in the anterior border of splenic swelling.
- Lower border is sharp as in a malignant liver swelling.

6. Intrinsic mobility test

- An intra-abdominal mass can be mobile if it has loose attachments or if it is not within the bony cage. Thus, liver, spleen, uterine mass are not mobile because of their location within bony cage.

Check for intrinsic mobility in different positions

- Carcinoma pyloric antrum can exhibit movements in different positions - left lateral or right lateral or even in the sitting position.
- Pancreatic carcinoma, advanced malignancies, lymph nodal masses also may not have intrinsic mobility.
- However, there are few swellings which have characteristic mobility.

Examples

A. Ovarian cyst is a freely mobile swelling which can be moved in all directions (Fig. 37.5A).

B. Mesenteric cyst moves at right angles to the direction of the line of mesentery (Fig. 37.5B).

C. Pseudopancreatic cyst may have a minimal side to side mobility (Fig. 37.5C).

D. Carcinoma transverse colon has vertical mobility unless it is advanced (Fig. 37.5D).

E. Eventhough pancreatic masses do not exhibit mobility, a cystadenoma of the pancreas because of the size and a narrow base, will exhibit **tree top mobility.**

F. Renal mass comes down during inspiration. As it comes down, it can be held back and can be pushed back to the renal pouch.

Key Box 37.1
INTRINSIC MOBILITY — MASS

- Side to side   —> Gall bladder
- Vertical   —> Transverse colon
- All directions   —> Ovarian cyst
- Right angle to the   —> Mesenteric cyst
  direction of mesentery
- Push back to renal   —> Kidney
  pouch
- Tree top mobility   —> Pancreatic cystadenoma

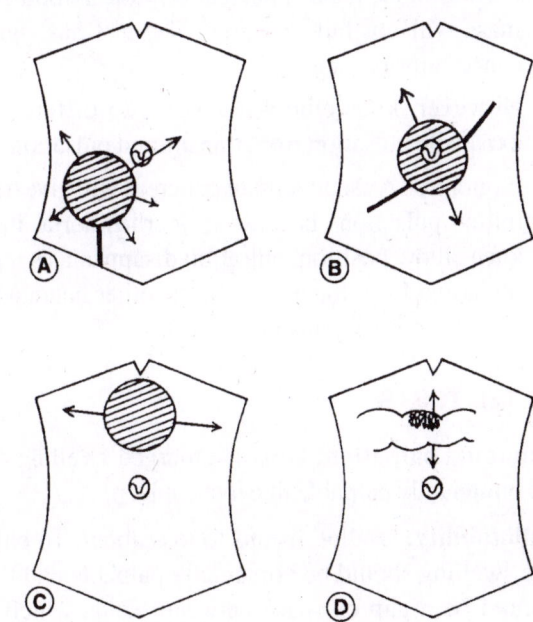

Fig. 37.5 (A-D) Intrinsic mobility

7. Plane of the swelling

A. Leg raising test or Head raising test

- The purpose of this test is to contract rectus abdominis muscles (also other abdominal wall muscles). Intraabdominal swellings become less prominent. On the other hand, abdominal wall swellings become more prominent, e.g. fibroma, neurofibroma, or lipoma in the abdominal wall.
- This test is done by asking the patient to raise his legs without bending at the knee (extended legs) or by raising the shoulders from the bed with arm folded over the chest.

B. Nose blowing test or straining test

- This test can be done by asking the patient to blow through the nose with mouth closed. The lateral abdominal muscles are more contracted with this test.
- It should be remembered that a swelling or the mass which moves with respiration is obviously an intra-abdominal mass.

C. Knee-elbow test

- This test differentiates an intraperitoneal mass from retroperitoneal mass. It is more useful when there is a mass in the centre of the abdomen - more so in the upper abdomen. To give a few examples, intraperitoneal cysts, intraperitoneal mass falls forwards. On the other hand, pancreatic mass, lymph node mass will not fall forwards. The test has significance only in 'selected' cases.
- However, knee-elbow test helps to differentiate expansile pulsation from transmitted pulsation.
- Examples: A pseudocyst of pancreas will give transmitted pulsations because it overlies aorta. In the knee elbow position, pulsation disappears as it gets separated from the aorta. On the other hand, aneurysms exhibit expansile pulsations.

SPECIAL TESTS

1. **Bimanual palpation:** Grossly enlarged swellings can be bimanually palpable like liver, spleen.

2. **Ballotability:** 'Ballot' means to toss about. To ballot, the swelling should be bimanually palpable and there should be a gap or space between hands which are kept anterior and posterior to the mass. Typically, renal swellings are **ballottable**. This test is done when patient is in the supine position, by keeping one hand anteriorly in the lumbar region over the swelling and the other hand posteriorly in the renal angle. A gentle push is given from behind and the swelling touches the hand which is placed anteriorly and it goes back. **Ballotability** is because of perirenal pad of fat.

3. **Murphy's kidney punch test** is elicited by applying pressure at the renal angle by the thumb.

PERCUSSION

1. To demonstrate mild ascites, the patient is put in a knee-elbow position and percussion is done around umbilicus. It gives a dull note if minimal fluid is present (normally area around the umbilicus is resonant).

Key Box 37.2

PERCUSSION

• Dull note	: Liver, spleen, renal angle
• Resonant	: Bowel anterior to the mass (E.g. Retroperitoneal mass)
• Impaired	: Stomach mass
• Shifting dullness	: Ascites

- Significant or moderate fluid in the abdomen is demonstrated by percussion of the centre and flanks of the abdomen in the lying down position and in the left or right lateral position.
- In the supine position flanks give a dull note due to fluid. However, in the lateral position, fluid shifts down and coils of bowel float up.

2. Liver dullness is elicited in the 5th intercostal space and the dullness is continuous with the mass, if it is arising from the liver.

3. Splenic dullness is elicited in the 9th intercostal space in the left midaxillary line.

4. **Percussion** over the mass:
   - Splenic and liver masses classically are **dull** to percuss.
   - Retroperitoneal masses may give **resonant** note because of intestines anterior to it. However, when they attain large size, eg,. Sarcomas, they push the bowel to one side and hence, they are dull to percuss.
   - Stomach mass may give **impaired resonant** note because of solid growth and due to the presence of air in the stomach.
   - **Renal angle percussion;** In cases of enlargement of kidney, there will be a band of resonance anteriorly due to the colon but posteriorly it gives a dull note.
   - **Hydatid thrill:** It is demonstrated by placing 3 fingers over the swelling and percussing the middle finger. Due to the fluid in the cyst, the fluid thrill (after-thrill) is felt by the other two fingers. This clinical sign is rarely demonstrable.

AUSCULTATION

1. Loud noisy sounds (Borborygmi) with or without peristalsis may indicate subacute obstruction. Such

patients may be having ileocaecal tuberculosis or carcinoma caecum. This should be done at right iliac fossa to hear for bowel sounds.

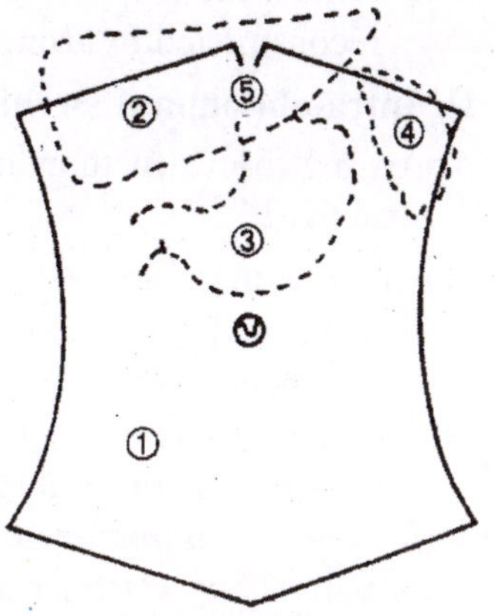

Fig. 37.6 Auscultation sites - 1-5 (Refer text)

2. Auscultation over the liver mass may reveal a **bruit** as a rapidly growing hepatoma.

3. **Succussion splash** is a splashing sound in cases of pyloric obstruction either due to carcinoma or due to chronic duodenal ulcer.

4. Perisplenitis and perihepatitis give rise to **friction rub** as in sickle cell anaemia due to repeated infarction and adhesions.

5. Aortic aneurysm will give a **continuous murmur** in the upper abdomen.

6. **Auscultopercussion** or auscultoscraping test is done to assess lower border of the stomach or greater curvature of the stomach.

RECTAL EXAMINATION

- Should be done in a case of intra-abdominal mass.

1. It can detect a carcinoma or a growth in the rectum in a case of secondaries in the liver.

2. It can detect pelvic secondaries in the rectovesical pouch.

VAGINAL EXAMINATION

- Should be done to rule out a carcinoma cervix or to detect lymph nodes in the pouch of Douglas.

Bimanual examination

- This should be done in cases of pelvic masses. One hand (left) is placed over the mass in the hypogastrium and right index finger or fingers inserted in the vagina or rectum in virgin females and the left hand is pressed downwards and backwards above the pubic symphysis. By this manoeuvre, details of the pelvic mass, solid or cystic, uterine or ovarian, free or fixed can be made out.

EXAMINATION OF LYMPH NODES

In cases of abdominal masses arising from lymph nodes, a thorough search of the body should be done to rule out other group of lymph nodes, such as axillary, iliac, inguinal, neck nodes, etc.

- **Left supraclavicular nodes** (Virchow's) are enlarged very often in visceral malignancies mainly from gastrointestinal tract. It indicates "inoperable" nature of the disease. Entire gastrointestinal lymph drains into the thoracic duct which joins the point of confluence of internal jugular vein and subclavian vein on the left side. This explains the significance of enlargement of Virchow's node. In 20% of cases, thoracic duct is single and 10-15% of cases it is double.

- **Significance of right supraclavicular node:** The lymphatics from the right mediastinal lymph trunk, and from the posterior right thoracic wall which form the right upper lymph trunk drain into the commencement of the right brachiocephalic vein.

SYSTEMIC EXAMINATION

Systemic examination should include respiratory system and cardiovascular system. Evidence of tuberculosis of the chest gives a clue about the mass in the abdomen, which may be a tubercular mass.

DIFFERENTIAL DIAGNOSIS: Students are requested to refer clinical books for details. However, mass arising from four different quadrants are discussed below.

MASS IN THE RIGHT ILIAC FOSSA

PARIETAL SWELLING

A. Parietal wall abscess
B. Desmoid tumour

INTRA-ABDOMINAL

A. Arising from normal structures
B. Arising from abnormal structures

FROM NORMAL STRUCTURES

I. Intestines

1. Appendicular mass
2. Appendicular abscess
3. Ileocaecal tuberculosis

4. Carcinoma caecum

5. Amoeboma

6. Intussusception

7. Actinomycosis

II. Lymph nodes

1. Acute lymphadenitis

2. Lymphoma

3. Secondaries

III. Retroperitoneal structures

1. Sarcoma

2. Aneurysm

3. Ileopsoas abscess

4. Chondrosarcoma

IV. In females

1. Ovarian cyst

2. Fibroid

3. Tubo-ovarian mass

FROM ABNORMAL STRUCTURES

1. Undescended testis — Seminoma

2. Unascended kidney

DIFFERENTIAL DIAGNOSIS OF MASS IN THE RIGHT ILIAC FOSSA

I. Parietal swelling: They are extra-abdominal. On head or leg raising test, they become more prominent. They are uncommon swellings.

A. Parietal wall abscess: It is a pyogenic abscess which can occur in a haematoma or pyaemic abscess which can occur as a part of pyaemia as in diabetic patients. Such abscesses are very tender, with warm surface, it is associated with fever with chills and rigors.

B. Desmoid tumour: It is an uncapsulated fibroma occurring in the abdominal wall.

- Occur in multiparous females. Repeated stretching of abdominal layers (due to pregnancy) is supposed to initiate tumour.

- It can also occur following abdominal wall injury including laparotomy.

- It is firm to hard swelling.

- It has no capsule. Hence, it should be treated with wide excision.

- It does not undergo sarcomatous change.

- After wide excision, the abdominal wall has to be reconstructed by using mesh.

II. Intra-abdominal swelling:

A. Arising from structures normally present in the right iliac fossa.

1. **Appendicular mass** (Fig. 37.8): It is a tender, soft to firm mass which develops after 48-72 hours following acute appendicitis. It is nature's attempt to limit the spread of infection by forming a mass consisting *of omentum, terminal ileum, caecum with pericaecal fat and inflammatory oedema.* It is managed conservatively by Oschner-Sherren's regime because an attempt to remove the appendix may result in faecal fistula. 6-8 weeks later, an elective appendicectomy can be done.

2. **Appendicular abscess:** It will be a very tender, firm, fixed mass. Such patients will have fever with chills and rigors.

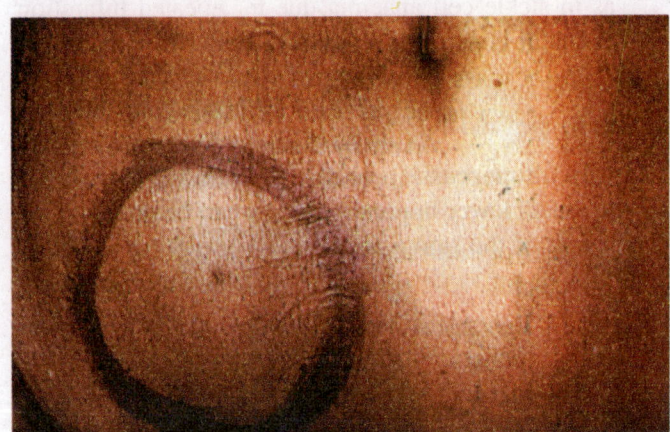

Fig. 37.7 Mass in the right iliac fossa

3. **Ileocaecal tuberculosis** (Fig. 37.9): Hyperplastic variety of tuberculosis forms a chronic cicatrising granulomatous reaction involving terminal ileum, caecum and part of ascending colon resulting in a mass in right iliac fossa. It is a chronic, nontender, firm, nodular mass, may have mobility, situated slightly (lumbar) higher side. Features of tuberculosis are usually present. It is treated by limited resection followed by ileocolic anastomosis.

4. **Carcinoma caecum** (Fig. 37.10, 37.11):

- More common in females, around 40-50 years of age.

- It produces bleeding per rectum, severe anaemia, etc.

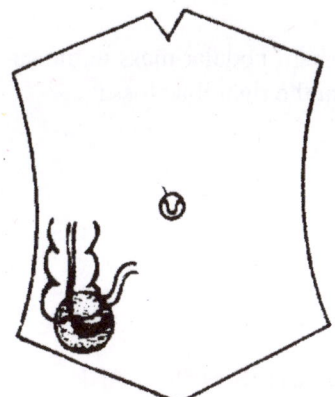

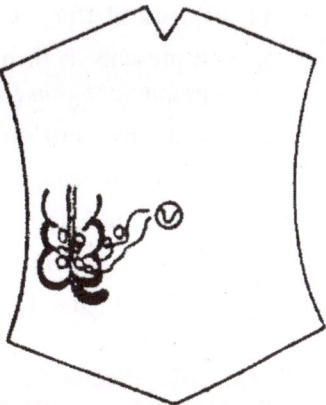

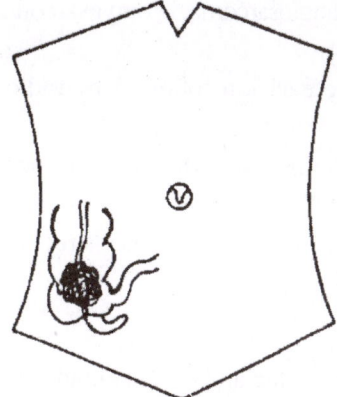

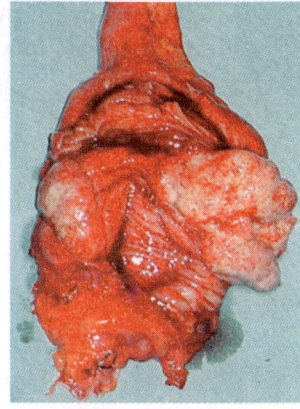

Fig. 37.8 Appendicular mass tender, laterally placed fixed mass

Fig. 37.9 Ileocaecal tuberculosis - caecum is pulled up

Fig. 37.10 Carcinoma caecum is an irregular non tender hard mass

Fig. 37.11 Proliferative lesions of carcinomas produce mass

- Hard, irregular mass in right iliac fossa with fixity or restricted mobility is a usual feature. Psoas spasm indicates infiltration into psoas muscle. It is treated by right radical hemicolectomy.

5. **Amoeboma:** Can be acute or chronic following chronic typhilitis (inflammation of the caecum). Amoeboma is tender and soft to firm. It is not common to find amoebomas nowadays because of effective treatment of amoebiasis with metronidazole tinidazole, etc.

6. **Intussusception:** Acute or chronic intussusception can give rise to a mass in the right iliac fossa which is tender and soft to firm. When acute intussusception occurs in children, it is described as idiopathic intussuception. Chronic intussusception may disappear spontaneously.

7. **Actinomycosis:** This is a rare mass in the right iliac fossa which usually develops 2-3 months after appendicectomy. A woody hard, indurated tender mass with multiple sinuses is characteristic of this condition. Sinuses discharge sulphur granules which can trickle down. Unlike tuberculosis, narrowing of lumen of the gut and lymph node enlargement do not occur.

8. **Lymph node mass:**
   a. Acute mesenteric lymphadenitis is common in children. It produces tender, nodular, firm, mass in right iliac fossa. Child usually has fever. Acute lymphadenitis can also involve external iliac nodes as in filariasis.
   b. Lymphoma involving external iliac nodes, nodular, firm to hard mass with involvement of other nodes, liver, spleen, etc.
   c. Secondaries in lymph nodes (external iliac) from carcinoma ovary, cervix, etc. Nodes are hard and fixity is a feature.

9. **Retroperitoneal sarcoma** (Fig. 37.12):
   - Common in young patients
   - Huge, nodular, fixed lump involving lumbar, umbilical and right iliac fossa. Recent increase in size brings about the attention of the patient.
   - Fixed to posterior abdominal wall
   - Later, obstruction of inferior vena cava results in oedema of legs.
   - Pressure on the ureter can give rise to hydronephrosis.
   - Liposarcoma is the commonest and may arise from pre-existing lipoma.

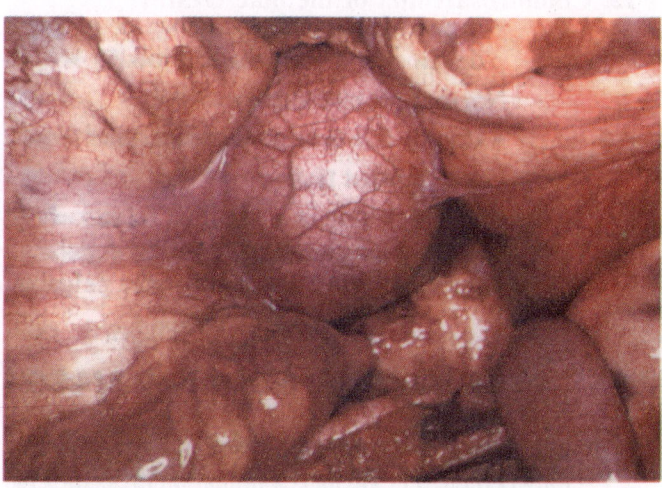

Fig. 37.12 Retroperitoneal sarcoma

- Fibrosarcoma, haemangiosarcoma, leiomyosarcoma are other sarcomas.
- It is treated by wide excision followed by radiotherapy.
- Chemotherapy is also helpful, when it is not possible to remove the entire mass.
- Debulking even if it is an advanced case is recommended.

10. **Aneurysm**

- Iliac artery aneurysm is rare and occurs in old aged patients. It produces a soft, pulsatile swelling in the right iliac fossa. Bruit or thrill is usually present.

11. **Iliopsoas abscess** (Fig 37.13):

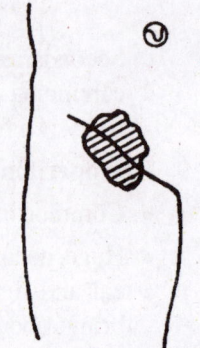

- It is the result of turberculosis of thoracolumbar spine. It should be suspected when a young patient complains of pain in the back referred to abdominal wall.

Fig. 37.13
Iliopsoas abscess

- Spine movements are limited.
- Gibbus is present.
- Initially, it forms paravertebral abscess and later it gravitates down beneath the medial arcuate ligament and forms psoas abscess. Psoas abscess burrows into the thigh under inguinal ligament and forms iliopsoas abscess.
- Fluctuation is present on both sides of the inguinal ligament. It is described as cross fluctuation test.

12. **Chondrosarcoma of the iliac crest:**

- It is a hard, fixed tumour which cannot be separated from the bone.

IN FEMALES

13. **Ovarian cyst**

- To start with the cyst develops in the pelvis and gives rise to discomfort in the lower abdomen. As cyst grows, it comes out of the pelvis and forms a mass in right iliac fossa. It has smooth surface, round borders, cystic, is *freely mobile* and can be pushed back into the pelvis. Sometimes, the cyst can attain huge size. Such freely mobile ovarian cysts have a long pedicle. Per vaginal examination gives the clue to the diagnosis.

14. **Fibroid of the uterus :**

- It presents as firm to hard nodular mass in the suprapubic region and in the right iliac fossa.

15. **Tubo - ovarian mass :**

- Is usually tender
- Pelvic infection is present
- It is soft to firm
- Can be bilateral

B. ARISING FROM STRUCTURES WHICH ARE NOT NORMALLY PRESENT

1. **Unascended kidney:**

- It can be either in the pelvis or in the iliac fossa. Such kidney is usually not very well developed. It presents as a lobular mass.

2. **Normal mobile kidney:**

- Can be felt in lumbar region, iliac fossa and it can be pushed back into loin.

3. **Undescended testis:**

- It is palpable in right iliac fossa *only* when it is involved by *Seminoma*. It is an intraabdominal testis and is hard, irregular, fixed mass. *Absent testis* in the scrotum clinches the diagnosis. Patient may have palpable para-aortic nodes, supraclavicular nodes, etc.

FIRM TO HARD NODULAR MASS IN THE UMBILICAL REGION

1. MASS ARISING FROM LYMPH NODES

a. **Metastasis or secondaries** is one of the common lymph node mass in the abdomen. Mass can be due to para-aortic nodes from testicular tumour, melanoma, carcinoma of ovary, carcinoma of penis, carcinoma of rectum, colon, stomach in late cases.

- The para-aortic lymph node mass has following features:

1. Fixed
2. Does not move with respiration
3. No intrinsic mobility
4. Does not fall forwards
5. Coils of bowel can be felt over the mass
6. Percussion may be resonant because of intestinal coils.

b. **Lymphoma:** The mass is enlarged para-aortic group of lymph nodes. It has all features of nodes mentioned above. Presence of lymph nodes in the neck, palpable liver and spleen clinches the diagnosis.

c. **Tuberculosis** can affect para-aortic nodes. However, it is uncommon.

2. RETROPERITONEAL SARCOMA

- Common in young patients
- Rapidly growing, enlarging mass in the abdomen of short duration
- It is firm, hard, nodular, fixed, does not fall forwards with intestinal coils anterior to it.
- Large sarcomas can cause compression on inferior vena cava or on the ureter, therefore pedal oedema and hydronephrosis can occur.
- Liposarcoma and fibrosarcoma are common
- Radical surgery should be attempted. However, many cases land up with debulking, radiotherapy, chemotherapy.

3. CARCINOMA BODY OF PANCREAS

- Cystadenocarcinoma of pancreas can attain a huge size. Otherwise, it is uncommon to get a large nodular pancreatic mass. However, carcinoma pancreas presenting as a palpable nodular mass indicates nonresectibility. Presence of **pulsations over the mass** (transmitted) clinches the diagnosis.

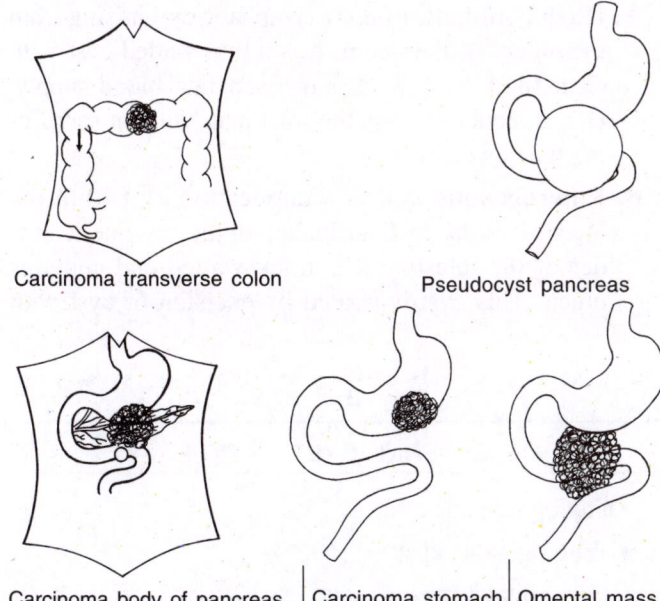

Carcinoma transverse colon

Pseudocyst pancreas

Carcinoma body of pancreas | Carcinoma stomach | Omental mass

Fig. 37.14 Mass in the umbilical region

- Men in the 6th decade are usually affected.
- Severe backache, loss of weight, recent development of diabetes suggests pancreatic pathology.
- Jaundice does not occur unless and until liver secondaries develop.
- It has all features of retroperitoneal mass.
- These cases are advanced with ascites. rectovesical deposits, etc.

4. CARCINOMA TRANSVERSE COLON

- Elderly patients present with constipation and bleeding per rectum.
- Firm to hard nodular mass occupying umbilical region may be found.
- It may have vertical mobility and being intra-abdominal it falls forwards.
- Caecum may be distended. Right to left peristalsis may be visible.

5. TUBERCULOUS ABDOMEN

- The mass can be rolled up omentum, with lymph nodes and coils of intestines which are matted.
- This is common in children and also occur in young adults in India.
- History of evening rise in temperature, loss of weight, loss of appetite, emaciation and improper digestion gives the clue to the diagnosis.
- Ascites is present in almost all cases.
- Features of subacute intestinal obstruction can also be present.

THE CYSTIC MASS IN THE ABDOMEN

Intra-abdominal cystic swellings are interesting swellings. They occur in young children, adults, middle-aged persons. There are many cases of cystic swellings which have given a surprise at laparotomy (notoriously cysts in females). In children cysts have confused many competent paediatricians!! Being intraabdominal cysts, it is not possible to elicit fluctuation and very often they are firm due to increased tension. The details of the important cystic swellings are given below :

1. **PSEUDOCYST OF PANCREAS** (see Chapter 25 for details): Tensely cystic upper abdominal mass may feel firm, tender and does not move with respiration.

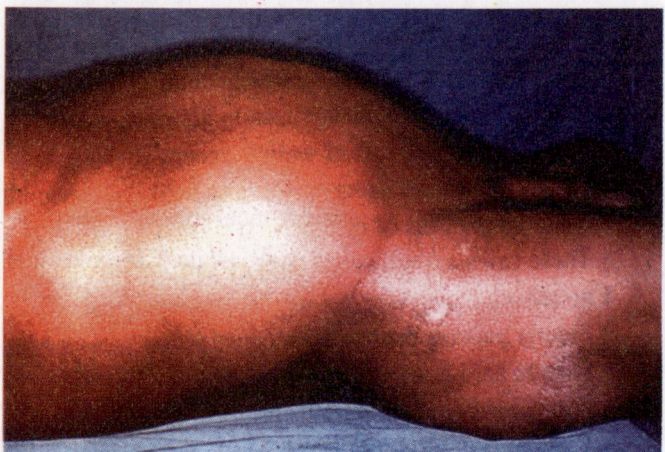

Fig. 37.15 Pseudocyst of pancreas (large).

Getting above the swelling is possible. Transmitted pulsations of the aorta can be felt over the mass which disappears on knee-elbow position. History of acute pancreatitis or blunt injury abdomen gives the clue to the diagnosis (Fig. 37.15).

2. HYDATID CYST OF LIVER

This swelling is of long duration, symptomless or dull pain in the upper abdomen. The cyst is spherical with smooth surface, rounded borders and feels firm. Since it is a mass arising from liver, it moves with respiration and getting above the swelling is not possible. Classical hydatid thrill, mentioned in the books, is rarely appreciated (Fig. 37.16). Simple cyst of the liver can also present as a cystic mass.

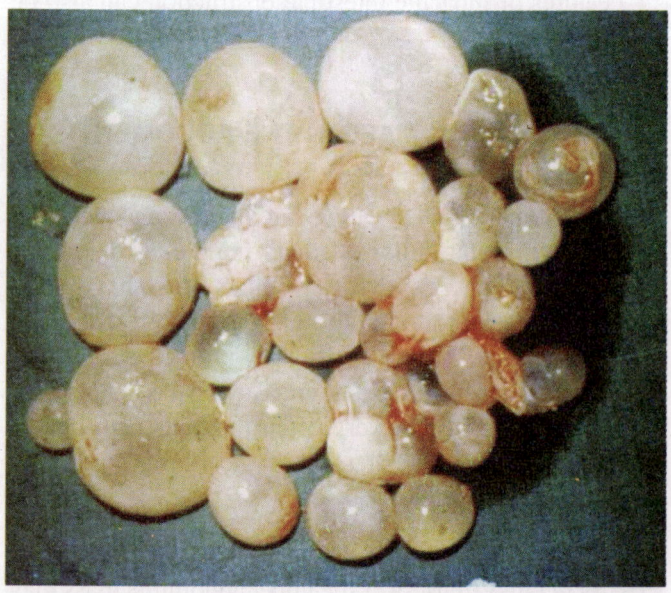

Fig. 37.16 Hydatid cyst

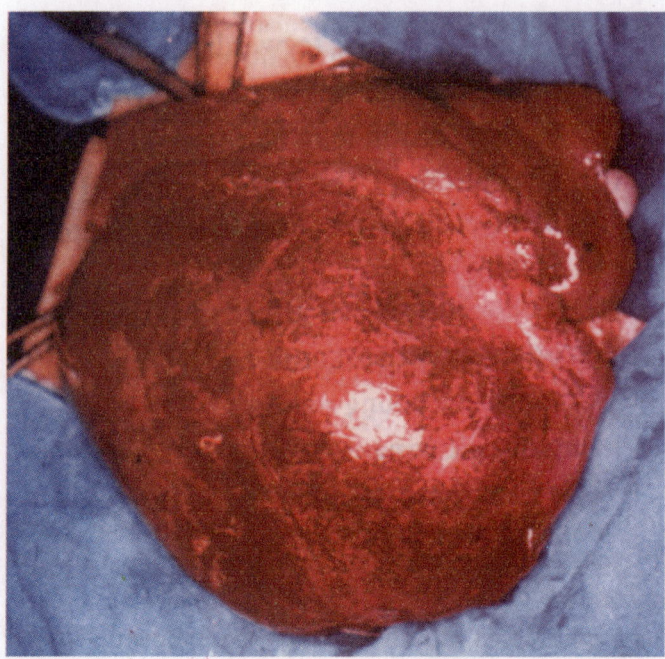

Fig. 37.17 Intra-abdominal cyst-serous cyst in the liver.

3. MESENTERIC CYST

These are congenital cysts, enterogenous or chylolymphatic, manifests in young children or during adolescence. Typically, the cyst is located in the umbilical region which moves at right angles to the direction of mesentery.

Types of Mesenteric Cyst (Figs. 37.18, 37.19 and 37.20)

A. **Chylolymphatic cyst** is a lymphatic cyst arising from mesentery of the ileum. It is a thin walled cyst with clear fluid or chyle. It has a separate blood supply. Hence, enucleation is the treatment without sacrificing the bowel.

B. **Enterogenous cyst** is a duplication cyst from the intestine or due to diverticulum of the mesenteric border of the intestine. It is thick walled and contains mucus. This cyst is treated by excision of cyst with

Key Box 37.3
MESENTERIC CYST —TYPES—
• Chylolymphatic cyst
• Enterogenous cyst
• Urogenital remnant
• Teratomatous dermoid cyst

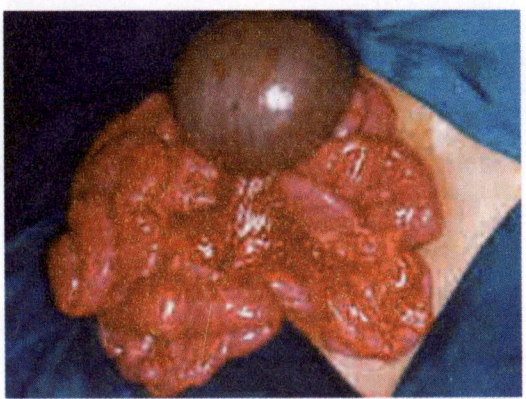

Fig. 37.18 Enterogenous cyst at surgery

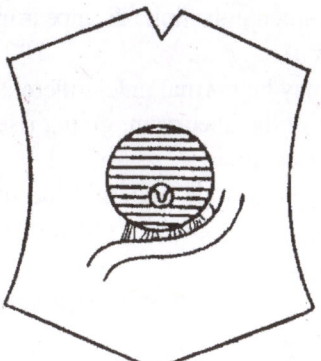

Fig. 37.19 Chylolymphatic cyst - it can be excised without resection of the bowel

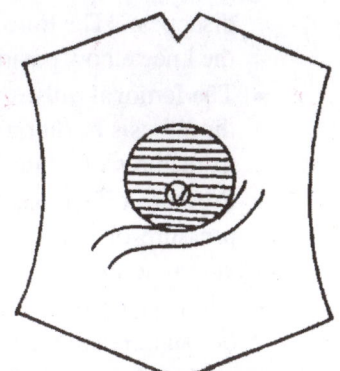

Fig. 37.20 Enterogenous cyst - it requires excision of intestine also along with the cyst

bowel segment because both share the same blood supply.

Complications

- Torsion of the cyst resulting in acute abdominal pain.
- Rupture of the cyst due to trauma.
- Haemorrhage into the cyst.

4. HYDRONEPHROSIS

Large hydronephrosis can attain a huge size without producing any symptoms. Bulk of the swelling is confined to one side of abdomen, with prominent bulge in the loin. It is difficult to elicit fluctuation in a tensely cystic intraabdominal mass. Bimanual palpation and ballotability give the clue to the diagnosis. One of the large cysts of polycystic kidney can present as a large renal cyst.

5. OVARIAN CYST

It is freely mobile, firm or soft mass in any quadrant of the abdomen. Such ovarian cysts, once they come out of pelvis will have free mobility. On pushing **the mass upwards there will be traction** on the pedicle, which may result in pain (Fig. 37.21). Any female patient who presents with lower abdominal mass, ovarian mass has to be considerd first, then mass consider other possibilities.

6. RETROPERITONEAL LYMPHATIC CYST

Retroperitoneal is one of the commonest of lymphatic cysts, which grows slowly to attain large size. Typically it is painless, seen in young patients and is tensely cystic. The bowel loop may be felt over the mass (retroperitoneal mass), or bowel loops may be pushed to the side.

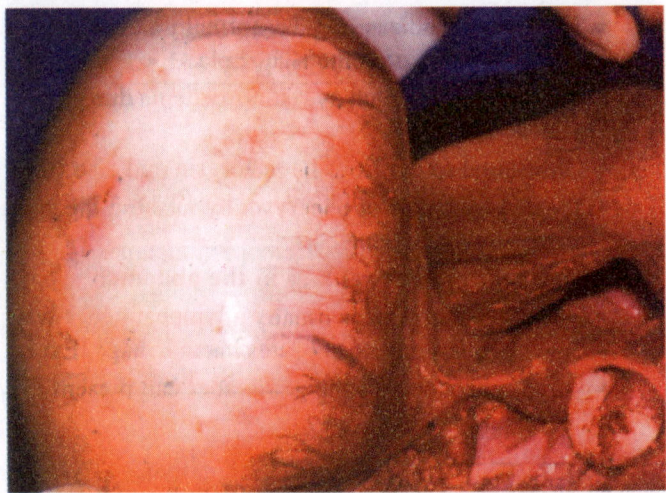

Fig. 37.21 Ovarian cyst

7. ENCYSTED ASCITES

This consists of ascitic fluid loculated by many loops of intestine along with omentum. Loss of weight, fever, anorexia, emaciation are the other features.

8. ABDOMINAL ANEURYSM

- Majority of cases are due to atherosclerosis and most of the aortic aneurysms are infrarenal. Hence, they present with a swelling in the umbilical region or epigastric region and with backache.
- Often they contain clotted blood, hence they feel firm, not compressible, fixed and tender.
- Characteristic feature of an abdominal aortic aneurysm is **expansile pulsation**. This can be appreciated by palpating the swelling gently all around. In the knee-elbow position, the pulsations do not

disappear. (The transmitted pulsations disappear in the knee elbow position).

- The **femoral pulses** may be normal unless there is thrombosis or rupture of the aneurysm, giving rise to features of acute ischaemia.

- Pressure effects such as **venous oedema** due to pressure on the inferior vena cava or erosion of vertebrae may be found.

- Ultrasound to confirm the aneurysm and also to rule out suprarenal aneurysm.

- Treated by repair of aneurysm, by incising the aneurysm and suturing a dacron graft end to end, inside the aneurysmal sac.

Key Box 37.4

AORTIC ANEURYSM

- Elderly males > 70
- Hypertensive
- Expansile pulsation +
- Anterior rupture : 20%—Hemoperitoneum
- Posterior rupture : 80%—Retroperitoneal haematoma
- > 6 cms size—dangerous

---

9. OTHER RARE CYSTIC SWELLINGS IN THE ABDOMEN (Fig. 37.22)

- **Omental cyst:** This is usually a lymphatic cyst which occurs in children and can attain a huge size. Sudden enlargement indicates haemorrhage. Excision is easy.

- **Large mucocoele** of the gall blader can present as a tense cystic, slighty tender mass in the upper abdomen.

CLINICAL NOTES

A female child, aged 6 years was examined by a paediatrician for generalised abdominal distension. All the investigations were normal. The child was put on antituberculous treatment, as the treating paediatrician diagnosed this case as tuberculous ascites. Child was brought back after 9 months with no improvement and abdominal pain since 2 days due to sudden increase in the size of the swelling. A paediatric surgeon was consulted, who palpated the abdomen and said she does not have ascites, but has a cyst and that the wall of the thin cyst can be felt. At exploration, a large cyst occupying all the 9

quadrants of the abdomen, was excised arising from omentum. Histopathological report was lymphatic cyst (Fig. 37.23).

One should not forget distended bladder in the lower abdomen as a cause of cystic swelling.

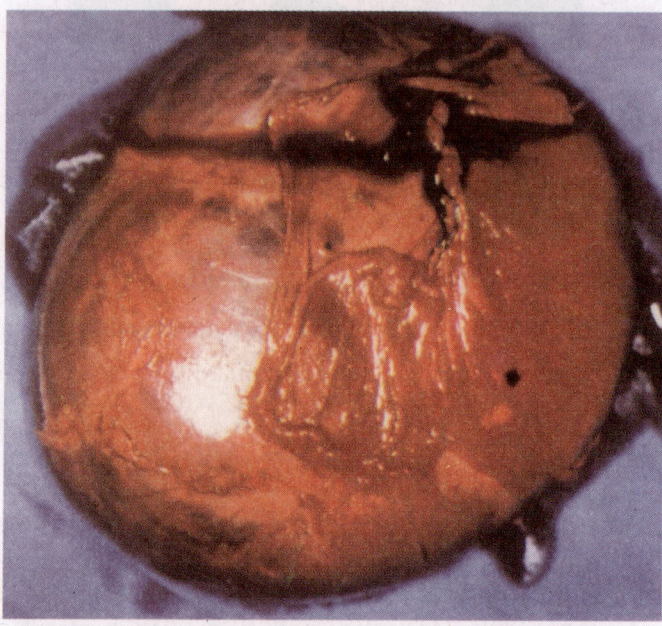

Fig. 37.22 Large lymphatic cyst arising from omentum

MASS IN THE EPIGASTRIUM

Mass in the epigastrium is one of the common long cases kept in the examination. Students should consider mass arising from liver and stomach first. Other possibilities must be considered later because common cases are common.

CLASSIFICATION

I) MASS ARISING IN THE ABDOMINAL WALL:

- First do the head raising test. If the mass becomes more prominent, it is extraperitoneal (abdominal wall).

- Lipoma, neurofibroma or desmoid tumour arising from the rectus sheath can present as a mass in the epigastrium.

- Also note epigastric hernia occurs in this region. It is a hernia, NOT A MASS.

Any hard subcutaneous swelling in the abdominal wall of recent origin can be a metastasis.

II) INTRAPERITONEAL MASS

1. MASS ARISING FROM THE LIVER

A. **Hepatoma:** Liver is enlarged, hard, irregular, nontender. However, rapidly growing hepatomas are tender, firm and even a bruit is heard over the swelling. Rapid deterioration of health in a cirrhotic patient is usually due to the development of a hepatoma.

B. **Secondaries in the liver:** Usually both lobes are enlarged, nodular surface without a bruit. Jaundice is a late feature in secondaries in the liver. The primary may be obvious as a colonic mass, a stomach mass or a testicular tumour etc. (Page 374)

C. **Hydatid cyst:** It is a benign swelling. History of contact with a dog is usually present. Epigastric swelling is due to enlarged liver which is smooth or irregular, nontender with rounded borders. Classical hydatid fremitus and thrill are rarely elicited. General health of the patient is usually good. (Page 366)

D. **Simple cyst** is not a clinical diagnosis but is mentioned here only for discussion. It is a serous cyst. Single big cyst can also be a part of Polycystic disease of the liver.

2. MASS ARISING FROM THE STOMACH

- For all practical purposes, the only mass arising from the stomach in the epigastrium is carcinoma stomach. It is hard, irregular and moves with respiration. Usually the patient is a male with loss of appetite and weight. Vomiting is a feature. If there is a growth in the pyloric antrum, visible gastric peristalsis can be seen in the epigastrium. Students are hereby requested not to offer lymphoma of the stomach or GIST of the stomach as a clinical diagnosis unless asked for by the examiner.

3. OMENTAL MASS

- Omentum gets involved in tuberculosis as a firm, nodular mass or in secondaries from intra-abdominal malignancies as a hard, nodular mass. Classically it moves with respiration.

- Rarely omental cyst can present as a tensely cystic mass in the epigastrium.

III) RETROPERITONEAL MASS

A. **Pseudopancreatic cyst:** It forms a tense cystic mass, felt as firm mass in the epigastrium. Its upper border cannot be made out. It does not usually move with respiration. It has smooth surface and round borders. H/O acute pancreatitis or H/O blunt injury abdomen is usually present. Pulsations over the mass (transmitted) suggests it is a mass close to the aorta. In such a case, it is a pseudocyst. Gurgle anteriorly suggests distended stomach.

B. **Cystadenoma:** Cystadenomas of pancreas are benign and can attain huge sizes. It can present as a mass in the epigastrium, left hypochondrium or umbilical region. They exhibit what is described as 'tree top mobility'.

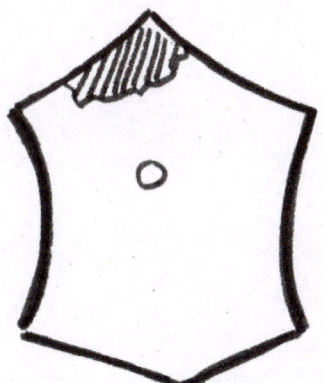 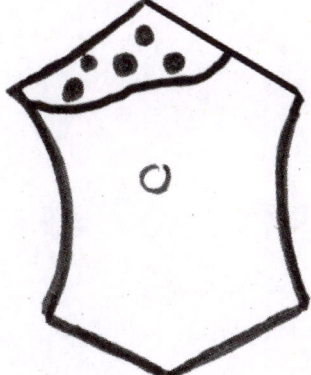 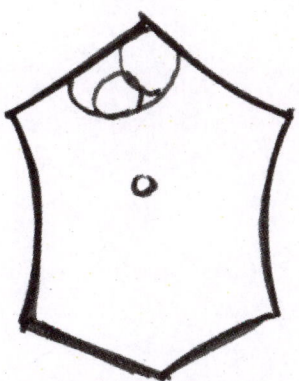 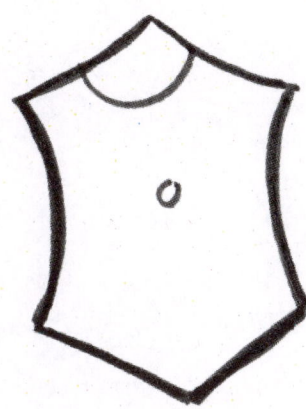

Fig. 37.23 Hepatoma   **Fig. 37.24** Secondaries in the liver   **Fig. 37.25** Hydatid cyst   **Fig. 37.26** Simple cyst

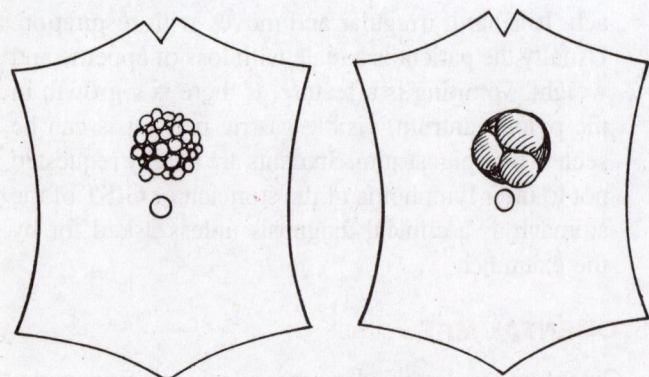

Fig. 37.27 Tuberculous abdomen   **Fig. 37.28** Lymph nodes

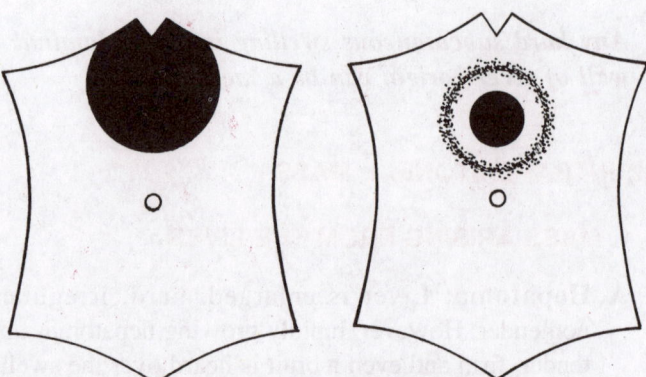

Fig. 37.29 Pseudocyst of pancreas   **Fig. 37.30** Abdominal aortic aneurysm

C. Carcinoma body of pancreas can present as a mass in the lower part of epigastrium or upper umbilical region. The mass is hard, irregular, fixed and does not move with respiration. Presence of severe backache and loss of weight are important features.

D. Abdominal Aortic Aneurysm (AAA):

An elderly patient, usually a hypertensive presents with features of abdominal pain, swelling or features of is-chaemia of the lower limb. On examination, tender swelling in the epigastrium with a characteristic expansile pulsation is present. Knee-elbow test will help differentiate it from transmitted pulsations. Presence of a bruit and weak or absent lower limb pulses (due to thrombus) also helps in establishing the diagnosis.

E. Lymph node mass (Page 600)

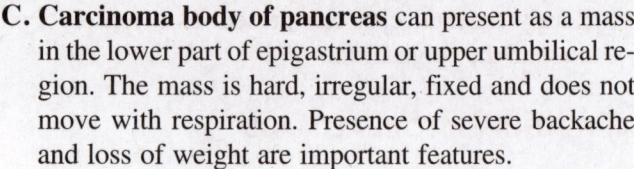

Investigations of the Urinary Tract

38

- Urine
- Blood
- Intravenous urogram
- Retrograde pyelography
- Renal arteriography
- Cystography
- Urethrography
- Ultrasonography
- Computed tomography
- Radioisotope scanning
- Endoscopy

INVESTIGATING A PATIENT WITH UROLOGICAL SYMPTOMS

URINE EXAMINATION

A. Urine routine

pH — Alkaline in renal tubular acidosis
Albumin — Nephrotic syndrome, physiological
Sugar — Diabetes
Deposits — Crystals, Casts
RBC — Glomerular and Nonglomerular
WBC — Infective and Sterile pyuria

B. Urine culture and sensitivity

C. Urine cytology — Positive in carcinoma

D. Urine AFB — Ziehl Neelsen staining

Fluorescent microscopy
AFB culture - LJ Medium
and radio-isometric culture
PCR studies for AFB

E. 24 hour studies - Stones, proteinuria

BLOOD EXAMINATION

- Renal function tests - Urea, creatinine
- Acid base Balance
- Metabolic studies for stones

IMAGING

- Today renal imaging is the most important part of investigating a case of urinary tract disease. There are many investigations, important ones being given below:

IVP: IVU (INTRAVENOUS PYELOGRAM, INTRAVENOUS UROGRAM)

Aim

1. To study renal function
2. To detect any pathology of kidneys, ureters and bladder
3. To study any anatomical variations of the renal system.

Procedure

- A fat-free, nonresidual diet is given for 2 to 3 days prior to the procedure to avoid intestinal gas shadows.

- Dimol 2 tablets 3 times daily for 2-3 days prior to the procedure to expel the gas.

- Patient should not take oral fluids 6 hours before the procedure.

- Radiological contrast dye: 45% sodium diatrizoate, 20-40 ml injected through median cubital vein.

Requirements before IVP

1. Blood urea (normal: 20-40 mg %): If blood urea is very high, the kidney does not excrete the dye. Hence, kidneys are not visualised. A high dose urography may be needed to delineate the kidney.

2. Plain X-ray kidney ureter bladder region (KUB) to look for a renal stone -90% of the renal stones are radio-opaque (Only 10% of gall stones are radio-opaque).

   • To distinguish between renal stones and gall-stones on plain abdominal radiograph, in case of doubt, take lateral film, stones anterior to the vertebral column are gall stones and lateral to it are renal stones.

Precautions while injecting the dye

1. The dye should be given very slowly
2. The dye should not extravasate
3. If bronchospasm occurs, hydrocortisone 100 mg I. V. and an antihistaminic I.V. should be administered.
4. In cases of urticaria and skin rashes, antihistaminic to be given.

Radiography

1. Early films taken after 2 or 5 minutes, demonstrates the kidney outline (nephrogram).
2. 5 minutes later, pelvicalyceal system is visualised.
3. 15-20 minutes later, ureter, bladder can be visualised.

4. Post-voiding picture is taken to demonstrate any residual contrast in the urinary bladder.

   • Abdominal compression has to be applied to demonstrate pyelograms better.

Contraindications for IVP

1. Idiosyncrasy to iodine: Test dose should be given before hand.
2. Renal failure: Kidneys fail to excrete the dye
3. Multiple myeloma: The dye precipitates myeloma proteins, blocks the ureter and kidney and causes anuria.
4. Hyperuricaemia: Uric acid crystals deposit in the renal tubules.
5. Sickle cell anaemia: Precipitates sickle cell crisis.
6. Dehydration.

Uses of IVU

1. Diagnosis of congenital abnormalities like polycystic kidney, horseshoe kidney, single kidney, duplication of kidneys and ureters.
2. Diagnosis of hydronephrosis, hydroureter, vesicoureteric reflux, ureterocoele (Fig.38.1).
3. Obstruction to pelviureteric junction, ureters-primary obstructed megaureter.
4. Diagnosis of renal, ureteric stones and bladder stones.
5. To diagnose renal tuberculosis, tumours.

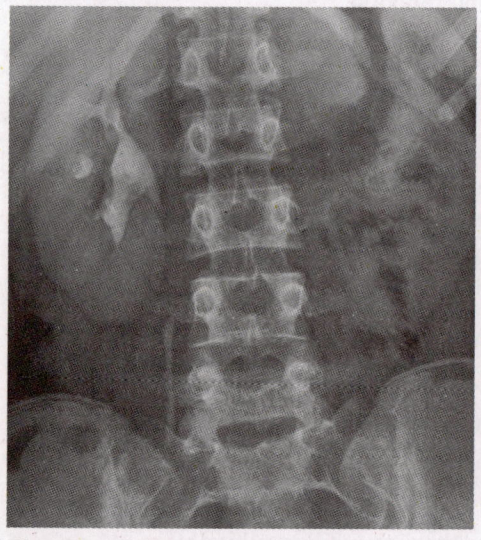

Fig. 38.1 IVU 5 minutes picture

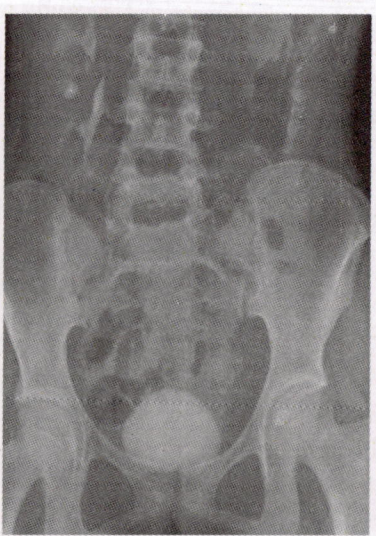

Fig. 38.2 IVU after 20 minutes

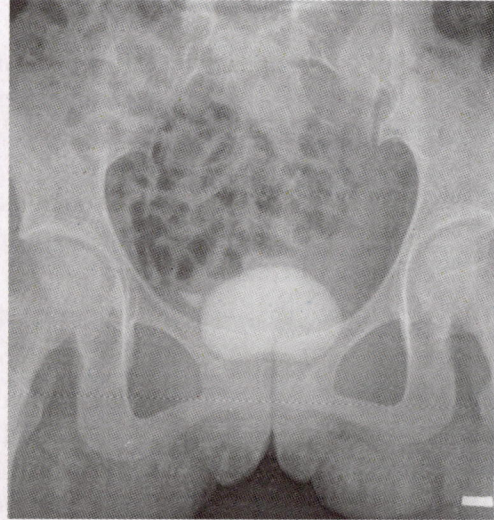

Fig. 38.3 Observe the bowel gas, inadequate preparation

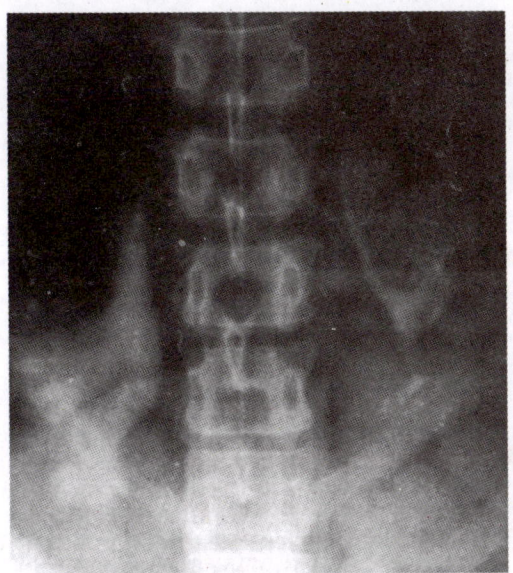

Fig. 38.4 IVU showing hydronephrosis

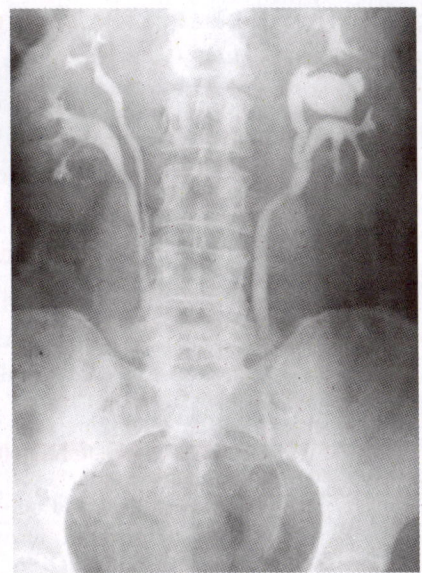

Fig. 38.5 IVU showing double ureter

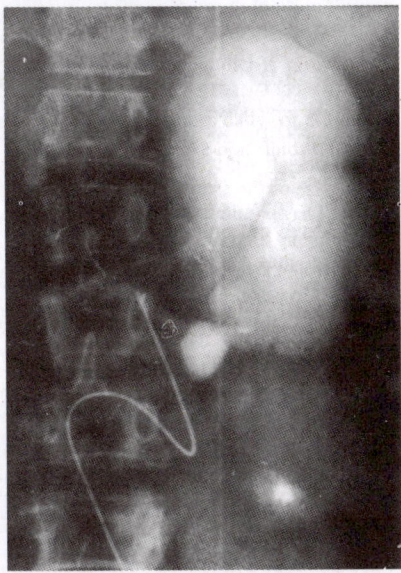

Fig. 38.6 RGP - retrocaval ureter with hydronephrosis

RETROGRADE PYELOGRAPHY: RGP

Indications

1. When the kidney is not visualised by IVU
   a. Gross hydronephrosis (Fig. 38.6)
   b. Very high blood urea
2. To collect selectively the urine sample from renal pelvis, e.g. Renal tuberculosis.
3. History of allergy to intravenous contrast materials
4. Prior to ureteroscopy

Procedure

- A cystoscopy is done first
- Ureteric orifices are identified and cannulated by a flexible catheter which is introduced upto the pelvis of kidney and the dye is injected. X-rays are taken at 5 minutes, 15 minutes, and 30 minutes.

Uses

1. Diagnosis of nonfunctioning kidney due to hydronephrosis.
2. Early diagnosis of renal tuberculosis.
3. Since the dye is injected directly into the pelvis, pelvicalyceal system can be identified better which helps in the diagnosis of early transitional cell carcinoma of kidney.

Complications of RGP

1. It is an invasive procedure and hence, urinary tract infection can occur. Prophylactic antibiotics are given before the procedure.
2. Rarely chances of perforation of the bladder or perforation of the ureters may occur.

RENAL ARTERIOGRAPHY

Technique

- There are two methods in which the test can be performed. The technique used now is the digital subtraction angiography (DSA).

1. Retrograde arteriography using Seldinger's technique. Selective renal angiography can be done by using a catheter over a guide wire passed into renal artery.
2. Translumbar aortography is done under general anaesthesia wherein aorta is punctured with a needle from behind, above the renal arteries at the level of 1st lumbar vertebra.

Dose

- For aortography 30 ml of contrast (hypaque) and for selective renal angiography 6-8 ml is used.

Uses

1. To demonstrate pathological anatomy of the renal artery when renal artery stenosis or aneurysm is suspected.

2. In renal cell carcinoma, tumour vascularity and extension of the tumour into the renal vein can be diagnosed during the venous phase.

3. Bleeding from the kidney due to trauma or arteriovenous malformation.

4. Therapeutic application:

   1. Transluminal angioplasty can be done by inflating the balloon in cases of renal artery stenosis.

   2. Embolization of bleeding vessels, aneurysms

Key Box 38.1
COMPLICATIONS
1. Tubular necrosis of the kidney
2. Paraplegia due to spasm of spinal arteries
3. Haematoma
4. Thromboembolism

MICTURATING CYSTOURETHROGRAPHY (MCU)

- In this procedure the dye is injected into the urinary bladder.

Indications

1. In children, to demonstrate vesicoureteric reflux
2. Posterior urethral valve
3. Vesical trauma
4. Vesicovaginal or vesicocolic fistula

Procedure

- A catheter is passed into the urinary bladder in a child and the dye is injected. The catheter is removed and the child is screened for vesicoureteric reflux during voiding of urine.

Complications

- Due to the invasive nature of the procedure, urinary tract infection can occur. Hence, prophylactic antibiotics should be used.

ASCENDING URETHROGRAPHY (ASU)

In the diagnosis of urethral stricture, to know the length of stricture, proximal dilatation or diverticulum, urethrography is used.

Indications

· Investigation of urethral stricture

Contraindication

· Urethral haemorrhage

Precaution

- Barium and Medium containing oil such as Lipiodol should not be used because if there is a urethral mucosal tear or breach, it can cause oil embolism. Conray 280 is injected slowly into the urethra.

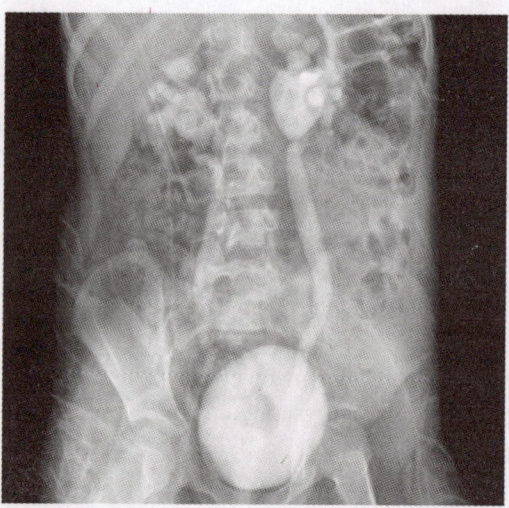

Fig. 38.7 MCU voiding phase - observe the dilated ureter due to reflux

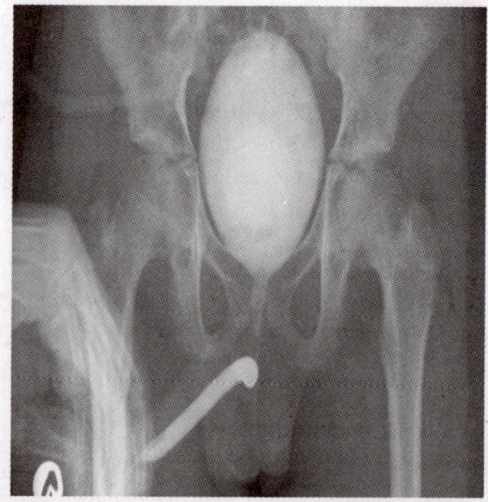

Fig. 38.8 Ascending urethrogram and micturiting cystourethrogram - stricture urethra

ULTRASONOGRAPHY (U.S.G.)

A. Fluid can be differentiated from solid tissue. Hence, cystic swellings can be made out.

B. Stones can be diagnosed

C. In an enlarged kidney thickness of cortex, disruption of the architecture of echoes can be made out as in hydronephrosis

D. Residual urine in the bladder can be found out, which may be an indication of enlarged prostate. The volume of the prostate can be measured (Key Box 38.2).

Ultrasonography has become the investigations of choice to diagnose fetal hydronephrosis due to various reasons. This has got dual advantages one the management of the disease causing hydronephrosis can be planned at the early stage thereby preventing damage to the kidney and secondly intrauterine interventions are also possible if the need arises.

Key Box 38.2
TRANSRECTAL ULTRASONOGRAPHY IN CARCINOMA PROSTATE
• Disruption of the architecture of echoes • Invasion of capsule • Biopsy - ultrasonography guided

COMPUTED TOMOGRAPHY (CT)

• It is more useful than **arteriography** to assess and display the images of the body at selected levels
• Thus, useful in the diagnosis of kidney tumour and its extent
• To stage cancer of prostate, bladder, kidney
• To stage testicular tumours

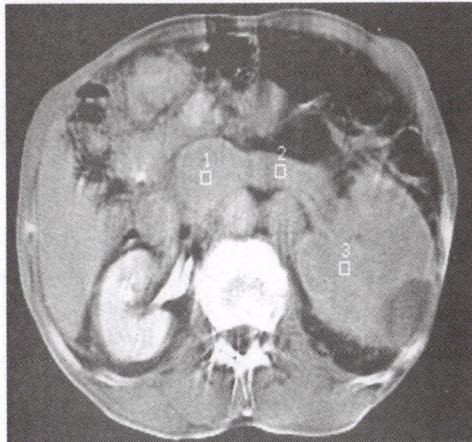

Fig. 38.9 CT scan showing left renal cell carcinoma

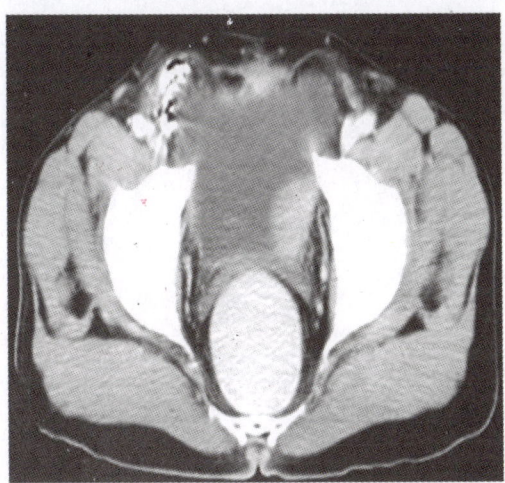

Fig. 38.10 CT scan showing bladder carcinoma

RADIO-ISOTOPE SCANNING

• Gamma camera screening following injection of Technetium 99^{m} will give information about proximal tubular function. To assess differential renal functions, 99^{m} TcDTPA (Diethylene triamine pentaacetic acid) or Tc^{99} DMSA (Dimercapto succinic acid) is used. It is filtered and secreted into the tubular lumen.

Tc 99^{m} DTPA

This scan is done to find out relative functions of both kidneys; it also tells about the total GFR and what percentage of total GFR is contributed by each kidney. Relative function of 45±2% is considered acceptable for each kidney. The main indication for DTPA is long term hydronephrosis. Examples are newborn with antenatally diagnosed hydronephrosis, children with posterior urethral valves etc.; and this scan is also useful in assessing the improvement in relative function of the kidney after surgery for above conditions. The yield of DTPA scan can be improved by injecting I.V. lasix. This is known as **diuretic renography.**

Key Box 38.3
RADIOISOTOPE SCANNING IN UROLOGY
• Tc 99m DTPA - Renal function, drainage • Tc 99m DMSA - Renal parenchymal images • Tc 99m Disphosphonate - Bone secondaries • I131 MIBG - Pheochromocytoma • Tc 99m Sestamibi - Parathyroid adenoma

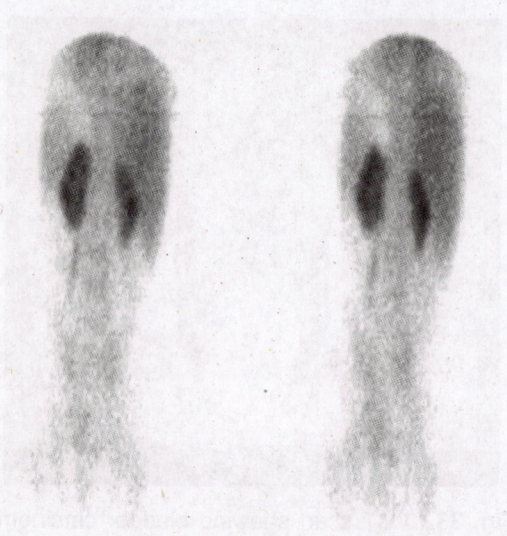

Fig. 38.11 DMSA scan

Tc 99^m DMSA

It is used most commonly for cortical imaging. It shows details of renal parenchyma. It is particularly useful when looking for segmental abnormalities of kidney (E.g. Renal scarring secondary to conditions like chronic pyelonephritis and renal tumours).

ENDOSCOPY

- Cystourethroscopy: Bladder and urethral mucosa can be visualised

- Procedure is done under surface anaesthesia

- Preparation: The external genitalia is cleaned with soap solution or an antiseptic agent and 1% lignocaine jelly is injected into urethra, to provide lubrication and ana-

esthesia. This should be left in place for 10 minutes for its action.

Uses of cystoscopy

1. Diagnosis of bladder cancer, papilloma, cystitis

2. Position and character of ureteric orifices - in tuberculosis involving the urinary bladder the ureteric orifices are shifted upwards and gaping.

3. **Indigocarmine test:** 7 ml of 0.4% dye is injected intravenously. Observe ureteric orifice through cystoscope. Unilateral delay in appearance of dye suggests obstruction. If there is bilateral delay, it indicates impaired renal function.

4. As a preliminary step to do RGP

5. To rule out involvement of bladder in gynecological cancer (e.g. cancer cervix)

6. To remove bladder stones

7. For transurethral resection of bladder tumour (TURBT) in early bladder cancers

URETHROSCOPY

1. Anterior urethroscopy is done in urethral stricture or in cases of chronic urethritis. It can rule out strictures due to granuloma.

2. Posterior urethroscopy: To visualise prostatic urethra and verumontanum

- Verumontanum is red in cystitis

- In chronic prostatitis, prostatic ducts may be seen discharging pus

- When lateral lobes of prostate gland are enlarged, they project into the internal meatus and produce an inverted 'V' appearance.

39

Kidney and Ureter

- Surgical anatomy
- Polycystic kidney
- Horseshoe kidney
- Renal stones
- Ureteric stone
- Hydronephrosis
- Renal tuberculosis
- Renal tumours
- Pyonephrosis
- Perinephric abscess
- Renal transplantation

SURGICAL ANATOMY OF KIDNEY

- Kidneys are the retroperitoneal organs, two in number on either sides of vertebral column. Each kidney is bean or reniform in shape.

  Owing to the presence of liver, right kidney is 1-2 cm lower than the left kidney extending from L_1-L_3 and the left kidney extends from T_{12}-L_3

- These relationships are very important for surgeons, as the structures, mentioned above may get injured during operations on kidney (Table 39.1). Also they may get directly involved by renal malignancies (local spread).

Table 39.1 Relations of kidneys

	RIGHT	LEFT
Anterior (Figure 39.1)	Below : Hepatic flexure of colon Medial : 2nd part of duodenum	Below : splenic flexure - pancreas and splenic vessels - below pancreas is jejunum - Above pancreas is stomach & spleen
Medial	Above : Adrenal Liver IVC Ureter	Above : Adrenal, DJ flexure, Inferior mesenteric vein, ureter
Lateral	Below : Ascending colon Above : Liver	Below : Descending colon Above : Spleen
Posterior	Same in both kidneys. Each kidney rests upon four muscles: psoas, transversus abdominis quadratus, diaphragm.	

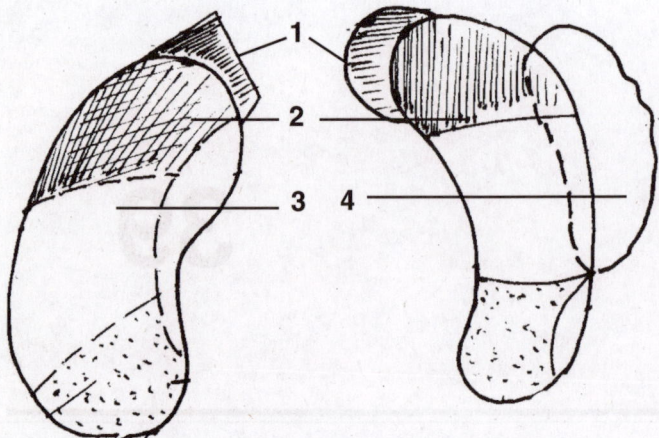

Fig. 39.1 Anterior relationships of the kidney
1. Adrenals 2. Gastric area 3. Colic area 4. Spleen

FASCIAL ATTACHMENTS

Both the kidneys and associated adrenal glands are surrounded by varying degrees of perirenal or perinephric fat and these together are loosely enclosed by the perirenal fascia, commonly called as Gerota's fascia.

The anterior and posterior sheaths of Gerota's fascia, become fused on three sides around the kidney laterally, medially and superiorly.

Superiorly

Gerota's fascia fuses with the diaphragm (as a result kidney moves with respiration). Students should remember here that movement with respiration is a characteristic feature of intraperitoneal organs and masses and many times this feature is used to support the diagnosis of intraperitoneal organ, however, kidney being the retroperitoneal organ also moves with respiration.

Medially

Gerota's fascia of one side crosses the midline and fuses with opposite gerota's.

Inferiorly

Gerota's fascia remains an open potential space, containing ureter and gonadal vessels.

- Gerota's fascia forms an important anatomical barrier and tends to confine pathological processes originating from the kidney; however because of deficiency inferiorly; the collection within Gerota's fascia may track down and extend into pelvis.

Some points to remember

- Renal artery is an end artery and the entire renal arterial system is composed of end arteries, without anstamosis and collateral circulation; occlusion of any branches of renal artery (with in kidney known as segmental arteries) results in infarction of area supplied by it.
- In contrast, the renal parenchymal veins anastomose freely with each other and even with perinephric veins.

POLYCYSTIC KIDNEYS (CONGENITAL CYSTIC KIDNEYS)

- This is an autosomal dominant disease transmitted through chromosome by anyone of the parents. Early onset congenital cystic kidneys are found to be autosomal recessive.
- More common in women

Associated lesions

- Congenital polycystic disease of liver (18%)
- Congenital polycystic disease of pancreas
- Congenital polycystic disease of ovary or testis
- Berry aneurysms

Pathology

- During development, some of the uriniferous tubules fail to join with the collecting ducts. Such uriniferous tubules develop into cysts. The important pathological features are as follows:
- Both kidneys are affected

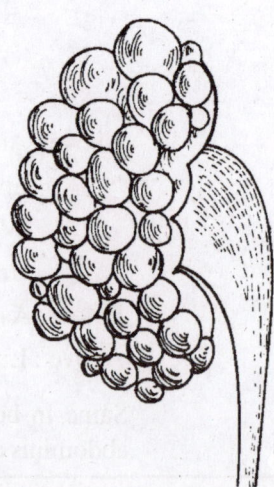

Fig. 39:2 Polycystic kidney

- They enlarge often to 3-4 times the normal size
- The kidneys are studded with multiple large cysts
- When the cyst ruptures into the pelvis of the kidney, it results in **hematuria.**
- As the disease progresses, cysts progress in size which lead to pressure atrophy of the functional renal parenchyma leading to renal failure.

Types

1. **Foetal type:** Autosomal recessive disease may cause intra-uterine death due to obstructed labour.

2. **Infantile type:** Autosomal recessive, early renal failure with death within 3-5 years of life.

3. **Adult type:** Autosomal dominant type. Presents in the 3rd or 4th decade with symptoms.

Clinical features

1. Eventhough congenital, it manifests at middle age around 40 years.

2. Dull aching pain in both loins is due to stretching of the renal capsule (dragging pain).

3. Microscopic or macroscopic **haematuria** in 70-80% cases.

4. **Hypertension** (secondary) (75%) is due to renal ischaemia which stimulates juxtaglomerular apparatus to secrete renin. It may also be related to a separate genetic factor.

5. **Bilateral renal mass**: Both kidneys are enlarged, surface is nodular or bosselated, firm to hard and sometimes cystic.

6. Features of **renal failure**: thirst, vomiting, abdominal distension due to paralytic ileus, anuria, uraemic smell, coated tongue, anemia.

7. Infection, pyelonephritis

Diagnosis

1. Urea and creatinine to rule out renal failure. Normal creatinine levels: 0.8-1.6 mg %. Normal urea: 20 to 40 mg %.

2. Plain X-ray KUB : Enlarged kidney can be seen because of changes in the density between the perirenal pad of fat and the kidney.

3. Abdominal USG to confirm the diagnosis.

4. IVU: The **spider leg deformity** of the calyces

Treatment

1. **Asymptomatic** polycystic kidney does not require any treatment.

2. Polycystic kidney with **hypertension**: Control of hypertension by drugs. When hypertension becomes uncontrollable, nephrectomy followed by renal transplantation should be done.

3. If the cyst is **infected or if pyelonephritis** develops, appropriate antibiotics are given and if necessary the cyst should be aspirated-ultrasound guided.

4. Polycystic disease with **renal failure**, emergency dialysis followed by renal transplantation is the treatment of choice.

HORSESHOE KIDNEY

- During the development, 2 mesonephric buds appear on the side of the future vertebral column and grows into metanephros. Mesonephric buds form ureter and metanephros kidneys.
- **If fusion occurs at lower pole**, it results in a classical **horseshoe kidney**.
- Rarely, upper polar fusion can occur giving rise to reverse horseshoe kidney.
- Inferior mesenteric artery crosses the isthmus at the level of L3-L4. Hence, **horseshoe kidney cannot ascend**. It is felt lower down in the abdomen.

Key Box 39.1
ASSOCIATED ANOMALIES
1. Spina bifida
2. Congenital hemivertebra
3. Turner's syndrome
4. Cleft lip and cleft palate

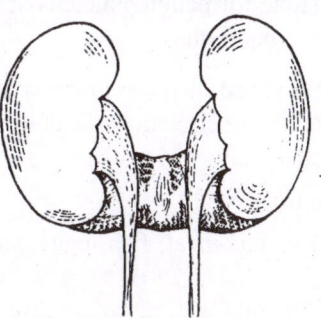

Fig. 39.3 Horseshoe kidney

Clinical features

1. It can be asymptomatic for many years.

2. A palpable mass below and to the right and to the left of umbilicus or umbilical region can be a horseshoe kidney.

3. **Recurrent urinary tract infection (UTI)** is common because the ureters are angulated over the isthmus resulting in kinking, stasis and infection.

4. As a result of stasis and infection, stones occur in the kidney.

5. They are more **prone for hydronephrosis** due to the angulation of ureters.

6. **Rovsing sign:** Hyperextension of the spine results in abdominal pain, nausea or vomiting due to stretching of the capsule.

Diagnosis

1. Ultrasonography (USG), to locate the kidney.

2. I. V.U.: Upper and middle calyx are directed laterally but **lower calyx is directed medially** where there is fusion, which is characteristic of horseshoe kidney.

3. CT scan or isotope renogram are confirmatory.

Treatment

• Indicated only when there are complications.

• Removal of the stone, or repair and reconstruction of the hydronephrosis are done in the usual manner.

RENAL STONES

AETIOPATHOGENESIS

1. **Infection:** Organisms such as Proteus, Pseudomonas, Klebsiella produce recurrent UTI. These organisms produce urea and causes stasis of urine which precipitate stone formation. Nucleus of the stone may harbour these bacteriae.

2. **Hot climates** cause increase in concentration of solutes, resulting in precipitation of calcium which forms calcium oxalate stones.

3. **Dietary factors**

   a. Diet rich in red meat, fish, eggs can give rise to aciduria.

   b. Diet rich in calcium, tomatoes, milk, spinach, rhubarb produce calcium oxalate stones.

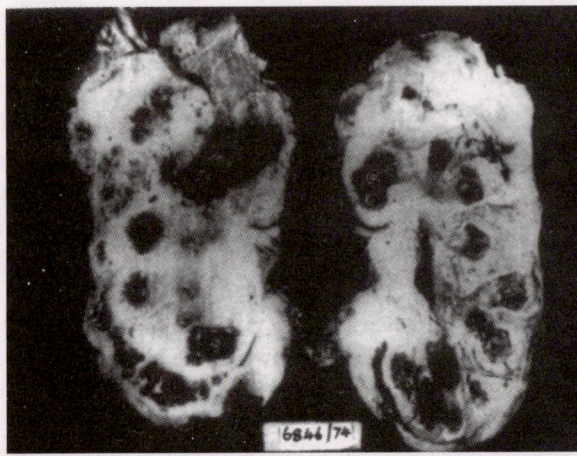

Fig. 39.4 Chronic pyelonephritis with multiple calculi (Prof. Sasidharan, Manipal)

   c. Diet lacking in vitamin A causes desquamation of renal epithelium which precipitates calcium and alters it and stone formation occurs.

4. **Metabolic causes**

   a. Hyperparathyroidism increases serum calcium levels resulting in hypercalcinosis and pelvic stones.

   b. Gout increases uric acid levels and causes multiple uric acid stones.

5. **Immobilisation:** Paraplegic patients secrete large amounts of calcium in the urine (they pass skeletons in urine) resulting in calcium oxalate stones.

6. **Decreased urinary citrate:** Citric acid (300-900 mg/ 24 hours) keeps the urinary pH low. When citric acid levels decrease, it promotes precipitation of urinary calcium. Citrate excretion is under hormonal control.

7. **Inadequate urinary drainage** as in cases of horseshoe kidney, unascended kidneys are more vulnerable for development of stones due to stasis.

8. **Randall's plaques:** Randall has suggested that initially a small erosion or an ulcer develops on the tip of renal papilla on which minute concretions or minor calcium particles get deposited and give rise to stone formation.

TYPES OF RENAL STONES

1. Calcium oxalate stone

• Called as mulberry calculi

• Common type of stone

• It is irregular having sharp projections

• Oxalate stone is hard and single

- Produce haematuria very early, resulting in deposition of blood over the stone giving a dark colour to the stone.
- It occurs in infected urine (Fig. 39.6).
- Contains alternate layer of calcium and bacterial vegetation. It is visualised in plain X-ray KUB.

2. Phosphate stone (Fig. 39.8, 39.9 and 39.10)

- Smooth, round
- Consists of triple phosphate of calcium, magnesium and ammonium.
- Dirty white to yellow in colour.
- Commonly occur in renal pelvis and tend to grow in alkaline urine.
- As it enlarges in the pelvis, it grows within the major and minor calyces and slowly forms **staghorn calculus**. This calculus produces recurrent urinary tract infection and haematuria and slowly damages the renal parenchyma (Fig. 39.5).

3. Uric acid stone (Fig. 39.7)

- Multiple, small, hexagonal, faceted, yellow coloured.
- Contain calcium oxalate which makes them opaque. Pure uric acid stones are radiolucent.
- Occur in acidic urine
- Common in patients who consume red meat

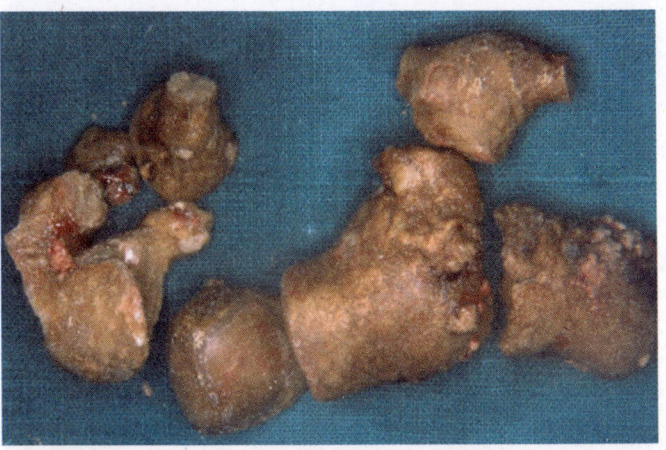

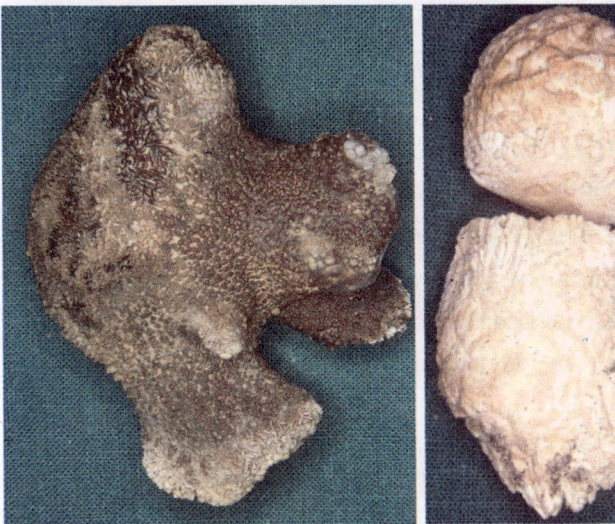

Fig. 39.8, 39.9 and 39.10 Staghorn calculi and phosphate calculi

4. Cystine calculus

- Cystinuria is an inborn error of metabolism which occurs due to decreased resorption of cystine from the renal tubules.
- Occurs in young girls at puberty.
- Increased excretion of cystine in urine results in cystine calculus.
- Stones are hard and radio-opaque due to sulphur content.

CLINICAL FEATURES

1. **Renal pain:** Dull aching to pricking type of pain posteriorly in the renal angle formed by the sacrospinalis and 12th rib. Murphy's kidney punch test demonstrates tenderness at renal angle. The same pain may some-

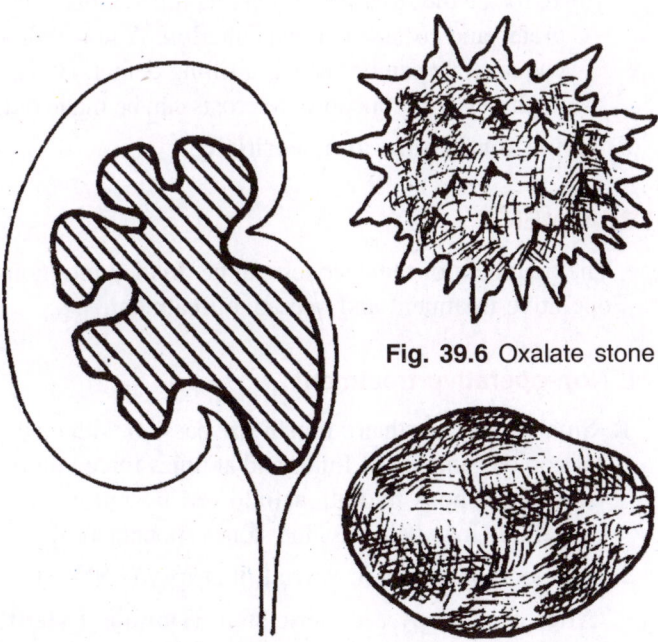

Fig. 39.6 Oxalate stone

Fig. 39.5 Staghorn calculi   **Fig. 39.7** Uric acid stone

times be felt anteriorly in the costal margin. Hence, it is described as costovertebral pain.

2. **Ureteric colic:** When the stone is impacted in the pelviureteric junction or anywhere in the ureter, it results in severe colicky pain originating at the loin and radiating to the groin, testicles, vulva and medial side of the thigh. This may be associated with strangury. The referred pain is due to irritation of the genitofemoral nerve.

3. **Haematuria:** is common with renal stone because the majority of the stones are oxalate stones. The quantity of blood lost is small but it is fresh blood.

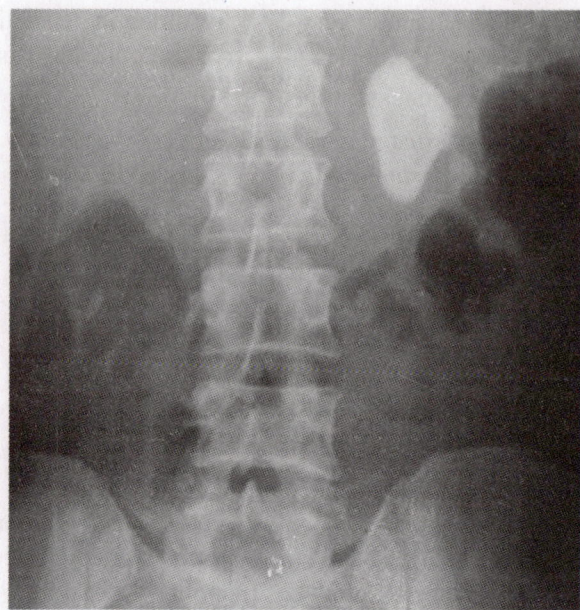

Fig. 39.11 Plain X-ray KUB showing large stone in the pelvis

Key Box 39.1

RENAL CONDITION - HAEMATURIA - CAUSES

1. Polycystic disease of kidney
2. Renal stone, ureteric stone
3. Renal tuberculosis
4. Carcinoma kidney
5. Papilloma of kidney
6. Renal infarction

---

4. **Recurrent U.T.I.:** Fever with chills and rigors, burning micturition, pyuria may occur, along with frequency of micturition.

5. **Guarding and rigidity:** of the back and abdominal muscles during severe attack of pain.

COMPLICATIONS

1. **Calculous hydronephrosis** occurs due to back pressure producing renal enlargement. Stretching of the renal capsule results in pain. In such cases, an associated palpable kidney mass, suggests hydronephrosis.

2. **Calculous pyonephrosis:** Infected hydronephrosis wherein the kidney is converted into a bag of pus.

3. **Renal failure:** Bilateral staghorn stones may not be symptomatic until they present with uraemia and renal failure.

INVESTIGATIONS

1. **Blood urea and creatinine** to rule out renal failure.

2. **Plain X-ray KUB:**
   - To diagnose stones 90% of the renal stones are radio-opaque.

   - Enlarged renal shadow can be made out

3. **USG**
   - Diagnosis of the stone and size can be made out.
   - Exact location of stone can be made out.
   - Can confirm the enlarged kidney due to dilatation of collecting system.

4. **IVP**
   - To locate the stone exactly in relation to kidney and ureter and to assess renal function. A non radio-paque stone can be seen as a filling defect. Hydronephrosis, hydronephroureterosis can be made out.

5. **Urine for culture and sensitivity**

TREATMENT

- The treatment of renal stones can be divided into non-operative treatment and operative treatment.

I. Non-operative treatment

1. Small stones less than 5 mm in size pass off with intake of copious amount of fluids and at times forced diuresis. Intravenous hydration followed by intravenous frusemide may help pass the stones spontaneously.

2. Extracorporeal Shock Wave Lithotripsy (**ESWL**)

   After cystoscopy a ureteric stent (**Double J stent**) is placed into the ureter on the side of a large renal stone. Shock waves are generated (around 500-1500

Key Box 39.2

ESWL

Advantages	Disadvantages
• No incision	• Cost factor
• No pain	• Availability
• Safe method	

shock waves) which blast the stone. The stones get crushed and most of the stones will come out by the side of the stent (Key Box 39.2).

II. Operative treatment

1. Endoscopic procedures
2. Open procedures
3. Special situations

1. Endoscopic procedures

Percutaneous nephrolithotomy (PCNL): RGP is done and stone is located in the pelvis of the kidney. With a small 1cm incision in the loin, the PCN needle is passed into the pelvis of the kidney and is confirmed by fluoroscopy. A guide wire is passed through the needle into the pelvis of the kidney. The needle is withdrawn with the guide wire within the pelvis. Over the guide wire the dilators are passed and a working sheath is introduced into the pelvis. A nephroscope is passed into the pelvis and if the stone is small it can be taken out. If it is big it may have to be crushed using ultrasound probes and the fragments are removed. Ultrasound or pneumatic energy is used for fragmenting.

Complications of PCNL

• Injury to the colon
• Injury to the blood vessels
• Urinary leak may persist for a few days
• Sepsis

2. Open surgical procedures

Depending upon the location of the stone, various types of procedures are done which are given below:

A. *Pyelolithotomy:* When there is extrarenal pelvis.

B. *Nephrolithotomy:* When there is intrarenal pelvis the stone has to be taken out through the kidney parenchyma.

C. *Extended pyelolithotomy:* By retracting the kidney parenchyma laterally, the incision over the pelvis can be extended over to the calyx and the stone can be extracted from the calyx, and even a large staghorn calculus can be removed.

D. *Pyelonephrolithotomy:* Stone is extracted through an incision in the pelvis as well as the renal parenchyma.

E. *Partial nephrectomy:* When the stone from a lower-most calyx is impacted, a lower pole nephrectomy can be done.

F. *Nephrectomy:* When the kidney is destroyed by pyonephrosis, following obstruction by stone.

3. Special situations

A. **Bilateral renal stones**: Kidney with better function has to be operated first. 1-2 weeks later, the opposite side can be operated.

B. If there is **pyonephrosis** with a severe degree of fever, pain and tenderness, **nephrostomy** is done and a tube drain is placed in the pelvis of the kidney for drainage of pus and urine. Once the pus is cleared, fresh assessment of renal function is done. If the kidney is nonfunctioning, nephrectomy is done. If the kidney is functioning ESWL/PCNL/open procedure is done. This is known as percutaneous nephrostomy (PCN).

Open procedures for the management of stone disease have become obsolete and are found in old surgery text books.

URETERIC STONE

Stones come down from pelvis of the kidney and may get impacted at any site of anatomical narrowing of ureter, namely:

1. Pelviureteric junction
2. Crossing of the iliac artery
3. Crossing of the vas deferens or broad ligament
4. Site of entry into the bladder wall
5. Ureteric orifice

This may lead to hydroureteronephrosis, renal parenchymal atrophy, infection and pyonephrosis.

Clinical features

1. Pain in the loin radiating to groin. Pain is severe, colicky, intolerable and lasts for a few hours. When stone descends into lower ureter, pain radiates to the testicles, labia majora and to the upper portion of thigh due to irritation of genitofemoral nerve. Colic lasts for about 4-6 hours and it is relieved by antispasmodics, narcotics and NSAID.

2. An attack of haematuria or pyuria

3. Guarding and rigidity of the abdominal wall if present on the right side, it is confused with acute appendicitis.

Investigations

- Same as renal stone

Treatment

1. Most of the ureteric stones pass via naturalis (urine). Patient is asked to consume a lot of water and antispasmodics.

2. **Flushing therapy:** Intravenous fluid about 2 litres, with 20-40 mg injection lasix (Frusemide). It can be repeated for a few days.

3. **Stone in the upper ureter:** ESWL is the ideal treatment.

4. **Middle ureteric stone:** ESWL, ureteroscopy basketing or open surgery (ureterolithotomy).

5. **Lower ureteric stone:** Ureteroscopic removal. With the usage of ureteroscope passed through the urethra, direct visualisation and manipulation of the stone even if it is impacted can be done. A laser lithotriptor or ultrasonic lithotriptor can be used to disintegrate the stone.

6. **Vesicoureteric junction:** Ureteroscopic removal or endoscopic meatotomy of vesicoureteric junction. For a stone impacted at uretero-vesical junction, cystoscopy is perfomed, ureteric orifice is identified and a cut is given at its mouth. Under fluoroscopic monitoring the stone can be manipulated and basketed out using a dormia basket or other types of baskets available.

7. **An impacted stone** which is not amenable to ESWL or fluoroscopic or ureteroscopic manipulation have to be extracted by ureterolithotomy (open surgical method).

Prevention of stone disease

1. Metabolic work up of urine and blood for identifying metabolic causes.

2. Fluid management

3. Dietary adjustments

4. Drug treatment
   - Xyloric, Soda bicarbonate - Uric acid stones
   - Potassium citrate - Calcium stones
   - Thiazides - Calcium stones
   - D-penicillamine - Cystine stones
   - Protease inhibitors - Infection stones

HYDRONEPHROSIS

DEFINITION

Aseptic dilatation of the whole or part of the pelvicalyceal system of the kidney due to partial or intermittent obstruction to the outflow of urine.

CAUSES OF UNILATERAL HYDRONEPHROSIS

I. Intraluminal (within the lumen)

1. Stones

II. Intramural (in the wall)

1. **Congenital:**

   A. Pelviureteric Junction (PUJ) abnormality (PUJ dyskinesia or achalasia of PUJ) is a congenital lesion where the hydronephrosis occurs due to failure of transmission of neuromuscular impulses through the narrow PUJ. It can also be bilateral. Female: Male Ratio = 2: 1.

   B. Ureterocoele, congenital narrow ureteric orifice.

2. **Acquired:**

   A. Carcinoma of the ureter, carcinoma of the bladder involving the ureteric orifice.

   B. Stricture of the ureter secondary to stone: After dislodgement of the stone there can be inflammatory stricture of the ureter.

   C. Tuberculosis of the ureter and bladder.

III. Extramural

1. Involvement of ureter by carcinoma cervix, rectum, bladder, the retroperitoneal tumours, primary or secondary deposits in lymph nodes.

2. Obstruction by aberrant vessels: Aberrant renal artery going to the lower pole of kidney can cause obstruction to the ureter causing hydronephrosis.
3. Retrocaval ureter
4. Horseshoe kidney
5. Idiopathic retroperitoneal fibrosis (Ormond's disease)

CAUSES OF BILATERAL HYDRONEPHROSIS

Lower urinary tract obstruction below the level of bladder neck will give rise to bilateral hydronephrosis (ORMOND's disease). Any of the causes for unilateral hydronephrosis when present bilaterally cause bilateral hydronephrosis.

I. Causes in children

1. Phimosis
2. Meatal stenosis
3. Posterior urethral valve
4. Bilateral vesico-ureteric reflux

II. In young adults

1. Stricture urethra is commonly due to gonococcal urethritis. Iatrogenic strictures following instrumentation of urethra, or a rupture urethra resulting in a stricture later is becoming more common.
2. Bilateral PUJ dysfunction.
3. Bilateral aberrant vessels : Many a time, these may be the branches of renal artery and vein which cross the ureters.

III. Causes in the middle age and above

1. Benign Prostatic Hypertrophy (BPH)
   • Common cause in middle age
2. Contracture of bladder neck

IV. Physiological: Pregnancy

• Due to growing foetus and partly due to the hormone progesterone.

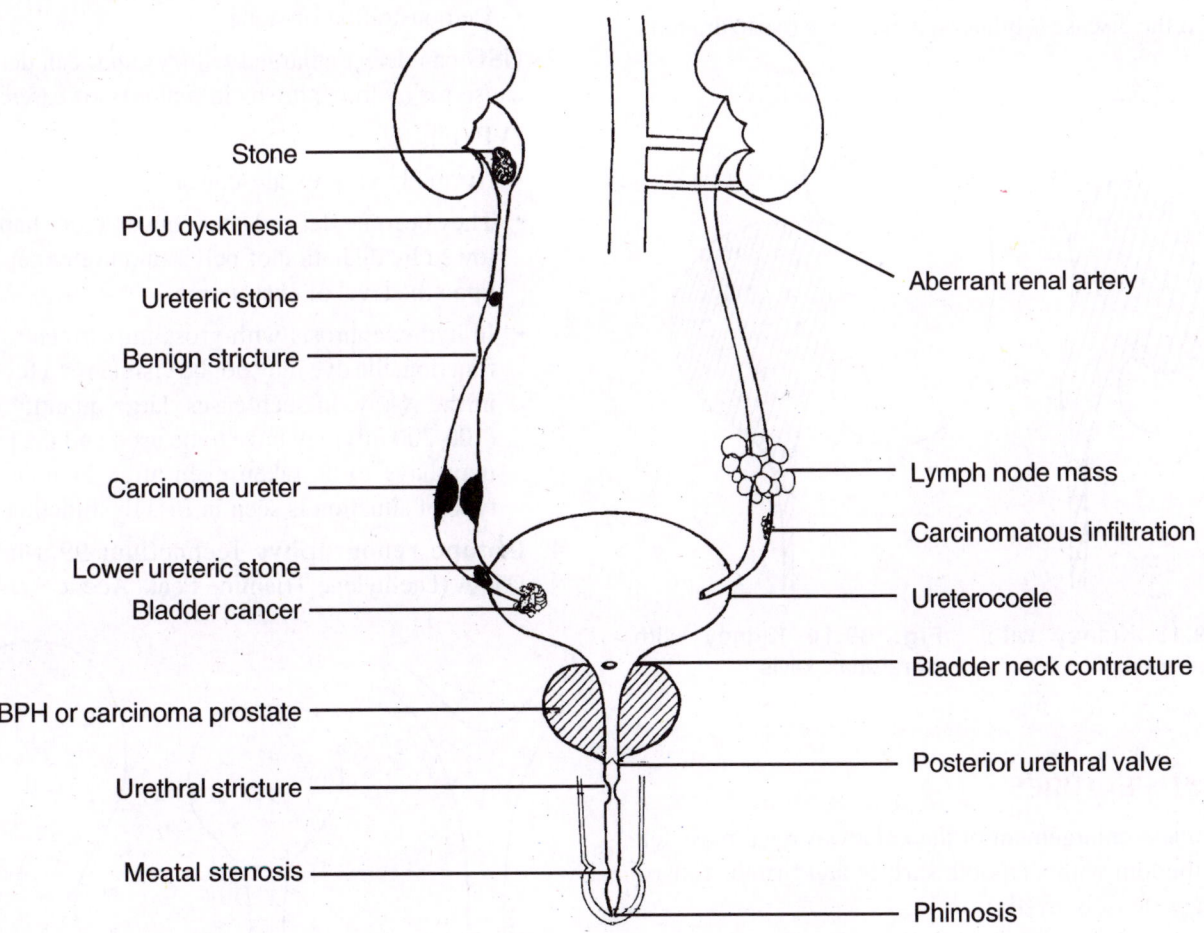

Stone
PUJ dyskinesia
Ureteric stone
Benign stricture
Carcinoma ureter
Lower ureteric stone
Bladder cancer
BPH or carcinoma prostate
Urethral stricture
Meatal stenosis

Aberrant renal artery
Lymph node mass
Carcinomatous infiltration
Ureterocoele
Bladder neck contracture
Posterior urethral valve
Phimosis

Fig. 39.12 Causes of hydronephrosis (bilateral)

PATHOGENESIS

The back pressure effect depends upon the type of the pelvis (Fig. 39.13 and 39.14).

1. In patients with intrarenal pelvis the kidney gets damaged very early. As the time goes on the urine gets diluted; all the salts are absorbed and is replaced by a watery type of fluid having a specific gravity of 1010.

2. Patients with extrarenal pelvis have minimal damage to the renal parenchyma for a long time.

3. Even if there is complete obstruction to the urinary flow in a hydronephrotic kidney, some amount of urine is secreted and some of it is absorbed by the renal pelvis and the collecting tubule and some by the lymphatics of the interstitial tissue of the kidney. The urine is thought to enter the interstitial space of the kidney from the pelvis through microscopic discontinuity (pyelo-sinus backflow - break) in the covering epithelium.

   • If the disease progresses further it leads to a non-functional kidney.

   • If the disease is bilateral it may give rise to uraemia.

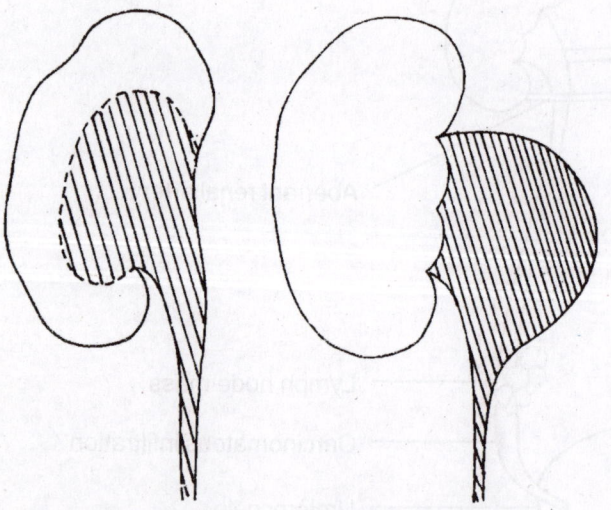

Fig. 39.13 Kidney with intrarenal plevis **Fig. 39.14** Kidney with extrarenal pelvis

CLINICAL FEATURES

1. Painless enlargement of the kidney. A renal mass felt in the loin with a smooth surface and firm in consistency (tensely cystic).

2. A dull aching pain in the loin

3. Previous history of calculus disease

4. Hypertension and haematuria are rarely seen in hydronephrosis.

5. **Dietel's crisis:**

   • It is intermittent hydronephrosis.

   • This is common in calculous hydronephrosis.

   • Following an attack of renal colic, ureteric obstruction occurs due to stone which results in enlargement of the pelvis of the kidney resulting in a palpable mass in the loin. After a few hours, the mass disappears due to the passage of a large quantity of urine due to reflux polyuria or due to slipping of the stone.

6. The symptoms of primary cause may be evident in the history e.g. colicky radiating abdominal pain due to stones and haematuria.

INVESTIGATIONS

1. **Plain X-ray KUB**

   • Enlarged renal outline can be made out

   • Demonstration of stone

2. **USG** can detect enlarged kidneys and can detect the cause for hydronephrosis in majority of cases.

3. **IVP** (Fig. 39.15)

   • Normally calyces are concave

   • They become flat and later convex/club shaped followed by dilatation of pelvis and ureter depending upon the level of obstruction.

   • In hydronephrosis with gross impairment of renal function, the dye may not be visible for a few hours in the X-ray. In such cases, large quantity of dye (100-200 ml) may have to be used and the pictures may have to be taken even after 24 hours. This type of situation is seen in PUJ dysfunction.

4. **Isotope renography:** Technetium 99m-labelled DTPA (Diethylene Triamine Penta Acetic Acid) scan

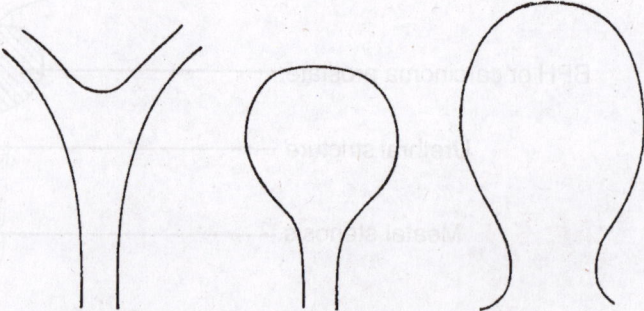

Fig. 39.15 Normal, flattened and club-shaped calyx

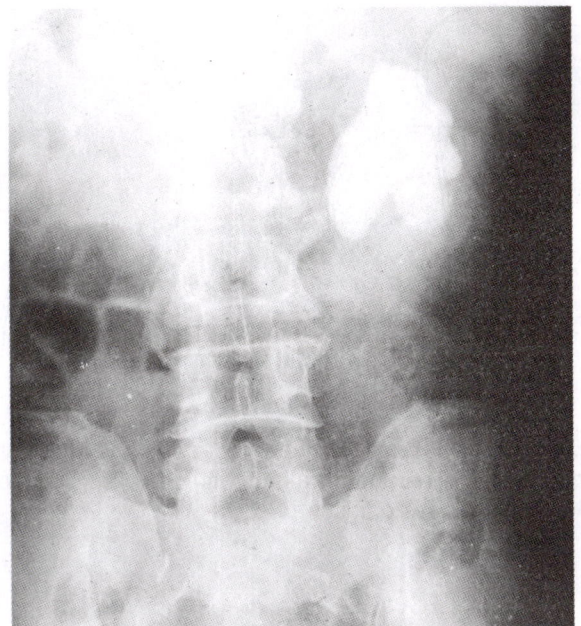

Fig. 39.16 Gross hydronephrosis due to PUJ obstruction

using a Gamma camera. The above Gamma Radiation emitter is injected intravenously and it can be detected to have been trapped in the urinary tract above the level of obstruction. It does not get washed off even after giving Frusemide injection.

5. **RGP**
   - When the IVP fails to demonstrate the kidneys, R.G.P is a useful investigation. This can be done just prior to definitive surgery for confirmation of the site of obstruction.
   - Less quantity of dye is required and better configuration of calyces can be made out.

6. **Blood urea, creatinine is estimated to rule out renal failure**

INDICATIONS FOR SURGERY

Key Box 39.4
INDICATIONS FOR SURGERY
• **P**ain • **A**trophy of kidney (damages) • **I**nfection • **N**ephrosis - hydronephrosis   Can be remembered as **PAIN**

TREATMENT OF HYDRONEPHROSIS

I . Hydronephrosis secondary to a cause

Treatment of the cause has to be done. Examples:

a. Stones: Pyelolithotomy, ureterolithotomy

b. Stricture: Stricturoplasty or excision and end to end anastomosis.

c. Aberrant vessel: Transection of the ureter and anastomosis in front of the vessel.

d. Phimosis: Circumcision

e. Meatal stenosis: Meatoplasty

f. Posterior urethral valve (PUV): Transurethral fulguration of the valve.

g. Benign prostatic hypertrophy (BPH): Transurethral resection of the prostate (TURP). Open prostatectomy.

h. Carcinoma of prostate: TURP + Bilateral orchidectomy + hormonal therapy. TURP in selected cases.

i. Stricture urethra: Visual internal urethrotomy or urethroplasty.

Principles of surgery

1. Non-functioning kidney with thinned out cortex with hydronephrosis/pyonephrosis-nephrectomy.

2. If the cortical thickness is adequate (0.5 cm) by ultrasonography, eventhough it is nonfunctioning kidney a preliminary nephrostomy to decompress the system has to be done. Reassessment of the renal function has to be done after a few days. If the renal function improves, definitive surgery for hydronephrosis has to be done. If it remains a non functioning kidney and the opposite kidney is normal, nephrectomy has to be done.

II. Patients with congenital hydronephrosis - PUJ dysfunction

Congenital hydronephrosis needs special mention here. With the increasing use of obstetric ultrasound, the incidence of antenatally detected fetal hydronephrosis is on the rise. In the present scenario, antenatal detection of fetal hydronephrosis has become the most common mode of presentation of congenital hydronephrosis.

Congenital hydronephrosis is defined as the antero-posterior diameter of renal pelvis > 10 cm at > 20 weeks of gestation; PUJ obstruction is the main cause. These fetuses undergo serial ultrasound monitoring during the rest of pregnancy and based on the increase or decrease in the pelvic diameter during this period, the postnatal management can be planned even before the child is born. Recently one study has graded antenatal hydronephrosis due to PUJ; on the basis of pelvic diameter and proposed the management guidelines (**Vikas Jain, Prof. Sasidharan et al -** KMC, Manipal).

Grades of Pelvic diameter

I   Mild   11-20 cm

II Moderate 21-35 cm

III Severe   >35 cm

- **Grade I hydronephrosis** can be managed conservatively by serial monitoring of pelvic diameter by ultrasound and renal functions by DTPA scan. This is known as conservative or nonoperative management. These kidneys improve over period of time.

- **Grade II hydronephrosis:** Majority (almost 80-90%) can be managed conservatively, however a close monitoring of the patient is required to detect any deterioration in renal function. Any deterioration in renal function is an indication for surgical intervention. In this group, 10-20% patients benefit from early surgery (patients with renal functions of involved kidney < 40%)

- All patients with grade III hydronephrosis should be operated early - Anderson-Hynes pyeloplasty to prevent permanent damage to kidney.

Types of pyeloplasty

1. Anderson-Hynes pyeloplasty

Principles

1. Excision of redundant pelvis

2. Disconnection of PUJ which is not functioning.

3. New ureteropelvic anastomosis is done in such a way that urine should drain by gravity.

- This is the most popular pyeloplasty called as dismembered pyeloplasty.

2. Non dismembered pyeloplasties

- They are Foley's Y-V plasty etc. also are being used. The PUJ is not transected. However, they are not very popular.

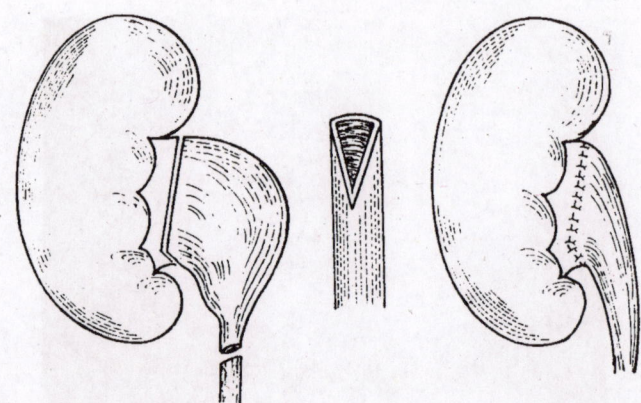

Fig. 39.17 Anderson - Hynes reduction pyeloplasty. **A** Excision of the redundant along with PUJ. **B.** Completed uretero-pelvic anastomoses

RENAL TUBERCULOSIS

- This is secondary to pulmonary tuberculosis/lymphatic tuberculosis. The primary focus is often difficult to identify.

- Common in males, in the age group 20-40 years

- Infection is always haematogenous

- Usually unilateral

PATHOLOGY (Fig. 39.18 to 39.25)

1. Tubercles develop and coalesce over the papilla which may ulcerate-**ulcerative form**.

2. The tubercles may caseate and rupture over the renal papilla and communicate with the pelvis **ulcerocavernous form**.

3. Attempt at healing produces calcification-**pseudocalculi** in the parenchyma of kidney.

4. Tubercular **hydronephrosis** is very rare. It is due to tubercular stricture of the pelvi-ureteric junction.

5. The opening of one of the calyces may get fibrosed leading to **hydrocalyx** which may distort rest of the calyces.

6. Tubercular **perinephric abscess** results due to cortical abscess which ruptures into the perinephric space. This may even point at the loin and rupture forming a sinus in the loin.

7. Tubercular **pyonephrosis** (Caseous kidney, putty kidney, cement kidney).

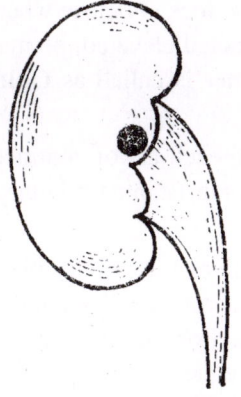

Fig. 37.18 Ulcerative form

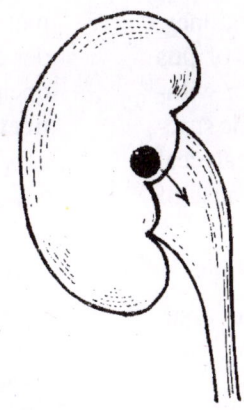

Fig. 37.19 Ulcerocavernous form

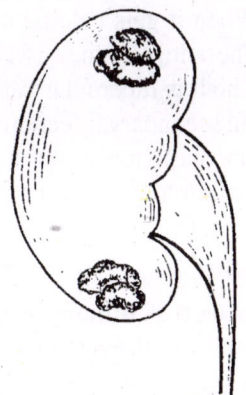

Fig. 37.20 Pseudocalculi

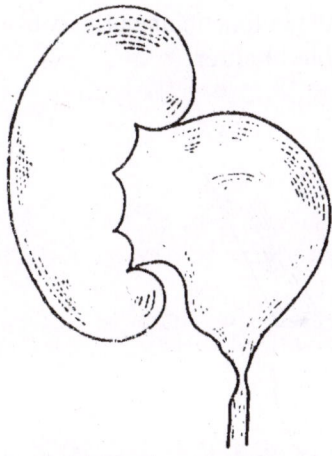

Fig. 37.21 Hydronephrosis

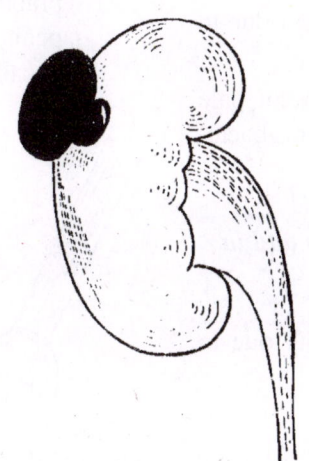

Fig. 37.22 Tuberculous perinephric abscess

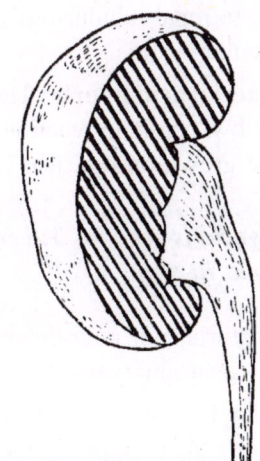

Fig. 37.23 Tuberculous pyonephrosis

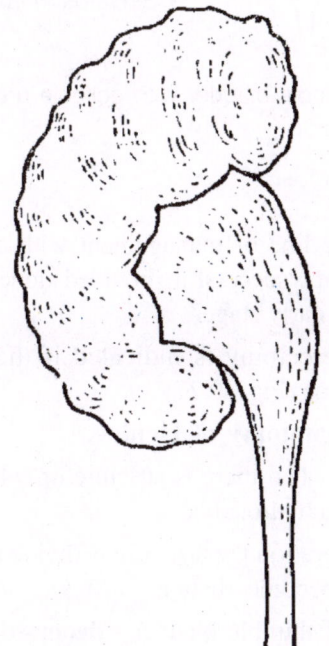

Fig. 37.24 Contracted kidney

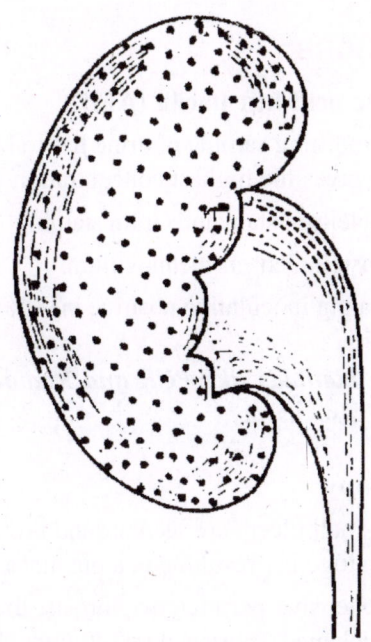

Fig. 37.25 Multiple tubercles - Miliary tuberculosis

- When it gets calcified, it is called cement kidney. The entire kidney is converted into a bag of pus which is tubercular caseous material with or without secondary infection. The complete ureteric stricture due to tuberculosis cutting off the pelvi-calyceal system may result in autonephrectomy because of fibrosis.
8. Small fibrosed, **contracted functionless kidney**
9. As a part of **miliary tuberculosis** - multiple small tubercles in the renal parenchyma

CLINICAL FEATURES

1. **Frequency** is the earliest symptom of tuberculosis. It is due to renal tubular inflammation and later due to tubercular cystitis.
2. **Abacterial acid pyuria:** The urine is opalescent, pale or yellow, acidic in reaction and no organisms/bacteria are grown on repeated culture.

Sterile pyuria is seen in Tuberculosis, Stones and in Carcinoma in situ.

3. Haematuria, not uncommon. Small quantity due to ulcerocavernous variety.
4. Evening rise of temperature.
5. Loss of appetite and loss of weight.
6. Evidence of pulmonary tuberculosis or lymphatic tuberculosis may be present.

INVESTIGATIONS

1. **Urine for acid-fast bacilli (AFB):**
   - Early morning sample of urine has to be examined which gives the highest concentration of AFB.
   - Ziehl-Neilsen stain and Gram staining
   - Lowenstein-Jensen media culture
   - Guinea pig inoculation positive in 90% of cases

Newer easy methods like PCR and Radioisometric culture are also used.

2. **Cystoscopy**

A. Initially small ulcers are seen around ureteric orifice. They join together resulting in a big ulcer.
   - Due to extensive periureteric fibrosis, the ureter becomes thickened, shortened and straight. The ureteric openings are lifted upwards and they are gaping which

means it does not contract/does not close when bladder contracts. Such contracted elevated, permanently opened lower end of ureter is called as **Golf hole-ureter.**
   - As a result of this with each act of contraction of bladder, there is reflux of urine into the kidney causing damage.

B. When the disease involves the urinary bladder, it results in fibrosis. It becomes small, contracted, ineffectively functioning. Storage capacity is lost resulting in intractable frequency, with few drops of urine. There is bleeding. Micturition is painful and is called strangury. There is also severe pain in suprapubic region which is referred to the tip of the penis. Such a small nonfunctioning urinary bladder is called as **thimble bladder.**

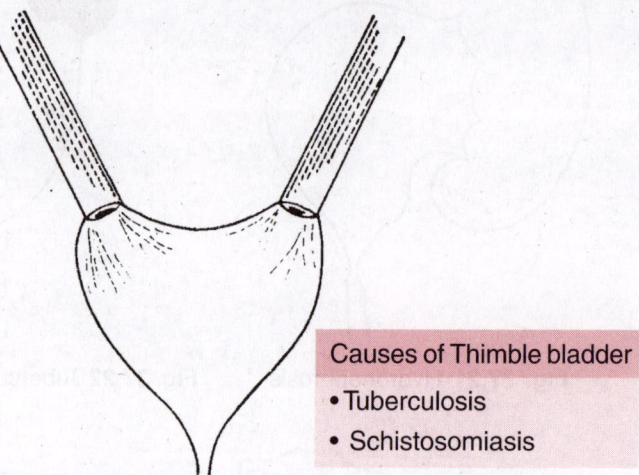

Causes of Thimble bladder
- Tuberculosis
- Schistosomiasis

Fig. 39.26 Thimble bladder with golfhole ureter (TB)

TREATMENT

1. Conservative line of management with antituberculous treatment is successful, provided kidneys are functioning as in early stages.
2. Nephroureterectomy is indicated if the kidney is nonfunctioning (Fig. 39.27)
3. **Renal cavernotomy of Henley:**
   - Indicated when there is stricture of calyces which results in a hydrocalyx.
   - In this operation the stricture is divided so that the drainage becomes better.
4. Treatment of thimble bladder - **ileocystoplasty.**
   - In this 10-15 cm of ileal loop is isolated based on

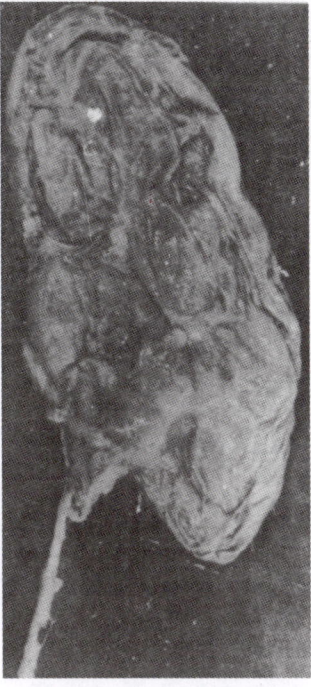

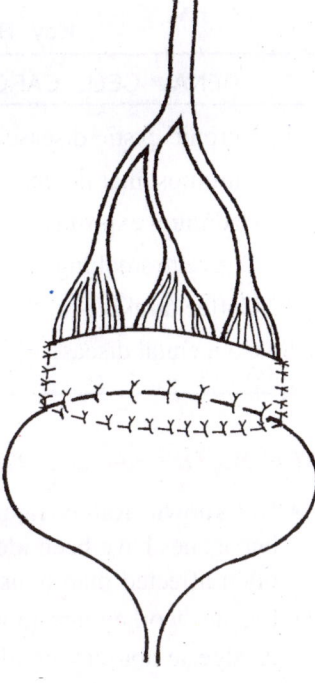

Fig. 39.27 Nephroureterectomy for renal tuberculosis (Prof. Sasidharan, Manipal)

Fig. 39.28 Ileocystoplasty

the blood vessels, the fibrosed bladder dome is excised, intestine is split open and sutured to urinary bladder (Fig. 39.28)

* This is to increase the capacity of bladder so as to store urine, and reduce frequency.

RENAL TUMOURS

CLASSIFICATION

* Benign: Adenoma, cortical adenoma; papilloma arising from pelvis, haemangioma
* Malignant: Nephroblastoma, renal cell carcinoma
* Transitional carcinoma (rare)
* Squamous cell carcinoma (extremely rare)

WILMS' TUMOUR (NEPHROBLASTOMA)

* This is a malignant tumour of the kidney occurring in children.
* The tumour is composed of epithelial and mesothelial elements. Thus, it may contain bone, cartilage, muscle, etc. Hence, it is called nephroblastoma (immature embryonic tissue).

* Tumour arises in one of the poles, distorting the reniform shape of the kidney. It is greyish white or pinkish white in colour. At places, there may be areas of haemorrhage/necrosis.
* Microscopic features include connective tissue elements cartilage, spindle cells, smooth striated muscle cells and epithelial elements.

CLINICAL FEATURES

1. Common in female children, around 2-4 years.
   * Less than 1 year of age carries good prognosis
   * Upper limit of age is 7 years
   * Rarely it may occur in adolescents
2. The child is brought with abdominal distension, due to hugely enlarged kidney which on palpation feels nodular.
3. Rarely, Wilms' tumour can be bilateral
4. Haematuria is a bad prognostic symptom, it is an indication of rupture of tumour into the pelvis of kidney. Most of such children are dead by 2 years of age.
5. Low grade fever can occur in rapidly growing tumour due to tumour necrosis, which releases pyrogens.
6. Rapid deterioration of health is characteristic.

INVESTIGATIONS

1. Abdominal USG can detect a solid tumour in the kidney. Ultrasound also rules out opposite kidney tumour.
2. CT scan to know extent of lesion and spread to the adjoining structures.
3. IVP is done to study distortion of calyces and to find out the function of the opposite kidney.
4. FNAC is done to confirm the diagnosis preoperatively.

DIFFERENTIAL DIAGNOSIS

1. Neuroblastoma arising from adrenals. This is more common than nephroblastoma.

SPREAD

1. Direct infiltration of the capsule
2. Lymphatic spread occurs to the hilar lymph nodes, para-aortic lymph nodes, mediastinal and left supra-clavicular lymph nodes.
3. Haematogenous spread occurs to the lungs, liver, bones, brain, etc. The tumour thrombus can extend to the renal vein and inferior vena cava.

TREATMENT

The anaemia has to be corrected at the earliest

1. For **tumours confined to renal capsule** or perirenal soft tissue not infiltrating the adjacent organs, radical nephrectomy followed by chemotherapy with actinomycin D and vincristine are given for 6 months.

2. For **tumours which have gone beyond renal capsule** and perirenal soft tissue, local infiltration to adjacent tissue, lymphatic metastasis, nephrectomy followed by local radiotherapy and chemotherapy is given with actimomycin D and vincristine for 15 months.

3. If the **tumour is found to be unresectable** by CT scan or magnetic resonance imaging (MRI), preoperative FNAC to confirm diagnosis is indicated followed by preoperative radiotherapy (1000 cGy) or chemotherapy and once the tumour regresses in size a nephrectomy has to be done. Post-operative chemotherapy is given with actinomycin D, vincristine and doxorubicin.

4. **Bilateral Wilms' tumour:** Side of the large tumour-radical nephrectomy, side of the small tumour - partial nephrectomy, should be done. As much of renal tissue as possible should be preserved after leaving a tumour free margin. Postoperatively the patient has to be treated with chemotherapy. If the surgery is not feasible only radiotherapy and chemotherapy has to be given.

Complications of radiotherapy

• Growth disturbances, cardiac and pulmonary toxicities.

RENAL CELL CARCINOMA (RCC)

• It is also called as **Hypernephroma - Grawitz tumour**.
• Commonly found in the age group 40-60 yrs.
• Male-female ratio: 2 : 1

Key Box 39.5

RISK FACTORS OF RCC

• Diabetes mellitus
• Chronic dialysis

Key Box 39.6

RENAL CELL CARCINOMA - ETIOLOGY

1. Chronic cystic disease
2. Chromosomal defect
3. Cadmium exposure
4. Cigarette smoking
5. Coffee drinking
6. Congenital disease - Von Hippel-Lindau disease

AETIOLOGY (Key Box 39.6)

• Not known. Rarely familial RCC is known. Specific oncogenes have been identified. Smokers are twice as often affected than nonsmokers.
• Leather workers are more prone for RCC.
• Analgesic abusers are also more prone.

PATHOLOGY

• Nearly all renal cancer in adults are adenocarcinoma.
• Cell of origin: Proximal renal tubular epithelium
• Starts in one of the poles, commonly in the upper pole and usually ruptures outside the capsule because of which reniform shape of kidney is maintained (Wilms' tumour grows within the capsule, hence the kidney shape is lost very early).
• On the outer surface, it is homogenous (Wilms' tumour is pleomorphic) and yellow in colour due to deposition of lipids.
• Few haemorrhagic areas are common because the tumour is very vascular.
• Microscopy: Clear cells and dark cells alternate.
• Tumour cells line the blood vessels which are responsible for early blood spread from renal cell carcinoma (like follicular carcinoma of thyroid-angioinvasion and capsular invasion).

CLINICAL FEATURES

I. Triad of renal cell carcinoma

1. Pain: Dragging or intermittent clot colic due to blood clot blocking the ureter.
2. Intermittent haematuria.
3. Palpable mass: Hard, nodular, ballotable or bimanually palpable, loin mass moving with respiration.

II. Other manifestations

1. **Pathological fractures**, e.g. fracture femur, humerus
   - Vascular, pulsatile, secondaries are common in the flat bones e.g. scalp, vertebra, rib, sternum because they contain red marrow for longer time.
2. **Anaemia** disproportionate to amount of haematuria is due to decreased production in erythropoietin.
3. Mild elevation of **temperature** is due to tumour necrosis producing pyrogens.
4. **Nephrotic syndrome** like features - rare.
5. **Endocrinal disturbances** are rare (paraneoplastic syndromes).
   a. Renin producing tumours are responsible for **hypertension**.
   b. **Polycythaemia** is due to increased erythropoietin secretion.
   c. Other hormones produced by the tumour are parathormone, ACTH, HCG, glucagon, prolactin.
6. **Hypertension**
7. **Liver dysfunction**. Non-metastatic liver dysfunction also known as Stauffer syndrome.

ROBSON'S STAGING OF RENAL CELL CARCINOMA

- Stage I : Tumour limited to kidney
- Stage II: Tumour invades perinephric tissues or adrenal gland, but does not extend beyond Gerota's fascia.
- Stage III : Tumour extends into major veins or lymph nodal involvement.
- Stage IV : Tumour invades beyond Gerota's fascia or distant metastasis.

TNM STAGING

TNM STAGING OF RENAL CELL CARCINOMA	
T_0	No tumour
T_x	Cannot be assessed
T_1	< 7 cms, within capsule
T_2	> 7 cms, within capsule
T_3	Extracapsular but within Gerota's fascia
T_{3a}	Into adrenal/ perinephric fat
T_{3b}	Extension into renal vein/ IVC
T_{3c}	Extension below diaphragm
T_4	Extension above diaphragm
N_0	No nodes
N_x	Cannot be assessed
N_1	Single < 2 cm
N_2	Single 2-5, multiple < 5 cms
N_3	> 5 cms
M_0	No metastasis
M_1	Distant metastasis +

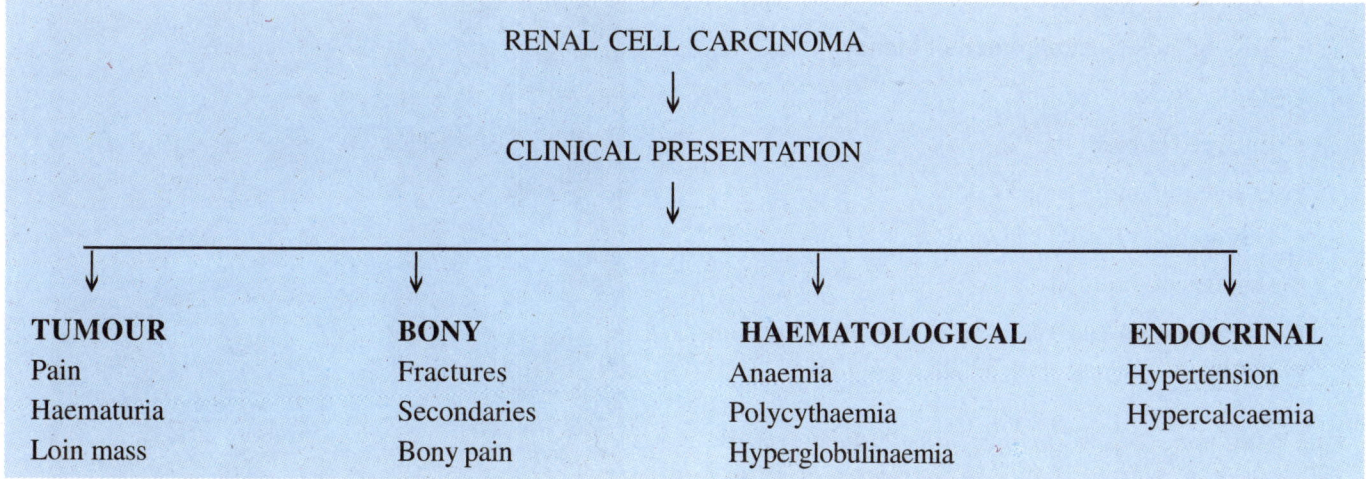

Fig. 39. 29 Flowchart of RCC showing clinical presentation.

STAGE GROUPING

Stage I	$T_1 N_0 M_0$
Stage II	$T_2 N_0 M_0$
Stage III	$T_1 N_1 M_0$
	$T_2 N_1 M_0$
	$T_3 N_1 M_0$
Stage IV	T_4 any $N M_0$
	Any $T N_2 N_3 M_0$
	Any T any $N M_1$

PATHOLOGICAL GRADES

G_1	:	Well differentiated
G_2	:	Moderate
$G_3 G_4$	:	Anaplastic or undifferentiated

INVESTIGATIONS

1. **Urine examination** is done when the patient has haematuria to see for malignant cells.

2. **Plain X-ray KUB** region: Enlarged kidney can be made out.

3. **IVP:**
   - Distortion of calyces
   - Missing of calyces
   - Loss of architectural pattern of kidney

4. **USG:**
   - Enlarged kidney
   - Locate tumour, site and extent
   - USG-guided FNAC can be done
   - Can detect thrombus in IVC

5. **Contrast enhanced CT scan is the investigation of choice** for staging (Fig. 39.30, 39.31).

Any renal mass which enhances after contrast on a CT scan in an elderly, should be considered as RCC until proved otherwise.

Key Box 39.7

CT SCAN

- Mixed density mass lesion
- Enhancement after contrast
- Secondary changes like tumour cell necrosis
- Local extent could be made out
- IVC thrombus and lymph node involvement identified.

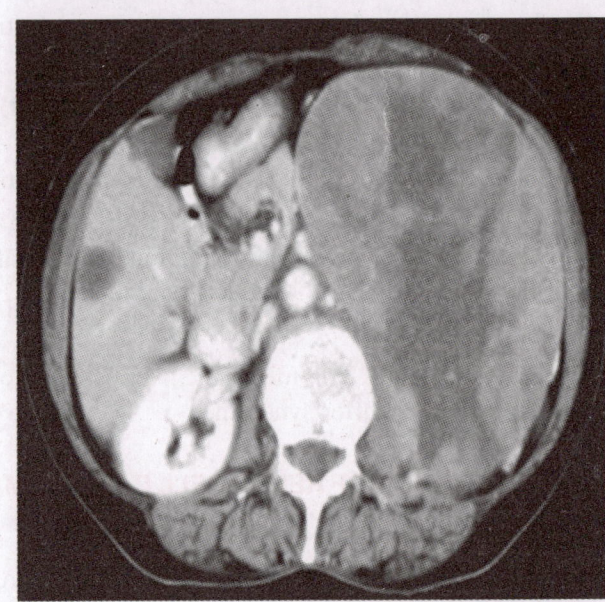

Fig. 39.30 CT scan showing left RCC

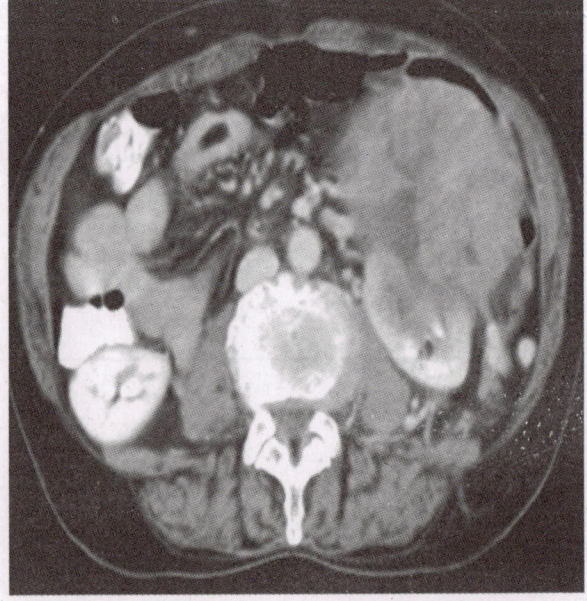

Fig. 39.31 Very extensive left RCC

6. **Renal angiography** is done by retrograde transfemoral approach. Features are given below.

   • **Neovascularization:** Tumour blush inside the tumour

   • **Venous phase** has to be observed to rule out tumour extension in the vein.

7. **MRI scan:** MRI scan is the investigation of choice to know the extent of IVC thrombosis (better than CT).

8. **Venacavogram:** It is done to know extent of tumour in IVC and presence of collateral circulation

TREATMENT

1. **Radical nephrectomy** (Fig. 39.32)

   • En bloc removal of entire Gerota' s fascia with its contents i.e. kidney, proximal ureter, adrenal gland.

   • Retroperitoneal lymph node dissection does not improve the survival rate.

2. **Extraction of tumour thrombus** (Fig. 39.33)

   • The tumour thrombus can extend along the renal vein into IVC and even into the right atrium.

   • Infradiaphragmatic tumour thrombus can be re-moved with proximal control over the vena cava. The supradiaphragmatic IVC thrombus requires cardiopulmonary bypass (Fig. 39.34).

   • In the absence of distant metastasis after removal of the thrombus these patients survive for a long duration.

3. **Therapeutic embolization**

   • This can be used as a palliative measure in advanced carcinoma to relieve symptoms. This can also be used preoperatively to regress the size of the large tumour.

   • A catheter is placed in the renal artery and substances like gel foam, blood clot, crushed muscle are injected; they block the lumen of the vessel and reduce size of the tumour so that radical nephrectomy can be undertaken later.

4. **Radiotherapy**

   • Not of much use. However, it is a good form of palliation for secondaries in the lung, bone and brain.

5. **Immunotherapy**

   • Administration of **interferon or interleukin-2** has been found to **improve the survival rate.**

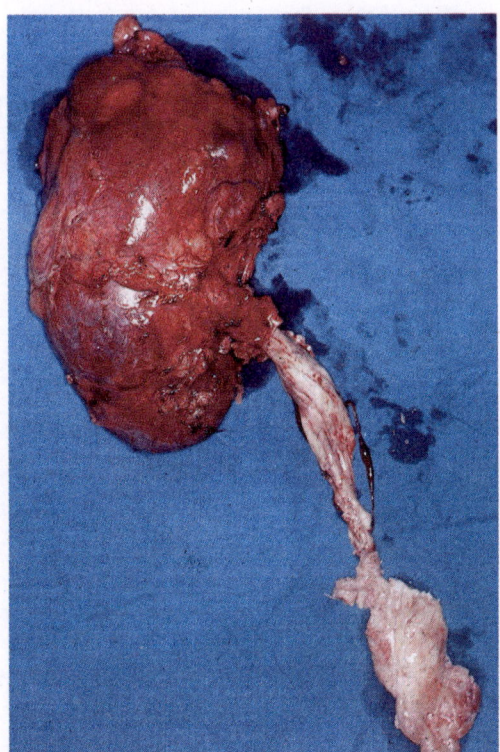

Fig. 39.32 Renal cell carcinoma - radical nephro ureterectomy specimen

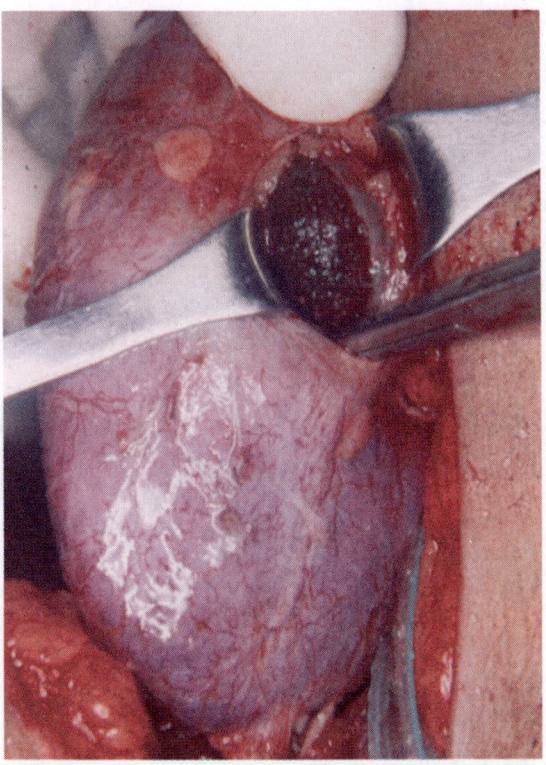

Fig. 39. 33 Radical nephrectomy with extraction of tumour thrombus

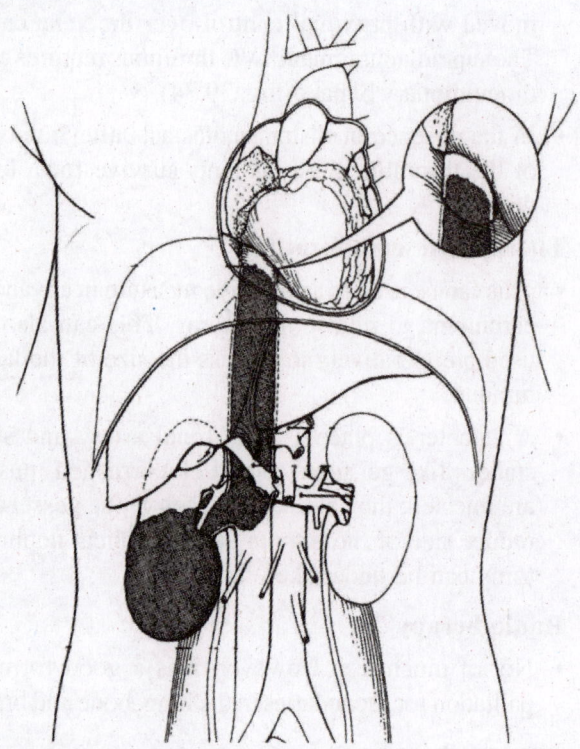

Fig. 39.34 Renal cell carcinoma with tumour thrombus in the renal vein, inferior venacava

TRANSITIONAL CELL CARCINOMA

Key Box 39.8
TRANSITIONAL CELL CARCINOMA PELVIS
• Uncommon tumour arises in the pelvis
• Multiple sites of urothelial mucosa involvement - often
• Low grade tumours
• Discovered late
• Haematogenous spread is common

RENAL MASS IN SURGICAL WARD (Table 39.2)

Clinical features of kidney mass

• Moves with respiration because the fascia of Gerota encloses the kidney and fuses above with the diaphragm

• Kidneys enlarge in the upward and downward direction.

• Bimanually palpable and ballotable.

• The colonic band of resonance is obliterated, when the kidney enlarges, where the colon is pushed laterally.

Table 39.2 Renal mass in surgical ward

		HYPERNEPHROMA	HYDRONEPHROSIS	POLYCYSTIC KIDNEY
1.	Chief symptoms	Haematuria, pain in the loin, renal mass	Asymptomatic distension, abdomen pain	Mass abdomen, hypertension, haematuria
2.	Age of the patient	More than 50 years	20-30 years	30-40 years
3.	Sex incidence	Common in males	Common in females	Common in females
4.	Anaemia	Present	Absent	May be present
5.	Features of renal failure	Absent	Can be present in bilateral cases (rare)	May be present
6.	Renal mass	Unilateral, nodular, hard, may be fixed, non-tender	Can be bilateral, smooth, cystic, feels firm, not fixed,. non-tender	Bilateral, bosselated, nodular, not fixed, non-tender
7.	Features of kidney mass	Ballotability, movement with respiration may be restricted or absent if an advanced malignancy	Present	Present
8.	I.V.U.	Irregular calyces	Gross dialation of pelvicalyceal system	Spider-leg deformity of calyceal system
9.	FNAC	Can give diagnosis	Not indicated	Not indicated
10.	Treatment	Radical nephrectomy	Pyeloplasty	Symptomatic, renal transplantation

ACUTE SURGICAL INFECTIONS OF THE KIDNEYS

PYONEPHROSIS

In this condition, the entire kidney is converted into a sac containing pus or purulent urine. Almost always the renal parenchyma is destroyed totally.

Causes

1. Renal **calculous disease** is the most common cause of pyonephrosis.
2. **Acute pyelonephritis** is more common in children and in females. Inadequately treated cases may develop into pyonephrosis, specially when pyelonephritis is associated with urinary tract obstruction.
3. **Infection** of a hydronephrosis

Clinical features

- Anaemia
- Fever
- Renal swelling
- Large swelling with high grade fever with chills and rigors suggest an imminent danger of septicaemia and calls for an immediate drainage of the pus.

Investigations

1. Urine examination may be positive for coliforms and other gram-negative organisms.
2. Plain X-ray KUB may reveal a stone or an enlarged renal outline.
3. Ultrasound can confirm hydronephrosis.
4. Intravenous urogram demonstrates poor function of the kidney on the diseased side. As a rule the opposite kidney is normal.

Treatment

- Broad spectrum **antibiotics** (parenteral) should be started immediately once the urine and blood is sent for culture sensitivity.
- Ultrasound - guided **aspiration** of pus or a percutaneous nephrostomy (better), and drainage of pus greatly improves the general condition of the patient.
- If any **obstruction or causative agent** is found such as a stone, it **should be removed**.
- **Nephrectomy** should be considered if the kidney is non-functioning with significant damage.

PERINEPHRIC ABSCESS

It refers to the collection of pus in the perirenal area.

Causes

1. Infection in a perirenal haematoma
2. Pyonephrosis when it ruptures
3. TB perinephric abscess
4. Pus from retrocaecal appendicitis can extend into loin, perinephric area and may present as abscess.

Clinical features

1. High swinging temperature
2. Rigidity, tenderness, fullness in loin
3. Oedema, in the loin

Investigations

1. Total count: Raised above 20,000 cells/mm^3
2. Urine analysis: No organisms are usually found
3. X-ray spine: Scoliosis with concavity towards abscess
4. Screening chest: Diaphragm is immobile and elevated on the diseased side.

Treatment

- Pus is drained by an incision in the loin, breaking all the loculi.

DIALYSIS

- In the end stage renal disease, until a transplantation is carried out, haemodialysis or peritoneal dialysis may be required.

1. Peritoneal dialysis

- Here a bag is worn by the patient and even when he is working dialysis continues. This is called as **Continuous Ambulatory Peritoneal Dialysis (CAPD)**.

Principle

- Fluid solution containing electrolytes and glucose is introduced into the peritoneal cavity and later it is drained by using a sterile, closed system. Sodium is the chief electrolyte.

Complications

1. Fluid and electrolyte abnormalities
2. Peritonitis

2. Haemodialysis: Principle

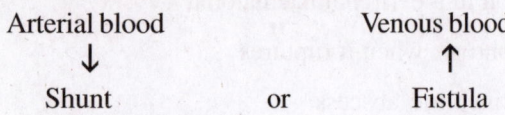

Arterial blood   Venous blood
$$\downarrow \qquad\qquad\qquad \uparrow$$
Shunt   or   Fistula

Shunt

Two sites are selected

1. **At the wrist:** Radial artery and cephalic vein are connected by insertion of teflon cannula.
2. **Ankle:** Posterior tibial artery and long saphenous vein.

These are examples of acquired A.V. fistula.

Complications of shunt

- Thrombosis
- Infection

RENAL TRANSPLANTATION

Preparation for transplantation

- Recipient is prepared by haemodialysis. It will also enhance the chances of success for a transplant.

Donors

Two sources

A. Cadaver kidney is got from 'brain dead patients' who are still living with mechanical support with ventilators. Consent should be taken from patient's relatives.
B. Living

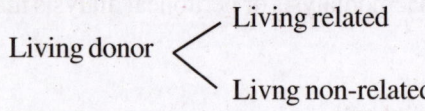

Living donor
     Living related
     Livng non-related

Criteria of an ideal donor

1. Less than 60 years of age
2. No previous renal disease
3. No diabetes
4. No hypertension
5. Adequate renal perfusion 50 ml/hr urine output is necessary.
6. No systemic infections, like hepatitis B, C, HIV infection.
7. No malignancy

Living related donors

- An identical twin
- Father or mother
- Son or daughter is ideal
- Brother or sister

Tests done before transplantation

- Blood group ABO compatibility
- Biochemical investigations
- Complete blood picture
- Renal function tests
- Rule out: Diabetes, hypertension, hepatitis B infections, hepatitis 'C' infection, HIV.
- Bilateral renal angiography to study vascular pattern
- Tissue typing

Recipient contraindication to renal transplantation is if the recipient is suffering from diseases such as heart disease or malignancy (advanced) which compromises his survival.

Operation technique

Donor operation

1. **Living related donor:** Donor nephrectomy with preserving as much length of the artery, vein and ureter.
2. **Cadaver donor:** Kidney is perfused with icy perfusion fluid and removed along with vena cava and aorta and packed in plastic bags surrounded by ice in an insulated box. It can be stored like this for 72 hours.

Perfusion fluid: It has high concentration of potassium (80 mmol/L) and high osmolarity (400 mosmol/kg). This is used during transplant anastomosis.

Recipient operation

- Kidney is transplanted in the right iliac fossa by anastomosing renal artery with internal iliac artery and renal vein with external iliac vein. Ureter is implanted in the bladder.

Postoperative management

1. Immunosuppression
   - Cyclosporin A is given alone or in combination with low doses of azathioprine and steroids.
2. Fluid balance

- Aim to maintain urinary output at the rate of 20 ml/hour. Even an anephric patient needs 500 ml of fluid/day to replace insensible loss. CVP is ideal for management of fluids in the postoperative period.

3. Postoperative oliguria

Causes

a. **Acute tubular necrosis (ATN):** Minimal ATN is common due to short ischaemic time. Hence, oliguria phase may be few hours.

b. **Rejection:** More likely on the 5th day. Twice weekly DTPA (Diethyl Triamine Penta-acetic Acid) isotope renography and gamma camera scan of the kidney confirms perfusion of the kidney when oliguria is present. Percutaneous needle biopsy can confirm the rejection.

Treatment of rejection

1. **Acute rejection:** Within 3 months, this responds to high doses of intravenous steroids. 90 mg methylprednisolone IV/day x 3 days.

2. Chronic rejection involves the vascular element. Does not respond to steroids.

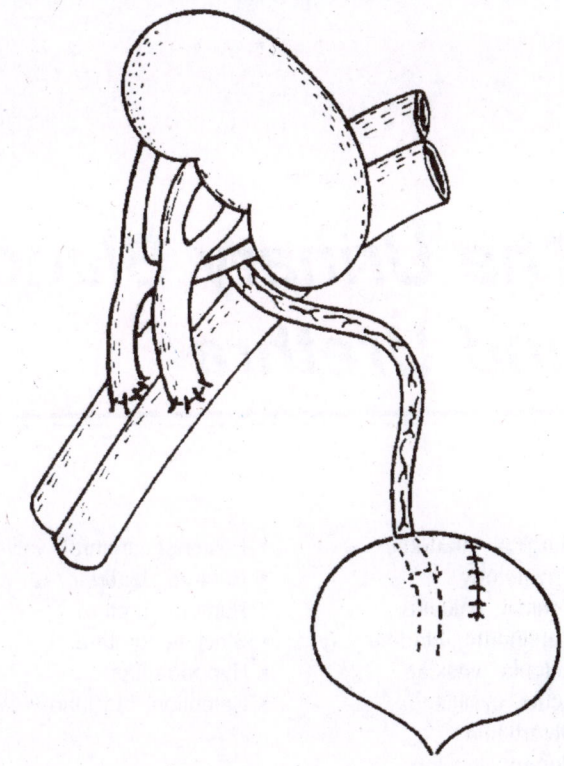

Fig. 39.35 Diagramatic representation of renal transplantation

Surgical complications

1. Haemorrhage manifests as oliguria, hypotension. Wound should be reexplored, and bleeding vessels should be ligated.

2. Renal artery thrombosis results in nonfunctioning of the transplanted kidney. It can be diagnosed by ultrasonogram and isotope studies. This is treated by nephrectomy.

3. Renal artery stenosis can develop later. It should be treated by an angioplasty.

4. Lymphocoele can develop due to perivascular dissection and increased flow of lymph. Such lymphocoele can lead to ureteric obstruction. Small collection needs to be observed, large ones need drainage.

5. Ureteric obstruction or urinary leakage due to disruption of ureteroneocystostomy can be due to ischaemia, necrosis of the distal ureter. During donor nephrectomy care should be taken not to remove too much of periureteric tissues and avoid too much dissection in the renal hilum to prevent ureteric ischaemia.

The Urinary Bladder and Urethra

40

- Surgical anatomy
- Physiology
- Vesical calculus
- Carcinoma bladder
- Ectopia vesicae
- Acute cystitis
- Diverticula
- Urinary fistulae
- Schistosoma haematobium
- Urinary diversion
- Posterior urethral valve
- Rupture bladder
- Rupture urethra
- Stricture urethra
- Hypospadias
- Retention of urine

SURGICAL ANATOMY OF THE BLADDER

Lining epithelium

- Urinary bladder is lined by transitional epithelium that covers a connective tissue known as lamina propria.

- Bladder cancers are **transitional cell carcinomas**. However, due to changes in the epithelium caused by chronic irritation (stone), one can get other malignancies such as squamous cell carcinoma.

- Bladder cancer can easily spread through lamina propria into the muscle coat (**detrusor muscle**).

Detrusor muscle

- It is a smooth muscle, fibres of which are intermingled. Hence, in cases of bladder neck obstruction, changes such as trabeculations/sacculations due to hypertrophy of this muscle is found.

Trigone

- It is a triangular area lying between the internal urethral orifice and the orifices of the ureter. It is the most sensitive part of the bladder, irritation of which is mainly responsible for frequency of micturition.

Bladder neck

- Internal sphincter is the smooth muscle which surrounds the bladder neck. It is innervated by α adrenergic fibres and it prevents retrograde ejaculation.

- Distal urethral sphincter is a somatic striated muscle which is supplied by S_2-S_4 fibres via pudendal nerves.

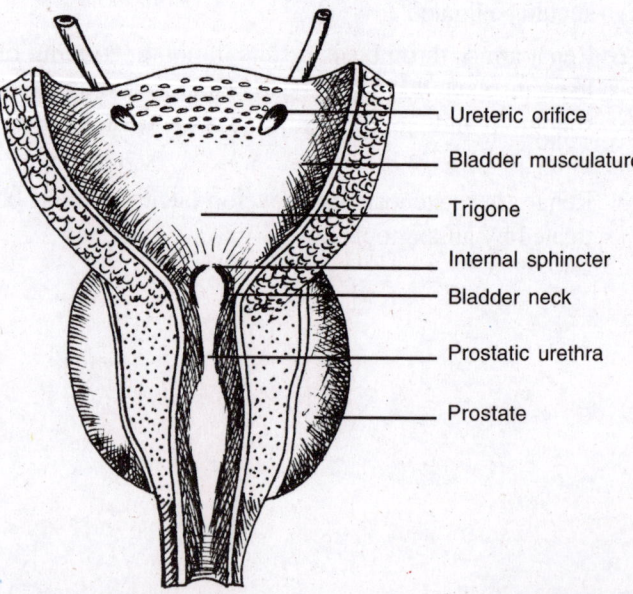

Ureteric orifice
Bladder musculature
Trigone
Internal sphincter
Bladder neck
Prostatic urethra
Prostate

Fig. 40.1 Surgical anatomy of the urinary bladder

Supports of the bladder

- Posteriorly **endopelvic fascia,** which is continuous with lateral ligaments of the rectum, need to be divided during radical cystectomy.
- Anteriorly **pubo-prostatic ligaments** also need to be divided during radical cystectomy.
- **False ligaments:** Urachus and obliterated hypogastric arteries together with the fold of peritoneum overlying these structures are called as false ligaments (median and lateral ligaments).

Blood supply

- **Superior and inferior vesical arteries** are derived from anterior trunk of internal iliac artery as the main source of arterial blood supply. Minor blood supply comes from obturator, inferior gluteal and in females from uterine and vaginal arteries also.
- **Veins** form plexus on lateral and inferior surfaces of the bladder. Hence during suprapubic cystostomy, these structures have to be avoided while entering into the bladder.
- **Vesical plexus** is continuous with prostatic plexus of veins in males which drain into the internal iliac vein.

Lymphatics

- Internal iliac nodes are the first level of lymph nodes.
- Obturator and external iliac lymph nodes get involved later.

Innervation

- **Parasympathetic** comes from anterior divisions of sacral nerves - $S_2S_3S_4$ through inferior hypogastric plexus. Following excision of rectum, disturbance of micturition and sexual function can occur due to damage to the pelvic plexus.
- **Sympathetic** supply comes from 11th thoracic to second lumbar segments.

VESICAL CALCULUS

- **Primary:** Stone which develops in sterile urine.

  They develop in the absence of bladder pathology. These also include renal stones which have migrated to the bladder.

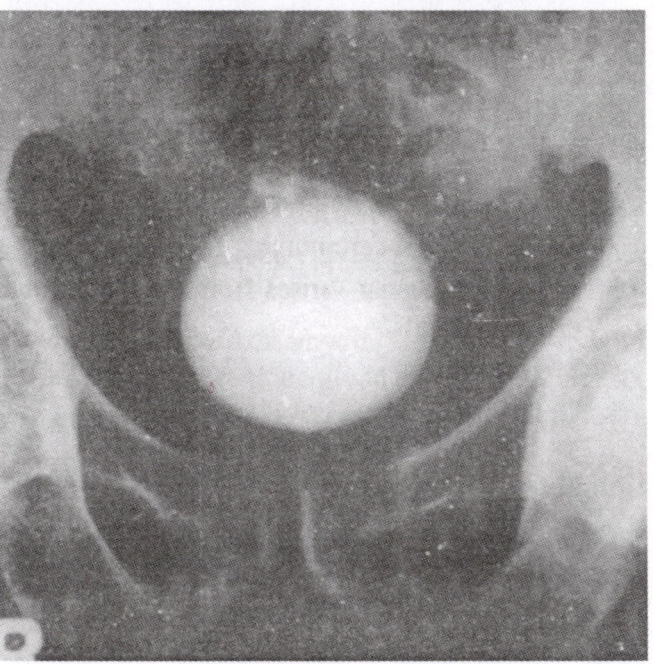

Fig. 40.2 Bladder Stone

- **Secondary:** Stone develops in presence of infection and stasis due to obstruction to the urinary flow.

  They develop secondary to bladder pathology.

TYPES

1. **Oxalate stone:** Moderate size, uneven surface, mulberry stone, is dark brown or black because of incorporation of blood pigment in it.

2. **Uric acid stone:** Round to oval, smooth, pale yellow, not opaque to X-rays. They are primary stones.

3. **Cystine:** Radio-opaque due to high sulphur content

4. **Triple phosphate:** These stones consist of ammonium, magnesium and calcium phosphates. They occur in **urine infected with urea-splitting organisms**. Sometimes, they grow rapidly. The nucleus of the stone can be made up of bacteria, desquamated epithelium or a foreign body. Dirty white in colour

CLINICAL FEATURES

1. **Frequency** of micturition is the earliest symptom of bladder stone. It is due to cystitis.

2. **Pain** at the end of micturition referred to tip of penis in young boys suggests bladder stone. In school-going

children, pain is aggravated by jumping and jolting. Pain is decreased on lying down because stone falls away from the trigone of the bladder. Typically, oxalate stones produce pain. Painful ineffective micturition is described as strangury.

3. **Haematuria,** is due to stone causing abrasions in the bladder mucosa.

4. **Acute retention of urine** due to the calculus obstructing the internal meatus.

5. **Males** are affected 8 times more frequently than females.

INVESTIGATIONS

1. **Urine:** Red blood cells may be present - microscopic haematuria

   • Envelope-like crystals: Oxalate stone

   • Hexagonal plates: Cystine calculi

2. **Radiography:** In 90% of the cases, the stone is visible. However, it is important to look for stones in the entire urinary tract.

3. **Cystoscopy:** Stone can be visualised.

   • A **click** can be heard when the stone comes into contact with the instrument.

TREATMENT

I. **Litholapaxy:** By introducing a cystoscopic lithotrite, stone is grasped firmly and broken. Small fragments of stone are evacuated by using evacuator.

   Contraindications for litholapaxy:

   1. **Urethra:** Obstruction like stricture, enlarged prostate.

   2. **Bladder:** Cystitis, contracted bladder, carcinoma.

II. **Suprapubic cysto-lithotomy:** Can be done (Page 813) when the stone is too big, too hard to crush or too soft.

CARCINOMA OF THE BLADDER

AETIOLOGY

1. Incidence is more in aniline dye workers. Products such as benzidine and 3-naphthylamine are carcinogenic.

2. Cigarette smoking

Key Box 40.1

**BLADDER CANCER
AETIOLOGY**

• Aniline dye workers
• Bilharziasis
• Chronic irritation
• Chronic smoking
• Cyclophosphamide

Key Box 40.2

**BLADDER CANCERS
HIGH RISK - OCCUPATIONS**

• Aniline dye workers
• Leather industry workers
• Paint industry workers
• Rubber industry workers

---

3. Chronic irritation by stones, catheter, also can produce carcinoma: 95% of the tumours originate in mucous membrane.

4. Bilharziasis or schistosomiasis increases the chances of bladder cancer (squamous cell carcinoma).

PATHOLOGY

1. **Malignant villous tumours:** They are transitional cell carcinomas. Multiple primaries are found in 25% of patients with bladder cancer.

   a. The villi are stunted, swollen and resemble cauliflower. They are slow growing.

   b. Can be sessile. Such tumours are high grade

   c. Bladder wall is more vascular.

   d. Submucous lymphatic nodules appear around the growth.

2. **Solid tumours are always malignant.** They are sessile, lobulated.

3. **Carcinomatous ulcer:** It arises in **leukoplakia.**

HISTOLOGICAL TYPES

1. Transitional cell carcinoma - 90% of tumours

2. Squamous cell carcinoma

3. Adenocarcinoma arises from urachal remnants and urethral glands

4. Mixed variety

5. Undifferentiated

CLINICAL FEATURES

1. In 90% of cases, initial symptom is **painless, intermittent haematuria.**

2. **Severe cystitis** like symptoms occur in carcinomatous ulcer.

3. Later painful, **blood stained micturition** can occur.

4. **Strangury:** Painful micturition with bleeding and incomplete emptying of bladder.

5. **Loin pain** is due to ureteric obstruction with hydronephrosis.

6. **Suprapubic pain,** groin pain, perineal pain are due to infiltration of nerves. This indicates the advanced nature of the growth.

INVESTIGATIONS

1. **Urine:** Cytology of a 3 hour specimen.

2. **IVP:** Filling defect in bladder, dilatation of ureter can be detected (Fig. 40.3).

3. **Ultrasound** is a very useful investigation which can detect a bladder carcinoma (Fig.40.4 and 40.5). It can also detect liver metastasis.

4. CT scan is the investigation of choice specially to know the spread of the disease (Fig. 40.6, 40.7 and 40.8).

   • Specially it is useful to know the infiltration of the muscle, perivesical tissue and also the prostate and pelvic wall.

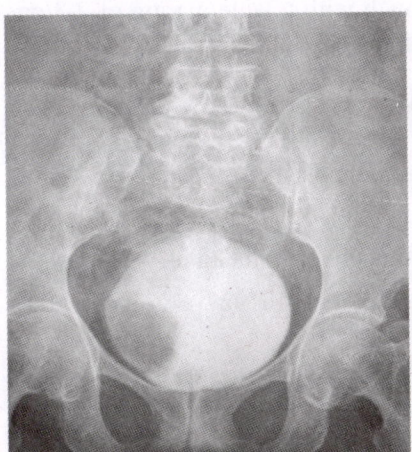

Fig. 40.3 IVU showing filling defect

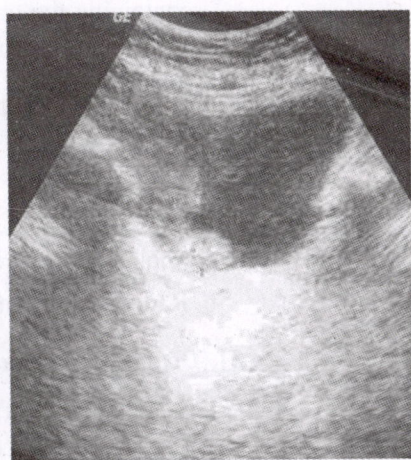

Fig. 40.4 Ultrasound suggesting carcinoma bladder

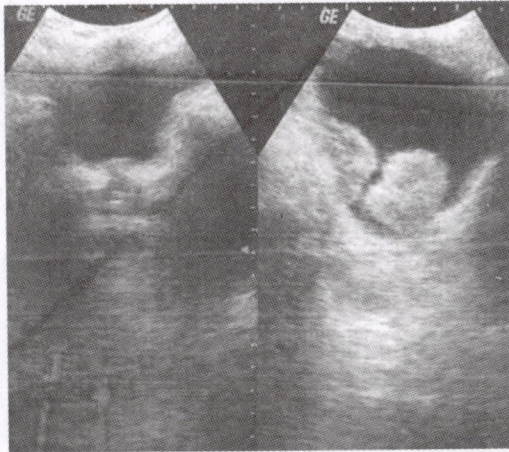

Fig. 40.5 Ultrasound suggesting carcinoma bladder

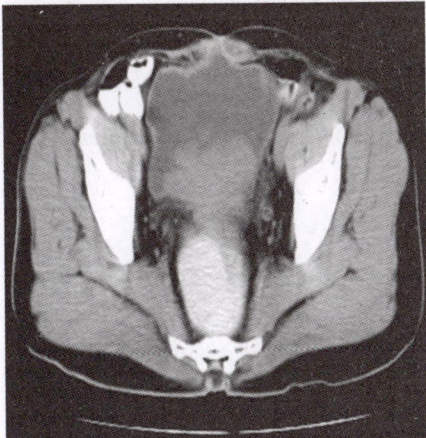

Fig. 40.6 Plain CT of the bladder

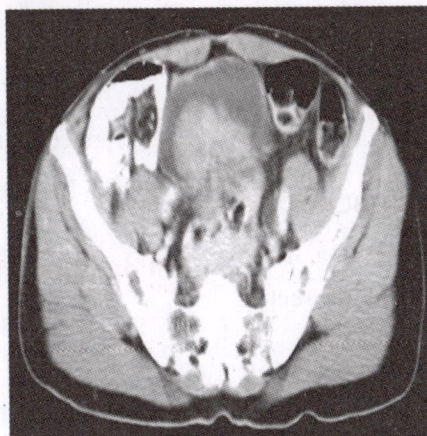

Fig. 40.7 Contrast CT of the bladder

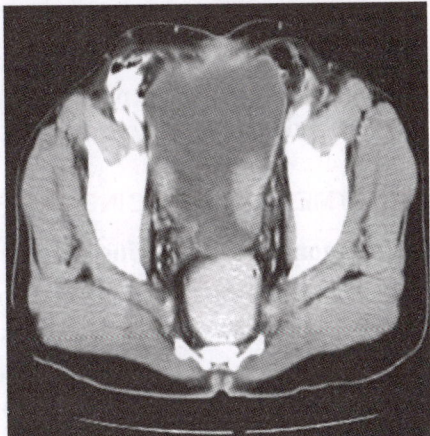

Fig. 40.8 Contrast CT of the bladder

5. **Cystoscopy:** To locate the lesion and to take biopsy

6. **Bimanual palpation,** rectoabdominally in males and vaginoabdominally in females is done under general anaesthesia. Thickening of bladder wall, mobility, fixity and hardness can be made out.

STAGING OF BLADDER CANCER

1. TNM

Tis Tumour in situ
Ta Tumour involving mucosa without invading the lamina propria
T1 Tumour involving mucosa invading lamina propria and submucosa
T2 Tumour involving the muscle layer
T3a Tumour involving the muscle layer throughout the thickness
T3b Tumour extending to the perivesical fat or peritoneum and involving the adjacent organs
T4 Involvement of the rectum and prostate
N0 No lymph nodes
N1 Lymph nodal metastasis
M0 No distant metastasis
M1 Distant metastasis present

2. Clinical Staging - Jewett, Strong and Marshall system

• Clinically the tumours are broadly classified into 3 groups - Superficial or non-invasive, infiltrating or invasive and carcinoma *in situ*.

TREATMENT OF CARCINOMA URINARY BLADDER

I. Carcinoma not involving muscle layer (Tis Ta, T1)

a. Transurethral resection (TUR) of tumour (resected base to be screened for tumour by microscopy).

b. Postoperative intravesical chemotherapy with Thiotepa/Adriamycin/Mitomycin retained inside the bladder for 1 hour. Such 6-8 courses at weekly interval are given to reduce recurrence.

c. BCG or interferon immunotherapy given postoperatively intravesically to prevent tumour recurrence.

II. T2-T4 lesions: Radical cystectomy followed by systemic chemotherapy (MVAC-Methotrexate, Vinblastine, Adriamycin, Cisplatin). (Vide infra)

Radical cystectomy

Removal of the bladder with pericystic fat and the prostate and seminal vesicles, urethra in men and bladder and pericystic fat, cervix, uterus, anterior vaginal vault, urethra and ovaries in women. It is a major surgery with 3 to 8% mortality rate.

III. Any T, N1, M0 or any T, N0, M1-**Systemic chemotherapy** (**MVAC**) followed by radiation therapy has to be given.

IV. Small lesion involving muscle in the vault of bladder or posterolateral wall of the bladder, **partial cystectomy** (segmental resection) of that part of the bladder containing the growth with a wide margin of 2-3 cm. This should be followed by intravesical chemotherapy.

ROLE OF RADIOTHERAPY

I. Local: If lesion is not anaplastic, is 4 cm or less, after open diathermy excision, radiotherapy can be given.

a. Implantation of radioactive Gold Grains-Au198
b. Radioactive Tantalum Wire-Ta192

II. Deep X-ray therapy

• Indication: Undifferentiated carcinoma
• By using Cobalt 60 or linear accelerator

ECTOPIA VESICAE (EXOSTROPHY OF THE BLADDER)

• A rare congenital anomaly seen in 1: 50,000 births
• Male: Female = 4 : 1

Aetiopathogenesis

• This occurs due to failure of development of lower abdominal wall and anterior wall of the urinary bladder.
• As a result, the posterior bladder wall is seen protruding out below the umbilicus. Hence, it is **exostrophy of the bladder.**

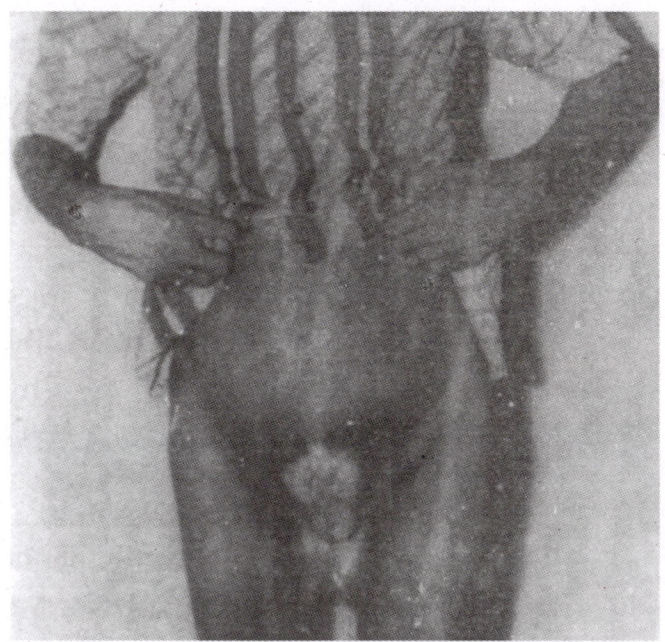

Fig. 40.9 A case of ectopia vesicae (Prof. Sasidharan, Manipal

Types

1. **Complete:** Pubic symphysis is not formed, complete epispadias in male or bifid clitoris in female.
2. **Incomplete:** Pubic symphysis, penis or clitoris are normal.

Clinical features

1. More common in male children
2. **Posterior bladder wall is seen in the lower abdomen** as a pink to red mucosa, partially inflamed.
3. Umbilicus is usually absent.
4. **Penis is rudimentary** and epispadias may be present.
5. Testis descends normally into a well developed scrotum.
6. **Pubic symphysis is widely separated,** it has the advantage in female patients in that it facilitates the delivery.
7. In female children-umbilicus is absent, external genitalia are poorly developed, and clitoris is bifid.
8. Constant dribbling of urine outside - therefore smell of the urine
9. Recurrent urinary tract infection (UTI)

Complications

1. Renal failure due to recurrent UTI

2. Adenocarcinoma of bladder at an early age
3. Ammoniacal dermatitis of the skin

Treatment

1. **Incomplete:** Reconstruction of the anterior wall of the bladder with reconstruction of the bladder sphincter.
2. **Complete:** Total cystectomy followed by urinary diversion by implantation of ureters in the sigmoid colon (**Ureterosigmoidostomy**) followed by reconstruction of anterior abdominal wall if the patient has urinary incontinence.

ACUTE CYSTITIS

Etiology and pathogenesis

Acute uncomplicated bacterial cystitis predominantly affects women. By definition these are infections occurring in the **absence of any anatomic or functional abnormality** of the urinary tract. The ascending fecal - perineal - urethral route is the primary source of infection.

- Men are somewhat protected from ascending infection because of:
1. Long urethra
2. Antibacterial properties of prostatic secretions

Causative organisms

- 80% of bladder infections in women are caused by E.Coli followed by other gram-ve organisms like klebsiella and proteus species.

Clinical features

- Irritative voiding symptoms (frequency, urgency, dysuria) are the hallmarks of cystitis. Low backache and suprapubic pain are other complaints. Fever and other constitutional symptoms are usually present.
- Physical examination is frequently unremarkable except for suprapubic tenderness.

Diagnosis

- **Urinary microscopy** is the mainstay of diagnosis. Diagnosis is strongly considered positive if microscopy shows >**5 WBCs**/high power field in females and 2-3 WBCs/high power field in males.

- **Urine culture** not only confirms the diagnosis but also identifies the causative organisms.
- Other tests and imaging studies are not indicated in an uncomplicated infection, unless patient presents with recurrent episodes.

Management

- Antibiotic therapy based on the culture and sensitivity report given for a period of 7-10 days, is curative.
- Symptomatic treatment in the form of anti-pyretics, urinary analgesics and anti-spasmodics may help.

DIVERTICULA OF THE BLADDER

Types

- **Congenital:** Rare and usually symptomless. They represent the **unobliterated vesical end of the urachus**. May require excision if chronic infection persists.
- **Acquired:** They are pulsion diverticulum and occur due to **bladder outflow obstruction.**

Pathology

- The diverticula is lined by bladder muccosa
- The opening (mouth) is situated above and to the outer side of one ureteric orifice.

Clinical features

- **Symptoms of recurrent urinary infection:** Suprapubic pain, frequency of micturition, fever with chills etc.
- **Symptoms of lower urinary obstruction:** Frequency, urgency, hesitancy etc.
- **Symptoms of pyelonephritis:** Backache, fever and renal angle tenderness etc.

Presence of diverticula is not an indication for surgery

Investigations

1. **Cystoscopy:** Full bladder distension is neccesary to search for diverticulum.
2. **Intravenous urography:** It can detect the site of diverticulum. It can also detect hydronephrosis.

3. **Ultrasonogram**
   - It can detect residual urine
   - It can detect diverticulum
   - It can detect associated stone

Treatment

- Combined intravesical and extravesical diverticulectomy

Complications

Key Box 39.4
COMPLICATIONS

- Recurrent urinary **infections**
- Bladder stone can cause **haematuria**
- **Hydronephrosis** and **hydroureter** occur due to peridiverticular inflammation and fibrosis
- **Neoplasm:** Squamous metaplasia and leukoplakia

URINARY FISTULAE

CLASSIFICATION

I. CONGENITAL

Key Box 39.5
CAUSES OF CONGENITAL URINARY FISTULAE

- Ectopia vesicae (Page 640)
- Patent urachus (Page 545)
- Association with imperforate anus (Page 510)

II. ACQUIRED

1. **Traumatic urinary fistula:** Perforating wounds or penetrating wounds or following surgery in the pelvis.
2. **Vesicovaginal fistula** (Given in detail below)
   Causes
   - Protracted or neglected labour
   - Gynecological operations such as total hysterectomy and anterior colporrhaphy

- Radiation causing avascular necrosis of the bladder
- Carcinoma cervix infiltrating into the bladder.

Leakage due to necrosis of tissues manifests usually after 7 days.

Clinical features

- Leakage of urine from vagina
- Excoriation of the vulva

Diagnosis

- Digital vaginal examination may reveal thickening on the anterior wall of vagina.
- **Vaginal speculum examination:** Dribbling of urine into vagina.
- **Swab test:** Methylene blue is injected into the urethra and if vaginal swab is coloured blue, it is vesicovaginal fistula.

Treatment

- **Low fistula:** Transvaginal repair
- **High fistula:** Suprapubic approach and repair

3. Fistula from renal pelvis to skin or gut

- Tuberculosis causes caseation and may result in fistula in the loin
- Large staghorn calculi
- Pyonephrosis
- Crohn's disease of the renal pelvis

INTERSTITIAL CYSTITIS

- It is also called as **Hunner's ulcer.**
- It is common in western female patients, many of them are psychiatric patients.
- There is severe fibrosis of the urinary bladder due to pancystitis, resulting in a **small thimble bladder.** (In India, tuberculosis to be considered)
- Frequency of micturition and pain due to decreased bladder capacity are the features.
- Cystoscopy and biopsy will confirm the diagnosis
- Treatment is difficult - hydrostatic dilatation, instillation

of dimethyl sulphoxide or surgical procedures such as ileo-cystoplasty have been tried.

SCHISTOSOMA HAEMATOBIUM

- It is called as urinary bilharziasis
- The disease is caused by embryos (cercariae) of schistosoma, which enter the body through penetration of the skin and reach the bladder via the portal vein in a retrograde manner. In the bladder, ova are released which via the urine are excreted back into the fresh water. Fresh water snail is the intermediate host.
- Multiple pseudotubercles, nodules, granulomas, fibrosis are the prominent pathological features.
- Diagnosis is suspected by painless terminal haematuria, initial cutaneous rashes, fever and eosinophilia
- Cystoscopy and biopsy to confirm the diagnosis.
- Treated by long term praziquantel and surgery may be required (ileo-cystoplasty)

It is a premalignant condition.

URINARY DIVERSION

Patients with lower urinary tract cancers or severe functional or anatomic abnormalities of the urinary bladder may require urinary diversion.

The most commonly used method of urinary diversion is by incorporating various intestinal segments into the urinary tract. Virtually every segment of the intestinal tract has been used.

1. **Ileal conduit:** 18-20 cm of ileum is used as a conduit. Ureters are directly implanted into it. The end of the ileal conduit is brought through lateral aspect of rectus abdominis muscle and stoma is made.

   This simply acts as a conduit carrying urine from the renal pelvis or ureter to the skin, where urine is collected in an appliance attached to the skin surface. It is not a continent mechanism.

2. **Uretero sigmoidostomy** is an example of continent urinary reservoir, wherein ureters are anastomosed into the sigmoid colon.

The most worrisome complication of this procedure is development of adenocarcinoma, at the site where ureters are implanted.

- Routine sigmoidoscopy is recommended annually, to be started after 5 years of procedure.
- Newer method of continent diversion - orthotopic bladder substitution.

3. **Nephrostomy:** It is required for drainage and decompression of the upper urinary tract and is indicated in following situations:

a. Retrograde ureteral catheterisation is not advisable (e.g: in sepsis secondary to ureteral obstruction).

b. Retrograde ureteral catheterisation is impossible (e.g: complete ureteral obstruction by stone, tumour or stricture).

- It is done by percutaneous methods.

4. **Uretero-ureterostomy**

Indications

a. Trauma to ureter

b. Ureteric involvement by neoplastic conditions. e.g: colonic carcinoma, which requires resection of ureter.

- Mainly indicated for upper and mid-ureteral involvement. The procedure of choice for lower ureteric involvement is bladder re-implantation.

RUPTURE OF THE URINARY BLADDER

CAUSES OF URINARY BLADDER RUPTURE

1. **Surgical** (iatrogenic) Bladder can be injured mostly during pelvic surgery i.e. excision of the rectum, or during gynecological procedures etc.

2. **Trauma:** Blunt injury abdomen due to road traffic accidents.
   - Kick or blow on abdomen.
   - Penetrating injury (very, very rare).

TYPES OF RUPTURE AND CLINICAL FEATURES

I. Intraperitoneal rupture

- When there is surgical trauma or trauma on a distended bladder the rupture will be intraperitoneal (Fig. 40.10A).

Clinical features

1. Sudden severe suprapubic pain, hypotension/syncope and shock.

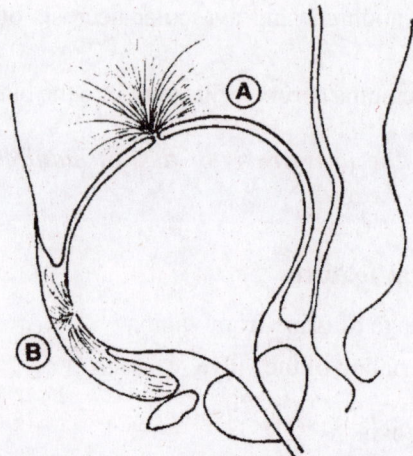

Fig. 40.10 Rupture bladder **A.** intraperitoneal; **B.** extraperitoneal

2. Lower abdominal guarding and rigidity occurs after few hours of injury.
3. Distension.
4. Eventhough the patient has not passed urine for a few hours there is no desire to micturate.
5. Shifting dullness may be elicitable.

II. Extraperitoneal rupture (Fig. 38.10B)

- Trauma either penetrating or blunt injury with fracture of pubis gives rise to this type of injury.
- Difficult to distinguish clinically from an injury to the membranous urethra.

INVESTIGATIONS

1. **Plain X-ray abdomen:** Lower abdomen shows ground glass appearance.
2. **IVP:** Extravasation of the dye into the peritoneal cavity or extraperitoneally.
3. **Retrograde cystourethrogram:** Confirms the site of leak.

TREATMENT

1. **Intraperitoneal rupture:** Laparotomy, repair of the bladder in two layers with vicryl. Drain the suprapubic space with a tube drain. An indwelling urethral catheter has to be placed for 10 days to two weeks to keep the bladder decompressed.

2. **Treatment of extraperitoneal rupture** Extraperitoneally expose the bladder with a suprapubic

midline incision and repair of the bladder. Drainage, as mentioned above, has to be carried out.

SURGICAL ANATOMY OF THE URETHRA

- Male urethra is divided into anterior urethra (bulbopenile) and posterior urethra (prostato-membranous urethra).
- Male urethra functions as a conduit for urine and semen. Anterior urethra is covered with erectile tissue of corpus spongiosum. Anterior urethra penetrates the urogenital diaphragm to enter the pelvic cavity as prostato-membranous urethra.
- Since its margins are attached to the perineal membrane it is vulnerable to tear at this point in pelvic bone fracture.
- Length of male urethra is about 14 -16 cms.
- Entire urethra is supplied by internal pudendal artery.
- Veins drain into Santorini's plexus around the bladder neck and prostate.
- Female urethra is short, drains only urine not vulnerable for injuries.

RUPTURE URETHRA

TYPES

I. RUPTURE BULBAR URETHRA

- The most common urethral injury
- Urethra angulates in the perineum, where it gets injured.

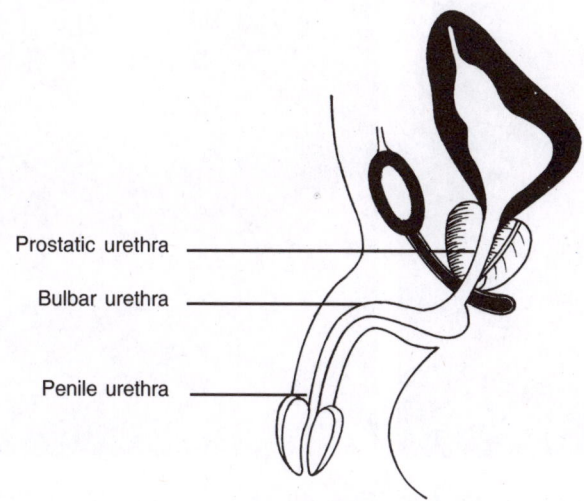

Fig. 40.11 Surgical anatomy of the urethra

Clinical triad of rupture of bulbar urethra

1. Perineal hematoma
2. **Urethral haemorrhage:** Blood at the urethral meatus
3. **Distended bladder:** Diagnosed by percussion over suprapubic region which gives dull note

Treatment

1. Advise the patient not to try to pass urine.
2. Urinary antibiotics
3. Should be shifted to the operation theatre and with aseptic precautions a catheter is passed gently, if it enters the bladder, it is kept in place for 2 weeks and perineal hematoma is drained.
4. If catheter does not reach the bladder, then, an incision is made in the perineum and the catheter is guided into the urethra.
5. If all the measures fail, emergency suprapubic cystostomy is done to drain the urine and later repair of urethra is undertaken.

II. RUPTURE MEMBRANOUS URETHRA-EXTRAPERITONEAL RUPTURE OF THE BLADDER

- Always associated with fracture of the pelvis.
- Occurs in major road traffic accidents.
- There may be disruption of pelvic bones, fracture symphysis pubis, with avulsion of the puboprostatic ligament leading to floating prostate.

Types of rupture membranous urethra

1. Complete transection results in floating bladder. In this condition, urethra is completely transected at the apex of the prostate. As the puboprostatic ligament is

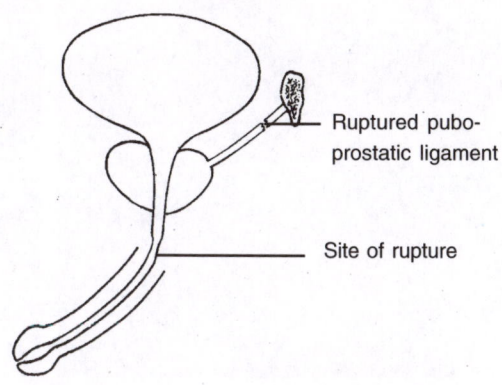

Fig. 40.12 Rupture membranous urethra with floating prostate. Note the ruptured pubo-prostatic ligaments

avulsed, the prostate falls back and migrates upwards. On rectal examination prostate is felt as though it is floating - **Floating prostate**.

2. **Incomplete transection**
3. Associated with injury to bladder: Extraperitoneal rupture of the bladder (intraperitoneal rupture of bladder occurs in a distended bladder).

Clinical features

1. History of injury
2. Features of shock due to significant blood loss (around 1-2 litres)
3. Haematuria
4. In cases of extraperitoneal rupture of the bladder, bladder will not be palpable due to extravasation of urine into perineum.
5. Suprapubic tenderness and dullness
6. **Rectal examination:** Floating prostate can be felt which is tender.

Investigations

1. X-ray pelvic bones may show a fracture or separation of pubic symphysis (Fig. 40.13).
2. Ascending urethrography (ASU) to confirm the rupture (Fig. 40.14, 40.15).
3. Once the stricture develops, vesicocystourethrogram (VCUG) is done to know the exact location of the stricture.

Treatment

- Urgent blood transfusion to treat shock

- Suprapubic cystostomy is done and degree of damage assessed.
- A bougie/sound is passed from above and another similar sound is passed through the external meatus (penis). When the two meet a click is made out. With both sounds in contact, the sound from bladder is withdrawn slowly. The lower one is advanced at this stage and 2nd sound appears in the bladder. A red rubber catheter is tied to it and the sound is withdrawn through external meatus.
- To this red rubber catheter which is seen outside, a Foley's catheter is tied and is drawn into the bladder and is kept in place for 15 days. This is called as **rail roading technique** (Fig. 40.16 - next page).
- Associated injuries like rupture bladder are treated by suturing.
- Antibiotics are given

Complications of rupture urethra

- Most dangerous complication being stricture urethra (Key Box 40.4)

Key Box 40.6
COMPLICATIONS OF RUPTURE URETHRA
1. Extravasation of urine into scrotum, beneath superficial fascia of the penis, beneath Scarpa's fascia
2. Urethral stricture
3. Haematoma
4. Recurrent urinary tract infection

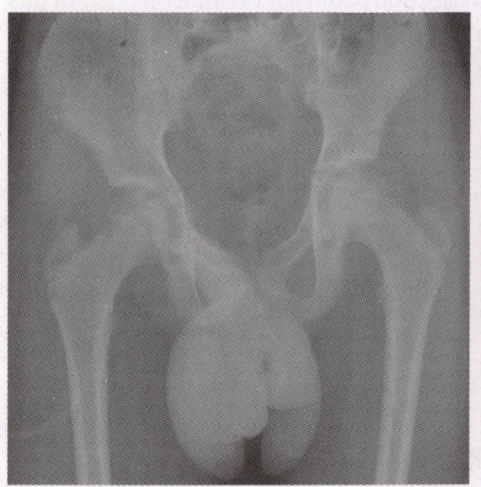

Fig 40.13 Plain Xray showing extravasation of the dye

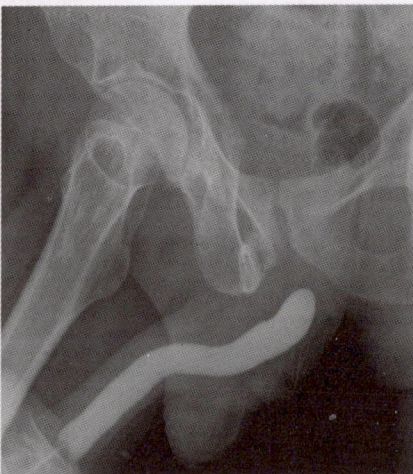

Fig 40.14 ASU total cut off stricture urethra

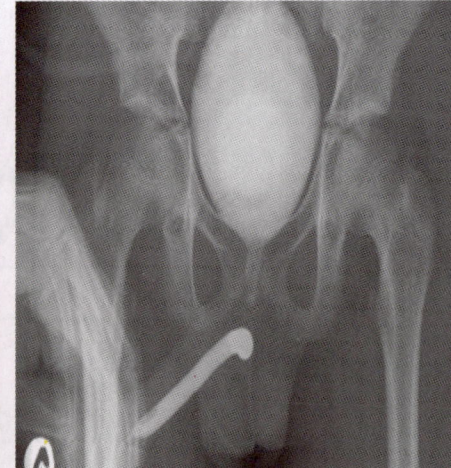

Fig. 40.15 ASU with MCU showing stricutre

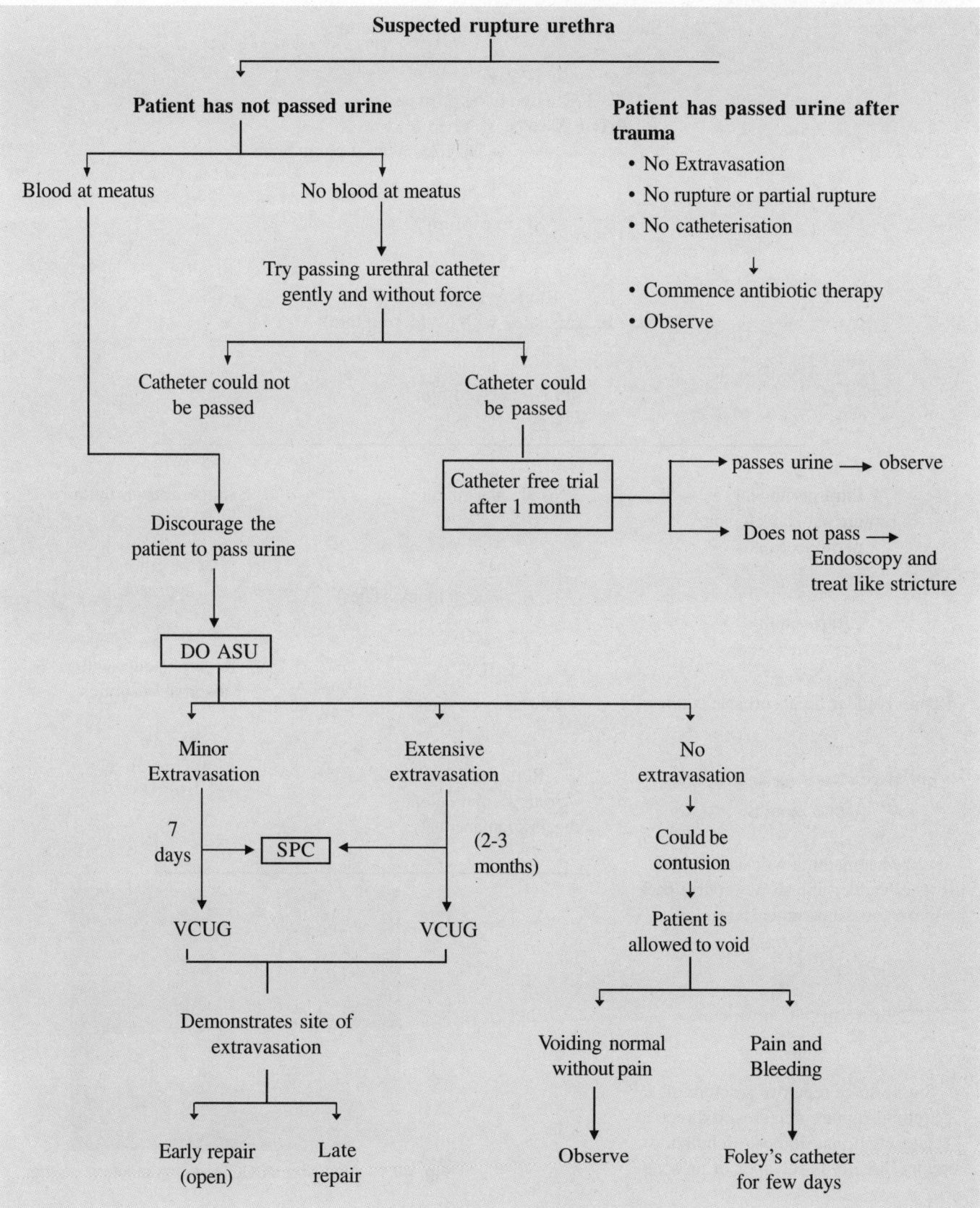

Fig 40.16 Algorithm for management of bulbar urethral rupture. Contributed by Dr. Vikas Jain, Asst. Prof., Dept. of Surgery, KMC, Manipal

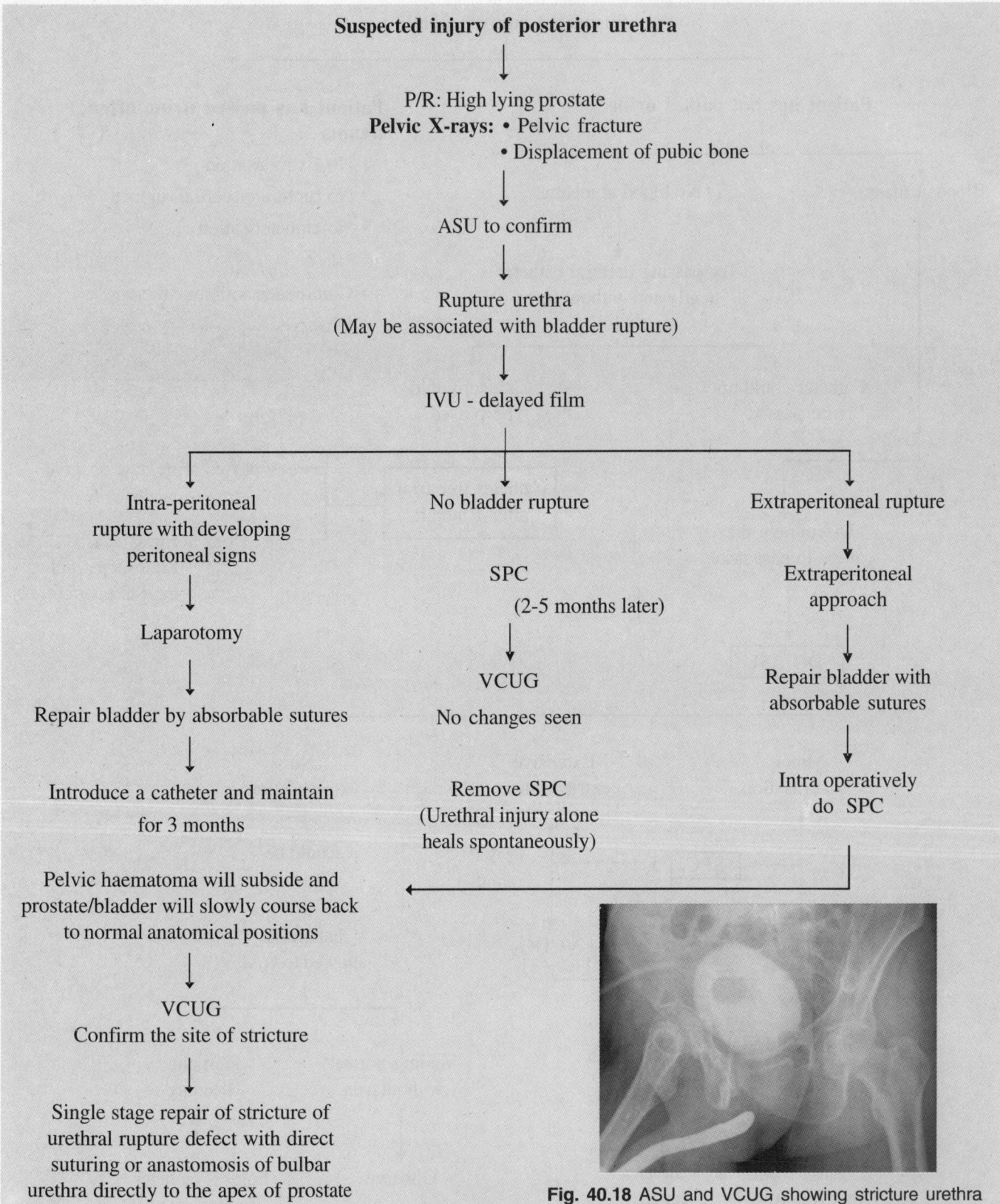

Suspected injury of posterior urethra

↓

P/R: High lying prostate
Pelvic X-rays: • Pelvic fracture
• Displacement of pubic bone

↓

ASU to confirm

↓

Rupture urethra
(May be associated with bladder rupture)

↓

IVU - delayed film

Intra-peritoneal rupture with developing peritoneal signs

↓

Laparotomy

↓

Repair bladder by absorbable sutures

↓

Introduce a catheter and maintain for 3 months

↓

Pelvic haematoma will subside and prostate/bladder will slowly course back to normal anatomical positions

↓

VCUG
Confirm the site of stricture

↓

Single stage repair of stricture of urethral rupture defect with direct suturing or anastomosis of bulbar urethra directly to the apex of prostate

No bladder rupture

SPC
(2-5 months later)

↓

VCUG
No changes seen

Remove SPC
(Urethral injury alone heals spontaneously)

Extraperitoneal rupture

↓

Extraperitoneal approach

↓

Repair bladder with absorbable sutures

↓

Intra operatively do SPC

Fig. 40.18 ASU and VCUG showing stricture urethra

Fig 40.17 Algorithm for management of posterior urethral rupture.   Contributed by Dr. Vikas Jain, Asst. Prof., Dept. of Surgery, KMC, Manipal

STRICTURE URETHRA

Causes

1. Congenital - very rare

2. Post - inflammatory

A. Post-gonococcal urethritis

- Within 48 hours of exposure to the venereal disease gonorrhoea, there is involvement of periurethral glands. They are concentrated more in the bulbar urethra. Hence strictures are more in bulbar urethra.

- It causes periurethral fibrosis, resulting in multiple dense strictures.

Key Box 40.7

ACUTE GONOCOCCAL URETHRITIS

- Pain during micturition
- Burning micturition
- Gleet : Early morning white flakes in the urine due to desquamated urethral epithelium

---

B. Tuberculosis

3. Post - instrumentation

- Catheterisation
- Dilatation
- Transurethral procedures

4. Postoperative

- Prostatectomy
- Repair of rupture urethra

5. Rupture urethra

6. Schistosomiasis

Clinical features

- Previous history of exposure to gonorrhoea or history of instrumentation or history of injury to urethra is usually present.
1. Common in young age 20-40 years
2. History of straining while passing urine
3. Suprapubic pain and swelling due to distended bladder

4. Stricture urethra may be felt in the perineum as a button hole.

Treatment

1. **Visual internal urethrotomy** (VIU) by using urethrotome

2. **Open method** is indicated in long strictures not responding to conventional treatment. They are grouped under urethroplasty

   a. Excision and end to end urethroplasty

   b. Reinforcement urethroplasty - Buccal mucosa

   c. Substitution urethroplasty - Buccal mucosa, skin

   d. Two step urethroplasty

3. **Regular dilatation** by using Lister's dilators

Complications

1. Acute retention of urine either following alcohol or due to postponement of micturition.

2. Secondary stones due to stasis of urine proximally.

3. Recurrent periurethral abscesses (multiple) which rupture and open externally in the perineal skin. When such a patient is asked to pass urine, urine can be seen coming out of multiple holes in the perineum **Watercan perineum**.

HYPOSPADIAS

In this condition some portion of distal urethra is not developed, as a result of which external meatus is situated in the undersurface of penis. Usually this is associated with chordee and hooded prepuce

Types (Fig. 40.19)

1. Glandular variety

- In this external meatus is situated few mm. away from normal site within the glans.

2. Coronal variety

- It occurs due to failure of development of urethra which runs in the glans penis.

- As a result of which urethra opens at the corona glandis-junction of glans and shaft of penis.

- Both these varieties do not give major problems functionally. It can be left alone without treatment.

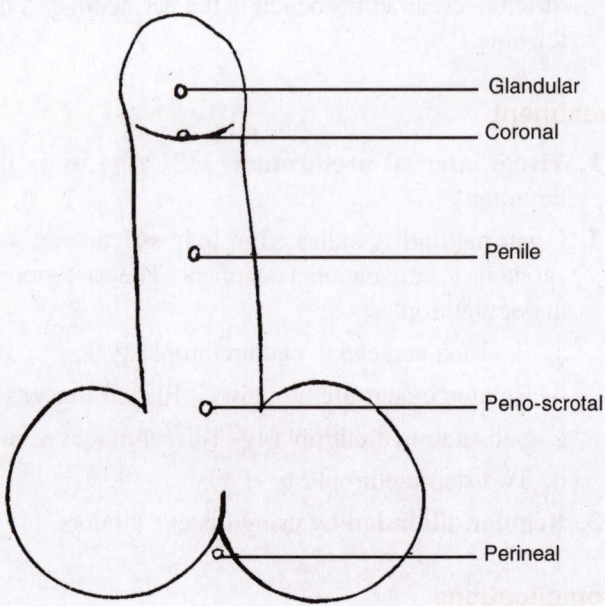

Fig 40.19 Various types of hypospadias

3. Penile hypospadias

- In this the external opening is situated somewhere in the under surface of the penis.

4. Peno-scrotal/perineal hypospadias

- In this condition, the entire urethra is not developed
- Penis is rudimentary
- Urethral opening is seen in between two halves of the scrotum and many times it is split
- Cases may be associated with undescended testes
- In such cases it is difficult to differentiate the sex of the child

Clinical features

1. Occurs in 1: 350 males.
2. Micturition: Stream is good, but it wets the clothes in 3rd and 4th varieties.
3. Chordee: Many of the cases are associated with bending of penis. Sexual intercourse will be difficult.

Treatment

1. One stage urethroplasty

- Chordee correction always confirm by inducing artificial erection
- Urethral tube formation by tubularising urethra
- Inner prepuceal island tube urethroplasty

2. Two stage urethroplasty

- When the child is 6 - 12 months old, chordee is corrected by straightening the penis. This is called as orthoplasty.
- When the child is 5-6 years old, reconstruction of the urethra is done by using locally available skin either from the prepuce or from penile shaft. This is called urethroplasty. Hence, circumcision should not be done in hypospadias.

DIFFERENTIAL DIAGNOSIS OF RETENTION OF URINE

CAUSES OF RETENTION OF URINE

I. Acute retention of urine

A) In males

- **Benign prostatic hypertrophy** (BPH) In elderly patients more than 50 years of age.
- **Stricture** urethra: In young patients
- **Post-operative retention** of urine: Operations like haemorrhoidectomy, fistulectomy, etc. produces reflex spasm of internal sphincter, which precipitates retention of urine. Management of such cases is given in the box.

Key Box 40.8
POSTOPERATIVE RETENTION OF URINE - TREATMENT
1. Hot water fomentation to the suprapubic region
2. Provide privacy
3. Run a tap nearby
4. Make the patient to stand and pass urine
5. Catheterisation should be done as the last resort

B) In Females

- Hysteria
- Retroverted gravid uterus
- Urethral stenosis

C) In children

- Meatal stenosis due to meatal ulcer with scab (due to scratching habit of child).

D) In general

- Spinal anaesthesia
- Spinal injuries
- Blood clot in the bladder following prostatectomy
- Bladder stone in school-going children: Pain referred to tip of penis
- Acute urethritis and acute prostatitis due to bacterial infection
- Faecal impaction in the rectum
- Contracture of the bladder neck
- Urethral calculus
- Drugs: Atropine, carbachol, bethanechol

II. Chronic retention of urine

- Benign prostatic hypertrophy
- Bladder neck contracture
- Stricture urethra

Key Box 40.9
CHRONIC RETENTION OF URINE
• BPH : Most common cause
• Painless
• Suprapubic dullness
• Slow decompression is recommended

Miscellaneous

POSTERIOR URETHRAL VALVE

- They are congenital, symmetrical valves in the posterior urethra.
- They are the most common cause of vesico-ureteric reflux and hydronephrosis in infants.
- Bladder wall is thickened due to obstruction and hypertrophy. The urinary bladder is palpable, hard and felt in the suprapubic region - **cricket ball bladder.**
- Due to stasis, recurrent urinary tract infection occurs commonly.

Investigations

- Micturating cysto-urethrography: Dilated proximal urethra is highly suggestive of posterior urethral valve.

Treatment

- Cystoscopic resection after initial suprapubic cystostomy (SPC).

Prostate and Seminal Vesicles

41

- Surgical anatomy
- Structural anatomy
- BPH
- Carcinoma prostate
- Prostatitis

- In benign prostatic hypertrophy the glands of the inner adenomatous zone hypertrophy and lead to urinary outflow obstruction. Carcinoma usually occurs in the outer non-adenomatous zone.

- New terminology for BPH arising zone is **transitional zone** and carcinoma arising zone is **peripheral zone**.

SURGICAL ANATOMY

- **Embryology:** The prostate develops around 12th week of intrauterine life. Primitive buds given from urethra form the glandular tissue and surrounding mesenchyme forms the fibromuscular stroma. Developmentally, the prostate has 5 lobes: Anterior, posterior, 2 lateral and one middle lobe.

- Middle lobe is situated in between the two ejaculatory ducts and the urethra. The enlargement of this lobe in benign hypertrophy of the prostate is responsible for the obstruction of urethra. This lobe enlarges upwards into the bladder (Fig. 41.1).

STRUCTURAL ANATOMY OF THE PROSTATE

- Prostatic urethra is surrounded by a fibroadenomatous gland.

- Urethral glands open into the prostatic urethra. These submucosal glands are responsible for BPH.

- When the prostate enlarges it compresses the outer zone resulting in a false capsule.

- The outer most zone is the zone of prostatic glands proper which is responsible for carcinoma of prostate (Fig. 41.2).

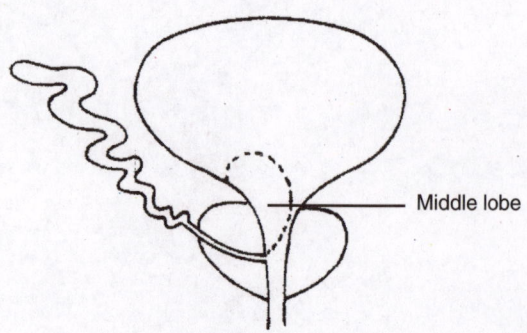

Fig. 41.1 Prostate - lobes

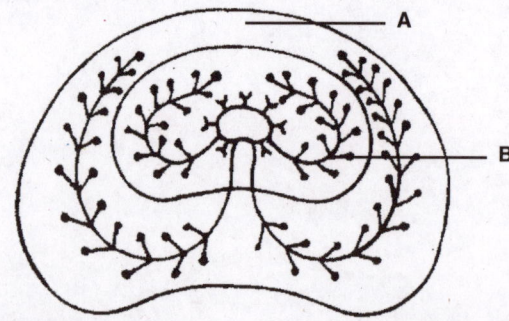

Fig. 41.2 Prostate - A. Outer carcinomatous zone, B. Inner adenomatous zone

- Surrounding this, there is fascia of Denon-villier which is a part of pelvic peritoneum.
- Between the anatomical capsule and pelvic peritoneum, prostatic venous plexus is present which may give rise to massive hemorrhage, if injured.

BENIGN PROSTATIC HYPERPLASIA (BPH)

AETIOPATHOGENESIS

There are 2 theories to explain BPH.

1. **Hormonal theory**
   - It has been compared to fibroadenosis in female patients.
   - As the age advances, the levels of androgens come down. There is a corresponding increase in the oestrogen which stimulates the prostate gland and produces BPH.
2. **Neoplastic theory**
   - According to this theory there is proliferation of all the elements of prostate: Fibrous, muscular and glandular resulting in fibromyoadenoma.

SECONDARY EFFECTS OF BPH

1. **Urethral changes**
   - Urethra gets compressed and gets converted into a narrow, longitudinal slit.
   - The effect is more with median lobe enlargement which is due to enlargement of subcervical glands.
   - Lateral lobes enlarge when there is involvement of submucous glands.
2. **Changes in the bladder** (Fig. 41.3)
   - As a result of obstruction, the bladder musculature undergoes hypertrophy. Very prominent thick bundles of the muscle can be seen, which are called as fasciculations or **trabeculations.**
   - In between the fasciculations, there are depressed areas which are called **sacculations.**
   - Since the sacculi are thin, as the pressure increases, herniation occurs outside resulting in diverticuli.
   - In the diverticuli, there is stasis of urine resulting in secondary infection and stone formation.
3. **Changes in the ureter and kidney**
   - Bilateral hydronephrosis and bilateral hydroureter are the end result of BPH which may result in renal failure (Key Box 41.1).

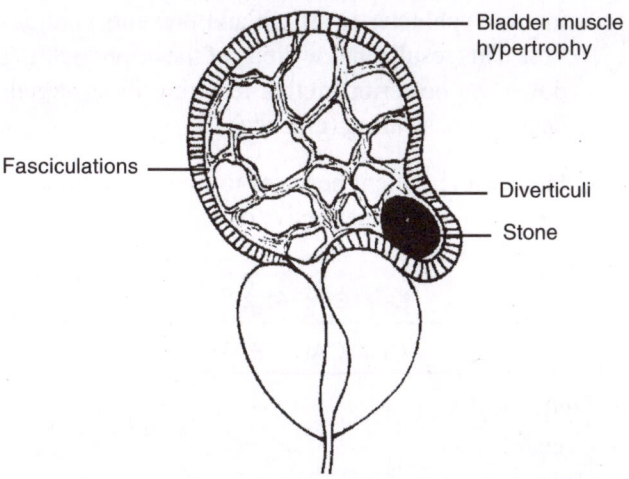

Fig. 41.3 Secondary changes in the urinary bladder due to BPH

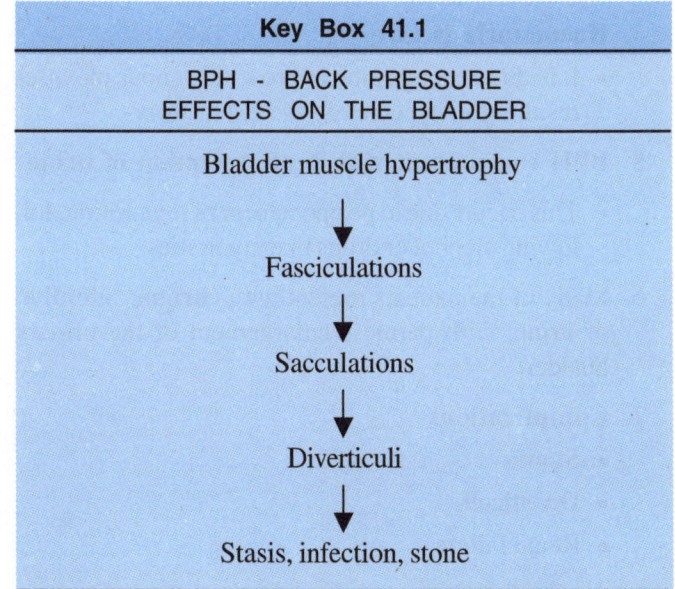

Key Box 41.1

BPH - BACK PRESSURE EFFECTS ON THE BLADDER

Bladder muscle hypertrophy
↓
Fasciculations
↓
Sacculations
↓
Diverticuli
↓
Stasis, infection, stone

CLINICAL FEATURES OF BPH (Key Box 41.2)

1. Frequency
2. Urgency
3. Hesitancy
   - **Frequency:** To start with, frequency is present during the day time followed by day and night (5-10 times during the night). It is due to ineffective emptying of the bladder. It results in residual urine in the bladder precipitating cystitis.
   - **Urgency:** As the prostate enlarges there is vesical introversion of sensitive mucous membrane of prostatic urethra within the bladder. This causes the

internal sphincter to stretch and prevents contraction. This results in few drops of the urine trickling down the posterior urethra resulting in an urgent desire to pass urine (urgency).

- **Hesitancy:** Patient hesitates to pass urine because micturition is so ineffective due to obstruction.

Key Box 41.2

BPH - CLINICAL FEATURES

- Frequency
- Urgency
- Hesitancy
- Acute retention of urine
- Chronic retention of urine

---

4. **Haematuria is rare**
   - It is due to congestion of prostatic venous plexuses resulting in hyperaemia and haematuria.

5. **BPH can present with acute retention of urine**
   - This occurs due to postponement of micturition, following alcohol or drugs like mydriatics.

6. Many of the patients present with **chronic retention** of urine, with painless enlargement of the urinary bladder.

7. **Complications**
   - Stones
   - Diverticuli
   - Renal failure

DIAGNOSIS OF BPH

Per rectal examination: Enlarged lateral lobes can be easily felt. Rectal mucosa is free. (In an enlarged prostate gland, in case of carcinoma of prostate, the mucosa of the rectum cannot be moved if it has infiltrated into the rectum).

INVESTIGATIONS

1. Blood urea and creatinine: The raised levels indicate renal failure.

2. **Uroflowmetry:** The person is asked to void urine from his full bladder into the flowmeter. The flow rate is assessed.

Peak flow rate

- Normal peak flow rate: 20 ml/sec.
- Doubtful peak obstruction: 10 to 15 ml/sec.
- Definite peak obstruction: Less than 10 ml/sec.
- Thus, the degree of bladder outlet obstruction (BOO) can be assessed by uroflowmetry in case of BPH.

3. **Ultrasonogram:** To assess the size and weight of prostate, to assess the residual urine and to look for hydroureteronephrosis.

4. IVP to study renal changes in selected cases

5. Cystoscopy as part of treatment

TREATMENT

- It can be classified into medical treatment and surgical treatment

I. Medical treatment of BPH

- If the patient has mere frequency of micturition and if the residual urine is not much (<150 ml), uroflowmetry shows more than 15 ml/sec of urine flow and if there are no back pressure effects on the kidney, the patient can be reassured and advised to avoid heavy alcohol consumption which may lead to prostatic congestion and acute retention of urine. To avoid over distension of the bladder, he has to void the urine as and when he feels the urinary sensation of micturition, and should not postpone micturition.

Drugs:

a. **Finasteride acetate** 5 mg daily for 6 months. It is a 5α- reductase inhibitor.

b. **α-adrenergic blocker:** It is supposed to relax the internal sphincter for better drainage of the bladder.

II. Surgical treatment

Indications for surgery

1. **Acute retention** of urine

2. **Chronic retention** of urine with postvoid residual urine more than 200 ml.

3. If **frequency** of micturition is so much that it disturbs the normal life style during day time.

4. **Complications** like haematuria due to congestion of prostatic venous plexuses, hydroureteronephrosis, prostatic diverticulosis, vesical calculus and recurrent infections.

Surgical methods

1. Transvesical suprapubic prostatectomy

- This method is now restricted to glands more than 100 gm in weight.
- Through an extraperitoneal approach the bladder is opened, prostate is enucleated with finger, bleeding is controlled by inflating the Foley bulb with about 30-50 ml of air and by ligatures.
- Bladder is drained by a Malecot's catheter which is wider than Foley so that it can drain well if the bleeding occurs in the bladder.
- During the process, the prostatic urethra is also avulsed.
- After about 7-10 days, a tract develops along the length of Foley's catheter which heals by granulation, fibrosis and forms the future prostatic urethra.

Disadvantages

1. Blind resection
2. Chances of hemorrhage are more
3. Stricture prostatic urethra

2. Transurethral resection of the prostate (TURP)

- This is the most popular method today.
- A resectoscope is passed through the urethra and under vision with constant irrigation with water or glycine, the prostate is resected into multiple pieces and removed.
- Haemostasis is obtained with the help of a cautery.

Advantages:

1. Post-operative recovery is smooth and rapid.
2. Incontinence is rare because the chances of damage to the internal sphincter are very low.

Disadvantages:

1. TURP syndrome with water intoxication and electrolyte imbalance, if water is used as irrigating fluid.
2. If there is BPH with diverticuli and stone, TURP has to be followed with litholapaxy.

3. Retropubic prostatectomy

- Done by extraperitoneal approach without opening the bladder, pushing the bladder to one side and excision of the prostate.

4. Perineal prostatectomy

- Not done nowadays

CARCINOMA OF THE PROSTATE

- Carcinoma of the prostate is common after the age of 65 years. The incidence increases with age.
- In Western countries, it is the second most common type of carcinoma after 65 years, following bronchogenic carcinoma.
- Prostatectomy done for BPH does not give protection for developing carcinoma of prostate because during prostatectomy the outer zone is left undisturbed (not resected).

CLINICAL FEATURES

1. **Histological surprise**
   - Prostatectomy done with diagnosis of BPH but histology reveals carcinoma of the prostate.
2. **Multiple bone pain,** confused for rheumatism, is due to multiple metastasis.
3. **Rectal examination:** Reveals a hard nodule on the anterior wall of the rectum, obliteration of median sulcus. The rectal mucosa cannot be moved over the prostate but it is not ulcerated (fascia of Denon-Villier prevents the spread of carcinoma prostate into the rectum).
4. Elderly man with **bilateral sciatica** with metastasis in the thoraco-lumbar vertebrae.
5. **Acute retention of urine** occurs in 5-10% of cases of carcinoma of prostate.
6. **Difficulty** in passing urine, painful micturition and sometimes with haematuria is due to involvement of prostatic urethra.

SPREAD (Key Box 41.3)

1. **Haematogenous**
   - This is due to retrograde tumour embolization which occurs through prostatic venous plexus which communicate through the emissary veins with the bone (paravertebral plexus of veins).

Peculiarities of secondary deposit from carcinoma of prostate:

- They are multiple
- Moth-eaten appearance
- Osteoblastic (in most other secondaries, they are osteolytic)

Key Box 41.3

THE BONES INVOLVED

1. Thoracolumbar vertebrae
2. Pelvic bone, iliac crest
3. Femur
4. Scalp
5. Ribs

2. Lymphatic spread

- Prostatic chain of lymphatics drain into internal iliac nodes.
- When spread occurs along seminal vesicle, external iliac nodes are enlarged.
- From this group of nodes para-aortic nodes, mediastinal nodes, followed by left supraclavicular nodes get involved.

3. Local spread

- On the medial side it can involve the prostatic urethra and give rise to retention of urine.
- When it spreads upwards, the bladder can get involved resulting in painful haematuria.
- Superiorly it can also involve seminal vesicle.
- Rectum is involved very late in carcinoma of prostate because of the tough Denon-Villier's fascia.

TNM staging of prostatic cancer

T_1	Tumours found incidentally during TURP
T_{1a}	Well or moderately differentiated tumour less than 5% of the resected specimen
T_{1b}	Poorly differentiated tumour or cancerous tissue more than 5% of resected specimen
T_2	Tumour confined to the prostate
T_{2a}	Tumour size less than 2 cm
T_{2b}	Tumour size greater than 2 cm
T_{2c}	Tumour size involving more than one lobe
T_3	Tumour extending to seminal vesicle or bladder
T_4	Tumour extending to rectum or pelvic wall
N_1	Single node less than 2 cm
N_2	Single or multiple nodes 2-5 cm in size
N_3	Nodes greater than 5 cm
M_0	No metastasis
M_1	Distant metastasis

INVESTIGATIONS

1. **Transrectal trucut biopsy**
   - Report-adenocarcinoma
2. **X-ray of bones**
   - Which are likely to be involved (already mentioned)

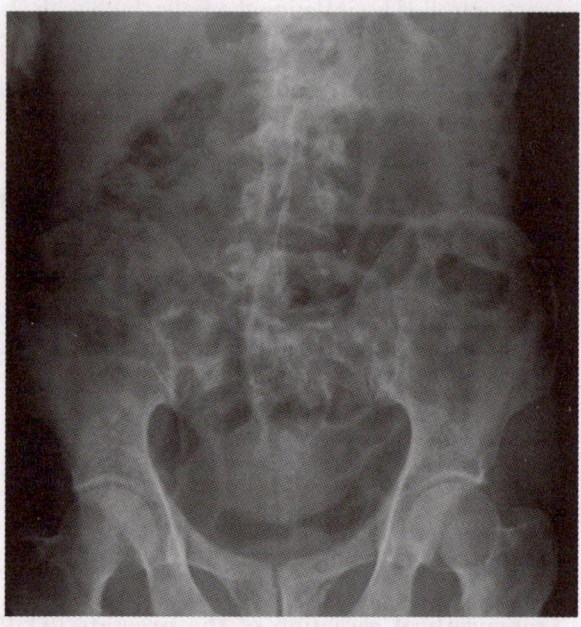

Fig. 41.4 Plain X-ray showing destruction of vertebrae

3. **Serum acid phosphatase** (Key Box 41.4)

   - The enzymes which split the organic phosphates are concentrated in the prostate which are responsible for acidic pH in the prostatic urethra.
   - Normally they are drained in the urine so that they are not detectable in the serum.
   - In carcinoma prostate because of the ductal blockage, it gets absorbed into the blood and thus high levels are reached specially with metastasis.
   - 1 to 3 King Armstrong units-suggestive of carcinoma of prostate.

Key Box 41.4

ACID PHOSPHATASE - INCREASED

1. Paget's disease of bone
2. Acute prostatitis
3. Cirrhosis of liver
4. Carcinoma prostate

Requirements before estimation of acid phosphatase

- Early morning blood sample
- On empty stomach
- Avoid fatty food
- Per rectal examination should not be done before drawing the sample of blood.

Significance of acid phosphatase

- Levels come down with the treatment of carcinoma of prostate especially when bone metastasis disappears.

4. Serum alkaline phosphatase

- It is increased if there is extensive liver metastasis or bone metastasis.

5. Prostate specific antigen (PSA)

- Prostate specific antigen (PSA) is a neutral protease, elaborated by columnar prostatic acinar epithelial cells.
- If it is more than 4 nmol/ml carcinoma is to be suspected; 10 nmol/ml is suggestive of prostatic carcinoma; 35 nmol/ml - Disseminated carcinoma.
- The highest concentration of PSA occurs in the lumen of the prostatic acini and ducts (upto million times greater than in systemic circulation). The prostatic luminal cells are normally surrounded by basal cells, prostatic basement membrane and prostatic stroma.
- A number of diseases disrupt some of the barriers to absorption resulting in elevation of serum PSA, **notably prostatic cancer, prostatic inflammation and infarction.** PSA is also transiently elevated (upto 24 hours) after ejaculation and cycling.

Thus PSA is organ specific but not cancer specific.

- PSA measurement is the most efficient screening test for prostate cancer and it increases further if the measurement is **combined with digital rectal examination (DRE)**
- PSA measurement is also vital in staging prostate cancer and assessing response to treatment.

6. Abdominal and transrectal USG

- For staging of the disease

7. CT scan or MRI scan

- These are done before proceeding on to radical surgery to assess the extent of the tumour.

8. Bone scan

- Is indicated in cases of carcinoma prostate especially with bony pain

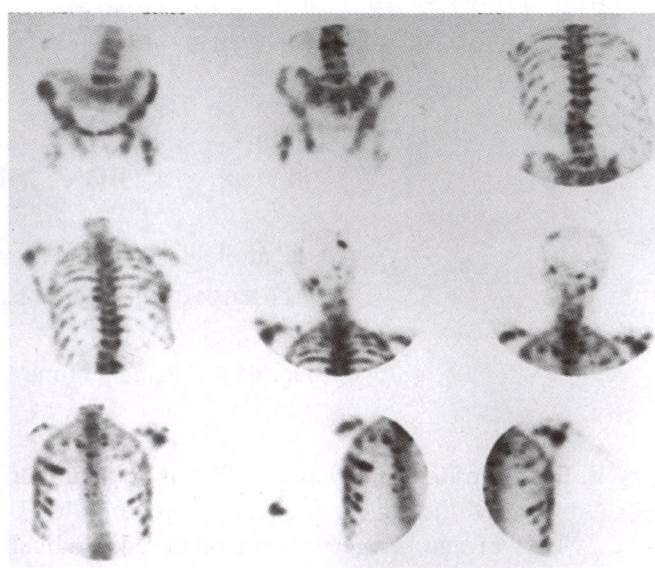

Fig. 41.5 Bone scan showing extensive metastasis

TREATMENT OF CARCINOMA OF PROSTATE

- It can be classified under following headings - early malignancy and late malignancy

I. Early malignancy

- It refers to - Tl or T2 N0 M0

    A. Early prostatic malignancy with PSA levels less than 20 nmol/ml

- If the life expectancy is more than 10 to 15 years, then **radical prostatectomy** is done which involves pelvic lymphadenectomy and removal of the prostate, seminal vesicles including the distal urethral sphincter followed by anastomosis of urethra to the bladder neck.
- Radical radiotherapy for prostate and pelvic nodes is given postoperatively.

Disadvantages of radical prostatectomy

- Impotence and stress incontinence may complicate the surgery.

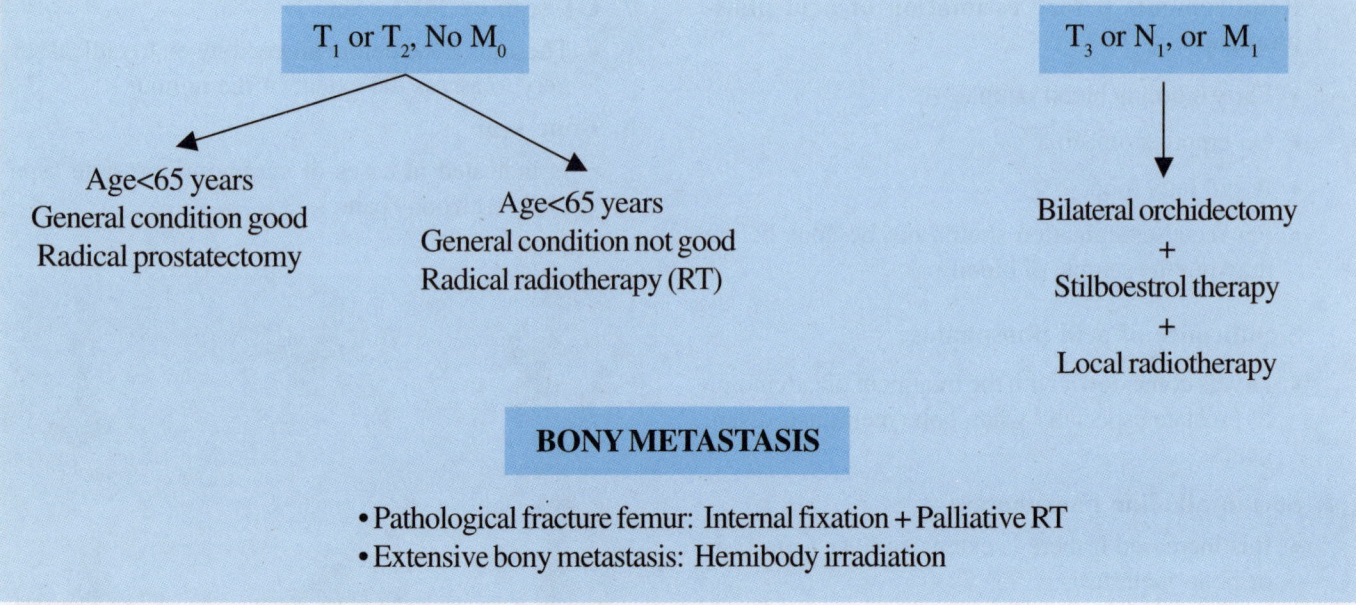

Fig. 41.6 Summary of the treatment of carcinoma prostate

B. Early prostatic malignancy if PSA is 20 mg/ml or more and the patient is already beyond 65 to 70 years of age, surgery is not favoured. Radical radiotherpy is given.

II. Late malignancy

- It means T3 lesions or involvement of regional nodes or presence of metastasis.

1. **Androgen ablation** in the form of bilateral orchidectomy is done as the tumour is androgen dependent followed by **anti-androgenic** measures.

2. For localised metastasis in bones or brain, **radiotherapy** relieves the symptoms.

   - For generalised metastasis, **hemibody irradiation** is excellent to improve the symptoms and the survival time.

   - If carcinoma of the prostate is diagnosed only by a biopsy of the prostate removed during TURP, no surgery needs to be done. Local radiotherapy to the prostatic bed is sufficient.

   - If the diagnosis of carcinoma of prostate is made on rectal findings, surgeons have no role to play because many a time it is an advanced cancer and there is a danger of bleeding from prostatic venous plexus. Hence, radiotherapy is administered by using linear accelerator (Cobalt).

3. **Anti-androgenic measures**

   i. **Bilateral subcapsular orchidectomy or low orchidectomy**

   - The testis is removed leaving behind tunica albuginea. This results in bleeding which becomes a clot and gives a feel of testis to the patient. Since this is a messy surgery, a low bilateral orchidectomy is done.

   ii. **Drugs**

   a. **Oral stilboestrol** therapy, dose 20-25 mg/day; phosphorylated diethyl stilboestrol (Honvon) given initially I.V. and then orally. Within 48 hours of treatment, dysuria improves, pain disappears, bone pains improve and metastasis may disappear.

   Disadvantages
   - Thromboembolism
   - Nausea and vomiting
   - **Gynaecomastia:** Can be prevented by pre-operative radiation to the breast-800 rads.

   b. **Phosphorylated diethylstilboestrol** is an excellent drug which can be given orally and I.V. and the drug is not broken down until it reaches prostate. Hence, systemic toxicity of stilboestrol does not occur. In the prostate it is broken down by acid phosphatase to release stilboestrol locally.

   - **Dose:** 100 mg I.V.

   - **Oral:** 100 mg/day after injection therapy is over.

4. **Palliative treatment of carcinoma prostate:** Chemotherapy

   i. Local radiotherapy to the enlarged para-aortic nodes and to the bone.

   ii. Chemotherapeutic drugs

   - Mitomycin and nitrogen mustard are being tried.

PROSTATITIS

The inflammation of the prostate can be acute or chronic. However in both types, in addition to the prostate, seminal vesicles and posterior urethra are involved.

ACUTE PROSTATITIS

Aetiology

- Causative organisms are Escherichia coli, Staphylococcus aureus and Staphylococcus albus.

- The infection is usually due to haematogenous spread from a distant focus or secondary to urinary tract infection.

- Instrumentation or invasive urological procedures are also factors.

Clinical features

1. The patient is ill with high grade fever, with chills and rigors.

2. Pain all over the body, more so in the back

3. Perineal heaviness or pain, rectal irritation and urethral discharge are also the features.

4. Pain on micturition is common and initial samples of urine contain 'threads'.

5. **Rectal examination finding:** Tender, boggy enlarged prostate. Fluctuation indicates prostatic abscess (rare).

Treatment

- Hospitalisation, intravenous fluids, antipyretics

- Antibiotics such as ciprofloxacin or norfloxacin should be given for 2-3 weeks. Otherwise, recurrent attacks of prostatitis can occur.

CHRONIC PROSTATITIS

Chronic prostatitis results due to inadequately treated acute prostatitis.

Clinical features

1. Elderly men are affected and they complain of perineal heaviness, perineal discomfort or pain on sexual intercourse.

2. Intermittent fever is also a feature

3. Rectal examination may reveal a boggy and tender prostate.

Diagnosis

- Prostatic massage is given by bidigital method- Index finger in the rectum and the thumb in the perineum to one side. Now the patient is asked to void urine. Presence of prostatic threads, or mucopus in the post-prostatic massage urine is diagnostic of chronic prostatitis.

Treatment

- Prolonged antibiotic therapy-Norflaxacin, trimethoprim and metronidazole are used.

Key Box 41.5

CHRONIC PROSTATITIS

- Follows recurrent prostatitis
- Elderly men are affected
- Symptoms - misleading
- Perineal heaviness, back pain
- Postprostatic massage - threads
- Pus cells and bacteria - prostatic fluid
- Prolonged antibiotics

Penis, Testis, Scrotum

42

- Surgical anatomy of the penis
- Phimosis
- Paraphimosis
- Carcinoma penis
- Differential diagnosis of ulcer penis
- Peyronie's disease
- Anatomy of the testis
- Hydrocoele
- Ectopic testis
- Undescended testis
- Varicocele
- Spermatocoele
- Epididymal cyst
- Torsion testis
- Testicular tumours
- Fournier's gangrene

SURGICAL ANATOMY OF THE PENIS

- It consists of two corpora cavernosa and one corpus spongiosum.

- **Corpora cavernosa** are vascular spaces wherein **arterioles open directly**. They are corkscrew shaped (**helicine arteries**) which allows their elongation in erection.

- **Corpora spongiosum** is perforated by urethra and continuous distally with the glans.

- Each corpora is enclosed by tough fibrous membrane - the **tunica albuginea** of the corpus.

- The fused fibrous sheaths are attached to the under surface of the symphysis pubis by a triangular sheet

of fibrous tissue called as **suspensory ligament**. It has to be divided during total amputation of the penis.

Blood supply

- The artery to the bulb supplies corpus spongiosum and the glans.

- Deep artery supplies corpus cavernosum alone - its sole function is erection.

- Dorsal artery supplies skin, fascia and glans

- Superficial dorsal vein drains into superficial external pudendal veins. Deep dorsal vein enters prostatic venous plexus.

Penile urethra

- Entire penile urethra is lined with transitional epithelium except dilated anterior part in the glans - fossa navicularis - lined by stratified squamous epithelium.

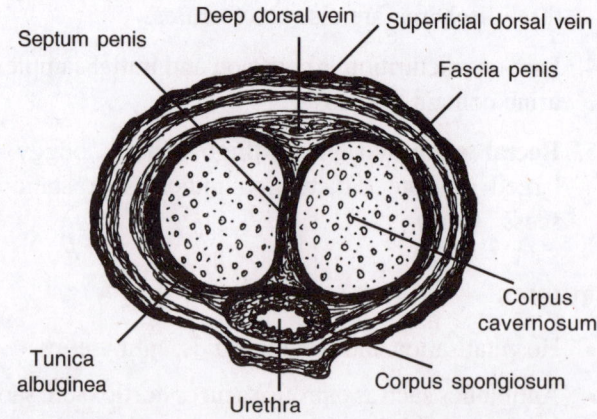

Fig. 42.1 Surgical anatomy of the penis

Lymphatic drainage

- Medial group of superficial inguinal nodes
- Some from glans pass directly to the node of cloquet

Nerve supply

- Parasympathetic nerves - nervi erigentes: stimuli resulting in erection of the external genitalia.
- Sympathetic system - hypogastric nerves: helps in ejaculation.

PHIMOSIS

Inability to retract the prepucial skin is described as phimosis.

Causes

1. **Congenital:** Most common type seen in young patients.
2. Secondary to **chronic balanoposthitis:** Balanitis means inflammation of glans penis and posthitis means inflammation of the prepuce. Balanoposthitis is common in diabetic patients.
3. **Chancre** also can cause phimosis
4. **Carcinoma** of the penis can present as a recent phimosis.

Key Box 42.1

PHIMOSIS - CAUSES

- Cancer
- Chancre
- Congenital
- Diabetes

Clinical features

1. Inability to retract the prepuce
2. In children, ballooning of the prepuce (second bladder) can be seen, which is diagnostic of phimosis.
3. Because of the phimosis, they are more prone for balanoposthitis because of inability to clean the glans.

Complications

1. Carcinoma of the penis
2. Paraphimosis

Treatment

- **Circumcision** - Removal of the prepuce

PARAPHIMOSIS

In this condition, the retracted skin of the glans penis (prepuce) cannot be pulled forwards. As a result of this, the retracted skin acts like a tight constricting agent which compresses the corona resulting in venous congestion. As venous congestion increases, glans swells up resulting in paraphimosis.

Causes

1. During catheterisation, if the retracted prepuce is not pulled forwards, it results in paraphimosis.
2. This can follow after a sexual intercourse.

Clinical features

1. Severe pain in the glans penis
2. Gross swelling of retracted prepucial skin and oedema of the distal glans penis.

Treatment

1. Sedation
2. Injection hyaluronidase 250 units in 10-15 ml of saline is injected into the constriction ring (prepucial skin which is retracted) 5-10 minutes later, when oedema is reduced, with gentle manipulation it is possible to reduce the paraphimosis.
3. Dorsal slit is given so that reduction can be done. Circumcision follows later.

Complications

1. Ulcers of glans
2. Gangrene of glans in later stages

CARCINOMA PENIS

PREMALIGNANT LESIONS

1. **Genital warts: Buschke-Lowenstein** tumour is a giant penile condyloma and resembles squamous cell carcinoma. It is a cauliflower-like lesion, may have foci of malignancy.

2. **Erythroplasia of Queyrat** or Paget's disease of penis-a persistent red, raw lesion which is a precancerous condition.

3. **Leukoplakia:** Persistent nonspecific patch in the glans or in the prepucial skin. Interestingly, leukoplakic patches are not white in the penis.

4. **Bowen's disease:** This presents as a small eczematous plaque. Carcinoma in situ is a complication which develops within this plaque.

AETIOLOGY

Phimosis

1. Extremely rare in Jews who practise it immediately after birth.

2. Carcinoma penis is rare in Mohammedans who practise circumcision few years after birth.

3. Carcinoma penis is common in Hindu and Christian population who do not practise circumcision. Due to the prepucial skin, smegma collects within, which is responsible for chronic irritation giving rise to carcinoma of penis.

CLINICAL FEATURES

1. Carcinoma penis is common in 6th decade. Majority of patients present with nonhealing ulcer.

2. Foul smelling discharge is common and occasionally it is blood stained.

3. Recent phimosis due to growth underneath the prepuce.

4. Haematuria, pain while passing urine indicate locally advanced tumours.

5. On examination, very often there is an ulceroproliferative growth with everted edges and induration of the base and edge. The induration is much more extensive than the lesion. Hence, entire shaft has to be examined for evidence of induration (Fig. 42.1).

6. Urethra is rarely involved in carcinoma of penis because it is protected by the tough Buck's fascia, which is a part of pelvic fascia. In large fungating lesions, it may be difficult to identify the external urinary meatus. In such situations the patient will point out at the external urinary meatus.

SPREAD

1. **Direct spread:** Involves the glans, prepucial skin and shaft

2. **Lymphatic spread:** Inguinal nodes are enlarged. 30% cases are due to infection. Nodes are firm and tender in infection. Hard nodes suggest metastases. Later, internal iliac and para-aortic nodes can also get enlarged. In advanced cases the lymph nodes may show fungation, as in Fig. 42.3.

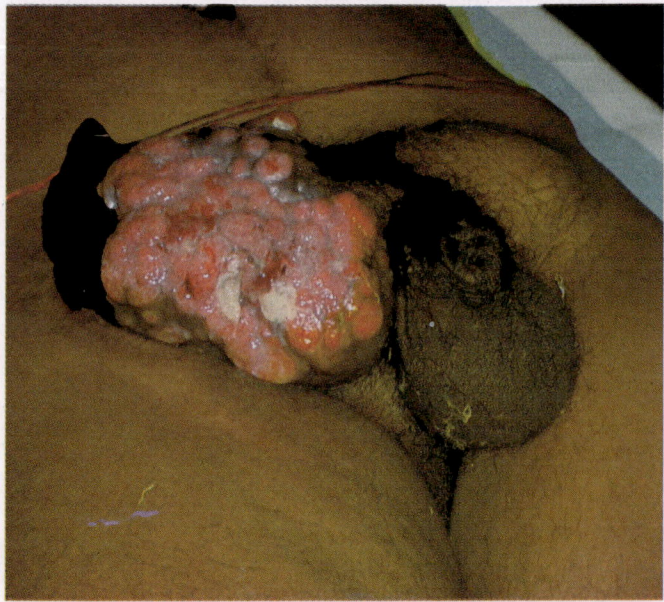

Fig. 42.2 This patient presented with fungating inguinal lymph nodes. Observe the penis - he has undergone partial amputation of the penis

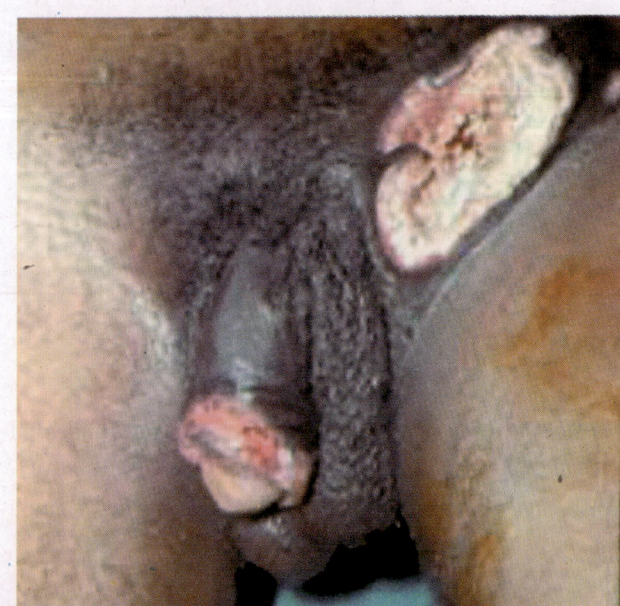

Fig. 42.3 This patient had a large foul smelling proliferative lesion in the glans penis with fungating inguinal lymph nodes

STAGING

I   Tumour confined to the glans or prepuce

II Tumour involving the penile shaft or corpora cavernosa

III Mobile regional nodal metastases, with stage I or II

IV Tumour beyond penile shaft, fixed regional lymph node or distant metastases

DIAGNOSIS

1. Wedge biopsy from the edge of the growth, proves the diagnosis of squamous cell carcinoma
2. FNAC of enlarged inguinal lymph nodes

TREATMENT

It can be divided into treatment of the primary and treatment of the secondaries.

I. Treatment of the primary

A. Surgical treatment

Stage I:

1. Growth confined to the prepuce - **circumcision**. Regular follow up is necessary.
2. Growth involving the glans: **Partial amputation** with at least 2 cm margin from the palpable indurated edge of the tumour.

Stage II:

1. **Partial amputation:** After having a macroscopic tumour-free, two cm margin proximally, if there is adequate length of penile shaft (minimum 2.5 cm) to carry out the sexual function and for directing the urinary stream, a partial amputation can be done.
2. **Total penectomy** with perineal urethrostomy, if adequate shaft cannot be retained. This is a major operation, patient has to be clearly instructed about the consequences and complications of perineal urethrostomy.

Complications of perineal urethrostomy

- **Ammoniacal dermatitis** of scrotum. To prevent this, patient has to lift the scrotum to pass urine.
- **Stricture of perineal urethra** which can be dilated by Hegar's dilators.

Stage III:

- Circumcision, partial amputation or total penectomy followed by ilioinguinal block dissection.

II. Treatment of inguinal lymph node secondaries in carcinoma penis

- Before discussing ilioinguinal block dissection, it is necessary to know the concept of **sentinel lymph node biopsy (SLNB).**

SLNB

- The concept of SLNB was first described by CABANA in 1977.
- Cabana, in 1977, demonstrated consistent drainage of the penile lymphatics into a sentinel lymph node or group of lymph nodes, located superomedial to the junction of saphenous and femoral veins in the area of superficial epigastric vein. He postulated that this sentinel lymph node is the first to get involved in the penile malignancy, and if this sentinel lymph node is negative for tumour, metastasis to other inguinal lymph nodes will not occur and metastasis to this lymph node will indicate the need for complete ilioinguinal block dissection.
- **Technique:** A dye, isosulphan blue, is injected at the site of primary tumour. After sometime, the inguinal dissection is done to expose the sentinel lymph node area and the lymph nodes which take up the dye, are sent for pathological examination. Based on the report, if node is positive for malignancy, a complete inguinal block dissection is indicated and in case of negative nodes, nothing else is required and patient is kept under regular follow up.
- Only 50% of patients presenting with palpable lymph nodes actually have metastatic disease, the remainder have lymph node enlargement secondary to inflammation. So, subjecting all patients with inguinal lymphadenopathy to surgery is not recommended. Hence, a course of antibiotics is given and wait for a period of 4-6 weeks, if the nodes are still palpable, block dissection is carried out. If the nodes are not palpable, and if primary tumour is poorly differntiated, superficial lymph node dissection is done and further treatment depends upon whether the nodes are positive or negative.
- Algorithm (Fig. 42.4) helps in the management of these patients is given in the next page.

Stage IV

- Radiotherapy + chemotherapy (cisplatin, methotrexate and bleomycin are the drugs used commonly).

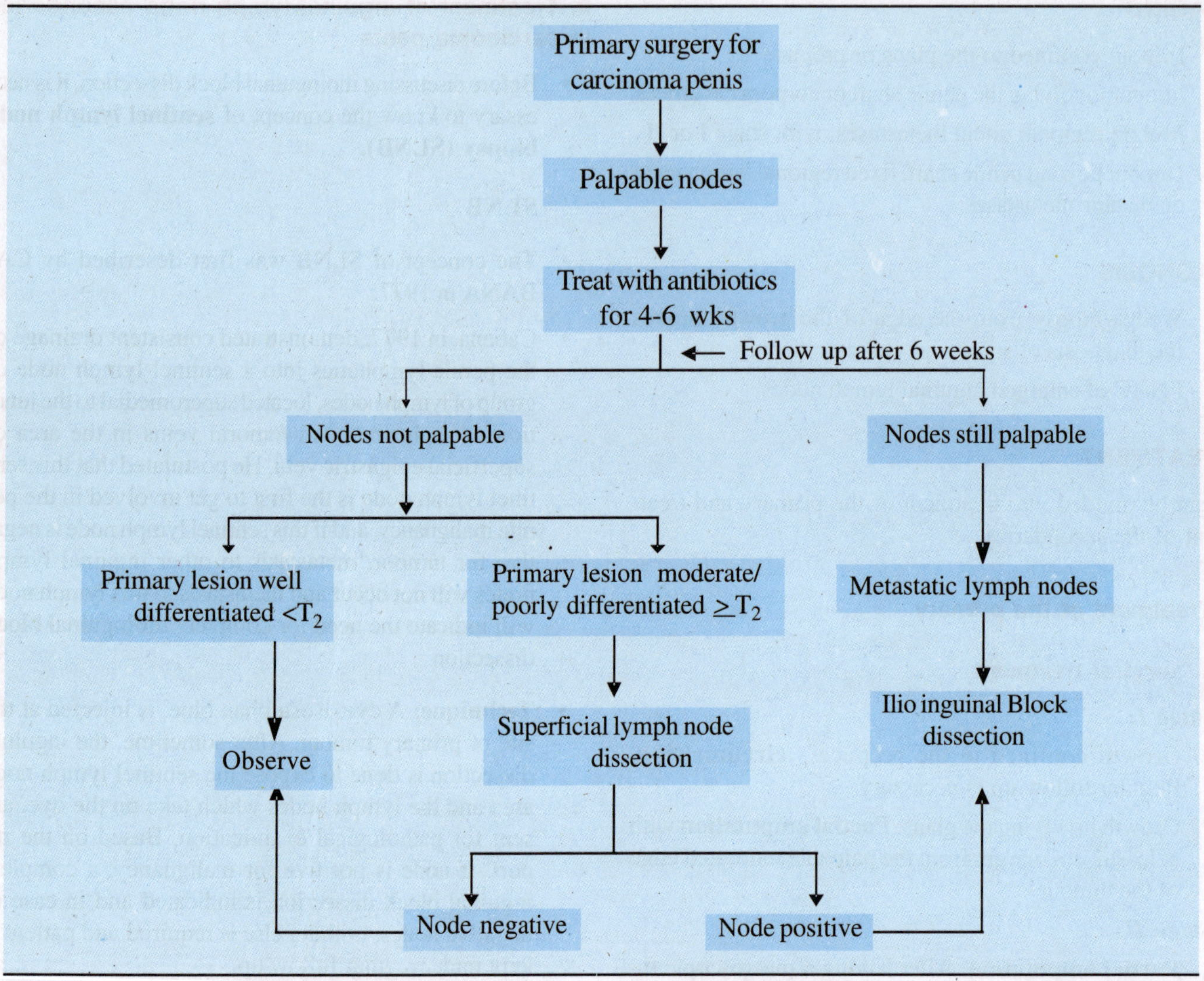

Primary surgery for carcinoma penis

↓

Palpable nodes

↓

Treat with antibiotics for 4-6 wks

← Follow up after 6 weeks

Nodes not palpable | Nodes still palpable

Primary lesion well differentiated <T₂ | Primary lesion moderate/ poorly differentiated ≥T₂ | Metastatic lymph nodes

Observe | Superficial lymph node dissection | Ilio inguinal Block dissection

Node negative | Node positive

Fig. 42.4 Algorithm of management of inguinal lymph node secondaries from carcinoma penis

B. Role of radiotherapy

Indications

1. Young patients who want to have a sexual life
2. Patient refuses surgery
3. Fixed/ulcerated inguinal metastasis

Types

1. External radiotherapy:
   - **Dose:** 4000-6000 rads which can include iliac and inguinal node also.
2. Interstitial radiotherapy: Iridium wires/tantalum wires are implanted within the glans.

Complication of radiotherapy

- Radionecrosis of penis

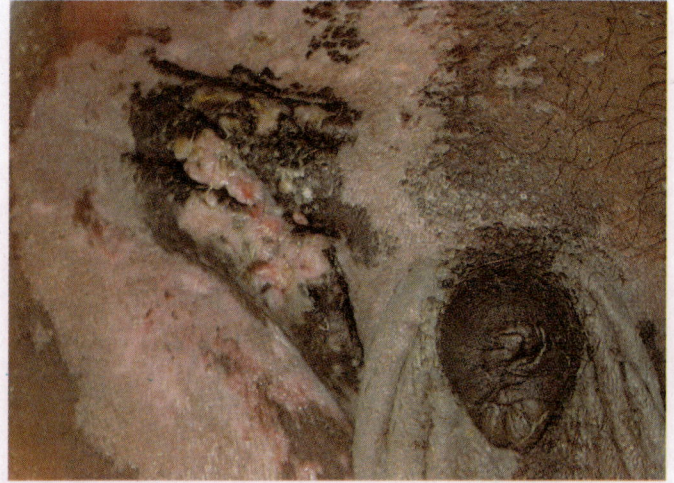

Fig. 42.5 Advanced lymph node secondaries treated with radiation

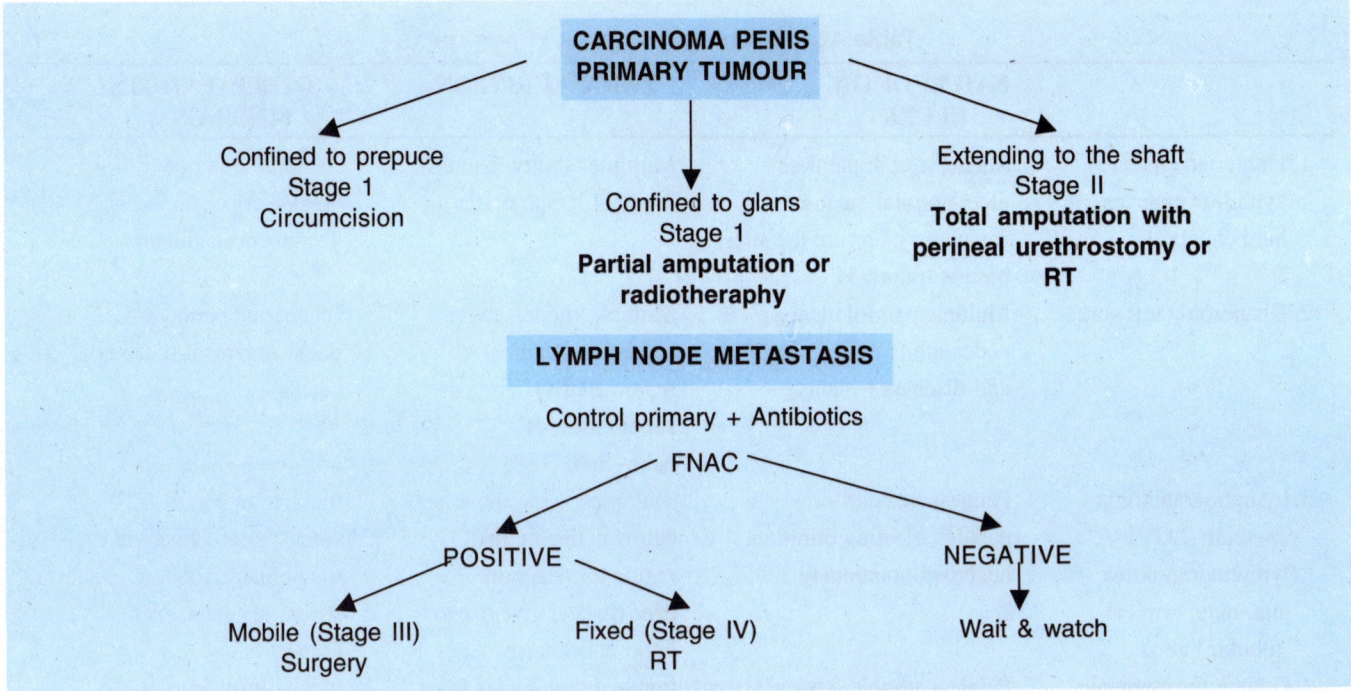

Fig. 42.6 Summary of the treatment of carcinoma of penis

- Summary of the treatment (Fig. 42.6)

PEYRONIE'S DISEASE

Aetiology

- Past trauma has been considered as one of the factors.
- Venereal diseases also have been blamed

Clinical features

- Hard plaques of fibrosis can be palpated along the length of the penis in the sheath of corpora cavernosa (induratio -penis -plastica).
- As a result of hard plaques, erection is not proper, and the erected penis tends to bend towards the side of the plaque.

Treatment

- Watch and observe some cases. It may regress after a few years.
- Straightening of the penis is recommended if the deformity is distressing.

DIFFERENTIAL DIAGNOSIS OF ULCER PENIS

- There are many causes of ulcer penis. The important ones being carcinoma and sexually transmitted diseases.
- The incubation period is an important clue followed by the nature of the ulcer for the diagnosis.
- Differential diagnosis is given in the next page (Table 42.1)

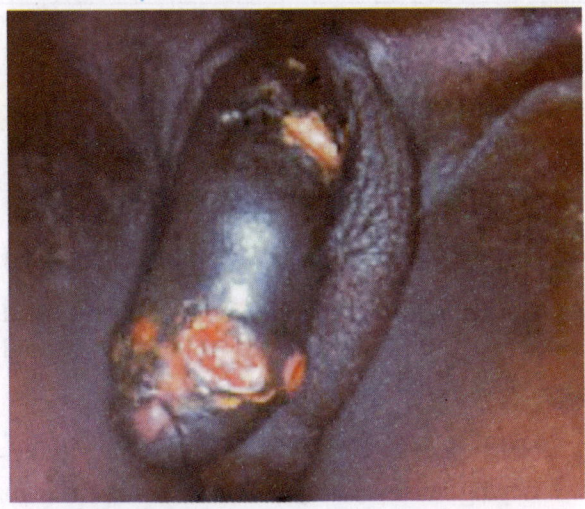

Fig. 42.7 Multiple painless ulcers due to chancroid

Table 42.1 Differential diagnosis of ulcer penis

	NATURE OF THE ULCER	INGUINAL REGION	OTHER FEATURES FINDINGS
1. Hunterian chancre (syphilitic chancre, hard chancre)	Single, round, painless ulcer-coronal sulcus, frenulum, glans are the sites; base is indurated	Multiple, shotty, painless inguinal lymph nodes	Incubation period-3 weeks; organism. Treponema pallidum
2. Chancroid (soft sore)	Multiple painful ulcers; oedematous edges, slough and discharge-plenty	Multiple nodes-above and below inguinal region-**BUBO**; suppuration of bubo--SINUSES	Incubation period 3-4 days; organism--Ducrey's bacilli
3. Lymphogranuloma venereum (LGV) (lymphogranuloma inguinale, tropical tubular bubo)	Painless vesicles or papules, fleeting duration, heals spontaneously	Multiple nodes above and below in the inguinal region form **sign of groove,** later give rise to bubo and sinuses	Incubation period 1-2 weeks; virus Chlamydia trachomatis; rubbery rectal stricture; can occur in females
4. Granuloma inguinale (granuloma venereum)	Painless vesicle, changes into an ulcer with exuberant granulation tissue; highly contagious ulcer; bleeds but painless	Inguinal region may be involved, but inguinal lymph nodes are not involved unless secondary infection supervenes	Incubation period-10-40 days; Organism-Donovania granulomatis (bacilli)
5. Balanoposthitis ulcers	Multiple, painful ulcers, difficulty in retracting prepuce	Lymph node enlargement uncommon	Recurrent balanoposthitis common in diabetic patients
6. Herpes progenitalis	Vesicles and pustules on the prepuce or on the glans	Inguinal lymph nodes are not enlarged	Neuralgic pain and itching occurs before the onset of ulcer
7. Carcinomatous ulcer	Painless, indurated ulcer with everted edges; bleeds on touch	Tender nodes, hard nodes. metastasis	Phimosis is one aetiological factor

ANATOMY OF TESTIS AND EPIDIDYMIS

TESTIS

- **Size:** 4x3x2.5cms found one each in both scrotal sacs.

- **Functional unit is a lobule:** 250 lobules filled with seminiferous tubules. It has following cells and their function is given below:

  Germ cells $\longrightarrow$ Sperm production

  Leydig cells $\longrightarrow$ Testosterone production

  Sertoli cells $\longrightarrow$ Oestrogen production

- The seminiferous tubules converge to form a rete testis, which is connected to the epididymis through 5-7 efferent ductules.

- Covered by thick inseparable covering of fibrous tissue - **tunia albuginea.**

- The serous space in front and lateral surface of testis is **tunica vaginalis.**

- **Blood supply** is by testicular artery - a branch of aorta. Veins form pampiniform plexus in the scrotum.

- **Lymphatics:** Para-aortic nodes lying along the side of aorta at the level of origin of the testicular arteries (L2) just above umbilicus.

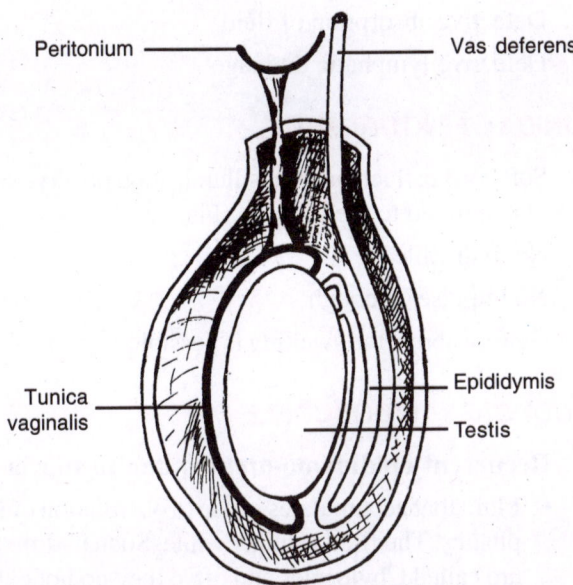

Fig. 42.8 Anatomy of the testis and epididymis

Epididymis

*   It is 6 mts. in length (20 feet long), highly coiled and packed and adherent to posterior surface of the testis.
*   It has following parts - head, body and tail. Head and body are commonly involved in tuberculosis resulting in posterior sinus formation.
*   It is lined by tall columnar epithelium
*   The head receives vasa efferentia from the rete testis and is firmly attached to the testis.
*   From the tail, the vas deferens (ductus deferens), a direct continuation of the canal of the epididymis, passes up medially.
*   Epididymis is supplied by branch of testicular artery

HYDROCOELE

Collection of excessive fluid in the tunica vaginalis sac (TV sac).

I. CONGENITAL HYDROCOELE

Occurs due to patent processus vaginalis sac either completely or partially.

Types

1. Vaginal hydrocoele (Fig.42.9)

*   Occurs when hydrocoele sac is patent only in the scrotum.
2. **Infantile hydrocoele** (Fig.42.10):
*   The sac from the scrotum is patent upto the deep inguinal ring.
3. **True congenital hydrocoele** (Fig. 42.11)
*   In this condition, the scrotal sac communicates with the peritoneal cavity. It is seen in infants, may be secondary to TB peritonitis. The scrotal swelling appears when the child assumes an erect posture for a long time and it may not reduce due to **Inverted ink bottle** effect. Hence, congenital hydrocoele is not reducible. It regresses in size if the child assumes supine position while sleeping.
4. **Encysted hydrocoele of the cord** (Fig. 42.12)
*   In this condition, the sac is obliterated above (inguinal canal) and below (scrotum) but patent at the root of the scrotum around spermatic cord.
*   It presents as a soft, cystic, fluctuant transilluminant swelling separate from testis, well above the testis.
*   Diagnosis is established by **traction test** - The swelling has got free mobility but when traction is applied to testis gently, the swelling becomes fixed and it moves down when testis is pulled down. This variety of hydrocoele is treated by excision of the sac.
5. **Hydrocoele-en-Bissac** (bilocular hydrocoele) (Fig. 42.13)
*   In this condition, the scrotal sac communicates with another sac underneath the anterior abdominal wall musculature. Diagnosis is made by eliciting **cross-fluctuation** test.
6. **Hydrocoele of canal of Nuck** (Fig. 42.14)
*   It presents as a swelling in the inguinal region in female.

II. ACQUIRED HYDROCOELE

a. Primary or idiopathic (Refer Table 40.2 for comparison).

b. Secondary hydrocoele

PRIMARY VAGINAL HYDROCOELE

This is the most common type of hydrocoele which is seen in young adults, middle age and beyond. It is due to following causes:

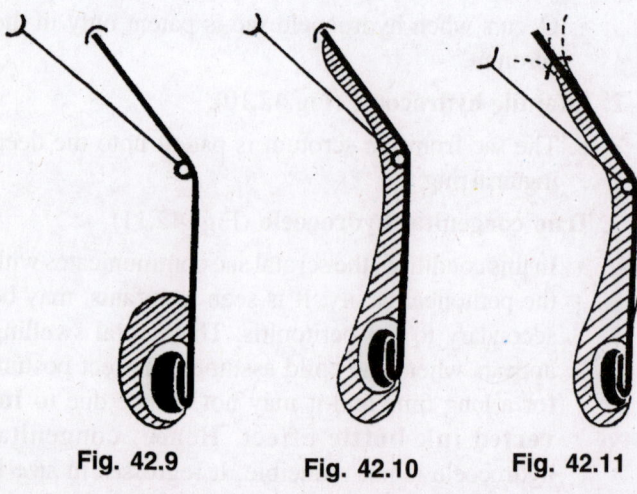

Fig. 42.9	Fig. 42.10	Fig. 42.11

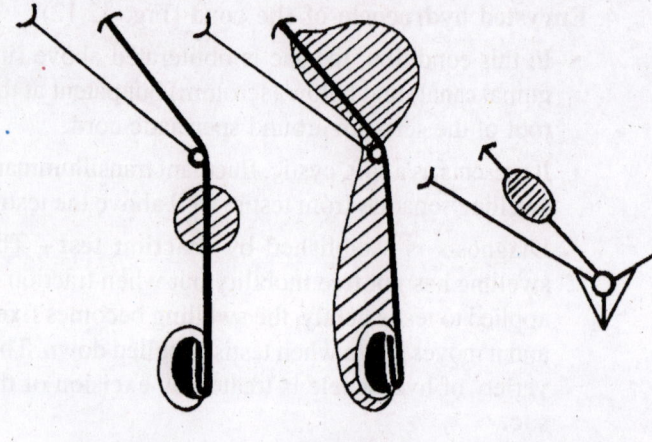

Fig. 42.12	Fig. 42.13	Fig. 42.14

Various types of hydrocoele

1. Defective absorption of fluid
2. Defective lymphatic drainage

CLINICAL FEATURES

* Soft, cystic, fluctuant, transillumination positive swelling confined to the scrotum (Fig. 42.15).
* Not reducible
* No impulse on cough
* Getting above the swelling is possible

SECONDARY HYDROCOELE

1. **Recurrent epididymo-orchitis due to filariasis**

   * Fluid that accumulates is due to obstruction of lymphatics. The fluid is milky white. Such hydrocoeles are called Chyloceles and often they do not exhibit transillumination. (See the key box)

2. **Tuberculous epididymo-orchitis** (Figs. 42.16, 42.17):

   * Retrograde infection from the seminal vesicles
   * **Craggy epididymis** refers to rough, hard irregular surface. This involves the epididymal head and causes fibrosis. So, the epididymis feels craggy. Vas deferens feels like beads, called as **beaded vas.** Secondary hydrocoele occurs in 30% of the cases. Eventually it forms **cold abscess** which ruptures and results in sinus posteriorly, in the scrotum.
   * It never involves the testis proper.

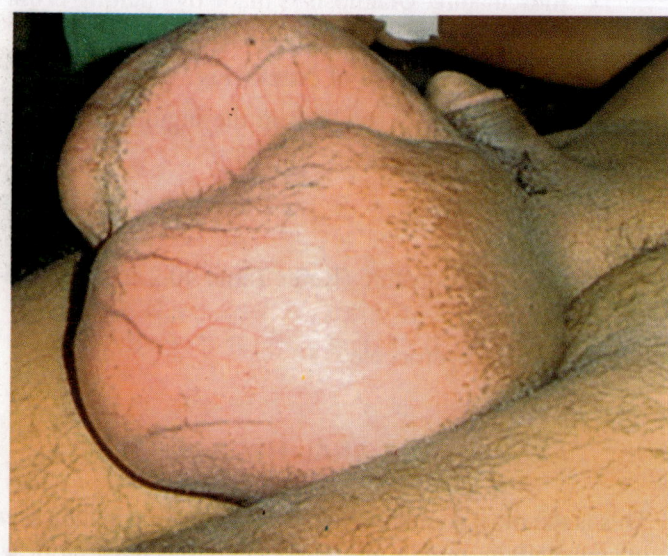

Fig. 42.15 Bilateral primary vaginal hydrocoele

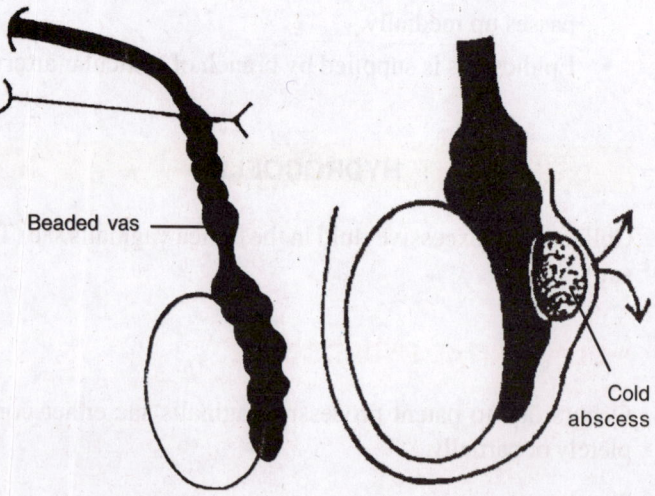

Beaded vas

Cold abscess

Fig. 42.16 and 42.17 Tuberculous epididymo-orchitis

Table 40.2 Comparison of primary hydrocoele with secondary hydrocoele

	PRIMARY HYDROCOELE	SECONDARY HYDROCOELE
Aetiology	Defective absorption of fluid	Excessive production of fluid
Examples	Vaginal hydrocoele, infantile hydrocoele, etc.	Filarial hydrocoele, secondary to malignancy of the testis, etc.
Size	Moderate, big	Small
Palpation of the testis	Difficult	Easily palpable
Transillumination	Positive in majority of the cases	Usually negative
Consistency	Tensely cystic	Lax, cystic
Treatment	Partial excision and eversion	Treatment of the primary

3. **Testicular tumours** can present with a swelling of the scrotum, often diagnosed as hydrocoele. Any young patient with a rapidly growing scrotal swelling-could be a testicular neoplasm. Fluid within the sac is haemorrhagic

4. **Pyocele:** Infected hydrocoele. Infection in a hydrocoele is rare because of the tunica vaginalis sac which is relatively avascular. However, few cases may get infected resulting in pyocele. These patients present with fever and chills and rigors.

5. **Haematocoele:** Trauma to the hydrocoele or spontaneous bleeding into the sac

---

Key Box 42.2

HYDROCOELE TRASILLUMINATION NEGATIVE

- Sac is very thick
- Sac is calcified
- Chylocele
- Haematocele
- Pyocele
- Malignancy testis - blood stained effusion

Comparison of primary and secondary hydrocoele is given in Table 40.2.

TREATMENT OF HYDROCOELE (Page 806)

1. **Lord's plication** is indicated in small hydrocoeles. The sac is opened and the cut edge of the sac is plicated to tunica albuginea. (It is the reflected portion of the processus vaginalis). As a result, the sac gets crumpled up near the testis. The testicular secretions get absorbed by subcutaneous lymphatics and venous system.

2. **Partial excision and eversion** of the sac: Jaboulay's operation. This is indicated in large hydrocoeles. The thick, large, sac is excised and is sutured behind testis.

3. **Aspiration** is a temporary method and there is a chance of introducing infection. It can be done only in high risk patients. This is a procedure to be condemned.

Key Box 42.3

TREATMENT

- Observe
- Lord's plication
- Jaboulay's operation

COMPLICATIONS OF HYDROCOELE

1. Haematocoele: Occurs due to minor trauma

2. Pyocoele: Infected hematocele

3. Calcification of hydrocoele sac

4. Rupture of hydrocoele sac-very rare

5. Hernia of the hydrocoele sac occurs when there is a small tear in the sac resulting in accumulation of fluid in the subcutaneous planes (Fig. 40.8).

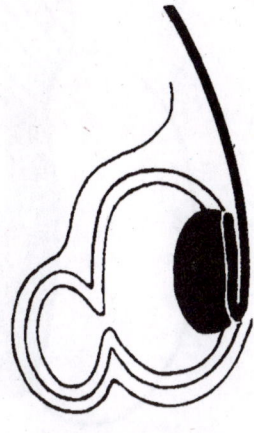

Fig. 42.18 Hernia of hydrocoele sac

Table 40.3 Comparison of epididymal cyst with spermatocoele

	EPIDIDYMAL CYST	SPERMATOCOELE
1. Aetiology	Cystic degeneration of the appendages of epididymis - **congenital**	Obstruction to the sperm conducting mechanism; **acquired** - retention cyst
2. Site	Behind and above the testis in the region of epididymal head	Behind the body of the testis
3. Loculi	Multilocular	Unilocular
4. Contents	Crystal clear, watery	Barley water - like
5. Transillumination	Brilliant (Chinese lantern pattern)	Poor transillumination-very often negative
6. Aspiration	Results in recurrence as the cyst is multilocular	May cure as the cyst is unilocular
7. Excision	Excision may be necessary if the cyst is large	May be excised if aspiration is not successful

CYSTIC SWELLINGS IN THE SCROTUM

I. Hydrocoele

II. Retention cyst

1. Spermatocoele (see Table 40.3 and Fig. 40.19)
2. Sebaceous cyst (skin of the scrotum)

III. Congenital cyst

1. Epididymal cyst (Fig. 40.20)
2. Cyst of the hydatid of Morgagni

IV. Tubercular epididymoorchitis

- Cold abscess with a sinus in the posterior aspect of scrotum.

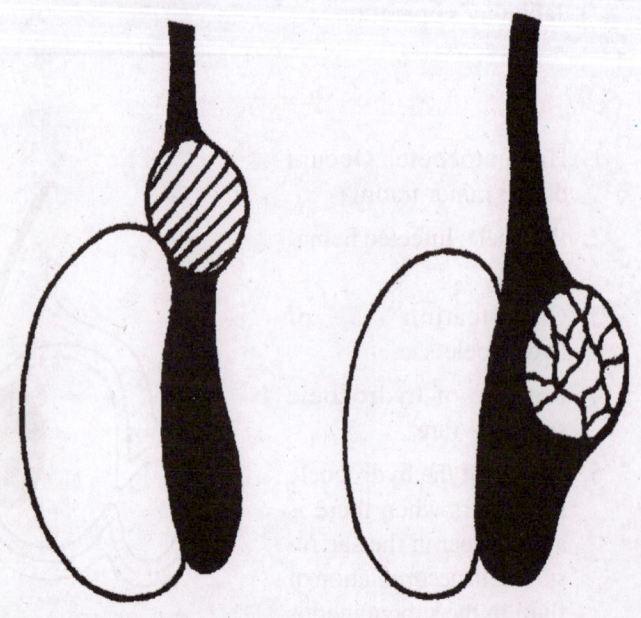

Fig. 42.19 Spermatocoele   **42.20** Epididymal cyst

UNDESCENDED TESTIS

When the testis is arrested somewhere in its normal pathway to the scrotum, undescended testis results.

DEVELOPMENT

- The testis develops in the retroperitoneum close to the posterior abdominal wall from the genital tubercles.
- It is guided to the scrotum by the gubernaculum.
- Around 7th month, it reaches the deep inguinal ring, 8th month inguinal canal and 9th month, superficial inguinal pouch. In normal situations, the testis reaches the scrotum at full term.
- As it comes down, it is surrounded by processus vaginalis sac. This sac gets completely obliterated in normal persons. The persistence of the processes vaginalis sac is responsible for development of a hernia and hydrocoele.

CAUSES

1. **Muscular hypotonia:** The descent of the testis depends upon muscular contractions of the anterior abdominal wall. Hence undescended testis is seen in children with poor muscle tone, e.g. Prune belly syndrome, Down's syndrome
2. **Gubernaculum dysfunction**
3. **Maternal human chorionic gonadotropin** (HCG) which causes development (maturation) of testis and also helps in descent of the testis. If there is deficiency of HCG, imperfectly developed undescended testis appears.
4. **Familial**

5. Retroperitoneal adhesions prevent the descent of the testis.

CLINICAL FEATURES

1. Right side is more often involved. Bilateral undescended testis is found in about 20% of cases.

2. **Cryptorchidism:** When both testis are impalpable as in cases of abdominal testis and inguinal testis.

3. **Retractile testis:** In this condition the scrotum is well developed, and the testis is palpable at the root of the scrotum and can be brought down to the scrotum. Retractile testis is harmless and spontaneously gets corrected within 1-2 years of age, without any treatment. The squatting position may help in such cases, in diagnosing the condition.

COMPLICATIONS (can be remembered as TESTIS)

T Trauma produces pain

E Epididymo-orchitis will mimic an acute abdomen

S Sterility: Histological changes start at the age of 2 years and by the age of 12 irreversible damage occurs to the spermatogenesis, due to atrophy of testes. Endocrine function will remain normal.

T Torsion

I Indirect hernia in majority of cases

S Seminoma of testis and other testicular malignancies are reported in greater frequency in undescended testis than in normal testis.

TREATMENT

1. **Treatment of choice is orchidopexy**

   - It can be done by open method or laparoscopic method.
   - It can also be a one stage or two stage procedure

   Procedure

   - Considering the psychological, functional . and malignant potential, 2 years is the ideal age in bilateral undescended testis and 4 years for unilateral cases. Testis is explored in the inguinal canal. It is mobilised by dividing the adhesions and brought down into the scrotum and fixed by using nonabsorbable suture material.
   - A dartos pouch can be formed and followed later by narrowing of the root of scrotum.
   - Associated hernial sac is excised

2. Orchidectomy is done after the age of 14 years because of malignant potential.

3. **Ombredanne's procedure:** Testis is brought down into the opposite scrotum through scrotal septum and kept in dartos pouch.

ECTOPIC TESTIS

- Testis is present in an **ectopic** site (not the route through which is desends).

- **Sites** of ectopic sites are:

  1. Superficial inguinal pouch
  2. Perineum
  3. Root of the penis
  4. Femoral triangle (thigh)

- Anatomically the size and physiologically, it functions normally.

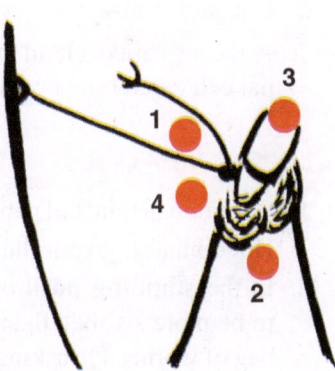

Fig. 42.21 Sites of ectopic testis

- **Embrology:** Testis reaches the scrotum by the scrotal tail gubernaculum. However, if this is weak, the other scrotal tail may pull it in a different direction, resulting in ectopic testis (**Lockwood theory**).

- **Complication:** It is more prone for injuries

- **Treatment:** Orchidopexy in a new scrotal pouch

VARICOCOELE

DEFINITION

- Dilatation of testicular veins with/without cremasteric veins which drain into testicular veins.

- Testicular veins which drain the testis and epididymis, form multiple veins in the scrotum which are called as pampiniform plexus of veins. As they travel the inguinal canal, they are reduced to 6-8 in number. At the level of deep ring, they are 2 in number and in retroperitoneum, it forms the single testicular vein.

- On the right side, the testicular vein drains into inferior vena cava (IVC) directly.
- On the left side, it drains into the left renal vein at right angles where there is a valve.

AETIOLOGY

1. Varicocoele is common on the left side (because left testis is at a lower level than the right). The flow of the blood from the left side is into the renal vein where it makes an angle of 90 degree.
2. Congenital absence of valves
3. A recent varicocele in an elderly patient suggests renal cell carcinoma invading the renal veins.

CLINICAL FEATURES

1. Common in thin, tall patients
2. Hot climates, favour the development of varicocoele.
3. In the **standing position**, the diseased side appears to be more swollen than the other side. It feels like a bag of worms. On asking the patient to cough, there is fluid thrill, due to regurgitation of venous blood. On the viable side, the scrotum is at a lower level.
4. On asking the patient to lie down, it is reducible (disappears).
5. Dragging pain in the scrotum is a feature, but it is nontender.
6. Testis may appear small and soft with diminished testicular sensation.
7. **Blow test:** On blowing, fluid thrill may be felt, it may increase in size (Valsalva manoeuvre).

COMPLICATIONS

OLIGOSPERMIA is the major but significant complication of varicocoele.

This occurs due to following reasons:
1. The **venous congestion** due to the varicocele results in increased temperature in the scrotum which is supposed to affect spermatogenesis.
2. **Reflux of the blood** from the renal vein brings powerful hormones secreted from adrenal glands like corticosteroids and adrenaline which may suppress spermatogenesis.

TREATMENT

1. **Inguinal approach:** Excision of pampiniform plexus

in the inguinal canal after ligating them. Testis still has a venous drainage through cremasteric veins.
2. **Retroperitoneal approach:** (Palomo's operation) In the retroperitoneum, testicular vein is single and is separate from vas deferans. Hence, it is ligated up in the retroperitoneum. This operation is better than inguinal approach since there is no danger of damaging the vas and ligation of testicular vein is easy.
3. **Sub-inguinal microscopic** varicocoelectomy for complete ligation

TORSION TESTIS (Torsion of spermatic cord)

Predisposing causes

1. **Inversion of testis** is the commonest cause where testis lies horizontally or upside down.
2. **High investment** of tunica vaginalis
3. In cases where the body of testis is separated from the epididymis.
4. **Sudden contraction** of spirally attached cremasteric muscle leads to rotation of testis around the vertical axis during straining at stools, lifting heavy weight, coitus.

Clinical features

1. Age: 10-25 years
2. Sudden agonising pain in the groin and lower abdomen and may be with vomiting.
3. **Scrotum is empty** and oedematous on the side of lesion.
4. Tender lump at the external abdominal ring - the testis is positioned high (**Deming's sign**)
5. Elevation of scrotum increases pain in torsion of completely descended testis (decreases pain in epididymoorchitis).
6. **Angell's sign:** Because of the presence of mesorchium, opposite testis lies horizontally.

Management

- Scrotal doppler to confirm the diagnosis
1. In the first hour untwist the testis manually
2. If this is not successful do urgent exploration of the scrotum and undo the torsion and viable testis should be fixed to the scrotum to prevent recurrence
3. Gangrenous testis should be removed
4. Opposite side testis should be fixed at an early date to prevent torsion

TESTICULAR TUMOURS

They constitute 1% of all malignant tumours in the males and almost all are malignant (more than 99%).

CLASSIFICATION

A. WHO CLASSIFICATION

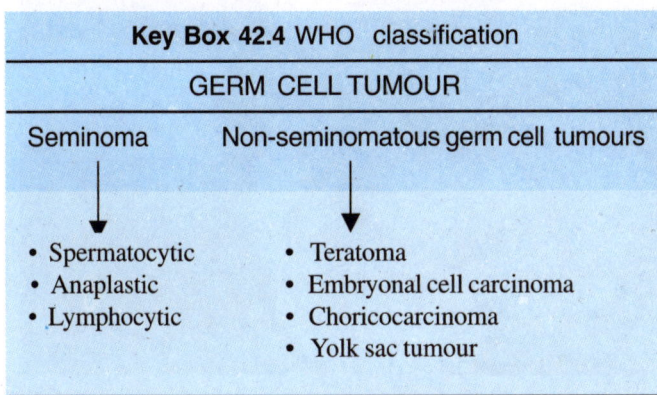

Key Box 42.4 WHO classification
GERM CELL TUMOUR

Seminoma →

Non-seminomatous germ cell tumours →

- Spermatocytic
- Anaplastic
- Lymphocytic

- Teratoma
- Embryonal cell carcinoma
- Choricocarcinoma
- Yolk sac tumour

B. OTHER CLASSIFICATION

I. Seminoma has the most common tumour incidence-50%

Types

1. Spermatocytic type-good prognosis
2. Lymphocytic type
3. Anaplastic type

II. Teratoma

- Incidence: 30% (subtype will be discussed later)

III. Combined

- 10 to 20%

IV. Interstitial cell tumours

 a. Leydig cell tumour

- It is prepubertal tumour
- Causes masculinisation
- Increased androgens

 b. Sertoli cell tumours

- They are feminising tumours
- Increased oestrogens
- Postpubertal tumour

V. Lymphoma of testis: Very rare

SEMINOMA

AETIOLOGY

1. **Undescended testis,** undoubtedly predisposes to seminoma.
   - 1 in 20 abdominal testis, 1 in 60 testis at the level of deep ring and 1 in 80 inguinal testis are prone for testicular tumours.
   - However, it should be noted that 25% of testicular cancers in patients with cryptorchidism occur in normal, descended testis.
2. **Trauma** to the testis is a coincidence. This may not precipitate a testicular tumour but brings to the attention of the patient.

PATHOLOGY

1. Seminoma arises from the seminiferous tubules. As the tumour grows, it compresses the (normal) testicular tissue. The cut surface is smooth, homogenous.
   - **Microscopy:** Round to oval cells with prominent nucleus. In few cases, lymphocytic infiltration can be found.
2. Teratoma arises from rete testis. The tumour contains totipotential cells and so can have ectodermal, mesodermal and endodermal elements (Key Box 42.5).

Key Box 42.5
TYPES OF TERATOMA

1. Teratoma differentiated: The most benign form of a malignant tumour - high orchidectomy
2. Malignant teratoma intermediate: The cells are mixture of differentiated and anaplastic cells
3. Malignant teratoma anaplastic: Highly malignant tumour
4. Malignant teratoma trophoblastic: Secretes HCG and it is similar to choriocarcinoma in a female

SPREAD

- Seminoma spreads by lymphatic route. Along the testicular vessels it spreads to paraaortic lymph node mass, through thoracic duct, to mediastinal nodes and left supraclavicular nodes.

- Malignant teratomatus tumours spreads predominantly by blood.

CLINICAL FEATURES OF TESTICULAR TUMOURS

I. Typical presentation

1. **Age:** Teratoma 20-30 years, seminoma 30-40 years

2. **Testicular swelling:** More often heaviness (Fig. 40.22) due to tumour rather than hypertrophy or if it is infiltrated with tumour but vas is never involved. This is called **sign of vas negative** (sign of vas positive in TB epididymo-orchitis where there is beading of vas).

5. **Haemospermia:** Blood in the semen, is rare

6. **Infertility:** Not uncommon

7. **Gynaecomastia** is seen in about 10% of the patients.

Key Box 42.6

TESTICULAR CANCER

- Irregular testis
- Indurated testis
- Nodular testis
- Nontender enlarged testis
- Young age testicular mass

II. Atypical presentation

1. Hurricane variety is the most malignant tumour. The tumour grows rapidly with pulmonary metastasis (cannon ball) and death in a few days.

2. Mimicking acute epididymo-orchitis : This variety presents as severe pain along with the swelling of the testis, but does not respond to antibiotics.

III. Symptoms mainly due to metastases

1. **Lymphatic spread**

- Para-aortic node mass-distension of the abdomen.
- Left supraclavicular node mass-swelling in the neck.
- Iliac node mass-swelling of the leg.

2. **Blood spread:** Extensive pulmonary secondaries occur from a malignant teratoma.

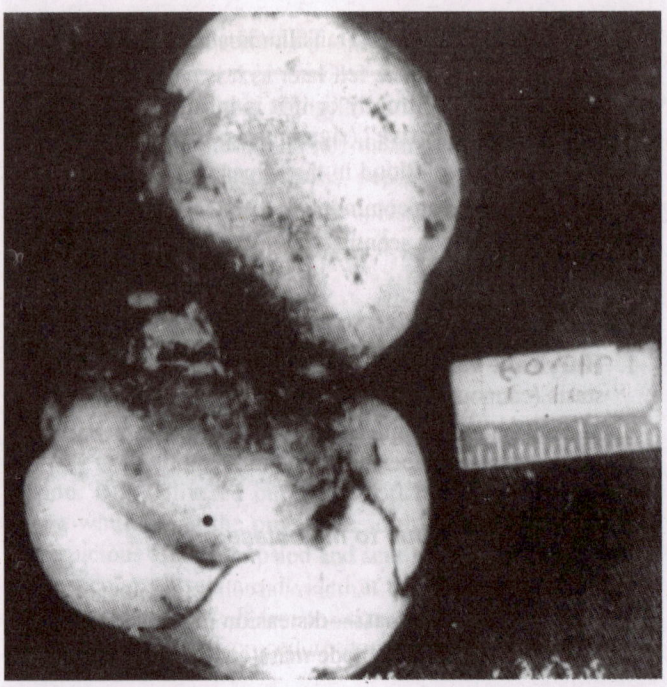

Fig. 40.22 Seminoma testis. Contributed by Prof. Sashidharan, KMC, Manipal

STAGING OF TESTICULAR CANCER

- Stage I Tumour confined to the testis only.

- Stage IIA Tumour and lymph nodes below the diaphragm-size less than 2 cm.

- Stage IIB Tumour and lymph nodes below the diaphragm-size more than 2 cm.

- Stage III Tumour and lymph nodes above the diaphragm.

- Stage IV Blood spread to lungs/liver/elsewhere.

INVESTIGATIONS

1. **No biopsy** should be done through scrotal route, because if the scrotal skin is involved, the spread occurs to inguinal lymphnodes opening up one more channel of lymphatics.

2. **Chest X-ray** To rule out cannon ball secondaries as in teratoma.

3. **IVP** to see back pressure effect on the kidney (hydronephrosis) due to enlarged paraaortic nodes).

4. **Abdominal ultrasonography** to see for enlarged lymph nodes, secondaries in the liver, or to detect a tumour in an undescended testis. However, CT scan is a better investigation.

5. 24 hours urine sample for HCG. (See the key box)
   - Normal levels-less than 100 IU
   - More than 1000 IV is diagnostic of choriocarcinoma
   - Hence, it is the tumour marker of choriocarcinoma

6. **Human chorionic gonadotrophin: Serum HCG:**
   - As the name suggests, it is made by chorionic elements.
   - The whole HCG (α- and β-HCG) may be increased in testicular neoplasm, melanoma, lymphoma, etc. It can also be raised in non-malignant conditions like cirrhosis, peptic ulcer disease, etc.
   - It is the β-HCG which is more important in diagnosing testicular neoplasms and also useful in the post-operative period to know residual tumour or recurrent tumour.
   - The blood levels of β-**HCG is 0 ng/ml.**

Key Box 42.7

β- HCG

- Never found in normal persons
- Choriocarcinoma - 100% cases
- Embryonal carcinoma - 65% of cases
- Seminoma - 10% of cases
- Increased levels after orchidectomy recurrence residual tumour.
- Tumour marker of teratocarcinoma

---

7. **α-fetoprotein:** Increased in non-seminomatous germ cell tumours.

8. **Lactate dehydrogenase (LDH):** Increased in non-seminomatous germ cell tumours.

9. **Placental alkaline phosphatase** is increased in seminoma testis.

MANAGEMENT

I. When a patient presents with rapidly growing testicular swelling and the neoplasm is doubtful, testis is explored through an inguinal incision. It is delivered out and a soft clamp is applied to the testicular vessels at the level of deep ring while doing the procedure so that tumour embolization does not occur. Testis is split open, the suspicious area is biopsied and sent for fro-

zen section. If the frozen section is positive, the cord and testicular vessels are divided at the level of deep ring and testis is removed. This is called as **high orchidectomy**. If frozen section is negative, the testis is sutured back and replaced back in scrotum. This kind of procedure done through inguinal route is called as **Chevasu's procedure**.

II. SEMINOMA

a. Stage I-IIA (Low stage)
- Radical orchidectomy (high orchidectomy) and radiotherapy to retroperitoneum (2500-3000 cGy) is the treatment of choice:
- 5-year survival rate is around 95%.
- Relapse after radiotherapy is managed by chemotherapy.

b Seminoma stage IIB, III, IV
- Radical orchidectomy + chemotherapy -PVB Regimen -Cisplatin, Vincristine, Bleomycin.

c. Treatment of residual disease in lymph nodes
- In Stage IIB and III, if there is residual lymph nodal mass 3 cm in size even after chemotherapy, then, a retroperitoneal lymph node dissection (RPLND) has to be done.
- Stage IIB and III : Survival for 5 years-75%
- Stage IV : Poor survival.

III. TERATOMA

a. Stage I, IIA (Low stage)
- Radical orchidectomy and RPLND 5-year survival-85%

b. Stage IIB, III
- Radical orchidectomy and Chemotherapy (PVB), post chemotherapy residual tumour in the retroperitoneum and if the tumour markers levels regress-RPLND should be done. 5-year survival rate is around 60%.

c. Stage IV
- Orchidectomy + Chemotherapy-poor prognosis

IV. INTERSTITIAL CELL TUMOUR
- It should be treated like teratoma

Table 42.5 Comparison of seminoma with teratoma

	SEMINOMA	TERATOMA
1. Cell of origin	Seminiferous tubules in the mediastinum of the testis	Totipotential cells in the rete testis
2. Incidence	35-40%	30%
3. Age group	30-40 years	20-30 years
4. Shape of testis	Retained	Not retained
5. Surface	Smooth	Irregular
6. Cut surface	Smooth	Variegated-nodules, cysts
7. Consistency	Firm	Firm or soft (cystic)
8. Spread	Mainly lymphatic	Predominantly blood
9. Tumour markers	---	HCG-malignant teratoma
10. Radiation response	Excellent-melts like snow	Less sensitive

- Comparison of seminoma with teratoma (Table 42.5)

FOURNIER'S GANGRENE (IDIOPATHIC GANGRENE OF SCROTAL SKIN)

AETIOPATHOLOGY

Even though Fournier's gangrene is called as idiopathic gangrene, certain factors precipitate the scrotal gangrene.

1. Low socio-economic group patients.

2. Unhygienic conditions

Following perianal abscesses, urogenital instrumentation a scratch, cut or bruise in the scrotal skin (instrumentation, injury, infection - Key Box 42.8).

CAUSATIVE ORGANISMS

- Microaerophilic Haemolytic streptococci
- Staphylococci
- E. coli
- Anaerobes-Clostridium welchii

(Can be compared to Meleny's ulcer -Synergistic gangrene - affecting abdominal wall skin).

CLINICAL FEATURES

1. Common in young apparently healthy individuals

2. Sudden appearance of scrotal inflammation-red, swollen, very painful. Patient is toxic with fever, prostration.

3. Within one/two days, extensive gangrene of the scrotal skin occurs resulting in sloughing of the scrotal skin exposing the testicles. In few cases, the gangrene can involve skin of the penis, anterior abdominal wall, medial side of thigh, perianal region. In such situations, it is described as perineal phlegmon.

4. Luckily, the testis does not get involved in Fournier's gangrene because of thick tunica albuginea.

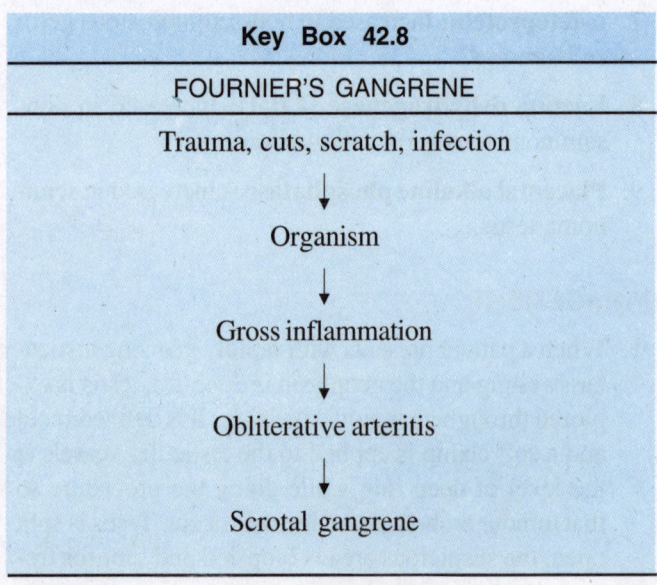

Key Box 42.8

FOURNIER'S GANGRENE

Trauma, cuts, scratch, infection

↓

Organism

↓

Gross inflammation

↓

Obliterative arteritis

↓

Scrotal gangrene

TREATMENT

1. Broad spectrum antibiotics are started, once pus is sent for culture and sensitivity, e.g.

   - Metronidazole for anaerobes
   - Gentamicin for gram-negative organisms
   - Ampicillin for gram-positive organisms
   - Cephalosporins may have to be added if required.

2. Gangrenous portion of the scrotum has to be excised, as soon as possible which brings a dramatic reversal of general condition of the patient from toxic to near normal.

3. If the testicles are exposed, they can be implanted in the thigh or once the inflammation subsides, skin grafting is done to cover testicles.

4. If penile skin is gangrenous, it is excised and covered with split skin graft later. Surprisingly, results are better than expected!!

Fournier's gangrene is classified under the heading of Necrotising fasciitis type I (Page 19).

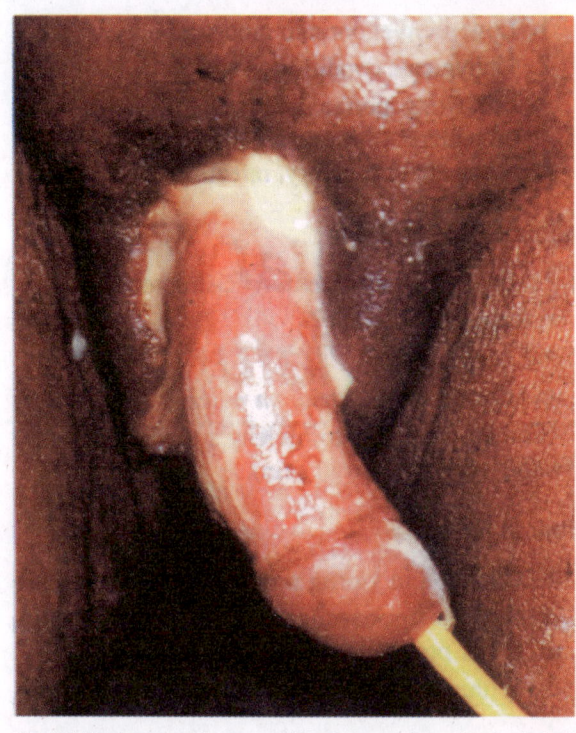

Fig. 42.24 Perineal phlegmon (Dr. Ramachandra L., Manipal)

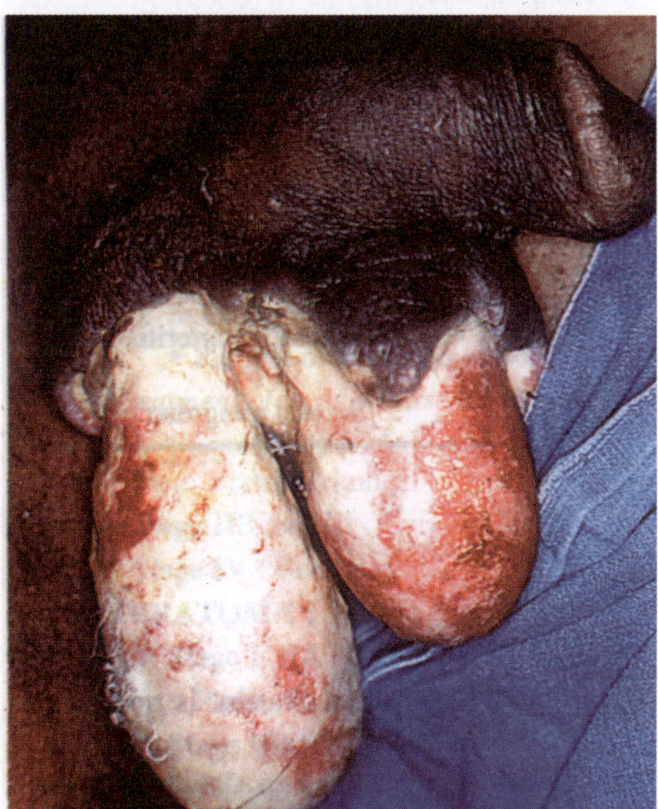

Fig. 42.23 Fournier's gangrene (Prof. U.S. Pai, Manipal)

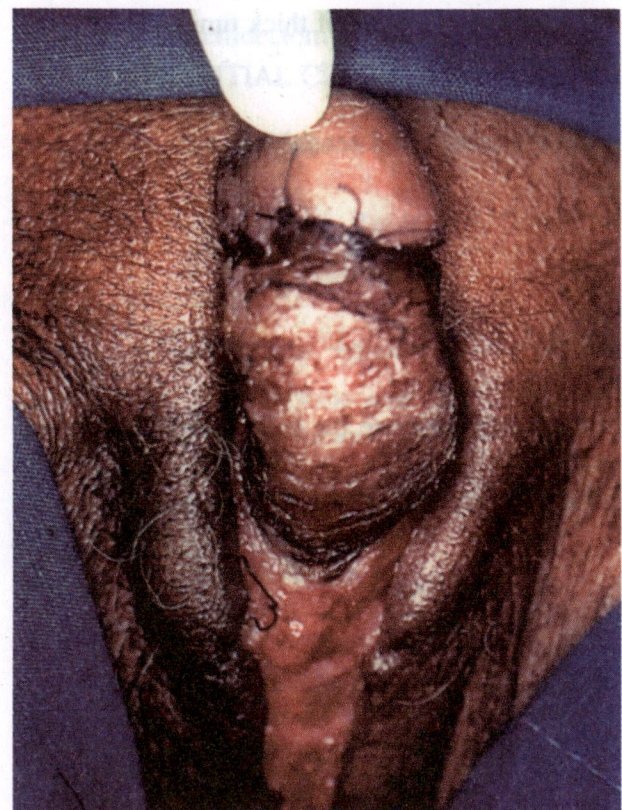

Fig. 42.25 Healing with skin grafting (Dr. Ramachandra L, Manipal)

Differential Diagnosis of Haematuria

43

- Causes
- Investigations
- History

CAUSES OF HAEMATURIA (Fig. 43.1)

I. In the kidney

1. **Infection**
   - Acute glomerulonephritis
   - Tuberculosis
2. **Infarction**
   - SBE with emboli causing renal infarction
   - Massive haemolysis with acute renal tubular necrosis
   - Mismatched blood transfusion
3. **Injury**
   - Stab/blunt injury
4. **Tumours**
   - Wilms' tumour-Nephroblastoma
   - Hypernephroma - Renal cell carcinoma (RCC)
   - Transitional cell carcinoma (TCC)
5. **Stones**
6. **Polycystic kidney**

II. In the ureter

1. Stone
2. Cancer-Rare

III. In the urinary bladder

1. Carcinoma of bladder
2. Carcinoma prostate
3. Cystitis
4. Tuberculosis
5. Bilharziasis
6. Stone-common in school-going children
7. Benign prostatic hyperplasia (BPH)

IV. Urethra

- Stone

V. Rare causes

1. Patients on anticoagulants
2. Sickle cell anaemia
3. Bleeding disorders

Key Box 43.1

HAEMATURIA

COMMON CAUSES
- Urolithiasis
- Tumours

UNCOMMON CAUSES
- Tuberculosis
- Cystitis
- Polycystic kidney

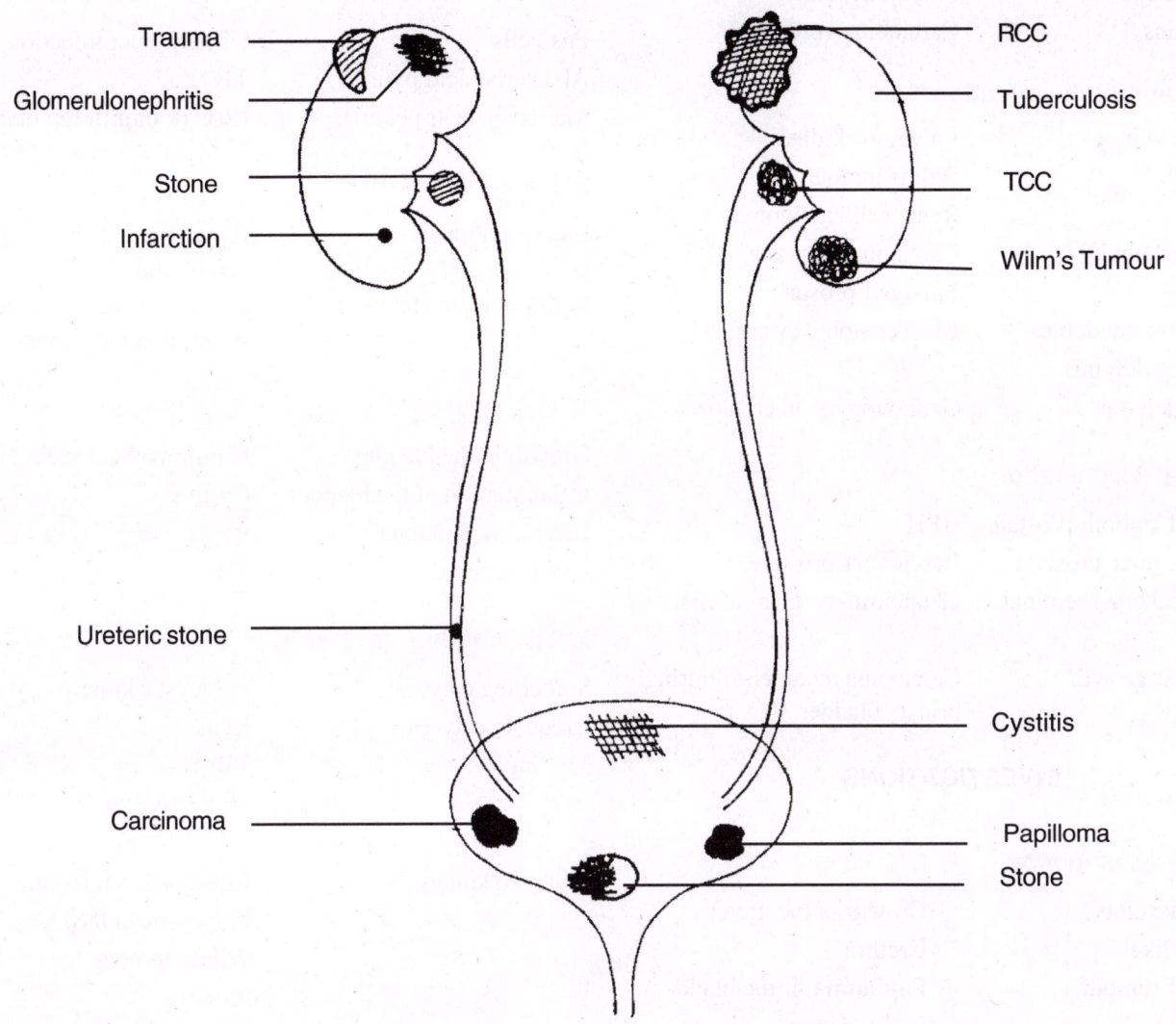

Fig. 41.1 Various causes of haematuria

HISTORY AND EXAMINATION

1. Age and sex

Young children	Vesical calculus
Young adults	Renal stones, tuberculosis (TB)
Elderly patients	Renal cell carcinoma (RCC)

2. Occupation

Aniline dye workers	Carcinoma bladder

3. Haematuria

Bright red	Lower urinary tract
Altered blood	Kidney
Profuse	Papilloma
Small quantity	Renal cell carcinoma, TB, stone
Beginning of micturition	Urethral pathology
End of micturition	Bladder pathology
Mixed with urine	Renal
Painless haematuria	Papilloma or carcinoma
Painful haematuria	Renal stone, bladder stone

4. General physical examination

Gross pallor	Significant blood loss
Gross pallor with minimal blood loss	Renal cell carcinoma

Hypertension	Polycystic kidney
Bony pains	Carcinoma (prostate)

5. Abdominal examination

Palpable kidney	Polycystic kidney
	Wilms' tumour
	Renal cell carcinoma
Distended bladder	Carcinoma prostate
	Enlarged prostate
Suprapubic tenderness	Bladder stone, cystitis
Craggy epididymis	
and beaded vas	Genitourinary tuberculosis

6. Rectal examination

Enlarged smooth prostate	BPH
Hard irregular prostate	Carcinoma prostate
Hard, thickened seminal	Genitourinary tuberculosis
vesicles	—
Advanced growth	Carcinoma rectum infiltrating urinary bladder

INVESTIGATIONS

1. Urine examination

Worm-like clots	Growth in the ureter
Flat disc-like	Urethra
Pieces of tumour	**Papilloma** of the bladder

2. Urine microscopy

Pus cells	Urinary tract infection
Abacterial acid pyuria	TB
Malignant cells positive	RCC or **papilloma** bladder

3. Plain X-ray KUB

Enlarged kidney	Polycystic kidney, renal cell carcinoma
Radio-opaque shadows	Renal stones, ureteric stones, bladder stone

4. Cystoscopy

Growth in the bladder	Papilloma bladder/TCC)
Inflammation of the bladder	Cystitis
Ulcers, hyperaemia, golf-hole ureter	TB

5. Intravenous urography

Spider leg calyces	Polycystic kidney
Irregular calyces	RCC
Missing calyces	TB

6. Ultrasound

Enlarged kidney	Renal cell carcinoma
	Polycystic kidney
	Wilms' tumour
	Stones

• *Differential diagnosis of haematuria is a major theory question in an undergraduate examination. I have given some idea how to evaluate these cases by analysing history, physical examination and investigations. This gives a good exercise to the students.*

44

Cardiothoracic Surgery

- Chest trauma
- Blunt trauma
- Pulmonary injuries
- Tracheobronchial injuries
- Surgical emphysema
- Mediastinal emphysema
- Patent ductus arteriosus
- Coarctation of aorta
- Coronary artery bypass graft
- Recent advances

In chest trauma, the mortality is very high unless it is promptly recognised and treated. The margin of safety is very slim and initial care dictates the final result. With varying degree of severity, chest injuries occur in almost 80% of road traffic accidents.

CHEST TRAUMA - MAIN AIMS OF RESUSCITATION

The standard method of resuscitation in all cases of polytrauma is as follows:

A. AIRWAY

- Aspiration of blood and secretions from oral cavity, pharynx and trachea
- Introduce plastic airway
- Intubation
- Cricothyroidotomy
- Tracheostomy

B. BREATHING

- Intubation
- Intercostal Chest Tube (ICT)
- Closure of any open chest wounds

C. CIRCULATION

- Control of major and life-threatening bleeding
- Volume infusion

D. DISABILITY

- Neurological

E. EXPOSURE

- All clothing to be cut open without moving the patient
- All the above steps are taken by the trauma centre team simultaneously and not one by one.
- Relieve pain. Do not sedate.

- All open wounds of the chest to be covered
- Life threatening injuries should be identified and treated immediately

The above two steps help in re-aerating the lung.

ASSESSMENT OF INJURY

History

- Time since the injury
- Details of the injury from the bystander or the police
- High Speed deceleration injury (aortic and cardiac rupture to be ruled out)
- Crushing accidents (tracheobronchial and oesophageal tear)
- Sudden abdominal compression (ruptured diaphragm)
- In stab injuries, length of the knife and direction of stab

Examination

- The clothing should be removed carefully without moving the patient.
- Palpate for clinical evidence of fractured ribs, surgical emphysema, any paradoxical movement of the ribs and auscultate for air entry in both lungs.
- Even if it is a trivial injury, the patient should be admitted and observed for a minimum of 24 hours before discharge.
- It is reasonable to do unilateral or bilateral closed tube thoracostomy (ICT) on suspicion of haemothorax or pneumothorax when the patient is in respiratory distress.

BLUNT TRAUMA TO THE CHEST

CAUSES

- Road traffic accidents
- Fall from a height
- Crush injuries
- Assault with blunt object

SIMPLE RIB FRACTURE

Rib fracture can be single or multiple.

Single rib fracture

- Often regarded as a trivial injury but should be treated with respect in elderly patients.
- Due to direct injury or excessive flexion.

- The common site is at the costal angle or middle of the shaft.
- Patients will have pain on breathing, coughing and on palpation.
- They are treated by analgesics, intercostal nerve block and assurance.

Multiple rib fractures

- When there are only multiple rib fractures, no pneumo- or **haemothorax** and no other organs are involved, intercostal nerve block and small amount of narcotics are required.
- Strapping is occasionally necessary in young adults.
- Elderly patients consider hospitalisation for observation, pain control and pulmonary toilet.
- Chest X-ray to be repeated after 24hrs and at the time of discharge, to rule out late onset pneumo- and haemothorax.
- Intermittent use of velcro belt rib support
- Inform the patient of deep breathing and coughing using the rib belt
- Epidural analgesia is becoming the standard of care for pain management in patients with multiple rib fractures

Key Box 44.2
POINTS TO REMEMBER

- First rib fracture is a marker for severe trauma - injury to brachial plexus, subclavian artery and vein
- Displaced fracture of 8th to 10th rib -injury to liver, spleen
- Fracture of 11th to 12th rib - injury to kidney
- Penetrating injury to left lower chest wall- injury to heart, lung, diaphragm, stomach and spleen

STERNAL FRACTURE

- Commonly due to steering wheel injury-blunt trauma
- Usually occurs at the sternal angle
- Associated with costochondral dislocations
- Classified as displaced and nondisplaced fractures
- Localised swelling, tenderness and deformity are the clinical findings.

Treatment

- Displaced fracture-requires surgical fixation
- Non-displaced fracture-conservative management

FLAIL CHEST

This results from severe chest injuries with multiple rib fractures.

Here there are fracture of four or more ribs at two places, anteriorly and posteriorly, so that certain segments of ribs will have no attachment to the chest wall. These ribs become indrawn due to intrathoracic negative pressure as the patient inhales and is driven outwards on expiration producing instability and paradoxical respiration resulting in hypoventilation, carbondioxide retention and respiratory failure.

Flail chest is of three types: anterior, posterior and lateral flail chest.

Anterior Flail

* Fracture of the costochondral junction at both right and left of the sternum

Posterior Flail

* Fracture ribs of posterior chest wall

Lateral Flail

* Fracture shaft of the ribs

TREATMENT

I. Commonly done procedures

1. **Anterior flail**

   Sea gull shaped prosthesis introduced to stabilise the flail segments.

2. **Posterior flail**

   No treatment is required as the scapula acts as a support to stabilise the flail segment.

3. **Lateral flail:** It is treated by chest-wall stabilization; reduction of the respiratory dead space; management of the pulmonary contusion; and pain control. Epidural analgesics are the pain-management agents of choice. Intercostal nerve blocks may also be used.

II. Other methods

* Surgical stabilization is rarely indicated i.e, open reduction of rib fracture or osteofixation.
* Recent method is to intubate and stabilise the flail segments with positive pressure ventilation, which has to be done for atleast one week. This is called as internal pneumatic fixation.
* Physiologic stabilization with intubation and IPPR to be initiated before hypoxia develops. IPPR produces satisfactory ventilation and helps the fractured ribs to unite in the position of inspiration, thereby reducing the deformity and improving the pulmonary function

STOVE IN CHEST

* Localized severe, blunt or crush injury producing depression of a portion of the chest.
* Treatment is same as that for flail chest; sometimes thoracotomy may be needed if there are internal injuries.

PULMONARY INJURIES

1. CONTUSION OF THE LUNG

* Deceleration injuries or crush trauma often produces extensive parenchymal damage. Haemorrhage and interstitial oedema, results in obliteration of alveolar spaces and consolidation of large areas of pulmonary tissue.
* Contusion of the lung can be unilateral or bilateral. The contusion can be in the form of a small area of damage with oedema and extravasation of the blood, or it may be a widespread damage. Haemoptysis and excessive tracheobronchial secretions give the clue to the diagnosis. Chest X-ray: Early patchy consolidation. To differentiate from adult respiratory distress syndrome (ARDS).

Key Box 44.3
PULMONARY INJURIES

* Contusion
* Pneumothorax, haemothorax
* Laceration
* Chest injuries

Treatment

* Fluid restriction
* Pulmonary care
* Chest physiotherapy
* Steroids and rarely ventilation

Usually self-limiting, if there are no other severe injuries

Complications

* Pneumonia
* Atelectasis
* Respiratory Failure
* ARDS

2. PNEUMOTHORAX

- Pneumothorax is the most common cause of respiratory insufficiency following chest trauma.
- Usually if there is a rib fracture and evidence of subcutaneous emphysema, pneumothorax is certainly present.
- Pneumothorax can be closed (simple), open and tension.
- Small simple pneumothorax does not need any treatment.
- A repeat chest X-ray after 12-24 hours is essential to confirm that it is not progressing.
- Small pneumothorax can be missed easily
- Bilateral pneumothorax is an emergency
- Late pneumothorax can also occur
- Open chest wound will produce complete collapse of lung and paradoxical shift of the mediastinum with each respiration (mediastinal flutter) causing hypoventilation and reduced cardiac output.
- Treatment is by closure of the wound, intercostal tube (lCT) and surgery.

Tension pneumothorax (Key Box 44.4, 44.5, 44.6)

- Injury to the lung results in continuous valvular air leak. The accumulating air, collapses the lung on the same side and pushes the mediastinum to opposite side. As a result of this tension, the intrapleural pressure increases, till at the time of expiration it is above atmospheric pressure. This **reduces the venous return** to the heart, as well as compromises the ventilation.
- Tension pneumothorax is **an emergency** which should be treated urgently with thoracocentesis in the second intercostal space in the mid clavicular line, to release the tension.
- **Thoracocentesis** converts TP to simple pneumothorax.

Key Box 44.4

TENSION PNEUMOTHORAX - CLINICAL FEATURES

1. **T**achypnoea
2. **T**achycardia
3. **T**ympanic note on percussion
4. **T**otal absence of breath sounds
5. **T**racheal shift

Key Box 44.5

TENSION PNEUMOTHORAX

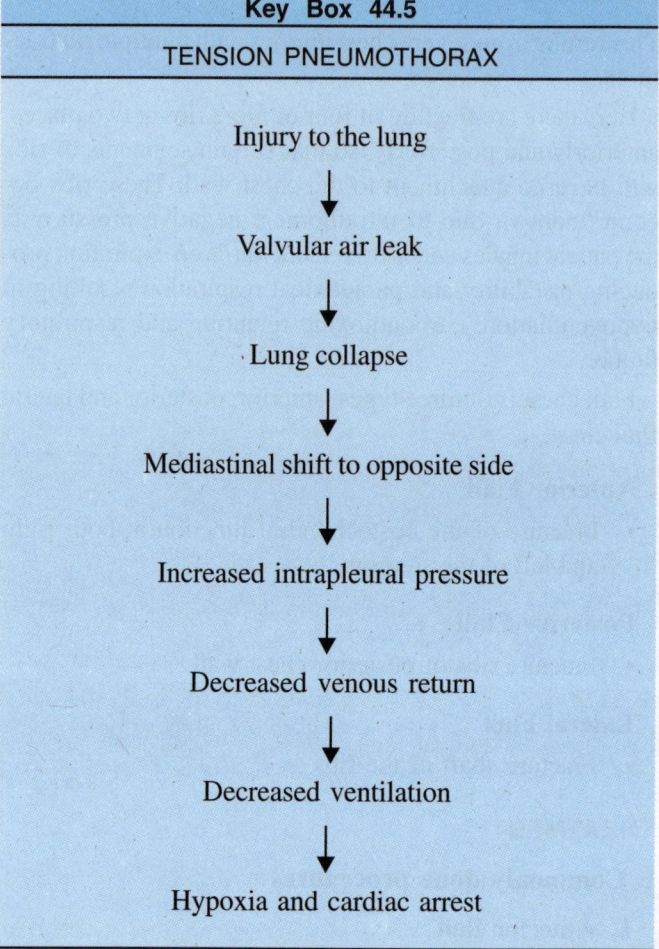

Injury to the lung
↓
Valvular air leak
↓
Lung collapse
↓
Mediastinal shift to opposite side
↓
Increased intrapleural pressure
↓
Decreased venous return
↓
Decreased ventilation
↓
Hypoxia and cardiac arrest

Key Box 44.6

TENSION PNEUMOTHORAX

- Immediate diagnosis to be done
- Do not wait for chest X-ray
- Thoracocentesis second ICS, MCL
- Then, intercostal chest tube

- Urgent intercostal tube insertion should be done and it should be connected to underwater seal (Page 685)
- Do not wait for chest X-ray

TENSION GASTROTHORAX

This occurs due to herniation of dilated and obstructed stomach into the mediastinum due to diaphragmatic tear resulting in haemodynamic compromise. It should be treated by reducing the hernial contents and repair of diaphragmatic tear.

3. HAEMOTHORAX

- May be missed in chest X-rays in the supine position.

- Results from injury to internal mammary artery, intercostal artery and vascular lung adhesions.

- Classical signs are: reduced chest expansion, dullness to percussion and absent breath sounds on affected side.

- Treated by intercostal chest tube insertion.

- If bleeding continues, or features of shock develop, thoracotomy has to be considered.

- The bleeding may be delayed or may recur after several days

Indications for thoracotomy

- Initial volume of blood loss is not as important as the amount of ongoing bleeding

- Drainage is more than 1000 ml or 100 ml each hour for 4 hours.

- Suspected clotted haemothorax (opacity persisting on chest X-ray even after ICT).

Complications

- Failure to adequately drain a haemothorax initially, results in residual clotted haemothorax and empyema or late fibrothorax

INTERCOSTAL CHEST TUBE (ICT) INSERTION (CLOSED TUBE THORACOSTOMY)

- Second intercostal space-Anteriorly midclavicular line is ideal for pneumothorax and sixth space in the midaxillary line for haemothorax.

- Can be introduced from sixth Intercostal space mid axillary line in pneumothorax also, but the chest tube should reach the apex of the lung.

- Infiltrate local anaesthesia upto the parietal pleura

- 2-3 cm incision - deepened, suture taken

- Insert the chest tube with trocar into the pleural cavity.

- Then the trocar is removed and the chest tube is connected to underwater seal.

- Observe for movement of the fluid column with respiration

- Take a check chest X-ray

Precautions with ICT

- All the holes in the plastic tube should be within the pleural space.

- The bottle should not be raised to a higher level than patient as it may result in contents of underwater seal entering into lungs (Figs. 44.1 and 44.2).

- Avoid kinking of the tube. do not clamp the ICT when there is air leak.

- ICT removal (Key Box 44.7)

Key Box 44.7
ICT - REMOVAL

- Chest X-ray-Lung fully expanded and drainage should be less than 100ml for two days and no air leak. Patient not on ventilator
- Clamp the tube for 24 hours
- Removal after 24 hours of clamping, provided the patient is comfortable and lung fully expanded

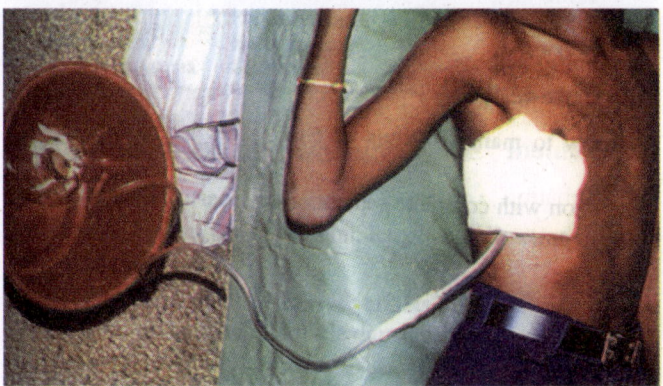

Fig. 44.1 Intercostal tube (ICT) connected to underwater seal

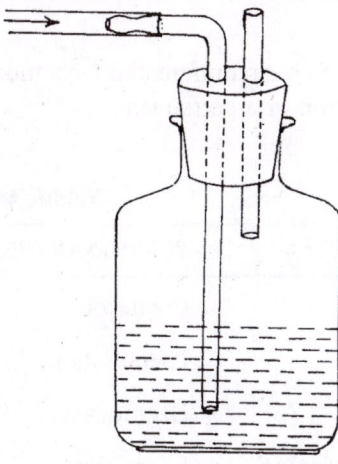

Fig. 44.2 Underwater seal (diagramatic)

LUNG LACERATION

- **Minor laceration:** Haemopneumothorax Usually intercostal chest tube is enough
- **Major laceration:** Haemopneumothorax:
  i. Introduce intercostal chest tube
  ii. Continuous air leak or bleeding through ICT and lung not expanding. Requires thoracotomy and repair or resection of lobe.

INJURY TO TRACHEA AND MAJOR BRONCHI

TRACHEAL INJURIES

- Injuries occur as a result of trauma sustained due to crush injuries
- Common in cervical trachea

Symptoms

- Acute airway obstruction
- Emphysema-mediastinal and cervical
- Pneumothorax
- Voice impairment

Treatment

- Intubation
- Tracheostomy
- Surgery and repair

MAJOR BRONCHIAL INJURIES (Refer Table 44.1)

- Blunt trauma produces stereotype injury to main bronchus of either side. Lobar bronchi are less commonly injured.
- Lesion is often a circumferential laceration with complete separation or a partial tear.

Symptoms

- Pneumothorax
- Uncontrolled air leak
- Haemoptysis
- Surgical emphysema
- Bronchoscopy for confirmation

Surgery

- Endobronchial intubation
- Bronchoplasty
- Injury to the lobar bronchus - Resection of the lobe of the lung.

INJURY TO THE DIAPHRAGM

Features

- Due to Crush injury
- Industrial-due to fall of heavy weights over abdomen
- Commonly, left diaphgram tear occurs
- Missed in chest X-ray in the supine position
- Diagnosed by ultrasound abdomen or chest X-ray reveals the Ryle's tube in the chest or coils of bowel (gas shadow) in the chest.

INJURY TO THE AORTA (Rupture of the Aorta)

- Deceleration injuries
- Gets avulsed at the region of ligamentum arteriosum
- Complete rupture-immediate death
- Incomplete rupture-shock, widening of mediastinum, unequal pulses

Surgery:

- Under cardiopulmonary bypass, the repair is done.

RIB FRACTURES	PULMONARY INJURIES	TRACHEOBRONCHIAL	DIAPHRAGM
Flail chest	Contusion	Mediastinal emphyscma	Breathlessness
Stove-in chest	Pneumothorax	Shock	Coils of bowel within thorax
Subclavian injury	Haemothrax	Airway obstruction	
Surgical emphysema	Laceration	Death	

Table 44.1 Summary of blunt chest injury

MYOCARDIAL CONTUSION

- Deceleration injuries
- Anterior chest impact
- Arrhythmias, reduced cardiac output, cardiac tamponade are the features.

SURGICAL EMPHYSEMA

Types

1. Localised
2. Extensive - from the eyelids to the scrotum, quite alarming in appearance. Indicates lung injury

Palpable crepitus is diagnostic of surgical emphysema

Treatment

- **Localised:** Not extending, no pneumothorax observation
- Pneumothorax - ICT
- **Extensive:** ICT to be introduced on the side where it is maximum
- Both sides ICT may be required
- Two ICT on the same side apical and basal, to be introduced if there is continuous air leak.
- The emphysema usually subsides within a week. Multiple incisions and expelling the air from the subcutaneous space manually are not required but may be carried out for cosmetic purposes or if patient has respiratory distress.

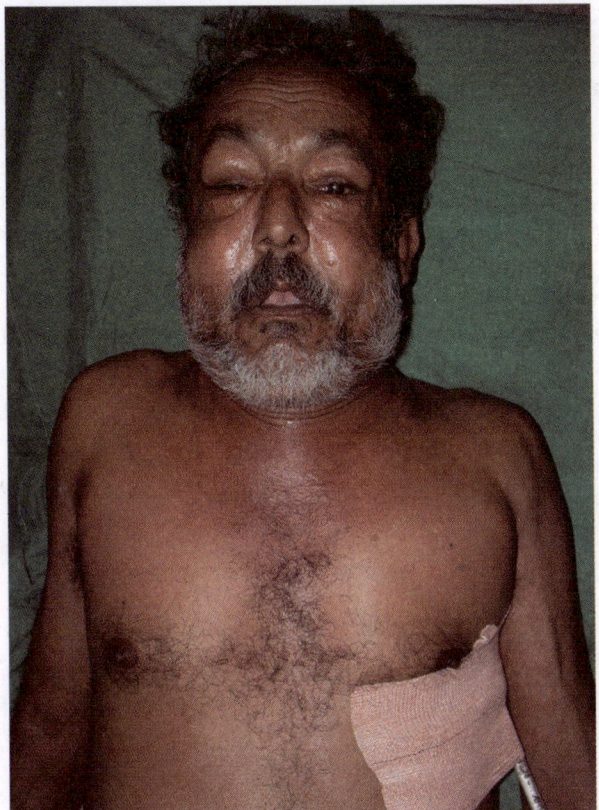

Fig. 44.3 Surgical emphysema

Key Box 44.8

SURGICAL EMPHYSEMA

- Air in the subcutaneous tissue
- Rib stabbing the lung
- Sometimes, can be gross
- Disfigurement is more than symptoms and signs
- Palpable crepitus
- Rupture of bronchus-mediastinal emphysema

PENETRATING THORACIC WOUNDS

Stab wounds

- They depend on type of weapon, length and direction of stab.

Projectile wounds

- Relatively low velocity revolver bullets, may perforate one or two lobes of the lung with little damage and only drainage of the pleural space is required.
- High velocity perforating wounds cause more damage to the tissue, adjacent to the tract. If the damage

---

Key Box 44.9

PENETRATING WOUNDS

- Represents mainly stab and gunshot wounds
- Immediately pack the wound
- Intercostal chest tube
- Thoracotomy mandatory

is extensive, lobectomy or pneumonectomy has to be considered.

- Bomb fragments, because of irregular shape, commonly carry with them pieces of ribs and are associated not only with **severe haemorrhage** and air leak from the torn pulmonary vessels and bronchus, but also with haemorrhage from irregular entry and exit wounds. Urgent thoracotomy is necessary.

- **Emergency Thoracotomy** is a life-saving procedure in the trauma centre. Thoracotomy for polytrauma has a poor prognosis than for isolated thoracic injuries.

Indications

- Decompression of cardiac tamponade
- Control of bleeding
- Allow for internal cardiac massage
- Clamping of descending thoracic aorta for exsanguinous bleeding in the abdomen

Surgery

- Anterolateral thoracotomy through 5th intercostal space, entered in 1-2 minutes.

MEDIASTINAL EMPHYSEMA

- The emphysema is mainly **suprasternal**
- On auscultation, pericardial crunching sounds synchronous with the heart beat, are heard.
- If there is haemodynamic instability, bilateral intrapleural ICT has to be introduced as a precaution against tension pneumothorax.
- Rule out oesophageal and tracheal injury.

PRINCIPLES OF MANAGING CHEST INJURIES

1. **Pulmonary physiotherapy:** Most important in all chest injury patients.
2. **Aspiration of secretions:** Tracheal aspiration, nasotracheal suction, aspiration of oral cavity and pharynx.
3. **Relieving pain:** Oral narcotics, parenteral narcotics, thoracic epidural analgesia, intercostal nerve block.

4. **Physiotherapy assistance**
   - Encourage coughing
   - Chest percussion and vibration
   - Deep inspiratory efforts
   - Humidification of air, nebulisation
   - Early mobilisation

5. **Treatment of pneumothorax or haemothorax**
   - Insertion of intercostal chest tube.

6. **Treatment of shock**
   - First of all the causes of shock in chest injuries has to be determined by thorough assessment of the patient. Once the cause (Key Box 44.10) is found out, depending upon the nature of the problem, patient is treated in an intensive care unit.

Key Box 44.10

CAUSES OF SHOCK

- Tension pneumothorax
- Massive haemothorax
- Cardiac tamponade
- Myocardial contusion
- Air embolism
- Ruptured diaphragm
- Injury to the great vessels

---

7. **FAST (Focussed Abdominal Sonography in Trauma) ultrasound:** Focused assessment with ultrasonography for trauma and rapid assessment for ruling out fluid collection in the abdomen, chest and pericardium

8. **Surgery** Depending upon the severity and location surgery is done

9. **Treatment of complications**
   - Thromboembolism
   - Tracheostomy complications
   - Prolonged ICU complications

Key Box 44.11

COMPLICATIONS

- Empyema
- Bronchopleural fistula
- Bronchial stenosis
- Chylothorax
- Clotted haemothorax
- ARDS
- Atelectasis

NON-TRAUMATIC RIB FRACTURES (Key Box 44.11)

Key Box 44.11
NON TRAUMATIC RIB FRACTURES
• Stress fractures • Metastatic disease • Metabolic disease such as hyperparathyroidism • Osteogenesis imperfecta • Consider child abuse, Battered baby syndrome • Older patients after violent coughing

PATENT DUCTUS ARTERIOSUS

Definition

- Persistence of the foetal ductus arteriosus in the post-natal period.

Embryology

- Derived from the 6th aortic arch
- Essential for the foetal circulation
- Blood ejected by right ventricle flows exclusively through the ductus to the lower extremity and placenta bypassing the high resistance pulmonary circulation in the foetus.

At birth

- Physiological closure occurs in 1-6 days
- Anatomical closure occurs in 2-3 weeks

Mode of closure

- Smooth muscle constriction in response to rising arterial oxygen tension.

Pathophysiology

- Shunt occurs across the ductus both in systole and diastole resulting in left ventricle overload and pulmonary plethora.
- Shunt depends on the size of the ductus and pulmonary and systemic vascular resistance.
- Continuous murmur is due to shunt during both systole and diastole.
- Incidence: M: F = 1:2

Occurs 1 in 5000 live births. 50% in premature babies

Clinical features

- It depends on the size of the ductus, pulmonary vascular resistance, age at presentation and associated anomalies.
- **a. Small ductus:** asymptomatic
- **b. Infants:** congestive heart failure
- **c. Children:** Dyspnoea on exertion, repeated respiratory tract infection

Examination

- Hyperdynamic precordium in large shunt and bounding peripheral pulses
- Machinery or continuous murmur(Gibsons murmur), Left second intercostal space, radiating to the left infraclavicular area.
- ECG: Left ventricular hypertrophy
- Chest X-ray: cardiomegaly
- Pulmonary congestion in large ductus and hilar dance on fluoroscopy
- 2 D echo is diagnostic - In supra sternal view the PDA is seen

Complications

- Reversal of shunt
- Infective endocarditis
- Congestive heart failure

Treatment

- It can be divided into surgical and nonsurgical methods.

1. Surgical methods

- Presence of PDA is sufficient indication for surgery even without symptoms.
- **In infants:** large PDA with congestive cardiac failure not responding to antifailure measures, surgery is indicated.

Surgery

- Triple ligation
- Division and suturing

- Right lateral position
- Posterolateral thoracotomy
- Thorax entered through 4th intercostal space.
- **It can also be done by thoracoscopy: VATS:** Video Assisted Thoracoscopic Surgery and clipping of PDA.

Care during surgery
- Left recurrent laryngeal nerve to be carefully preserved.

Complications during surgery
- Haemorrhage
- Left recurrent laryngeal nerve palsy
- Chylothorax

II. Nonsurgical methods

- **Pharmacological closure:** In preterm infants - Indomethacin
- **Transcatheter Closure:** (Interventional Cardiology)
- Double umbrella device - Rashkind
- Gianturco Coils
- Lock Clamshell Occluder

COARCTATION OF AORTA

Definition
Congenital narrowing of the descending thoracic aorta usually occurring just distal to the left subclavian artery origin, adjacent to the site of insertion of the ductus arteriosus.

Incidence
- 0.2- 0.6 per 1000 live births
- 5-8% of all cases of congenital heart diseases

Aetiology
- **Flow theory** - Reduced flow in the aorta due to multiple abnormalities in the heart during the foetal period.
- **Ductal sling theory** - When there is isolated coarctation this theory is applicable. Abnormal extension of contractile ductal tissue into the adjacent aorta which results in coarctation.

Types
- Infantile - preductal
- Adult- juxtaductal

Key Box 44.12
ASSOCIATED CONGENITAL ANOMALIES
- Ventricular septal defect
- Bicuspid aortic valve
- Patent ductus arteriosus
- Mitral valve abnormalities

Classification
- Group I - Isolated coarctation
- Group II - Coarctation with VSD
- Group III - Coarctation with complex intracardiac anomalies.

Clinical features
Depend on
- Age and symptoms at presentation
- Location and severity of the coarctation
- Associated anomalies

Symptoms
- Visual disturbances
- Exertional dyspnoea
- Upper extremity hypertension
- Headache
- Epistaxis
- Claudication of the lower limbs

Examination
- Systolic murmur heard over the precordium and posteriorly between the scapula.
- **Feeble femoral pulses**
- Enlarged collateral vessels seen (Suzzmans sign) and palpable between scapulae and bruit heard here.
- Systolic gradient between arm and leg blood pressure.

Collaterals
- Subclavian and its branches

- Internal mammary artery
- Intercostal artery
- Scapular, cervical, vertebral, epigastric and spinal arteries.

Investigations

- **ECG:** LVH with LV strain
- **CHEST X-RAY:** Notching of the ribs (Docks sign) from third rib onwards, above four years of age.

> *Classic three signs: Dilated left subclavian artery, narrowing of the coarctation and the post-stenotic dilatation of aorta.*

Diagnosis

- 2 Decho
- Cardiac catheterisation
- TEE
- Angiogram

Complications

- Circle of Willis aneurysm rupture
- Aortic dissection
- Early coronary atherosclerosis
- Bacterial endocarditis
- Congestive heart failure
- Spontaneous rupture of aorta

Treatment

A. Nonsurgical: Balloon dilatation in infants

B. Surgery

- Left posterolateral thoracotomy
- Thorax entered through fourth intercostal space
- Arterial line in the right upper limb
- Preserve the vagus and RLN
- Arterial line in the lower limb
- Lower limb pressure during cross-clamping of aorta, to be kept above 45 mmHg
- If the pressure is low, then create a shunt from the aortic arch to the descending thoracic aorta with the help of a cannula.

Complications of surgery

- Haemorrhage
- RLN injury
- Phrenic nerve injury
- Horner's syndrome
- Chylothorax
- Paradoxical hypertension
- Paraplegia
- Stroke

Late complications

- Recoarctation
- Aneurysm
- Left arm ischaemia (when subclavian flap aortoplasty is done)

Pseudocoarctation

Rare condition which results from congenital elongation of the aortic arch which leads to redundancy and kinking of the aorta and may appear similar to coarctation but there is no obstruction to blood flow.

CORONARY ARTERY BYPASS SURGERY

Introduction

Often simply called bypass surgery, is the most commonly performed open-heart surgery all over the world. The incidence of coronary artery disease is rapidly rising in the developing countries.

A vein graft from the lower limb or an arterial graft (Internal mammary artery or the radial artery) is used to bypass the obstructed coronary artery. The bypass is done from the root of the aorta to the distal coronary artery. The obstruction or the block is not touched.

HISTORY

- 1946 - Vineberg implanted IMA into the heart
- 1967 - Kolesov anastomosed IMA to LAD
- 1967 - Rene Favalaro anastomosed Reversed SVG to coronary arteries
- 1977 - Gruntzig - PTCA

INCIDENCE

- Least in Japan and highest in Finland

INDICATIONS FOR SURGERY

1. **Stable angina**
   - Triple vessel disease
   - Double vessel disease involving LAD
   - Single vessel disease involving LAD
   - Left main stem disease

2. **Unstable angina**
   - Severe angina not responding to medications

3. **Failed Percutaneous Trans-Coronary Angioplasty - PTCA**

4. AMI with complications like VSD, MR and ventricular aneurysm

5. **Post MI angina**

> *With Interventional cardiology progressing rapidly the indications for surgery are getting blurred.*

Risk factors

I. Non modifiable
- Age
- Sex
- Family history

II. Modifiable, Controlled or treated by medicines:
- Smoking
- Uncontrolled diabetes
- Uncontrolled hypertension
- Obesity and over weight
- Individual response to stress
- High blood cholesterol or lipid abnormalities
- Lack of physical exercise

Investigations

- ECG
- 2D Echocardiogram
- Holter monitoring
- Thallium scan-201 or Technetium -99m
- Stress test
- Coronary angiogram

SURGERY

- Bypass surgery with vein or artery graft

- Endarterectomy
- Venous patch
- Transmyocardial laser revascularisation (TMLR)

Bypass surgery

Technique of bypass

- Cold cardioplegia with moderate hypothermia with cardiopulmonary bypass
- Ischaemic cross-clamp with moderate hypothermia with cardiopulmonary bypass
- Empty beating heart, normothermic with cardiopulmonary bypass
- Beating heart surgery, NO heart lung machine

Grafts

- Veins   - Lower limbs (Long Saphenous Vein)
- Upper limb (Cephalic vein) rarely used
- Arteries - Radial
- Internal Mammary Artery both right & left (IMA)
- Gastroepiploic
- Inferior Epigastric
- Inferior Mesenteric

Non-Autogenic Conduits

- Cryopreserved human saphenous vein allograft
- Processed bovine sacral artery
- Polytetrafluoroethylene graft (Gortex)

STANDARD SURGICAL PROCEDURE

- Median sternotomy
- Internal mammary artery dissection done
- Pericardium opened
- Systemic heparinisation 3mgs/kg
- Aortic and venous cannulation
- Cardiopulmonary bypass started
- Aorta cross-clamped and cold K^+ rich solution given in the aortic root
- Heart arrested in diastole to achieve immobile surgical field
- Distal anastomosis completed
- Proximal anastomosis done with the heart beating
- Weaned off CPB

- Protamine given and decannulation carried out
- Sternum closed
- Extubation 6-8 hrs later

Arterial graft advantages

- It is artery to artery anastomosis
- Compatible size
- Flow adaptation
- IMA advantages: No vasovasorum
- Dense non-fenestrated intact internal elastic lamina that inhibits cellular migration and subsequent initiation of hyperplasia.
- Thin medial layer with few smooth muscle cells which provide little vasoreactivity.
- Produces more prostacyclins which is a vasodilator and platelet inhibitor

Complications of surgery

- Perioperative MI
- Stroke
- Reinfarct
- Wound infection
- Bleeding
- General debility and weakness
- Mortality 1-3%

Prognosis

- Ability to return to normal life style
- Improvement in ventricular function
- Work capacity better than preoperative
- Risk of arrthymias unchanged
- Minimal medications
- Complete and dramatic relief of chest pain

Patency

Year	Artery	Vein
1	97	90
5	95	60
10	90	40

RECENT ADVANCES

- Age limitation changed (CABG done in 80 yr old also)
- Improved myocardial preservation
- TMLR
- Composite arterial grafts
- Sutureless anastomosis
- Endoscopic vein harvesting
- Intracoronary injections of vascular endothelial growth factor (VEGF)
- All major cities have the centres and expertise

TMLR (TRANSMYOCARDIAL LASER REVASCULARISATION)

- Severe CAD not treated by PTCA or CABG
- Emulates reptilian circulation in the mammalian heart
- No CPB
- CO_2 or Excimer laser
- Limited thoracotomy
- Creation of channels 1mm in size in the myocardium from epicardium to endocardium
- Allows perfusion of blood directly from the LV cavity to the intramyocardium
- Creation of intramyocardial channels, neoangiogenesis and denervation are the factors which improve perfusion to the ischaemic myocardium.

COMPOSITE ARTERIAL GRAFTS

- Arterial grafts have long term patency
- Patients with total arterial grafts may not require future surgery
- Arterial grafts are used in the shape of T or Y
- Can revascularise almost all blocked major vessels
- OPCAB: Off Pump Coronary Artery Bypass surgery
- Beating heart surgery
- No heart lung machine
- Sternotomy
- Stabilization devices used
- Short acting beta blockers to reduce the HR
- Proper positioning of the heart with mechanical stabilization device for proper visual presentation

- CPB standby
- All vessels can be bypassed by proper position of heart
- Quick recovery
- Early extubation
- No CPB, less trauma
- Reduce risk of bleeding and kidney failure
- Reduced hospital stay

ENDOSCOPIC VEIN HARVESTING

- Only two small incision
- With help of a subcutaneous tunnel the vein is dissected
- Requires expensive equipment
- Major branches tied and smaller ones controlled by pressure
- Cosmetic advantage
- Takes longer time

Symmetric aortic bypass system connection

- Stapler for proximal anastomosis
- Fast
- More precise anastomosis
- No clamping of aorta
- Very few complications

Future problems

- Atherosclerosis is a progressive disease
- Diet restriction and exercise to continue even after bypass surgery
- Early disease in males in developing countries in 2nd - 3rd decade

Future advances

- Robotic bypass surgery (endothoracic CABG) ETCAB
- Biodegradable stents
- Intravascular laser ablation
- Rotablator
- Gene therapy

45

Neurosurgery

- Classification
- Primary lesions
- Secondary damage
- Extradural haematoma
- Fracture skull
- CSF rhinorrhoea
- Pott's puffy tumour
- Chronic subdural haematoma
- Hydrocephalus
- Brain tumours

Head injuries derive their importance because of the fact that many patients who die or who are disabled belong to the younger age groups. Head injuries account for 1% of all deaths, one fourth of deaths due to trauma and they are responsible for **half of all deaths** from road traffic accidents. Majority of the patients are young, adult males.

HEAD INJURIES

CLASSIFICATION

I. Based on clinical type

1. Open
2. Closed

II. Based on type of Injury

1. Blunt injury—acceleration, deceleration
2. Missile injuries

- The term **open head injury** is used to denote a type of injury in which there is a **fracture of the skull associated with tear of the dura and arachnoid,** resulting in cerebrospinal fluid leak either to the external environment or into one of the potentially infective areas in the base of the skull, e.g. Cerebro Spinal Fluid - CSF rhinorrhoea or otorrhoea.

- **A closed head injury** is one where there is **no such leakage.** The advantage of this classification is that it helps the treating physician to recognise a group of patients who are likely to develop an infective complication following the head injury and he can initiate measures to prevent it.

- **Blunt injuries** depending on the severity of impact can result in an open or closed head injury. Missile injuries tend to result in an open head injury most often.

- The brain is protected by a bony box which has a **vault** and **base of the skull.** The **base** of skull in contrast to the vault is a **rough terrain** due to the various **bony prominences, ridges** and **foraminae.**

- This factor is important in causing extensive brain damage to the brain in acceleration/deceleration type of injuries. In addition to the linear acceleration/deceleration, **rotational acceleration** is also capable of producing damage to the brain as the **brain swirls about** inside the skull, such injuries result in maximal damage at interfaces between structures of different densities such as **grey matter-white matter junctions.**

PATHOLOGY

- The pathological changes due to trauma to the brain can be classified into primary and secondary

Primary lesions

- Diffuse neuronal damage
- Shearing lesions
- Contusions and lacerations

Secondary lesions

- Swelling
- Haemorrhage
- Extradural
- Subdural
- Intracerebral
- Infection

PRIMARY LESIONS

- Diffuse neuronal damage is the most constant feature of blunt injuries. Immediately after an injury no changes may be seen. But changes begin **after 14 hours of injury and maximum effects** may last upto **one week**. Prolonged unconsciousness may follow injuries which produce only diffuse neuronal damage without any obvious macroscopic changes. Shearing lesions of the nerve fibres account for some severe injuries without any conspicuous changes to naked eye examination of the brain (**cerebral concussion**). **Wide spread degeneration of white matter** occurs without much changes in the cortex or brainstem. These patients have spasticity in all four limbs after injury and when they regain consciousness they are found to be severely demented.
- **Contusion** and **lacerations** are the obvious naked eye changes seen after injuries and were thought to be the

---

Key Box 45.1

CEREBRAL CONCUSSION

- Temporary physiological paralysis of the nervous system
- Loss of consciousness
- Post-traumatic amnesia
- Recovery may be complete
- Some can develop complications

Key Box 45.2

PRIMARY LESIONS

- Diffuse neuronal damage
- Cerebral contusion
- Cerebral laceration

---

main injuries before diffuse neuronal damage and shearing lesions were described. Contusions are seen on the summit of the gyri which get injured against the bone. The overlying pia is torn and the blood seeps into the subarachnoid space. A bleeding cortical vessel may result in the formation of an **acute subdural haematoma or intra-cerebral haemorrhage. Brain oedema** which develops surrounding the contusion and lacerations is the one that determines the outcome. Most often contusions are seen at the **tips of the frontal and temporal lobes; under surface of frontal and temporal lobes; over corpus callosum, superior and anterior surfaces of cerebellum and anterior surface of brain stem.**

SECONDARY LESIONS

Brain swelling

- This is a vague term applied to increase in brain bulk due to both oedema and venous congestion. It is aggravated by hypoxia or respiratory insufficiency which may be due to associated lung injury or obstruction to upper respiratory passages. Sometimes such a swelling can lead to severe brain compression which is difficult to relieve, since there is no single mass lesion.

Intracranial haemorrhage

- Extradural or subdural haemorrhages may develop as a clean cut secondary event, even though bleeding may have started at the time of injury. These cause compression of brain, secondary rise in intracranial pressure and can cause death if not detected and treated early.

Infections

- All open head injuries are liable to result in intracranial infection either as generalised meningitis or focal infection such as subdural empyema or brain abscess, osteomyelitis of skull. After closed head injuries, infection of a subpericranial blood clot may result in **Pott's puffy tumour**. When infection supervenes on

Key Box 45.3

SECONDARY LESIONS

1. Brain swelling
   - Oedema
   - Venous congestion
   - Hypoxia
2. Intracranial haemorrhage
   - Extradural
   - Subdural
3. Infections
   A. Open head injury
      - Generalised meningitis
      - Subdural empyema
   B. Closed head injury
      - Pott's puffy tumour

an already injured brain, it may retard the recovery or may even lead to death. Hence, it becomes mandatory to treat all infections vigorously.

CAUSE OF DEATH IN HEAD INJURIES

- It is instructive to consider the pathological findings in fatal cases and to speculate the **deaths** which might have been prevented. For example, earlier, many deaths which had occurred due to aggravation of brain swelling **due to hypoxia** could have been prevented by **ventilation** and **anti-oedema measures**. It should be emphasised that the role of the treating physician is to anticipate and take appropriate measures to prevent the patient from succumbing to the secondary changes. In extensive primary damage to the brain, apart from supportive treatment, one may have to wait and hope.

- Extensive injury to vital areas like diencephalon, or patients with **diffuse damage** are **not likely to survive.** These are patients who are unconscious from the time of injury with bilateral, dilated, fixed pupils, flaccidity in all 4 limbs and autonomic disturbances.

- Sometimes a head injury associated with extensive injuries to chest, abdomen or the limbs by their sheer severity can cause death.

- Whereas intracranial complications like haematomas, brain swelling, infection and extracranial complications like chest injury/metabolic abnormalities if recognised and treated early, can go a long way in saving the life of the patients.

INTRACRANIAL HAEMATOMA

- Most of the head injuries, are mild or minor and however they are managed the patient recovers on his own. All those who are unconscious, no matter how briefly, run the risk of respiratory obstruction, some of the so called trivially injured run the risk of developing an intracranial haematoma. Hence, all head injuries must be taken seriously. A **complicated head injury** is one where anyone of the **secondary pathological changes** may occur and threaten the life of the patient. **Uncomplicated** head injury is one where no **such events** occur. However, it could be a severe one where the unconsciousness is prolonged.

- These haematomas could develop in any one of the planes intracranially. Extradural (epidural), subdural, intracerebral haematoma, or a haemorrhagic contusion.

- The clinical presentation of these haematomas are due to either increase in the intracranial pressure or due to signs of cerebral compression. In the case of acute subdural haematoma or intracerebral haematoma, the clinical picture and the outcome of treatment is also dependent on associated brain damage.

EXTRADURAL/EPIDURAL HAEMATOMA

- The clot collects between the dura and the inner table of skull. A majority of them occur in the **middle cranial fossa,** since injury to **middle meningeal vessels (vein and artery) is the commonest cause.** However, about 20-25% of the extradural haematomas can occur in the frontal, parietal regions, at the vertex or in the posterior fossa. Injury to the dural venous sinuses or a large diploic venous channel are the other causes for the formation of a haematoma. Depending upon the source of bleeding the haematoma could collect rapidly (hyperacute type) or slowly over a period of few hours to few days and present as a **chronic lesion.** 60-80% of these patients have an associated fracture of the skull bone and only a few of them may present with classical symptoms with **LUCID INTERVAL.** In the remaining patients, the initial picture can vary from an unconscious state to a fully conscious person with or without a history of post-traumatic amnesia. With the widespread availability and use of CT scan, the diagnosis has become much simpler now-a-days. However, a few clinical features are worth mentioning.

1. DETERIORATING CONSCIOUSNESS LEVEL

- This is one of the hallmarks for the diagnosis of intracranial haematoma. The term **lucid interval** is used when a patient recovers from an initial period of unconscious state. Though in earlier days this was said to be associated with intracranial haematomas it can occur in other conditions like brain oedema, multiple constusions etc. To assess the consciousness level properly, instead of using vaguely defined terms like semiconscious, obtunded etc., the **Glasgow Coma Scale** has been used widely, thereby avoiding observer errors in the observation of such patients (Page 699).

- Restlessness in a previously quiet patient indicates increasing intracranial pressure, which again needs to be investigated or at the earliest appearance of focal neuronal deficit, patient has to be taken up for exploratory burrholes.

- Progressive neurological deficit, indicates cerebral compression and the manifestation may depend on the area of the brain affected.

2. PUPILLARY ABNORMALITIES

- These are to be considered as a late manifestation. It is due to pressure by the **herniating temporal lobe on the ipsilateral third nerve at the tentorial hiatus**. In the **early stages** due to irritation of the nerve, there is **constriction.** Due to the transient phenomenon, the early constriction most of time goes unnoticed and the patients are detected in the **next stage of pupillary dilatation** - caused by **paralysis of pupillo-constrictor fibres in the third nerve**. However, if the cerebral compression is unrelieved, this may go on to bilateral pupillary constriction. Pupillary dilatation is due to **ischaemia of third nerve nucleus** at the midbrain which is caused by pressure on the posterior cerebral artery. These series of pupillary changes have been termed as paralysis of 3rd nerve **Hutchinsonian pupils.** The dilated pupil has a definite localising value that if at all an exploratory burr-hole has been decided upon, it should be carried out on the side of the initially dilated pupil.

3. AUTONOMIC DISTURBANCES

- Bradycardia, though said to be a definite sign, is a late and not an early sign. Initially, there may be a rise in the pulse rate (tachycardia) which may progress to bradycardia, when the systolic blood pressure increases. At times there may be a rise in the diastolic pressure also. These **changes are brought about due to changes in the cerebral blood flow as a consequence of increased intracranial pressure**. Respiration becomes deep, with slow rate (bradypnoea) and later patients may develop Cheyne-Stokes ventilation due to brain stem ischaemia.

- Local scalp swelling is seen in more than half of the cases. Thus, examination of the head for any such swelling becomes important.

- Some of these patients may have a stiff neck either due to increased intracranial pressure or due to associated injury to neck muscles. Mild fever may, at times, occur and this sometimes confuses the observer in which case the patients must be investigated with a definitive investigation like CT scan or if not much time is available, one should not hesitate to proceed to exploratory burrholes or a trauma craniotomy flap has to be employed to rule out a haematoma.

- Though in adults, 'SHOCK' is a rare complication of head injury, in children with intracranial haematoma and associated cephalohaematomas, due to volume depletion, 'SHOCK' may be encountered. Even in adults, if there is a large scalp injury which is not sutured immediately, shock can occur.

- Posterior fossa haematomas in any plane are dangerous because of the lesser space available for the haematomas as a result of which rapid brain stem compression can occur which may prove fatal. Though the availability of CT scan has made detection of these so called unusual haematomas more frequently in a suspected case, even if **facilities are not available,** the treating physician should **explore the posterior fossa**, if the clinical features suggest haematoma or if the skull X-rays show a fracture line extending across the occipital bone towards the foramen magnum.

INVESTIGATIONS

As has been pointed out earlier, the advent of CT scan of the head has made the diagnosis easier and more specific,

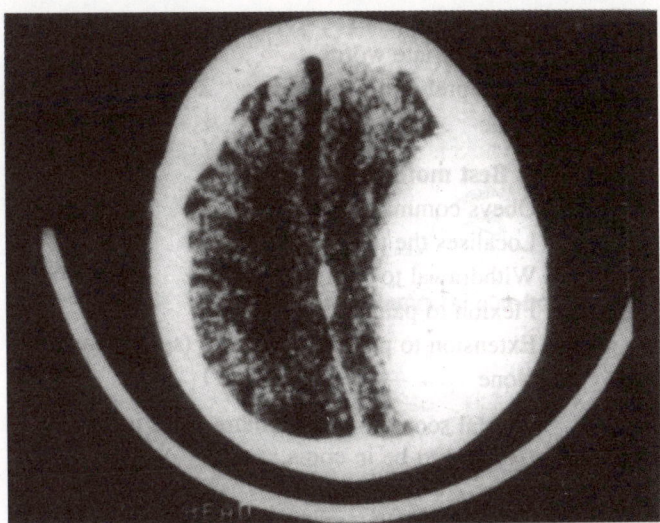

Fig. 45.1 CT scan showing extradural haematoma

it should be emphasized that **in the absence of CT scan** if adequate clinical features point out to the **possibility of an intracranial haematoma**, the patient must be taken up immediately for an exploratory surgery rather than wait and allow him to develop irreversible brain stem damage. Since 60-80% of patients with an intracranial haematoma have a skull bone fracture, immaterial of the consciousness level, the patient has to be observed for at least 24-48 hours. Occasionally one may have to resort to old investigations like angiography not only to establish the haematoma but also to rule out associated dural venous sinus injury etc.

Key Box 45.4

INDICATIONS FOR SKULL RADIOLOGY

- Loss of conciousness
- Obvious depression on the skull
- Compound fracture
- Laceration or contusion of the scalp
- Focal neurological signs

TREATMENT OF HEAD INJURIES IN GENERAL

I. Resuscitation and support

1. Admission is indicated when:

   a. Definite history of unconsciousness

   b. Fracture temporal bone

   c. Person who cannot be attended to by the doctors immediately i.e. no medical facilities nearby.

2. Casualty reception

   a. **Airway**

- Mouth gag—to prevent tongue falling backwards.
- Endotracheal intubation with positive pressure ventilation. Hypoxia is an important cause of cerebral oedema which worsens the level of consciousness.

   b. **General assessment of patient**:

- To rule out abdominal injuries like splenic rupture.
- Haemothorax—may need an intercostal tube.
- Long bone fractures.

   c. **General assessment** of the degree of shock by pulse, BP monitoring and treatment.

   d. **Neurological assessment by GLASGOW-COMA SCALE.**

     1. Eyes open

Spontaneously	4
To speech	3
To pain	2
None	1

     2. Best verbal response

Oriented	5
Confused	4
Inappropriate words	3
Incomprehensible sounds	2
None	1

     3. Best motor response

Obeys commands	6
Localises the pain	5
Withdrawal to pain	4
Flexion to pain	3
Extension to pain	2 (severe damage with increase of ICP)
None	1

- Total score is 15; minimum score is 3. Any patient who has a coma score of 7 or less than 7 is said to be in coma.

II. Care of unconscious

a. Ryle's tube aspiration or feeding
b. Care of the eyes - padding
c. Catheter for drainage of urine
d. Change of position to avoid bed sores

III. Surgical treatment for extradural haematoma

Immediate surgery for removal of haematoma and relief of cerebral compression is a must. Extradural haematoma especially is a neurosurgical emergency and whether the patient lives or dies will depend upon the speed with which the compression is relieved. It is not an exaggeration to state that even if one has to do decompression with unsterile instruments at the bedside, it may be worth the effort. In every neurosurgeon's career, at least once such an opportunity might have occurred and a live patient may justify the means employed. Once the consciousness is lost, pupil dilates or decerebrate rigidity and periodic breathing develop it may be only a matter of few minutes that may be available to save the life of the patient and one should not wait and waste time. In the case of extradural haematoma the **outcome is dependent on the size of the haematoma and the stage at which** the patient was taken up for surgery. While in the case of acute subdural and intracerebral haematoma, it depends on associated brain damage. If the associated brain damage is very severe, patients succumb to it (Key Box 45.5, Fig. 45.2).

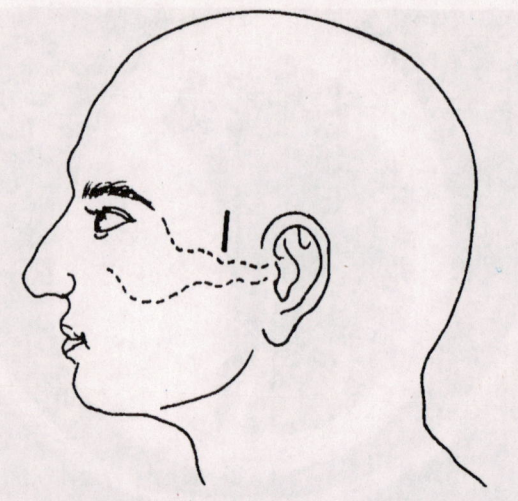

Fig. 45.2 Site of temporal burr-hole

2. Fracture may extend to the orbit—subconjunctival haemorrhage.
3. Olfactory nerve involvement - partial anosmia
4. Optic nerve may be contused or fracture may involve the optic foramen resulting in partial or total loss of vision.
5. Rarely 3rd nerve palsy giving rise to dilated pupil

Middle cranial fossa fracture

1. Epistaxis due to fracture venous/sphenoid sinuses
2. CSF from the ear: CSF with blood, hence does not clot
3. 7th nerve palsy
4. Rarely 6th and 8th nerves also involved

Posterior cranial fossa fracture

1. Extravasation of blood in the suboccipital region causing boggy swelling in the nape of the neck
2. 9th, 10th, 11th cranial nerves may be involved
3. Battle's sign : Discolouration of skin and collection of blood occur in the region of mastoid process.

Key Box 45.5

EXTRADURAL HAEMATOMA

- 3 cm vertical incision immediately above the midpoint of zygoma
- Strip the pericranium
- Burr hole with Hudson's brace
- Evacuate 'black-currant jelly' clot
- Extend the burr-hole and control bleeding middle-meningeal artery by bipolar diathermy
- Dural hitch sutures to prevent stripping of dura

MISCELLANEOUS

FRACTURE SKULL

Anterior fossa fracture

1. Fracture cribriform plate can result in CSF rhinorrhoea.

CSF RHINORRHOEA

- There should be a communication between the intradural cavity and the nose. (subarachnoid space)
- It indicates tear of the dura mainly in the basal region,

and a fracture involving paranasal sinuses— frontal, ethmoidal, sphenoidal.

- There is always an injury to a small portion of the brain. It (the portion of brain) plugs the tear, preventing the dura from healing, thus the rhinorrhoea persists for many days.

- This leads to complication i.e. infection and meningitis.

Treatment:

- Prophylactic antibiotics

- If the rhinorrhoea persists, repair of the dural defect alone or at times with a shunt procedure will be needed.

POTT'S PUFFY TUMOUR

- This is **subperiosteal infection** usually caused by **osteomyelitis of the underlying skull**.

- It is common in the frontal region and the frontal bone is commonly involved.

- The cause of infection is through **frontal sinusitis**. Another common cause of infection of a sub- pericranial haematoma at times, is following needle aspiration.

- It can also follow **chronic suppurative otitis media**.

- Pus collects in the subpericranial space and extradural plane, which communicate with each other (dumb-bell type abscess).

- It causes a boggy swelling in the frontal region and tenderness over the scalp.

- Pitting oedema over the scalp is conclusively called as Pott's puffy tumour.

- Severe headache, vomiting and blurring of vision should clinch the diagnosis.

Treatment

- CT scan to confirm the diagnosis

- A **burrhole and aspisration of pus** can be done, followed by 6-8 weeks of antibiotics.

- In chronic cases, the wall of the abscess may have to be removed and the associated osteomyelitic skull bone requires a radical removal under cover of antibiotics which have to be given for 6-8 weeks period.

CHRONIC SUBDURAL HAEMATOMA

- Common in old people.

- Because of the shrinkage of the brain, the distance between the dura and the skull increases and due to a minor trauma, cortical veins are torn resulting in collection of blood.

- Bleeding is never progressive and the blood in the subdural space slowly compresses the brain causing features of raised ICT.

Clinical features

1. Old aged patients
2. History of minor trauma
3. Bilateral headache
4. Mental apathy
5. Slowness
6. Confusion - later alteration in the level of consciousness may progress to unconsciousness.
7. Waxing and waning of the level of consciousness is seen in some patients - if such a history is elicited, one should always suspect chronic subdural haematoma.

Diagnosis

- CT scan or, if feasible, MRI scan are the ideal investigations. Cerebral angiography had been used and is still being used in some centres where access to the latest imaging facilities are not available.

Treatment

- Burrhole and drainage of the haematoma under local anaesthesia or under general anaesthesia occasionally, is the often practised mode of treatment. At times, one may have to resort to two or more burrholes to ensure adequate evacuation. If the brain fails to expand and obliterate the cavity, especially in older people - or persons with a very thick inner membrane, a large craniotomy and wide excision of the subdural membrane has to be carried out to remove the constricting effect. Adequate bed rest and plenty of fluid administration are also important postoperative measures.

HYDROCEPHALUS

This is a condition which occurs due to disturbances of CSF flow and imbalance between CSF production and absorption - resulting in the accumulation of CSF and dilatation of ventricles.

CSF PRODUCTION

CSF is mainly produced by the choroid plexus of lateral ventricles by an active autoregulated process.

Daily production: 140 ml

CSF CIRCULATION

Lateral ventricle

↓ Via Foramen of Monroe ①

3rd ventricle

↓ Via Aqueduct of Sylvius ②

4th ventricle

↓

CSF leaves the 4th ventricle by Foramen of Luschka and Magendie to circulate over the convexity where it is finally absorbed over arachnoid granulations.

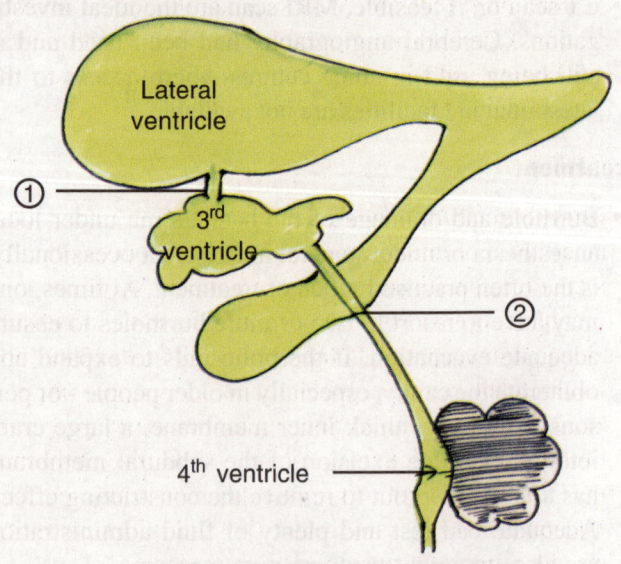

Fig. 45.2 Ventricular system

AETIOPATHOLOGY

Hydrocephalus occurs due to **two reasons:**

• If there is over production of CSF, or
• If there is decreased absorption

• **Over production:** True over production is rare and occurs in cases of **choroid plexus papilloma.**

• **Decreased absorption:** Failure of CSF absorption is much more common due to following factors:

- Infection
- Haemorrhage
- Structural abnormality occurring in CSF pathway- Tumour, congenital malformation such as aqueduct stenosis etc.

TYPES

1. Communicating: Due to obstruction in subarachnoid space

2. Non-communicating: Due to obstruction in ventricular system.

CLINICAL FEATURES

I. Infantile hydrocephalus

1. Difficulty in delivery of large head (Key Box 45.6)
2. Craniofacial disproportion
3. Increase in head circumferance more than 2 cm/month
4. Scalp is thin, shiny and prominent veins
5. Fontanelles: Bulging and tense especially during crying
6. Sutures: open
7. Excessive irritability
8. Inability to retain feeds
9. Mental retardation, delayed milestones
10. **Sun-set sign**
    • Weakness of upward gaze
11. Hypothalamic disturbances

Key Box 45.6	
DIFFERENTIAL DIAGNOSIS OF LARGE HEAD	
1. Megalencephaly	- Intracranial pressure is normal
2. Chronic subdural haematoma	- Enlargement of parietal region
3. Cerebral atrophy	- May cause ventricular enlargement
4. Cerebral tumours	

II. Childhood /Adult Hydrocephalus

- By this time fontanelles have closed

1. Features of increased intracranial pressure
   - Headache
   - Nausea
   - Vomiting
2. Irritability
3. Indifference
4. Apathy
5. Drowsiness
6. Blindness is due to papilloedema and ophthalmoplegia
7. Bradycardia, systemic hypertension, altered respiratory rate is due to distortion of brainstem. Untreated cases also develop unilateral or bilateral abducens palsy or upward gaze palsy.

TREATMENT

Aim

1. **To decrease CSF production** by using pharmacological agents:
   - Acetazolamide
   - Frusemide
   - Isosorbide
   - Glycerol
2. **Direct removal** of cause of obstruction
3. **Diversion** of CSF to another viscus for reabsorption by means of various shunt procedures.

Shunts
- Ventriculo-peritoneal shunt
- Ventriculo-atrial shunt

Complications of shunts

1. Shunt obstruction
2. Shunt inflammation
3. Seizures
4. Extracerebral fluid collection
5. Subdural Haematoma
6. Spontaneous pneumocephalus
7. Ascites

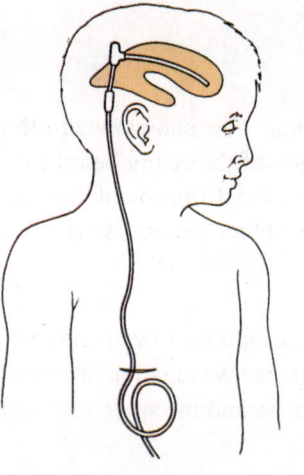 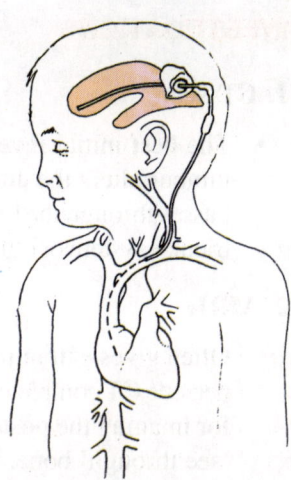

Fig. 45.3 Ventriculo-peritoneal shunt   **Fig. 45.4** Ventriculo-atrial shunt

BRAIN TUMOURS

8 % of all primary cancers arise in the CNS. In adults it constitutes the sixth largest group of cancers and in children the CNS is the commonest site for solid tumours.

Most adult brain tumours are supratentorial, but 60% of those in children arise in the posterior fossa.

PRESENTING FEATURE

1. **Progressive neurological deficit:** in upto 2/3 patients, a focal motor weakness is the most common presentation. This deficit arises from the direct neuronal damage or the effects of tumour compression on brain or cranial nerves. Sudden change may be due to haemorrhage into a pre-existing tumour.

2. **Headache:** occurs in over 50 % of patients caused by raised ICP. Only 10% patients have the classic presentation of early morning worsening of headache associated with nausea and temporary relief by vomiting.

3. **Generalised or focal seizures** occur in 25%. Focal seizures may help to localise the site of tumour. A high index of suspicion is required for patients past the second decade with recent onset epilepsy.

4. **Other presentations** include visual disturbances, visual field defects, mental changes etc. depending on the site of tumour.

INVESTIGATIONS

1. CT scan

- The best initial investigation. This shows where the tumour alters the attenuation of the X-ray beam as it passes through the brain and also distortion of the ventricular system or obliteration of the pattern of the sulci.

2. MRI:

- Often gives extra information and may eventually supersede CT completely. It is the investigation of choice for imaging the posterior fossa and the spine as it can 'see through' bone.

3. X-rays:

- X-rays are only of anecdotal interest picking up incidental calcification or erosion of the skull.
- Newer imaging modalities including SPECT and PET scans are increasingly being used in higher centers.

SPECIFIC TYPES OF BRAIN TUMOURS

Astrocytoma

- This is the **most common primary brain tumour** arising from the supporting glial cells and diffusely infiltrates brain tissue early on.
- **Two grading systems** are available - WHO and St Anne/Mayo. Grade 1 and 2 (low grade) tumours are slow growing and compatible with good quality survival. Grade 3 and 4 are rapidly growing. Grade 4 tumours which are also called glioblastoma multiforme are highly radio and chemo resistant with median survival of only 12 months even with optimal treatment.
- Even low-grade astrocytomas may evolve over time into secondary glioblastomas.

Oligodendroglioma

- This type of glioma is usually a slow growing tumour and over half arise in the frontal lobes.
- There may be a history of epilepsy or even focal neurological signs of many years duration.
- They may show calcification both microscopically and macroscopically.

Ependymoma

- These glial tumours arise from cells, which line the

ventricles of the brain and the central canal of the spinal cord.

- They are most common in the fourth ventricle in children and young adults where they block CSF flow and often present with hydrocephalus.

Embryonal Tumours

- Primitive neuroectodermal tumours (PNET) are a group of highly malignant tumours of which the cerebellar PNET or medulloblastoma is the archetype.
- Commonest in children and young adults and may originate from primitive cell rests which have undergone malignant transformation. Medulloblastoma is the most common brain tumour in children.
- The patient presents with truncal ataxia, headache, vomiting and sometimes diplopia. All PNETs are prone to spread within the CNS producing sugarcoating metastasis which are best seen on MRI of the spine.

Schwannoma (neurilemmoma)

- Peripheral neurons get their myelin sheaths from schwann cells. Occasionally these form slow growing benign tumours on cranial or spinal nerves.
- The cranial nerve most affected is the vestibular division of the 8th cranial nerve and the tumour is then usually called as acoustic neuroma.

Even though it does not arise from the acoustic division and is not a neuroma - it is still called as acoustic neuroma.

- It causes progressive deafness, hydrocephalus and ataxia. It is slow growing. Less often it may involve the trigeminal or the vagus nerve.

Meningioma

- These tumours arise from the arachanoid layer from the meninges and the arachanoid villi. They are commonest over the falx and the convexity of the skull but rarely may also arise from the skull base (especially from the sphenoid wing and olfactory groove) or inside the lateral ventricle.
- Commonest in middle aged women and may occur at the site of a previous radiation field. Most are benign and slowly growing. Signs occur based on the site of tumour.
- They tend to provoke endosteal hypertrophy or

exostosis of the overlying skull which is still occasionally detected on an incidental skull film or even by palpation of the skull. Patient with Neurofibromatosis Type 2 often have multiple meningiomas. Rarely they are malignant.

Other tumours

- They are pineal region tumours, pituitary adenomas, craniopharyngiomas, choroid plexus tumours etc

METASTASES

One fourth of all cancer patients have intracerebral metastases at the time of death. Common primary sites include the bronchus (50%), breast (15%) and melanoma (10%).

TREATMENT

- They can be divided into medical and surgical line of treatment

I. Medical

- Acutely raised ICP is treated by I.V. Mannitol 1g/kg body weight.
- Hydrocephalus can be relieved using a CSF diversion system (closed external ventricular drainage or a ventriculo-peritoneal shunt).
- Seizures are treated with lorazepam and phenytoin commonly and maintained on phenytoin.
- Corticosteroids, especially dexamethasone 4mg QID is given to reduce symptoms of raised ICP, which may make surgery easier.

II. Surgery

- This is the mainstay of treatment. The aim of surgery is to obtain as complete a tumour excision as possible without producing a neurological deficit.
- This is not always possible due to the site of the tumour, in which cases compromises must be made and a **debulking procedure** is done.
- Any residual tissue may be observed or treated with adjuvant radiotherapy.
- **Stereotactic guided surgery** is now a well established concept in brain surgery allowing more targeted treatment of the lesion with minimal surrounding damage.

III. Radiotherapy

- Intracranial tumours are relatively radioresistant, and radiotherapy is primarily a palliative treatment

IV. Chemotherapy

- No definite benefit of chemotherapy for the treatment of brain tumours. Temozolomide is a promising new drug for the treatment of brain tumours.

OUTCOME

Surgery offers good prospects for the treatment of benign brain tumours such as meningioma or pituitary adenoma, but outcome of treatment of malignant tumours is still poor.

Principles of Radiology

46

- Barium swallow
- Barium meal
- Barium meal follow through
- Barium enema
- Enteroclysis
- Angiography
- Splenoportography
- Sialography
- Computed tomography
- Ultrasonography
- Magnetic resonance imaging
- Peripheral venography
- Myelography
- Interventional radiology
- PET scan
- Virtual colonoscopy

BARIUM STUDIES

This is the study of the gastrointestinal tract by instillation/ingestion of barium suspension made from pure **barium sulphate**.

BARIUM SWALLOW (Fig. 46.1)

It is the contrast study from the oral cavity upto the fundus of the stomach.

Indications

- Dysphagia and obstruction
- Odynophagia
- Assessment of mediastinal masses
- Motility disorders of oesophagus—achalasia, scleroderma

Relative contraindications

- Tracheo-oesophageal fistula
- Perforation

Procedure

- One mouthful of contrast media is given, and fluoroscopic observation of the act of deglutition is observed. After a mouthful of barium, films are exposed to the region of interest.

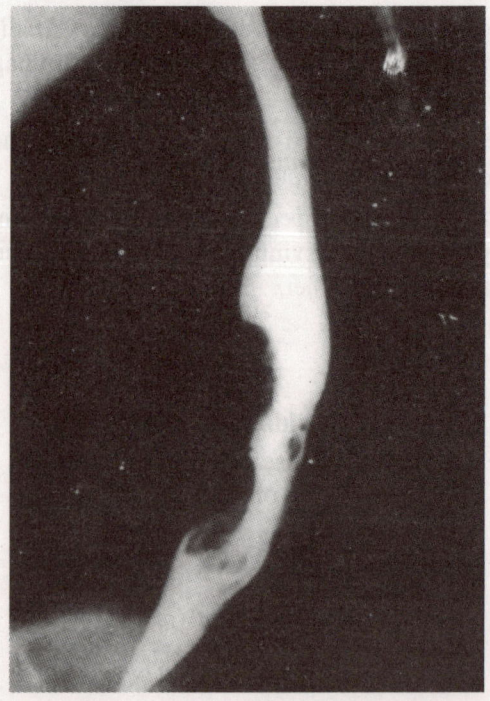

Fig. 46.1 Barium swallow: Opacified thoracic oesophagus showing a intraluminal mass with mucosal irregularity in its lower third suggestive of malignancy

Interpretation of study

1. Malignant obstructions are seen as annular constrictions, shouldering cranial and caudal to the lesion, mucosal destruction, ulceration and fistulae formation.

2. Benign strictures are long segment narrowings with no mucosal abnormalities.

3. Achalasia cardia is evident as rat tail appearance of the lower end of the oesophagus, with gross dilatation of the oesophagus proximally and thin streaks of contrast entering the stomach.

4. Scleroderma shows dilatation, atonicity, poor or absent peristalsis and free gastro-oesophageal reflux.

BARIUM MEAL (Fig. 46.2)

This is the radiological study of oesophagus, stomach, duodenum and proximal jejunum.

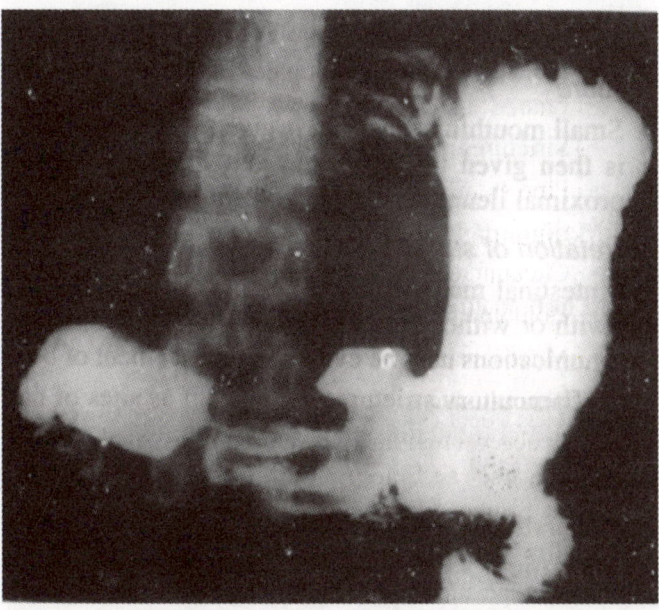

Fig. 46.2 Barium meal: Contrast opacified stomach demonstrating a projection from lesser curvature due to a benign gastric ulcer (niche)

Indications

* Symptoms of vomiting, epigastric pain, heartburn, dyspepsia
* Upper abdominal mass
* Gastrointestinal haemorrhage
* Gastric or duodenal obstruction
* Malignancies

Contraindications

* Suspected perforation
* Suspicion of aspiration
* Large bowel obstruction.

Procedure

* An undiluted barium suspension is given and deglutition is seen under fluoroscopy. Once the barium reaches the stomach, the patient is rotated so as to coat the entire stomach and filming is done. More barium is given to distend the stomach wall. Filming is done as contrast enters the duodenum and opacifies proximal jejunum.

Interpretation of study

1. **Hiatus hernia** is evident as presence of the stomach above the oesophageal hiatus. In addition gastro-oesophageal reflux will be evident. Mucosal ulceration and strictures may be demonstrable in long-standing cases.

2. **Gastric and duodenal ulcers** appear as projections from the normal contour with pooling of contrast. Benign **ulcers** usually **project out** and have the mucosal folds radiating upto the edge of the ulcer. Deformity of the stomach and duodenal cap are seen in chronic stages.

3. **Bezoars of stomach** are seen as radiolucent masses in the stomach and the barium fills the crevices between the particles forming a characteristic appearance.

4. **Infantile hypertrophic pyloric stenosis** : Thin **streak** of barium is seen extending across pylorus. Indentation of barium-filled antrum is seen.

BARIUM MEAL FOLLOW THROUGH

This the radiographic examination of the GIT—oesophagus, stomach, small bowel and ileocaecal junction, by oral administration of contrast media.

Indications

* Symptoms of small bowel disease like diarrhoea, abdominal pain, weight loss, Crohn's disease.
* Small bowel obstruction (Chronic)
* Gastrointestinal bleeding
* Palpable mass possibly involving the small bowel
* Malabsorption

Contraindications

- Colonic obstruction
- Suspected perforation

Procedure

- A small mouthful of barium is given and the stomach is studied and films are taken. 500-800 ml barium is then given to the patient and filming is done after 15-20 minutes to demonstrate the jejunum and proximal ileum. Subsequently, films of the ileum and ileocaecal junction are taken.

Interpretation of study

1. Intestinal malignancies such as lymphomas are evident as strictures which may be short or long segment with or without proximal dilatation. The mucosa shows irregularity and ulcerations and fistulous communications may be evident. Displacement of bowel loops in large extraluminal masses may be seen.

2. Inflammatory strictures are evident as sites of narrowing with mucosal abnormality and ulceration, proximal dilatation and mucosal fold thickening.

Complications

- Perforation of the bowel
- Aspiration

BARIUM ENEMA

This is the radiographic study of the large bowel by administration of contrast media through the rectum.

Types

- Single contrast barium enema and double contrast barium enema

Indications

- Change in the bowel habit:
- Melaena
- Mass suspected to be arising from colon
- Features of large gut obstruction (Subacute)

Contraindications

- Toxic megacolon
- Pseudomembranous colitis
- Rectal biopsy done recently (procedure withheld for 7 days)

Procedure

- Bowel is prepared with low residue diet, purgation and cleansing water enema. High density barium suspension is allowed to flow upto the ileocaecal junction and reflux into the terminal ileum. Single contrast filming is done- Patient is asked to evacuate the barium and a post evacuation film is taken. Once barium is evacuated properly, air insufflation is carried out so as to distend colon upto the ileocaecal junction.

- Filming is done to demonstrate the double contrast of large bowel with additional spots of hepatic, splenic flexures and rectosigmoid junction in oblique positions so as to open up these regions.

Interpretation of study

Few example are given below:

1. **Ulcerative colitis**
   - Loss of haustral pattern
   - Fine granularity of mucosa
   - Fine ulcerations resulting in spiking of colonic surface
   - Strictures
   - Pipe stem colon, increase in presacral space.

2. **Malignant lesions**
   - Circumferential/accentric growth narrowing the lumen
   - Hold up of barium proximal to the lesion
   - Mucosal abnormality—ulcerations

3. **Tuberculosis**
   - Ileocaecal region is the commonest site. Deformed, elevated caecum, stricture and ulceration involving ascending colon and ileum.

4. **Crohn's disease**
   - Multiple ulcerations, thickening and distortion of valvulae conniventes, short or long strictures, cobblestone pattern and separation of bowel loops are the features.

5. **Malabsorption**
   - Dilution of barium, segmentation of the column of barium, Moulage sign (barium in a featureless tube) and jejunal dilatation are the findings.

SMALL BOWEL ENEMA OR ENTEROCLYSIS (Fig. 46.3)

This is the radiological study of the small bowel (from jejunum to the ileocaecal junction) by intubation of the jejunum and instillation of contrast media through the tube.

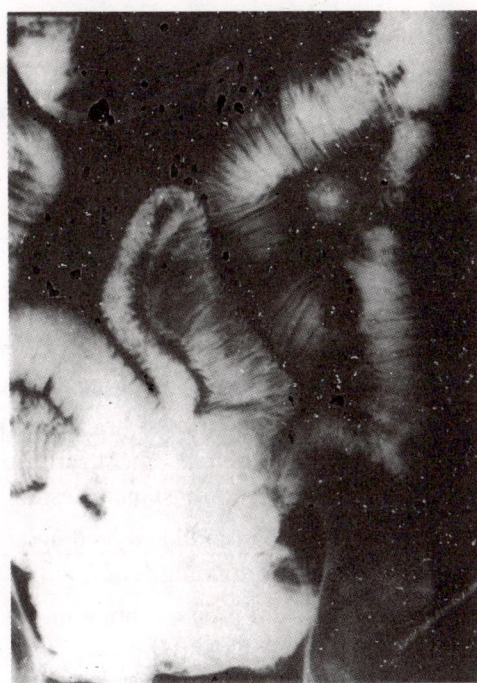

Fig. 46.3 Small bowel enema showing stricture terminal ileum. Contributed by Dr. Vijayalaxmi, Sri Venkateshwara Institute of Medical Sciences, Tirupati

Procedures

- Bilboa Dotter tube is inserted with the guide wire through one of the nostrils and advanced caudally with the swallowing action till the tip reaches the stomach. The tube is then advanced through the antrum of the stomach to the pyloric canal. Then it is advanced under fluoroscopic guidance to about 4-5 cm distal to the Trietz ligament (duodenojejunal junction).

- 200 ml barium suspension is injected at a rate of 75 ml/min followed by 5% of methylcellulose at a rate of 100 ml/min. The head of the barium column is followed with intermittent fluoroscopy and films exposed wherever necessary.

Key Box 46.1
INDICATIONS
• Mechanical obstruction • GIT bleeding • Tumours of small intestine • Unexplained abdominal pain • Diarrhoea

Key Box 46.2
CONTRAINDICATIONS
• Complete obstruction • Suspected perforation • Massive dilatation of small bowel • Duodenal obstruction • Gastrojejunostomy

- Ileocaecal spot films are taken when the junction is opacified and distended.

Interpretation of study

1. Normal small bowel shows a decrease in calibre from jejunum to ileum and the change of prominent valvulae conniventies to featureless ileum is evident.

2. Malignancies and lymphomas show evidence of strictures, proximal dilatations and mucosal abnormality. Large mesenteric nodal masses displace the bowel loops.

3. Strictures and ulceration of terminal ileum. Dilatation of the segment proximal to the narrowed segment and conical shrunken caecum are seen in Ileocaecal tuberculosis. In later stages, ileal strictures, fistulae, etc. may be seen.

Complications

- Perforation
- Inspissation of barium
- Transient bacteraemia

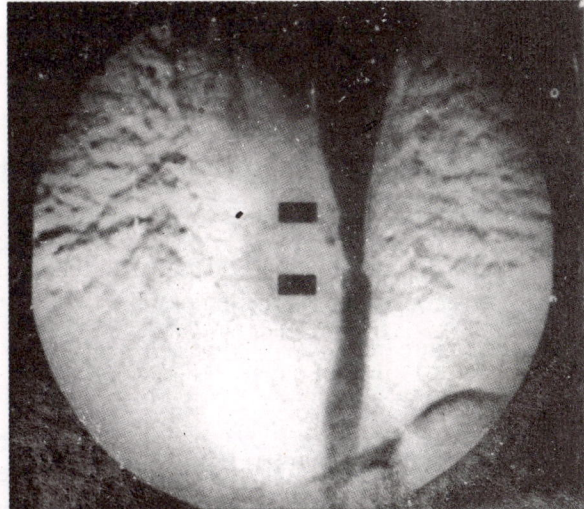

Fig. 46.4 Aortogram: Contrast in the thoracic aorta showing narrowing at D_8-D_9 level

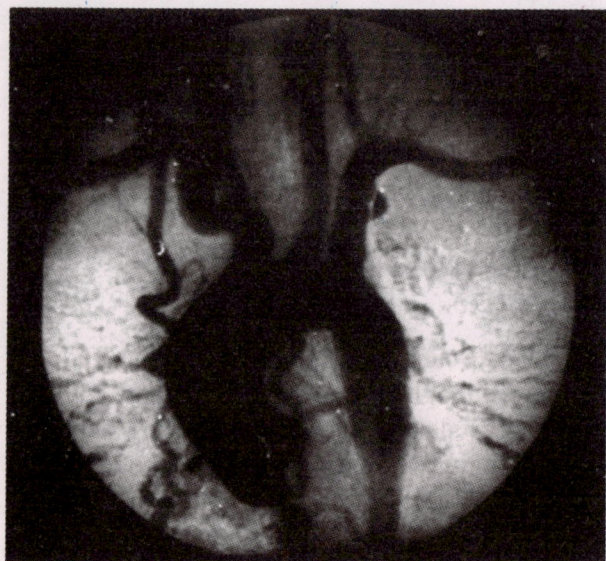

Fig. 46.5 Arch aortogram: Contrast in the arch of aorta demonstrating the major vessels arising from it

ANGIOGRAPHY (Figs. 46.4 and 46.5)

Definition

- This is the study of the blood vessels by injection of a contrast medium containing iodine into the vessel.

Indications

- Primary vascular diseases like vaso-occlusive disease, aneurysm, AVM, etc.
- Vascularity assessment of a tumour
- Congenital vascular conditions like coarctation
- Percutaneous interventional vascular procedures

Contraindications

- Bleeding tendencies
- Skin infections at site of entry
- Cardiovascular disease like recent myocardial infarction, overt congestive cardiac failure
- Hepatic failure

Procedure

- Local anaesthesia at site of puncture is preferred except in children or restless patients, wherein general anaesthesia is preferred. Using a Seldinger needle the artery is punctured.

- The catheter of appropriate dimension is placed into the artery and negotiated into the desired vessel to be studied. Contrast is injected and filming is done.

Puncture sites

- Femoral artery, axillary artery, brachial artery

Interpretation of study

1. Aneurysms are seen as focal dilatations of vessel or projecting from the main vessel through a neck.
2. Tumour vessels show abnormal branching pattern, vascular encasement, displacement, arteriovenous shunting and pooling of contrast in the lesion.
3. AVM shows evidence of a dilated feeding artery/abnormal blush and early draining vein.
4. Vascular occlusions are seen as abrupt or gradual tapering of vessel with collateral supply distally.

Complications

- Damage to arterial walls at the site of puncture
- Severe hypotensive reactions
- Thrombosis of arteries, catheter clot embolus, haematoma at puncture site
- Vagal inhibition
- Allergic reactions to contrast
- Damage to nerves and to organs

SPLENOPORTOGRAPHY (Fig. 46.6)

This is the contrast study of the portal venous system, percutaneous splenic puncture.

Indications

- Demonstration of the anatomy of the portal system in patients with portal hypertension prior to surgery
- Check the patency of a portosystemic anastomosis

Contraindications

- Abnormal prothrombin time
- Ascites

Procedure

- Splenoportography needle is introduced into the spleen in the midaxillary line under local anaesthesia. After confirming the placement of needle in the splenic pulp,

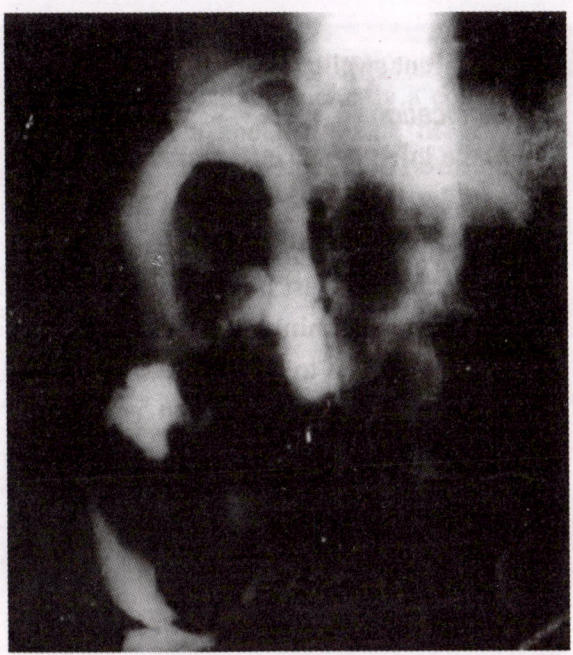

Fig. 46.6 Splenoportography showing dilated splenic vein

injection of iodine containing contrast media is done and films are taken to include the splenic vein, portal vein and the portal radicles in liver.

Interpretation of study

- Contrast injected into the splenic pulp drains into the hilum through the splenic radicles and then through the splenic vein and portal vein into liver.

- Thromboses are seen as filling defects in the contrast opacified splenic and portal vein.

- In severe portal hypertension multiple collaterals are seen as branching channels from the normal pathway.

Complications

- Haemorrhage
- Perforation of adjacent structures (Pleura, colon)
- Splenic rupture
- Infection

SIALOGRAPHY

This is the contrast opacification of the duct and the glandular acini by cannulating the ducts of salivary glands.

Indications

- Pain
- Recurrent swelling

Contraindications

- Acute infection or inflammation

Procedure

- The orifice of the parotid duct or submandibular duct is cannulated depending on the indication. Iodine containing contrast medium is injected.

- Injection is terminated **immediately if any pain is experienced.**

- Films are taken to demonstrate the duct and the glandular branching pattern.

- Post-secretory films are taken 5 minutes after administration of a sialogogue to demonstrate sialectasis.

Interpretation of study

1. Stones in the gland are identified as filling defects and those in the ductal system result in proximal obstruction and dilatation.

2. Glandular enlargement due to inflammation result in pooling of the contrast injected.

3. Tumours of the salivary gland result in irregular filling defect with duct distortion and pooling of contrast medium.

Complications

- Pain
- Damage to duct orifice
- Rupture of ducts
- Infection

COMPUTED TOMOGRAPHY (CT)

This is an imaging procedure where detailed information is obtained from thin sections in collimated X-rays.

Indications

- Structural evaluation of intracranial lesions (Fig. 46.7)
- Detailed evaluation of lung, mediastinal pathologies
- Intra-abdominal and pelvic masses where exact site of origin and relation to adjacent structures can be evaluated.

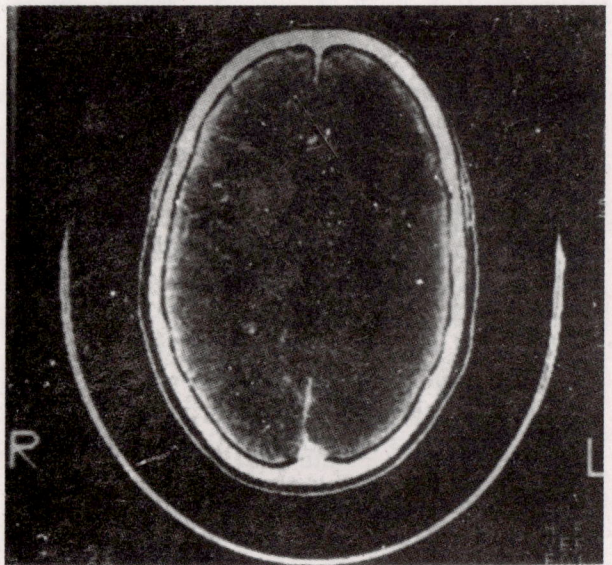

Fig. 46.7 Cranial CT: Hypodensity of the left (L) fronto-parietal cerebral parenchyma suggestive of a (L) middle cerebral artery territory infarct

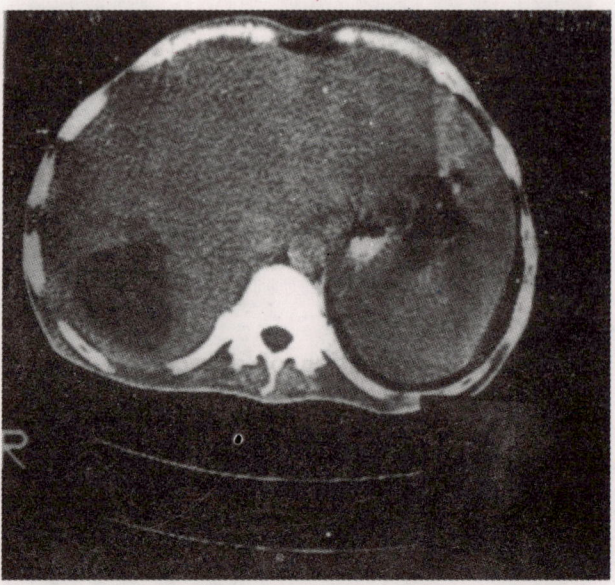

Fig. 46.8 CT scan of abdomen: Contrast enhanced scan demonstrating a hypodense lesion in right lobe of liver posteriorly due to an abscess

- Extra-osseous and soft tissue extension of bone tumours.
- Vascularity of the normal organ and the abnormal tissue can be evaluated and compared.

Contraindications (relative)

- Pregnancy
- Restless patients

Interpretation of images

- Structures imaged appear densely white to densely black depending on the absorption of X-rays and the emerging resultant X-rays which are detected. **The composite picture is actually a collection of Hounsfield numbers.** Each Hounsfield number being assigned a specific shade of gray, thus producing a picture that might be easily understood. Some of the common densities to be encountered in practice are as follows (Hounsfield units = HU) :

Air	-1000 HU
Fat	-50 to -100 HU
Water	0 HU
CSF	0 to +3 HU
White matter	+22 to +32 HU
Grey matter	+36 to +46 HU
Clotted blood	+60 to +80 HU
Calcification, bone	+80 to +1000 HU

- In order to increase the contrast that may exist between the structures in the body, **intravenous contrast (iodine containing) is administered.** Certain tissues show enhancement of their density and various pathologies also show fairly characteristic contrast uptake patterns (Fig. 46.8).

- In abdominal scanning, **oral contrast** is administered to the patient before the procedure, to enable the operator to accurately separate the bowel loops from the other intra-abdominal structures.

- The advantages of CT over conventional radiology are that it can visualise an extremely small pathology not evident on conventional films and is cost effective as multiple X-ray films and procedures can be avoided. It is non-invasive and the radiation levels applied to the patient are extremely low.

ULTRASONOGRAPHY (Fig. 46.9)

Principle

- This imaging modality is based on the **Piezo-electric effect** which is the property of certain substances to convert **electrical energy to sound energy.** These are the active portions of the ultrasonic transducers. **The commonly used substance in the transducer is lead zirconate titanate.**

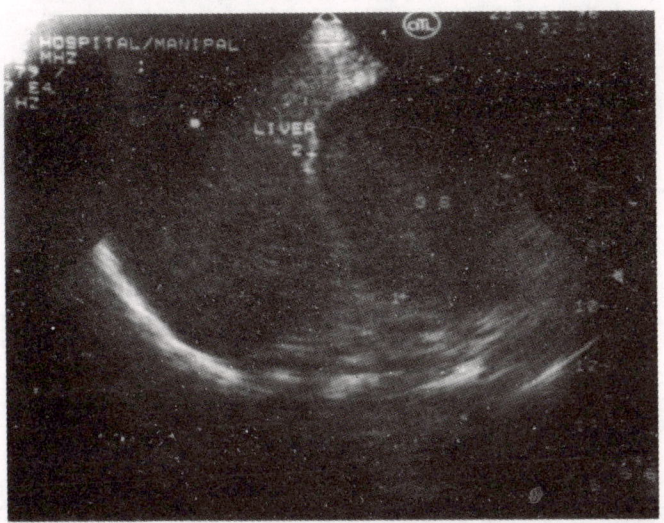

Fig. 46.9. Ultrasound of liver and gall bladder demon- strating an isoechoic mass lesion occupying the lumen of gall bladder which was due to malignancy

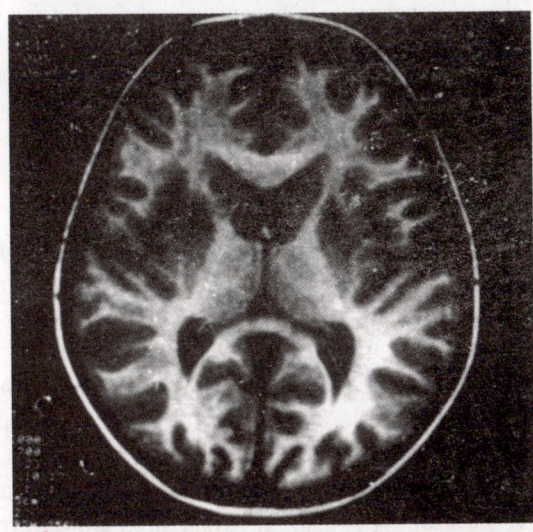

Fig. 46.10 MRI: T_1 and T_2 weight axial and coronal scans of normal brain

Applications

- Ultrasonic beam of **high frequency** gives excellent resolution images of only superficial structures. This is used for study of musculoskeletal system, joints, thyroid, scrotum, etc.

- For imaging **deeper structures of abdomen a low frequency** probe with greater **penetrancy** is used.

Interpretation of images

- Images are dependent on the **intensity of echoes** received back by the transducer.

- Structures which reflect all the sound waves back are depicted as **bright echoes** and **termed hyperechoic.**

- Structures which reflect **moderate** level of sound waves appear of uniform grains and are **termed isoechoic.**

- Fluid filled structures which transmit all the sound waves, **do not reflect any echoes and are termed hypoechoic.**

- The reflection of sound waves in the form of echoes depends on the density of the organ and the transmission of sound through the same.

Advantages of ultrasonography

1. It is a cost effective investigation
2. It is widely available
3. Non-invasive

4. Owing to the relatively small size of the apparatus, it is fairly portable, and can thus be brought to the bedside of the moribund patient.

5. It does not involve the use of ionising radiation, and can therefore be safely used in a pregnant patient and can be repeatedly used as a follow-up modality.

Limitation of ultrasonography

1. Its use is limited in thorax
2. Limited use in the abdomen when there is gaseous distension
3. Operator expertise is important
4. It cannot image bone

MAGNETIC RESONANCE IMAGING (MRI) (Fig. 46.10)

Principle

Certain atomic nuclei, which possess unpaired protons or neutrons, possess an inherent spin. The nucleus is positively charged and therefore creates a small magnetic field around itself, when it spins. The human body contains in abundance such spinning nuclei in the atoms of hydrogen which is found in water and lipids.

When the tissues containing these nuclei are within a strong magnetic field, the nuclei tend to align themselves along the lines of the force field. The spinning protons now tend to process i.e. wobble about the axis of the main magnetic field. Now a radiofrequency is applied, being of the same frequency as the processing but at right angles to the main magnetic field. This excites the protons at low energy states into higher energy states. Thus, an absorption of energy is taking place, which is used as the excited protons 'relax' back to their original energy level when the radio-frequency is switched off.

The relaxation of protons back to equilib E and lower energy state is termed the **spin relaxation** or **longitudinal relaxation**. It is exponential and referred to by the time **constant** T_1. When the RF pulse is applied the protons process together in synchronism or in phase with each other. During relaxation, however, they quickly get out of phase due to small variations in local magnetic fields. This loss of phase is termed **spin-spin relaxation** or **transverse relaxation**. It is also an exponential and referred to by the time constant T_2 depending on the type of tissue under study, the T_1 and T_2 relaxation times will differ, thus giving rise to differences in the image.

The MRI image depends upon 4 main factors:

1. The T_1 relaxation time
2. The T_2 relaxation time
2. The proton density
3. The blood flow

Depending on the characteristics of the above four parameters, the signal intensity of the image will vary, thus deciding the appearance that any given tissue will finally cast.

Advantages of MRI

1. It is non-invasive.
2. It does not involve the use of ionising radiation, hence is safe in that respect.
3. It gives high intrinsic contrast
4. Direct transverse, sagittal and normal imaging possible
5. No bone/air artefact
6. It has no known biological hazard

Disadvantages of MRI

1. The imaging time is long, hence movement of the patients may produce artefacts.
2. Due to variety of protocol options during scanning, the final image is highly operator dependent and this requires expert technical staff.
3. Expensive

4. Poor bone and calcium detail
5. **Patients with pacemakers, and critically ill patients cannot be scanned.**

PERIPHERAL VENOGRAPHY

This is the contrast study of the veins of the limbs.

Indications

- Deep venous thrombosis
- Demonstration of incompetent perforators
- In case of suspected venous obstruction by tumour
- To outline venous malformations

Procedure

- Tourniquet is applied just above the ankle or elbow to occlude the superficial venous system.
- A 19 g butterfly needle is inserted into a distal vein and contrast media (iodine containing) is injected.
- Filming is done upto the region of interest.

Interpretation of study

1. Thrombosis of deep veins are seen as filling defects.
2. Incompetent perforators are evident as refluxing of contrast from deep to superficial system and prominent tortuous collaterals.
3. Displacement of the opacified veins are seen at sites of tumour. Tumour encasement of veins and thrombosis also may be demonstrable.

Complications

- Complications due to contrast media
- Thrombophlebitis
- Tissue necrosis due to extravasation of contrast
- Pulmonary embolus due to dislodged clot.

MYELOGRAPHY (Fig. 46.11)

Definition

- This is the study of the spinal canal and spinal cord by injection of contrast medium into the thecal subarachnoid space.

Indications

- Suspected intraspinal or nerve root abnormalities

Contraindications

- Papilloedema
- Recent lumbar puncture, since CSF collected outside the thecal space may be tapped.
- Previous adverse reactions to intrathecal injection of contrast medium.

Procedure

- Lumbar puncture is most preferred. Puncture done at L2-L3 level.
- Once good flow of CSF is obtained low osmolar non-ionic contrast media is injected.
- Filming is done of lumbar region and with adequate tilt towards head end, thoracic and cervical regions are also filmed.
- Cisternal puncture is done when lumbar puncture is a failure.

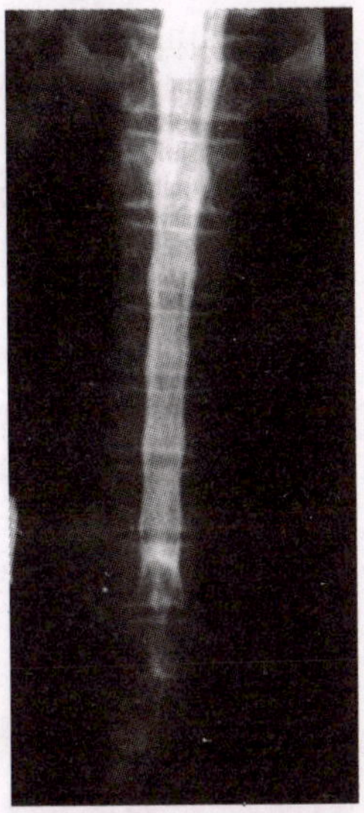

Fig. 46.11. Thoracic myelogram: Contrast in the thecal sac showing a total interruption in the flow of contrast cranially due to an intradural mass lesion

Interpretation of study

1. Disc lesions are seen as impressions on contrast column and cut off of the nerve roots at a particular level.
2. Intraspinal tumours cause widening of the contrast column with or without total obstruction to flow.
3. Vertebral and paravertebral lesions result in displacement of the contrast column and cut off at particular level.

Complications

- Headache
- Convulsions—rare
- Transient increase in lumbar or sciatic pain
- Hypotension
- Spinal cord damage in cisternal puncture

INTERVENTIONAL RADIOLOGY

The role of radiology was limited as only a diagnostic art until mid 1970's. However, now radiology has taken on an exciting new aspect and has entered the field of Intervention Radiology. Two main types of interventional procedures: vascular and non-vascular.

Vascular

1. **Angioplasty:** This is performed by the use of intraluminal balloon catheters and may be performed for almost any diseased vessel in the body. The more commonly treated vessels are the coronaries, renals, peripheral limb vessels, etc.

2. **Embolisation:** This procedure is performed either preoperatively to reduce the vascularity of certain tumours or as a curative treatment for vascular malformations, aneurysms, GI bleeding etc. Temporary embolisation being achieved by using gel foam, autologous clots and permanent embolisation by using balloons, steel coils, ethanol, etc. Inferior vena cava (IVC) umbrella placement, IVC membranotomy, etc.

3. **Intravascular ultrasound:** The use of ultrasound inside a blood vessel to visualize the interior of the vessel in order to detect problems inside the blood vessel.

4. **Stent placement:** A tiny, expandable coil called a stent, is placed inside a blood vessel at the site of a blockage. The stent is expanded to open up the blockage.

- **Important types of stents and stent selection**

  Self expanding stents - are compressed within a catheter device and released by removing a constraining sheath or membrane. The final diameter of the stent is a function of the outward elastic load of the stent and the inward recoil of the elastic wall.

  Ballon expandable stents: are mounted on angioplasty ballons in a compressed state and then deployed by balloon inflation. These stents retain the diameter imposed by angioplasty balloon unless externally compressed.

5. **Foreign body extraction:** The use of a catheter inserted into a blood vessel to retrieve a foreign body in the vessel.

6. **Needle biopsy:** A small needle is inserted into the abnormal area in almost any part of the body, guided by imaging techniques, to obtain a tissue biopsy. This type of biopsy can provide a diagnosis without surgical intervention.

7. **Blood clot filters:** A small filter is inserted into a blood clot to catch and break up blood clots.

8. **Injection of clot-lysing agents:** Clot-lysing agents, such as tissue plasminogen activator (TPA), are

injected into the body to dissolve blood clots, thereby increasing blood flow to the heart or brain.

9. **Catheters insertions:** A catheter is inserted into large veins for giving chemotherapeutic drugs, nutritional support, and haemodialysis. A catheter may also be inserted prior to bone-marrow transplantation.

10. **Cancer treatment:** Administering cancer medications directly to the tumour site.

Nonvascular

1. **Hepatobiliary**: (PTBD) Percutaneous transhepatic biliary drainage is widely accepted in cases of biliary obstruction, along with percutaneous biliary calculus removal. Biliary stent placement across a malignant lesion in inoperable cases as a palliative procedure is widely being done.

2. **Urinary**: Percutaneous nephrostomy, percutaneous stenting and percutaneous nephrolithotomy are being performed.

3. **Guided biopsy**: Fluoroscopy, ultrasound or CT guided biopsy of various lesions are now part of routine technique.

4. **Other interventional procedures**: Percutaneous gastrostomy, catheter drainage of abscesses, pseudocysts, ultrasound guided intra-uterine foetal surgeries, etc.

Advantages of interventional procedures

1. Patient compliance is high as surgery is avoided

2. Cost effectiveness is high

3. Infection rates are low

4. Can be repeated as it is relatively non-invasive

5. Certain untreatable conditions are treated palliatively with interventional procedures.

MISCELLANEOUS

POSITRON EMISSION TOMOGRAPHY (PET Scan)

• PET scan is a medical imaging technique that combines computed tomography (CT) and Nuclear Scanning. It is used to determine the metabolic or biochemical activity in the brain, heart and other organs by tracking the movement and concentration of a radioactive tracer injected into the blood stream.

• A camera records the tracer's signal as it travels through the body and collects in organs. A computer then converts the signals into 3D images of the examined organ, which provide a clear view of an abnormality.

• One of the main differences between PET scan and other imaging tests like CT or MRI is that the PET scan reveals metabolic and functional changes occuring at the cellular level in an organ. A PET scan often detects these changes very early whereas CT or MRI detect changes a little later - as the disease begins to cause structural changes in organs or tissues.

VIRTUAL COLONOSCOPY

• It is a recently developed technique that uses a CT scanner and computer virtual reality software to look inside the body without having to insert a long tube (conventional colonoscopy) into the colon or without having to fill the colon with liquid barium (Barium enema).

• More formally known as three dimensional CT colonography, the virtual procedure allows radiologists to obtain 3D images from different angles, providing a sort of movie of the colon's interior without having to insert an endoscope into the bowel.

ADVANTAGES

• Noninvasive procedure

• Well-tolerated by patient

• Requires no sedation

• Less time consuming

• Useful in elderly who are frail and infirm

• Useful when a tumour is large enough to block passage of scope.

DISADVANTAGES

• Exposure to radiation

• Less detail of inner lining of colon

• Small polyps are located more reliably by colonoscopy

• Strictly a diagnostic procedure (unlike colonoscopy)

Principles of Clinical Radiation Oncology

47

- Radiation
- Dose fractionation
- Sources and methods
- Measurement
- Clinical uses
- Curative treatment
- Palliative treatment
- Radiotherapy reactions
- Advances in radiation therapy

RADIATION

The term radiation applies to the emission and propagation of **Energy** through space and material medium. Radiation travels with the speed of light in a vacuum and interacts with living or nonliving matter resulting in varying degrees of energy transfer to the biological medium. This process of deposition of energy within the cells is brought about by **Ionization** (removal of an orbital electron) of atoms and molecules. Ionizing radiations are very high frequency (3 x 10^{21} Hertz) and short wavelength (10^{13} m) electromagnetic waves. Ionization can occur within the nuclear DNA molecule of a cell (**Directly acting**) or interaction with other molecules, mainly water (H_2O) to produce **Free Radicals (Indirectly)**, which in turn can damage DNA and result in cell death or mutagenesis.

By damaging DNA, radiation interferes with cell division and can result in **reproductive** death of a cell. This process in a malignant tumour could mean the loss of its ability for uncontrolled cell division or proliferation. This process is unselective; it occurs both in cells of normal tissues and in those of tumours. Therapeutic usefulness of radiotherapy, therefore, depends on the differential sensitivity of tissues (Normal vs Tumor cell), on careful treatment planning and dose prescription to minimize normal tissue damage, and the patients tolerance to radiation.

DOSE FRACTIONATION

The five 'R's of radiobiology provide the basis for fractional radiotherapy. In clinical practice dividing a dose into a number of fractions has the following advantages:

1. The **acute effects** of single dose of radiation can be decreased with fractionation. The patients symptomatic tolerance improves with **fractional radiation.**

2. Fractionation exploits the difference in **recovery rate** between normal tissues and tumours. Effects on normal tissues are less because of the repair of sublethal damage between dose fractions and normal cellular **repopulation.**

3. Radiation induced **redistribution** of cells within the cell cycle tends to sensitize the rapidly proliferating cells, which is seen more in tumours

4. **Radiosensitivity** of cells depend markedly on the phase of the cell cycle at which they receive the radiation. Cells in **Mitosis and G2 phase are the most sensitive** and cells in early Gl and late S phases are the most resistant.

Key Box 47.1
FRACTIONAL R.T. BASIS
• Repair • Redistribution • Reoxygenation • Repopulation/Recovery • Radiosensitivity

5. Reduction in the number of hypoxic cells is brought about through cell kill and **reoxygenation**. Also blood vessels compressed by a growing cancer are decompressed as the cancer shrinks, permitting better oxygenation.

Oxygen effect

The biologic effects of ionizing radiations are greatly influenced by the presence of normal oxygen concentration within the cells. The absence or low oxygen content conveys a resistance to radiation requiring about three times the dose to produce the same biologic effects. Certain solid tumours and large tumours are likely to contain 10-15% of hypoxic cells.

For routine practice the "Conventional or Standard" Dose fractionation schedule is followed. This consists of 180-200 cGy fraction per day and 5 fractions per week over 4-6 weeks(depending on the total dose). The choice of optimal dose/time/fractionation schedules for various tumours should be individualized according to the cell kinetic characteristics and clinical observations.

RADIOCURABILITY refers to the eradication of tumour at the primary or regional site and reflects the direct effect of irradiation, which may or may not parallel the patients ultimate outcome.

PROBABILITY OF TUMOUR CONTROL (Fig. 47.1)

It is axiomatic in radiation therapy that higher doses of radiation produce better tumour control, and numerous dose-response curves (sigmoid in shape) in a variety of tumours have been published (Fig 47.1).

For every increment of dose a certain fraction of cells will be killed. Therefore the total number of surviving cells will be proportional to the initial number present and the fraction killed with each dose. Thus it is apparent that **various levels of irradiation yield a different probability of tumour control**, depending on the extent of lesion or number of clonogenic cells present.

For **subclinical disease** (10^{3-4} cells) in squamous cell carcinoma of the upper respiratory tract or for adenocarcinoma of the breast, doses of 4500-5000 cGy result in control of disease in over 90% of patients.

For **microscopic residual disease** or cell aggregates greater than $10^6/10^9$ are required for the pathologist to detect them. Therefore, these volumes must receive higher doses of radiation in the range of 6000-6500 cGy in 6-7 weeks for epithelial tumours.

For **clinically palpable tumours (Gross disease)**, does of 6000 cGy (for Tl) to 7500 cGy to 8000 cGy for T4 tumours) are required (200 cGy/day/5 fractions weekly). This dose range and probability of tumour control have been documented for various tumors.

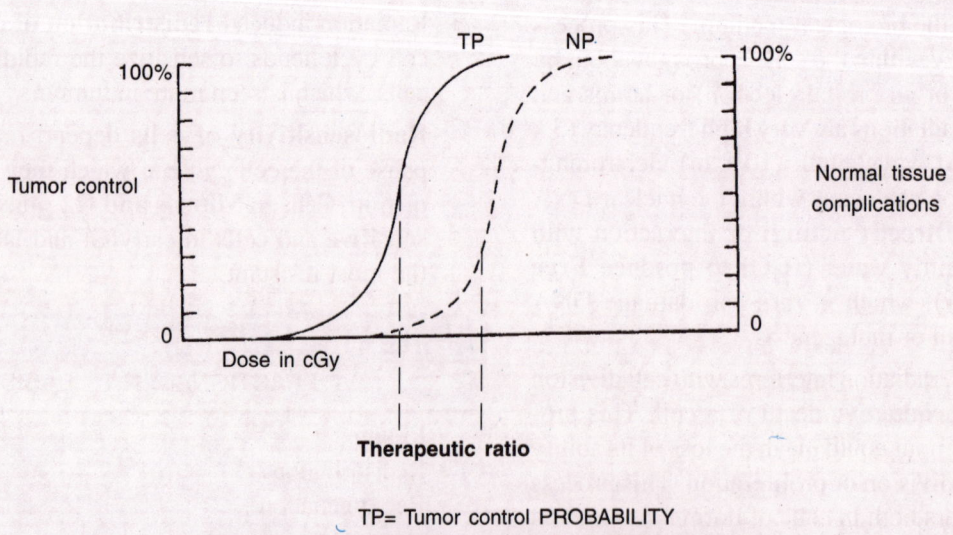

TP= Tumor control PROBABILITY

NP= Normal tissue complication PROBABLITY

Fig. 47.1 The graph showing tumour probability control

RADIOTHERAPY—SOURCES AND METHODS OF DELIVERY

Radiotherapy is the therapeutic use of high-energy ionizing radiation in the treatment/management of malignant disease.

These are either electromagnetic waves, X-rays, gamma rays or corpuscular (subatomic particles) electrons, protons, neutrons, alpha particles, or heavy ion nuclei. Ionizing radiation penetrates tissues to different depths according to its type of energy and physical nature. Radiotherapy treatment planning is an important part of the radiation oncologist's work.

SOURCE OF RADIATION (Fig. 47.2 on Page 721)

Gamma and beta rays from radioactive isotopes (Cobalt-60, Caesium 137, Indium 197) and X-rays and electrons from a high energy X-ray machine (Linear accelerator). Protons, neutrons, and heavy ion nuclei from Cyclotrons.

X-rays and gamma rays are identical in properties but are produced by different sources. Ionizing radiations can be classified according to their density of ionizations per unit length of the distance in the absorbing media as Low and High LET (Linear energy transfer) radiation.

IONISING RADIATION

- Low LET—X-rays, gamma rays, electron.
- High LET—Neutrons, protons, a-particles and negative ions.
- High LET radiation has a mass heavier than electrons, hence cause dense ionization and are biologically more effective (damaging) than low LET radiation. They are also less dependent on repair of sublethal damage, Cell cycle phases, and oxygen content of the cells for radiosensitivity.
- High LET radiation is available in limited cancer centres around the world, require expensive equipment to produce and are undergoing clinical trials.

METHODS OF DELIVERY

Ionizing radiations may be delivered clinically in three ways:

1. External beam Irradiation

From sources at a distance (usually 80-100 cm) from the body surface. This includes 60 Co Teletherapy Units and X-ray sources, such as linear accelerators (Fig. 47.3 on Page 721)

Advantages of megavoltage beam RT

1. Deeper penetration
2. Sharp beam edges
3. Skin sparing
4. Equal absorption in bone and soft tissues
5. Improved dose distribution within tissue

II. Brachytherapy

Brachytherapy refers to use of radiation sources in or close to the tumour.

Use of sealed (closed containers) radioactive sources for radiation treatment from a short distance.

Types of brachytherapy

1. **Intracavitary** (within a cavity) e.g. uterine cavity, Vaginal cavity, oesophageal and bronchial lumen.

Key Box 47.2
ADVANTAGES OF BRACHYTHERAPY
1. High localized dose to limited volume
2. Minimal dose to adjacent tissues
3. Spares deeper normal tissues
4. Continuous RT in a single course
5. Short overall time (high dose rate)
6. Alone : Rarely (early stage)   Combined : Often (as boost)

2. **Interstitial** when radioactive needles or wires are inserted into and around a tumour.
3. **Surface moulds or plaques** as radioactive surface applicators, e.g. skin cancer, eye cancers.

With this mode of therapy a high dose can be delivered locally to the tumour with rapid dose fall off in the surrounding normal tissue. In the past. brachytherapy was carried out mostly with Radium or Radon sources. Currently, use of artificially produced radionuclides such as Cs^{137} (Caesium 137), Ir^{192} (Iridium 192), Au^{198} (Gold 198), and I^{125} (Iodine 125) is rapidly increasing.

New technical developments have stimulated increased interest in brachytherapy:

1. Introduction of improved artificial isotopes

2. Manual after loading devices to reduce personnel exposure

3. Remote after loading, high dose rate (HDR) machines, have increased accuracy, improved dosimetry, reduced (short) treatment time, treatment on OPD basis and have improved patient compliance.

Brachytherapy is used very often. **Combined** with **external beam treatment** and **rarely alone** (early stage). The rationale behind combining the two is to treat the primary site and regional spread(very often subclinical disease) with external RT and to deliver a higher dose (boost) to the primary (gross disease) with brachytherapy. Aim is not to exceed the normal tissue tolerance and at the same time the tumour should receive adequate curative dose. Brachytherapy can also be used as palliative therapy e.g. bronchial and oesophageal obstruction.

III. Internal or systemic irradiation

From unsealed radioactive sources (i.e. I^{131}, P^{32}, Sr^{89}) administered enterally, intracavitarly or intravenously, for diagnostic (nuclear medicine) and therapeutic purposes, e.g. carcinoma thyroid, bone tumours and thyrotoxicosis.

MEASUREMENT OF IONIZING RADIATION

1. The **Roentgen** is a unit of exposure. It is a measure of ionizations produced per unit volume of air by X-rays and gamma rays and cannot be used for photon energies above 3 MeV.

   • The SI unit for exposure is Coulomb per kilogram (C/kg)

   • $1 R = 2.58 \times 10^4$ C/kg air

2. **Radiation absorbed dose (RAD):**

   • Absorbed dose is a measure of the biologically significant effects produced by ionizing radiation. Absorbed dose = De/dm, De is the mean energy imparted by the ionizing radiation to material of mass dm. The old unit of dose is rad and represents the absorption of 100 ergs of energy per gram of absorbing material.

   • 1 rad $==$ 100 ergs/g $= 10^2$ J/kg

   • The SI unit of absorbed dose is Gray (Gy) and is defined as

   • 1 Gy = 1 J/kg

Thus the relationship between rad and gray is 1 Gy = 100 rad or 1 cGy = 1 rad.

ELECTRON BEAM THERAPY

Source

• Mainly linear accelerators

Energy

• Most useful range for clinical use is 6 to 20 MeV

Use

1. Superficial tumours upto a depth of 5 cm

2. Local boost

Advantages

1. Characteristic sharp dose fall off beyond the tumour

2. Dose uniformity within the target volume

Principle applications

1. Treatment of skin and lip cancers
2. Chest wall irradiation for breast cancer
3. Boost dose to nodes and tumour bed
4. Head and neck cancers

Table 47.1. Difference between radical and palliative radiotherapy

PALLIATIVE RADIOTHERAPY	RADICAL RADIOTHERAPY
• Treatment is intended to eradicate all clonogenic malignant cells.	• Treatment is intended to control symptoms to improve quality of life.
• High dose curative courses of RT needed and considerable normal tissue morbidity (acute) may be associated.	• Minimum doses of RT to achieve maximum control with minimal side effects.
• Late side effects of adjacent normal tissues may be dose limiting.	• Short patient survival times, less concern with long term limiting, morbidity.
• Patient often needs high doses and long courses of treatement.	• Patient prefers few hospital visits, so short courses of treatment, treatment used.

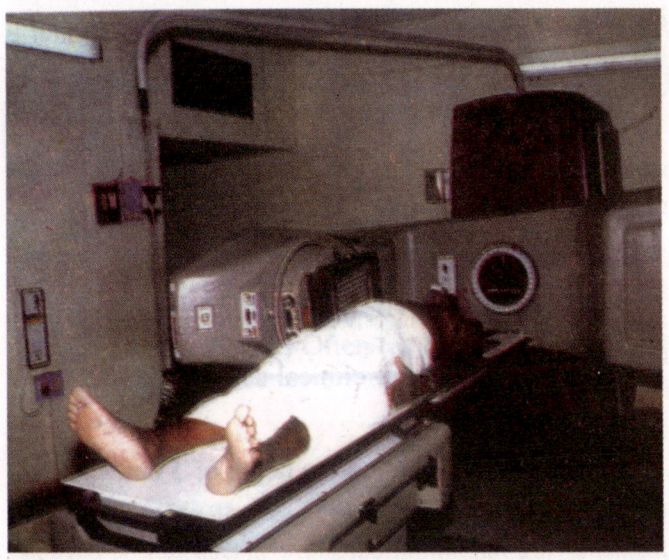

Fig. 47.2 Cobalt teletherapy unit

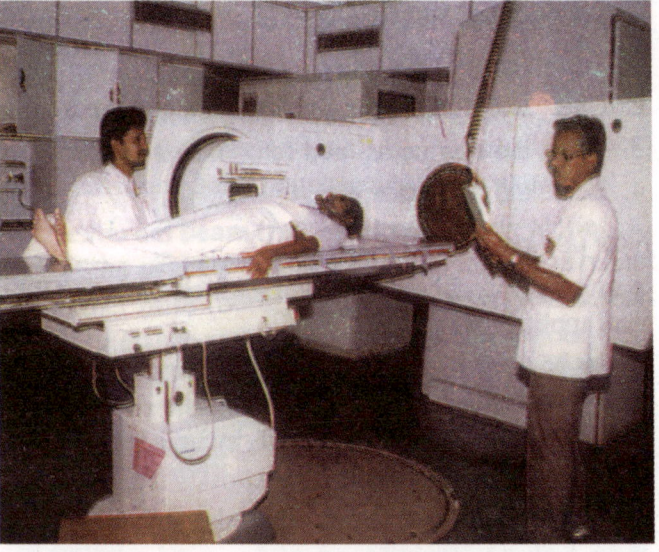

Fig. 47.3 Linear accelerator

Clinical use of radiotherapy

Like surgery and chemotherapy, radiation therapy (RT) has definite indications and contraindications for its application.

It can be used alone to cure or, in combination with other methods, as an adjuvant. Currently 50-60% of all patients with cancer receive RT during the course of their illness. If properly used, 50% of these patients could get cured. For the other half, incurable by any current method, palliation of specific symptoms and signs can improve quality of life.

Before treating a patient with radiotherapy, the radiotherapist must be satisfied that the working diagnosis is correct, pretreatment investigations and staging have to be complete. Then the radiation oncologist must address two questions:

1. Is the treatment intent CURATIVE or PALLIATIVE?

2. What is the best approach to achieve this goal?

The first question is vital, for there are important differences between radical and palliative radiotherapy.

The second question recognizes that cancer can be treated by surgery, radiotherapy, and drugs. In many instances, radiotherapy is the best approach. In view of the increasing complexity of curative cancer management for many tumours, with different combinations of surgery, radiotherapy, and chemotherapy for different stages of the disease, require a coordinated **Multi disciplinary** approach. The correct initial choice gives the best prospect for cure or good palliation.

AS A PRIMARY CURATIVE MODALITY

A. **RT frequently may be the sole agent used with curative intent** for anatomically limited tumours of the retina, optic nerve, brain (craniopharyngioma, medulloblastoma, ependymoma), spinal cord (low grade glioma), skin, oral cavity, pharynx, larynx, oesophagus, uterine cervix, vagina, prostate and reticuloendothelial system (Hodgkin's disease, stages I, II and III A).

B. **When no other potentially curative treatment exists.** Some cancers remain localized for all or much of their natural history. These cancers might also be unresectable by virtue of their anatomical location or because of local infiltration into surrounding normal/vital structures, which would mean that surgery will severely affect physiological function e.g. locally advanced head and neck cancer, cervical cancers stage IIb-III, medulloblastoma (alternative to surgery for inaccessible and inoperable malignancies).

Key Box 47.3
RADIOTHERAPY USE IN FOUR SETTINGS
1. As a primary **CURATIVE** modality
2. As an **ADJUVANT** for curative therapy (combined modality)
3. As **PROPHYLACTIC RADIATION**
4. As **PALLIATIVE** treatment

C. **Where alternative therapy is considered more "toxic".** Carcinoma of the larynx, anal canal, ar breast can all be managed by ablative surgery and in each case the anatomy and physiology of the respective organ is lost. Each of these cancers can be managed by irradiation with preservation of anatomy and function.

Preservation of organ and its function (larynx, breast, anal canal, limbs, cervix, tongue, bladder)

Key Box 47.4

INDICATIONS FOR CURATIVE RT

Stages I and II:

Testis	Seminoma
Ovary	Dysgerminoma
Skin	Basal cell and squamous cell carcinoma
Lymphatic	Hodgkin's lymphoma
Cervix	Cervix, uterus, vagina
Bladder	Transitional cell ca
Prostate	Adenocarcinoma
Anal canal	Carcinoma
Head and neck	Cancers
Oesophagus	Cancer
Lung	Non-small cell cancer
Brain	Medulloblastoma

Key Box 47.5

ADJUVANT RT (SURG+RT+/-CT)

- Head and neck cancer locally advanced
- Brain tumours
- Breast cancer
- Rectal cancer
- Soft tissue sarcoma
- Bone sarcoma
- Endometrial Ca.
- Paediatric solid tumours (Wilms', rhabdomyosarcoma, neuroblastoma)

ADJUVANT FOR CURATIVE THERAPY (COMBINED MODALITY)

RT is combined with Surgery for advanced cancers of the head and neck, cancers of the lung, uterus, breast, urinary bladder, testis (seminoma), and rectum, and soft tissue sarcomas and primary bone tumours.

RT is an adjuvant to chemotherapy for some patients with lymphomas, lung cancers, and cancer in children (rhabdomyosarcoma, Wilms' tumour, neuroblastoma).

In some clinical situations the combined benefits of surgery, RT and chemotherapy might be exploited. It has been most useful in the management of breast cancer, bone sarcoma, Wilms' tumour.

COMBINED TREATMENT (SURGERY AND RADIATION THERAPY)

In many situations radiation therapy alone is inadequate for achieving maximum cure levels. This can be because the number of tumour stem cells is too large, some or all of the cancer cells are radio-resistant, or tolerance of the contiguous normal tissues is too low. The rationale for combining surgery and radiation therapy is the differing mechanisms of the two disciplines. Radiation therapy fails at the centre of the tumour where the concentrations of the tumour cells is the largest and the conditions may be hypoxic (less sensitive to RT).

Surgical resection fails because the tumour extends further than the margins of excision, infesting contiguous tissues with undetectable microscopic foci. Radiation therapy is efficient in the sterilization of these tumour cell numbers that are well vascularized, and the surgical resection is efficient in removing the gross necrotic tumour masses.

Radiation can be combined with surgery either preoperatively or postoperatively.

Aims and advantages of preoperative RT

1. Unresectable cancer to resectable cancer
2. Prevent iatrogenic metastases
3. Reduction of size and vascularity
4. Destroys microscopic foci beyond surgical margin

Disadvantages

1. Delay in surgical (primary) treatment
2. Delay in wound healing
3. Pathologic downstaging to influence other adjuvant treatment
4. Alters anatomical staging (precise pathological extent)
5. Inability to tailor RT to high risk areas

Post-operative RT

Aim and advantages

1. Exact disease extent known so as to tailor the treatment individually

2. Operative margins are well-defined- gross or microscopic.

3. Less post-operative complications- wound healing intact.

4. GI anastomoses and ileal conduits can be done in a non-irradiated field.

5. Potential for unnecessary irradiation in some patients is reduced

Disadvantages

1. Delay in RT due to postoperative complications—delay wound healing

2. Decreased radiosensitivity due to vascular supply of oxygen

3. Postoperative adhesions of organs/structures

4. No effect on dissemination during surgery

5. Volume of normal tissue to be irradiated is more usually all tissue planes potentially contaminated by surgery.

Clinical situations may indicate different sequences but such combinations of surgery and radiation therapy improve the local tumour control rate for many advanced cancers. Combined therapy may also improve the cure rate at the same time reducing the morbidity associated with more aggressive single modality treatment.

COMBINATION OF RADIOTHERAPY WITH CHEMOTHERAPY

In general, chemotherapy is used in an adjuvant way to control subclinical disease elsewhere in the (body or in an additive way to enhance the local effects of the radiation to achieve higher rate of local control. Many other agents will act in both ways.

Agents of choice are those whose toxic effects are in organs not included in the radiation target volume An example is the combination of the Cisplatin compounds with radiation therapy for Head and Neck cancers. Here the toxicity of chemotherapy is primarily hematogenous and renal; the toxicity of RT is on the oral mucosa.

Chemotherapy could be combined with RT in three main ways

1. Neo-adjuvant : 1-3 courses before definitive RT.

2. Adjuvant: After completion of definitive RT

3. Concurrent: During a course of radiotherapy

4. Combinations of the above

PROPHYLACTIC CRANIAL RADIATION

Certain cancers have a high incidence of developing brain (CNS) metastases even after their primary disease is controlled as the CNS, because of the blood brain barrier, can act as a sanctuary site for relapse. Among such patients it is possible to reduce their local CNS relapse rate and improve survival by treating the CNS by prophylactic cranial RT ± intrathecal chemotherapy. The total dose needed is low (18-24 Gy) and has minimal side effects e.g.: acute lymphoblastic leukemia/high grade lymphomas.

Palliative treatment

Objective of palliative irradiation include relief of pain, usually from metastases to bone, relief of headache nd neurological dysfunction from intracranial metastases, relief of obstruction, such as tumours involving ureter, oesophagus,bronchus, lymphatic and blood vessels; Promotion of healing of surface wounds by local tumour control. Hemostatic for cervical/bladder cancers.

MANAGEMENT: RADIOTHERAPY REACTIONS (Table 47.2)

The incidence of systemic symptoms from radiotherapy is variable. In broad terms, the larger the treatment field, the fraction size, and the total given dose, the greater will be the chance of the patient developing problems. The dose of radiation that can be delivered is limited by acute reactions and by late irreversible organ/tissue damage. Each organ has a known tolerance which should not be exceeded. But in order to achieve a given level of tumour control probability certain amount of normal tissue sequelae are unavoidable.

During a course of radiotherapy mild to moderate grade acute reactions occur frequently and can be usually conservatively managed and might require a short break in the treatment.

Where as Chronic reactions are usually the Dose limiting complications and severe grade reactions should be avoided using proper time dose fractionation regimens, accurate treatment planning and execution. Some of the important acute reactions following RT, their threshold doses and management are shown in Table 47.2.

Table 47.2 Complications and management of RT

ORGAN	TOXICITY	APPROX. DOSE THRESHOLD Gy	SPECIFIC MANAGEMENT POINTS
Skin	Erythema	10-12	No specific treatment required
Skin	Dry desquamation	40-50	Proflavine and emollients may produce symptomatic relief
Shin	Moist desquamation	45-55	Keep the affected area dry: gentian violet may be helpful in drying the affected area
Mucous	Mucositis	30-40	Topical benzydamine hydrochloride mouth rinse or spray; stop smoking; mucaine for esophageal mucositis; always exclude candidiasis
Hair	Alopecia	30-40	Warm patient prior to starting treatment; advise a wig fitting
lung	Pnuemonitis with cough, dyspnea	20	Consider systemic corticosteroids
GI tract	Nausea, vomiting	Any dose	Regular antiemetics may be required
GI tract	Diarrhea	30-40	Advise low-fiber diet when starting treatment; antidiarrheal preparations may be required for symptomatic relief
Bladder	Urinary frequency and dysuria	40-50	Exclude urinary tract infection and consider antimuscarinic drugs
Bone Marrow	Suppression especially of white blood cells and platelets during wide-field radiotherapy	10-20	Check full blood count regularly

ADVANCES IN RADIATION THERAPY

Current research in radiation oncology is of such significance that it promises a new standard of care for patients with cancer. Recent advances in radiation therapy include efforts to improve the effectiveness of radiation and to improve the quality of life of treated patients. Innovations in radiobiology, imaging technology, computer technology and treatment machine technology have resulted in marked changes in the way radiotherapy is practised at present. The newer methods aim at increasing the accuracy of treatment planning and dose delivery using the highly sophisticated features offered by the modern day equipment.

Some of these include

1. 3D-Conformal Radiotherapy (3-Dimensional)

2. IMRT (Intensity Modulated Radiation Therapy)

3. SRS / SRT (Stereotactic Radiosurgery and Radiotherapy)

4. Intravascular brachytherapy

1. **3D CONFORMAL RADIOTHERAPY** (Three-Dimensional Treatment Planning and Conformal Dose Delivery). In 3-D CRT, patient immobilization, image-guided treatment planning, and computer-controlled treatment delivery, can create a radiation dose distribution that conforms to the shape of the tumor volume. The tumor volume containing the cancer and areas of potential cancer is much more accurately outlined as are normal tissues to be avoided. The target radiation dose can be increased when necessary without increased toxicity to normal tissue. This is accomplished by using volumetric CT data in a 3-D treatment planning computer.

2. **IMRT:** IMRT is an advanced form of 3D-CRT. It is one of the technologically most advanced treatment methods available in external beam radiation therapy. IMRT allows very precise external beam radiotherapy treatments. Rather than having a single large radiation beam pass through the body, with IMRT the radiation is effectively broken up into thousands of tiny pencil-thin radiation beams of varying intensity with millimeter accuracy, these beams enter the body from many angles and intersect

on the cancer. This results in a high dosage to the tumor and a lower dose to the surrounding healthy tissues.

Intensity modulation radiotherapy can allow us to treat tumors to a higher dose, re-treat cancers that have previously been irradiated, and safely treat tumors that are located very close to delicate organs like the eye, spinal cord, or rectum. Simply put, this can translate into a higher cancer control rate and a lower rate of side effects.

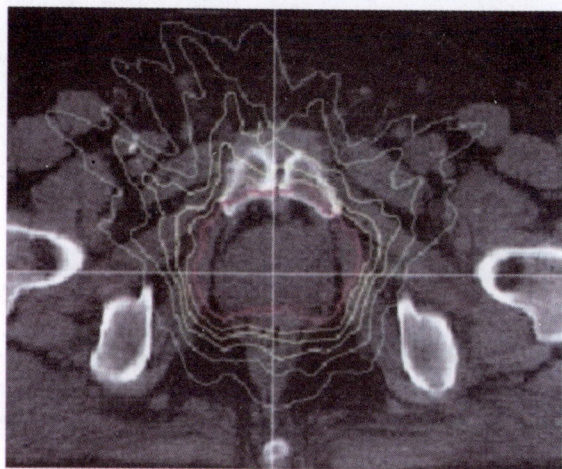

Fig. 47.4 IMRT is a wonderful treatment option for prostate cancer. IMRT can provide a high radiation dosage to the prostate gland while reducing the dosage which reaches the rectum and bladder

Key Box 47.6
CANCERS BEING TREATED WITH IMRT

- Prostate cancer, Pancreatic tumors, Lung cancer
- Metastatic brain tumors, Primary brain tumours (glio-blastomas, gliomas etc)
- Liver tumors (metastatses, hepatocellular carcinoma)
- Head & neck cancer (larynx, tongue, sinus, base of skull, mouth etc)
- Radiosurgery (single fraction) and stereotactic radiation therapy (Fractionated)

3. SRS/SRT (STEREOTACTIC RADIOSURGERY AND RADIO-THERAPY)

High-dose highly focused radiation therapy for small (SRS= Single fruction, SRT=Multiple Fractions) target lesions (<2 - 4cm) can be accomplished by either gamma knife(multiple, fixed, precisely aimed cobalt teletherapy beams) or stereotactic radiation therapy (multiple rotational arcs of photon beams from a linear accelerator). Both techniques are similar in their use of standard energy photon beams for treatment and rely on meticulous patient immobilisation to deliver treatment to a precisely localised target within a coordinate mapping system. These techniques have been widely used and well described for the treatment of intracranial neoplasms (meningiomas, acoustic neuromas, and metastatic tumors) and for the ablation of arteriovenous malformations and ocular melanomas. [Equipment used: 1. Gamma Knife (Multiple cl^{60}sources) or 2. X- knife (modified linear accelerator)]

4. INTRAVASCULAR BRACHYTHERAPY

ARTERIAL renarrowing after angioplasty,or restenosis, occurs in 30 to 40 percent of patients and results from neointimal pro-liferation and constrictive remodeling of

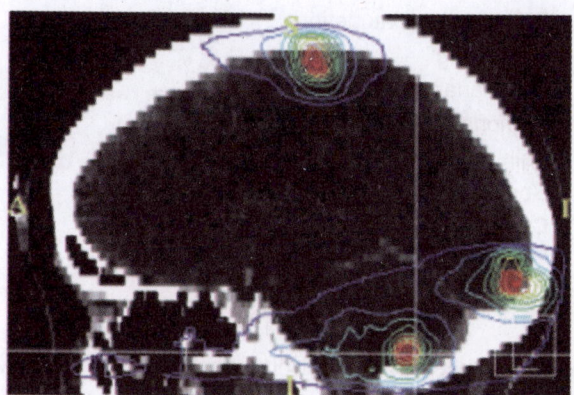

Fig. 47.5 Stereotactic radiosurgery brain (Metastatsis)

the angio-injured artery. Coronary stenting has led to a 30 to 50 percent decrease in the rate of restenosis,primarily by preventing the constrictive remodeling of the artery,but at the cost of an increase in neointimal proliferation. The system used for intraarterial beta-radiation therapy has yttrium-90 beta- ray-emitting source (half-life, 64 hours; maximal energy, 2.284 MeV), a centering balloon,and an automated delivery device. An 18-Gy dose not only prevents the renarrowing of the lumen typically observed after successful balloon angioplasty, but actually induces luminal enlargement.(N Engl J Med 2001; 344:243-9.).

Drawback (all techniques)

1. High cost of treatment (expensive equipment + Time and labor intensive)
2. Lack of long term data (survival / late morbidity)

Principles of Anaesthesiology

48

- Preoperative assessment
- General anaesthetic agents
- Muscle relaxants
- Endotracheal intubation
- Monitoring
- Local anaesthetics
- Regional anaesthesia
- Pain relief
- Complications
- Cardiopulmonary resuscitation

Surgery has been practised for ages. However, the advent of modern techniques of anaesthesia has allowed surgery to develop by leaps and bounds. A good understanding of the physiology and pharmacology, complemented by continuous and vigilant monitoring has made the practice of anaesthesia safer. Safe practice of anaesthesia comprises of the following steps: a good rapport with the patient, a thorough preoperative preparation and premedication, monitoring and perioperative care.

PREOPERATIVE ASSESSMENT AND PREMEDICATION

Every patient is anxious when he comes into the operating room. The causes of anxiety can be varied: fear of the disease condition, of surgery and its course, of the anaesthetic, whether it will work or whether he will wake up. A good rapport developed between the patient and the anaesthesiologist can build up his confidence and help allay many of these fears.

Anaesthesia can be associated with changes in the internal homeostasis. Normally these are well tolerated by the different systems. However, if the patient has a pre-existing preoperative derangement, his capacity to withstand wide fluctuations in haemodynamics may be limited. It is thus very important to know the preoperative condition of the patient.

History

A detailed history of the patient with symptoms pertaining to the various systems must be elicited.

CVS: H/O dyspnoea, angina, syncope, palpitations, leg swelling, h/o being diagnosed to have a cardiac problem, exercise tolerance

RS: Cough, fever, breathlessness, chest pain, recent onset upper respiratory tract infection

Central nervous system: Consciousness level, convulsions, orientation, ability to walk, speak, movement of all four limbs, bowel and bladder movements, any paraesthesia or altered sensation in the limbs.

Renal: Any h/o of decreased urine output, haematuria

Hepatic: Any h/o jaundice

Haematology: Any h/o easy bruising, increased blood loss with trivial injuries

Musculoskeletal: H/O weakness in the limbs

H/O allergy to any drug or other substances

H/O any previous surgeries/ anaesthetics, any problems during the previous experience

H/O smoking, alcohol, drug abuse

H/O hospitalisation in the past

H/O tuberculosis, asthma, diabetes, hypertension, epilepsy

H/O current medications, steroid intake in the last 6 months

Last menstrual period or possibility of pregnancy (in female patients)

Any relevant family history

Physical examination

A detailed physical examination is done and the relevant history specially borne in mind. The baseline blood pressure, heart rate, temperature and respiratory rate are recorded. Evidence of anaemia, cyanosis, raised jugular venous pulse and clubbing are looked for. The airway is carefully examined to detect any difficult airway (see the section on endotracheal intubation). The spine of the patient is then examined to rule out infection over the skin covering the spine, tenderness, stiffness or fractures of spine.

Various systems

A detailed examination of the various systems is then carried out and relevant findings noted.

Investigations

There is no place for routine investigations to be ordered before any surgery. However, the commonest investigations ordered and which can be considered basic are a haemoglobin estimation and routine urinalysis. An electrocardiogram, blood sugar estimation, blood urea and serum creatinine may be considered necessary in patients above 50 years or in diabetics. A white cell count is ordered if infection is present or suspected. A chest X-ray is requested if a major abdominal or thoracic surgery is planned, postoperative ventilation is expected or cardiorespiratory disease is suspected. Other advanced investigations such as stress test, echocardiogram, pulmonary function test or a blood gas analysis are requested if considered necessary. Blood grouping and cross matching are requested if the surgery is expected to be associated with major blood loss.

Informed consent

The patient is explained in detail about the anaesthetic planned, anticipated problems, if any, and alternatives, if requested in the patient's own language and a written and informed consent is obtained.

Preoperative instructions

The patient is kept 'Nil by mouth' for solids and milk for 6 - 8 hours, for clear fluids for up to 3 hours prior to surgery. This may be relaxed for neonates and infants where a four-hour fast for breast milk is sufficient. Formula feeds and milk from any other source are treated as solids. If the last food intake contained a considerable amount of fat, gastric emptying time may be delayed.

Premedication

1. **To allay anxiety:** Certain degree of anxiety is felt by most patients before surgery. A good rapport developed between the patient and the anaesthesiologist helps relieve this anxiety to some extent. More often, the patients are given benzodiazepines to allay anxiety. Tab Diazepam in the dose of 0.1 - 0.2 mg/kg body weight may be given one hour prior to surgery with a sip of water. Lorazepam 2 - 4 mg may be given orally as an alternative.

   Midazolam 0.5 mg/kg may be mixed with 5 ml of any sugary syrup and administered orally half an hour prior to the procedure in children enables easy separation from parents. Triclofos syrup, in a dose of 100 mg/kg body weight may be given as an alternative to midazolam for premedication in children.

2. **To relieve pain:** If the patient has any painful condition, a narcotic is usually added to reduce the pain during shifting from the ward. Morphine 0.1 - 0.2 mg/kg or pethidine 1 mg/kg may be given intramuscularly one hour prior to surgery.

3. **To dry secretions:** An anticholinergic such as atropine (0.01 mg/kg) or glycopyrrolate is usually added if a fibreoptic intubation is planned so that oral secretions do not hinder vision. Local anaesthetic agents produce better local anaesthesia of the upper airway when the mucosa is dry. The anticholinergic agent may be given intravenously just prior to surgery in ENT surgeries, plastic surgery of the lip and palate, if an LMA insertion is planned or induction with ketamine is contemplated.

4. **To help anaesthesia induction:** Premedication with a narcotic provides analgesia and helps induce anaesthesia more smoothly.

5. **To blunt baroreceptor reflexes:** A small dose of beta blockers, clonidine or captopril may be given to blunt baroreceptor reflexes.

6. **To reduce gastric volume and acidity:** Some patients are at risk of regurgitation of gastric contents and aspiration. They may be premedicated with a

prokinetic such as metoclopramide (10 mg) and a H_2 blocker such as ranitidine (150 mg orally). The consequences of aspiration of gastric contents depends on its quantity and acidity. Metoclopramide reduces residual gastric content by hastening gastric emptying and ranitidine reduces the acidity. Particulate matter causes major problems and hence the requirement to fast before induction of anaesthesia. Sometimes, a nonparticulate antacid such as sodium citrate may be given to neutralise existing gastric acid.

ASA Physical Status Classification

The patient's preoperative physical status can be classified into five different categories. The American Society of Anaesthesiologists' classification of Physical Status is as follows:

ASA I   -   Healthy patient, no medical problems

ASA II   -   Mild systemic disease

ASA III   -   Severe systemic disease, but not incapacitating

ASA IV   -   Severe systemic disease that is a constant threat to life

ASA V   -   Moribund, not expected to live 24 hours irrespective of operation

A suffix E is added if the surgery is of emergent nature. A sixth category called ASA VI is given to the patient who is brain dead but is being operated on as an organ donor.

The risks associated with anaesthesia in a patient with concurrent diseases must be explained to the patient in detail. Algorithms by different organisations are available to help decision-making in individual patients: e.g., American Heart Association recommendations for evaluation of ischaemic heart disease in a patient posted for noncardiac surgery. The goal of preoperative assessment and preparation is thus to ensure that the patient is in the best possible condition prior to surgery and anaesthesia.

INDUCTION OF ANAESTHESIA

The choice of anaesthesia depends on several factors: the site of operation, duration of operation, general condition of the patient, expertise of the anaesthesiologist and preference of the patient. Anaesthesia can be classified into two main categories: general anaesthesia and regional anaesthesia. During general anaesthesia, the patient is unconscious and there is a generalised and reversible depression of the central nervous system. Regional anaesthesia involves injection of local anaesthetic agents in close proximity to the nerves or nerve bundles supplying the site of operation. When regional anaesthesia is induced by injecting the local anaesthetic agents around the spinal cord, it is called central neuraxis block.

GENERAL ANAESTHETIC AGENTS

General anaesthetic agents induce unconsciousness, amnesia, analgesia and to some extent muscle relaxation. They are mainly of two types: inhalational anaesthetic agents or intravenous anaesthetic agents.

INHALATIONAL ANAESTHETIC AGENTS

- **Volatile anaesthetics:** The volatile anaesthetic agents need a vaporiser to calibrate and deliver the vapour accurately in measured doses, e.g., halothane

- **Nonvolatile anaesthetics:** e.g., nitrous oxide

Classification

I   Agents of mainly historical interest

1. Ethyl chloride

2. Chloroform

3. Trichloroethylene

4. Cyclopropane

5. Methoxyflurane

II. Agents in occasional use

1. Diethyl ether

2. Enflurane

III. Agents in clinical use

1. Halothane

2. Isoflurane

3. Sevoflurane

4. Desflurane

5. Nitrous oxide

IV Agent undergoing research - Xenon

HALOTHANE

It is a colourless liquid with a pleasant smell. It is non-inflammable.

Clinical effects

Central nervous system (CNS)

- Halothane produces rapid and progressive depression of the CNS. The recovery is also fast.

Respiratory system (RS)

- Halothane is non-irritant and **pleasant to breathe**. There is a rapid loss of pharyngeal and laryngeal reflexes. It is a **bronchodilator**. It also causes a dose-dependent decrease in minute ventilation.

Cardiovascular system (CVS)

- Halothane is a **potent depressant** of myocardial contractility and depresses cardiac output. The arterial pressures and heart rate decrease. **Arrhythmias** are common during halothane anaesthesia.

Gastro-intestinal tract (GIT)

- Gastrointestinal motility is inhibited. Postoperative nausea and vomiting are seldom severe.

Uterus

- Halothane relaxes uterine muscle.

Skeletal muscle

- Halothane causes skeletal muscle relaxation. Postoperatively, shivering is common.

Halothane - associated hepatic dysfunction

On extremely **rare** occasions (widely quoted incidence 1:35,000), the administration of halothane may be associated with the production of hepatic dysfunction. This entity, known as halothane hepatitis is largely a diagnosis of exclusion. Causative theories include the toxic metabolites, particularly fluoride ions. The risk of halothane hepatitis is enhanced with obesity, hypoxia, repeated administration as well as when the patient is on enzyme-inducing drugs such as phenobarbitone.

ISOFLURANE

It is a halogenated ether. It has a **pungent** smell and hence is not popular for inhalation induction. Isoflurane causes less cardiac depression and less cerebral vasodilatation than halothane. Hence it is **preferred** over halothane for use **in patients with cardiac disease and patients with raised intracranial pressure.**

SEVOFLURANE

It is a newer general anaesthetic agent and has a **sweet smell**. Induction and recovery with sevoflurane are **faster** than with halothane. It produces minimal myocardial depression. It is **popular for induction in children**. It is also a useful agent for induction of anaaesthesia in patients with difficult airways.

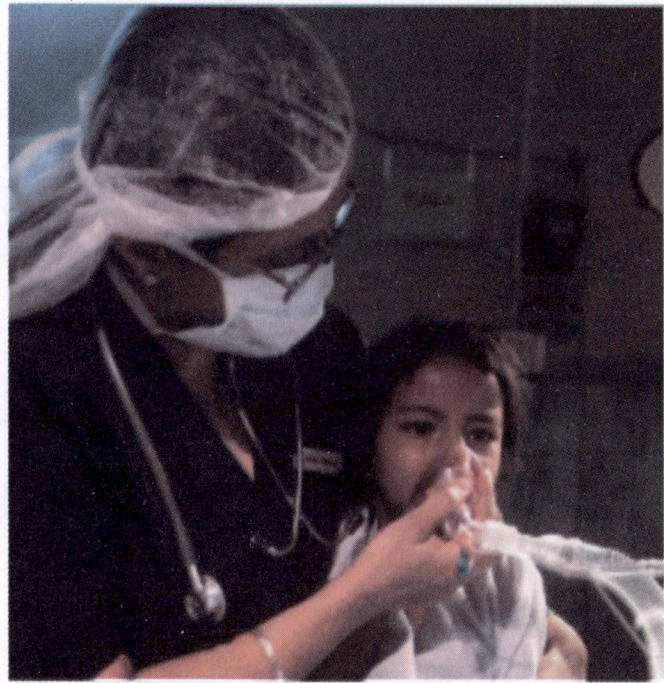

Fig. 48.1 Inhalation induction of anaesthesia in a child using sevoflurane

DESFLURANE

It is another new volatile anaesthetic agent. It also maintains cardiovascular stability. Induction and recovery are very fast. However, it is irritant to the respiratory tract and hence is not suitable for inhalational induction. It is highly volatile and is the only agent that is used with a specially constructed heated vaporiser.

NITROUS OXIDE

It is an anaesthetic gas which is compressed and supplied as a liquid in cylinders. It is sweet smelling and non-irritant. It is a good analgesic but a weak anaesthetic. Nitrous oxide alone is insufficient to produce an adequate depth of anaesthesia but enhances induction of anaesthesia with the volatile anaesthetics and reduces their requirement. It does not produce significant depression of the cardiovascular system.

Side-effects

1. It can diffuse into closed gas spaces such as pneumothorax, in the intestines, sinuses and middle ear. The volume of a cavity can increase 3 to 4 times within 30 minutes. This is easily reversed by administration of 100% oxygen.

2. Its use is associated with increased incidence of postoperative nausea and vomiting.

3. In prolonged administrations, it can affect Vitamin B12 synthesis causing megaloblastic anaemia.

4. **Teratogenicity:** This has been observed in pregnant rats exposed to nitrous oxide for prolonged periods but not proved in human beings. Nitrous oxide is best avoided in early pregnancy.

INTRAVENOUS ANAESTHETIC AGENTS

Intravenously administered anaesthetic agents are more popular for induction of anaesthesia because it is more rapid and smooth than that associated with inhalational agents. They can also be used for maintenance of anaesthesia, sedation during regional anaesthesia, sedation in the ICU and treatment of status epilepticus.

Classification

Rapidly-acting (within one arm-brain circulation time)	*Slower-acting (more than one arm-brain circulation time)*
1. Barbiturates	1. Ketamine
2. Etomidate	2. Benzodiazepines
3. Propofol	3. Large dose opioids

THIOPENTONE SODIUM

It is an ultra-short acting barbiturate, available as yellowish powder. It is used as a 2.5% solution (25 mg/ml). It is used in a dose of 4 - 5 mg/kg intravenously.

Clinical effects

CNS:

• Generalised depression of the CNS is observed within 15 to 20 seconds of intravenous injection of thiopentone. It is a potent **anticonvulsant**.

• It is not an analgesic. To the contrary, it increases pain sensation (**antianalgesic**). Consciousness is regained within 5 to 10 minutes.

CVS

• It produces myocardial depression, **peripheral vasodilatation and hypotension** especially when large doses are administered rapidly. Profound hypotension may occur, especially in a patient with hypovolaemia or cardiac disease. It may induce tachycardia.

RS

• It reduces respiratory drive. A short period of apnoea is common.

Skeletal muscle

• There is poor muscle relaxation with thiopentone.

Uterus and placenta

• There is little effect on resting uterine tone. It crosses placenta rapidly, although foetal blood concentration is far less than that observed in the mother.

Eye

• It reduces intraocular pressure. The corneal, eyelash and eyelid reflexes are abolished.

Side effects

1. Hypotension

2. Respiratory depression

3. Irritant to veins and can cause thrombophlebitis. If it extravasates, can cause tissue necrosis.

4. Intra-arterial injection: Usually inadvertent, can cause severe arterial spasm and pain. This may be treated with vasodilators and heparin.

5. Allergic reactions: Very rare.

Contraindications

Absolute	*Relative*
1. Airway obstruction	1. Hypovolaemia
2. Acute intermittent porphyria	2. Asthma
3. Previous hypersensitivity reaction	

PROPOFOL

This drug became commercially available in 1986. It is comparable to thiopentone but is five times more expensive. It is highly lipid soluble and is formulated in a white, aqueous emulsion containing soy bean oil and egg phosphatide. It is used in a dose of 2 to 2.5 mg/kg intravenously. The dose should be reduced in the elderly and in haemodynamically unstable patients.

CNS

- Propofol depresses the central nervous system within 20 to 40 seconds of injection. Loss of verbal contact is used as an end-point. **Recovery is rapid** and there is a minimal 'hang-over' effect even in the immediate post-anaesthetic period.

CVS

- The arterial pressure decreases more than with thiopentone. This is due to peripheral vasodilatation. The degree of hypotension can be reduced by slowing the rate of administration. Heart rate increases slightly.

RS

- After induction, apnoea occurs commonly and for a longer duration than with thiopentone. It causes ventilatory depression, particularly with opioids. It has no effect on bronchial muscle tone.

GIT, uterus and placenta:

- Propofol has no effect on GI motility and minimal and transient decrease in hepatorenal function.

Adverse effects

1. Cardiovascular depression
2. Respiratory depression
3. Pain on injection
4. Allergic reactions

ETOMIDATE

Etomidate is a rapidly acting intravenous anaesthetic agent with a short duration of action of 2-3 minutes. **It is very cardiostable**. It depresses the synthesis of cortisol by the adrenal gland and impairs the response to ACTH. Hence, continuous infusions are not advisable. It is used in a dose of 0.2 - 0.3 mg/kg IV.

Adverse effects

1. Suppression of synthesis of cortisol
2. Excitatory phenomena: Involuntary movements, cough, hiccoughs during induction.
3. Pain on injection
4. Nausea and vomiting
5. Venous thrombosis

KETAMINE HYDROCHLORIDE

Ketamine differs from other intravenous anaesthetic agents in many respects and produces dissociative anaesthesia, rather than generalised depression of the central nervous system. It is used in a dose of 2 mg/kg IV or 5 - 10 mg/kg IM.

CNS

- It induces anaesthesia within 30 - 60 seconds of intravenous injection and lasts for 10 - 20 minutes. It is effective within 3 -4 minutes of intramuscular injection and lasts for 15 - 25 minutes. It is a **potent analgesic**. Vivid and unpleasant hallucinations are known with ketamine and can be prevented by prior injections of benzodiazepines. It increases cerebral blood flow and intracranial pressure.

CVS

- The heart rate, blood pressure and cardiac output increase.

RS

- Respiration is usually well-maintained with ketamine although transient apnoea may occur occasionally. Ketamine is a good **bronchodilator**.

Skeletal muscle

- There is increased muscle tone and spontaneous movements may occur.

GIT

- Increased salivation can occur and can be prevented using anticholinergic agents.

Eye

- Intraocular pressure increases.

Uterus and placenta

- It readily crosses the placental barrier and hence should be given in lower doses.

Adverse effects

1. Emergence delirium
2. Hypertension and tachycardia
3. Increased intracranial pressure
4. Increased secretions

Uses

1. Patients in severe hypotension, shock
2. Paediatric anaesthesia

3. Analgesia and sedation

4. Bronchial asthma

5. **Difficult locations:** Accident sites, war casualties

ENDOTRACHEAL INTUBATION

Endotracheal intubation is one of the most basic skills acquired by an Anaesthesiologist. Endotracheal intubation involves introduction of a tube into the trachea for purposes of maintaining the patency and protecting the airway as well as to ensure adequate oxygenation and ventilation. It is also the most definitive way of maintaining the airway in patients who require muscle paralysis and intermittent positive pressure ventilation. Whenever general anaesthesia is induced and needs to be maintained for long periods, endotracheal intubation is done.

Indications

1. To administer general anaesthesia for long (> 1- 2 hours) periods

2. To maintain patency of the airway in unconscious patients

3. To protect the lungs from aspiration of regurgitated gastric contents

4. To ensure delivery of adequate tidal volumes to the lungs

5. To clear excessive and retained secretions from the lungs

Contraindications

When the upper airway integrity is lost as in extensive maxillofacial injury with bilateral fractures of mandible and maxillae, injuries to the neck with laryngeal rupture, large tumours of the upper airway, endotracheal intubation may be extremely difficult and even dangerous. In such situations, a tracheostomy may be a better choice.

EQUIPMENT

Laryngoscopes (Fig. 48.2) - These consist of a handle and a blade. The handle contains batteries. The blade has a flange to push the tongue towards the left side. This ensures more room for visualisation of the glottis. A bulb nearer the tip of the blade lights up when the handle and blade are at right angles to each other and electrical contact is made.

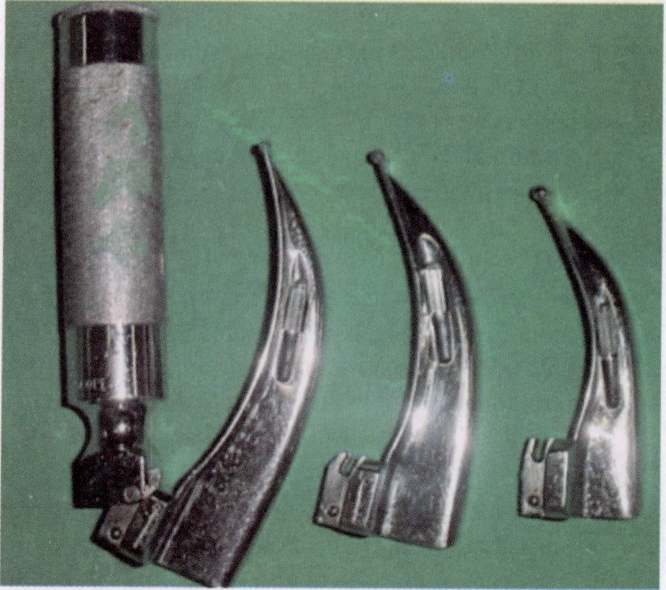

Fig. 48.2 Macintosh laryngoscope. Note the curved blade. Sizes 1, 2 and 3 are displayed

The Macintosh type blade is curved and is popular for use in adults. The Miller blade is straight and is used in children and in adults with difficult airway. Laryngoscopes with short handles are available for use in difficult airways, e.g., pregnant women, obese patients. A variety of laryngoscopes are available for use in special situations.

Endotracheal tubes (Fig. 48.3)

It is a 'C' - shaped tube and is commonly made of polyvinyl chloride (PVC). The machine end has a standard 15 mm diameter connector. The patient end is **bevelled** and has an opening on the side just proximal to the tip called the **Murphy's eye**. This ensures patency of the tube even if the bevelled tip is against the tracheal wall.

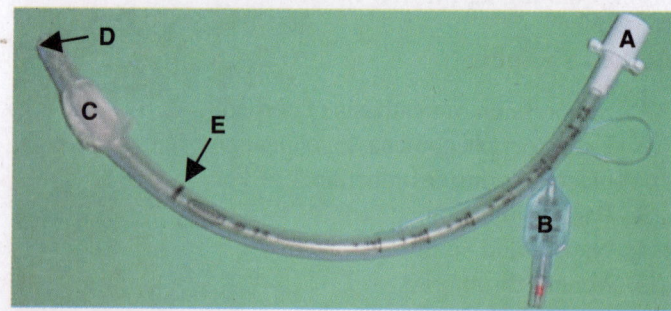

Fig. 48.3 Endotracheal tube. A) Standard 15 mm connector B) Pilot balloon C) Inflatable cuff D) Bevelled patient-end E) Black line to indicate optimum positioning of the tube. This line is usually placed just above the glottis.

Endotracheal tubes are available in different sizes. Their size is indicated as the internal diameter in mm. An 8 or 8.5 mm internal diameter tube is used for adult men and a 7 or 7.5 mm ID for adult women. For children, an approximate size is given by the following formula:

Age/3 + 3.5 mm for children below 6 years and

Age/4 + 4.5 mm for children above 6 years.

However, the correct size will depend on the growth of the child. The distance of several points on the tube from the patient end is marked in cm along the tube. The tube is fixed at 22 or 23 cm in adult men and at 20 or 21 cm in adult women. In children, the following formula is used: Age/2 + 12 cm.

ASSESSMENT OF AIRWAY

Whenever a person becomes unconscious, the tongue and epiglottis fall back on to the pharynx and obstruct the airway. A general anaesthetic involves making people unconscious and it is the Anaesthesiologist's duty to ensure that the patient's airway is maintained. Hence, assessment of the airway becomes important before a patient is made unconscious.

The assessment is done as follows

'The 1-2-3 test'

When a person opens his mouth, one should be able to insinuate one finger in the temporomandibular joint. There should be at least two finger breadths' distance between his incisors. There should be at least three finger breadths' distance between the chin and the thyroid cartilage (thyromental distance) of the patient.

Mallampati test (Fig. 48.4)

The patient is made to sit upright, open his mouth wide and protrude his tongue. The structures visualised are classified as follows:

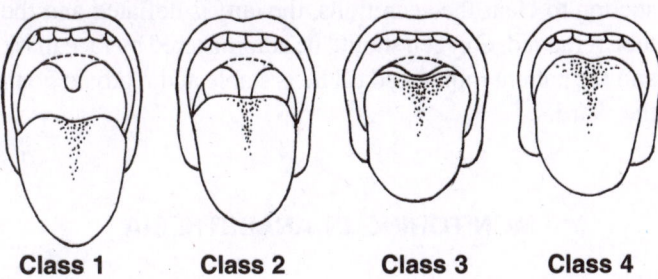

Class 1   **Class 2**   **Class 3**   **Class 4**

Fig. 48.4 Mallampati classification of the airway

These classes are roughly correlate with the following grades of laryngoscopic views (Fig. 48.5). The anaesthesiologist is alerted by Mallampati Class III and IV and needs to anticipate difficult intubation.

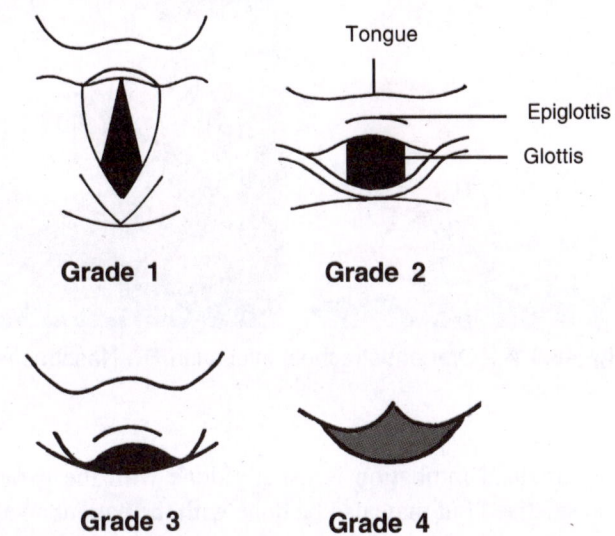

Figure 48.5 Modified Cormack and Lehane grading of laryngoscopic view

Neck movements

A full range of neck movements including flexion and extension makes endotracheal intubation easier.

Technique

Position - A pillow (7 - 10 cm) under the patient's head enables mild flexion at the cervical spine. The head is then extended at the atlanto - occipital joint. This is called the intubating position or "sniffing position".

Procedure

Route - Endotracheal intubation can be done either orally or nasally (Fig. 48.6 A & B). It can be done either under direct vision or indirectly using a fibreoptic scope. It may need to be done blindly when visualisation of the glottis by direct means is not possible and a fibreoptic scope is not available. In such cases, if the regular antegrade technique (mouth or nose to larynx) or a retrograde intubation (larynx to mouth) may be tried. In the retrograde technique, a guide wire is passed from the cricothyroid membrane upward into the mouth or nose and the endotracheal tube is guided over it into the larynx.

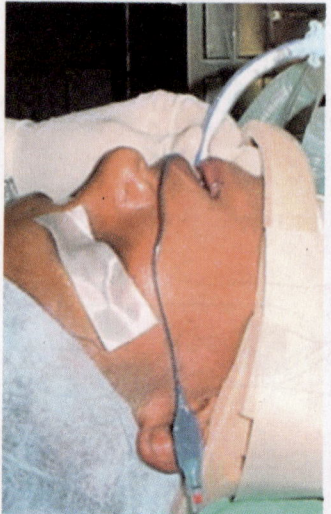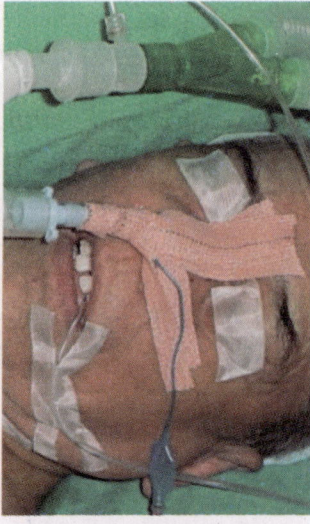

Fig. 48.6 A - Oral endotracheal intubation **B** - Nasotracheal intubation

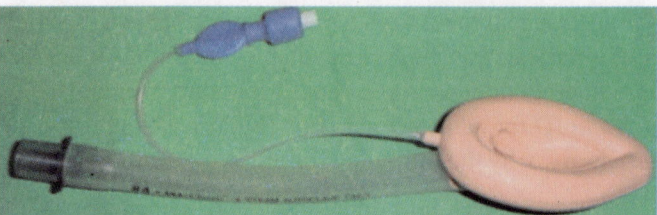

Fig. 48.7C Laryngeal mask airway

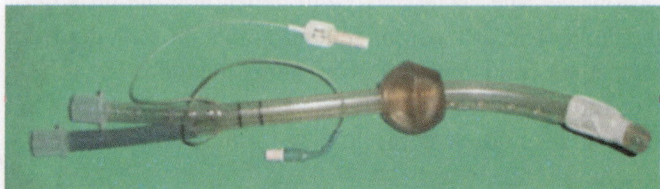

Fig. 48.7D Combitube®

Endotracheal intubation is usually done with the patient anaesthetised but may also be done with the patient awake after administering local anaesthesia to the upper airway when a difficult intubation is anticipated. Many airway adjuncts are available for use when a difficult airway is encountered, especially when it is unanticipated. These include oropharyngeal airway, nasopharyngeal airway, laryngeal mask airway and Combitube® (Fig. 48.7).

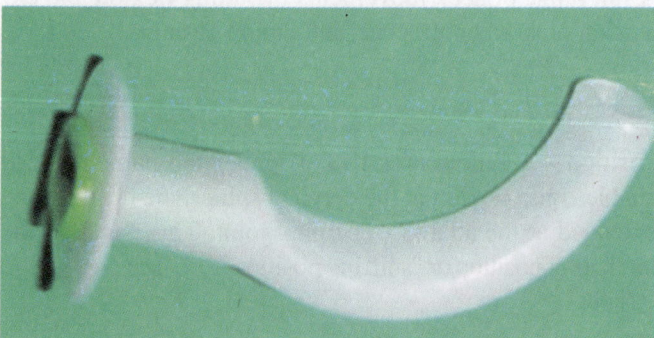

Fig. 48.7A Oropharyngeal airway

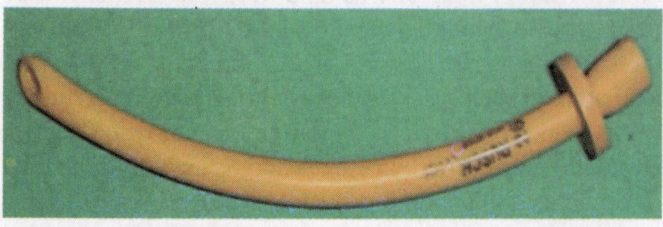

Fig. 48.7B Nasopharyngeal airway

Complications

The complications of endotracheal intubation may be classified as follows:

Immediate

- Trauma to the teeth, lips, tongue, pharynx or larynx
- Haemodynamic changes - tachycardia, hypertension, myocardial ischaemia
- Misplaced tube - accidental extubation, oesophageal intubation

Delayed

- Laryngeal granuloma, laryngeal or subglottic stenosis

Endotracheal extubation

Endotracheal extubation is as important as intubation. The patient's level of consciousness and ability to maintain his airway, presence of a good cough and haemodynamic stability are necessary before extubation is considered. Equipment for reintubation and personnel skilled in intubation should be readily available. After a good oropharyngeal suction to clear the secretions, the cuff is deflated and the tube removed. Oxygen should be administered by face mask and the patient monitored till he is stable and ready to go to the ward.

MONITORING IN ANAESTHESIA

The administration of anaesthesia is associated with changes in the internal homeostasis of the patient, especially the cardiac and respiratory systems. Constant monitoring of the various body systems is necessary to ensure the well-being of the patient and prompt recovery from anaesthesia at the end of surgery. Identification and prompt treatment of any untoward changes should alleviate complications due to anaesthesia.

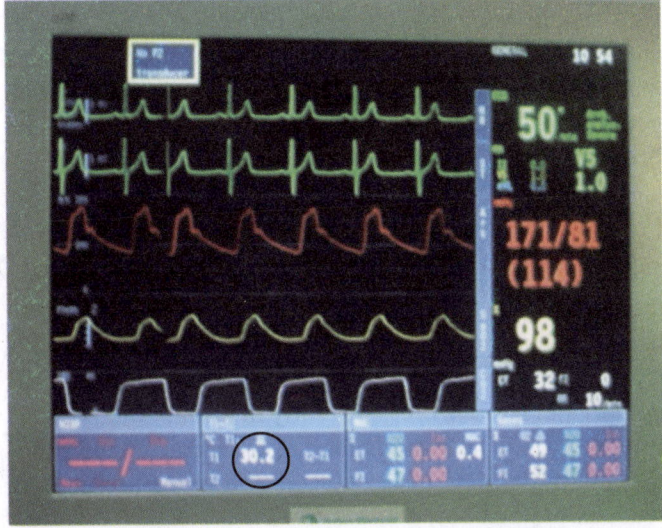

Fig 48.8 Monitoring of a patient under anaesthesia. The monitor displays the electrocardiogram (Lead II and V5), heart rate, invasive arterial blood pressure, oxygen saturation, temperature, capnogram and anaesthetic gas analysis

Monitors used in anaesthesia may be classified into noninvasive and invasive monitoring. The extent of monitoring depends on the patient's preoperative condition, the extent of surgery, the type of anaesthesia and the facilities available. Most patients are noninvasively monitored. Invasive monitoring becomes necessary when considerable haemodynamic instability exists or is expected to occur perioperatively. Constant monitoring of the electrocardiogram, noninvasive blood pressure and pulse oximetry are considered mandatory monitoring for a patient undergoing any type of anaesthesia.

CARDIOVASCULAR MONITORING

Basic noninvasive monitoring includes clinical observation of the patient and monitoring of the patient's haemodynamic parameters. Adequate cardiac output is associated with good urine output, warm and well-perfused peripheries and good capillary refill. Heart rate may be monitored with a finger on the pulse. Blood pressure may be measured using a standard sphygmo-manometer. More conveniently and accurately, heart rate and rhythm are continuously monitored using the electrocardiogram and blood pressure using automated non-invasive blood pressure monitoring systems.

Baseline readings of the heart rate, blood pressure and oxygen saturation prior to induction of anaesthesia are recorded. After induction, the patients are continuously monitored and a record of these is made at least every five minutes thereafter. When a patient undergoes an extensive or a long procedure associated with large fluid shifts, his urinary bladder is catheterised so that hourly urine output can be measured. A normal person produces at least 0.5 - 1 ml/kg/hour of urine output.

ELECTROCARDIOGRAM (ECG)

The objectives of electrocardiographic monitoring (Fig. 48.9) are to monitor heart rate and rhythm and to look for myocardial ischaemia. Lead II is monitored commonly as it is best for identifying arrhythmias. V5 detects left ventricular ischaemia. Hence, both Lead II and V5 should be monitored continuously for patients with suspected ischaemic heart disease. Subtle changes in the electrocardiogram on the monitor must be confirmed by a 12 lead - ECG.

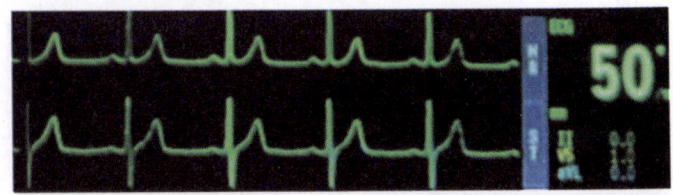

Fig. 48.9 ECG monitoring Lead II and V5

NONINVASIVE BLOOD PRESSURE (NIBP)

Most automated devices use an oscillotonometric technique and as a result the most accurate pressure is the mean arterial pressure. They tend to overestimate at low pressures and underestimate at high pressures. They may also give erroneous results in patients with atrial fibrillation or with other arrhythmias. The cuff width (Figure 48.10) is the most important determinant of the accuracy of the pressure reading. The cuff width should be 40% of the mid-circumference of limb (the length should be twice the width). Cuffs which are too narrow tend to overestimate BP while those which are too wide tend to underestimate BP.

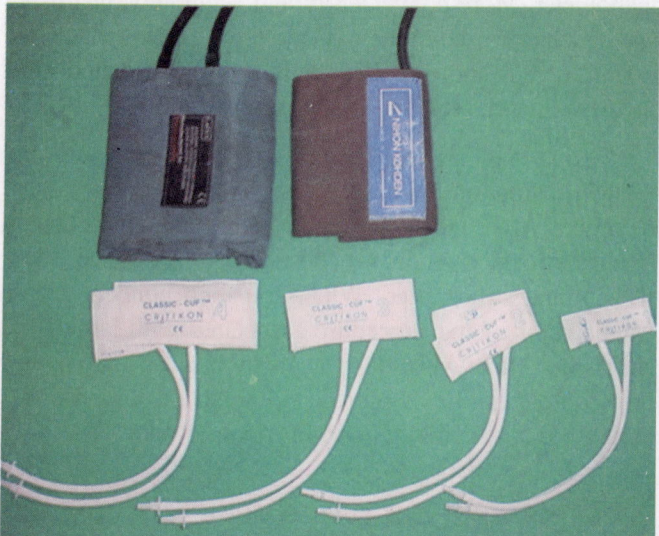

Fig. 48.10 Blood pressure cuffs of various sizes

DIRECT ARTERIAL PRESSURE MONITORING

Direct arterial pressure monitoring is preferred whenever haemodynamic instability exists or is expected to occur perioperatively. In such situations, invasive measurement enables beat to beat monitoring of arterial pressure.

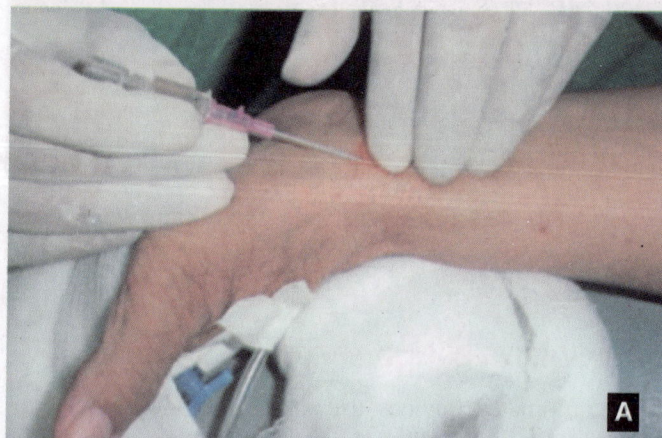

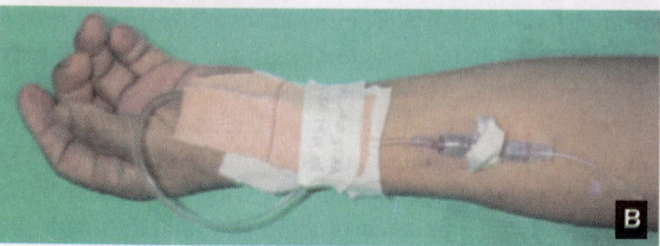

Fig. 48.11 Radial arterial cannulation a) Cannulation b) Catheter securely taped in place and labelled (Arterial line - Do Not Inject!)

Sites

Radial arterial cannulation (Fig. 48.11) is most often performed. When these are inaccessible or they have already been used, dorsalis pedis arteries also can be used. If the peripheral circulation is sluggish, blood pressures are too low and the radial arteries are not felt, cannulation of brachial or femoral arteries may be considered. However, these sites should be changed to more peripherally placed catheters as early as possible to avoid complications such as distal ischaemia. The distal circulation must be assessed periodically by capillary refill time, colour of the digit, nail bed, pulse oximetry etc.

What information is obtained?

The invasive arterial pressure monitoring provides not only the systolic, diastolic and mean blood pressures but also the heart rate and rhythm (Fig. 48.12). In mechanically ventilated patients, positive intrathoracic pressure increases LV output (and systolic pressure) early in inspiration, which is followed a few heart beats later by a decrease. This variation in arterial pressure is exaggerated in the presence of reduced preload.

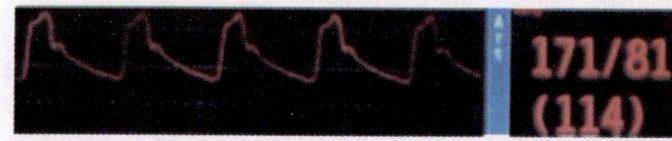

Fig. 48.12: Arterial pressure waveform. This helps beat to beat monitoring of arterial blood pressure, rate and rhythm. The slope of the upstroke indicates myocardial contractility. Changes in the systolic blood pressure with respiration may be correlated with the left ventricular end-diastolic blood volume (preload)

What size cannula?

A 20 gauge cannula may be used for the radial, brachial or dorsalis pedis arteries but a long 18 or 16 gauge non-kinking cannula is preferred for femoral lines.

Complications

- Ischaemia distal to cannula- Normally collateral circulation is adequate to maintain perfusion distal to the arterial cannulation site. Occasionally major sequelae may occur and are associated with low cardiac output, shock, sepsis, prolonged cannulation and vasculitis

- Exsanguination- In case of accidental disconnection,

flows through 18 FG cannula can cause blood loss of up to 500 ml/min

- Spurious result - wrong position or calibration of transducers
- Infection
- Intra-arterial injection of drugs

CENTRAL VENOUS PRESSURE MONITORING

Indications

1. To guide fluid therapy as in hypovolaemia, low cardiac output states, renal failure
2. For total parenteral nutrition
3. To infuse potent drugs such as antibiotics, vasopressors, chemotherapeutic agents
4. When peripheral venous access is not available
5. To enable pulmonary artery catheterisation and cardiac output measurement

Sites of insertion

CVP can be monitored through catheters placed in the internal jugular or subclavian veins (Figure 48.13). Peripherally placed central venous catheters may also be useful in measuring CVP if the tip of the catheter is intrathoracic. Femoral vein catheters may also be used provided the tip of the catheter is close to the diaphragm in the inferior vena cava.

CVP as a guide to fluid replacement

CVP is used as a guide to right ventricular filling (7-3 rule). A baseline record of CVP is made and then fluid is infused (50 - 200 ml of colloid over 10 minutes) if hypovolaemia is suspected. A lower volume is selected if the baseline CVP is more than 8 - 10 mmHg. If the CVP rises by < 3 mmHg from baseline in response to the fluid challenge, more fluid loading may be required. If the CVP rises by > 7 mmHg, fluid loading is then probably maximal. However, should the CVP return to within 3 mmHg of its original value within 10 minutes after an initial rise by more than 7 mmHg, the risk of pulmonary oedema is only moderate; nevertheless no further filling is required.

Limitations

Right ventricular pressures are measured as an alternative to measurement of right ventricular volumes. This would be acceptable only if the ventricular compliance is normal. However, an isolated CVP reading is of limited value without knowledge of ventricular compliance. Compliance varies from patient to patient, and with time in the same patient. Thus, dynamic changes in CVP are more useful than absolute values.

PA catheter

These are long catheters placed through the central veins, right atrium and right ventricle to end in the pulmonary artery. The tip of this catheter ends in a small distal branch of the pulmonary artery. When the balloon on its distal tip is inflated, the pressure distal to the catheter reflects the left

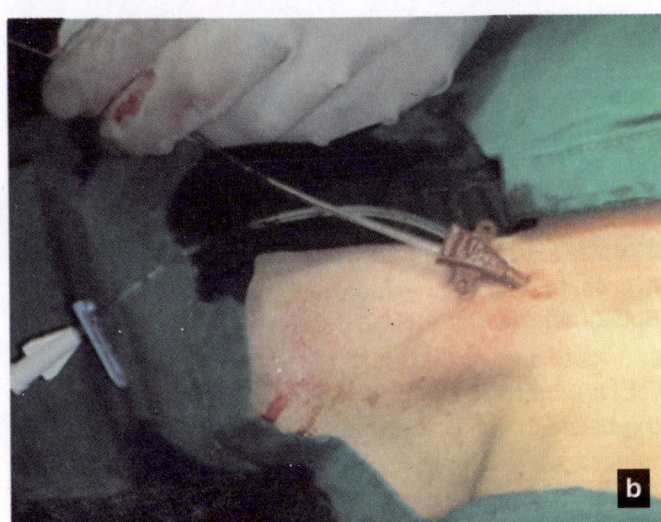

Fig. 48.13 Subclavian venous cannulation a) Locating subclavian vein b) A double lumen catheter in place

atrial pressure which may reflect left ventricular end-diastolic pressure and hence the preload more truthfully. However, the insertion of the pulmonary artery catheter is also associated with a number of complications and its utility is a subject of debate.

Complications of central venous catheterisation

Associated with insertion

- Bleeding
- Carotid artery puncture
- Pneumothorax
- Haemothorax
- Air embolism
- Arrhythmias

Associated with use

- Sepsis
- Disconnection, leading to bleeding or air embolism
- Pleural or pericardial effusion due to misplaced catheter

RESPIRATORY MONITORING

Pulse oximetry

The pulse oximeter displays the oxygen saturation of haemoglobin continuously, noninvasively and in real-time (Fig. 48.14 and 48.16). Its use has revolutionised the way patients are monitored. The pulse oximeter works on the principle of Beer-Lambert's law. This law states that the amount of light absorbed by a solution is directly proportional to the amount of solute in it.

The pulse oximeter consists of two light emitting diodes

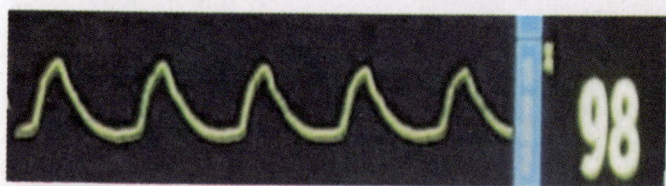

Fig. 48.14 The plethysmograph and oxygen saturation (SpO2) obtained by a pulse oximeter

(LEDs), emitting light at around 660 nm and 940 nm. Oxyhaemoglobin absorbs more of light at 940 nm whereas reduced haemoglobin absorbs more light at 660 nm. The amount of oxyhaemoglobin in tissues increases with each pulse wave. The differential absorption of light by oxyhaemoglobin and reduced haemoglobin and the varying concentration of these two substances with arterial pulsa-

tions are utilised in the construction of the pulse oximeter.

The pulse oximeter has one LED on, then the other on, then both off. This happens several times a second. The ratio of absorption of these two wavelengths of light by oxyhaemoglobin and reduced haemoglobin is related to the oxygen saturation using a nomogram. The normal oxygen saturation of a person breathing room air is around 98 - 100%. If the saturation dips below 90% or lower, hypoxia is said to exist. Hence, the inspired oxygen concentration is adjusted to maintain a SpO_2 of > 93 - 95% during anaesthesia.

Sites of monitoring

Fingers, toes, ear lobes; soles and palms may be used in neonates and infants.

Limitations

- **Movement:** The pulse oximeter may not be reliable when there is movement of the part monitored.
- **Electrical interference** may occur with concurrent use of diathermy.
- **Vasoconstriction:** It may fail to pick up a pulse with profound vasoconstriction as in hypothermia or low cardiac output.
- **COHb:** It may over-read in patients with significant carboxyhaemoglobin concentrations.
- **Meth-Hb:** It may under-read in patients with significant methaemoglobin concentrations.

CAPNOGRAPHY

The amount of carbon dioxide in the exhaled gases can be measured using a capnograph. The capnograph (Fig. 48.16) passes infrared light through the gases to be analysed. The carbon dioxide in the gases absorbs the infrared light in proportion to its concentration. This absorption is measured and the carbon dioxide concentration is displayed according to a nomogram. When the carbon dioxide concentration is displayed against time, a capnogram is obtained.

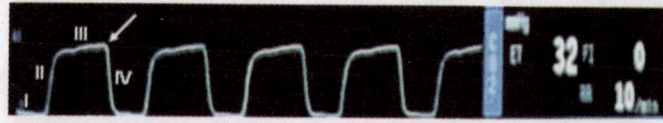

Fig. 48.15 The normal capnogram: Phase I - Dead space gases, Phase II - Mixed dead space and alveolar gases, Phase III - Alveolar gases, Phase IV - Inspiration. The arrow is pointing towards the end-tidal carbon dioxide concentration (ETCO2)

The normal capnogram has four different phases as illustrated in Figure 48.15. Phases I, II and III represent expiration and Phase IV, inspiration. The carbon dioxide concentration at the end of expiration is called end-tidal carbon dioxide concentration [normal range: 35 - 40 mmHg] which represents the alveolar carbon dioxide concentration. Normally, the arterial carbon dioxide concentration is nearly equal to this end-tidal carbon dioxide concentration.

Information obtained

Carbon dioxide is excreted from the body only through one organ in the body, i.e., lungs. A normal capnogram obtained from the exhaled gases helps identify the correct position of the endotracheal tube.

- If the capnograph registers zero levels of carbon dioxide, the endotracheal tube is malpositioned as in oesophageal intubation or accidental extubation. Artificial ventilator disconnection also results in zero $ETCO_2$ levels.
- The end-tidal carbon dioxide levels may also reduce to near zero levels if no carbon dioxide returns to the lungs from the tissues as in profound hypotension and an impending cardiac arrest may be suspected.
- However, the $ETCO_2$ will register zero if the patient is in cardiac arrest since there is no circulation and no carbon dioxide is brought to the lungs. In such situations, a capnograph cannot be used to identify the cor-

rect position of endotracheal tube. However, a capnograph is extremely useful in assessing the effectiveness of CPR. If the $ETCO_2$ is more than 15 mmHg during CPR, the chances of successful resuscitation are higher.

Limitations

When there is an increase in dead space ventilation (that part of ventilation that does not take part in gas exchange), the arterial to end-tidal carbon dioxide concentration gradient increases (Normal: 0 - 5 mmHg).

MUSCLE RELAXANTS

Physiology of neuromuscular transmission

When a nerve impulse arrives at the neuromuscular junction through the motor neuron, acetylcholine (ACh) molecules are liberated from the nerve endings into the junctional cleft. Acetylcholine molecules act as neurotransmitters by interacting with the ACh receptors on the postjunctional muscle membrane at the motor end plates. This induces the opening of the ionic channel of the receptor to allow ionic (sodium, calcium) flux into the muscle. The sudden influx of sodium results in depolarisation and muscle contraction.

Acetylcholine receptor

The acetylcholine receptor is flower-shaped with five petal-like structures. These five subunits are named $\alpha(2)$, $\beta(1)$, $\gamma(1)$ and $\delta(1)$. Each alpha subunit must be occupied by an acetylcholine molecule to open the channel. This acetylcholine receptor at the neuromuscular junction is nicotinic in nature and thus different from those in the rest of the body.

Muscle relaxants

These are drugs that interfere with the combination of acetylcholine molecules with their receptors. These block neuromuscular transmission, cause relaxation of the muscle resulting in muscle paralysis. The neuromuscular blockers are of two types: depolarising and non-depolarising muscle relaxants.

Depolarising muscle relaxant

Succinylcholine is the only drug of this category in clinical use. It has a molecular structure similar to acetylcho-

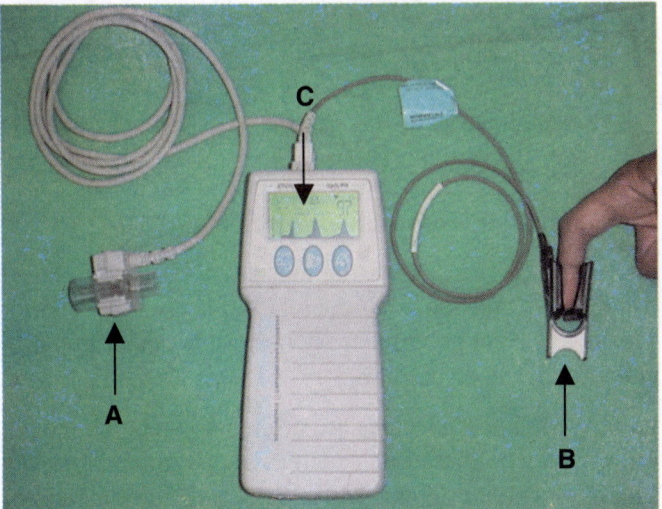

Fig. 48.16 A portable pulse oximeter and capnograph. A) The capnograph and adaptor B) Pulse oximeter probe C) Graphical display window that can be programmed to show either a plethysmograph (as seen in the photograph) or a capnogram

line. It combines with the alpha subunit of the ACh receptor and produces muscle contraction. However, unlike acetyl choline, it has a prolonged action. Continued depolarisation of a muscle results in 'accommodation blockade' and the muscle relaxes.

Dose: 1 - 1.5 mg/kg intravenously.

Onset of action: Within 60 seconds

Duration of action: 3 - 5 minutes

Metabolism: By plasma cholinesterase

Adverse effects

1. **Muscle pains:** The initial depolarisation that occurs due to succinylcholine causes unco-ordinated contraction (fasciculations) of different groups of muscle fibres. This can cause severe muscle pain postoperatively.

2. **Bradycardia,** especially if a second dose of succinyl choline is given. This is easily avoided by pre-treatment with atropine.

3. **Hyperkalaemia** in patients with renal failure, burns, massive crush injury, etc.

4. **Increase in intracranial pressure**

5. **Increase in intraocular pressure**

6. **Prolonged action** in patients deficient in pseudocholinesterase (plasma cholinesterase). This occurs as a genetic problem in a small number of patients but may be an acquired problem as in severe liver disease.

7. **Malignant hyperthermia** in susceptible patients. Those with a family history of anaesthetic mishaps, neuromuscular diseases such as muscular dystrophy may be susceptible to this disorder and succinylcholine is best avoided in these patients. It is not always possible to identify latent muscular dystrophies in infants and children. Administration of succinylcholine in these patients can be disastrous. Hence, the use of succinyl choline should be avoided in children less than 2 years unless an indication such as a full stomach exists. Even then, alternatives such as rocuronium may be considered.

Uses

Succinyl choline is the only muscle relaxant which has the shortest time to onset of action (60 seconds) and lasts for 3 - 5 minutes. It is used:

1. To facilitate endotracheal intubation in 'full-stomach' patients. It is useful in patients with difficult airway because it gives very good relaxation to facilitate intubation but if intubation fails, the patient is likely to resume spontaneous breathing early and avoid hypoxic injury.

2. To maintain paralysis for short procedures

Non-depolarising muscle relaxants

Pancuronium, vecuronium, atracurium and cisatracurium are drugs belonging to this group in clinical use. The nondepolarising muscle relaxants combine with the ACh receptors but do not have any intrinsic effect on the muscle. They cause muscle paralysis by preventing the acetylcholine molecules that are released from the nerve terminal to combine with the acetylcholine receptors on the postsynaptic membrane to produce their action (competitive inhibition). Even if one alpha subunit is combined with a molecule of nondepolariser muscle relaxant, the muscle cannot contract in response to a nerve impulse and gets paralysed. The muscle regains its power when the muscle relaxant gets metabolised.

The nondepolarising muscle relaxants can be classified according to their duration of action as follows:

- Short-acting (10-20 minutes) - Mivacurium, Doxacurium

- Intermediate-acting (20-30 minutes) - Atracurium, Vecuronium.

- Long-acting (>45 minutes) - Pancuronium, Pipecuronium.

Uses

1. To facilitate endotracheal intubation

2. To maintain paralysis during anaesthesia and in the intensive care unit.

Reversal of neuromuscular blockade

At the end of anaesthesia, the muscle relaxation produced by the nondepolarising muscle relaxant is usually reversed. This is to ensure good recovery of muscle power to maintain airway and respiration.

Acetylcholine molecules are broken down by cholinesterases. Anticholinesterases such as neostigmine block the action of cholinesterase, thus increasing the amount of acetylcholine in the neuromuscular junction. The block produced by the nondepolarising muscle relaxants is competitive. Neostigmine is the only anticholinesterase in clinical use. Its dose is 0.05 - 0.08 mg/kg body weight. Neostigmine increases the amount of acetylcholine not only at the neuromuscular junction but also in the entire body. It can cause the muscarinic effects of acetyl choline such as bradycardia, bronchoconstriction etc. Hence, neostigmine is always combined with atropine (0.025 mg/kg) or glycopyrrolate (0.0125 mg/kg) to counter these effects.

When acetyl choline molecules are greater in number due to the action of anticholinesterase, and the number of molecules of the nondepolarising muscle relaxant are reduced due to metabolism, muscle power returns.

Clinical criteria of recovery from neuromuscular blockade:

- Opening of eyes without furrowing of forehead
- Good hand grip
- Raising arms against gravity
- Good cough
- Ability to lift head against gravity (Sustained head-lift) for at least five seconds

Objective criteria

The amount of neuromuscular blockade can be checked using a nerve stimulator. The nerve is stimulated and the response of the muscle is checked. If there are good muscle contractions in response to the nerve stimulation, the muscle power is assumed to have returned.

The patient is allowed to breathe spontaneously and his trachea extubated when there is clinical evidence of complete recovery from neuromuscular blockade. If there is inadequate recovery of muscle power, the patient may need to be ventilated artificially till the muscle power is normal.

LOCAL ANAESTHETICS

Local anaesthetics are drugs when injected around the nerves block impulse conduction distal to the site of injection and produce analgesia and anaesthesia in that area.

CLASSIFICATION

Local anaesthetics consist of a hydrophilic tertiary amine group linked to a lipophilic aromatic group. They are classified into two main categories based on this linking group: the aminoamides and the aminoesters.

- **Aminoesters:** Procaine, chloroprocaine, tetracaine
- **Aminoamides:** Lignocaine, bupivacaine, ropivacaine

MECHANISM OF ACTION

A nerve impulse is transmitted by progressive opening of sodium channels across the membrane and sudden influx of sodium into the intracellular fluid. Local anaesthetics block the fast sodium channels and the sodium influx, thus blocking all impulse transmission across the membrane. Local anaesthetic exists in two forms: ionised and nonionised. The nonionised form is lipophilic and crosses the phospholipid membrane more easily. The ionised form blocks the channel in the open state and blocks nerve transmission (use-dependent blockade). The drug blocks the channel from the intracellular direction.

FACTORS INFLUENCING ACTIVITY

Lipid solubility

Higher the lipid solubility, higher is its ability to penetrate the lipoprotein membrane and hence greater is its potency.

pKa

The pKa of a drug is the pH at which the ionised and nonionised portions of the drug are equal. The lower the pKa, lower is the degree of ionisation for any given pH. The nonionised portion is lipophilic and crosses the cell membrane more easily hastening the onset of nerve blockade. For e.g., lignocaine has a pKa of 7.9 and acts faster than bupivacaine with a pKa of 8.1.

pH

Acidosis decreases the proportion of the nonionised drug and reduces the amount of drug able to cross the membrane.

Protein binding

The degree of protein binding reflects the ability of the drug to membrane proteins: the greater the binding, longer is the duration of action.

CHOICE OF LOCAL ANAESTHETIC AGENTS

- **Lignocaine** - Skin infiltration - 0.5%,

  Minor nerve block - 1%

  Epidural - 1.5 - 2%

  Spinal anaesthesia-5%, heavy (hyperbaric)

Two topical preparations are available: 2% lignocaine jelly and 4% lignocaine spray for the mucosal surfaces of the body.

Note: 1% means each ml contains 10 mg of the drug, 2% - 20 mg/ml and so on.

- **Bupivacaine** - Skin infiltration, epidural - 0.25%, 0.5%

    Spinal anaesthesia - 0.5%, heavy (hyperbaric)

Maximum recommended doses of local anaesthetics for infiltration and blocks

- Lignocaine - 5 mg/kg
- Lignocaine with adrenaline - 7 mg/kg
- Bupivacaine - 2 - 3 mg/kg
- Lignocaine when used as an antiarrhythmic agent is given IV, in a dose of 1 - 2 mg/kg.

Caution: Adrenaline containing preparations should not be used for nerve blocks of fingers, toes and penis as it can cause ischaemia. Bupivacaine is not for intravenous use.

CLINICAL EFFECTS

Local effects

Local anaesthetics block the sodium channels in the neuronal membrane and thus the propagation of impulses across it.

Systemic effects

These drugs can produce systemic effects when high plasma levels of the drug are achieved. This may be deliberate as when lignocaine is used as an antiarrhythmic agent. It is classified as Class Ia drug (sodium channel blockers) in the Vaughan Williams classification of antiarrhythmic agents.

When high plasma concentrations of local anaesthetics are achieved, either due to accidental intravenous injection of the drug or due to intravascular absorption of large amount of drug infiltrated in a region, systemic toxicity can occur.

TOXICITY OF LOCAL ANAESTHETICS

Systemic toxicity

If significant amount of local anaesthetics reach the tissues of heart and brain, they exert the same membrane stabilising effect as on peripheral nerve, resulting in progressive depression of function. The toxicity of local anaesthetics is dose-dependent. These drugs always produce **central nervous system (CNS) toxicity first. As the plasma level rises, cardiovascular toxicity and collapse occur**.

The plasma levels of lignocaine required to produce cardiovascular collapse (CVS toxicity) is seven times that required to produce convulsions (CNS toxicity). Bupivacaine requires only three times the plasma level to produce cardiac toxicity as for CNS toxicity. Thus, bupivacaine has a greater potential for cardiotoxicity.

Clinical features of local anaesthetic toxicity are related to plasma level of the local anaesthetic. The clinical effects and their relation to plasma level of lignocaine are given in the table 48.1.

The likelihood of toxicity of local anaesthetics depends on several factors:

1. Amount of drug injected
2. Site of injection - Vascularity
3. Addition of vasoconstrictors
4. Rapidity of injection
5. Nature of drug given
6. Presence of associated conditions such as low cardiac output or renal failure

Amount and nature of drug injected

Lignocaine is mostly used to produce peripheral neural conduction blockade. It can be used in doses not exceeding

PLASMA CONCENTRATION (μg/ml)	CNS TOXICITY	CVS TOXICITY
5	Tingling, numbness, tinnitus, light-headedness.	
5 - 10	Slurred speech, muscle twitching	
10	Loss of consciousness	
10-15	Convulsions	
15	Coma	Myocardial depression
20	Respiratory arrest	Cardiac arrhythmias
25		Ventricular arrest

Table 48.1 The clinical effects and their relation to plasma level of lignocaine

5 mg/kg body weight for plexus blocks or infiltration. When combined with vasopressors such as adrenaline, the dose can be increased up to 7 mg/kg. The intravenous dose of lignocaine is 1 - 1.5 mg/kg when used as an antiarrhythmic. However, even a small dose such as 20 mg in an adult may be sufficient when injected accidentally into the carotid artery to produce convulsions.

Bupivacaine is used only for nerve blocks or infiltration. It is not an antiarrhythmic drug. Bupivacaine is cardiotoxic and care should be taken not to exceed the prescribed doses. Circulatory collapse and cardiac arrest due to large doses of bupivacaine can be very resistant to resuscitation. It can be used in a dose of up to 2 mg/kg body weight.

Ropivacaine is a newer amide local anaesthetic agent which is similar to bupivacaine but with less cardiotoxic. A levo-isomer of bupivacaine, called levobupivacaine is also less cardiotoxic and has been put into clinical use recently.

Site of injection

Certain sites are very vascular as compared to others. A higher plasma level of local anaesthetics is reached when they are injected for multiple intercostal nerve block. Brachial plexus block produces lower plasma levels of local anaesthetics as compared to intercostal blocks.

Prevention of toxicity

- Do not exceed recommended doses
- Aspirate to rule out presence of the needle tip in a vessel before injecting the drug.
- Slow injection, especially the first few ml and watch for signs of toxicity.

TREATMENT OF LOCAL ANAESTHETIC TOXICITY

The toxicity of local anaesthetics manifests initially as CNS depression and convulsions. Maintenance of airway, breathing and circulation must be a priority. These convulsions generally last for a short period of time.

- Patency of the airway must be maintained
- Oxygen by face mask
- Ventilation, if apnoea occurs
- Convulsions are treated with intravenous diazepam or thiopentone in incremental doses.
- Cardiovascular collapse with ephedrine, inotropes and vasoconstrictors, and CPR as needed.
- Arrhythmias must be treated appropriately.

SPINAL AND EPIDURAL ANAESTHESIA

Injection of local anaesthetics around the spinal cord to produce a reversible blockade of impulses that pass through it is called central neuraxial blockade. When the local anaesthetic is injected into the cerebrospinal fluid bathing the spinal cord, it is called spinal anaesthesia (subarachnoid block). When the local anaesthetics are injected into the epidural space to block the nerves that emerge from the spinal cord, it is called epidural anaesthesia.

SPINAL ANAESTHESIA

Physiological effects

Nervous system

The local anaesthetics spread from the site of injection by mixing with the cerebrospinal fluid (CSF). They reach the nerve fibres in the spinal cord and block transmission of all impulses below the highest level of spread. The concentration of the drug reduces with increasing distance from the site of injection. The smaller fibres (C and Aδ) need a lower concentration of the drug whereas the thick motor fibres (Aα) require a larger concentration to get blocked. Thus, a differential blockade occurs after a spinal anaesthetic. The sensory level of block is generally two segments above the level of motor block. Sympathetic fibres (smallest) are blocked about two to four segments above the level of sensory block.

Cardiovascular system

Due to the blockade of sympathetic nerves below the level of spinal block, there is profound vasodilatation in the affected areas. A relative hypovolaemia occurs and hypotension is usually seen. The extent of hypovolaemia depends on the preoperative volume status, level of block and the ability to compensate for the vasodilatation. The vessels in the upper limbs constrict to compensate for the vasodilatation in the lower limbs. This is described as "pink trousers, blue jacket" phenomenon.

Respiratory system

When the level of spinal anaesthesia ascends, the intercostal nerves are gradually blocked. The diaphragm is not easily paralysed as the phrenic nerve is a thick and strong nerve. The respiration is usually maintained till the level of block is high. In high spinals, the alveolar ventilation reduces and may lead to hypoxia and hypercarbia.

Gastro-intestinal system

Unopposed parasympathetic activity leads to constriction of gut with increased peristaltic activity. Nausea, retching or vomiting may occur and may be the symptom of impending hypotension. These symptoms disappear when the hypotension is corrected. Occasionally, it may need administration of an anticholinergic or an antiemetic agent. However, since the bowel is contracted and small, and the skeletal muscle relaxation produced is greater, the surgeons find it easier to operate on such a gut.

Techniques of spinal anaesthesia

The spinal anaesthetic may be administered with the patient in lateral, sitting or prone position. The prone position is rarely used for procedures on the perineum (pilonidal sinus excision).

Procedure

A pre-procedure check of the anaesthesia equipment, resuscitation equipment and drugs is made. An intravenous line is placed and baseline monitoring established. The patient is then positioned for spinal anaesthesia.

Lateral position

The patient lies either in the left or right lateral position. The back should be parallel to the edge of the operating table and perpendicular to the ground. The legs should be flexed at the hips as much as possible.

Sitting position

The patient sits on the table, with the back bent forward. He is allowed to rest his arms on pillows. The back is cleaned with spirit and betadine and draped. Under aseptic precautions, the vertebral spines are identified in the lumbar region. The highest point of the iliac crest corresponds to L3-4 space. The L2-3, L3-4, L4-5 intervertebral spaces can also be used. A space higher than this is not used as the spinal cord ends at L1 in adults. This point is lower in children and should be borne in mind in paediatric spinals.

Approach

The subarachnoid space may be approached either from the midline or by a paramedian technique. A subcutaneous weal of local anaesthetic is raised in the chosen intervertebral space.

In the midline approach, the lumbar puncture needle (23,

25 or 29 # needle) is inserted in the midline, midway between the spines and perpendicular to the skin. The spinal needle passes through the following structures to reach the subarachnoid space:

1. Skin
2. Subcutaneous tissue
3. Supraspinous ligaments
4. Interspinous ligaments
5. Ligamentum flavum
6. Dura and arachnoid

In the paramedian technique, the needle is inserted a finger-breadth lateral to the spine and advanced in a slightly cephalad direction towards the midline. This approach helps access the subarachnoid space in those patients whose interspinous and supraspinous ligaments are calcified or in patients unable to bend enough to open the interspaces well.

The correct position of the needle is identified by obtaining a free flow of CSF. The local anaesthetic is now injected into the CSF, taking care not to displace the needle.

INDICATIONS

Any surgery below the level of umbilicus

CONTRAINDICATIONS

- Patient refusal
- Infection at the site of injection
- Hypovolaemia
- Bleeding tendencies
- Severe stenotic valvular heart disease

Drawbacks

- Limited duration of block

COMPLICATIONS

These may be classified into Minor and Major based on the reversibility and seriousness of the complication.

Minor

Hypotension

This is treated with intravenous fluids to compensate for the vasodilatation. If necessary, incremental doses of a vasoconstrictor may also be used.

Bradycardia

If the cardioaccelerator nerves (T1-T4) are blocked. This is usually easily treated with an anticholinergic such as atropine or glycopyrrolate. If profound, a small dose of adrenaline may be required (very rare).

Postdural puncture headache (PDPH)

The incidence of PDPH depends on the size of the needle used, number of punctures made, fluid status and ambulation. With finer (25 and 26# needles) and good hydration of the patient, PDPH is uncommon. This may be treated with rest, increased fluid intake, plenty of coffee and NSAIDs. Rarely, an epidural patch may be required.

Respiratory depression

If the level of spinal anaesthesia is high and all intercostal muscles are paralysed, respiratory depression may occur. However, diaphragm, the principal muscle of respiration is supplied by the thick phrenic nerve which does not get blocked easily. The respiratory depression seen during spinal anaesthesia is more due to hypoperfusion of the respiratory centre (due to hypotension). This can be treated with respiratory support as required and stabilisation of blood pressure.

Retention of urine

Backache: This is not a problem of spinal anaesthesia *per se* but may be due to faulty positioning during surgery.

Major

1. **Infection:** Arachnoiditis, meningitis
2. **Nerve injury:** Cauda equina syndrome

EPIDURAL ANAESTHESIA

In this type of central neuraxial blockade, local anaesthetic is injected in the space around the dura (epidural space). The local anaesthetic blocks the nerves as they emerge through the intervertebral foramen. Some of it diffuses through the meninges into the spinal cord and acts on the spinal cord.

Procedure

A pre-procedure check of the anaesthesia equipment, resuscitation equipment and drugs is made. An intravenous line is placed and baseline monitoring of heart rate, electrocardiogram, blood pressure and oxygen saturation is established.

Position

The epidural puncture can be done with the patient in sitting position or in the lateral decubitus position.

Technique

The patient's back is cleaned with an antiseptic and then draped. Under aseptic precautions, epidural puncture is done using a 16 or 18# Tuohy needle. This needle has a blunt tip to reduce the risk of dural puncture. The needle is inserted either in the midline or by a paramedian approach. It passes through the same tissues as during a lumbar puncture but not into the subarachnoid space.

The needle is inserted along with its stylet and always advanced slowly from skin onwards. Once the subcutaneous tissue is entered, the stylet is removed. A 2 ml or 5 ml syringe with a freely moving plunger and containing either air, saline or both is then connected to the needle hub. A gentle attempt at injection of this air or saline is made as the needle advances through the tissues. The entry of the needle into the epidural space is heralded when it penetrates the ligamentum flavum and there is a loss of resistance to injection of air or saline. This is taken as the end-point.

An epidural catheter is passed through this needle and advanced to about 3-4 cm into the space. The needle is removed and the catheter taped and fixed to the back. A bacterial filter is attached to the injection port of the catheter (Fig. 48.17).

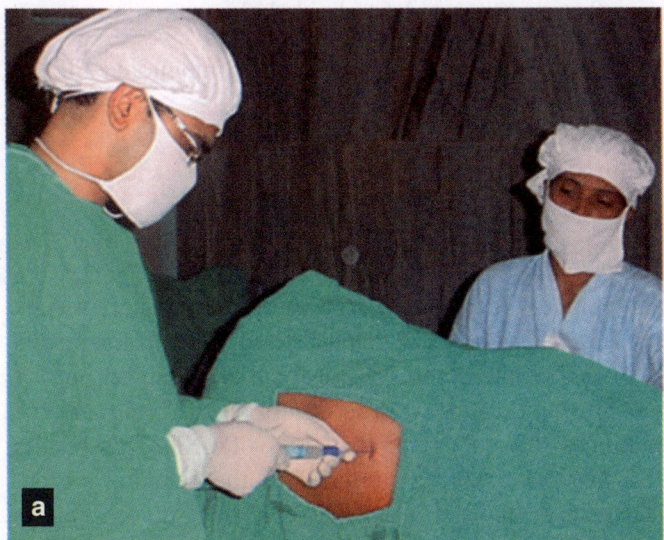

Fig. 48.17 Epidural anaesthesia **A.** Epidural puncture with 18# Tuohy needle

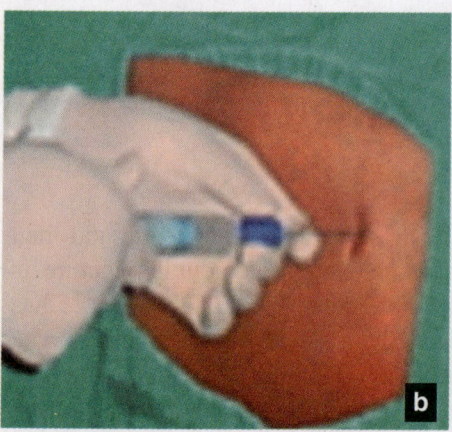 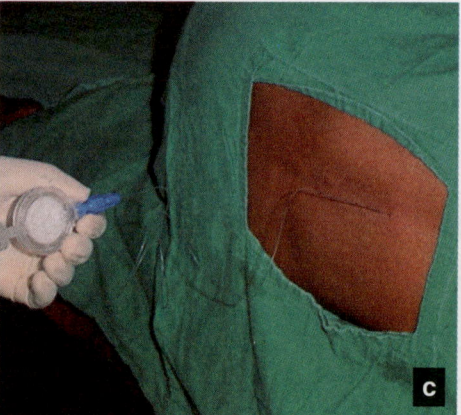 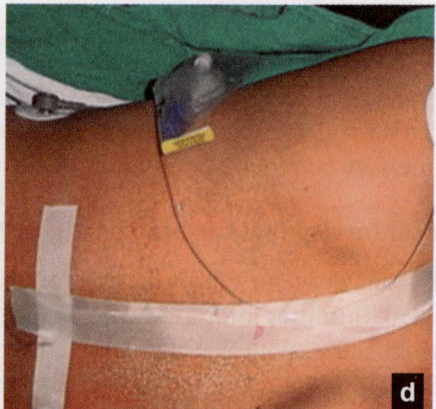

Fig. 48.17 Epidural anaesthesia **B.** Eliciting loss of resistance to air **C.** Epidural catheter attached to bacterial filter **D.** Epidural catheter taped to the back

The epidural needle or catheter may accidentally enter an epidural vein or the subarachnoid space. To avoid injecting a large dose of local anaesthetic into either of these spaces, a test-dose containing a small amount of local anaesthetic (3 ml of 2 % lignocaine) and 15 μg of adrenaline is injected. Any sensory or motor block following this dose would suggest an accidental dural puncture resulting in spinal anaesthesia. An accidental intravascular injection is identified by an increase in the heart rate and blood pressure within a minute of the injection due to intravascular injection of adrenaline. In either situation, the epidural catheter may need to be withdrawn or replaced. If neither response is seen, an epidural placement is assumed and the full dose of local anaesthetic is injected in divided doses.

The patient should be continuously monitored till the block wears off.

COMPLICATIONS

1. Postdural puncture headache (PDPH)

The epidural needles are large and dural puncture results in a larger leak of cerebrospinal fluid (CSF). This results in low CSF pressures. Whenever the patient sits up or becomes ambulatory, a drag occurs on the brain and the meninges due to gravity and loss of CSF. This results in a headache typically referred to the occipital region. The pain disappears when he lies down supine. This is more common in obstetric patients. It may occur up to 2 to 7 days after lumbar puncture and may persist for up to 6 weeks.

Treatment

Plenty of oral fluids may increase CSF production. Rest, plenty of coffee and NSAIDs may also help. Rarely, an epidural patch may be required.

Epidural patch: If the headache is very severe or disabling, an epidural blood patch may be given. 10 to 15 ml of patient's own blood is drawn under aseptic precautions and immediately injected into the same space as the previous epidural puncture. The injected blood clots in the epidural space to seal the puncture hole. This is nearly 100% effective in relieving the headache.

2. Total spinal block

When a large dose of local anaesthetic is injected intrathecally inadvertently, all spinal nerves are inadvertently blocked, causing profound hypotension, bradycardia and collapse. If the patient is continuously monitored and treated promptly, this is completely reversible.

Treatment

- Volume infusion and vasopressors
- Endotracheal intubation and ventilation as necessary.

3. Urinary retention

4. Meningitis: If aseptic precautions are not followed

5. Cauda equina syndrome, adhesive arachnoiditis

This neurological complication is very devastating but extremely rare.

Table 48.2 Comparison of spinal and epidural anaesthesia

SPINAL ANAESTHESIA	EPIDURAL ANAESTHESIA
1. Done in the lumbar region only	Can be done in the lumbar, sacral (caudal), thoracic or cervical regions.
2. Confirmation of correct placement of needle by ensuring free flow of CSF	Placement confirmed by using loss of resistance to injection of air, saline or both
3. A small amount of local anaesthetic is used	Larger mass of local anaesthetic is injected
4. 23 - 25 # LP needles used	Larger needles (18-20 #) are required
5. Test doses not required	Use of test doses advisable
6. Onset of neural blockade is fast. So also side-effects	Onset slow as drugs have to penetrate the dura. So, less hypotension
7. All the nerves are blocked below the level of anaesthesia	The local anaesthetic spreads both caudad and cephalad. Segmental block can be achieved
8. Limited duration	Epidural catheters are routinely introduced and hence duration of anaesthesia can be prolonged with repeated boluses or continuous infusion through catheters
9. Postdural puncture headache possible	PDPH not seen, unless dura is inadvertently punctured
10. No such problem	Inadvertent intrathecal or intravascular injection of large amount of drugs possible, with consequent complications such as total spinal blockade and local anaesthetic toxicity respectively.

OTHER REGIONAL TECHNIQUES

CAUDAL ANALGESIA

This is a very popular technique in providing postoperative analgesia in children. Caudal analgesia involves injection of local anaesthetics with or without opioids in the caudal epidural space.

Procedure

Position

The patient is positioned in lateral position with the knees flexed and the back perpendicular to the ground. The area over the sacrum, coccyx and the gluteal region is cleaned and draped.

Needles

A 22 G hypodermic needle or a scalp vein set is used to administer the block. Technique: The needle is inserted at the apex of the sacral hiatus at a 60° angle to the skin. A distinct 'pop' or a 'give way' is felt as the needle punctures the sacrococcygeal membrane. The angle of the needle is then changed to about 15° to 20° to the skin and advanced a little further into the sacral epidural space. The latter step is optional and has to be done with caution as the dural sac may end relatively low in infants. After careful aspiration to rule out blood or CSF, a small dose of local anaesthetic is injected. There should be no resistance to injection. A subcutaneous injection should also be ruled out.

Drugs

0.25% bupivacaine in a dose of 0.5 ml/kg is sufficient for perineal and low sacral procedures, 1 ml/kg for lumbosacral procedures and 1.5 ml/kg for lower abdominal procedures. However, a total volume of 20 ml and a total dose of 2 mg/kg of bupivacaine may not be exceeded.

Indications

Postoperative pain relief in children and adults for perineal and lumbosacral procedures.

Contraindications

Absence of consent from parents/patients, local infection, bleeding tendencies.

Complications

Intrathecal injection, intravascular injection of large dose of local anaesthetics.

BRACHIAL PLEXUS BLOCK

Injection of local anaesthetics injected around the brachial plexus produces analgesia and even surgical anaesthesia in the upper limb. The brachial plexus can be blocked by four different approaches: interscalene, supraclavicular, infraclavicular or the axillary. Of these, the supraclavicular and axillary techniques are the most popular.

I. Supraclavicular brachial plexus block

Position

The patient is positioned in supine position with the head turned to the opposite side of the block. The area over the lower part of the neck is cleaned and draped.

Needles

A 22 G hypodermic needle, a scalp vein set or an insulated needle with an internal nerve stimulator may be used to administer the block.

Technique

The needle is inserted at a point 1 to 1.5 cm above the midpoint of the clavicle. The subclavian arterial pulsations are felt with the thumb of one hand and the needle advanced posterior to it with a medial and caudad direction. Paraesthesia must be sought in the upper limb and the injection of local anaesthetic made at the point of paraesthesia. Undue pain during injection suggests intraneural injection. Careful aspiration for absence of blood to rule out intravascular injection is mandatory before injection of the local anaesthetic.

Drugs

Plain lignocaine not exceeding 5 mg/kg or bupivacaine not exceeding 2 mg/kg may be used.

Indications

Intraoperative analgesia, anaesthesia and postoperative pain relief in children and adults for procedures on the upper limb.

Contraindications

Absence of consent from parents/patients, local infection, bleeding tendencies.

Other regional blocks such as wrist block and popliteal nerve blocks are beyond the scope of this book.

Complications

Haematoma, intravascular injection of local anaesthetics, pneumothorax.

II. Axillary brachial plexus block

Position

The patient is positioned in supine position with the arm abducted to a right angle and the elbow bent at right angles to the arm. The area over the axilla is cleaned and draped.

Needles

A 22 G hypodermic needle, a scalp vein set or an insulated needle with an internal nerve stimulator may be used to administer the block.

Technique

The needle is inserted at a point just above the point of maximum pulsations of the axillary artery but parallel to the artery. This point should be as high in the axilla as possible. Paraesthesia must be sought in the upper limb and the injection of local anaesthetic made at the point of paraesthesia. Undue pain during injection suggests intraneural injection. Careful aspiration for absence of blood to rule out intravascular injection is mandatory before injection of the local anaesthetic. A single injection of the local anaesthetic can be made at this point. Alternately, half the total volume of injection can be made at a point on the other side of the artery.

Drugs

Either bupivacaine not exceeding a total dose of 2 mg/kg; lignocaine plain 5 mg/kg or with adrenaline 7 mg/kg may be used. A volume 35 - 40 ml may be required.

Indications

Intraoperative analgesia, anaesthesia and postoperative pain relief in children and adults for procedures on the upper limb.

Contraindications

Absence of consent from parents/patients, local infection, bleeding tendencies.

Complications

Haematoma, intravascular injection of local anaesthetics

ANKLE BLOCK

This is a very popular technique in providing intraoperative and postoperative analgesia in adults undergoing procedures on the foot. Ankle block involves injection of local anaesthetics to block all five nerves supplying the foot: posterior tibial, sural, saphenous, superficial peroneal and the deep peroneal nerves.

Procedure

Position

The patient is positioned in the supine position. The foot is raised by an assistant and the area around the ankle is cleaned and draped.

Needles

A 22 G hypodermic needle is used to administer the block.

Technique

The posterior tibial nerve is blocked with 3-5 ml of local anaesthetic at a point midway between the medial malleolus and the heel, just behind the posterior tibial arterial pulsations. The sural nerve may be blocked at a point midway between the lateral malleolus and the heel, just lateral to the Achilles' tendon. The deep peroneal nerve is blocked at a point midway between the lateral and the medial malleoli lateral to the tendon of extensor hallucis longus and the atherior tibial artery. The saphenous nerve and the superficial peroneal nerves are easily blocked by raising a subcutaneous weal of local anaesthetic between the malleoli anteriorly.

Drugs

Lignocaine plain not exceeding 5 mg/kg or bupivacaine not exceeding 2 mg/kg may be used.

Indications

Postoperative pain relief in adults for procedures on the foot.

Contraindications

Absence of consent from patients, local infection, bleeding tendencies.

Other regional blocks such as wrist block and popliteal nerve blocks are beyond the scope of this book.

Introduction

One of the main anxieties of undergoing an operation is the pain that is anticipated along with it. An anaesthesiologist's responsibilities do not end with providing safe perioperative care. He must also ensure that the pain associated with the surgery is relieved adequately so that the surgery itself is not so unpleasant an experience.

Definition

Pain is defined as an unpleasant sensory and emotional experience associated with actual or potential tissue damage, or described in terms of such damage. Pain can be acute or chronic. The pain that is seen immediately after surgery is acute postoperative pain and is easier to treat. The mechanism of perpetuation of chronic pain is less well understood and is more difficult to treat.

Pain pathways

Pain begins with injury to the tissue. Both the peripheral and the central nervous systems are involved in the ultimate pain perception (Fig. 48.18).

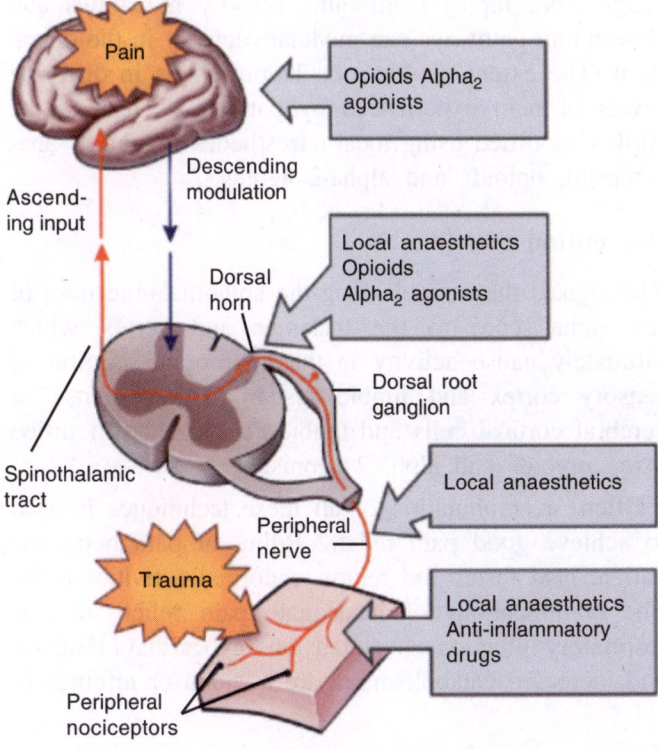

Fig. 48.18 Pain pathways and their modulation using drugs

Acute pain

Four basic mechanisms are involved in the final appreciation of pain: transduction, transmission, modulation and perception. Pain relief can be achieved by blocking each of these steps.

Transduction

The transduction of noxious stimuli begins with peripheral nociceptors. These nociceptors (transducer) convert the stimulus of injury (heat, pressure, mechanoception) to pain sensation. This is also assisted by the production of prostaglandins and leukotrienes in response to the injury. Nonsteroidal anti-inflammatory analgesics can be used to reduce their production. Local application of local anaesthetics also reduces transduction.

Transmission

Signals from these nociceptors travel along myelinated Aδ and unmyelinated C fibers. Their axons synapse in the dorsal horn of the spinal cord, where the neurons of laminae (of Rexed) I, II and V are most involved in the perception of pain. These fibres can be blocked at the nerve plexus level using local anaesthetics.

Modulation

Large fibre inputs from other sensory modalities and descending pathways can modulate activity in the dorsal horn. The extent of this modulation results in differing levels of pain experienced by patients. This can be further modified using local anaesthetics (epidural anaesthesia), opioids and alpha-2 agonists.

Perception

The signals then travel along the spinothalamic tract of the spinal cord to the thalamus and cortex which ultimately cause activity in the appropriate portion of sensory cortex and limbic system. The response of cerebral cortical cells and limbic cells can be modified using opioids and alpha-2 agonists.

Often, a combination of all these techniques is used to achieve good pain relief. Relief of pain helps the patient heal faster and return to normal activities early. The complications of inadequate pain relief such as respiratory infections, hypertension, myocardial infarction and increased catabolism etc are avoided or minimised.

Assessment of pain

Pain is more difficult to measure as compared to other parameters such as temperature or heart rate. The measurement of pain is mainly dependent on the patient's perception of it and may be done in any of the following ways:

1. **Visual Analogue Scale (VAS):** the pain is assessed along a 100 mm scale where 0 corresponds to no pain at all and 100 to the worst imaginable pain. The patient scores his pain at any point he finds appropriate. The pain relief is assessed thereafter from this point. The VAS is the most popular tool used to assess pain and its relief.

2. **Category rating scale:** Pain is rated as none, mild, moderate or severe.

3. **Wong-Baker Faces pain rating scale:** A scale with different faces, a happy face at one end and a face in severe pain and crying at the other with four other faces in between may be used for children.

4. **Biological measures** such as tachycardia, hypertension, tachypnoea or inadequate breathing are relatively inaccurate but useful estimates of pain.

Chronic pain

The initial response to a noxious stimulus is brief and correlates with the sharp, well-localised initial pain. The second phase of the response is more prolonged and correlates with the dull, diffuse pain experienced after the initial injury. This second phase is associated with a growing region of hypersensitivity around the point where the noxious stimulus was initially applied and is said to result in chronic pain. The response to noxious stimuli can be modulated by their repeated application. Peripheral nociceptors become more responsive with the repeated application of noxious stimuli. Their sensitivity can be further enhanced by many tissue factors and inflammatory mediators released in the course of tissue injury.

The process through which the neurons of the dorsal horn of the spinal cord become sensitised by prior noxious stimuli is often referred to as **windup** or **central sensitisation**. Much less is known about pain-induced sensitisation of the supraspinal components of the CNS. This phenomenon leads to chronic pain where the patient experiences pain, often, excruciating, and long after the stimulus that initially caused the pain is removed.

The relief of chronic pain is more difficult. Various techniques used to treat chronic pain are as follows:

Nonpharmacological techniques

- Transcutaneous Electrical Nerve Stimulation (TENS)
- Acupuncture

Pharmacological techniques

- Paracetamol
- Nonsteroidal analgesics
- Opioids

Sympathetic blockade

- Sympathetic ganglion blocks - Stellate ganglion block, Coeliac plexus block etc
- Epidural local anaesthetics
- Epidural neurolytic such as phenol, alcohol injections.

COMPLICATIONS IN ANAESTHESIA

The practice of anaesthesia has become very safe due to better preoperative evaluation and preparation, careful choice of patients, better monitoring, availability of safer drugs and safer anaesthetic techniques. The incidence of complications has come down drastically. However, complications can still occur. The perioperative (pre-, intra-, and postoperative periods) complications can be classified as follows:

Respiratory

- Airway obstruction
- Bronchospasm
- Respiratory failure

Cardiovascular

- Hypertension
- Hypotension
- Arrhythmias
- Shock
- Cardiac arrest

Central nervous system

- Postoperative drowsiness
- Postoperative nausea and vomiting
- Neurologic complications of regional blockade

Renal failure

Hepatic failure

I. RESPIRATORY COMPLICATIONS

1. Airway obstruction

Airway obstruction may occur during the induction of general anaesthesia. When a person becomes unconscious, the tongue and the epiglottis fall back and can obstruct the airway. The patency of the airway is usually maintained fairly easily by the anaesthesiologist by using chin lift or jaw thrust manoeuvres. A definitive airway such as an endotracheal tube may then be inserted into the trachea.

Occasionally, the chin lift or jaw thrust manoeuvres are inadequate to maintain a patent airway as in patients with abnormal airways. Insertion of an endotracheal tube may also prove to be difficult in certain individuals. An oral or nasopharyngeal airway may be inserted to overcome this obstruction and maintenance of the airway for a short duration. If the difficulty in inserting the endotracheal tube is due to supraglottic causes and oral or nasopharyngeal airway is not sufficient to relieve the obstruction, insertion of a laryngeal mask airway or a Combitube® may be attempted. If the problem is at the glottis or subglottis and the airway is obstructed, an emergency cricothyrotomy or a tracheostomy may be required.

Perioperative airway obstruction may also be due to any of the following causes:

- Trauma - maxillofacial, head injury
- Foreign body aspiration
- Infection - Ludwig's angina, retropharyngeal abscess
- Oedema - Postoperative laryngeal/pharyngeal oedema, laryngeal oedema of anaphylaxis
- Neurological - Recurrent laryngeal nerve injury
- Endocrine - Thyroid enlargement
- Tumour - Malignancy of the airway (tongue, cheek, larynx or the pharynx)

A thorough assessment of the airway must be done preoperatively and a management plan formulated. Plan B and Plan C also should be considered in the eventuality of failure of Plan A. Generally loss of life occurs not because of inability to intubate but due to an inability to oxygenate and ventilate the patient. This situation, also called, 'cannot intubate - cannot ventilate' (CVCI) is one of the most dreaded situations faced by an anaesthesiologist.

2. Bronchospasm

Bronchospasm may occur in a patient under anaesthesia. The possible causes are as follows:

- Irritable airways as in a known asthmatic, chronic obstructive airways disease - i.e., exacerbation of preexisting bronchospastic disease
- Endobronchial intubation and carinal stimulation

- As part of allergic reaction to anaesthetic drugs, antibiotics
- Aspiration of regurgitated gastric contents
- Pneumothorax
- Upper airway obstruction and laryngospasm can reflexly stimulate bronchospasm

Treatment involves treatment of the precipitating cause and bronchodilators.

3. Respiratory failure

A patient is said to be in respiratory failure if he is unable to maintain adequate oxygenation and ventilation, i.e., arterial blood gas tension of oxygen is less than 60 mmHg (when the patient is breathing 60% oxygen) and of carbon dioxide more than 50 mmHg.

Causes

Central

- Awareness
- Head injury
- Depressant drugs - Anaesthetics, opioids
- Hypoxic encephalopathy
- Metabolic causes such as hyponatraemia, hypoglycaemia, hyperglycaemia

Peripheral

- Prolonged effect of muscle relaxants
- Weakness of muscles, e.g., myasthenia gravis

Treatment

- Treat the cause
- Intermittent positive pressure ventilation till the patient improves.

II. CARDIOVASCULAR COMPLICATIONS

Hypertension, hypotension and arrhythmias occur perioperatively due to various reasons such as inadequate preoperative treatment, surgical stress, inadequate anaesthesia, metabolic or endocrine causes or even drug interactions. Brief periods of haemodynamic instability, although common are well-tolerated by healthy individuals. Continuous and appropriate monitoring and prompt treatment should avoid long-term complications.

Hypotension may be due to decreased preload, reduced

contractility or increased afterload to the left ventricle. If not identified or treated in time, it may progress to shock and cardiac arrest. Hypovolaemic shock is the commonest type of shock encountered during surgery. However, cardiogenic shock due to perioperative myocardial infarction, anaphylactic shock due to allergic reaction to anaesthetics or neurogenic shock due to vasovagal attack, high spinals may also occur in susceptible individuals.

For more details on shock and cardiac arrest, refer appropriate sections in the manual.

III. CENTRAL NERVOUS SYSTEM COMPLICATIONS

1. Awareness

This is one of the most dreaded complications by both the anaesthesiologist and the patient. This is more likely to occur if the patient's haemodynamics are very unstable (as in postpartum haemorrhage, trauma) and the anaesthesiologist fears further cardiac depression with the use of inhalation agents. The use of opioids and nitrous oxide may provide analgesia but not the amnesia and anaesthesia required. The awareness of this complication among anaesthesiologists coupled with the use of benzodiazepines and modern anaesthetic agents which are more cardiostable, the incidence of this must be reduced. A new monitor called BIS index monitor provides some information of the conscious state of the patient but is not widely available yet.

2. Postoperative drowsiness

A patient may be slow to awaken after anaesthesia due to persistent effect of the anaesthetic agents or opioids administered during the anaesthesia. However, other causes such as hypoxia, hypothermia, hypo- or hypernatraemia, hypo- or hyperglycaemia may also occur. If all these causes are ruled out and the cause of prolonged drowsiness is still unclear, a neurological consultation is obtained to rule out any space-occupying lesions in the central nervous system, stroke or hypoxic encephalopathy.

3. Postoperative nausea and vomiting (PONV)

PONV is a frequent complication of anaesthesia. It is common in women, after laparoscopic surgeries, squint surgeries and is associated with the use of nitrous oxide and opioids or even early oral intake postoperatively. It may be treated with metoclopramide (10 mg), ondansetron (4 - 8 mg) or dexamethasone (4 - 8 mg) in an average adult.

4. Nerve injuries

Nerve injuries may arise as a complication of regional blockade. Complications such as adhesive arachnoiditis, cauda equina syndrome or paraplegia have been reported after spinal and epidural anaesthesia but are extremely rare. The use of tourniquet, if prolonged or if very high pressures are used, can also cause nerve injuries.

Peripheral nerve injuries may occur perioperatively due to improper positioning under regional or general anaesthesia. The common peroneal nerve and the sciatic nerve can be injured during lithotomy position. The ulnar and the radial nerves may be affected in the arm or at the elbow due to inadequate attention to positioning. Brachial plexus stretch injury can occur if the arms are allowed to be abducted more than ninety degrees. Injury to optic nerves or the retina may occur in prone position due to compression of the eyeball. Corneal injury may occur due to exposure in an unconscious patient.

IV. RENAL FAILURE

Renal failure, usually prerenal is associated with large fluid shifts or major haemodynamic instability. Direct injury to the kidneys (acute tubular necrosis) may occur if adequate attention is not given to prerenal failure. Methoxyflurane, an inhalation anaesthetic agent can cause renal failure but is no longer in use. Renal failure can also occur as part of hepatorenal syndrome or after a mismatched blood transfusion.

V. HEPATIC FAILURE

A patient with compromised hepatic function may proceed to hepatic failure perioperatively, e.g., cirrhosis of liver, obstructive jaundice. Hepatic failure may also occur due to infective complications such as hepatitis or sepsis. Massive hepatic necrosis has been reported after repeated use of halothane. The incidence of this is very rare and must be a diagnosis of exclusion.

CARDIOPULMONARY RESUSCITATION (CPR)

Cardiac arrest is an inevitable and natural event in every one's life. However, this event may have been precipitated prematurely due to some underlying but treatable cause. If prompt intervention is made and the patient's heart and respiration are supported at this stage, precious time may be gained to treat this precipitating cause. Many victims of cardiac arrest may lead normal lives once this calamity is tided over. This is the basis of Cardiopulmonary Resuscitation (CPR).

CPR when given without the help of any equipment is called Basic CPR (also called Basic Life Support - BLS). When equipment and drugs are used in CPR, it is called Advanced CPR (Advanced Cardiac Life Support - ACLS).

CPR must be given promptly and in the correct manner to be effective. Basic CPR is given in the field by bystanders whereas Advanced CPR is administered by paramedical personnel or in the hospital setup by doctors and nurses. **Hence, knowledge of CPR is mandatory for all medical and paramedical personnel.**

Points to note

- CPR is only a symptomatic therapy. Attention must be given to the precipitating cause and must also be treated
- The best of CPR can deliver only one-third of the normal cardiac output. Hence, it is important to get the patient's heart beating spontaneously as early as possible.
- It is important to differentiate between respiratory arrest and cardiac arrest.

Respiratory arrest

The patient stops breathing due to a primarily respiratory cause. The heart continues to beat till all the oxygen in the lungs is removed. The heart will stop once hypoxia occurs. This may take up to a minute to occur. If the respiration is assisted promptly, it is possible to avert cardiac arrest. However, this is possible only in a witnessed respiratory arrest.

Cardiac arrest

The heart stops beating and there is no circulation. Oxygen delivery to the tissues stops. Within 15 seconds of a cardiac arrest, a person loses consciousness. The brain stops functioning within 3 minutes. This is called survival time. If resuscitation is not done in another five minutes, brain death occurs. This is called revival time. Many factors influence this survival and revival times. The important 'take home' message is that prompt and effective treatment is necessary for successful resuscitation.

BASIC CPR

Approach to CPR is always done in the following order: A,

B, and C, A for Airway, B for Breathing and C for Circulation. There are seven steps in Basic CPR.

STEP 1: ASSESS UNCONSCIOUSNESS 'SHAKE GENTLY AND SHOUT LOUDLY'

A conscious person cannot be in cardiac arrest. On shaking gently, if there is no response, turn the patient in to a supine position. Take care to turn the head, neck and body together in a trauma victim who may possibly have a cervical spine injury.

STEP 2: 'CALL FOR HELP AND DEFIBRILLATOR'

The chances of resuscitation are lower with Basic CPR and it is important to get help (in the form of ambulance services for advanced CPR) as early as possible. It is also difficult for a single rescuer to administer CPR for long periods. The rescuer may take up to a minute to call for help (Fig. 48.19).

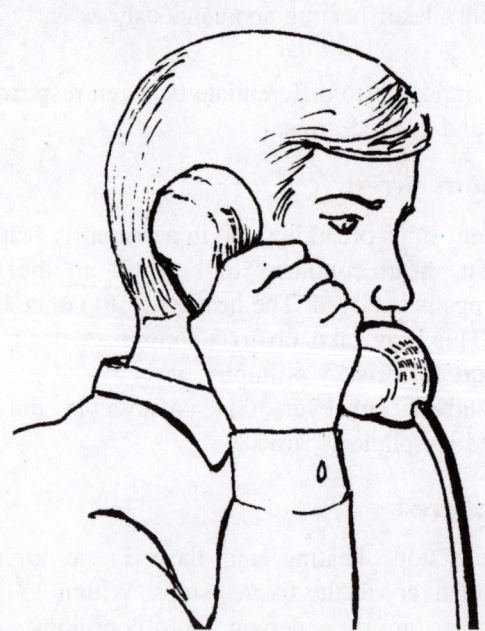

Fig. 48.19 Call for help and defibrillator

STEP 3: 'OPEN AIRWAY'

When a person loses consciousness, the muscles of the tongue, epiglottis and pharynx relax. The tongue and the epiglottis fall back and obstruct the glottis. Unless the airway is opened, it is not possible to check accurately whether respiration is present or not and if present, whether it is adequate or inadequate. The airway is

opened using a "head-tilt and chin-lift method". The palm of one hand is placed on the forehead of the patient and the head tilted posteriorly to extend the head as much as possible. The chin of the patient is lifted up manually with the thumb and fingers of the other hand so that the lower incisors of the victim override the upper incisors. The tongue and the epiglottis are attached to the mandible and are lifted up with the chin lift (Figure 48.20).

STEP 4: LOOK, LISTEN AND FEEL FOR THE PATIENT'S RESPIRATION

The rescuer takes his face close to the patient's mouth to listen and feel for the patient's breath. Looking tangentially at the chest, the rescuer can visually check for breathing (Fig. 48.20).

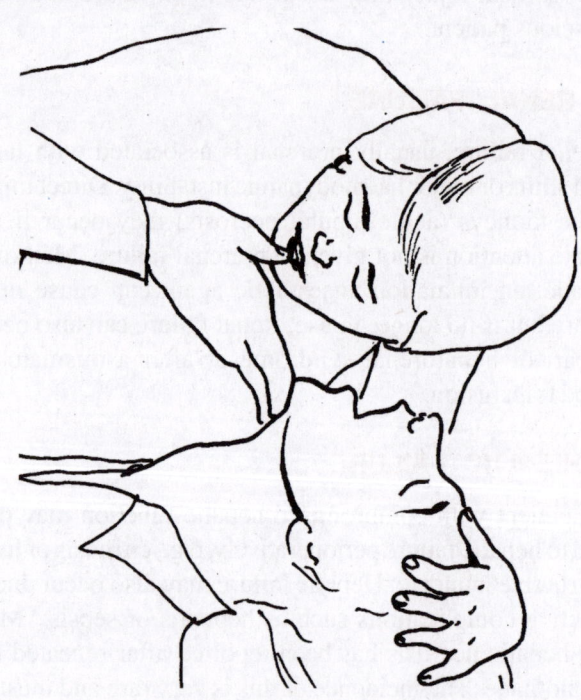

Fig. 48.20 Open airway. Then, "Look, Listen and Feel"

STEP 5: GIVE TWO BREATHS

The rescuer opens his/her mouth wide, makes a mouth to mouth seal and delivers a large breath into the victim so as to expand the chest adequately. He/she takes a breath in from the atmosphere and gives another breath to the victim. Take two seconds to deliver each breath. If the victim's chest does not expand, reopen the airway and try again (Figure 48.21).

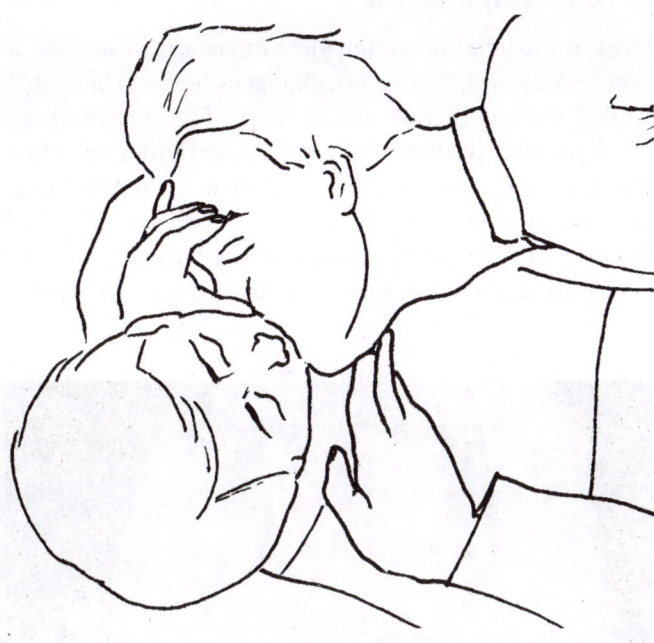

Fig. 48.21 Give two breaths

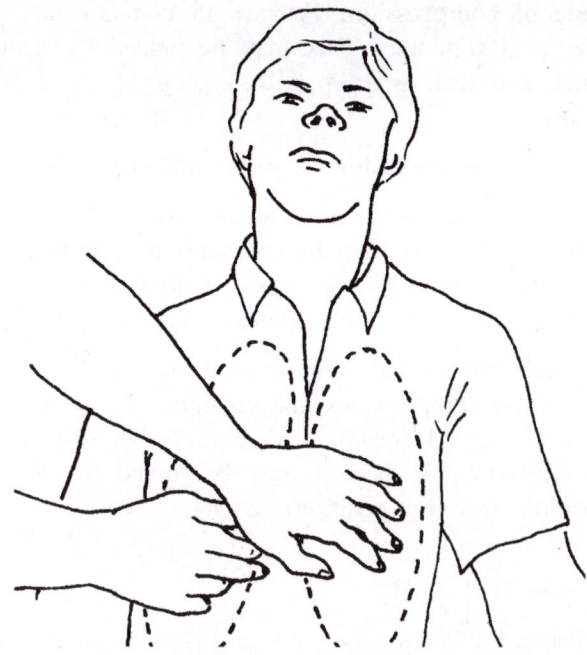

Fig. 48.22 Position hands

STEP 6: FEEL CAROTID PULSE FOR NOT MORE THAN 10 SECONDS

Check for pulse or other signs of circulation such as coughing, movement in response to the rescue breaths). When circulation is inadequate, the body tries to conserve circulation to the vital organs as long as possible. Thus, the carotid artery pulsations are the last to disappear when cardiac output gradually reduces. Hence, it is important to feel the carotid pulse to identify cardiac arrest. Infants and neonates have short necks and it is difficult to feel their carotids. In them, the brachial artery may be used to identify cardiac arrest. If no pulse is felt, the patient is in cardiac arrest.

STEP 7: GIVE CARDIAC COMPRESSIONS

Feel the subcostal margin and trace it to the xiphoid process.

Site of compression

Place the heel of one hand two-finger breadths on the sternum between the nipples. Care should be taken not to compress on either side of the sternum as it may cause rib fractures (Fig. 48.22).

Technique

Clasp this hand with the heel of the other hand; keep the elbows straight and the shoulders directly above the sternum. Compressions are given using body weight by allowing the movement to occur at the rescuer's hips (Fig. 48.23). Only one hand may be used in children less than 8 years of age.

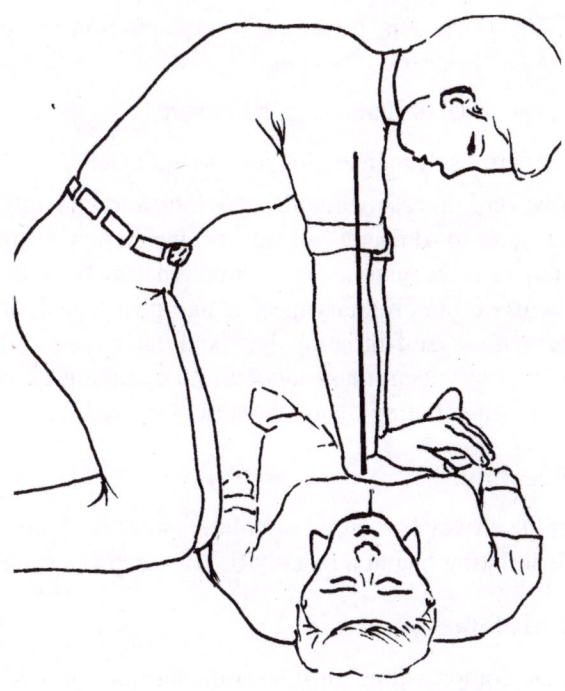

Fig. 48.23 Start cardiac compressions

Rate of compression: Provide 15 compressions at a rate of 100/minute. This may be helped by using a mnemonic such as "a, b, c, d, e, f, g, h, i, j, k, l, m, n, off."

Depth of compression: 2 inches (5 cm) in an adult.

Cycles of compression: Provide cycles of 15 compressions and two breaths (4 cycles in a minute) and then check pulse to see whether circulation has been restored. If not, continue compressions and ventilations.

Check pulse every few minutes. If a pulse returns, stop chest compressions and continue rescue breathing as necessary (1 breath every 5 seconds). If breathing also returns, the patient may be turned to a lateral position (recovery position) and monitored.

ADVANCED CPR

Advanced CPR involves using airway adjuncts, other equipment and drugs for resuscitation. The priority of treatment remains the same as Basic CPR, i.e., Airway, Breathing and Circulation.

A. Airway

Airway is best maintained with endotracheal intubation. The route of choice for intubation is through the mouth because it is faster and involves less trauma. Endotracheal intubation has the following advantages:

1. The trachea is protected from aspiration of regurgitated gastric contents.

2. The tidal volume can be assured

3. There is no distention of the stomach.

However, in case endotracheal intubation is difficult either due to difficult airway or inexperience in the technique, oxygenation and ventilation can be achieved by the use of an oropharyngeal or nasopharyngeal airway along with a self-inflating bag and face mask. Occasionally a laryngeal mask airway or a Combitube® along with a self-inflating bag may also be used.

B. Breathing

After the airway is secured, ventilation must be done using a self-inflating bag at a rate of 10 - 12 breaths per minute.

C. Circulation

Cardiac compressions must be commenced as in BLS.

The initial ABC's must be followed by the following steps:

D. Drugs/Defibrillation

Most of the adult nontraumatic cardiac arrests are due to ventricular fibrillation/ventricular tachycardia. If untreated, VF/VT will degenerate into asystole. The only treatment of ventricular fibrillation is electrical defibrillation which should be done as early as possible. Hence, a monitor must be connected to view the rhythm. Three cardiac arrest rhythms are described: Ventricular Fibrillation/Ventricular Tachycardia, Pulseless Electrical Activity and Asystole.

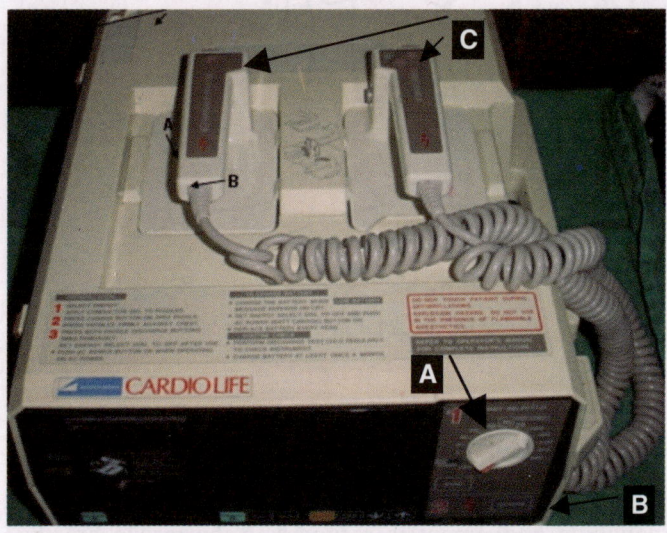

Fig. 48.24 Defibrillator. A. Select energy **B.** Charge button **C.** Paddles. The discharge buttons on each of the paddles have to be depressed simultaneously to discharge the energy.

VENTRICULAR FIBRILLATION/VENTRICULAR TACHYCARDIA

1. If the rhythm shows ventricular fibrillation or ventricular tachycardia (Fig. 48.25 A and B), the following algorithm must be followed:

A. Ventricular fibrillation (VF)

B. Ventricular tachycardia (VT)

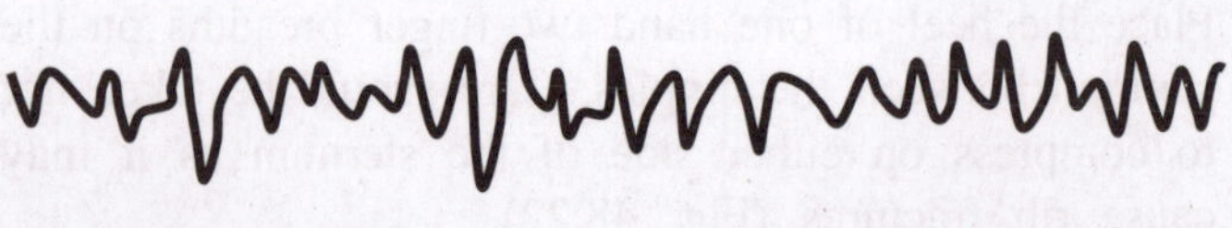

Fig. 48.25A ECG rhythm showing ventricular fibrillation. Note the saw tooth shaped waves that are irregular and chaotic in pattern

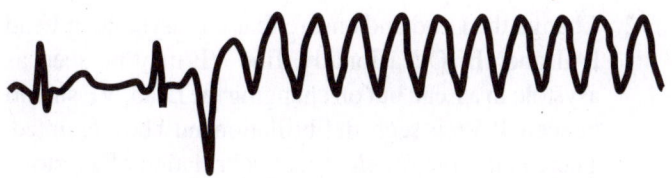

Fig. 48.25B ECG rhythm showing ventricular tachycardia which is more regular and shows wide QRS complex with inverted T waves.

Take care of Airway, Breathing and Circulation till the debrillator arrives. Once the rhythm is confirmed, deliver three stacked shocks as needed to the patient (200 J, 300 J and 360 J). The second and the third shocks are delivered only after the rhythm is checked and the VF/VT is seen to be still persisting. There is no need for ventilation or cardiac compressions between these three shocks. If the VF/VT persist after three shocks, the trachea is intubated, cardiac compressions are started and an intravenous access is secured.

Drugs used in CPR

1.Adrenaline

This is the drug of choice in cardiac arrest. It is given in a dose of 1 mg, diluted to 10 cc (1:10,000) intravenously every 3 - 5 minutes. This should be followed by at least 20 cc of chaser solution (0.9% saline or Ringer lactate). The drug should be injected in a central line if present. In the absence of any intravenous access, adrenaline may be injected through the endotracheal tube (2 - 5 mg diluted to 10 cc). Intracardiac administration of adrenaline is not advisable because of the following reasons:

a. Possible injury to coronary arteries

b. Injury to the pleura

c. Accidental injection into the myocardium can precipitate resistant ventricular fibrillation

d. The injection is made into the right ventricle which is anterior and it has to traverse the pulmonary circulation to reach the coronary arteries. This may well be achieved by an intravenous injection, running it in a drip and avoiding the complications of intracardiac injection.

2. Vasopressin

This is a potent vasoconstrictor that can be given as a single dose of 40 IU and as an alternative to adrenaline in a patient with VF/pulseless VT. The vasoconstriction produced raises the coronary perfusion pressure during CPR.

3.Amiodarone

If the VF/Pulseless VT persist in spite of adrenaline/ vasopressin followed by a DC shock of 360 J, amiodarone may be given in a dose of 300 mg intravenously. Other drugs that may be used are: Lignocaine: 1 - 2 mg/kg body weight intravenously or Magnesium sulphate: 1 -2 g intravenously. Not more than two antiarrhythmic drugs may be used to treat an arrhythmia as all antiarrhythmics are also proarrhythmics and may produce myocardial depression.

4. Sodium bicarbonate

It is an alkalinising agent used when there is documented metabolic acidosis, the cardiac arrest is due to hyperkalaemia or the arrest period is prolonged beyond 10 minutes. The dose is 1 -2 mmol/kg intravenously.

5. Calcium chloride/gluconate

Calcium is given only if the cardiac arrest is due to hyperkalaemia, there is documented hypocalcaemia or the patient has been on calcium channel blockers. Thus, both calcium and sodium bicarbonate are indicated when there is hyperkalaemic cardiac arrest. Their routine use in any cardiac arrest is not indicated as they can cause more harm.

Remember

- The drugs used to treat VF/VT must be followed by a DC shock of 360 J about 30 seconds after their injection.
- Cardiac compressions and ventilation must continue between these shocks.

PULSELESS ELECTRICAL ACTIVITY (PEA)

If the monitor showed no VF/VT, but a discernible rhythm, sinus or nonsinus with the patient manifesting no pulse (no carotid pulsations), it is termed Pulseless Electrical Activity (PEA). This means that electrical activity is present while mechanical activity is absent.

The causes of PEA are as follows

1. Massive myocardial infarction where the myocardial necrosis results in absent contractions. It may also be called **"Electro-Mechanical Dissociation (EMD)".**

2. A PEA may also be caused by the following factors

which may result in ineffective contractions while electrical activity is still present. This is called **'pseudo-EMD'**. In pseudo-EMD, the causes are reversible. If the cause is identified and treated promptly, the chances of successful resuscitation are high.

The causes of PEA can be remembered as 5 H's and 5 T's.

5 H's	**5 T's**
1. Hypoxia	1. Tension pneumothorax
2. Hydrogen ions (acidosis)	2. Tamponade (Cardiac)
3. Hypovolaemia	3. Thrombosis (Pulmo nary)
4. Hyper/hypokalaemia	4. Thrombosis (Coronary)
5. Hypo/hyperthermia	5. Toxins

3. Whenever a PEA is seen, look for a treatable cause and treat promptly. As the basic cause is being treated, the patient also needs to given CPR. The airway must be secured and, ventilations and cardiac compressions given. This must be followed by adrenaline (standard dose as mentioned in the VF/VT section) every 3-5 minutes as necessary till return of spontaneous circulation is achieved. Sodium bicarbonate and calcium chloride/gluconate may also be given if indicated (as mentioned above).

ASYSTOLE

If the monitor shows a flat line, it is asystole. Whenever aystole is seen on a monitor the following things should be done. Confirm that it is asystole and then commence therapy.

1. Check whether all leads are connected correctly. Improper connections may manifest as asystole.

2. Change the Lead and ensure that it is asystole in Lead I, II and III. Occasionally, fine VF may be seen as asystole in a Lead but on changing the Lead, VF should be seen. If VF is seen, defibrillation must be attempted. There is no role for electrical debrillation of asystole.

3. **CPR** must be commenced with **A, B and C.** The airway must be secured, ventilations and cardiac compressions given.

4. This must be followed by **adrenaline** (standard dose as mentioned in the VF/VT section) every 3-5 minutes as necessary till return of spontaneous circulation is achieved.

5. **Atropine:** Atropine is injected in a dose of 0.6 - 2 mg intravenously. Asystole often follows a bradycardia due to vagal overactivity.

6. A **transcutaneous pacemaker** may be used to pace a rhythm.

7. If there is no response to resuscitation in spite of all the above efforts and given for a reasonable period of time, consider abandoning resuscitation efforts.

Postresuscitation care

If return of spontaneous circulation is achieved, it is important to ensure it is sustained. Cardiac compressions are stopped when the pulses begin to be felt without the compressions. An infusion of an inotrope such as adrenaline or dopamine may be required. The patient needs intensive care where respiratory and renal support can be provided. It is important to preserve cerebral function by maintaining normal blood pressures, normal blood gases and pH, and normal cerebral perfusion pressures. Hence, CPR is also called CPCR (Cardio-Pulmonary Cerebral Resuscitation).

Nuclear Medicine in Surgery

49

- What is nuclear medicine?
- Radionuclides used in thyroid diseases
- Radionuclide tests of thyroid
- Solitary thyroid nodule
- Thyroid cancer
- Other organ-systems

WHAT IS NUCLEAR MEDICINE?

Nuclear medicine uses small amounts of radionuclides to diagnose and treat a variety of diseases. Nuclear medicine determines the cause of the disease based on the function of the tissue and thus it differs from x-ray, utrasound or other radio- diagnostic test that determines the presence of disease based on structural appearance. In a nuclear medicine test, the radioactive material is tagged to a organ-specific pharmaceutical compound and introduced into the body by injection, ingestion or inhalation. A gamma camera is used to take pictures of the body. The camera detects the distribution of radiopharmaceutical in the organ being imaged and records this information on a computer screen or on film. Generally, nuclear medicine tests are not recommended for pregnant women . Nuclear medicine tests are non-invasive and provide minimum radiation exposure to the patient.

THYROID

The thyroid, an endocrine gland consists of two lobes connected by a narrow isthmus. It is situated anterior to the trachea, just below the larynx deep to the sternocleidomas-toid muscles of the neck at the level of C5-T1 vertebrae. The thyroid produces triiodothyronine (T3), thyroxine (T4), and calcitonin. The production of T3 and T4 are stimulated by TSH, (thyroid-stimulating hormone) from the pituitary gland and is involved in growth and metabolism. Calcitonin is involved with calcium uptake and calcium blood levels.

Thyroid disorders are among the most common endocrinological diseases for nuclear medicine studies.

Thyroid diseases can be of three types

1. **Decreased production of thyroid hormones**
   - Hashimoto's thyroiditis (myxoedema)
   - Nontoxic goitre (iodine deficiencies)
   - Neonatal goitre or cretinism
   - Riedel's thyroiditis

2. **Increased production of thyroid hormones**
   - Thyrotoxicosis (Graves' disease)
   - Toxic nodular goitre
   - Iatrogenic hyperthyroidism

3. **Tumours**
   - Thyroid carcinoma

RADIONUCLIDES USED IN THYROID DISEASES

Iodine- 123 (I^{123}) and Iodine - 131(I^{131}), the isotopes of iodine and Technetium -99m Pertechnetate (Tc 99m) are used for thyroid imaging. Iodine-125 is not used for imaging. It is primarily used for radioimmunoassays and other in vitro procedures.

Iodine-123 has a physical half-life of 13.6 hours gamma energy of 159keV. Dose: 200-400 uCi. **Iodine-131** has a physical half-life of 8.05 days and emits high-energy gamma (364 keV) and beta particles with average energy =192 keV, max energy = 607 keV. Beta energy is deposited within 2.2mm of its site of origin. Diagnostic dose: 2-5 mCi; Therapeutic dose:10-15 mCi for Graves' disease, Autonomously functioning toxic nodule and Toxic multinodular goitre; 50-250 mCi for Carcinoma thyroid.

Technetium-99m Pertechnetate has a physical half-life of 6 hours and gamma energy of 140 keV. Dose=3-10 mCi.

Iodine-125 has a physical half-life of 60.2 days and emits gamma energy of 35 keV.

RADIONUCLIDE TESTS OF THYROID

1. THYROID SCAN

The thyroid gland traps iodine and uses this to make thyroid hormone. Radioactive Iodine-123 and Iodine-131 are trapped by the thyroid gland by an active transport mechanism and further organified in the follicular cells similar to the stable iodine. Approximately 10% to 35% of a dose of radioactive iodine, given orally, is taken up by the thyroid gland within 24 hours.

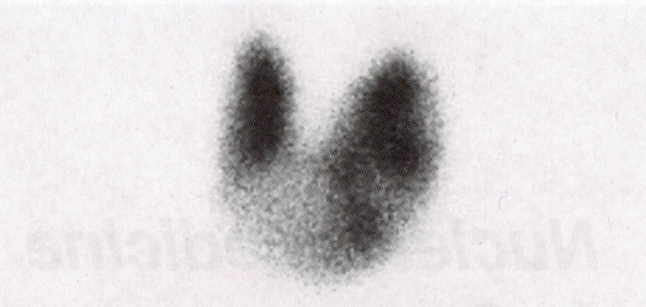

Fig. 49.2 Toxic multinodular goitre

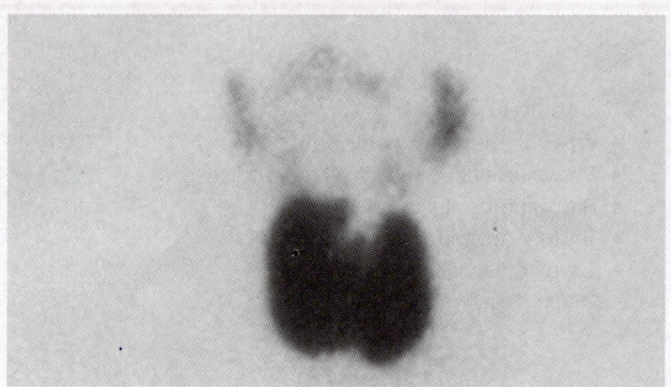

Fig. 49.3 Diffuse toxic goitre

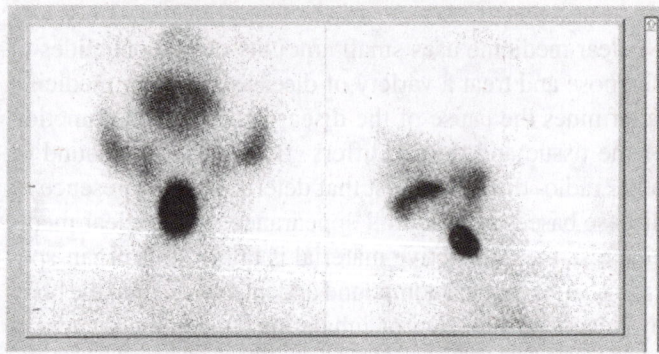

Fig. 49.4 Ectopic (lingual) thyroid

Technetium-99m Pertechnetate is trapped by the thyroid gland in the same manner as iodine (an active transport mechanism) but it does not undergo organification. It is administered intravenously. Only 2-4% of the administered dose is trapped in the thyroid and the maximum uptake occurs at 20 minutes after injection.

The test is safe since the radiation dose is very small. The gland is imaged by a gamma camera and the distribution within the gland of the radioisotope recorded (Fig. 49.1). The scan also gives an idea of the shape and size of the thyroid gland and can be used for patients with thyroid nod-

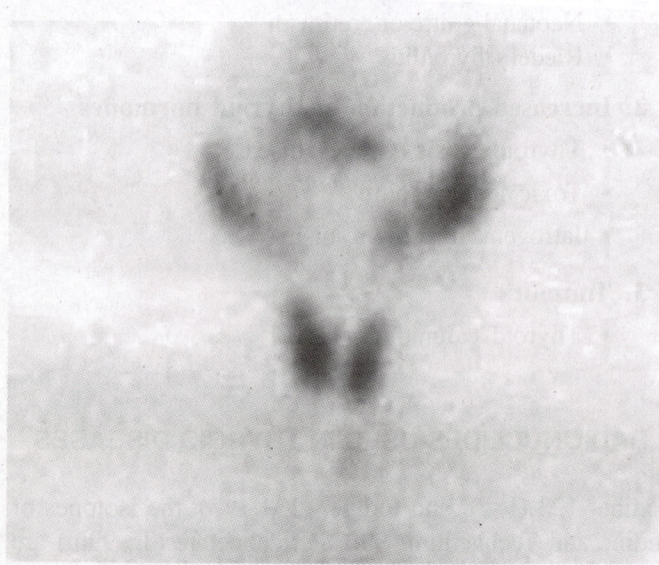

Fig. 49.1 Normal 99ᵐ Tc thyroid scan

ules to determine whether the nodule is functioning(Fig. 49.2). A hypofunctioning gland appears less intense than the salivary glands, a normal gland equal to the salivary glands, and a hyperfunctioning thyroid appears more intense than the salivary glands (Fig. 49.3). Ectopic thyroid tissue can be beautifully located by a thyroid scan (Fig. 49.4).

The normal distribution of iodine, and therefore its radio-isotopes is in the thyroid, salivary glands, gastric mucosa, small and large bowel, urinary bladder, liver, and breast (especially during lactation). Iodine undergoes both renal (up to 75% in 24 hours) and gastrointestinal excretion.

Pregnancy is an absolute contraindication to thyroid scanning, especially after the 12th week of gestation when the foetal thyroid begins to trap iodine. Both Iodine and Technetium isotopes cross the placenta easily. Breast feeding is a relative contraindication. Both Iodine and Technetium are secreted in the breast milk of lactating women, so nursing should be delayed for 48-72 hours following Tc99m, and for 2-3 weeks following I-131 imaging- essentially this translates to discontinuance of breast feeding.

Technetium-99m Pertechnetate is the preferred imaging agent when:

- Patient has been taking thyroid blocking agents (Propylthiouracil). Thiouracil blocks oxidation and organification of iodide following its uptake by the thyroid gland, but will not interfere with trapping of pertechnetate.

- Patient is unable to take medication orally

- The study must be completed in < 2 hrs

- Thyroid function (uptake measurement) is not necessary

2. RADIOACTIVE IODINE UPTAKE TEST (RAIU)

RAIU can be determined using either I-131 or I-123.

Dose: I-131 (25 μCi); I-123 (200-300 μCi).

A thyroid uptake probe is used to measure the radioactive counts over the thyroid-bed in the neck and also the background counts over the thigh region.

Normal 2-4 hour RAIU is generally between 5% to 15%. Normal 24 hour RAIU is between 15% to 35%.

% Uptake= [(net neck counts - net thigh counts) x 100] / (net standard counts)

The RAIU test provides a useful assessment of thyroid function: the higher the iodine uptake, the more active the gland as seen in Graves' disease.

In patients with hypothyroidism such as Hashimoto's disease, the % uptake may be low, normal or high depending on the steps affected in thyroid hormone synthesis. This is therefore of no value in establishing the diagnosis of hypothyroidism.

Indications

RAIU test may be helpful in the following clinical conditions:

1. To confirm hyperthyroidism
2. To calculate therapeutic dose of I-131
3. To determine autonomous thyroid tissue (i.e. toxic nodules, combined with thyroid scan)
4. To determine the cause of thyrotoxicosis*

* Thyrotoxicosis refers to a state of excess thyroid hormone in the body which may be due to overactivity of the thyroid gland (hyperthyroidism), or other causes such as inflammation of the gland (thyroiditis) or ingestion of excess thyroid hormone. In hyperthyroidism, RAIU uptake will be high while thyrotoxic patients with thyroiditis (Fig. 49.5) or who abuse thyroid hormones will have a low RAIU.

Factors decreasing RAIU uptake

Patient's iodine pool:

- **Dietary variations:** RAIU can be falsely elevated in patients who are iodine deficient.

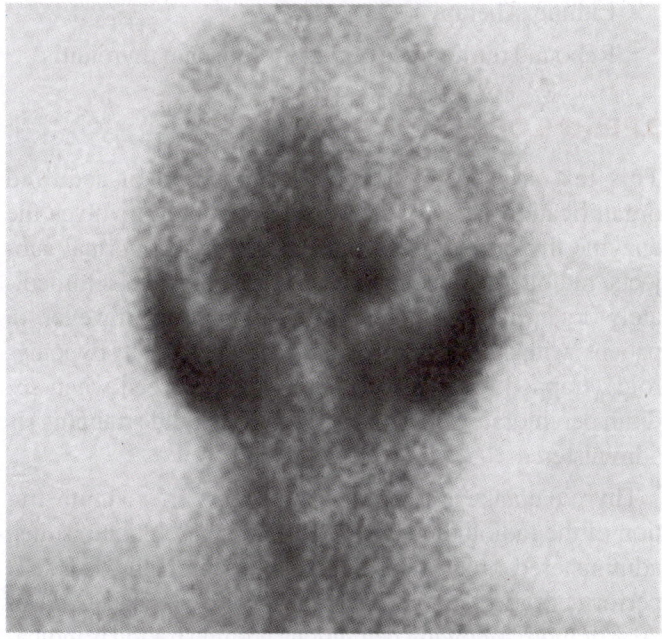

Fig. 49.5 Acute thyroiditis - no uptake

- **Renal function:** Poor renal function results in decreased excretion of iodine, the larger iodine pool will compete with the radiopharmaceutical for uptake thus falsely lowering RAIU.
- **Recent iodine contrast study:** The excess iodine will falsely lower the RAIU.

Medications:

- Antithyroid drugs: Propylthiouracil and methimazole result in a poor 24 hour scan because they block iodide oxidation and organification. Because the agents do not inhibit iodine trapping, a pertechnetate scan may be technically adequate.
- Thyroid hormone
- Amiodarone

Factors increasing RAIU uptake

- Hyperthyroidism (Graves' disease or TSH-secreting pituitary adenoma)
- Rebound following abrupt withdrawal of antithyroid medication
- Long term antithyroid therapy: Prolonged therapy may result in decreased circulating levels of T4, hence TSH levels will increase. This will accentuate radioiodine uptake.
- Enzyme e.g. thyroid peroxidase defects (high 2-4 hour uptake; low 24 hour uptake)
- Iodine starvation
- Lithium Therapy
- Rebound during recovery from subacute thyroiditis

3.PERCHLORATE WASHOUT TEST

This test is used to identify a congenital or acquired organification defect which most commonly involves the enzyme thyroid peroxidase or its activity. In normal subjects, radioiodine when taken up by the thyroid is immediately organified and bound to thyroglobulin. However, in patients with defects in peroxidase activity (usually hypothyroid), trapped radioiodine is rapidly discharged when sodium perchlorate (an inhibitor of thyroid iodide trapping) is administered.

Thyroid uptake is determined at 2 hours after administration of the radioiodine dose. Potassium perchlorate is then administered orally and a repeat measurement of RAIU performed after another 2 hours. A decrease in RAIU of 20% or more following perchlorate administration is indicative of organification defect.

SOLITARY THYROID NODULE

A palpable solitary thyroid nodule is a discrete swelling within a thyroid gland. The lifetime risk of developing a palpable thyroid nodule is 10%. By autopsy series, there is up to a 50% incidence of single or multiple nodules. Approximately 5% of palpable thyroid nodules are malignant.

EVALUATION OF THYROID NODULE

Thyroid nodules are evaluated because they may be malignant, cause hyperthyroidism or cause local compressive symptoms.

Work-up of a nodule includes the following:

I. Clinical Evaluation

a. History

Rate of nodule enlargement

Local compressive symptoms such as dysphagia, dyspnoea, cough, pain, hoarseness.

Symptoms of hyperthyroidism or hypothyroidism

History of radiation exposure

b. Physical examination

Vital signs- pulse, blood pressure, body weight

Thyroid examination

Evidence of local compressive symptoms

Presence of cervical lymphadenopathy

II. Lab Evaluation

1. Blood tests -

Serum TSH

Serum anti-thyroid peroxidase antibodies

Serum calcitonin

III. Thyroid imaging

a. Thyroid scintigraphy: Commonly thyroid scintigraphy is done with Tc-99m, I-123, and I-131. I-123 is often used because it is physiologic (both transported and organified) and it gives a reasonably low total body dose, but patient has to return at 24 hours making it a two-day procedure. Tc-99m has an advantage that images can be obtained the same day and the radiation dose is low. Occasionally there is the problem of discordant nodule when using Tc-99m (tumors may be hot on Tc-99m, cold on I-123). The possibility of discordant nodule arises because Tc-99m is only transported and not

Table 49.1 CURRENT APPROACH TO THYROID NODULE

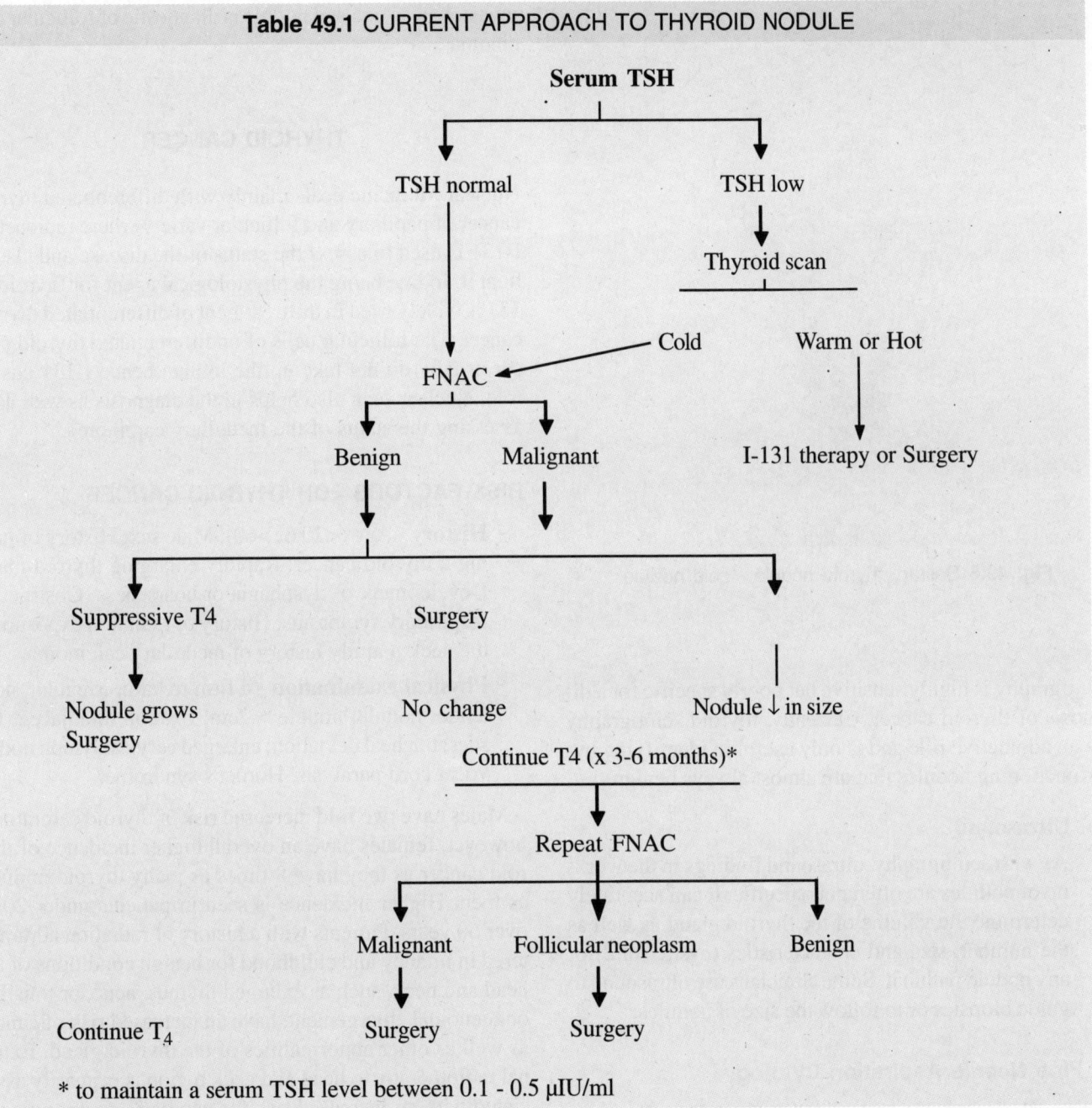

Serum TSH

TSH normal → FNAC

TSH low → Thyroid scan

Thyroid scan → Cold → FNAC

Thyroid scan → Warm or Hot → I-131 therapy or Surgery

FNAC → Benign, Malignant

Benign → Suppressive T4 → Nodule grows → Surgery

Malignant → Surgery → No change

→ Nodule ↓ in size

Continue T4 (x 3-6 months)*

Repeat FNAC

Malignant → Continue T$_4$

Follicular neoplasm → Surgery

Benign → Surgery

* to maintain a serum TSH level between 0.1 - 0.5 µIU/ml

organified, and some tumors can transport Tc-99m. I-131 is avoided for normal thyroid imaging because of the high radiation burden and poor imaging characteristics.

Scintigraphic findings

- Focal area of decreased radioisotope uptake is called a cold nodule (Fig. 49.6). Approximately 80% to 85% of nodules are cold. A cold nodule is of concern because it may be malignant. The likelihood

of carcinoma for a given cold nodule is considered to be between 15% to 20%.

- Multiple cold areas with regions of increased isotope uptake indicates a multinodular gland where there is a low incidence (<5%) of associated malignancy (Fig. 49.2)

- A focal area of increased uptake is called a hot nodule. A hot nodule almost never (<1%) harbours malignancy and instead represents either autonomous or hypertrophic adenoma.

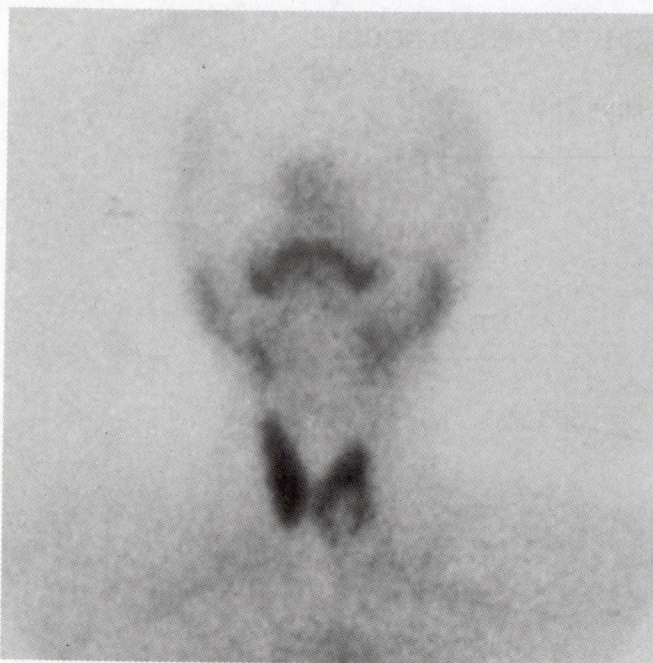

Fig. 49.6 Solitary thyroid nodule - cold nodule

Scintigraphy is highly sensitive but poorly specific for a diagnosis of thyroid cancer. Currently, thyroid scintigraphy has an adjunctive role and is only useful in identifying hyperfunctioning nodules that are almost always benign

b. Ultrasound

- As with scintigraphy, ultrasound findings in the workup of nodules are often non-specific. It can accurately determine the volume of the thyroid gland as well as the number, size and characteristics (cystic/solid) of any nodule within it. Some clinicians use ultrasound to guide biopsies or to follow the size of nodules.

IV. Fine Needle Aspiration Cytology

Fine needle aspiration cytology (FNAC) yields a diagnosis in 85% of specimens, with 75% being benign, 5% malignant and 20% suspicious of malignancy. The remaining 15% of specimens are nondiagnostic i.e., unsatisfactory for cytological interpretation. The sensitivity of FNAC for detection of a malignant lesion is approximately 83%, and the specificity is about 92%. Problems with FNAC include difficulty in differentiating follicular adenoma from carcinoma, false positives in Hashimoto's thyroiditis, and false negatives due to inadequate sampling.

Histopathological evidence of capsular and/or vascular invasion in an excised nodule is diagnostic of follicular carcinoma.

THYROID CANCER

Nuclear Medicine deals mainly with differentiated thyroid cancer of papillary and follicular variety where radioactive I-131 is used to assess the status of the disease and also to treat it. Iodine being the physiological agent for thyroid, I-131 is widely used in the treatment of differentiated thyroid cancer. The follicular cells of undifferentiated thyroid cancer usually do not take up the iodine; hence I-131 has no role. Nuclear scan also helps in the diagnosis as well as in assessing the status of the medullary carcinoma.

RISK FACTORS FOR THYROID CANCER

- **History** - Age (<20 or >60); Male sex; History of having a thyroid cancer; Rapidly enlarging thyroid mass; Development of dysphagia or hoarseness; Obstructive respiratory symptoms; History of radiation exposure to the neck; Family history of medullary carcinoma.

- **Physical examination** - a firm to hard, irregular, non-tender nodule; nodule > 2cm; fixation to adjacent tissues; tracheal deviation; enlarged cervical lymph nodes, vocal cord paralysis, Horner's syndrome.

Males have two fold increased risk of thyroid carcinoma; however, females have an overall higher incidence of thyroid cancer as they have 8 times as many thyroid nodules as men. Higher incidence is seen in patients under 20 or over 60 years. Patients with a history of radiation administered in infancy and childhood for benign conditions of the head and neck, such as enlarged thymus, acne, or tonsillar or adenoidal enlargement, have an increased risk of cancer as well as other abnormalities of the thyroid gland. External radiotherapy to head and neck region is primarily associated with an increased risk for papillary carcinoma, and to a lesser degree follicular carcinoma. Exposure as a consequence of nuclear fall-out has also been associated with a high risk of thyroid cancer, especially in children.

PROGNOSTIC FACTORS

Poor prognostic factors for differentiated thyroid cancer:

- Patient age >40 yrs. at diagnosis
- Large tumours (>4.0 cm)
- Male sex

- Advanced tumor grade
- Tumors with local extension
- Bilateral cervical or mediastinal lymph node metastases
  - Distant metastasis
  - Extensive vascular and capsular invasion

Thyroid cancer commonly presents as a painless nodule with the features discussed above. The diagnostic work-up of solitary thyroid nodule has been discussed in the previous section of Solitary Thyroid Nodule.

Radionuclide imaging identifies the nodule as functioning or non-functioning. About 15% of the nodules are functioning nodules. Remaining 85% are non-functioning nodules, also called as cold nodules. Incidence of carcinoma in solitary cold nodules ranges from 5% to 40%. Functioning nodules have a very low probability of thyroid malignancy i.e., ~ 1%.

For the definitive diagnosis of thyroid cancer Fine Needle Aspiration Cytology is a simple, less time consuming and the most cost-effective tool. The sensitivity of FNAC to diagnose papillary carcinoma is high whereas lowest for follicular carcinoma due to its inability to differentiate cytologically benign from malignant follicular growth. Examination of paraffin sections (after performing Excision Biopsy) is required to demonstrate capsular and vascular invasion by follicular cells and to diagnose follicular carcinoma.

Usually, papillary carcinomas metastasise via the lymphatic system while the follicular carcinomas metastasise via the haematogenous route.

MANAGEMENT

Management of all follicular carcinomas and of papillary carcinomas is total thyroidectomy followed by radioiodine ablation.

Post-thyroidectomy, patient should be advised to avoid intake of any iodine containing medication (including thyroxine) or application of any iodine containing topical agents for six weeks. This is to elevate the serum TSH level beyond 30 µU/ml prior to therapy. If the TSH level is less than 30, functioning thyroid metastasis may not be identified on diagnostic scans, and may not accumulate sufficient I-131 during therapy. Serum TSH level of more than 30 µU/ml will stimulate iodine uptake in functioning metastasis. TSH stimulation with human TSH should be considered for patients with TSH values less than 30 µU/ml.

I-131 Imaging

- **Pre thyroidectomy:** Thyroid carcinomas almost invariably appear as cold areas on routine thyroid scanning. Dose of I-131 = 100 µCi.
- **Post thyroidectomy:** Whole body I-131 imaging to detect the residual (Fig. 49.7) as well as metastatic thyroid tissue. Dose of I-131 = 2 - 3 mCi.
- Follow-up of the patients after radioiodine therapy.

I-131 Ablation

The ablation therapy with I-131 is performed to destroy the residual thyroid tissue and also the functioning metastatic tissue simultaneously. A dose of 30,000 rads is needed to be delivered to the residual thyroid tissue.

I-131 Ablation therapy Protocol

Fixed amounts of I-131 may be given accordingly:

- Residual thyroid bed: 100 mCi
- Regional Metastasis (Cervical Nodes): 150-175 mCi
- Lung Metastasis: 175-200 mCi
- Skeletal Metastasis: 200 -250 mCi

Guideline for maximum dose administration

- Blood dose should be no more than 200 rads to reduce marrow toxicity. Doses of this level are associated with mild, transient decrease in blood cell counts without permanent suppression.
- Retained whole body activity of no more than 120 mCi at 48 hours (or 80 mCi in patients with lung metastasis to avoid potential pulmonary fibrosis)

Following high dose I-131 administration, patients are hospitalized in isolation until the retained radioactivity is less than 15mCi or the radiation exposure rate from the patient is less than 2.5 mR/hr at one meter. At the time of discharge from the hospital, whole body scan should be performed. It can detect new lesions because of higher I-131 dose administered for therapy (Fig. 49.8) Whole body scans can detect new lesions in up to 15% of patients. Post therapy, patients are advised to avoid close contact with anyone for two weeks. This is to avoid unnecessary radiation exposure to the public.

Benefits of I-131 Therapy

- Decreases local recurrence
- Improves survival in patients following local recurrence

- Prolongs survival in patients with lung or bone metastasis
- Eliminates the thyroid gland as source of thyroglobulin

Side effects of I-131 Thyroid Ablation Therapy

- **Oedema** - painless swelling of the neck occurs within 24 - 48 hrs. When there is a substantial mass of residual tissue as after a hemithyroidectomy or a considerable mass of inoperable recurrence of thyroid cancer. It responds well to large doses of corticosteroids and is transient lasting for 3 - 4 days.
- Sialoadenitis
  - **Acute sialoadenitis** - pain, tenderness and swelling of the salivary glands occurring within 24 hours when the competing thyroid remnant tissue is minimal. The use of sialogogue in the form of hard sour candies or lemon reduces this effect.
  - Chronic sialoadenitis - dryness of mouth, altered taste.
- **Thyroid storm** - May occur with extensive follicular metastasis due to release of large amounts of thyroid hormone, typically seen 2 to 10 days post treatment.
- **GI symptoms** - nausea and vomiting.
- Radiation effect on gonads and fertility
  - **Male gonadal function** - Short-term infertility has been documented. It is transient and dose dependent. Good hydration and frequent voiding (every 2 hours) minimizes the testicular dose.
  - **Female gonadal function** - Transient amenorrhea has been documented. I-131 therapy has not been shown to reduce fertility of treated patients or increase the risk of congenital abnormalities in their offspring especially if an interval of 2 to 3 years has elapsed after treatment.
- **Minimal bone marrow suppression** - Transient pancytopenia with a nadir at about 6 weeks post therapy especially when the dose delivered to the blood cells is no more than 200 rads. Recovery is spontaneous.
- **Radiation pneumonitis and pulmonary fibrosis** - may be a complication in patients with lung metastasis. The risk can be decreased by restricting the whole body retention at 48 hours to less than 80 mCi.
- **Cerebral oedema or spinal cord compression** - in patients with metastasis to the central nervous system.
- Radiation sickness - headache, nausea, vomiting - occurs in Dose > 200mCi.
- Malignant neoplasm

- **Leukemia** - The risk for Acute myelogenous leukemia is only minimally increased above the general population with a peak incidence 2 to 10 years post therapy (0.5% increased risk). Patients at risk are generally above the age of 50 and have received a cumulative dose of more than 800 mCi. The risk is greatest when this large dose has been given over a short period of time (few months). These patients have usually received a blood dose greater than 200 rads. The lifetime risk of leukemia is so small that it does not outweigh the benefit of treatment with I-131. Moreover the mortality from tumour recurrence exceeds that from leukemia by 4 to 40 fold.
- **Bladder carcinoma** - There may be a slight increased incidence of bladder carcinoma.
- **Other malignancies** - breast carcinoma, salivary carcinoma, melanoma. These have probably an increased risk in the general population rather than a consequence of I-131 therapy.

Post-Therapy Hormonal Treatment

Thyroid hormone (T4) suppression therapy is effective in the management of differentiated thyroid carcinoma and doses sufficient to suppress TSH, decrease the risk of recurrence. This is because well differentiated thyroid cancer responds to TSH stimulation, and grows more slowly in the absence of TSH.

Follow-up Post-Ablation Screening

Post-therapy follow-up whole body I-131 scans and serum thyroglobulin assays can detect the presence of residual or metastatic disease and should be done at not less than 6 months after I-131 ablation therapy. Thyroid gland being the only source of thyroglobulin production in the body, serum thyroglobulin appears to be the most sensitive test for determining the presence of persistent or recurrent well differentiated thyroid cancer. Thyroglobulin levels should be undetectable in post ablation patients. Thyroid hormone (T4) suppression therapy has to be stopped for 6 weeks before a whole body I-131 scan. Withdrawal of thyroxine therapy results in an increase of endogenous thyroid stimulating hormone (TSH) and increased functional activity of any residual as well as metastatic thyroid tissue (thyroglobulin synthesis, I-131 uptake). However, withdrawing thyroxine induces hypothyroidism, which may not be well tolerated by the patient, and prolonged elevation of serum TSH levels may theoretically stimulate the growth of metastasis. As an alternative to hormonal withdrawal, exogenous

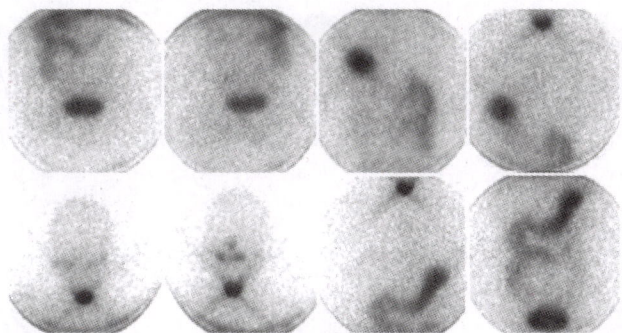

Fig. 49.7 Carcinoma thyroid - pretherapy whole body scan

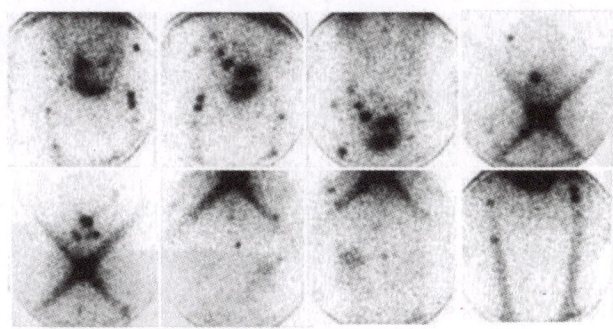

Fig. 49.8 Carcinoma thyroid - post therapy whole body scan of the same patient as in Fig. 49.7

TSH can be used to elevate serum TSH levels. Recently, a highly purified, recombinant form of the naturally occurring human protein TSH (Thyrogen) has been developed for use in elevating TSH levels in patients prior to both radioiodine scanning and thyroglobulin testing, while remaining on their hormone replacement therapy. A thyroglobulin level of >10 ng/ml is seen in patients with residual or metastatic lesions.

(Repeat high dose I-131 therapy)

High dose I-131 therapy is planned if the follow-up whole body scan show any I-131 concentrating tissue and a serum thyroglobulin level of more than 10 ng/ml.

If follow-up whole body scans do not show any I-131 concentrating tissue and the serum thyroglobulin level is less than 10 ng/ml, the patient can be left on suppressive doses of thyroxine with six-monthly or annual check-up on serum thyroglobulin only. Subsequently, a serum thyroglobulin level of more than 5 ng/ml is taken as an indicator of recurrence of thyroid cancer.

Medullary carcinoma of thyroid

Medullary carcinoma arises from the parafollicular C-cells and accounts for only 1 to 5% of all thyroid malignancies. The role of nuclear medicine in medullary carcinoma thyroid is limited to diagnosis only. Imaging with 20 mCi of 99mTc-**DMSA** (V) detects the thyroidal carcinoma in the neck as well as the extrathyroidal spread.

LIVER AND SPLEEN

Liver and spleen have wide functions. Radionuclide imaging depends on the function common to both i.e., phagocytosis.

The most commonly used agent is 99m Technetium sulphur colloid, with an average particle size of 0.3-1 μm.

The administered activity is usually 4-5 mCi for planar imaging and 8-10 mCi for Single Photon Emission Computer Tomography (SPECT.)

Uptake and distribution of sulphur colloid in the liver reflect both the distribution of functioning reticuloendothelial cells and the distribution of hepatic perfusion.

In normal scan there is homogenous distribution of 99mTc Sulphur Colloid throughout the organ (Fig. 49.9). **Evaluation of the liver spleen includes**

1. Size, shape and position of the liver and spleen
2. The homogeneity of the activity within the organs
3. The presence of any focal defects in activity
4. The relative distribution of colloid among the liver spleen and bone marrow.

Any localized space occupying process in the liver may present as a focal area of decreased activity (referred to as a defect).

Differential diagnosis of focal hepatic lesions on 99mTc Sulphur Colloid scans

Decreased Uptake

- Metastasis (especially colon)
- Cyst
- Hepatoma
- Adenoma
- Haematoma
- Haemangioma
- Abscess

Increased Uptake

- Focal Nodular Hyperplasia

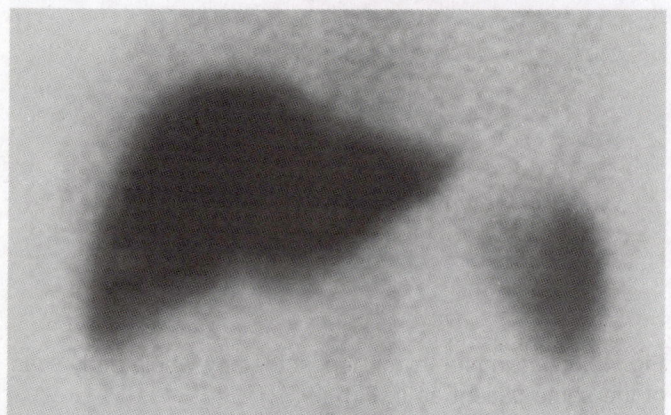

Fig. 49.9 Normal liver and spleen scan

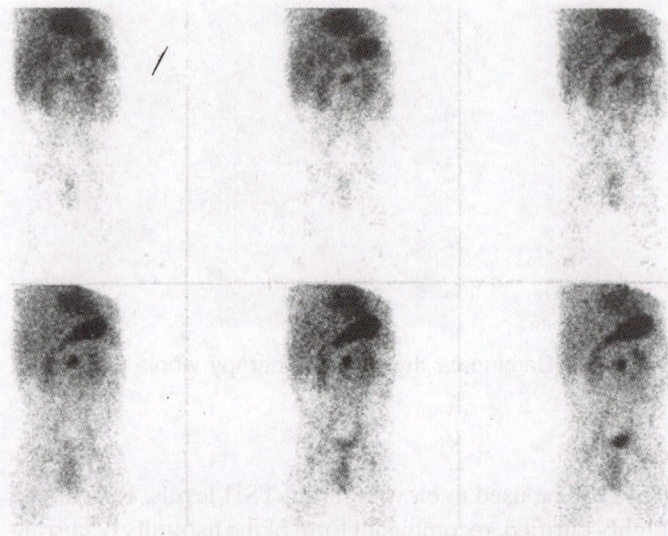

Fig. 49.10 Meckel's diverticulum

- Cirrhosis with Regenerating Nodule
- Budd Chiari Syndrome
- Superior Vena Caval Obstruction.

Splenic Imaging

On the posterior and anterior views of a technetium colloid scan the normal spleen exhibits homogenous activity equal to or less than that of the liver.

Solitary or multiple spleenic defects may be produced by a number of abnormalities. Therefore, careful correlation with the clinical history is necessary.

Isotope imaging of the spleen is also possible with 99mTc or 51Cr labeled heat damaged red cells which are sequestered by the spleen.

MECKEL'S DIVERTICULUM

Meckel's diverticulum occurs in about 2% of the population. The most common presentation in a child is painless rectal bleeding. Nearly in all cases of bleeding, ectopic gastric mucosa with or without ulceration can be seen in the diverticula.The investigation is based on the visualisation of the ectopic mucosa with intravenously administered 99mTc pertechnetate. The study consists of intravenous administration of 10-15 mCi of pertechnetate in case of adults and 200-300μCi/kg in children. Anterior images of the abdomen are acquired for 45-60 min. A typical positive scan consists of a focal area of increased activity in the right lower quadrant or in the mid abdomen which does not move with time as in case of GI bleed (Fig. 49.10)

Several pharmacological interventions have been tried to increase the sensitivity of this imaging. These include the use of cimetidine to block the release of pertechnetate from the ectopic gastric mucosa, pentagastrin to enhance the mucosal uptake of the tracer, and glucagons to prevent the small bowel movement.

GASTROINTESTINAL BLEEDING

A variety of radiopharmaceuticals can be used in the detection of gastrointestinal bleed .The commonest of these are the 99mTc red blood cells and the 99mTc Sulphur Colloid. The accuracy of endoscsopy in making the diagnosis of the upper GI bleed is around 90%. Significant background activity in the upper abdomen and the diagnostic efficacy of endoscopy in the upper GI have primarily limited nuclear imaging techniques to lower GI bleed.

Preoperative localisation of the bleeding site (Fig. 49.11) helps better in angiography and surgical intervention.

The commonest causes of lower GI bleeding in adults are diverticular disease, angiodysplasia, neoplasms, and inflammatory bowel disease which at times are intermittent in nature. Angiography may be negative in patients who are having intermittent bleeding or bleeding rates below 1ml/min. With radionuclide techniques bleeding as low as 0.1ml/min can also be visualized. The technique is most suited for patients who have active but intermittent bleeding.

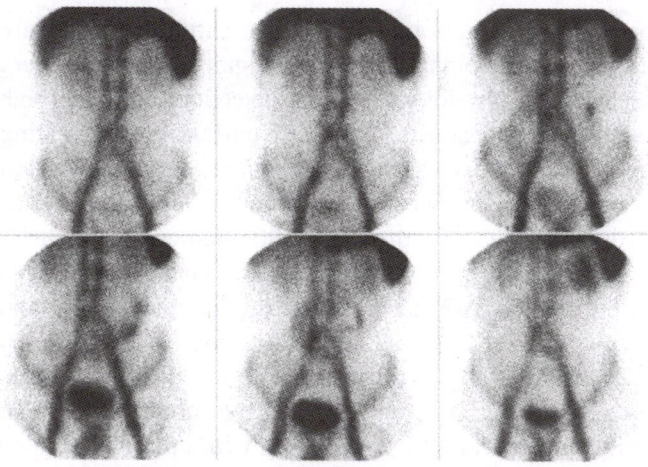

Fig. 49.11 Gastrointestinal bleed

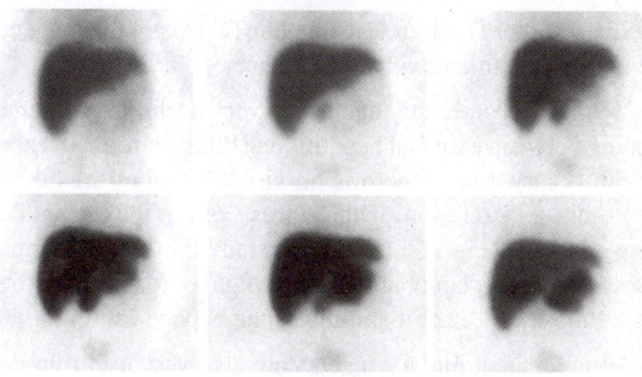

Fig. 49.12 Normal hepatobiliary scan

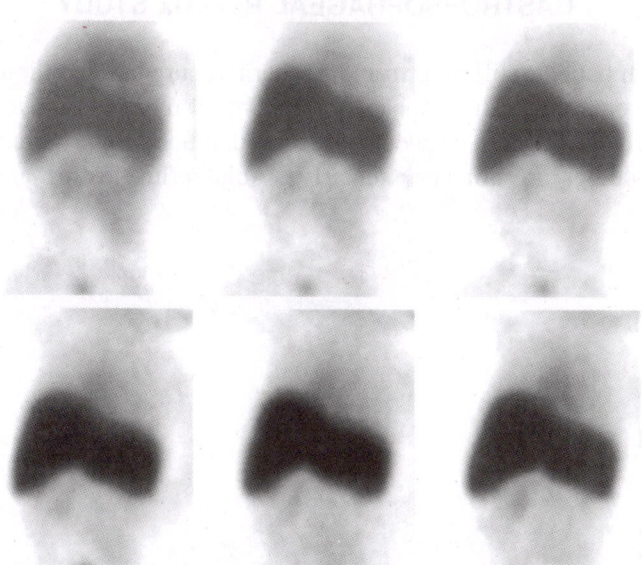

Fig. 49.13 Biliary atresia

99mTc labeled red blood cells are the agents of choice for a patient who has intermittent bleeding with a sensitivity of greater than 90%. With red blood cells most bleeding sites will show increased concentration of the tracer at the site of bleed which progresses distally in the bowel. If the activity remains static then vascular anomalies like aneurysm or vascular angiodysplasia should be suspected.

HEPATOBILIARY IMAGING

Development of 99mTc labelled hepatobiliary agents enables accurate and convenient imaging in acute and chronic biliary disease. Common indications are for acute (calculous, acalculous) cholecystitis, biliary patency, identification of biliary leak and in neonates differentiation of biliary atresia from neonatal hepatitis. **99mTc Mebrofenin is the most commonly used pharmaceutical nowdays.** It can demonstrate biliary visualisation with bilirubin level upto 30-40 mg/dl. Mebrofenin uptake and excretion follows the same pathway as bilirubin only it does not get conjugated like bilirubin.

For elective studies the patient is given nothing by mouth beginning at midnight the night before the study. Subsequent to the intravenous injection of 3-10 mCi of 99mTc mebrofenin sequential anterior images of the abdomen are acquired, with the patient in the supine position. In a normal patient sufficient mebrofenin is present in the liver by 5 min to allow good visualisation of the liver. After 10 -15 min there is gradual clearance of the pharmaceutical from the liver. The major hepatic ducts and the common ducts are visualized first, next the gall bladder is visualized as the labelled

bile flows through the cystic duct. In the presence of a patent common duct, activity flows promptly into the duodenum and proximal small bowel. So normal visualisation of these structures is complete by 1 hour (Fig. 49.12)

Hepatobiliary study is of great importance in the diagnosis of acute cholecystitis. Usually there is no visualisation of the gall bladder over a period of 4 hours after injection in a case of acute cholecystitis. Delayed visualisation of the gall bladder but within 4 hours suggests the presence of chronic cholecystitis. **Accuracy of the diagnosis of acute cholecystitis by scintigraphy is more than 95%.**

Lack of visualisation of the biliary tree with good visualisation of the liver is seen in cases of acute complete obstruction of the common bile duct.

The localisation and confirmation of the biliary leak after

biliary surgery or trauma using 99mTc hepatobiliary agents can be done in a noninvasive manner.

99mTc hepatobiliary agents are very useful in differentiating between neonatal hepatitis and biliary atresia. In cases with biliary atresia there is no visualisation of the biliary tree or any excretion of the tracer even in the 24 hrs delayed image (Fig. 49. 13) In this study it is better to prime the liver with phenobarbitol 5mg /kg/day for 5-7 days before the study since it stimulates the hepatic excretion .

99mTc hepatobiliary agents are also very useful in detecting hepatobiliary leaks after surgery or trauma.

GASTROESOPHAGEAL REFLUX STUDY

In patients suffering from heartburn, regurgitation, bilious vomiting, gastroesophageal reflux have to be investigated so that they can be adequately treated. Fluoroscopic barium studies are not very sensitive. Acid reflux testing and oesophageal manometry, require intubation and are uncomfortable for the patients. Scintigraphy studies are very sensitive and physiological for the detection of reflux in both pediatrics and adults. An adult patient comes fasting overnight to the department, he is made to drink 150 ml of orange juice combined with 150 ml of 0.1 Molar normal hydrochloric acid (with around 500 microcuries of 99mTc Sulphur colloid), an additional 30 ml of plain water is given to the patient and placed under the gamma camera and serial images acquired with the abdominal binder at 0,20,40,60,80, and 100 mm of Hg. Position, pressure, presence of acid are all used to aggravate reflux. **In children the tracer is given along with milk** (also called Milk Scan), abdominal binders are not used.

It is a very sensitive method of studying pulmonary aspiration. This study being noninvasive is used in the detection as well as in the evaluation of various therapeutic modalities.

50

X-rays

- Plain X-rays
- Barium meal
- Barium swallow
- Barium enema
- T-tube cholangiography
- ERCP
- Aortography
- Splenoportography

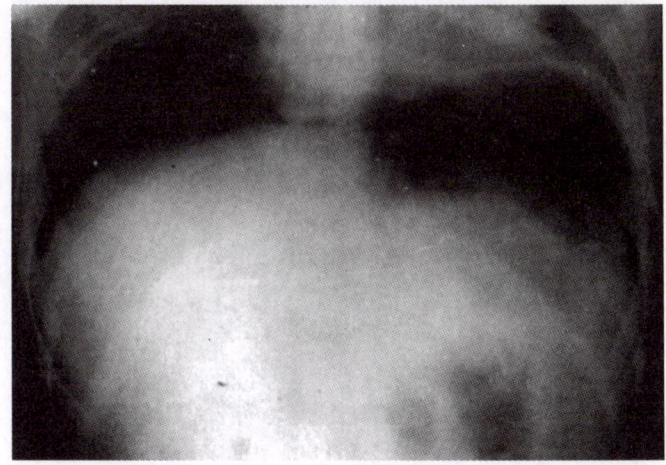

Fig. 50.1 Plain X-ray abdomen showing collection of free gas under the right dome of the diaphragm

I. PLAIN X-RAY ABDOMEN SHOWING COLLECTION OF FREE GAS UNDER THE RIGHT DOME OF THE DIAPHRAGM

Normally, fundic air bubble is present on the left side. Hence, importance is given to the gas on the right side.

1. What are the causes of free gas under the right dome of the diaphragm?

1. Perforation of hollow viscus. Examples:
   - Duodenal ulcer, gastric ulcer
   - Perforation of enteric ulcer
   - Perforation of Meckel's diverticulum
   - Malignant ulcers—colonic, gastric
   - Perforation of the tuberculous ulcer—ileum

2. Abdominal stab injury

3. Laparotomy

4. Tubal insufflation test done for tubal patency

2. Any other finding in the X-ray?

- **Ground glass appearance** indicates significant fluid in the peritoneal cavity.

3. How do you manage a case of perforated duodenal ulcer?

- With antibiotic coverage, Ryle's tube aspiration and early resuscitation with intravenous fluids, exploratory laparotomy is done. Identify the site of perforation which is in the first part of the duodenum and perforation is closed by using non-absorbable sutures. Omentum can be used to reinforce the suture line. This is called as **Roscoe Graham** operation. Corrugated red rubber drain or tube drain is used to drain peritoneal cavity.

4. Will you do elective surgery like G.J, and vagotomy or HSV at this stage?

- Since the **general condition** of the **patient is very**

very poor, because of hypovolaemic and septic shock, elective surgery is not done.

5. *What are the stages of duodenal ulcer perforation?*

   • Stage of chemical peritonitis

   • Stage of illusion or dilution

   • Stage of bacteria peritonitis

II. PLAIN X-RAY ABDOMEN SHOWING MULTIPLE GAS AND FLUID LEVELS

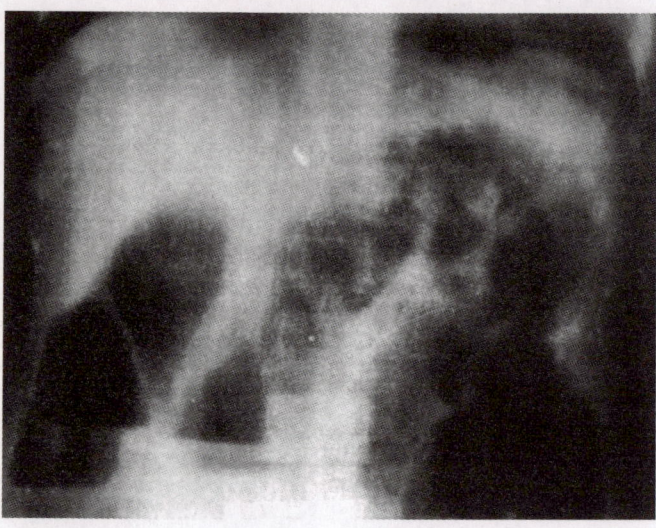

Fig. 50.2 Plain X-ray abdomen showing multiple gas and fluid levels

1. *What is the diagnosis?*

   • Since jejunal loops are prominently seen and loops are centrally located, it is probably terminal ileal obstruction.

2. *What are the common causes of terminal ileal obstruction ?*

   1. Tuberculous stricture

   2. Bands - congenital

   3. Adhesions

   4. 'Worm Ball' in children

   5. Obstructed hernia

3. *How do you identify jejunum, ileum and colon in a plain X-ray?*

   • Jejunum—valvulae conniventis—regularly placed mucosal folds placed opposite each other.

   • Ileum — No character — CHARACTERLESS LOOP OF WANGENSTEEN

   • Colon—HAUSTRATIONS— large incomplete mucosal folds NOT PLACED opposite each other.

4. *How do you treat tuberculous strictures?*

   • Resection and end to end anastomosis.

5. *Any other surgical procedure can be done?*

   • **Stricturoplasty** (like pyloroplasty)

III. PLAIN X-RAY SHOWING RADIO-OPAQUE SHADOW IN THE RIGHT UPPER ABDOMEN

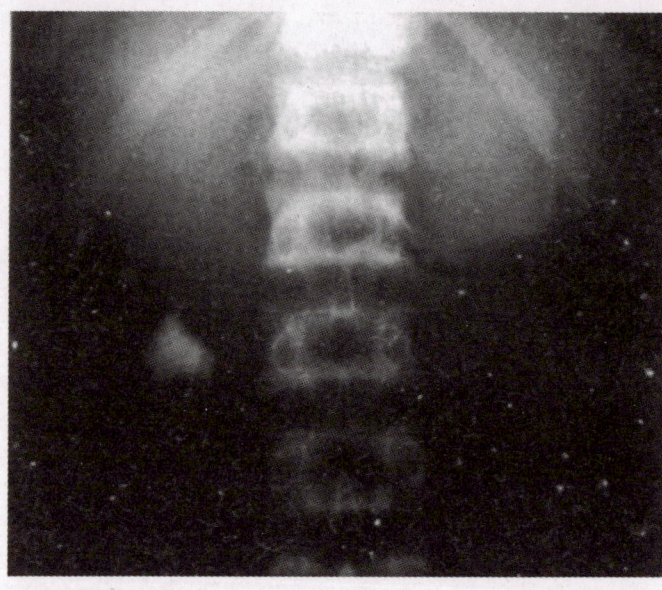

Fig. 50.3 Plain X-ray abdomen showing radio-opaque shadow in the right upper abdomen

1. *What is the diagnosis?*

   • Probably renal stone

2. *Why is it not a gallstone?*

   • The location of the stone is at lower level when compared to gall stone

   • The shape of the stone suggests that it is a stone in the pelvis growing within calyces.

3. *What do you call such a stone ?*

   • Staghorn calculus

4. *What type of X-ray is ideal to distinguish renal stone from gall bladder stone?*

   • Lateral view

5. What will be the findings in case of renal stones in a lateral picture ?

- Renal stones are found superimposed on vertebral bodies. On the other hand, gall stones are found anterior to it.

IV. PLAIN X-RAY ABDOMEN SHOWING RADIO-OPAQUE SHADOWS IN THE REGION OF GALL BLADDER

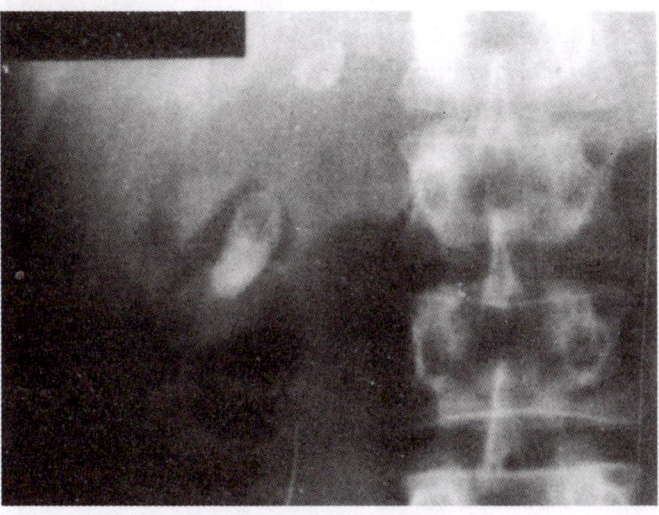

Fig. 50.4 Plain X-ray abdomen showing radio-opaque shadows in the region of gall bladder

1. What is the diagnosis?

- Probably gallstone

2. What percentage of gall stones are visible in a plain X-ray?

- Only 10%

3. What is the reason for that?

- The calcium content in gall stones is very less.

4. What are the causes of radiopaque shadow in the abdomen ?

- Gall stones
- Renal stones
- Pancreatic stones
- Renal tuberculosis
- 'Chip' fracture of the transverse process of the vertebrae.
- Calcified lymph nodes—tuberculosis.
- Faecoliths
- Phleboliths

5. What is the treatment of symptomatic gall stones?

- Cholecystectomy.

V. X-RAY CHEST P/A VIEW SHOWING MULTIPLE ROUND SHADOWS IN BOTH LUNG FIELDS

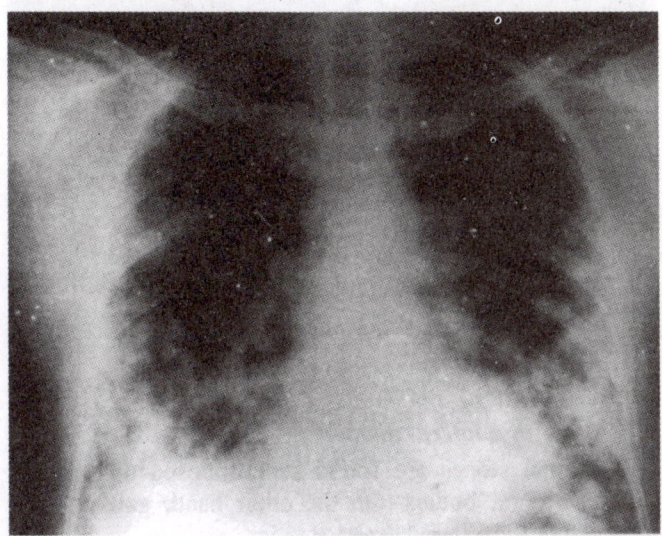

Fig. 50.5 X-ray chest PA view showing multiple round shadows in both lung fields

1. What is the diagnosis?

- Bilateral chest secondaries

2. What are they called?

- **Cannon ball** secondaries

3. Why are secondaries in the lung round?

- Lung is an elastic tissue, it has resilience. Hence during the act of inspiration and expiration, equal amount of pressure is exerted on secondaries, which are growing. Hence, they tend to become round.

4. What are the common causes of chest secondaries?

1. Carcinoma breast
2. Carcinoma testis
3. Malignant melanoma
4. Hepatoma
5. Renal cell carcinoma
6. Sarcoma

5. Any other differential diagnosis?

- Miliary tuberculosis: The shadows will be very small and numerous.

VI. X-RAY CERVICAL VERTEBRAE WITH UPPER RIBS SHOWING BILATERAL CERVICAL RIBS

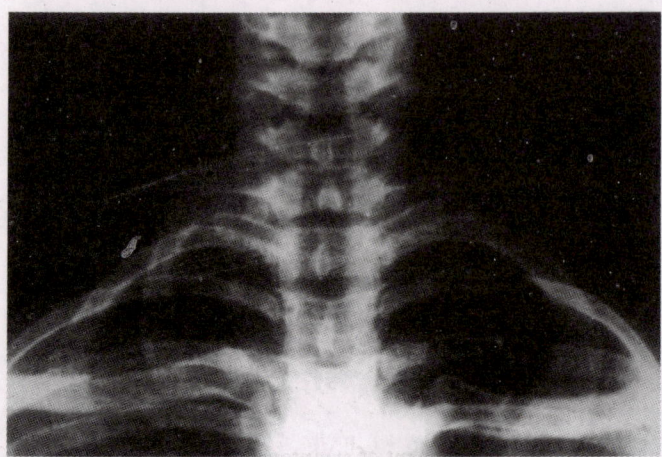

Fig. 50.6 X-ray cervical vertebrae with upper ribs showing bilateral cervical ribs

1. What is a cervical rib?
- It is an extra rib arising from 7th cervical vertebra.

2. What are 4 types of cervical rib?
- Incomplete bony
- Complete bony with anterior expanded bony end
- Partly fibrous, partly bony
- Complete fibrous band

3. What variety gives rise to vascular symptoms?
- The fibrous band variety

4. What is your finding here?
- On the right side, it is complete variety and on the left side, it is incomplete.

5. If cervical rib is symptomatic, what is the treatment?
- Extraperiosteal excision of cervical rib which means removal of the rib along with the periosteum. Some surgeons also do cervical sympathectomy to decrease vasomotor tone of vessels.

VII. BARIUM SWALLOW SHOWING INTRINSIC, IRREGULAR, PERSISTENT, FILLING DEFECT IN THE LOWER OESOPHAGUS

1. What is the diagnosis?
- Carcinoma lower one-third of oesophagus

2. What are the other findings?
- Proximal shouldering is very characteristic of malignancy.

3. How do you confirm the diagnosis ?
- Oesophagoscopy and biopsy

4. If biopsy report is adenocarcinoma, what is the treatment?
- Operable—oesophagogastrectomy
- Inoperable—To relieve dysphagia, metallic stents can be introduced thus one can avoid surgery

5. What are the pre-malignant conditions?
- Achalasia cardia
- Reflux oesophagitis
- Corrosive stricture
- Plummer-Vinson syndrome

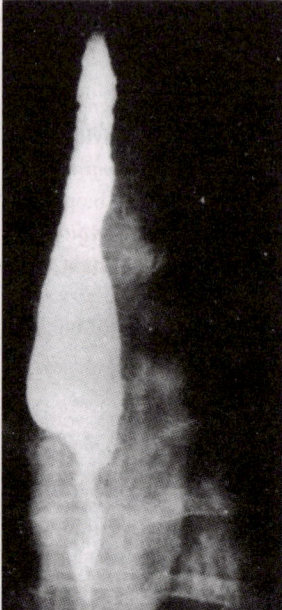

Fig. 50.7 Barium swallow showing intrinsic, irregular, persistent filling defect in the lower oesophagus

VIII. BARIUM SWALLOW SHOWING AN EXTENSIVE, IRREGULAR, FILLING DEFECT INVOLVING MIDDLE ONE-THIRD OF OESOPHAGUS

1. What is the diagnosis?
- Carcinoma middle one-third of oesophagus

2. How do you confirm the diagnosis?
- Oesophagoscopy and biopsy

3. What will be the biopsy report?
- Squamous cell carcinoma

4. What other investigations are necessary in such case?
- Bronchoscopy to see infiltration into the bronchus

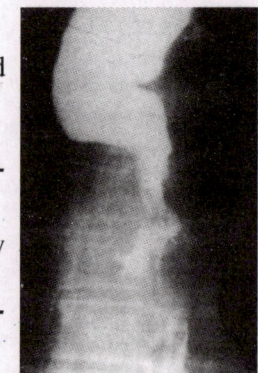

Fig. 50.8 Barium swallow showing an extensive, irregular filling defect involving middle one-third of oesophagus

5. *Looking at this advanced lesion, what is probably the best treatment for this patient?*

   • Radiotherapy followed by dilatation of the oesophagus, since chances of fibrosis and narrowing of the lumen following radiotherapy are high.

IX. BARIUM MEAL SHOWING INTRINSIC, IRREGULAR, PERSISTENT, FILLING DEFECT INVOLVING PYLORIC ANTRUM

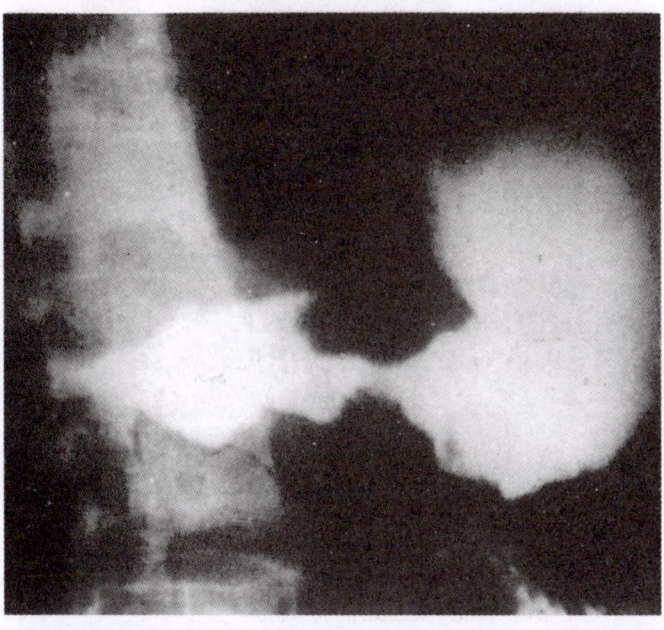

Fig. 50.9 Barium meal showing intrinsic, irregular, persistent filling defect involving pyloric antrum

1. *What is the diagnosis?*

   • Carcinoma pyloric antrum

2. *How do you confirm diagnosis?*

   • Gastroscopic biopsy

3. *What will be the. biopsy report?*

   • Adenocarcinoma

4. *What is the treatment, if it is operable?*

   • Lower radical partial gastrectomy

5. *What structures are removed in the operation?*

   • Growth along with 60-70% of distal stomach, omentum, enlarged regional nodes such as prepyloric, suprapyloric, infrapyloric, left and right gastric nodes, are removed, followed by gastrojejunal anastomosis.

X. BARIUM MEAL X-RAY SHOWING ENORMOUS DILATATION OF THE STOMACH AND FAILURE OF BARIUM TO FILL INTO THE DISTAL INTESTINE

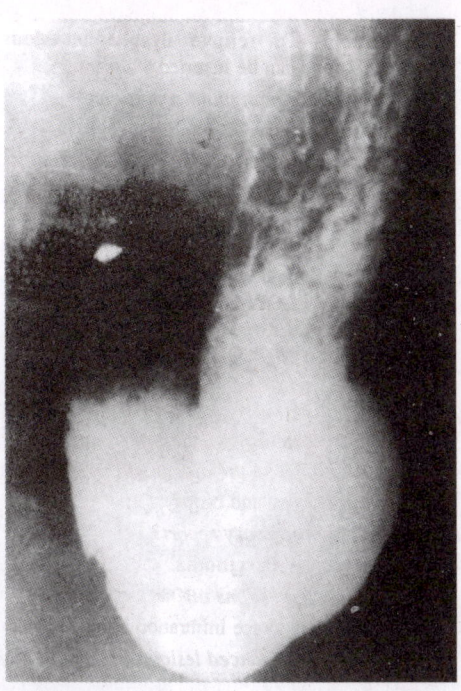

Fig. 50.10 Barium meal showing enormous dilatation of the stomach and failure of barium to fill into the distal intestine

1. *What is the diagnosis?*

   • Gastric outlet obstruction due to chronic cicatrised duodenal ulcer (Pyloric stenosis is an old terminology).

2. *Why is it not due to carcinoma pyloric antrum?*

   • There is no filling defect in the pyloric antrum.

3. *How do you treat this case?*

   • With a pre-operative stomach wash, adequate intravenous fluids, total truncal vagotomy with GJ is the treatment of choice.

4. *Why GJ and vagotomy?*

   • After vagotomy, motility of the stomach is lost and in pyloric stenosis, there is already obstruction at the pyloric antrum. Hence, gastrojejunostomy is the drainage procedure of choice.

5. *Why not pyloroplasty or highly selective vagotomy?*

   • Pylorus is scarred and deformed. Hence, it is not safe to do pyloroplasty. HSV is contraindicated in the presence of pyloric obstruction.

XI. BARIUM ENEMA SHOWING THE LEFT COLON, TRANSVERSE COLON AND A PART OF ASCENDING COLON

XII. BARIUM ENEMA SHOWING INTRINSIC, IRREGULAR, PERSISTENT FILLING DEFECT IN THE ASCENDING COLON

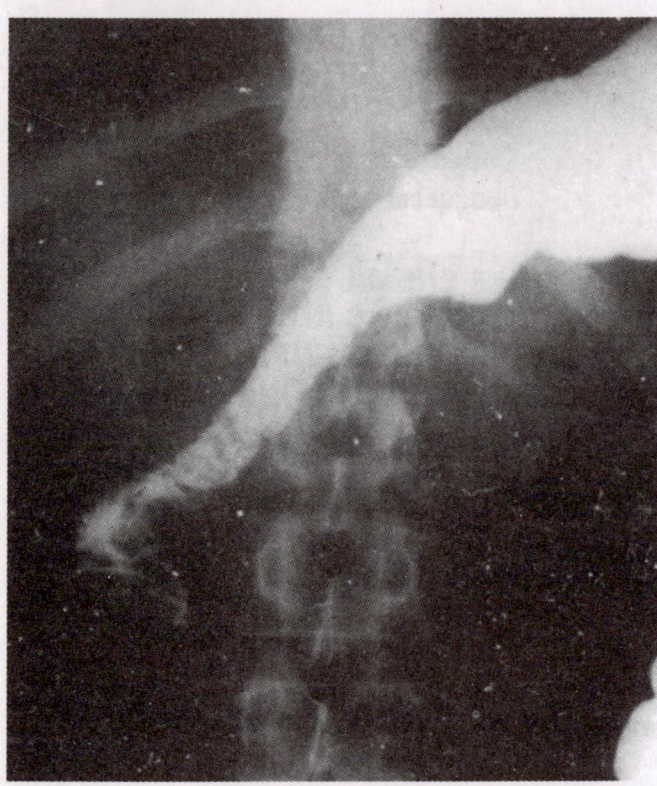

Fig. 50.11 Barium enema showing the left colon, transverse colon and a part of ascending colon

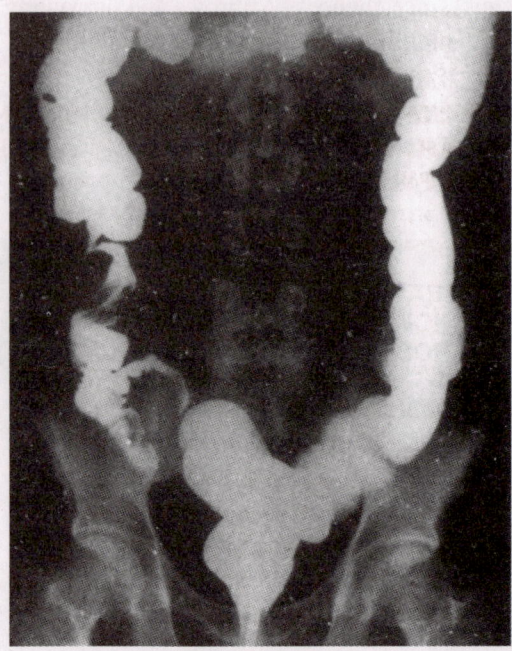

Fig. 50.12 Barium enema showing intrinsic, irregular persistent filling defect in the ascending colon

1. What is the diagnosis?
- Carcinoma ascending colon

2. What is the confirmatory investigation?
- Colonoscopy and biopsy

3. What is the report, if it is carcinoma?
- Adenocarcinoma

4. What is the treatment?
- Right radical hemicolectomy if it is operable. Structures removed in this operation include terminal ileum (6-8 cms), caecum including appendix, ascending colon and 1/3 of right transverse colon. If it is inoperable, part of ileum is anastomosed to the transverse colon to prevent or relieve intestinal obstruction (side to side). One need not remove two feet of ileum.

5. What is the differential diagnosis?
- Ileocaecal tuberculosis: In this condition:
  1. Irregular filling defect is not seen.
  2. Caecum is usually pulled up and then ileocaecal angle becomes **obtuse**.

1. What is the diagnosis?
- ILEOCOLIC intussusception

2. Why do you say so?
- The 'claw' like ending or pincer ending is typical of intussusception.

3. What are the causes of intussusception in adults?
- Submucous lipoma, or polyps
- Meckel's diverticulum
- Growth in the caecum
- Leiomyoma of the ileum

4. In a child, what are the causes?
- Weaning of the diet or viral infection

5. What is the treatment of adult intussusception?
- Resection because there is a precipitating cause

XIII. BARIUM ENEMA SHOWING LOSS OF HAUSTRATIONS IN THE LEFT COLON, AND SMALL, MULTIPLE, REGULAR FILLING DEFECTS DUE TO PSEUDOPOLYPOSIS

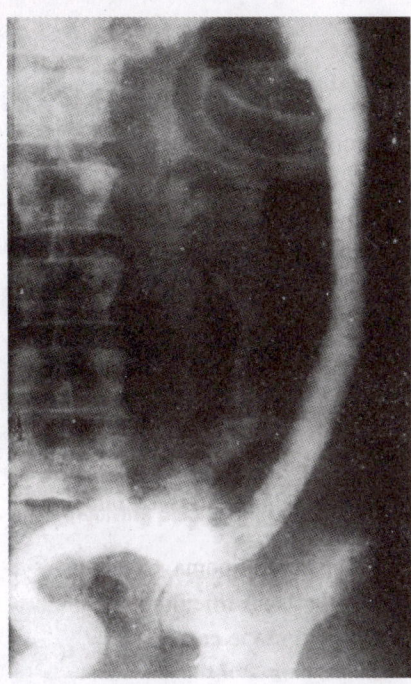

Fig. 50.13 Barium enema showing loss of haustrations in the left colon and small multiple, regular filling defects due to pseudopolyposis

1. What is the diagnosis?
- Ulcerative colitis

2. What are pseudopolyposis ?
- An attempt at healing in between the ulcers produces granulation tissue which have the appearance of polyps. Hence, pseudopolyposis.

3. What are the dangerous complications of ulcerative colitis?
- Haemorrhage, toxic megacolon, perforation and malignancy.

4. What are the drugs used in the treatment of ulcerative colitis?
- Salazopyrines and corticosteroids.

5. What are the surgical treatments?
- Total colectomy with permanent ileostomy. OR
- Total colectomy, creation of a pouch with anastomosis of the pouch to the anal canal.

XIV. X-RAY LATERAL VIEW OF THE SKULL SHOWING A LARGE SWELLING WITH EROSION IN THE PERICRANIUM

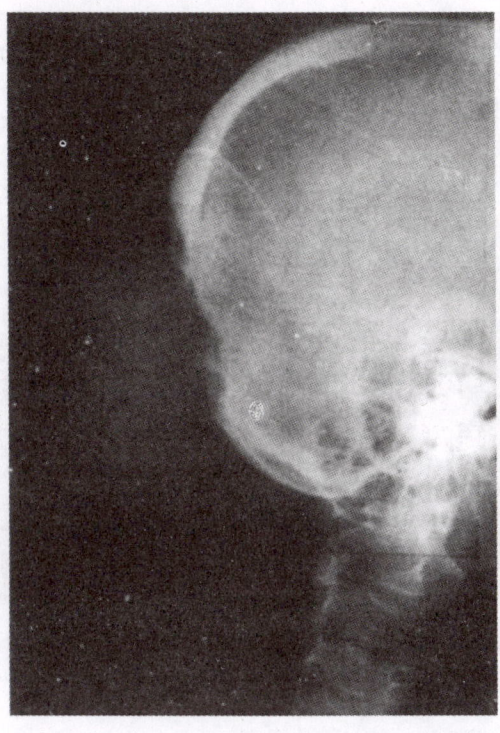

Fig. 50.14. X-ray lateral view of the skull showing a large swelling with erosion in the pericranium

1. What is the diagnosis?
- Secondary deposit in the skull

2. Why is it not a lipoma or neurofibroma ?
- Erosion of the bone is seen in malignancy. not in benign tumours.

3. If this patient is a female aged 40 years, what are the causes?
- Follicular carcinoma thyroid
- Carcinoma of the breast
- Renal cell carcinoma

4. What is the treatment if this is follicular carcinoma thyroid?
- Near total thyroidectomy, radio-iodine therapy and external radiotherapy.

5. How do you diagnose follicular carcinoma thyroid histologically?
- Angioinvasion and capsular invasion

XV. ENDOSCOPIC, RETROGRADE CHOLANGIO-PANCREATOGRAPHY (ERCP) SHOWING THE BILIARY AND PANCREATIC SYSTEM

XVI. T-TUBE CHOLANGIOGRAPHY SHOWING A FILLING DEFECT IN THE LOWER END OF THE COMMON BILE DUCT (CBD)

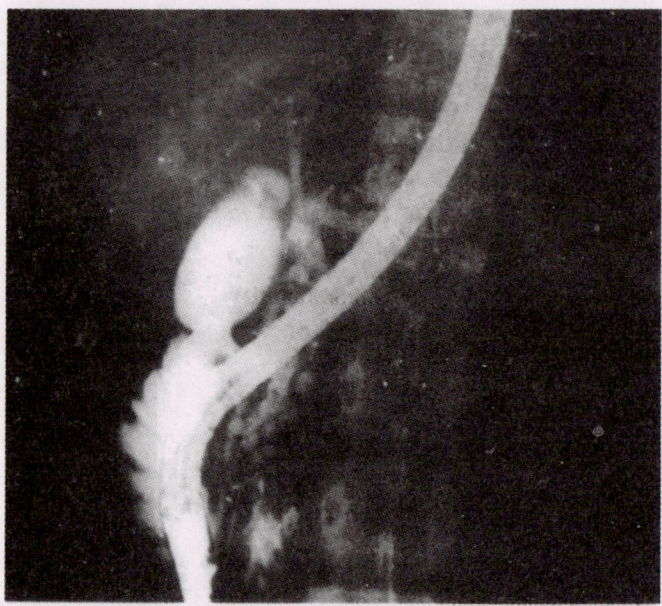

Fig. 50.15 Endoscopic retrograde cholangio-pancreatography (ERCP) showing the billary and pancreatic systems

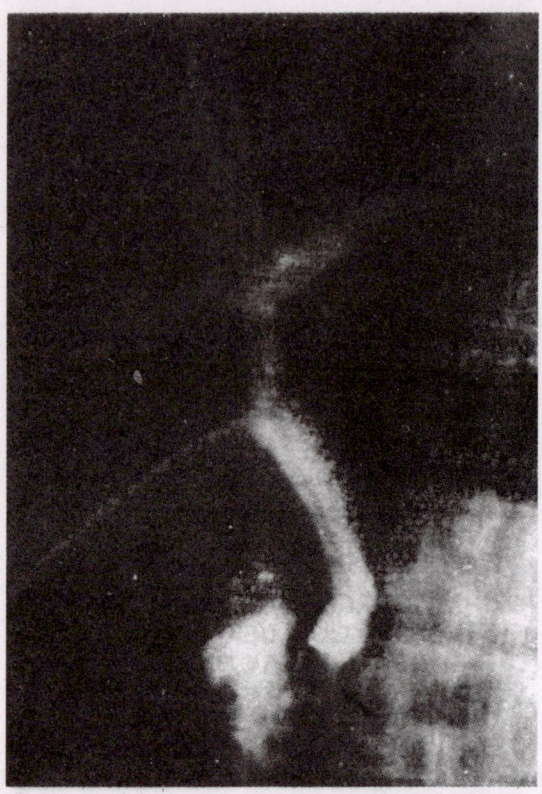

Fig. 50.16. T-tube cholangiography showing a filling defect in the lower end of the common bile duct (CBD)

1. What is the diagnosis?

- Chronic pancreatitis

2. Why do you say so?

- Extensive calcification involving head, body and tail of pancreas.

3. What is the simple investigation to diagnose chronic pancreatitis?

- Plain X-ray abdomen, showing calcification

4. Why is ERCP done in this patient?

- To know whether the pancreatic duct is dilated or not.

5. If pancreatic duct is dilated more than 8 mm in a patient with severe abdominal pain with chronic pancreatitis, what is the treatment?

- Longitudinal pancreaticojejunostomy—Puestow's operation. In this operation, pancreatic duct is laid open, strictures are divided and the duct is anastomosed to jejunum.

1. What is the diagnosis?

- Post cholecystectomy - Residual stone in the CBD

2. What is the surgery done for this patient?

- Cholecystectomy and choledocholithotomy

3. Why do you insert a T-tube after CBD exploration?

- In case of distal obstruction by a residual stone, the bile starts leaking from the suture line on the CBD and may result in biliary peritonitis. In such situations, T-tube helps in drainage of the bile.

4. What material is T-tube made of?

- Latex

5. How do you treat this patient in order to extract the stone?

- Endoscopic sphincterotomy and extraction of the stone.

XVII. SPLENOPORTOVENOGRAPHY (SPV) SHOWING EXTENSIVE COLLATERALS IN THE REGION OF SPLEEN

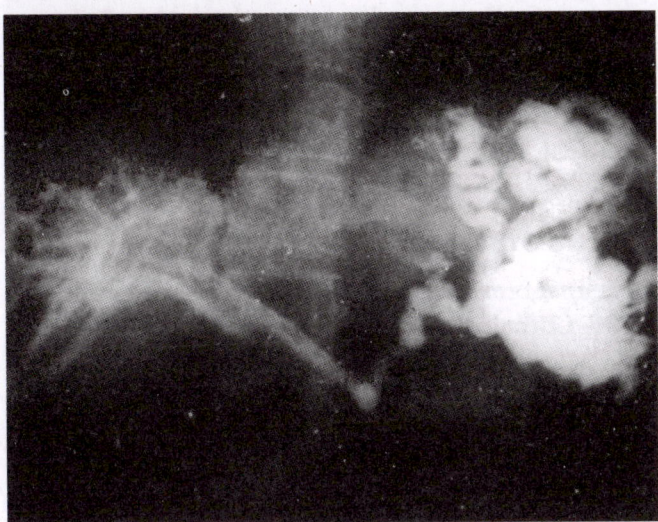

Fig. 50.17 Splenoportovenography (SPV) showing extensive collaterals in the region of spleen

XVIII. RETROGRADE ANGIOGRAPHY SHOWING OCCLUSION OF FEMORAL ARTERY ON THE LEFT SIDE

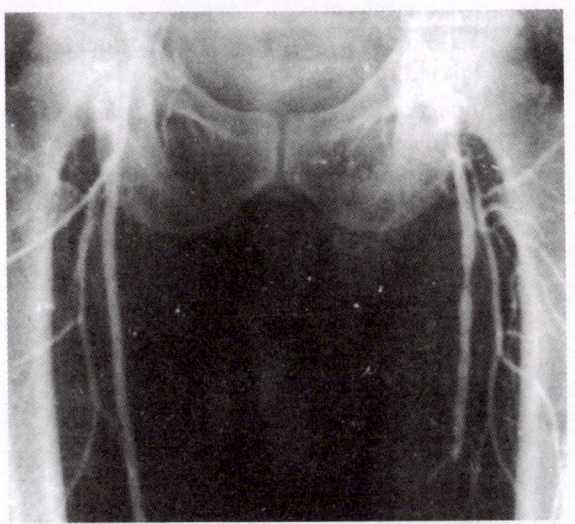

Fig. 50.18. Retrograde angiograophy showing occlusion of femoral artery on the left side

1. What is the diagnosis?
- Portal hypertension

2. What is the type of portal hypertension?
- Hepatic type

3. Why do you say so ?
- Splenic vein, portal vein and its branches within the liver are visualised.

4. What is the probable cause in this patient?
- Cirrhosis of the liver

5. What is the first line of specific treatment for bleeding oesophageal varices?
- Endoscopic sclerotherapy/banding
- Perivariceal or intravariceal injection of 2% solution of sodium tetradecylsulphate.
- Sclerotherapy is given at multiple sites and in multiple sittings.
- Banding is a better alternative but needs more expertise.

I. What is the technique employed in this angiography?
- Seldinger's technique—percutaneous, transfemoral, retrograde.

2. What is the probable cause in our country?
- Buerger's disease (Thrombo Angitis Obliterans)

3. Why do you say so ?
- Buerger's disease affects a medium- sized vessel and narrowing of femoral artery is segmental in this radiograph.

4. What is the surgical treatment for Buerger's disease?
- Lumbar sympathectomy

5. How does lumbar sympathectomy help these patients?
- By reducing the sympathetic tone of the lower limb, arterioles and capillaries get dilated allowing cutaneous ulcers to heal.

51

Instruments

- Forceps
- Retractors
- Occlusion clamps
- Dialators
- Tracheostomy set
- Rubber tubes
- Catheters
- Sengstaken tube

1. ARTERY FORCEPS (HAEMOSTAT)

- It is also called **Spencer Well's artery forceps.** It has a ratchet and two blades with uniform serrations.

- It is used to control bleeding, not only from arteries but from the veins and capillaries. Once the bleeding points are caught, they are coagulated or ligature is applied.

- The curved artery is commonly used (Fig- 51.1 B).

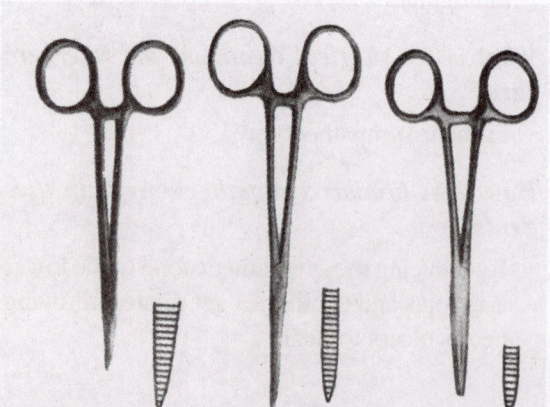

Fig. 51.1A- Mosquito forceps **B-** Curved artery forceps **C-** Straight artery forceps

- The smaller version of this is called Mosquito forceps (Fig. 51.1A). This is extremely useful in repair of hare-lip, cleft palate or other plastic surgery operations.

- It is also available as straight artery which is used to hold the stay sutures (Fig, 51.1C).

2. ALLIS TISSUE HOLDING FORCEPS (Fig. 51.2)

- It has a ratchet and triangular expansion at the tip, where the serrations are present.

- It can be used to **hold tough structures** such as fascia, aponeurosis etc.

- Eventhough it can cause trauma, because of its better grip, it can be used to hold the duodenum for duodenal closure during gastrectomy.

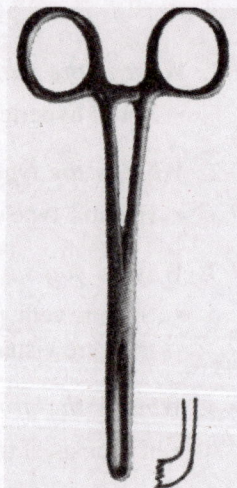

Fig. 51.2 Allis forceps

3. KOCHER'S FORCEPS (Fig. 51.3)

- This is similar to an artery forceps with serrations. It is available as curved and straight.

- There is a sharp tooth at the tip of the instrument. Hence, it has a better grip.

- Kocher's forceps can be used to **hold tough structures** such as **aponeurosis, fascia** etc.

- During thyroidectomy, it can be used to hold the strap muscles for dividing them.

Key Box 51.1
REMEMBER

- Kocher's forceps
- Kocher's test
- Kocher's thyroid dissector
- Kocher's vein
- Kocher's subcostal incision
- Kocher's gland holding forceps

- Theodor Kocher, German surgeon got the Nobel prize for his contribution to thyroid surgery.

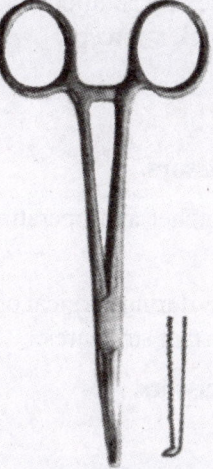
Fig. 51.3 Kocher's forceps

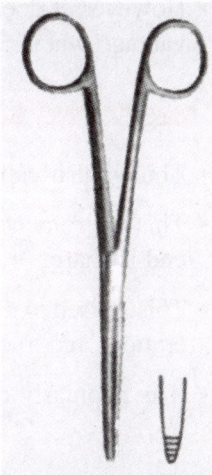
Fig. 51.4 Sinus forceps

4. SINUS FORCEPS (Fig. 51.4)

- This is like an artery forceps which has NO RATCHET.
- Serrations are confined to the tip so as to hold the wall of an abscess cavity, for biopsy.
- In Hilton's method of drainage of an abscess, once the incision is made, the sinus forceps is thrust into the abscess cavity and by opening the blades in all directions, the loculi are broken. To facilitate free opening of the blades, sinus forceps has no ratchet.

5. SWAB HOLDING FORCEPS (Fig. 51.5)

- This has a ratchet and two long blades.
- Operating end is rounded with serrations.
- It is used to hold the swab (gauze pieces) to prepare the parts with antiseptic agents at the time of surgery.
- This instrument can also be used as a blunt 'dissector' with the swab, while dissecting at a depth, e.g. lumbar sympathectomy, vagotomy, etc.

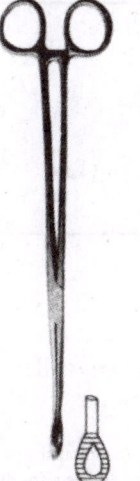
Fig. 51.5 Swab holding forceps

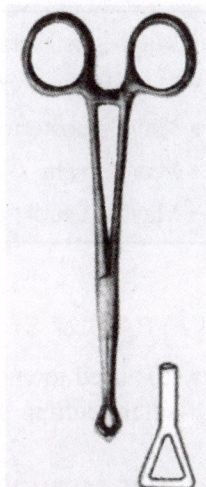
Fig. 51.6 Babcock's forceps

6. BABCOCK'S FORCEPS (Fig. 51.6)

- An instrument with a ratchet and a triangular expansion with fenestrations at the operating end. It does not have any teeth. Thus, it is used to hold intestines during anastomosis or resection.
- This instrument can also be used to hold many other structures such as thyroid gland, mesoappendix, uterine tubes, etc.

7. LANE'S FORCEPS (Fig. 51.7)

- This is similar to Babcock's forceps but the tip is more broad, expanded with a bigger opening.
- It is used to hold the appendix.

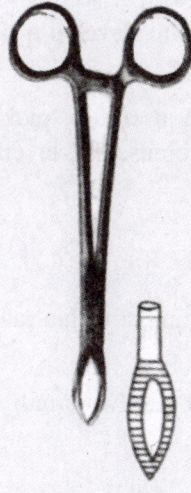
Fig. 51.7 Lane's forceps

- However, it does not seem to have any additional advantage when compared to Babcock's forceps.

8. DISSECTING SCISSORS (Fig. 51.8)

- This is also called as **Mayo's scissors.**
- This instrument does not have ratchet and operating end is sharp.
- This is used to dissect tissue planes during surgical operations and to cut or divide important structures.
- It is popularly called as **tissue scissors.**

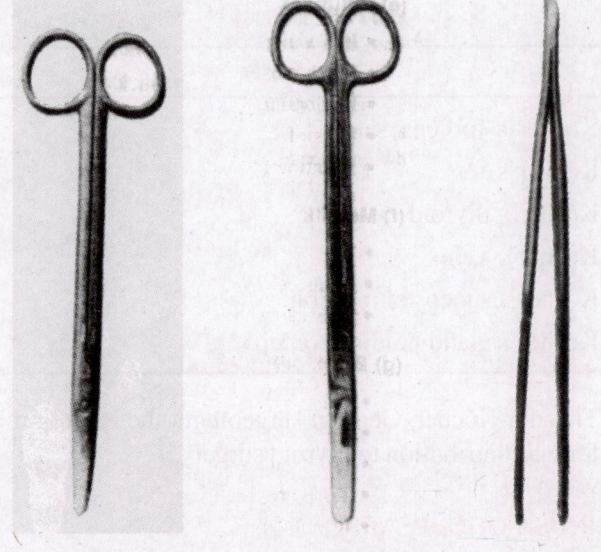

Fig. 51.8 Mayo's dissecting scissors

Fig. 51.9 Straight scissors

Fig. 51.10 Dissecting forceps

Key Box 51.2
REMEMBER
• Mayo's scissors • Mayo's herniorrhaphy • Mayo's posterior G J • Mayo's vein • Mayo's needle (Used for hernia repair)

9. STRAIGHT SCISSORS (Fig. 51.9)

- It is used to cut the sutures or knots. Hence, called as suture-cutting scissors.

10. DISSECTING FORCEPS (Fig. 51.10)

- This is a toothed forceps. It is also available as non-toothed forceps.
- Dissecting forceps with dissecting scissors makes good 'tool' for a surgeon to **develop a tissue plane** in majority of surgeries.
- The forceps is very useful to 'pick' individual layers such as serosa, seromuscular, layers mucosa etc. during anastomosis.

11. NEEDLE HOLDER (Fig. 51.11)

- This is a long instrument with a ratchet at non-operating end.
- The operating end has two small blades with serrations.

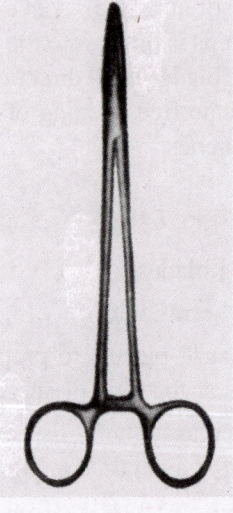

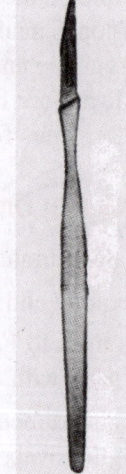

Fig. 51.11 Needle holder **Fig. 51.12** Scalpel with blade

- The instrument is used to **hold the curved needles** which are used to suture the parts.
- A **firm grip** is essential to apply proper sutures.

12. SCALPEL WITH BLADE (Fig. 51.12)

- Popularly called as the **surgeon's knife.**
- This is used to incise the skin and subcutaneous tissue.
- Due to the sharp nature, it can be used to divide a major vascular pedicle once ligatures are applied.

---

1. Mayo clinic is in Rochester. After whom the umbilical nodule in visceral malignancies is named?

13. CHEATLE'S FORCEPS (Fig. 51.13)

- It is a long instrument having a curved shaft.
- The **handle has no lock**
- It is kept dipped in antiseptic solutions
- This instrument is used to pick sterilized articles like sponges, gauze pieces or other instruments and to transfer to the instrument trolly.

14. DEAVER RETRACTOR (Fig. 51.14)

- This is popularly called **Deaver Liver retractor**
- It has a long blade and operating end is curved
- It can be used to retract the liver during vagotomy cholecystectomy or gastrectomy etc.
- Since it has long blades, it can be used to retract the kidney upwards, during lumbar sympathectomy or to retract the urinary bladder during surgery on the rectum.

15. MORRIS RETRACTOR (Fig. 51.15)

- This is a long instrument with broad operating end.
- This is used t**o retract the abdominal wall,** once the peritoneum is opened.
- However, if a self-retaining retractor is used to widen the laparotomy wound, the use of Morris retractor gets limited.

16. CZERNY RETRACTOR (Fig. 51.16)

- This is a double hooked retractor on one side and a single blade on the other side.
- This is a **superficial retractor,** can be used to retract layers of the abdominal wall, muscles etc. Thus, during appendicectomy, herniorrhaphy or thyroidectomy, this instrument is very useful.

17. LANGENBECK RETRACTOR (Fig. 51.17)

- This instrument has only **one blade.**
- The uses of this are similar to that of Czerny's retractor.

18. MOYNIHAN'S STRAIGHT OCCLUSION CLAMP (Fig. 51.18)

- This is a long instrument with a ratchet. The operating end has two long blades with serrations in the line of blades.
- This instrument is used to **occlude the intestinal**

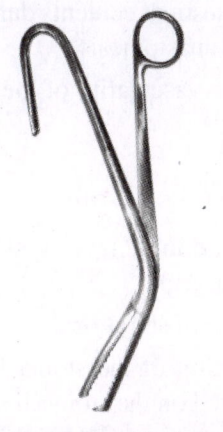
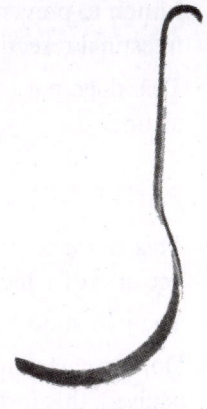

Fig. 51.13 Cheatles's forceps   **Fig. 51.14** Deaver retractor

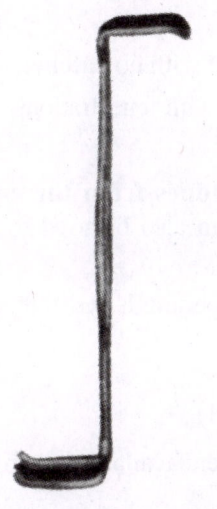
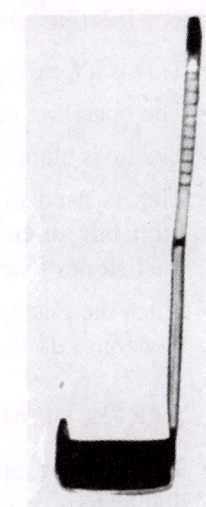

Fig. 51.15 Morris retractor   **Fig. 51.16** Czerny retractor

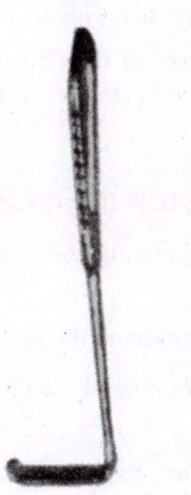
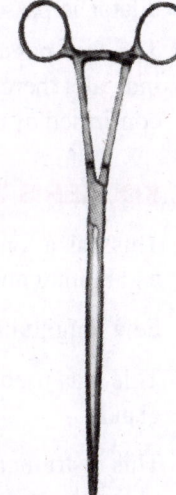

Fig. 51.17 Langenbeck retractor   **Fig. 51.18** Moynihan occlusion clamp

lumen to prevent spillage of intestinal contents during intestinal resection or intestinal anastomosis.

- This does not interfere with the vascularity of the intestine.

19. PAYR'S CRUSHING CLAMP (Fig. 51.19)

- This is a heavy instrument with **double lever system,** because of which it has a better grip.
- The two short blades have uniform serrations
- During gastrectomy, when portion of the stomach is excised, this instrument is applied on the stomach side so that the stomach, with this instrument is excised.

20. DESJARDIN'S CHOLEDOCHOLITHOTOMY FORCEPS (Fig. 51.20)

- This is a long curved instrument with no **ratchet.**
- The operating end is expanded with fenestrations.
- The tip is blunt.
- This is used to **extract the stones from the common bile duct.** However, it can also be used to extract stones from the ureter.
- Since there is no ratchet, free opening is possible, and the stones do not get crushed.

21. BAKE'S DILATOR (Fig. 51.21)

- This is a long malleable instrument available in various diameters.
- It has a handle, long body and the tip is blunt.
- Once common bile duct exploration is completed, this dilator is passed **to assess for any distal obstruction.**
- The free passage of Bake's dilators of different sizes indicate, there is no distal obstruction (However, to be confirmed by cholangiogram)

22. KOCHER'S THYROID DISSECTOR (Fig. 51.22)

- This has a long handle and the operating end is small and blunt with an opening.
- Few longitudinal serrations are present at the tip.
- This was used to dissect the upper pole of the thyroid gland.
- This instrument can also be used to dissect the isthmus of the thyroid gland from the trachea.
- **A silk thread can be fed** into the opening so as to ligate the vascular pedicle or isthmus.

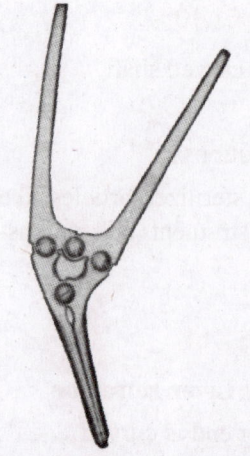 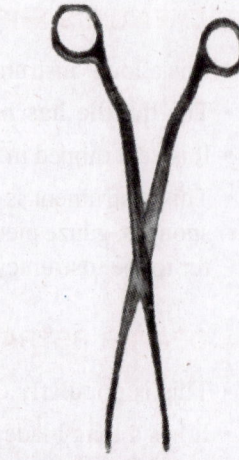

Fig. 51.19 Payr's crushing clamp   **Fig. 51.20** Desjardin's forceps

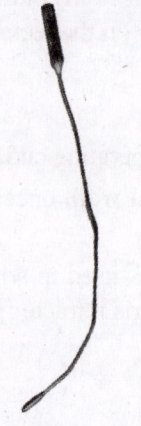 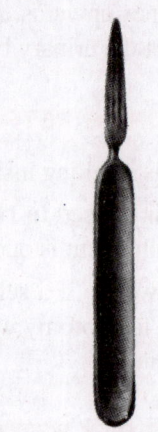

Fig. 51.21 Bake's dilator   **Fig. 51.22** Kocher's thyroid dissector

- With the availability of the right angled forceps, this instrument is not in routine use nowadays.

23. ANEURYSM NEEDLE (Fig. 51.23)

- This is a long instrument with an 'EYE' at the operating end.
- It is called as aneurysm needle because it was used to ligate the feeding artery in an aneurysm. However today, this instrument is of limited use.
- During **venesection or cut down,** the silk suture can be threaded within the 'EYE', passed round the vein and it is tied.

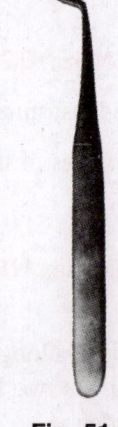

Fig. 51.23 Aneurysm neddle

24. TROCAR AND CANNULA (Fig. 51.24)

- This has two parts. The inner sharp part is the trocar and outer blunt part is cannula.

- It is used to drain hydrocoele fluid.

- Once hydrocoele sac is delivered, it is punctured with trocar and cannula, the trocar removed and the fluid drained.

- Make sure that trocar and cannula should match, otherwise injury to the deeper structures (Testis) can occur.

25. HUMBY'S KNIFE (Fig. 51.25)

- This instrument has a handle and a long sheath.

- When in use, a disposable blade can be attached to it.

- The instrument is used to take skin graft. Hence, it is also called skin grafting knife.

- To facilitate the exact thickness of the skin to be removed, there is a screw at the operating end, with which, prior adjustment should be done.

26. MYER'S METAL STRIPPER (Fig. 51.26)

- This is a long metallic chain or a stripper used in varicose vein surgery.

- It has a handle which is T shaped and the 'advancing' end which enters the vein. This is blunt. Once this end comes out of the cut end of the vein, a medium sized head is connected to it.

- With gentle force, (traction) exerted on the handle, the varicose vein can be stripped.

- Hence, it is also called vein stripper.

27. SELF-RETAINING RETRACTOR (Fig. 51.27)

- It is a strong, heavy instrument with two blades.

- This is used to spread the laparotomy wound. Hence, it is called as self- retaining retractor.

28. RIB SPREADER (Fig. 51.28)

- This is also a strong heavy instrument with two long blades.

- Once an incision is deepened through the intercostal spaces and the pleura is opened, the rib spreader is used and by rotating the latch handle, the ribs are spread over.

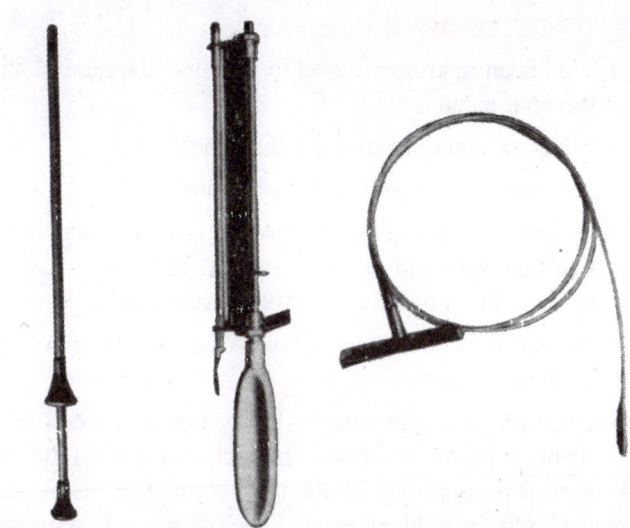

Fig. 51.24 Trocar and cannula

Fig. 51.25 Humby's knife

Fig. 51.26 Myer's metal stripper

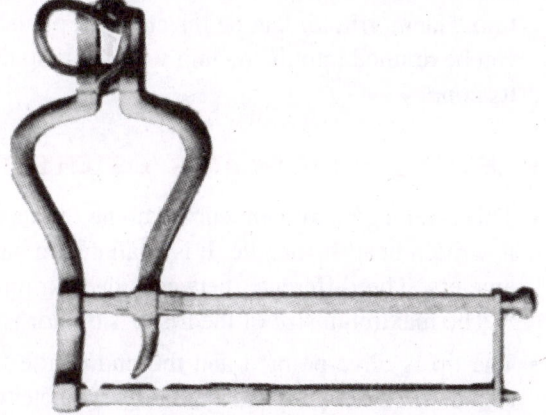

Fig. 51.27 Self-retaining retractor

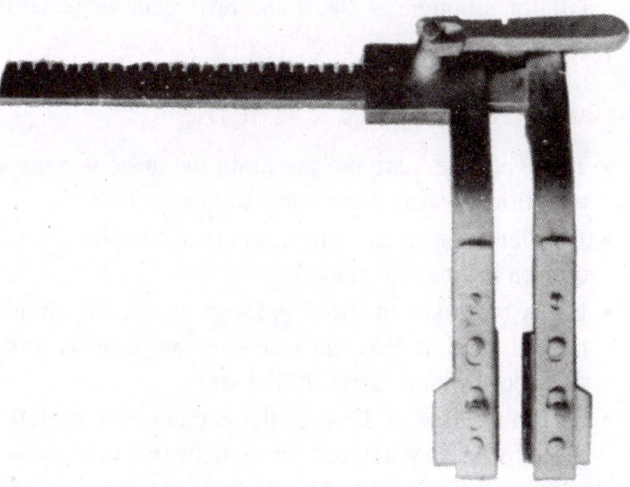

Fig. 51.28 Rib spreader

29. PROCTOSCOPE (Fig. 51.29)

- This is an instrument used to visualise the rectum and the anal canal.

- It has an outer sheath with the handle (A).

- An inner blunt pan is called obturator (B).

- Before introducing the proctoscope one must make sure that obturator and the outer sheath must match. Lubricate the instrument well before introducing.

- In painful conditions like fissure-in-Ano, proctoscopy is contraindicated.

- Once rectal examination is done, proctoscope is held firmly with the left hand, (buttocks separated) the obturator is supported by the right hand. The instrument is slowly introduced inside. The obturator is removed and rectum is visualised using light source.

- Proctoscope is used to diagnose haemorrhoids, carcinoma rectum or rectal ulcers etc. Biopsy can be taken with a biopsy forceps in nonhealing ulcers of the rectum. Haemorrhoids can be injected and pelvic abscess can be drained into the rectum with the help of a proctoscope.

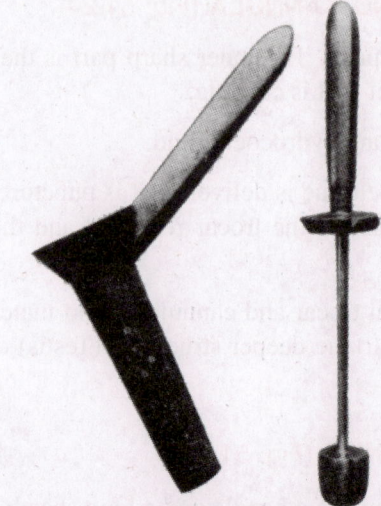

Fig. 51.29 Proctoscope

30. LISTER'S METAL DILATOR (LISTER'S BOUGIE)

- This is a long instrument curved at the tip. Its diameter is written near the handle. It is available in various diameters. The difference between the two numbers is 3. The maximum size of the Lister's dilator is 9/12.

- The tip is olive-pointed and the end of the handle is round. The minimum and maximum diameter of the instrument is written on the handle. The other type of bougie is Glutton's bougie with a plain tip and the end of the handle is trapezoid. The maximum size of Glutton's bougie is 24/28 and difference between the two numbers is 4.

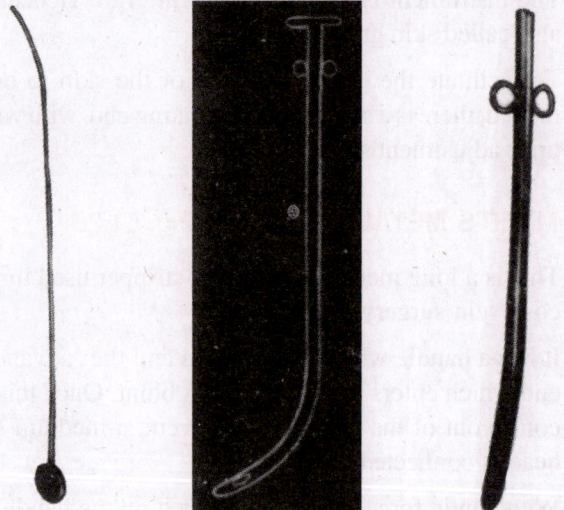

Fig. 51.30 Lister's dilator   **Fig. 51.31A** Male metallic catheter   **Fig. 51.31B** Female metallic catheter

31.A: MALE METALLIC CATHETER

- These catheters are used to drain the urine in cases of retention of urine when rubber catheter fails.

- It is a long instrument which is curved because the male urethra is long and curved.

- It has two eyes at the distal end which are situated laterally and at different levels so that the instrument does not become weak at that spot.

- Once the urine is drained, the catheter can be left in place by passing a thread through the two rings present at the proximal end and fixing them to patient's thigh.

- Due to the fear of false passage, injury to the urethra

and introducing infection, this catheter is not used nowadays. It is replaced by trocar suprapubic cystostomy.

31.B: FEMALE METALLIC CATHETER

- Used to drain urine in females.

- This is a short and straight instrument because the urethra is short and straight in females.

- It has multiple holes at the tip.

- Indications for usage of this catheter is very rare because acute retention of urine is rare in females and even if it occurs, a red rubber catheter can be passed.

- Emptying the bladder is mandatory before any gynaecological examination of the patient.

32. TOWEL CLIP (Fig. 51.32)

- This instrument has a ratchet and the operating end is sharp.
- This is available in different sizes.
- Once the part is cleaned and draped the clips are used to hold the towels in place.

33. RIGHT ANGLED FORCEPS—LAHEY'S FORCEPS

- This is a long instrument with right angle at the operating end.
- This instrument is extremely useful in **ligating the major vascular pedicles**, e.g. superior thyroid pedicle— Thyroidectomy
- Cystic artery—Cholecystectomy
- Lumbar veins—Lumbar sympathectomy.

34. HUDSON'S BRACE AND THE BURR

- This is a heavy instrument with a brace and the burr (drill).
- This is used to create **openings into the cranium** so as to get an access to the structures within.
- Thus once a 'burr' is made, drainage of blood or fluid or pus can be done.

35. CRICOID HOOK (Fig. 51.35)

- This has a broad handle and a thin shaft with a hook at the operating end.
- This is used to stabilise the trachea by hooking the cricoid cartilage 'up'.
- This step is essential in children wherein veins are very superficial and can get injured easily when child moves the head and neck. By stabilising the trachea, it is easy to incise the trachea, without injuring the vessels.

36. TRACHEAL DILATOR (Fig. 51.36)

- This is an instrument with **no ratchet** at the non-operating end.
- The operating end is blunt and curved.
- The peculiarity of this instrument is that **when the handle is opened**, the **operating end closes** and **when the handle is closed, the operating end opens.**
- Tracheal dilator is used in the **post-tracheostomy period,** when the tube has to be changed due to blockage. In such situations, once the tube is removed, tracheal dilator is introduced, the opening in trachea is kept open, and the new tube is introduced. However, once the track is formed, tracheal dilator need not be used.

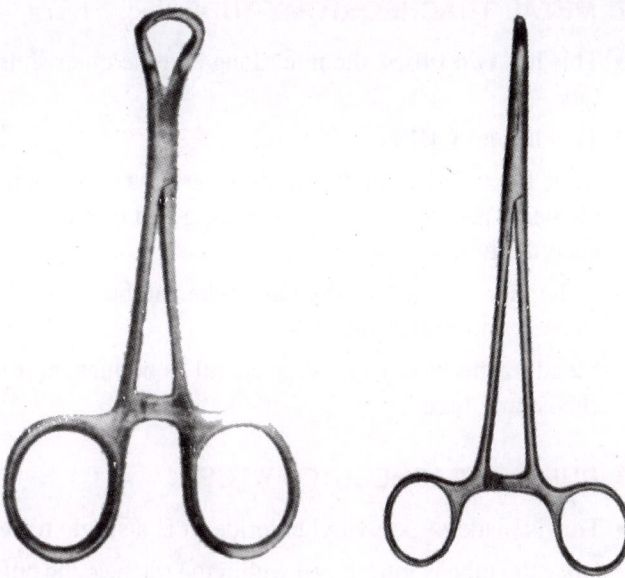

Fig. 51.32 Towel clip   **Fig. 51.33** Right-angled forceps

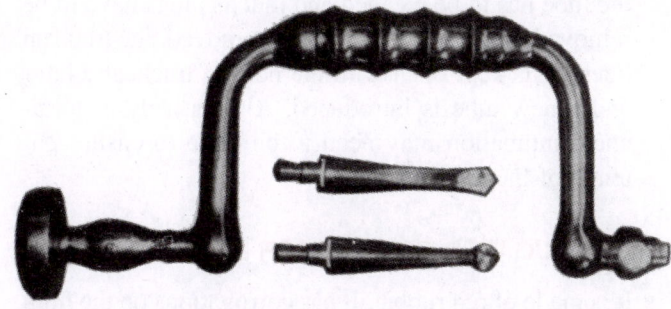

Fig. 51.34 Hudson's brace and the burr

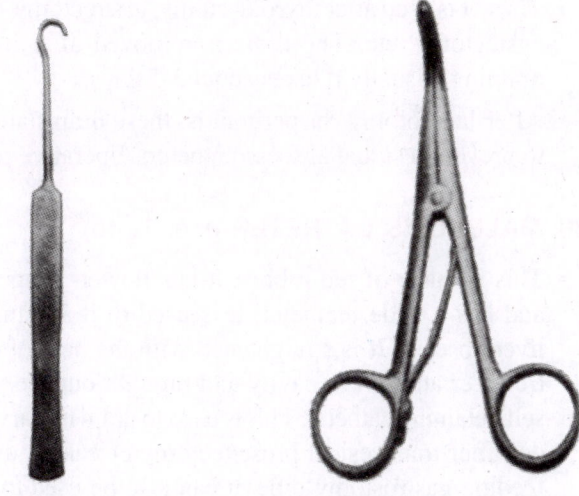

Fig. 51.35 Cricoid hook   **Fig. 51.36** Tracheal dilator

37. METAL TRACHEOSTOMY TUBE (Fig. 51.37)

- This has **two tubes**, the inner long and the outer short tube.

- This has no **CUFF.**

- Once the tube is introduced, the tape is passed around the neck, passed through the opening and tied so as to keep the tube in place.

- If the tube is blocked, the inner tube can be removed, cleaned and reintroduced.

- Metal tracheostomy tubes are useful as permanent tracheostomy tube.

38. CUFFED TRACHEOSTOMY TUBE

- This is made of polyvinyl chloride. It is a **single tube.**

- Once the tube is introduced within the trachea, the cuff is inflated by using 3-5 ml of air.

- The cuff prevents leakage of air and prevents **acid aspiration syndrome (Mendelson's syndrome).**

- If this tube is blocked, it is an emergency. In such cases, the tube has to be cleaned and mucus plugs have to be removed. Otherwise, the tube is removed, the tracheal opening is kept open with the help of tracheal dilator and a new tube is introduced. Alternatively endotracheal intubation may need to be done to ensure patency of the airway.

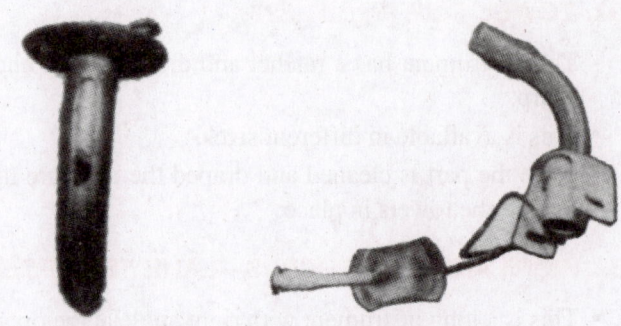

Fig. 51.37 Metal tracheostomy tube   **Fig. 51.38** Cuffed tracheostomy

39. CORRUGATED RED RUBBER DRAIN (Fig. 51.39)

- It is made of red rubber. It has corrugations on the both sides. Whenever a major surgery is done, some amount of blood loss or anastomotic leakage is expected. This drain is used so that **fluid can escape freely outside**.

- Thus, it is used after thyroidectomy, gastrectomy, cholecystectomy, etc. The drain is removed after it stops draining. Usually it takes about 3-5 days.

- After laparotomy for peritonitis, these drains are used to prevent residual abscess in the postoperative period.

40. MALECOT'S CATHETER (Fig. 51.40)

- This is made of red rubber. It has flower-shaped end and has a wide diameter. It is used to drain amoebic liver abscess. It is straightened with the help of an introducer and left in cavity and brought outside. It is a self-retaining catheter. This is used to drain urinary bladder after transvesical prostatectomy or can be used as feeding gastrostomy tube. It can also be used to drain empyaema thoracis.

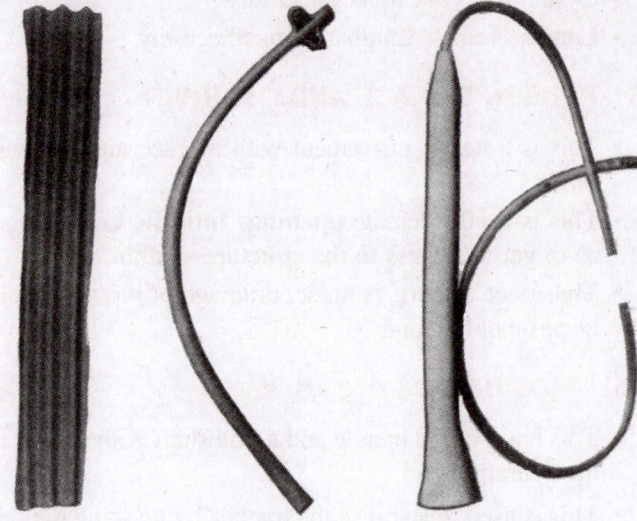

Fig. 51.39 Corrugated red rubber drain   **Fig. 51.40** Malecot's catheter   **Fig. 51.41** Mousseau Barbin's tube

41. MOUSSEAU BARBIN'S TUBE (Fig. 51.41)

- This is also called as M.B, Tube. It is a funnel shaped tube with Ryle's tube like attachment. It is used in inoperable cases of carcinoma oesophagus to palliate dysphagia. It is stitched to the Ryle's tube which is brought out through the mouth and it is slowly drawn in by pulling the other end of Ryle's tube which is in the stomach, after doing a gastrotomy.

- Once the tube is below the level of growth, it is cut at a sufficient distance and is stitched to the stomach wall.

- With the availability of laser coagulation of the growth, and considering discomfort caused by the tube including its migration, the MB tube is not popular and not preferred.

42. FOLEY'S SELF-RETAINING URINARY CATHETER (Fig. 51.42)

- This is made of **latex with silicon coating**. At the tip, there is a bulb, capacity of which is written at the other end (Fig. 51.42A).

- Before inflating the bulb, one must make sure that **catheter is in the urinary bladder, not in the urethra.** This is assessed by free flow of urine.

- After introducing the catheter, bulb is inflated using saline. Thus, it becomes self retaining. After the usage, it is removed by deflating the bulb. It can also be used to drain peritoneal cavity as in biliary peritonitis. Inflated bulb compresses the prostatic bed & controls bleeding after prostatectomy.

43. RED RUBBER CATHETER (Fig. 51.43)

- This is used to drain urine temporarily. It causes urethritis if it is left long in the urinary bladder. Once the urine is emptied, it is removed. It is not a self-retaining catheter. Not routinely used nowadays because of availability of Foley's catheter. It is more stiff than Foley's catheter. Hence, **in cases of stricture urethra,** where **Foley's catheter cannot be passed, red rubber catheter may be used.**

44. RYLE'S TUBE (Fig. 51.44)

- This is also called as **Nasogastric Tube.** At the end of this tube there are **lead shots.** After introducing within the Stomach, its position is confirmed by pushing 5-10 ml of air and auscultating in the epigastrium or aspirating gastric juice. It is a long tube having 3 marks. When the tube is passed upto the 1st mark, it enters the stomach. Usually it is passed upto 2nd mark. **Life-saving use of Ryle's tube is in acute gastric dilatation.**

- **In volvulus of the stomach, it is impossible to pass Ryle's tube.** Ryle's tube is used to aspirate as in intestinal obstruction or pyloric stenosis, used in the diagnosis of G.I. haemorrhage, also used to feed coma or tetanus patients.

45. T-TUBE (KEHR'S) (Fig. 51.45)

- This is a flexible tube made of latex with a long vertical limb and a short horizontal limb.

- Whenever the **common bile duct (CBD) is incised**, it is sutured after inserting the T-tube. The short horizontal limb is placed vertically within the common bile duct after making 2-3 holes within. Some surgeons slit open the entire length of the short limb.

- The long limb is brought to the exterior from the most dependent part of the common bile duct and connected to a sterile container.

- Presence of the T-tube may prevent peritonitis due to biliary leakage in cases of residual stones blocking the lower end of the CBD.

Removal of the tube

About 7-10 days later, a T-tube cholangiogram is done and the T-tube is removed with a gentle pull, provided following criteria are fulfilled.

1. The dye flows freely into the duodenum
2. No filling defects in the CBD
3. After clamping the tube for 24 hours, the is no abdominal pain or fever
4. Patient is passing normal coloured stools.

Once the tube is withdrawn, some amount of biliary leak may persist for 2-3 days and it stops by itself provided there is no distal obstruction.

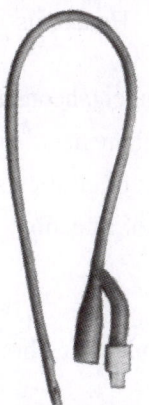

Fig. 51.42 Foley's catheter

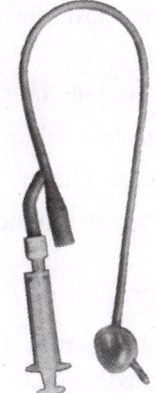

Fig. 51.42A Distended bulb

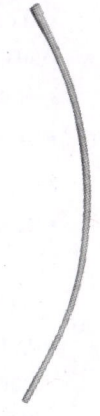

Fig. 51.43 Red rubber catheter

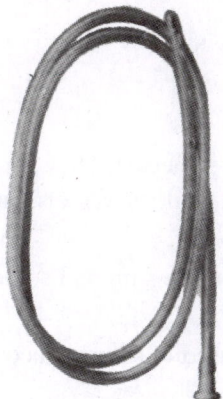

Fig. 51.44 Ryle's tube

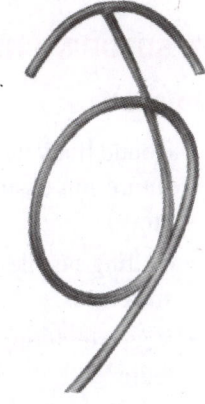

Fig. 51.45 T-tube (Kehr's)

46. SENGSTAKEN BLAKEMORE DOUBLE BALLOON TRIPLE LUMEN TUBE (Fig. 51.46)

- It is used in controlling bleeding **oesophageal varices.** It has 3 lumens and 2 balloons, A gastric balloon and an oesoph-ageal balloon.

- **Gastric balloon is in-flated** with about **200-250 ml** of air and oesoph-ageal balloon is inflated with about **40-60 ml of air**. It is pulled upwards so as to snugly fit at the oesophagogastric junction and thus it acts by internal tamponade.

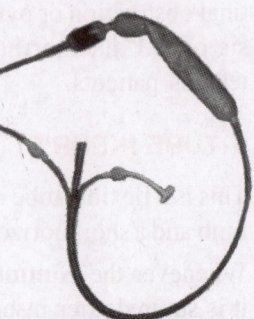

Fig. 51.46 Sengstaken Blackmore double ballon triple lumen tube

- Sengstaken tube should not be kept in place for more than 48 hours, because it can cause pressure necrosis of oesophagus.

- It should be deflated for few minutes after 24 hours.

- Sengstaken tube should be used by an experienced phy-sician. Oesophageal secretions and saliva cannot be aspirated while using this tube, and if gastric balloon is deflated suddenly, it slides up and causes choking- The oesophageal balloon should be immediately deflated in such situations.

- **Modification of Sengstaken tube is called as Min-nesota tube or 4 lumen tube.** It has 4 lumens. One to inflate oesophageal balloon, one to inflate gastric bal-loon, one to aspirate like a Ryle's tube, and the 4th lu-men is used to aspirate oesophageal secretions. If there is any difficulty in breathing while using Sengstaken tube or Minnesota tube, bulb should be deflated or tube should be Cut.

47. SUTURING NEEDLES

Traumatic

- Round body needle is an eyed needle. They are used to suture soft tissues, muscles, tendons, vessels, intestines etc.

- Cutting needle is used to suture slim and some tough structures.

- Reverse cutting needle is used to suture muco-perios-teum.

These needles have an eye. The eye is wider than body of the needle, so tissue trauma is more.

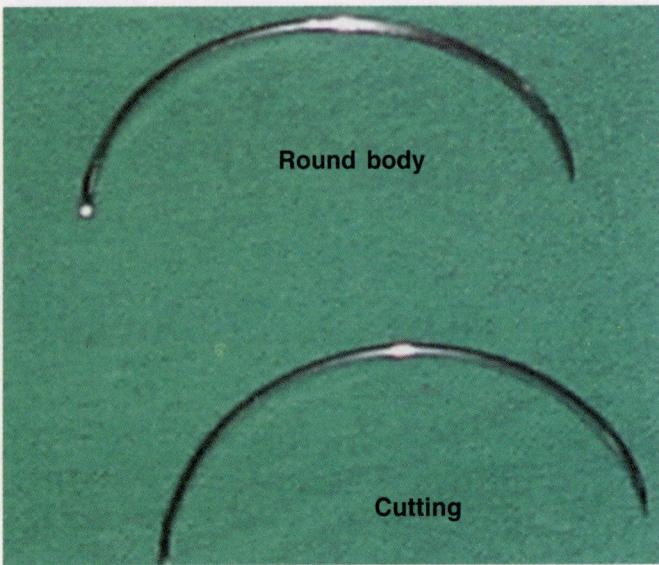

Fig. 51.47 Suturing needles

Atraumatic

- These needles have no eye. Suture is attached to the needle by a process called as swaging. Tissue trauma is less, hence used in suturing vessels or to repair a small tear in the bowel etc.

48. SUTURE MATERIALS (Fig. 51.47)

ABSORBABLE

1. Plain catgut (7 day catgut)

- The word catgut is derived from KIT-GUT, which means the violin strings.

- Catgut is derived from the submucosa of the sheep in-testines.

- It is the oldest suture material known.

- The plain catgut lasts for **7-10 days**. Hence, its uses are minimal.

- It can be used to put 'fat stitches' (subcutaneous fat).

- It is biological, absorbable and monofilament.

- Sheep's submucosa has a rich content of elastic tissue

- It should not be used in the presence of infection.

2. Chromic catgut (21 day catgut)

- When plain catgut is mixed with chromic salts, chromic catgut is obtained,

- **The strength of the chromic catgut is about 15-25 days**.

- Chromic catgut is widely used in intestinal anastomosis, closure of urinary bladder, closure of common bile duct, ligature of cystic artery stump, etc.
- Catgut is biological, absorbable, monofilament suture material.
- Chromic catgut is packed along with round body needle.
- The number 2-0 refers to the thickness of the suture.
- Knotting property is good.
- The catgut is preserved in 70% alcohol and is kept soft due to 5% glycerine.

3. Vicryl (Polyglactin)

- This is a copolymer of glycolide and lactide.
- It is a synthetic and absorbable suture.
- Unlike catgut, this is absorbed by hydrolysis.
- Since the strength and reliability is more than catgut, vicryl is being used more and more for small intestinal and colonic anastomosis.
- Being synthetic, tissue reaction is less than that of chromic catgut.
- This has also replaced catgut while suturing common bile duct.
- Knotting property is good.
- Vicryl can be used in the presence of infection.

4. Dexon (Polyglycdic acid)

- Synthetic absorbable
- Braided
- Used like vicryl

5. PDS (Poly Dioxanone suture)

- Like vicryl
- Costly
- Creamy in colour

NONABSORBABLE

1. Prolene

- This is polypropylene and nonabsorbable.
- It is monofilament, artificial and uncoated. Does not harbour micro-organism. Hence the chances of infection are less.
- Since it is nonabsorbable, prolene can be used for abdominal closure, repair of hernias, repair of incisional hernia, etc.
- It has high memory (Recalling tendency after removal from the pocket) requires many knots.

Key Box 51.3	
COLOUR	SUTURE MATERIAL
• Yellow	Plain catgut
• Brown	Chronic catgut
• Violet	Vicryl
• Creamy yellow	Dexon
• Creamy	PDS
• Blue	Prolene
• Black	Silk
• White	Cotton

2. Sutupack

- It is a monofilament or multifilament polyamide.
- Black in colour.
- It is braided, uncoated and nonabsorbable.
- Uses of sutupack are similar to prolene.
- Knotting property is not very good. Hence, it is mandatory to put 4-5 knots.

3. Mersilk

- This is nonabsorbable, braided silk, black in colour.
- It is provided with a round body. This can be used in ligating bleeding points or anastomosis, etc.

4. Black silk

- This is a nonabsorbable suture material.
- It is biological and derived from the **cocoon of the silkworm larva.**
- It is braided, coated with wax to reduce capillary action. Tissue reaction is much more with black silk because it is a foreign protein.
- In spite of this, it is widely used because of its easy availability and is cheap.
- Knotting property is excellent.

5. Cotton

- White in colour
- Multifilament - infection rate is high
- Nonabsorble, cheap

52

Specimens

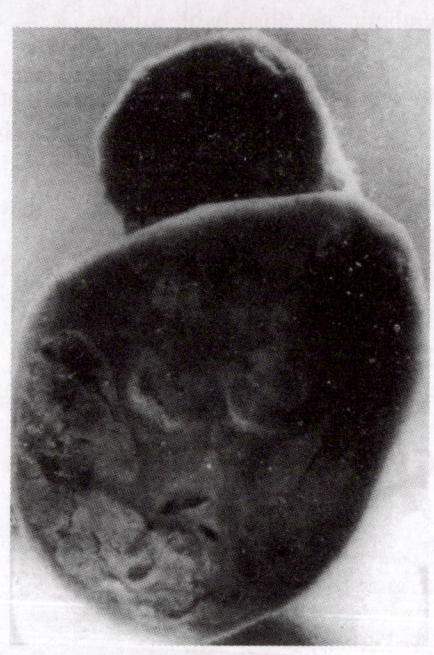

Fig. 52.1 Tuberculous (TB) lymphadenitis

I. TUBERCULOUS (TB) LYMPHADENITIS

1. What is this specimen?

- Specimen of lymph nodes which are matted. Cut surface shows caseation. Hence, it is tuberculous lymphadenitis.

2. What is the microscopic picture?

- Central caseation surrounded by epitheloid cells, Langhans type of giant cells.

3. What are the stages of TB lymphadenitis?

- Stage of lymphadenitis

- Stage of matting

- Stage of cold abcess

- Stage of collar stud abscess

- Stage of sinus formation

4. Why is matting seen in TB lymphadenitis?

- It is because of periadenitis

5. What is the treatment of COLD ABSCESS?

- Non-dependent aspiration by using wide bore needle, to avoid sinus formation.

II. LYMPHOMA

1. What is the diagnosis?

- Multiple lymph nodes which are discrete and not matted. Cut surface does not show caseation. It is homogeneous. Hence, this is a specimen of Hodgkin's lymphoma.

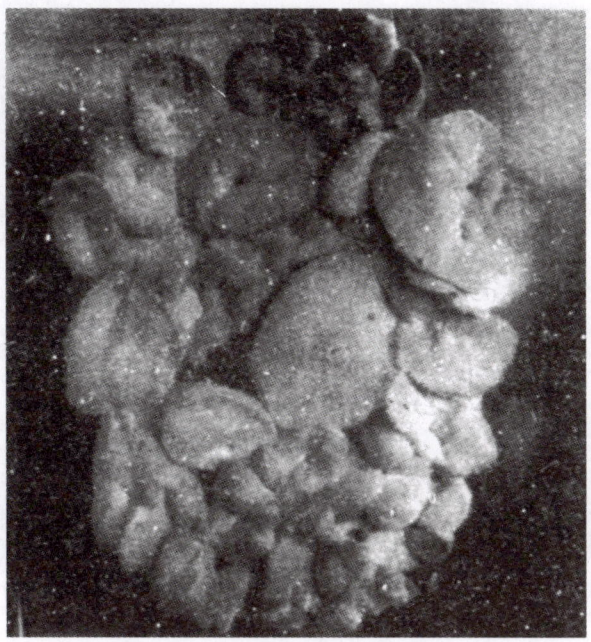

Fig. 52.2 Lymphoma

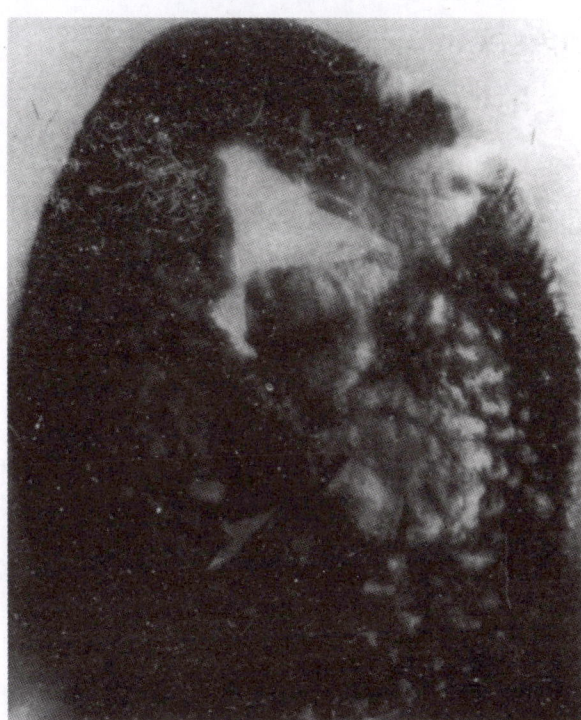

Fig. 52.3 Marjolin's ulcer

2. How do you confirm the diagnosis?

- Lymph node biopsy

3. What is the microscopic picture?

- Cellular pleomorphism: Lymphocytes, histiocytes, eosinophils, monocytes with giant cells containing mirror image nuclei—Reed-Sternberg cell.

4. What are the common lymph nodes involved in Hodgkin's lymphoma?

- Cervical, axillary, para-aortic, iliac and inguinal lymph nodes.

5. Is Waldeyer's ring involvement seen in Hodgkin's lymphoma ?

- No. It is usually seen in Non-Hodgkin's lymphoma.

III. MARJOLIN'S ULCER

1. What is this specimen?

- Wide excision specimen, showing ulcerated growth arising from the scar. It has everted edges, and there is extensive scarring.

2. What is the diagnosis?

- Squamous cell carcinoma arising in scar tissue is called as Marjolin's ulcer.

3. What are the common causes of Marjolin's ulcer?

- Burns
- Snake bite
- Varicose ulcer

4. What are the peculiarities of Marjolin's ulcer?

- It grows very slowly because of scar tissue
- It is painless as nerves have been destroyed
- It does not spread by lymphatics as they are also destroyed.

5. What is the treatment?

- Wide excision followed by split skin grafting

IV. SQUAMOUS CELL CARCINOMA

1. What is the specimen?

- Specimen of wide excision showing ulcerated growth with everted edges arising from skin.

2. What is the diagnosis?

- Squamous cell carcinoma

3. What is the microscopic picture?

- Mitotic figures with keratin pearls or epithelial pearls

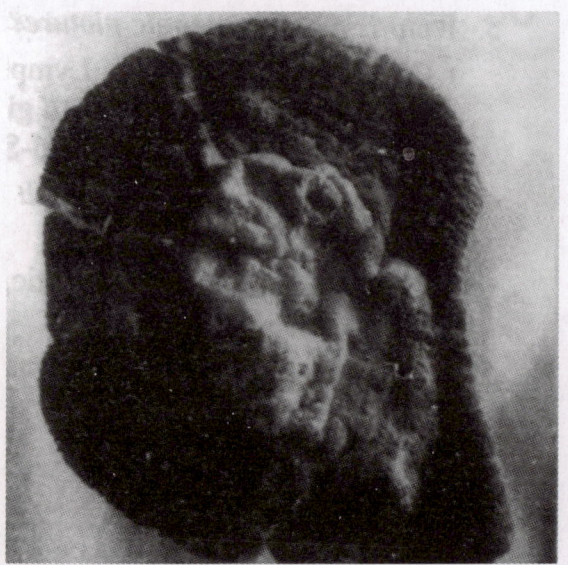

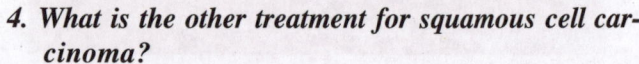

Fig. 52.4 Squamous cell carcinoma

4. What is the other treatment for squamous cell carcinoma?

- Radiotherapy

5. What are the common causes of squamous cell carcinoma?

- Leukoplakia
- Radiation dermatitis
- Bowen's disease
- Congenital skin conditions like xeroderma pigmentosa and albinism
- Chronic scar

V. SPECIMEN OF HEMIGLOSSECTOMY WITH HEMIMANDIBULECTOMY

1. What is this specimen?

- Specimen showing growth arising from the tongue and infiltrating the mandible.

2. What is the diagnosis?

- Advanced carcinoma tongue.

3. Is radiotherapy indicated in this situation ?

- No, because chances of radionecrosis of the mandible are high.

4. What type of X-ray is taken to see for involvement of the mandible?

- *ORTHOPANTOMOGRAM*

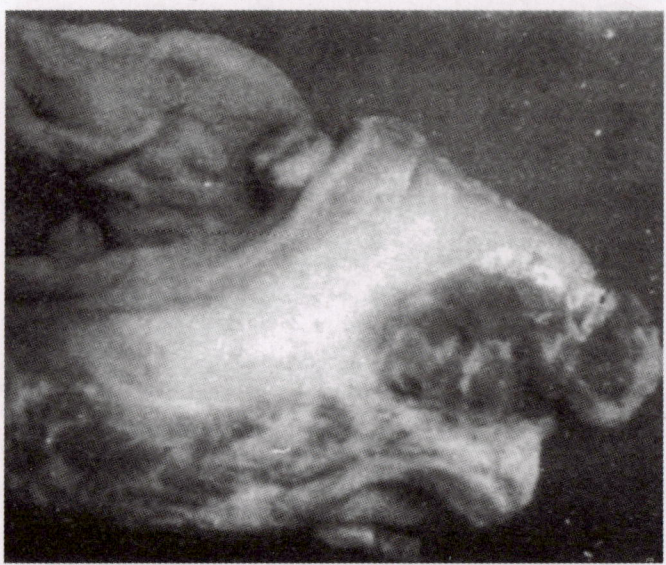

Fig. 52.5 Specimen of hemiglossectomy with hemimandibulectomy

5. What is Commando's operation?

- Hemiglossectomy with excision of the floor of the mouth, hemimandibulectomy, with radical block dissection of the neck done in a single stage, with en bloc removal.

VI. CHRONIC GASTRIC ULCER

1. What is this specimen?

- Specimen of the stomach showing rugosity of the stomach. There is a deep ulcer crater along the lesser curvature.

2. What is the diagnosis?

- Benign gastric ulcer

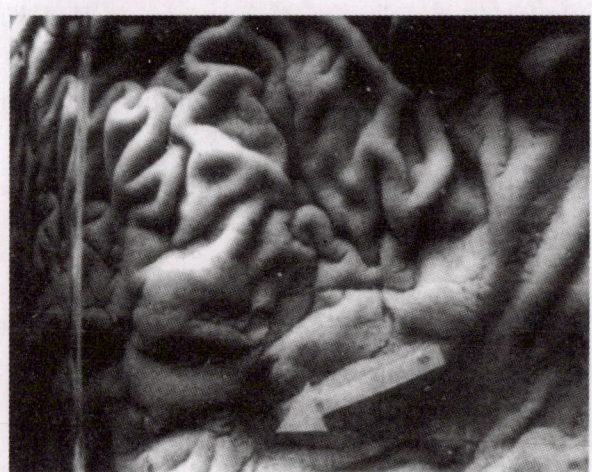

Fig. 52.6 Chronic gastric ulcer

3. Why is it a benign gastric ulcer?

- Since the rugae are of converging type. It is benign gastric ulcer

4. How do you rule out malignancy in a gastric ulcer?

- Endoscopic biopsy

5. What is the incidence of gastric ulcer turning into malignancy?

- 0.5 to 5% (2%)

VII. LINITIS PLASTICA

1. What is this specimen?

- Specimen of the stomach showing loss of normal rugosity. There is a nodular extensive infiltrating lesion along the entire length of the stomach.

2. What is the diagnosis ?

- Linitis plastica — Leather bottle stomach

3. What is linitis plastica?

- It is an extensive fibrosis involving entire submucosa of the stomach initially and also involves other layers later.

4. What is the treatment for linitis plastica?

- Radical total gastrectomy

5. What is the prognosis?

- Very poor

VIII. INTUSSUSCEPTION

1. What is this specimen?

- Specimen of intestine showing one portion of bowel invaginated within the other.

2. What is the diagnosis?

- Intussusception

3. What is the common type of intussusception?

- Ileocolic.

4. What are the parts of intussusception?

- Intussusceptum, intussuscipiens, neck and apex.

5. What is the treatment in children?

- Hydrostatic reduction or operative reduction.
- If there is gangrene - resection followed by end to end anastomosis

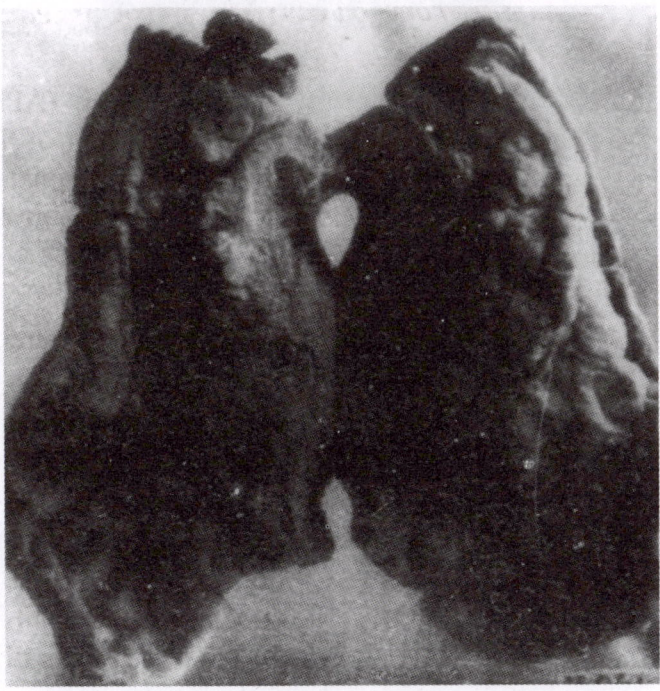

Fig. 52.7 Linitis plastica

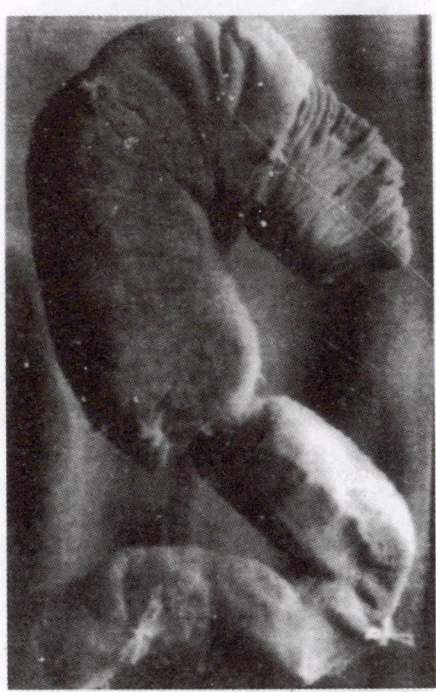

Fig. 52.8 Intussusception

IX. CARCINOMA RECTUM

1. *What is this specimen?*

- Specimen of rectum showing ulceroproliferative growth in the middle of the rectum. Specimen also shows entire rectum and anal canal.

2. *What is the diagnosis?*

- Carcinoma rectum

3. *What is this surgery called?*

- Abdomino-perineal resection (excision) (APR). In this operation, entire rectum, anal canal, part of the sigmoid colon, fat, fascia, lymphatics and regional nodes are removed en bloc followed by permanent colostomy in the left iliac fossa.

4. *What are the indications for APR?*

- Growth in the middle and lower rectum wherein sphincter cannot be saved.

5. *What is the position of the patient in APR?*

- Supine with lithotomy called as Lloyd Davis position.

X. GANGRENOUS APPENDICITIS

1. *What is this specimen?*

- It is an appendicectomy specimen showing blackish discolouration of the appendix.

2. *What factors cause gangrene of the appendix?*

- Gangrenous appendicitis occurs usually in old aged patients, where there is decreased vascularity due to atherosclerosis. It can also occur when the lumen is blocked due to faecolith, thereby causing ischaemia.

3. *What is the one simple investigation which is useful in diagnosing the appendicitis?*

- Total WBC count. Above 10,000 cells/cumm of blood with increased neutrophil count.

4. *What are the complications of acute appendicitis?*

- Appendicular mass (in untreated cases)
- Perforation with an abscess
- Perforation with generalised peritonitis
- Pylephlebitis, portal pyaemia
- Septicaemia, gram-negative shock

5. *How do you treat an appendicular mass?*

- Conservative line, Oschner-Sherren regime—Aspiration, antibiotics, intravenous fluids, etc.

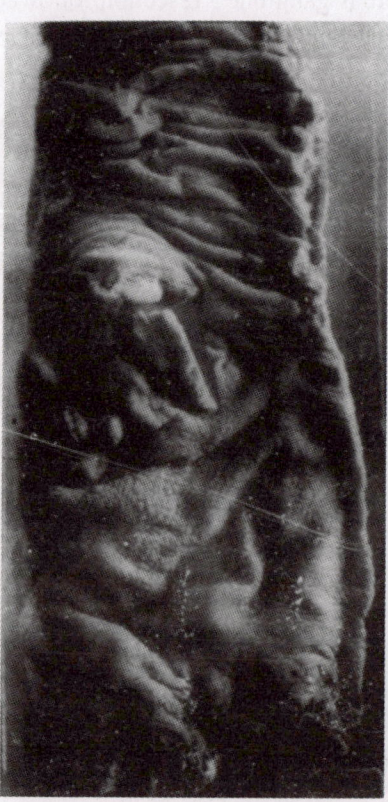

Fig. 52.9 Carcinoma rectum

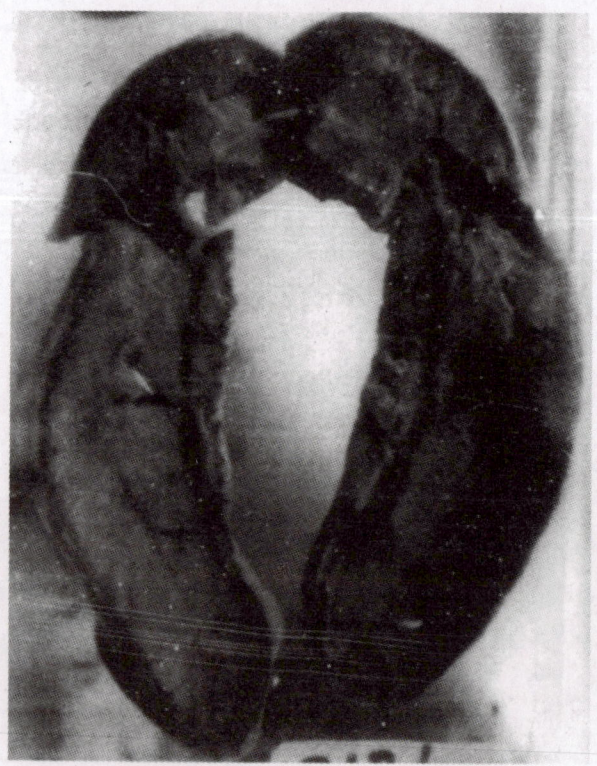

Fig. 52.10 Gangrenous appendicitis

XI. CARCINOMA ASCENDING COLON

1. What is this specimen?

- Specimen of terminal ileum, caecum and right colon with removal of involved lymph nodes fat and fascia. Nowadays, only 4-6 cms. of ileum is removed.

2. What is it called?

- Right radical hemicolectomy done for growth in the ascending colon

3. How will you identify colon?

- Taenia coli and appendix is seen, The colon has larger diameter compared to small intestine

4. What are the investigations?

- Barium enema will show persistent filling defect. However, colonoscopy is the investigation because one can visualise the growth and biopsy can be taken.

5. What do you mean by limited resection?

- It is done for ileo-caecal tuberculosis wherein diseased segment is removed.

XII. MECKEL'S DIVERTICULUM

1. What is the specimen?

- Resected specimen of intestine showing a diverticulum, hence Meckel's diverticulum

2. Why do you say it is Meckel's diverticulum?

- Because it is a single diverticulum arising from antimesenteric border of the intestine.

3. What are common symptoms?

- Bleeding per rectum, abdominal pain due to inflammation, intestinal obstruction and peritonitis due to perforation

4. What is the cause and what are the types of bleeding?

- Ulcer in the ectopic gastric mucosa. Bleeding can be occult or small quantities and rarely can be massive.

5. How do you diagnose Meckel's diverticulum?

- Radio-nuclear (99m Tc pertechnetate) scan is helpful when there is active bleeding (Page 770)

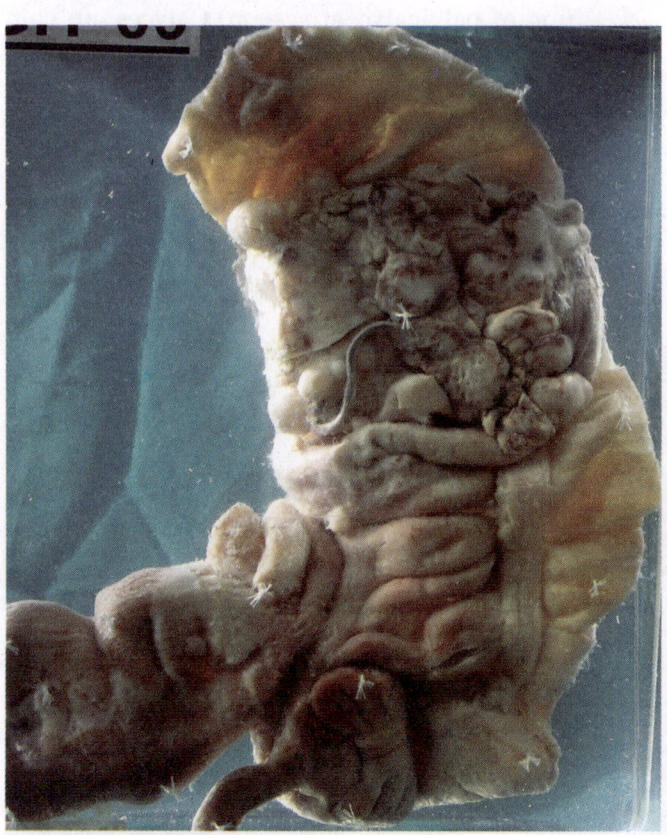

Fig. 52.11 Carcinoma ascending colon

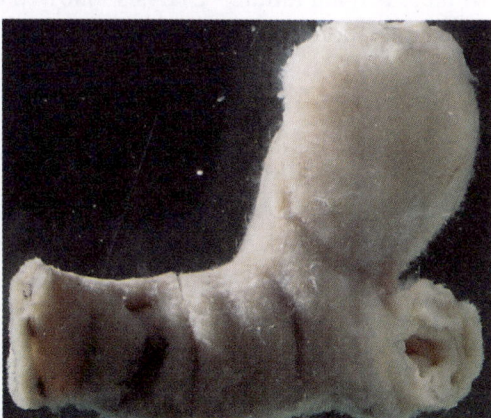

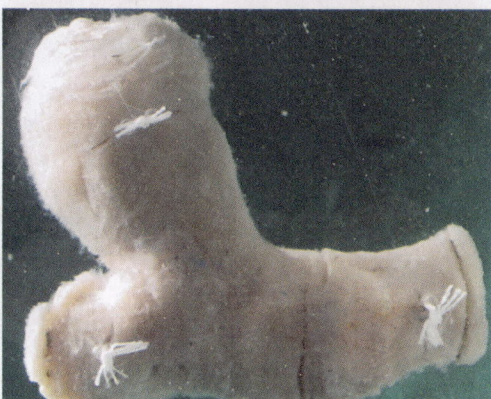

Fig. 52.12 Meckel's diverticulum

XIII. POLYCYSTIC KIDNEY

1. What is this specimen?

- Specimen of kidney with multiple cystic lesions. Entire kidney is involved.

2. What is the diagnosis?

- Polycystic kidney

3. Why do you say it is polycystic kidney?

- Kidney is grossly enlarged
- Outer surface is bossellated
- Multiple cysts are present

4. What are clinical features of polycystic kidney?

- Women : 30-50 years
- Bilateral renal mass
- Hypertension
- Haematuria
- Renal failure

5. What is the treatment?

- If there is no renal failure, control hypertension.
- If there is renal failure - Dialysis followed by renal transplantation.

XIV. RENAL CELL CARCINOMA

1. What is this specimen?

- Specimen of the kidney because it is reniform shaped, ureter and calyces are seen.

- In the upper pole, there is destruction of the calyces with solid mass. Cut surface is smooth.

2. What is the diagnosis?

- Renal cell carcinoma

3. What is the microscopic picture?

- Cuboidal or polyhedral clear cells with deeply stained rounded nuclei—Clear cell carcinoma. Sometimes, dark cells can coexist. In some cases, walls of blood vessels are lined by tumour cells.

4. How does it spread?

- Lymphatic and blood spread.

5. What are the primary malignant tumours which spread by blood?

- Renal cell carcinoma, follicular carcinoma thyroid, carcinoma prostate, carcinoma breast, bronchogenic carcinoma.

XV. HYDRONEPHROSIS

1. What is this specimen?

- Specimen of the kidney with ureter showing dilatation of pelvicalyceal system. Calyces are club shaped.

2. What is the diagnosis?

- Hydronephrosis—probably PUJ obstruction

3. Why do you say it may be PUJ obstruction?

- Ureter is not dilated

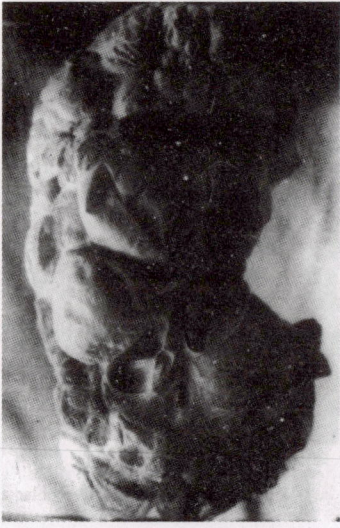

Fig. 52.13 Polycystic kidney

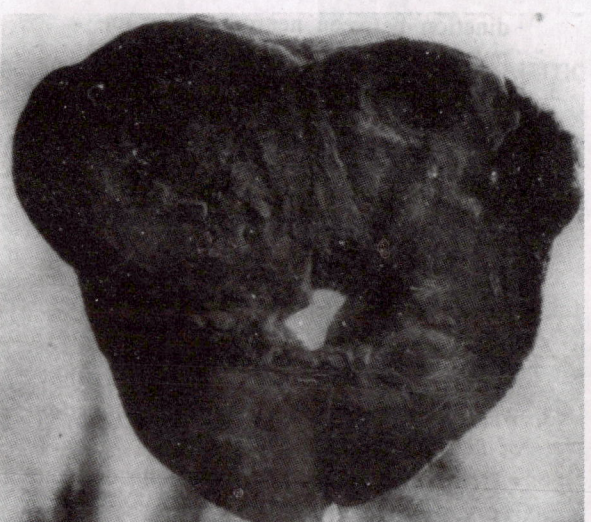

Fig. 52.14 Renal cell carcinoma

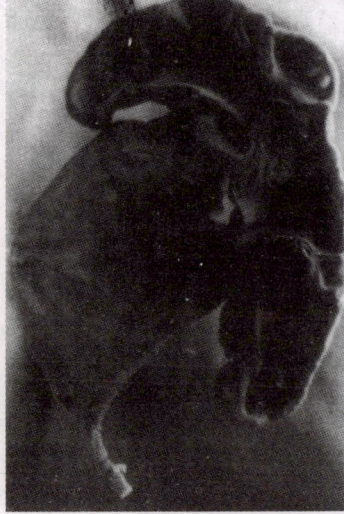

Fig. 52.15 Hydronephrosis

4. What are the common causes of obstruction at PUJ?

- Stone in the pelvis
- Aberrant vessels—a lower polar artery or vein arising from the main vessels in an aberrant position obstructs the upper ureter.
- PUJ dyskinesia—Occurs due to incoordination between neuromuscular impulses and pelvis.

5. What is the treatment of PUJ dyskinesia?

- Anderson-Hynes pyeloplasty

XVI. CARCINOMA PENIS

1. What is this specimen?

- Specimen of penis, showing the glans. Prepuce is cut open showing the growth.

2. What is the diagnosis ?

- Partial amputation done for carcinoma penis

3. What are the indications for partial amputation of the penis?

- Growth confined to the glans penis or to the prepuce

4. What is the treatment if the shaft is involved?

- Total amputation of penis followed by perineal urethrostomy.

5. What are the complications of perineal urethrostomy?

- Bleeding, dermatitis and stenosis. The stenosis should be dilated by using Hegar's dilators.

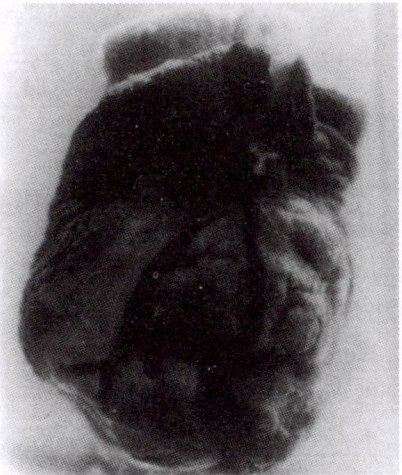

Fig. 52.16 Carcinoma Penis

XVII. SEMINOMA TESTIS

1. What is this specimen ?

- Specimen of testis showing spermatic cord. Cut surface of the testis is smooth and homogeneous with a tumour in the upper port.

2. What is the diagnosis?

- Seminoma

3. Why is it not a teratoma?

- Teratoma—Cut surface is not homogenous

4. How does seminoma spread?

- Mainly by lymphatics

5. What type of orchidectomy is done for testicular tumours and why?

- High orchidectomy, through an inguinal incision. If scrotum is incised, chances of alternate pathway of lymphatics opening up are high. Hence, inguinal exploration is the choice.

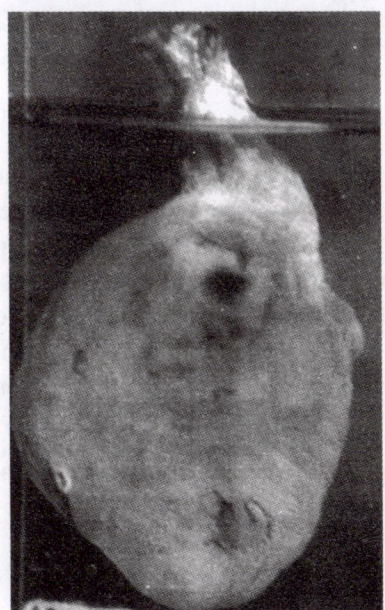

Fig. 52.17 Seminoma testis

Useful Tips

- Please look into the specimen carefully
- Please see both sides of the specimen
- Think which is the most likely organ involved
- Think what is the probable diagnosis

53

Operative Surgery

- Appendicectomy
- Herniorrhaphy
- Partial excision and eversion of sac
- Incision and drainage
- Breast abscess drainage
- Venesection
- Vasectomy
- Tracheostomy
- Suprapubic cystostomy
- Thyroidectomy
- Amputation
- Accessories
  - High frequency electro surgery
  - Cryosurgery
  - Lasers in surgery
  - Staplers in surgery

STEPS OF OPERATIVE SURGERY

1. Indication
2. Contraindication
3. Position of the patient
4. Anaesthesia
5. Preparation of parts
6. Procedure
7. Closure
8. Post-operative treatment
9. Post-operative Complications
10. Advice at discharge

ANTISEPTIC AGENTS

- Povidone iodine
- Spirit 70%
- Savlon

Over a period of time, the number of operations which an undergraduate should know has become less and less. Today no M.B.B.S. doctor is supposed to do a surgical procedure because of availability of surgeons even in a village. Hence, I have discussed very few surgical procedures in this chapter. These are the common surgical procedures, which are of help for an undergraduate student.

Every operation has been discussed under certain basic steps which are given below and the key words used are given in the key box.

Key Box 53.1
POST-OPERATIVE PAIN RELIEF

- Opioids
- Non-steroidal anti-inflammatory drugs
- Local anesthetics through epidural catheter

Key Box 53.2
KEY WORDS

S.A	Spinal anaesthesia
G.A	General anaesthesia
L.A	Local anaesthesia
OT	Operation theatre
NPO	Nil per oral
IV	Intravenous
RT	Ryle's tube

Autoclave and sterilisation (Kindly refer *Manipal Manual of Surgery for Dental Students* for details)

Table 53.1 Sterilisation	
AGENTS FOR STERILISATION	**COMMON OT ITEMS**
1. Autoclaving	Linen, Operative instruments, syringes
2. Dettol or phenol	Sharp instruments (scissors, needles, blades)
3. Glutaraldehyde	Endoscopy/Laparoscopy equipments
4. Ethylene oxide gamma radiation	Surgical catgut, heart lung machine syringes
5. Formaldehyde	Disinfect rooms like OT

APPENDICECTOMY

Appendicectomy can be one of the easiest and sometimes one of the most complicated surgeries.

1. INDICATIONS

- Acute appendicitis-Emergency appendicectomy
- Recurrent appendicitis-Elective appendicectomy

2. CONTRAINDICATIONS

- Appendicular mass

3. POSITION OF THE PATIENT

- Supine

4. ANAESTHESIA

- This surgery can be done either under GA or regional anaesthesia (spinal or epidural).

5. PREPARATION

- Parts are cleaned with iodine and spirit, from the level of umbilicus above to the upper part of thigh below.

6. PROCEDURE

Incision

1. McBurney's grid-iron incision is the most popular incision. It is at right angles to spino-umbilical line placed at McBurney's point. It is about 6-8 cm in length (Fig. 53.1)

2. **Lanz** Incision is a curved transverse incision, placed at the McBurney's point. Cosmetically, it is a better incision (Fig.53.2)

3. Right paramedian incision is made when diagnosis is in doubt as a part of EXPLORATORY LAPAROTOMY. This is also preferred in females where there

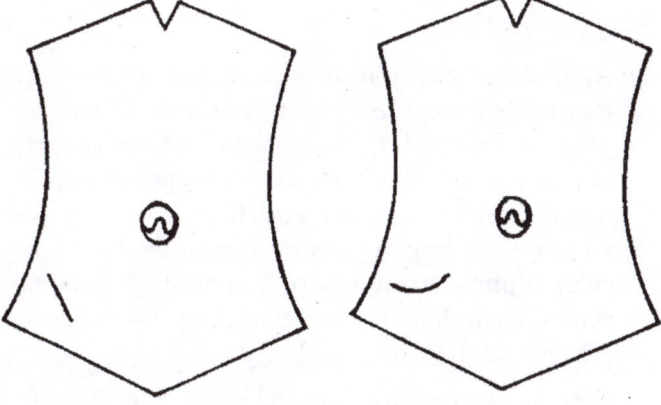

Fig. 53.1 Grid iron incision   **Fig. 53.2** Lanz incision

is a gynec pathology like ovarian cyst which may be the cause of right iliac fossa pain (Fig.53.3).

Layers opened

- Skin
- Two layers of subcutaneous tissue - superficial fatty (Camper's), deep membranous (Scarpa's). (C : comes first, S : later). There is no deep fascia in the abdomen.

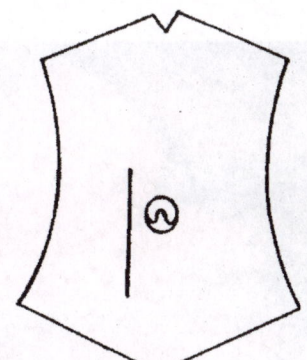

Fig. 53.3 Right paramedian incision

- External oblique aponeurosis is seen running downwards and medially. It is incised in the direction of its fibres.
- Internal and transverse abdominal muscles are split (Grid Iron- right angle to each other).
- Peritoneum is incised.

Feature of acute appendicitis at operation are

- Inflamed, turgid appendix
- Pus in the right iliac fossa
- Presence of omentum in the right iliac fossa
- Black or green appendix (gangrenous)
- Faecolith

Location of appendix

- Trace taenia coli, it will lead on to the base of appendix (ALL ROADS LEAD TO ROME).

Surgical procedure

- Appendix is gently held at mesoappendix by using Babcock's forceps and blood vessels in the mesoappendix are divided. These include appendicular artery, branch of ileocolic artery (Accessory appendicular artery of Seshachalam, is a branch of posterior caecal artery). Once appendix is freed upto the base (caecum), a **purse string suture** is applied all round appendix, taking bites from caecum, using 2-0 atraumatic silk (Fig. 53.4).

- Appendix is crushed at base and is held 1 cm above the crush. A tight silk ligature is applied at the crushed site and appendix is cut in between. Stump is cleaned with spirit and is invaginated and purse string is tightened. This is called as burial of the stump. Perfect haemostasis is obtained (53.5).

> *Look for Meckel's diverticulum, which may be the cause of right iliac fossa pain.*

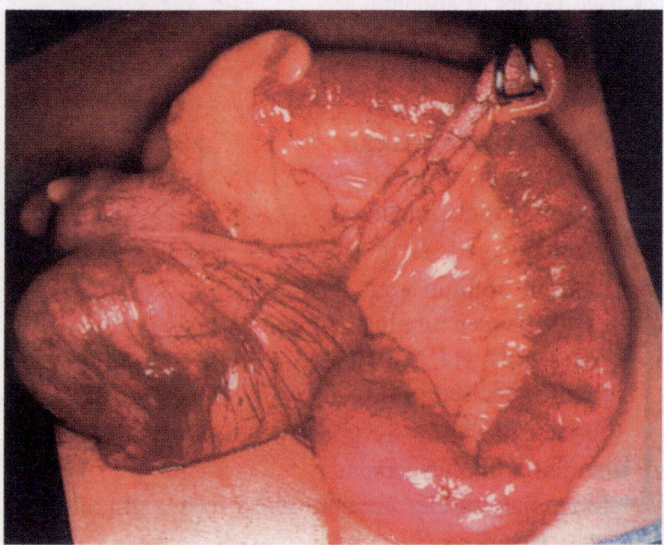

Fig. 53.5 Appendix at surgery

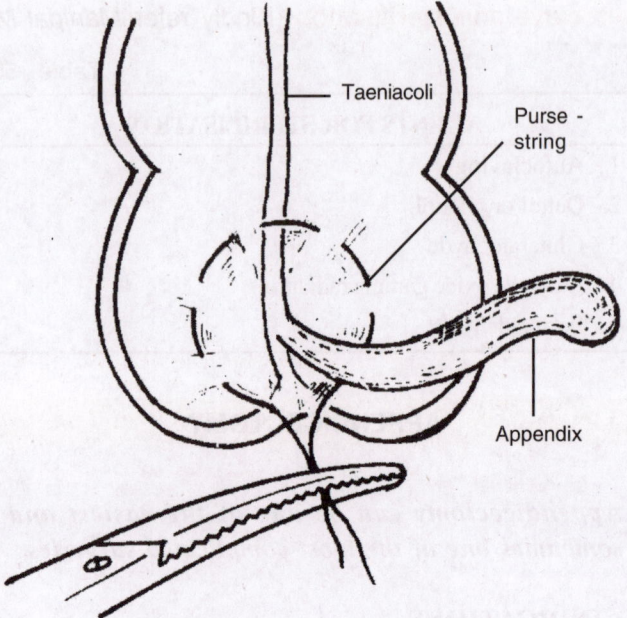

Fig. 53.4 Purse - string suture

7. CLOSURE

- Peritoneum-Continuous 2-0 chromic catgut
- Split muscles-Sutured together by few interrupted chromic catgut.
- External oblique with chromic catgut
- Subcutaneous fat with plain catgut
- Skin with interrupted silk. (Instead of chromic catgut, 2-0 silk can also be used to close the layers.)
- Corrugated red rubber drain is not kept routinely, unless there is gangrenous appendicitis or lot of pus in the peritoneal cavity.

8. POSTOPERATIVE TREATMENT

- RT aspiration for one or two days
- I.V. fluids 2.5 litres/day for one-two days
- Oral fluids are allowed once abdomen is soft and bowel sounds are heard
- Appropriate antibiotics to cover Gram+ve, Gram-ve and anaerobic organisms
- Suture removal by 7-10 days

9.COMPLICATIONS AFTER APPENDICECTOMY

1. **Postoperative fever** can be due to various factors. Thrombophlebitis, urinary tract infection and I.V. fluids are common causes. In the absence of these, wound infection or intraperitoneal abscess secondary to gangrenous appendicitis, may have to be considered.

- Change of antibiotics according to culture and sensitivity reports of urine, pus and blood help in treating postoperative fever.
- Elderly patients may have co-existing pulmonary disease. Respiratory tract infection also has to be considered.

2. **Wound infection**

3. **Intra-abdominal abscess** needs drainage

4. **Faecal fistula-causes:**

   a. Gangrene spreading into caecum

   b. Persistent infection

   c. Carcinoma caecum (elderly patients)

   d. Ileocaecal tuberculosis

   e. Actinomycosis (RARE)

   f. Crohn's disease (rare in India)

> *Most of the faecal fistulae will stop by themselves provided there is no distal obstruction.*

5. Septicaemia, portal pyaemia, Gram-negative shock in late cases of peritonitis due to perforated appendicitis are the uncommon but dangerous complications.
   - Mortality of appendicular perforation and peritonitis is around 2%.

10. ADVICE AT DISCHARGE

- Rest for 15 days

HERNIORRHAPHY-BASSINI'S

This means herniotomy and approximation of conjoined tendon to inguinal ligament to strengthen the posterior wall of the inguinal canal.

1. Indication

- Indirect or direct hernia with good muscle tone

2. Contraindication (relative)

- Serve cardiopulmonary insufficiency

3. Position of the patient

- Supine

4. Anaesthesia

- Regional anaesthesia or G.A
- **Local anaesthesia** may be preferred in **high risk patients**.

5. PREPARATION OF THE PARTS

- Parts are cleaned with iodine and spirit, from the level of umbilicus above to the upper part of thigh below.

6. PROCEDURE

Incision

- 6-8 cm incision is made parallel to the inguinal ligament at the level of deep ring in the medial two thirds of the inguinal ligament.

Layers opened

1. Skin
2. Two layers of superficial fascia
3. External oblique is incised in the line of direction of fibres, till external ring is slit open.
4. Thin cremasteric box is opened.
5. Identification of the sac-glistening white colour.
   - Isolation of the card from the sac by blunt and sharp dissection and cord is held separately by using cord holding forceps (Fig. 53.6)

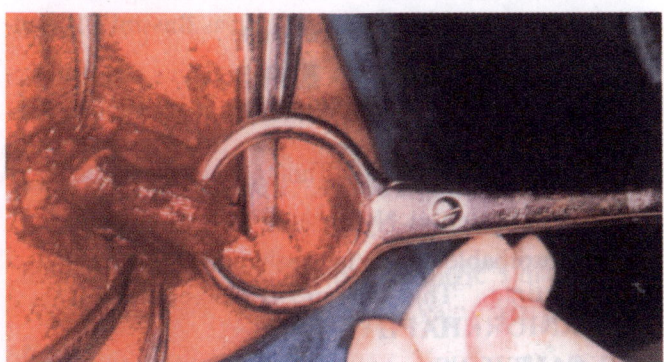

Fig. 53.6 Spermatic cord held with cord holding forceps

- Mobilise the sac up to the deep ring. Mobilisation is complete when inferior epigastric artery pulsations and extraperitoneal pad of fat are seen.
- **Open the sac and see for contents.**
- **Reduce the contents.**
- **Twist the sac** so as to avoid injury to the contents of the sac (Fig. 53.7).
- **Transfixation ligature** is applied as high as possible at the neck of sac and it is tightened.
- **Excision of the sac :** After excision, see the excised sac whether omentum or intestine have been

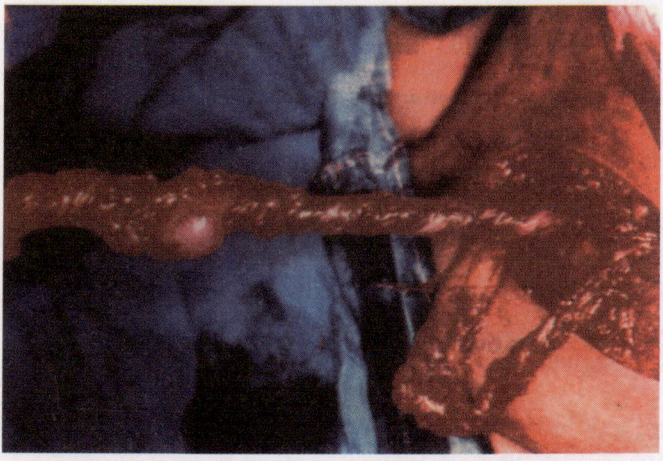

Fig. 53.7 Twisted hernial sac ready for trasfixation

injured or not. Upto this stage, it is called as **herniotomy**.

Repair

- Conjoined tendon above is approximated to the inguinal ligament by using nonabsorbable suture such as nylon, silk or polypropylene.
- Nonabsorbable suture is used to that strength remains for long time. This repair is called as **Bassini's Herniorrhaphy.**

Precautions

1. Ilioinguinal nerve should not be caught in ligature
2. Conjoined muscles should not be strangulated
3. There should not be any tension on the suture lines

7. CLOSURE

- External oblique is sutured with chromic catgut or silk
- Subcutaneous fat with absorbable catgut suture
- Skin with silk

Key Box 53.3
HERNIORRHAPHY
• Identification of the sac • Isolation of the sac • Mobilisation of the sac • Open the sac • Reduce the contents • Trasfixation ligation of the sac • Repair

8. POSTOPERATIVE MANAGEMENT

- NPO for 6-8 hours, oral fluids and soft diet later
- Analgesics
- Antibiotics-Not always necessary
- Scrotal support if the dissection is more (complete hernia)
- Suture removal after 7-10 days

9. POSTOPERATIVE COMPLICATIONS

1. Immediate: Haematoma due to the injury to the pampiniform plexus of veins or improper haemostasis. It may need reexploration.
2. Wound infection may result in discharging pus which is the cause of postoperative fever. Infection is the chief cause of recurrence.
3. Severe periostitis pubis (to avoid this nowadays, the repair need not be done by taking the bites through pubic bone). It is managed by analgesics and in intractable cases, injection of corticosteroids locally may help the patient.
4. Nerve entrapment causing pain

10. ADVICE AT DISCHARGE

- Not to strain or lift heavy weights (bucketful of water) or to carry load on the shoulders for 3 months.
- If there is any precipitating cause such as chronic cough or difficulty in passing urine etc., they have to be treated first, otherwise hernia will recur once again.

Dissecting an inguinal canal and performing a good repair is a good exercise for a postgraduate because he has to dissect various anatomical layers, preserve nerves, vessels, the vas deferens and do a good repair. Various steps of herniorrhaphy teaches a postgraduate basic fundamental principles of surgery.

SURGERY FOR HYDROCOELE

1. Indication

- Vaginal hydrocoele. (This procedure is described for vaginal hydrocoele.)

2. Contraindication

- Secondary Hydrocoele due to testicular tumours, they

contain haemorrhagic fluid. BIGGEST BLUNDER can be done here by incising the scrotum mistaking it to be a vaginal hydrocoele.

3. POSITION OF THE PATIENT

• Supine

4. ANAESTHESIA

• S.A or G.A
• It can also be done by using local infiltration anaesthesia

5. PREPARATION OF THE PARTS

• Savlon and spirit. (Iodine is better avoided because it can cause severe scrotal dermatitis and excoriation of skin, which can cause more discomfort to the patient than hydrococle surgery.)

6. PROCEDURE

Incision

• Hydrocoele is held tense by an assistant and 5-6 cm incision (depending upon size) is made over the most prominent part of the swelling parallel to the median raphe of the scrotum.

Layers opened

• Skin
• Dartos
• External spermatic fascia
• Cremasteric fascia
• Internal spermatic fascia

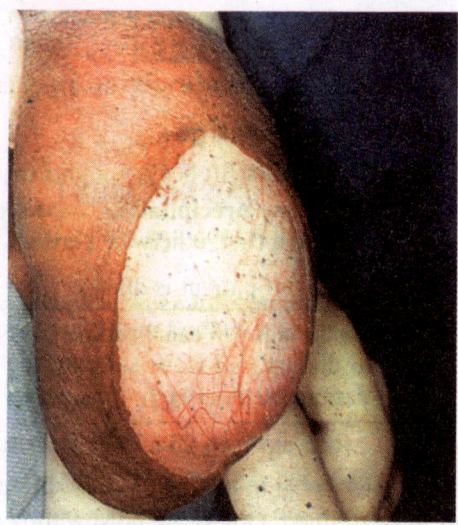

Fig. 53.8 Hydrocoele sac being delivered

Key Box 53.4

HYDROCOELE SURGERY

• Aspiration - Not advised
• Lord's plication - Small hydrocoele
• Jaboulay's - Large hydrocoele

At this stage hydrocoele sac is visible and is delivered outside the incision (Fig. 53.8).

Hydrocoele fluid is drained by using trocar and cannula. An opening is made in the tunica vaginalis sac and it is enlarged. All fluid is sucked out. Testis and epididymis is inspected for any pathology, e.g. Craggy epididymis can be found in tuberculosis. Depending on the size of the hydrocoele, thickness of the wall of the sac, two types of surgery can be done.

Surgery

1. Small tunica vaginalis sac (T.V. sac): The redundant tunica vaginalis is plicated by interrupted sutures. The sac gets crumpled up and surrounds the testis. This is called as 'LORD'S PLICATION **(Fig. 53.9)**.

2. Sac is large and thick: Partial excision and eversion of sac is ideal treatment. In this operation, after excision of the sac cut edge of the sac is everted and sutured behind the testis. This is called as JABOULAY'S OPERATION. By eversion of the sac, the secreting surface of the testis becomes anterior and secretions are absorbed by subcutaneous lymphatics **(Fig. 53.10)**.

7. CLOSURE

• A corrugated red rubber drain is kept in the scrotum

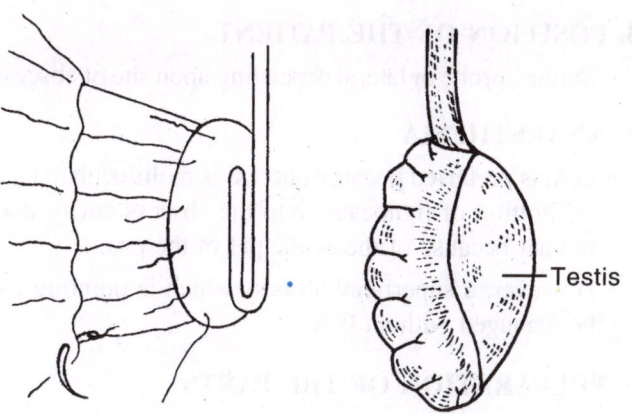

Fig. 53.9 Lord's plication   **Fig. 53.10** Jaboulay's operation

and brought out separately by making a stab incision and is anchored to the scrotal skin by white thread.

- Subcutaneous layer by using 2-0 chromic catgut.
- Skin—interrupted thread (White)
- Scrotal support is given to reduce oedema and bleeding.

8. POSTOPERATIVE MANAGEMENT

- NPO for 6 hours followed by soft diet
- Antibiotics and analgesics
- Suture removal after 7-8 days

9. POSTOPERATIVE COMPLICATIONS

1. Haematoma : If it is large and increasing, wound should be reopened urgently and bleeders have to be ligated. It may be due to injury to the testicular artery, vein or pampiniform plexus of veins.

2. Wound infection can result in pyocoele. Testis can undergo necrosis.

3. Injury to the spermatic cord

10. ADVICE AT DISCHARGE

- Rest for about a week

Even though surgery for hydrocoele is minor, it should not be taken lightly.

INCISION AND DRAINAGE (I and D)

1. INDICATIONS

- Pyogenic abscess

2. CONTRAINDICATION

- Cold abscess

3. POSITION OF THE PATIENT

- Supine, prone or lateral depending upon site of abscess.

4. ANAESTHESIA

- G.A. is preferred because abscess is multiloculated and infiltration of lignocaine into the abscess cavity does not act because of the acidic pH of the pus.
- However, a superficial abscess which is pointing can be managed without G.A.

5. PREPARATION OF THE PARTS

- Iodine and spirit

Key Box 53.5

I & D — POSITION

- Ischiorectal —LITHOTOMY
- Pilonidal — JACK-KNIFE
- Axillary — Abducted arm
- Back — Lateral

6. PROCEDURE

Incision

- A STAB INCISION is made over the most prominent part of the swelling (which is red, skin is thinned out and is pointed).
- Pus comes out and is sent for culture-and sensitivity.

Procedure

- A sinus forceps or finger is introduced within the abscess cavity and all the loculi are broken. When fresh blood oozes out, it indicates the completion of the procedure.
- Cavity is irrigated with H_2O_2 solution or Iodine solution.
- If the cavity is large, it is packed with roller gauze soaked in iodine and it is removed after 24-48 hours. Packing helps in controlling the bleeding and because of the pack the opening of the abscess cavity does not close. By 7-10 days, the cavity collapses, granulation tissue fills up the cavity and thus, healing takes place.

7. CLOSURE

- An abscess should not be closed, as it contains pus, bacteria etc.

8. POSTOPERATIVE MANAGEMENT

- Antibiotics
- Control of diabetes (If patient is diabetic)
- Regular dressing of the wound with antiseptic agents.

9. POSTOPERATIVE COMPLICATIONS

1. During the process of breaking the loculi, vessels underneath may be injured causing haematoma which needs to be drained. Otherwise no specific complications.

2. Injury to the vessels or the nerves can occur if basic principles of drainage of an abscess are not followed. When an abscess is located over the major vessel, as in axilla or neck, DO NOT MAKE A STAB INCISION. An incision is made on the skin and subcutaneous tissue and sinus forceps is introduced. Later, it is treated like treatment of abscess. This method is followed to avoid injury to major vessels. It is also indicated in parotid abscess to avoid damage to facial nerve. This is called as Hilton's method of drainage.

10. Advice at discharge

• Control of diabetes (if present).

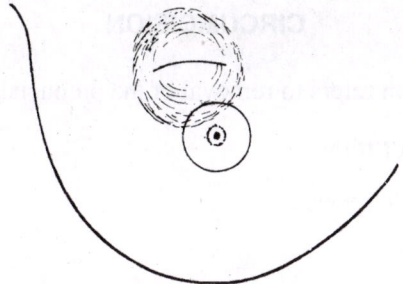

Fig. 53.11 Incision for breast abscess

I and D OF BREAST ABSCESS

1. INDICATION

• Breast abscess

2. CONTRAINDICATION

• None

3. POSITION OF THE PATIENT

• Supine

4. ANAESTHESIA

• G.A.

5. PREPARATION

• Iodine and spirit

6. PROCEDURE (Figs. 53.11 and 53.12)

Incision

• A semicircular incision about 5-6 cm is made over the swelling where there is maximum tenderness.

Procedure

• It is drained just like pyogenic abscess. Another stab incision is made in the dependent position and corrugated rubber drain is brought out through this incision.

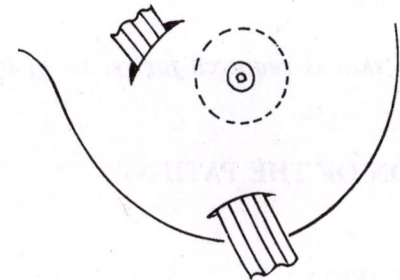

Fig. 53.12 Drainage and usage of corrugated rubber drain

7. CLOSURE

• If infection is very severe, DO NOT CLOSE THE INCISION.
• Otherwise, main wound is sutured and corrugated red rubber drain is brought down at the dependent position. Drain is removed, once the drainage is minimal.

8. POSTOPERATIVE MANAGEMENT

• NPO for about 6 hours
• Antibiotic of choice is CLOXACILLIN 500 mg 6th hourly because the common organism is Staphylococcus aureus.
• It may take 7-15 days for complete healing.
• One should not wait for fluctuation to develop in a breast abscess. If pain and tenderness does not subside by 48 hours, breast abscess is incised. Otherwise, breast tissue gets damaged.

9. Postoperative complications

• Haematoma needs evacuation.

10. Advice at discharge

• Lactating women should clean the nipple after every breast feed and keep it clean.

Do not use radial incision in breast surgery.

Key Box 53.6
BREAST ABSCESS DRAINAGE
• G.A is preferred • Do Not wait for fluctuation • Throbbing pain is an indication for surgery • Semicircular incision • Keep in mind, mastitis carcinomatosa

CIRCUMCISION

Circumcision refers to removal of the prepucial skin.

1. INDICATION

   a. Ritual: Religious

   b. Phimosis

2. CONTRAINDICATION

- Hypospadias

Prepuceal skin is required for repair of hypospadias

3. POSITION OF THE PATIENT

- Supine

4. ANAESTHESIA

   a. In children-G.A.

   b. In adults-L.A.

5. PREPARATION OF THE PARTS

- Savlon and spirit

Use plain lignocaine (Without adrenaline) for L.A. during circumcision Dose: 2% Lignocaine 10-15 ml.

6. PROCEDURE

In adults (Fig. 53.13)

- Skin of the tip of the penis is held in two places by using fine scissors, prepuce is separated from the glans and is slit up in mid-dorsal line to a point a little beyond the middle of the glans.

- Prepuceal layers are trimmed away in a line parallel to the corona. On the ventral surface, frenular artery needs to be ligated by using figure of 8 stitch. Two layers of prepuce are united by interrupted fine chromic catgut sutures. Dressings are applied.

In children (Fig. 53.14)

- Prepuce is held by two artery forceps and gentle traction is applied. A small artery clamp is applied distal to the glans and skin distal to the clamp is removed.

- Once clamp is removed, bleeding points are identified and ligated.

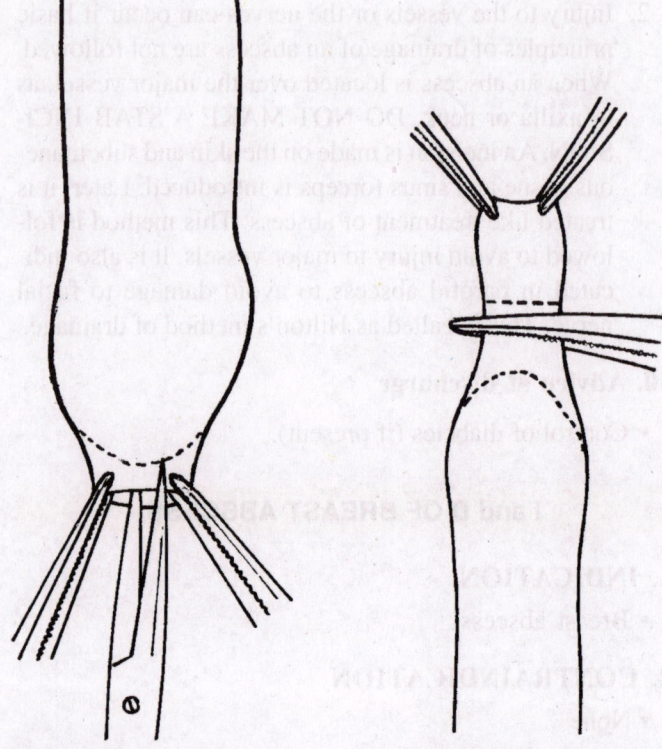

Fig. 53.13 Circumcision in adults   **Fig. 53.14** Circumcision in children

7. CLOSURE

- Two layers of prepuce are approximated by using chromic catgut.

8. POSTOPERATIVE MANAGEMENT

- Sedatives and analgesics.
- Antibiotics
- Removal of sutures is very painful. Hence, DO NOT USE NONABSORBABLE SUTURES.

9. POSTOPERATIVE COMPLICATIONS

1. Injury to the glans penis can occur when there are extensive adhesions between prepuce and glans. It needs suturing.

2. **Haematoma :** Due to injury to the corpora cavernosa or due to the bleeding from cut edges.

3. **Tension at suture line** if too much skin is removed. This may cause painful erection at a later date.

10. ADVICE AT DISCHARGE

- This surgery in adults is done on an out-patient basis. Patients are discharged within a few hours. Hence patients are advised to report if there is bleeding and also not to wet the area for 2-3 days.

VENESECTION OR CUT DOWN

1. INDICATION

- Shock : Hypovolaemic, haemorrhagic, burns etc.,
- When peripheral veins are not visible due to shock, burns or massive haemorrhage, an incision is made in the anatomical sites of the vein and vein is identified, isolated and cannulated for transfusion of fluids. This procedure is called as venesection or cut down.

2. CONTRAINDICATION

- None

3. POSITION OF THE PATIENT

- Supine

4. ANAESTHESIA

- Local infiltration by using 2% lignocaine 3-5 ml.

5. PREPARATION

- Iodine and spirit

6. PROCEDURE

- Cephalic vein cutdown is the most popular and an ideal procedure. A transverse incision about 5 cm is made in the deltopectoral groove. Cephalic vein is isolated and distal end of vein is ligated so that venous blood does not leak. A nick is made in the vein, through which a sufficient sized cannula (infant feeding tube can be used) is introduced. A silk ligature is applied above, just tight enough to hold the cannula in place. Free flow of venous blood in the cannula indicates that it is inside the vein. Cannula is advanced further for about 10-15 cm. It is connected to I.V. line containing fluid (Fig. 53.15).

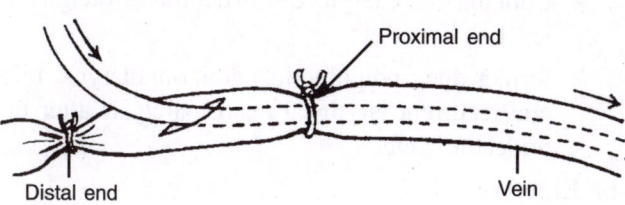

Fig. 53.15 Venesection

Precautions

1. **Neither air bubbles should be injected** nor should they be present in the drip set, to avoid air embolism.
2. **Upper ligature should not be tight.** It may obstruct the flow of fluids.
3. **Strict antiseptic principles** to be followed to avoid septicaemia.

Other veins selected for cut down are

- Basic vein in arm
- Cubital vein at the elbow
- Long saphenous vein in the leg. Avoid leg veins as far as possible to prevent deep vein thrombosis.

7. CLOSURE

- Skin - Interrupted silk

8. POSTOPERATIVE MANAGEMENT

- Antiseptic methods
- To avoid air bubbles in the drip set

9. POSTOPERATIVE COMPLICATIONS

1. Infection chills, rigors and septicaemia
2. Air embolism

10. ADVICE AT DISCHARGE

- Nil

Advantages of cephalic vein cut down

1. Reliable vein and easy to do
2. If cannula is advanced into the right heart, CVP can be measured.
3. Mobility of the patient is not restricted.
4. Substances which cannot be given in a peripheral vein, such as 50% dextrose, lipids, amino acids etc. can be given without risk of thrombosis of the vein, for hyperalimentation purposes.

Cannulate vein, not an artery for venesection.

VASECTOMY

Division of the vas deferens is vasectomy.

1. INDICATIONS

- Family Planning

- To prevent epididymoorchitis after prostatectomy. (Nowadays not routinely done).

2. CONTRAINDICATION

- **Relative :** TB epididymoorchitis. The incision may result in a nonhealing sinus. Hence, control of tuberculosis is done first followed by vasectomy.
- **Absolute :** Suspicion of testicular malignancy.

3. POSITION OF THE PATIENT

- Supine

4. ANAESTHESIA

- Local anaesthesia using 3-5 ml of 2% Lignocaine

5. PREPARATION OF THE PARTS

- Savlon and spirit
- Better avoid iodine

6. PROCEDURE

Feeling the vas deferens

- After cleaning and draping, VAS is felt, at the root of scrotum between the index finger and thumb. It feels like a CORD. Lignocaine is infiltrated and wait for 1-2 minutes for lignocaine to act.

Incision

- An incision of 2-4 cm is made in root of scrotum and it is deepened through layers of scrotum. An **Alli's forceps** is introduced within the incision and spermatic cord is held. During this step, fingers of the other hand help in guiding/locating/stabilising the cord. The coverings of the cord are incised.

Precaution

- Not to damage testicular vessels
- Vas is separated. It is confirmed by its white colour, and it feels like a cord.
- Division of vas by three clamp method (Fig. 53.16).
- Vas is cut in two places A and B so that a piece of vas is removed, which can be sent for histopathology to confirm that it is vas.
- Since a piece of vas is removed, reunion of the cut ends will not occur.
- The two cut ends of vas are doubly ligated by using silk.

7. CLOSURE

- The skin is closed by interrupted **White Thread** so that removal is easy. (Catgut can also be used).

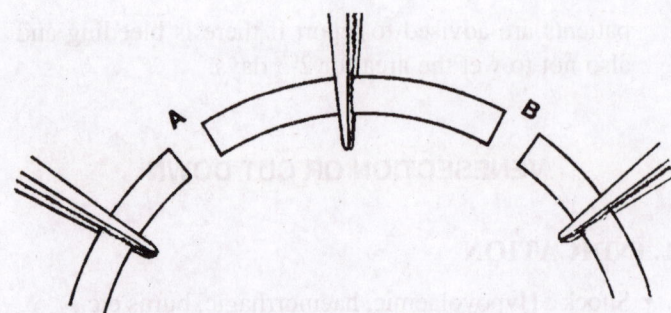

Fig. 53.16 Division of vas deferens by 3-clamp method

8. POSTOPERATIVE TREATMENT

- Rest for few hours
- Antibiotics and analgesics

The procedure is repeated on the other side.

9. POSTOPERATIVE COMPLICATIONS

1. Injury to the vessels, resulting in large haematoma
2. Infection
3. Testicular atrophy can occur few years later. It is due to immunological reaction rather than disuse atrophy.

10. ADVICE AT DISCHARGE

- To use family planning device for two months while having sexual intercourse, as some sperms may be present in the distal end of the vas and seminal vesicle.

Vasectomy being a part of family planning project, every student should be familiar with this.

TRACHEOSTOMY

An opening made in the trachea is tracheostomy.

1. INDICATIONS

a. Emergency

- Choking of the larynx due to dentures, foreign bodies, fish bones etc.
- Stridor due to diphtheria, carcinoma larynx, bilateral recurrent laryngeal nerve paralysis after thyroidectomy etc.

b. Elective

- Coma

- Tetanus
- Barbiturate poisoning
- Head injuries
- Pulmonary insufficiency

2. CONTRAINDICATIONS

- Anaplastic carcinoma thyroid patients presenting with stridor due to infiltration of growth into trachea. It may not be possible to do tracheostomy or an attempt to do tracheostomy may result in growth fungating through the incision (which is not worth it) In such patients, **endotracheal intubation** is done if possible. Otherwise, they are left alone for a merciful end.

3. POSITION OF THE PATIENT

- Supine with extension of neck and head by keeping a sandbag or a pillow under the shoulders.

4. ANAESTHESIA

- Local infiltration anaesthesia

5. PREPARATION OF THE PARTS

- Iodine and spirit

6. PROCEDURE

Incision

- Transverse curved incision for about 6 cm is made at the level of 2nd tracheal ring

Layers opened

- Skin, subcutaneous tissue and deep fascia are incised.

Procedure

- Isthmus of thyroid is separated.
- A transverse cut is made in the 2nd tracheal cartilage and edge of the cartilage is held with Alli's forceps and a small cuff of cartilage is removed. 'Cricoid hook' can be used to stabilise the trachea (found more useful in children).
- A suitable sized tracheostomy tube is introduced within.
- The cuff of tracheostomy tube is inflated by using 2-5 ml of air and it is held in place by passing a tape around the neck.
- Confirm that the **tube** is in the **trachea**, not in the subcutaneous plane.
- Confirm **air entry** on both sides of lung.

7. CLOSURE

- Few interrupted skin sutures by the side of the tracheostomy tube and dressing is applied.

8. POSTOPERATIVE ADVICE OR TREATMENT

- Suction of tracheostomy tube, regular dressing
- Humidification of air
- Check for air entry

9. POSTOPERATIVE COMPLICATIONS

1. Wound infection
2. Air leakage
3. Improper air entry
4. Cricoid stenosis (high tracheostomy)

CLOSURE OF TRACHEOSTOMY

- Once the foreign body is removed, trachestomy is blocked for few hours, if there is NO RESPIRATORY DISTRESS, cuff is deflated and the tube is removed. A few skin sutures can be put or dressing is applied. It closes automatically.

10. ADVICE AT DISCHARGE

- Tracheostomy done after laryngectomy is permanent. Patients should learn to use metal tracheostomy, cleaning the tubes etc.

Confirm air entry well once the tracheostomy tube is introduced within the trachea.

SUPRAPUBIC CYSTOSTOMY (SPC)

In this operation, urinary bladder is drained to the exterior by inserting a Malecot's catheter into the bladder.

1. INDICATIONS

- Retention of urine due to any cause where a catheter or a dilator cannot be passed through the urethra to empty the bladder. However this operation is rarely done now a days since suprapubic catheterisation with a trocar and cannula has simplified the procedure.

2. CONTRAINDICATION

- Carcinoma bladder

3. POSITION OF THE PATIENT

- Supine

4. ANAESTHESIA

- S.A or G.A

5. PREPARATION OF THE PARTS

- Iodine and spirit

6. PROCEDURE

Incision (Fig. 53.17):

- A vertical incision of 6-8 cm is made below the umbilicus in the midline.

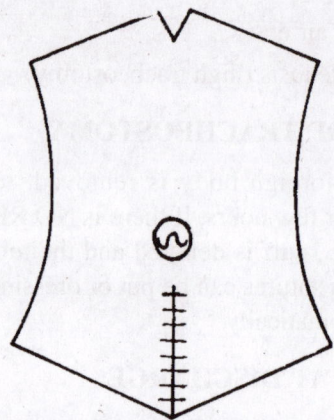

Fig. 53.17 Incision for SPC

Layers Opened

- Skin, subcutaneous tissue, and linea alba in the upper part of incision. (**Below the semilunar line** there is **NO LINEA ALBA**).

- Rectus muscle is split in the midline (separated).

- Extraperitoneal tissue with fat is seen.

- With blunt dissection, fat and peritoneum is swept upwards so that anterior wall of the bladder is seen with its peritoneal covering. The bladder is identified by perivesical plexus of veins or by aspiration of urine with syringe and needle.

- Two stay sutures are applied on the anterior bladder wall. The bladder is incised and urine drained out. The opening is enlarged and a Malecot's catheter is introduced within. It is brought outside from the upper part of the incision and connected to a closed bag (Urosac) (Fig. 53.18).

- Urinary bladder is closed with absorbable 2-0 chromic catgut sutures.

- A Corrugated drainage tube is kept in the prevesical space.

7. CLOSURE

- Split rectus muscles are approximated by using catgut sutures.

- Anterior rectus sheath/linea alba - By nonabsorbable sutures.

- Subcutaneous tissue - chromic catgut

- Skin - Silk

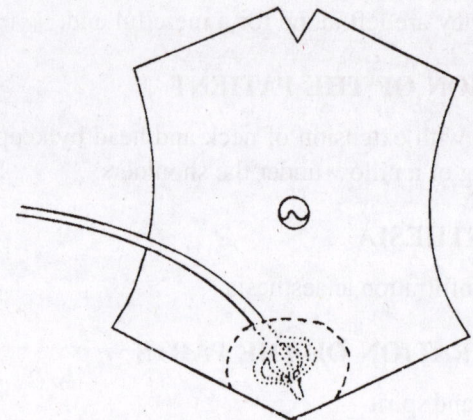

Fig. 53.18 Completion of SPC

8. POSTOPERATIVE MANAGEMENT

- Antibiotics

- Analgesics

9. POSTOPERATIVE COMPLICATIONS

1. Wound infection

2. Haemorrhage : Bladder wash is given till the contents are clear. Rarely, it may need re-exploration and control of the bleeding.

3. If urinary leakage occurs it is usually minor.

10. ADVICE AT DISCHARGE

- If urinary leakage continues or if postoperative fever persists to report to the hospital

This operation has become less popular because of suprapubic catheterisation which is a simple procedure.

THYROIDECTOMY

1. INDICATIONS

- All goitres with symptoms-MNG, toxic goitres, colloid goitres and malignant goitres.

2. CONTRAINDICATIONS

- Asymptomatic Hashimoto's thyroiditis

3. POSITION OF THE PATIENT

- Supine with extended neck by keeping a sandbag under the shoulders.
- Head end of the patient is elevated to about 30^0 to reduce venous congestion. This position is called as **anti-Trendelenberg position**.

4. ANAESTHESIA

- G.A

5. PREPARATION OF THE PART

- Iodine and spirit

6. PROCEDURE

Incision (Fig. 53.19):

- 6-8 cm collar neck incision or crease incision.

Layers opened

- Skin, platysma, subcutaneous tissue in the line of incision
- Deep fascia is incised vertically
- Strap muscles are separated (can be cut in very large goitres)
- Pretracheal fascia is incised
- Thyroid gland is mobilised by using blunt dissection

- Assess the entire gland to know whether it is a solitary nodule or multinodular goitre.
- One of the lobes is mobilised by dividing middle thyroid vein (single, short, thin, vein).
- Then, upper pole is dissected. This pedicle contains superior thyroid artery and veins- They are ligated and divided in between. **Please apply double ligature proximally.**
- Upper pole should be ligated as close to the gland as possible to avoid damage to external laryngeal nerve.
- Inferior thyroid artery can be ligated which has a horizontal course. It is thick and pulsatile. It is ligated in continuity. (By chance, even if ligated structure is recurrent laryngeal nerve, ligature can be removed later, hence ligate in continuity). Multiple veins, present in the lower pole are ligated and divided.
- Isthmus is separated from trachea, both above and below.
- In subtotal thyroidectomy, the entire isthmus, parts of the right and left lobes are removed in flush with tracheal surface, leaving behind tissue in the tracheo-oesophageal groove to protect recurrent laryngeal nerve and parathyroid gland. Cut edges of thyroid gland are sutured by using chromic catgut sutures (Fig. 53.20)

PRECAUTIONS

- Any structure directly entering the gland can be cut.
- Recurrent laryngeal nerve enters the thyrohyoid membrane, after running a vertical course, in the tracheo-oesophageal groove.

7. CLOSURE

- A corrugated red rubber drain or suction drain is kept in the thyroid bed.

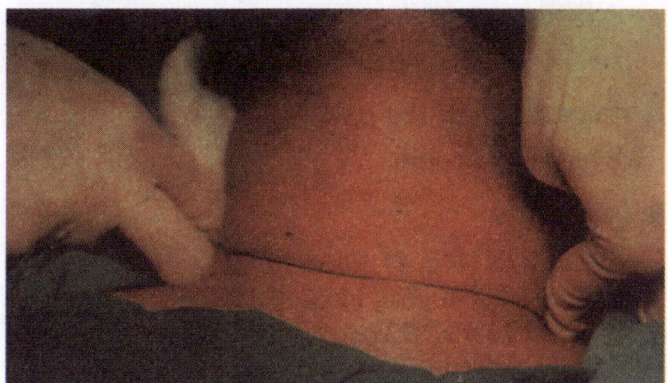

Fig. 53.19 Position and incision for thyroidectomy

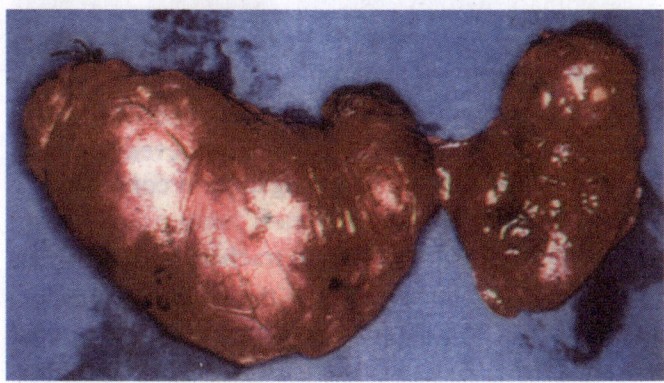

Fig. 53.20 Subtotal thyroidectomy for MNG

- Deep fascia—Continuous catgut.
- Subcutaneous fat—Chromic catgut.
- Skin—Interrupted silk.

8. POSTOPERATIVE MANAGEMENT

- NPO for 6-8 hours followed by liquid diet
- Antibiotics not always necessary
- Head end to be elevated to reduce oedema of the wound.
- In toxic goitres, propranolol to be continued after surgery, and slowly tapered.
- Blood transfusion depending upon blood loss.
- Drain removal after 2-3 days
- Suture removal after 4-5 days

9. POST-OPERATIVE COMPLICATIONS (For details refer chapter 19)

1. **Haemorrhage: Tension haematoma.** Reactionary haemorrhage is due to slipping of ligature due to coughing, hypertension etc. If it is alarming, sutures have to be opened, haematoma drained and haemostasis to be achieved.

2. Thyrotoxic crisis in toxic goitre patients

3. Wound infection

4. Hypothyroidism

5. Recurrent laryngeal nerve paralysis

6. Hypoparathyroidism

7. Tracheomalacia

* Different types of thyroidectomy - Table 53.1

	Table 53.1		
DISEASES	**BEFORE SURGERY**	**AFTER SURGERY**	**NAME OF THE OPERATION**
1. Solitary nodule (benign)			**Hemithyroidectomy:** means removal of one lobe with isthmus (Page 267)
2. Multinodular goitre			**Subtotal thyroidectomy** (Page 251)
3. Toxic multinodular goitre			**Subtotal thyroidectomy** (Page 254)
4. Primary thyrotoxicosis			**Subtotal thyroidectomy** (Page 255)
5. Malignant neoplasm			**Near-total thyroidectomy:** (Page 260)
6. Malignant neoplasm- high grade carcinoma			**Total thyroidectomy:** (Page 261)

10. Advice at discharge

- This depends on the type of indication for thyroid surgery, e.g. those who undergo subtotal thyroidectomy for thyrotoxicosis have to be closely followed for recurrent thyrotoxicosis or hypothyroidism. If calcium levels are low, it has to be supplemented.

This is an operation which provides a surgeon to an opportunity to demonstrate his skills and 'meticulous' capacity.

AMPUTATIONS

Indications

1. Vitality of the parts are destroyed by injury or disease- Dead limb

2. Life of patient is threatened by spread of a local condition - Deadly limb

   Examples : Gas gangrene , extensive melanoma

3. Patient may be better served by an artificial limb because of deformity or paralysis . Deformed limb

Optimum levels of amputation

- Level of amputation depends not only upon the extent of disease but also function desired in the remaining stump. This differs markedly in the upper and lower limbs.

LOWER LIMB AMPUTATIONS

TRANS METATARSAL AMPUTATION

- All toes are disarticulated at Metatarso - phalyngeal joint and head of all metatarsals are removed
- Long volar flap is created and rotated and sutured to the dorsal skin.
- Sutures are removed after 14 days

TARSO METATARSAL AMPUTATION

- Foot is shortened through the base of the metatarsals.
- Long volar flap is created if possible and sutured to the dorsal skin.

MID TARSAL AMPUTATION

- Long volar and short dorsal flaps are raised

- Disarticulation of foot is completed through talo-navicular joint and through calcaneo-cuboid joint

SYME'S AMPUTATION

- The tibia and fibula are divided at or immediately above the level of ankle joint and their ends are covered with a single flap obtained from heel.
- The end of stump is at height of about 6-8 cm from the ground.
- 50% of people will be able to walk on the stump without prosthesis.
- It is of value in patients who do not have access to modern artificial limbs.
- Pirgroff's modification of Syme's amputation retains a small portion of calcaneum in the flap obtained from heel.

BELOW KNEE AMPUTATION

- It is the operation of choice when it is not possible to preserve the foot or heel
- The ideal length of the tibial stump is 14 cm.
- Minimum length required to fit an artificial leg is 8 cm, stump shorter than this tends to slip out of the socket of an artificial limb.
- Stump is covered by creating long posterior flap
- This is commonly done amputation in patients who are in severe sepsis involving the leg with   uncontrolled diabetes and in whom life is in danger.

AMPUTATIONS THROUGH THIGH

- Ideal length is 25-30 cm as measured from tip of trochanter.
- It is done when it is not possible to save at least 8 cm of tibia as in some cases of diabetes spreading infections of the leg and when muscles involved are not bleeding at surgery
- When this amputation is done in children as much length as possible should be preserved (Growing epiphysis of femur is at lower end)

UPPER LIMB AMPUTATIONS

GENERAL PRINCIPLES

- Conserve as much tissue as possible
- Skin closure should not be under tension

- Soft tissue cover over bony stump is desirable otherwise painful adherent scar will result.
- Amputation through middle or terminal phalynx is preferred to disarticulation at inter- phalangeal joints since attachment of flexors tendons is there by preserved.
- Every effort should be made to preserve as much as possible.

AMPUTATION THROUGH FOREARM AND UPPER ARM

- Ideal stump is 16-20 cm measured from olecrenon
- Stump less than 8 cm is useless for transmitting movement to an artificial elbow joint.
- A stump measuring 20 cm from acromion is ideal for fitting prosthesis

ACCESSORY EQUIPMENT

HIGH FREQUENCY ELECTRO SURGERY

Principle involves passage of electric current through tissue by means of potential difference (Voltage). The resultant flow of electrons excites the tissue molecules, notably water, creating heat energy, which causes water evaporation and tissue coagulation. HF electro surgery can be monopolar or bipolar. Here, the current escapes from electrode tip into receptive tissue and exits through the grounding pad.

Unmodulated continues sine wave in voltage range 200-500 for electrocutting.

Uses of electrocautery

1. To achieve haemostasis
2. Removal of skin tags
3. Treating very small early basal cell carcinoma
4. Treatment of erosions of cervix
5. Treatment of condylomata, acanthoma, warts etc.

Bipolar electrocautery

Heat energy is concentrated between two electrodes and does not dissipate thorughout the tissue. Hence,

- Small volume of tissue is injured
- Less risk of burning injury
- Safe with pace makers
- Excellent for obtaining haemostasis in areas that may be in close proximity to delicate structure. e.g. head and neck surgery.

Effective in wet fields, uses coagulation current only

Monopolar electro-cautery

Head energy and thus tissue injury can extend for some distant away from the point of contact. Hence it should not be used with.

- Direct contact with a hollow viscus as this may lead to perforation
- Closed proximity to a major blood vessel as it may cause vessel wall injury

Not effective in wet fields, uses both lutting and co-agulation current, therefore dissecting is possible.

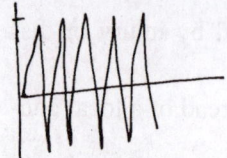

Electro cutting
(Voltage 200-500)

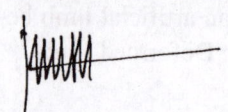

Soft co-agulation
(Voltage range<200)
Unmodulated current

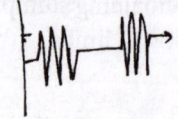

Forced co-agulation
(Modulated HF voltages peak value high enough to produce electric areas)

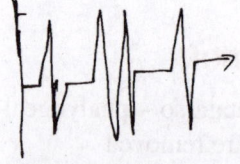

Spray co-agulation
(Strongly modulated HF voltages of a few kilo volts to produce long electric areas)

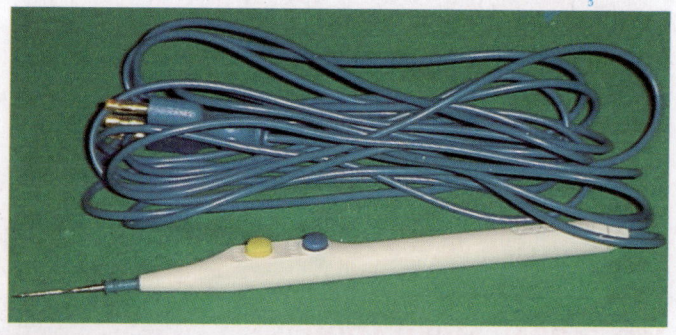

Fig. 53.21 Cautery chord - yellow button is for cutting current and blue is for coagulation

CRYOSURGERY

Definition

- The application of a freezing problem to the living tissues is called as **Cryosurgery**.

Mechanism of tissue destruction

- Freezing procedures ice crystal formation within all resulting in cell membrane rupture and death
- Also as the crystals grow, water is removed from neighbouring cells leading to an increase in the concentration of electrolytes. These soon reach toxic levels, initiating cell death by osmotic shock.

Methodology and instrument used

- **N_2 system** can achieve a probe tissue temperature of around -70^0C. It works with the principle of rapid expansion of a gas producing refrigeration (Jule - Thomson effect)
- **Liquid Nitrogen:** N_2 system can achieve a probe temperature of around -190^0C

Uses

1. Haemorrhoidectomy
2. Cutaneous lesions - Excision or biopsy

LASERS IN SURGERY

- **L**ight **A**mplification by **S**imulated **E**mission of **R**adiation
- Molecules which are placed in a compact are activated when power is passed through.
- As a result of this they move in different directions, they hit each other, releasing energy. This energy is used as LASER to the area whenever required.
- The laser energy goes by the name of the medium which may be solid, liquid or dye. Hence, lasers are known as CO_2 laser, Argon laser, NdYAG laser or dye laser.

Types

1. Argon laser
2. Neo-Dynium yttrium Aluminium Garnet Laser (ND-YAG Laser)
3. CO_2 laser
4. Neon laser

Advantages

- Most important advantage being blood less field - specialy useful in head and neck surgeries and ENT surgeries.
- It is quick and causes less tissue trauma

Precautions

- To avoid injuries to normal tissues, all reflecting instruments should be avoided so that laser should not get reflected.

All should wear protective spectacles for their eyes.

Disadvantages

- Cost

Clinical applications

1. **Vascular malformation** of the GIT
2. Endoscopic laser for **advanced carcinoma oesophagus** to relieve obstruction and dysphagia
3. **Obstructed colorectal cancer**
4. **Liver resections:** NdYAG laser combined with CUSA can be used for liver resections
5. CO_2 laser and NdYAG laser can be used for **haemorrhoidectomy**

Key Box 53.7	
Argon laser :	Retinal photocoagulation
NdYAG laser :	Debulk obstruction in GIT
	Coagulate bladder tumour
CO_2 laser :	Used as a cutting and vapourising instrument

STAPLERS IN SURGERY

Principle

- They are used for opposition of tissues

Types

1. Cutaneous staplers

- Used after thyroidectomy. It is quick and gives clean apposition

- Needs a special instrument for removal
- Cosmetic results are better

2. Linear staplers

- Used to close the bowel partially or completely
- Used for transection of visera in conjunction with a scalpel

3. Circular staplers

- Are also called as EEA stapler- End to End Anastomosis
- Uses in surgery:

  a. After low or high anterior resection done for carcinoma rectum

  b. After oesophagogastrectomy

  c. Any other intestinal resection

4. GIA staple

- Gastrointestinal anastomosis stapler: used for side to side anastomosis.

5. Endostapler

- With the increasing use of laparoscopic surgeries for facilitating a quick, safe anastomosis, endostaplers are used for intestinal anastomosis
- Endovascular staplers are used to ligate vascular pedicles - Example: Renal pedicles during laparoscopic nephrectomy.
- Adrenal veins during laparoscopic adrenalectomy.

Advantages of staplers

- Saves operating time

- The low rectal and oesophageal anastomosis have higher incidence of leakage rates. However it can be decreased by using staplers.

Disadvantages

- Costly
- Improper apposition results in leakage

Parts

1. Handle
2. Shaft
3. Head detachable anvil + a staple cartridge

The staples (approximately 15 in number) are present in the cartridge. The cartridge also has a circular knife.

The doughnuts (rings of excised tissue) should be complete after the stapled anastomosis. Incomplete doughnuts means incomplete wound closure.

Contraindications

1. If the tissues which have to be approximated are under tension, they should not be stapled
2. Different lumen diameters should not be stapled end to end
3. If the circular head is of greater diameter than the lumen, it should not be used.

- *The last four chapters are important for viva voce examination in general surgery. The questions given in these chapters are most commonly asked. This does not mean, however, that they are the only questions asked. As the subject is vast, the number of questions that can be asked can be unlimited. The purpose of viva voce section is to see how much the student knows as well as the depth and understanding of the subject.*

- AUTHOR

Index